PEDIATRIC
AIDS

The Challenge of HIV Infection in Infants, Children, and Adolescents

SECOND EDITION

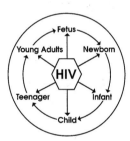

PEDIATRIC
AIDS

The Challenge of HIV Infection in Infants, Children, and Adolescents

SECOND EDITION

EDITED BY

PHILIP A. PIZZO MD

Chief of Pediatrics
Head, Infectious Disease Section
National Cancer Institute
National Institutes of Health
Professor of Pediatrics
Uniformed Services University of the Health Sciences
Bethesda, Maryland

CATHERINE M. WILFERT MD

Professor of Pediatrics and Microbiology
Chief, Pediatric Infectious Diseases
Department of Pediatrics
Duke University Medical Center
Durham, North Carolina

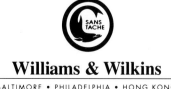

Williams & Wilkins

BALTIMORE • PHILADELPHIA • HONG KONG
LONDON • MUNICH • SYDNEY • TOKYO

A WAVERLY COMPANY

Editor: Jonathan W. Pine, Jr.
Managing Editor: Molly L. Mullen
Copy Editor: Therese J. Grundl
Designer: Wilma E. Rosenberger
Illustration Planner: Ray Lowman
Production Coordinator: Barbara J. Felton

Accurate indications, adverse reactions, and dosage schedules for drugs are provided in this
book, but it is possible that they may change. The reader is urged to review the package information data of the manufacturers of the medications mentioned.

Printed in the United States of America

First Edition 1991

Library of Congress Cataloging-in-Publication Data

Pediatric AIDS: the challenge of HIV infection in infants, children, and adolescents/edited
   by Philip A. Pizzo, Catherine M. Wilfert. — 2nd ed.
     p. cm.
   Includes bibliographical references and index.
   ISBN 0-683-06895-4
   1. AIDS (Disease) in children. I. Pizzo, Philip A. II. Wilfert, Catherine M.
   [DNLM: 1. HIV Infections—in infancy & childhood. 2. HIV
Infections—in adolescence.   WD 308 P371 1993]
RJ387.A25P43   1993
618.92'9792—dc20
DNLM/DLC
for Library of Congress

        93-36389
        CIP
   93 94 95 96 97
  1 2 3 4 5 6 7 8 9 10

*To all who have joined in the effort to improve the lives of children
and their families throughout the world who are facing the challenge of HIV.*

Perspectives

From a Parent—Elizabeth Glaser

From a Child—Hydeia Broadbent

From the Health Care Community—Margaret C. Heagarty

From the Federal Government—Antonia C. Novello

Perspective from a Parent

Elizabeth Glaser
Cofounder, Pediatric AIDS Foundation

I have been infected with HIV since 1981. In 1988, I lost my daughter to AIDS. My son, who is 9, has been infected since birth. I am in the middle of this epidemic.

As the 1990s move along my greatest concern is that we don't become complacent about HIV, that we keep fighting as hard as we can to find different and complicated answers. That we remember the urgency of families like mine—families struggling to keep their hope alive.

Each year we have new information. This book reminds all of us that we must stay on the cutting edge of this devastating epidemic.

The information here will help children and families around the country and the world. But, these facts are only partially helpful. We must also know that people, our doctors, our government, our neighbors, our families, care. That along with medicine and treatment comes compassion and love. Then hope is within reach of us all.

Perspective from a Child

Hydeia Broadbent
Las Vegas, Nevada

My life has been a little different than other children that I have known. I was born with AIDS. Some people think it's not okay to have AIDS. And some people know that it's okay to have AIDS because you are still a normal person. I would like to tell you what is important. I would also like to tell you what has been the best parts about living with AIDS and what are the scariest parts.

WHAT IS IMPORTANT

Friends and family are important especially when you have a deadly disease. I am very important to my mommy and daddy and all the rest of the people that know that I have AIDS. Some kids don't understand that if they play with me they can not get AIDS. Some kids even know more than their parents. When I have a new friend and she or he finds out I have AIDS and they do not know a lot about it, I will help them understand. My life is fun because I have a big sister who understands a lot. I also have two very special friends. One helps me a lot when I need her. She is my social worker. The other one acts like a kid even though she is grown. She is a volunteer. But my very, very special friend is my mom. She helps me when I need her and I help her when she needs me. Even though I might die before her I will never stop loving her and she will never stop loving me.

THE BEST PART ABOUT LIVING WITH AIDS

AIDS is in a way good. Because some people learn alot like I did. I learned to help other people deal with it by explaining to them what it really is. Actually many people do not know a lot about what AIDS is, and it is in a way good for me because I can help people learn and I can educate people. When I educate people I feel happy because they listen to me because an 8-year-old may know more than a 30-year-old person. It is good to have a child that's been living with this disease all their life to tell people what is safe and what is not safe. Because no one that's not lived with AIDS can tell other people what it is really like. And I get more and more friends and a whole lot of love. So AIDS is not so bad at all.

THE SCARIEST PART ABOUT LIVING WITH AIDS

There are times that are scary though. Getting shots and having new procedures done is frightening. I don't look forward to those times. Sometimes when I am sick and in the hospital I get worried about getting sicker. If I got sicker I would die. You could die from AIDS. When you do your mommy and daddy will be very sad because they wouldn't have a child anymore. But you will always be remembered. My mommy and daddy would always think of me and they will keep all my stuff in my room like my toys and pictures and my books. I always want them to remember me saying "I love you." They will always remember me sucking my thumb and wanting me to "STOP."

WHAT I WANT THE WORLD TO KNOW

I would like everyone to like everyone and respect others. This is very important. Many people may be sick and not feel good and by not being nice to them you might hurt their feelings. No one likes it very much when someone hurts their feelings.

I also don't think it is very nice when people tease you. People have teased me because of my catheter and my backpack. I like when people treat me nice, and I don't like when people tease me. It is not funny. Having AIDS is not fun, and I want the world to know that sometimes it makes you not feel very good and not want to do very much. We should not be teased about that either.

THE FRIENDS I ONCE KNEW

I never worry about dying anymore. I used to worry about dying but I don't anymore. The reason I don't worry anymore is because I know so many children with AIDS who have died, and I know they are all in Heaven. I often wonder what Heaven is like. I think there is angels all over, baby angels and grown up angels. We can always remember our friends who are in Heaven. They are standing by us. When I get there, Cory and Ezra and Dougie and Blayne and other children I once knew will be there for me to play with. I think I will be happy in Heaven.

This is not like the other poems I have written because the others help educate people. This one tells you how I feel. Thank you for listening. The End.

Perspective from the Health Care Community

Margaret C. Heagarty
Professor of Pediatrics
Columbia University College of Physicians and Surgeons

The first child with AIDS was admitted to the Harlem Hospital, a New York City municipal hospital located in an urban disadvantaged community more than 10 years ago. At the time those of us involved in the struggle to provide health care for the poor children of this community were mercifully unaware of what was to follow. We did not foresee that we would be forced to become scientific and clinical pioneers in one of the most serious epidemics in children of this century, nor did we understand how difficult it would be to get the larger, more affluent community interested and concerned about these children and their families.

We, like our young patients and their families, faced this epidemic unprepared. But we had experience in the difficulties of providing health care for the poor, for all health professionals concerned with children, no matter where we are, cope daily with the results of the absence of a national, universal, and comprehensive system of health care. All of us caring for the poor, by necessity, have long since become ingenious, crafty, and frustrated manipulators of a health care system that does not meet the needs of these children.

Now more than 10 years later and with the advantage of hindsight, several things become clear. First, it is probably just as well that we did not recognize early the scope of the epidemic and the complexity of care for children and families with AIDS. If we had, we all might have given up before we started. Because children with HIV infection are for the most part from the most disadvantaged families in our communities, the provision of medical care, complicated as it is, in many ways is the least of the problems. So we who provide the care have had to try, with precious little outside support, to find ways to help these children and their families deal not only with the emotional consequences of a serious, chronic, and ultimately lethal disease but also with the realities of poverty and often of drug addiction.

Second, from the vantage of more than 10 years, the process of the development of care of children with this disease resembles a bit of a muddle, that is, an evolutionary process invented by human beings struggling to find answers, not only answers in the laboratory but also at the bedside. And in that muddle, that human process, lies whatever comfort and satisfaction there is to be found for those engaged in the care of children with AIDS. Over the years, care of these children has demanded that we use every ounce of imagination, energy, creativity, not to say moral indignation, we possess. We have sometimes failed—many children have died despite our best efforts—but those engaged in this care will, I think, agree that when we have done our best, have used all we have, then we are most nearly human and have come closest to the ideals that led us to the health care professions.

Perspective from the Federal Government

Antonia C. Novello
Former United States Surgeon General

It began, like so many epidemics, with a few isolated cases, a whisper that caught the ear of only a few in medical research. Today, that whisper has become a roar heard around the world. AIDS is now the epidemic of our generation, invading our lives in ways we never imagined—testing our scientific knowledge, probing our private values, and sapping our strength. AIDS no longer attracts our attention—it commands it.

In this second decade of AIDS, HIV infection continues to spread, despite the fact that most people know how to prevent it. Too many people continue to take chances, and too many of them become infected. Adolescents are a special concern. More and more adolescents are becoming infected with HIV.

As parents we cannot stand idly by while AIDS threatens our children's future. It is painful to think about the temptations and dangers adolescents face every day. But sex and drugs are facts of life; we can no more ignore them than death itself. We must prepare our children to face the realities of AIDS in their lives. The urgency for action stems from the growing scope of the problem.

Although adolescents aged 13–19 comprise less than 1% of total AIDS cases in the United States reported through March 1993, individuals aged 13–29 make up more than 20% of total AIDS cases. Given the period of roughly 10 years between infection with HIV and the onset of symptoms, it can be assumed that many of these individuals were infected as adolescents. This distressing growth of adolescent AIDS may herald the future profile of HIV infection in the general population.

To respond to this pressing challenge, we must come to grips with the fact that the teenagers of today are not the teenagers we were back in the hazy days before AIDS, condoms, and MTV.

If HIV/AIDS prevention in adolescence is truly our number one priority, it can no longer be conducted in a didactic or moralistic vacuum. Books and sermons are simply not enough in today's imperiled world.

Simply put, we can no longer afford to allow debates regarding the appropriateness of teenage sexuality to paralyze our efforts to address the spread of HIV infection among our adolescent population.

If we are to respond to the challenge of HIV/AIDS, we must acknowledge that adolescents are not adequately served by programs designed for adults or children. A comprehensive and well integrated system of care for HIV-infected adolescents will be most effective if the services provided are family centered, community based, culturally sensitive, and developmentally appropriate. This comprehensive strategy must integrate education, testing, counseling, and preventive and treatment services under one roof.

If latex condoms are the preferred and sanctioned mode of such prevention in the community, then the mechanism by which they are made available must respect local concerns and, in addition, address the shared responsibility of protection by each partner.

Above all, it must reflect a continuum of care—with case management as a focal point. It should also include a core set of services: pharmacy and laboratory, health guidance, vocational training, job counseling, legal services, food and nutritional assistance, shelter, parenting education, and, where needed, child care.

All these offerings should be augmented by services relevant to HIV-infected youth: specialized education, counseling and testing, mental health care, substance abuse treatment, education services, basic support services (including housing and transportation), social and legal services, and access to clinical research and appropriate treatment protocols.

If we are to halt the spread of HIV/AIDS in adolescents, we all must advocate the urgent health needs of adolescents and redouble our efforts to ensure that prejudice, complacency, isolated agendas, and political expediency do not deter us from dealing with the reality of teenagers and AIDS.

Ultimately, the success or failure of our effort to address HIV infection in adolescents will depend less on the precise technical components of our initiatives than on the political will needed to carry them out.

Preface to the Second Edition

The first cases of AIDS in children were described a decade ago. Since then, HIV infection has become one of the leading causes of death in children. It has destroyed the lives of men, women, children, families, and communities throughout the world. It has stirred political debate, discrimination, lawsuits, and moral accusations. It has splintered medical communities by recrimination and fear. It has stressed the economic resources of individuals, families, communities, cities, and nations. And, sadly, it has not always been taken seriously enough by governments and leaders who could make a difference.

At the same time, HIV infection has galvanized communities and has empowered children, parents, and people infected or impacted by HIV to become advocates for change. It has mobilized a new work force of dedicated health care providers and researchers who have contributed fundamental discoveries in basic science and clinical research. It has created a new dialogue and cooperation in the drug development process for children and engendered a new collaboration among health care providers, policy makers, and social services. Still, the strains of living with AIDS and caring for people with HIV infection take an ever increasing toll. There is never enough time, money, effective therapies, or people to make the difference for which we all seek and hope. And there are always so many new findings, recommendations, and controversies to sift through, digest, and implement.

The Second Edition of *Pediatric AIDS: The Challenge of HIV Infection in Infants, Children, and Adolescents* is not a solution to these ills or problems. It is an attempt to provide the community of care providers with the information needed to understand the nature and impact of this pandemic, to define the current principles of care and management, and to forecast the future research

agenda and challenges. This Second Edition has been fully revised and expanded, keeping pace with the explosion of new information that has taken place since the First Edition of just three years ago.

This Second Edition is divided into six parts. It begins with "Evolving Epidemiology of HIV," updating what changes have occurred in the United States and Europe. Chapter 3 provides a clear warning to developed nations that heterosexual transmission can become a dominant mode of infection and gives a sobering insight of the horrible reality of HIV infection in developing nations. A new chapter on the impact of HIV on women has also been added to help bridge the gap into family centered care. As serious a toll as HIV infection is taking in many of our urban centers, it cannot compare to enormity of the problem in the developing world.

The "Etiology, Pathogenesis, and Transmission" of HIV are detailed in Section II. The basic principles of retrovirology and pathogenesis are presented against the backdrop of immune ontogeny and its impact on virus replication and restriction. The timing of infection and the factors that lead some fetuses or infants to become infected are among the most important questions that can be asked. They are considered from various perspectives, including the impact of the placenta on transmission of infectious agents, information that has been learned from various experimental models, and the current state of knowledge about the clinical dimensions and features of the prenatal transmission of HIV.

Section III, "Diagnostic Challenges in Fetus and Infant," delineates the unique and specific problems that relate to making the diagnosis of HIV infection in infants born to seropositive mothers before the onset of symptoms. The sensitivity, specificity, advantage, and limitations of current and future virus specific diagnostic tests and procedures are reviewed in detail along with the formulation of specific diagnostic guidelines.

Section IV, "Clinical Manifestations in Infants, Children, and Adolescents," embodies 20 chapters and delineates the multidimensional infectious and noninfectious complications that occur with HIV infection. Each chapter presents updated information on the epidemiology, patterns of disease, diagnosis, management, and prevention strategies in a practical format that will help with the daily care of the HIV-infected child. A new chapter on sexually transmitted diseases and an expanded chapter on mycobacterial infections are also included.

Section V focuses on the "Medical Management and Treatment" of the HIV-infected infant, child, and adolescent. A detailed discussion of the development of drugs active against HIV and their clinical pharmacology is coupled with a comprehensive review of current and future antiretroviral, pharmacological, and biological strategies. Both the basic principles and their practical applications are stressed and amplified by how they apply to vertically infected infants, children with transfusion or coagulation associated HIV infections, adolescents, and pregnant women. Because medical treatment and psychosocial support must be closely aligned, detailed discussions on the nursing care, psychosocial support, and respite care of children and their families are covered in detail.

Finally, Section VI addresses the important "Prevention, Education, and Public Policy Issues" that impact the HIV-infected child and family. Advances in the development of vaccines against HIV are discussed in the context of current and future discoveries and their implications. So too is the use of passive immunization strategies, particularly in relation to the prospect for blocking the perinatal transmission of HIV infection. The use of immunizations to prevent common bacterial and virus infections is also delineated. Because of the emotional, medical, and legal issues that accompany HIV infection, detailed and authoritative reviews of the common medical

and legal issues that arise in the care of the HIV-infected child in the hospital, home, day care, school, and community are fully detailed. Understanding the perceptions of our communities along with developing strategies for training future care providers, expanding the access to health care, and empowering parents as advocates are integral to the ultimate translation of medical therapies to those in need and are covered in depth in this edition. Further, knowing what resources are available and how to access them is critical and is also fully considered.

Although the facts and figures that describe the blueprints for care are important, understanding the impact of this disease on the children and families who are infected is the heart and soul of the matter. A unique and special chapter is included that permits children to speak with drawings, writings, and stories about the impact of AIDS on themselves and their siblings, friends, and families. Our usual stereotypes about what children "understand" are broken down, keeping our focus on what our true purpose must be—finding solutions to improve the lives of our children and their families.

The production of *Pediatric AIDS: The Challenge of HIV Infection in Infants, Children, and Adolescents* required enormous dedication and efforts by its many contributors and collaborators. Each of the world-class authorities has given freely of his or her time, energy, knowledge, and wisdom, and we are deeply indebted to them. We thank Marie Priest for outstanding assistance in facilitating the flow of this project. We also thank the very special working relationship we have had with Williams & Wilkins in the production of this Second Edition. Jonathan Pine, Molly Mullen, Barbara Felton, and the excellent staff at Williams & Wilkins provided caring support and superb professionalism.

It has been a privilege to edit both editions of *Pediatric AIDS: The Challenge of HIV Infection in Infants, Children, and Adolescents.* Our greatest pleasure would be that a third edition would not be necessary.

Philip A. Pizzo MD
Catherine M. Wilfert MD
September 1993

Preface to the First Edition

AIDS has reset all of our preconceived agendas and timetables. This volume is no exception. As the disease has accelerated its toll around the world, the pace of research and care has been trying to keep up. Although children currently constitute only 2% of the recognized cases of AIDS in the United States, the incidence of infection is increasing rapidly. Indeed, in the early 1990s, between 10,000 and 20,000 cases of HIV infection in children are anticipated. The vast majority of these children will have acquired HIV perinatally, most commonly from mothers who were infected as a consequence of intravenous drug use or sexual contact with an IV drug-using partner. Pediatric AIDS is a disease affecting children in minority groups, often in cities where there is a high incidence of IV drug use. At the same time, children who are HIV infected, either perinatally or as a result of blood product transfusion, can be found throughout the United States and Europe. In many developing countries, children constitute nearly a quarter of the cases of AIDS. Although the number of adolescents with symptomatic AIDS is relatively small, the rapid increase in AIDS in young adults means that many of these individuals became infected as adolescents.

Thus, pediatric HIV infection represents a condition that is relevant to a wide range of medical specialists, including neonatologists, pediatricians, and adolescent specialists as well as obstetricians, perinatologists, and internists along with pediatric and medical infectious disease specialists and oncologists. Because the diagnosis, management, and prevention of HIV infection include a focus on mothers, infants, and families, frequently in a setting of social disruption and poverty, the involvement of epidemiologists, nurses, social workers, psychologists, and rehabilitation specialists as well as health administrators, sociologists, community workers, and advocacy groups along with local, state, and federal policy makers will all be essential. Either directly or indirectly, pediatric AIDS has touched or will touch large segments of our society and those of nations around the world.

Although this is a rapidly advancing field, and while new information is accumulating at an astounding rate, it seems appropriate to formulate a blueprint of our current knowledge as a foundation for future information exchange and utilization. This volume is an attempt to integrate the ingredients and components that are essential to current and future strategies aimed at the management and prevention of this ever-increasing problem. Indeed, we hope that *Pediatric AIDS: The Challenge of HIV Infection in Infants, Children, and Adolescents* will serve as a template for current and future communications.

Our initial commitment to this project arose as a consequence of an assignment at an Editorial Board meeting for *The Pediatric Infectious Disease Journal* to develop a series for the *Journal* on pediatric AIDS. As we developed this concept, the possibility of putting the series together in a monograph was considered. But such a monograph would only be useful if it could be compiled and published within a very short production time. The 2 to 3 years it usually takes to produce a multiauthored reference was unacceptable. But could a meaningful, comprehensive text be produced more rapidly—closer to the timetable for a medical journal? In August, 1989, we met with Laurel Craven and John Gardner, editors at Williams & Wilkins and set a publication schedule that seemed consonant with the challenge of AIDS. Our goal would be to produce a comprehensive, authoritative text on pediatric AIDS that would be published within 6 months after it was assembled. Obviously, this would require nearly missionary zeal and effort by the contributing authors, the publisher and, of course, editors. This book is a testimony to everyone's joint efforts and mutual commitment.

Contributing authors were sought and signed on to this project in September 1989, and detailed outlines of their respective chapters were submitted, reviewed, and returned by October. Draft chapters were due in December 1989 and were reviewed extensively by the editors and then revised by the authors so that final manuscripts were returned to the editors between February and March 1990. All of the final and edited manuscripts were delivered to the publisher at the end of March, enabling *Pediatric AIDS* to stay on its production schedule for publication in October 1990.

Clearly, a timetable that enabled the production of an entire book on a schedule that was faster than many journals can publish articles is evidence of the commitment of everyone involved in this project. We want to express our deepest thanks and appreciation to all who were involved in this effort. Of course, the contributing authors deserve our highest praise. Already overwhelmed with their individual battles against AIDS, they each took the time to write outstanding state-of-the-art chapters. Not only did they meet a very demanding schedule, but they also accommodated, with grace and patience, our unrelenting demands for more data, more tables, etc.

Without their cooperation and efforts, this volume would not be possible. Happily, many of the authors felt that writing their chapters had helped to raise important research questions and to stimulate new avenues of investigation. We hope that this is true and that this will result in improvements in the care of children with AIDS.

We owe deep gratitude to Marie Priest, who helped with the coordination of this ambitious effort in Bethesda, and to Ruth Robinson, who facilitated the Durham connection. Both made personal sacrifices to help keep everyone on track.

There was also enormous help from the Williams & Wilkins staff. Laurie Craven, Victoria Vaughn, and Barbara Felton became colleagues in this project and were ably assisted by Becky Himmelheber. In every way, the production of *Pediatric AIDS* formed new families and became a family affair.

Clearly this book is not a treatment or a cure. But it is a frame of reference and a guidepost for what we know and don't know. It is our hope that the contributing authors have learned as they were teaching. It is our dream that *Pediatric AIDS* might serve as a stimulus for new ideas and that it might stimulate new insights that will help overcome the challenge of HIV infection in infants, children, and adolescents.

Philip A. Pizzo, M.D.
Cathy M. Wilfert, M.D.
July 1990

Contributors

Arthur J. Ammann MD, Director, Ariel Project for Prevention of HIV Transmisson from Mother to Infant, Novato, California

Clark L. Anderson MD, Department of Internal Medicine, Ohio State University College of Medicine, 2054 Davis Research Center, Columbus, Ohio

Warren A. Andiman MD, Professor of Pediatrics and Epidemiology, Yale University School of Medicine, Director of Pediatric AIDS Program, Yale-New Haven Hospital, New Haven, Connecticut

Ann Armstrong-Dailey, Founding Director, Children's Hospice International, Alexandria, Virginia

Frank M. Balis MD, Head, Pharmacology and Experimental Therapeutics Program, Pediatric Branch, National Cancer Institute, National Institutes of Health, Bethesda, Maryland

Anita L. Belman MD, Associate Professor, Department of Neurology, State University of New York, Stony Brook, New York

Aprille Best, Parent, Jacksonville, Florida

Mary G. Boland RN, MSN, Director, AIDS Program, Children's Hospital of New Jersey, Associate in Pediatrics, University of Medicine and Dentistry, New Jersey Medical School, Newark, New Jersey

Pim Brouwers PhD, Visiting Scientist, Pediatric Branch, National Cancer Institute, National Institutes of Health, Bethesda, Maryland

Carolyn Keith Burr RN, MS, Associate Director, National Pediatric HIV Resource Center, Newark, New Jersey

Stephen Chanock MD, Senior Staff Fellow, Infectious Disease Section, Pediatric Branch, National Cancer Institute, National Institutes of Health, Bethesda, Maryland

Edward M. Connor MD, Associate Director, Division of Allergy Immunology and Infectious Diseases, Associate Professor of Pediatrics, University of Medicine and Dentistry of New Jersey, Newark, New Jersey

Ruth I. Connor PhD, Postdoctoral Research Fellow, Aaron Diamond AIDS Research Center, New York, New York

Lawrence Corey MD, Professor, Laboratory Medicine, Microbiology and Medicine, University of Washington, Seattle, Washington

Deborah Cotton MD, MPH, Assistant Professor of Medicine, Harvard Medical School, Infectious Disease Unit, Massachusetts General Hospital, Boston, Massachusetts

Judith S. Currier MD, Associate in Medicine, Division of Infectious Diseases, Beth Israel Hospital, Boston, Massachusetts

Gordon B. Cutler Jr. MD, Chief, Section on Developmental Endocrinology, Developmental Endocrinology Branch, National Institute of Child Health and Human Development, National Institutes of Health, Bethesda, Maryland

Lawrence J. D'Angelo MD, Chairman, Adolescent and Young Adult Medicine, Professor, Pediatrics, Medicine, and Health Care Sciences, George Washington University Medical Center, Washington, DC

Marinos C. Dalakas MD, Chief, Neuromuscular Diseases Section, Medical Neurology Branch, National Institute of Neurological Disorders and Stroke, National Institutes of Health, Bethesda, Maryland

Barry Dashefsky MD, Associate Professor, Department of Pediatrics, University of Pittsburgh School of Medicine, Pittsburgh, Pennsylvania

Billie Davison-Fairburn DVM, Clinical Veterinarian, Tulane Regional Primate Research Center, Covington, Louisiana

Marc D. de Smet MD, CM, FRCSC, Visiting Scientist, Laboratory of Immunology, National Eye Institute, National Institutes of Health, Bethesda, Maryland

Ann Duerr MD, PhD, MPH, Chief, HIV Section, Women's Health and Fertility Branch, Centers for Disease Control and Prevention, Atlanta, Georgia

Anne-Marie S. Duliège MD, MS, Associate Director, Biocine Clinical Research, Chiron Corporation, Emeryville, California

L. Jean Emery MSW, ACSW, LICSW, Director, HIV/AIDS Program, Child Welfare League of America, Washington, DC

Leon Epstein MD, Professor, Department of Neurology, Pediatrics, Microbiology, and Immunology, Rochester, New York

M. Elaine Eyster MD, Professor of Medicine, Chief, Division of Hematology, Department of Medicine, Milton S. Hershey Center, Pennsylvania State University, Hershey, Pennsylvania

Cindy Fair MSW, MPH, Doctoral Student, Maternal and Child Health, School of Public Health, University of North Carolina, Chapel Hill, North Carolina

Anthony S. Fauci MD, Director, National Institute of Allergy and Infectious Diseases, National Institutes of Health, Bethesda, Maryland

John C. Fletcher PhD, Director, Center for Biomedical Ethics, Professor of Religious Studies and Clinical Ethics, University of Virginia, Charlottesville, Virginia

Henry Friedman MD, Associate Professor of Pediatrics, Division of Hematology/Oncology, Duke University Medical Center, Durham, North Carolina

Donna Futterman MD, Assistant Professor of Pediatrics, Albert Einstein College of Medicine, Medical Director, Adolescent AIDS Program, Montefiore Medical Center, Bronx, New York

Jonathan C. Goldsmith MD, Head, Children's AIDS Center, Director, Hemophilia Comprehensive Care Center, Children's Hospital, Los Angeles, California

Laura T. Gutman MD, Director, Pediatric STD Program, Division of Infectious Diseases, Duke University Medical Center, Durham, North Carolina

Alexandra Halpern MA, AT, Art Therapist, Pediatrics, National Cancer Institute, National Institutes of Health, Bethesda, Maryland

Neal Halsey MD, Professor and Division Director, International Health, Division of Disease Control, Joint Appointment, Department of Pediatrics, Johns Hopkins University, Baltimore, Maryland

Karen Hein MD, Professor of Pediatrics, Albert Einstein College of Medicine, Director, Adolescent AIDS Program, Montefiore Medical Center, Bronx, New York

David D. Ho MD, Director, Aaron Diamond AIDS Research Center, Professor of Medicine and Microbiology, New York University School of Medicine, New York, New York

Rod Hoff DSc, Chief, Vaccine Trials and Epidemiology Branch, Vaccine Trials Section, Division of AIDS, National Institute of Allergy and Infectious Diseases, National Institutes of Health, Bethesda, Maryland

Marc E. Horowitz MD, Associate Professor of Pediatrics, Division of Hematology-Oncology, Texas Children's Hospital, Baylor College of Medicine, Houston, Texas

Walter T. Hughes MD, Chairman, Department of Infectious Diseases, St. Jude Children's Research Hospital, Professor of Pediatrics and Biostatistics and Epidmiology, University of Tennessee College of Medicine, Memphis, Tennessee

Robert N. Husson MD, Assistant Professor of Pediatrics, Division of Infectious Diseases, Children's Hospital, Harvard Medical School, Boston, Massachusetts

Cheryl Jay MD, Clinical Associate, Neuromuscular Diseases Section, National Institute of Neurological Disorders and Stroke, National Institutes of Health, Bethesda, Maryland

Sue Jue MD, Pediatric Infectious Disease Fellow, Department of Pediatrics, Microbiology, and Medicine, University of Alabama, Birmingham, Alabama

David L. Katz MD, JD, Associate, Arnold and Porter, Washington, DC, Lecturer on Psychiatry, Harvard Medical School, Boston, Massachusetts

Samuel L. Katz MD, Wilburt C. Davison Professor of Pediatrics, Duke University School of Medicine, Durham, North Carolina

Richard A. Koup MD, Staff Investigator, Aaron Diamond AIDS Research Center, Assistant Professor of Medicine, Department of Medicine and Microbiology, New York University School of Medicine, New York, New York

Andrea Kovacs MD, Assistant Professor, Departments of Pediatrics and Pathology, Los Angeles County and University of Southern California Medical Center, Los Angeles, California

Keith Krasinski MD, Associate Professor, Department of Pediatrics, New York University Medical Center, New York, New York

Michael D. Lairmore DVM, PhD, Assistant Professor, Ohio State University, Center for Retrovirus Research and Department of Veterinary Pathobiology, Columbus, Ohio

Daniel V. Landers MD, Associate Professor, Department of Obstetrics, Gynecology, and Reproductive Sciences, San Francisco General Hospital, University of California, San Francisco, California

Louisa Laue MD, Assistant Professor, Department of Pediatrics, Georgetown University School of Medicine, Washington, DC

Linda L. Lewis MD, Medical Officer, Pediatric Branch, National Cancer Institute, National Institutes of Health, Bethesda, Maryland

Steven E. Lipshultz MD, Associate in Cardiology, Children's Hospital, Director, Pediatric Cardiology, Boston City Hospital, Assistant Professor of Pediatrics, Harvard Medical School, Boston, Massachusetts

Ian T. Magrath MD, Head, Lymphoma Biology Section, National Cancer Institute, National Institutes of Health, Bethesda, Maryland

M. Juliana McElrath MD, Director, AIDS Vaccine Evaluation Unit, University of Washington, Seattle, Washington

Kenneth McIntosh MD, Chief, Division of Infectious Disease, Children's Hospital, Professor of Pediatrics, Harvard Medical School, Boston, Massachusetts

Tracie L. Miller, Assistant in Medicine, Department of Gastroenterology, Children's Hospital, Boston, Massachusetts

Howard L. Minkoff MD, Professor, Department Obstetrics and Gynecology, State University of New York Health Science Center, Brooklyn, New York

Charles D. Mitchell MD, Associate Professor, Division of Pediatric Immunology and Infectious Diseases, Unversity of Miami School of Medicine, Miami, Florida

Lynne M. Mofenson MD, Associate Branch Chief for Clinical Research, Pediatric, Adolescent, and Maternal AIDS Branch, National Institute of Child Health and Human Development, National Institutes of Health, Bethesda, Maryland

Brigitta U. Mueller MD, Visiting Associate, Pediatric Branch, National Cancer Institute, National Institutes of Health, Bethesda, Maryland

Michael Murphey-Corb PhD, MS, BS, Senior Research Scientist, Department of Microbiology, Tulane Regional Primate Research Center, Tulane University, Covington, Louisiana

Marie-Louise Newell MB, PhD, Lecturer in Epidemiology, Department of Epidemiology and Biostatistics, Institute of Child Health, London, United Kingdom

Robert B. Nussenblatt MD, Chief, Laboratory of Immunology, National Eye Institute, National Institutes of Health, Bethesda, Maryland

James Oleske MD, MPH, Francois-Xavier Bagnoud Professor, Department of Pediatrics, New Jersey Medical School, Newark, New Jersey

Margaret J. Oxtoby MD, Chief, Pediatrics Family Studies Section, Division of HIV-A, Centers for Disease Control and Prevention, Atlanta, Georgia

Catherine S. Peckham MD, Professor, Paediatric Epidemiology, Institute of Child Health, London, United Kingdom

Larry K. Pickering MD, Professor and Vice Chairman for Research, Department of Pediatrics, Director, Center for Pediatric Research, Eastern Virginia Medical School and Children's Hospital of the King's Daughters, Norfolk, Virginia

Peggy Daly Pizzo MEd, Affiliate Faculty, Bush Center in Child Development and Social Policy, Yale University, New Haven, Connecticut

Philip A. Pizzo MD, Chief of Pediatrics, Head, Infectious Disease Section, National Cancer Institute, National Institutes of Health, Professor of Pediatrics, Uniformed Services University of the Health Sciences, Bethesda, Maryland

David G. Poplack MD, Elise C. Young Professor of Pediatric Oncology, Head, Hematology-Oncology Section, Chief, Hematology/Oncology Services, Texas Children's Hospital, Baylor College of Medicine, Houston, Texas

Neil S. Prose MD, Assistant Professor of Medicine and Pediatrics, Department of Medicine/Dermatology, Duke University Medical Center, Durham, North Carolina

Thomas C. Quinn MD, MSc, Professor of Medicine, Department of Medicine, Johns Hopkins University School of Medicine, Baltimore, Maryland

Martha F. Rogers MD, Chief, Epidemiology Branch, Division of HIV/AIDS, Centers for Disease Control and Prevention, Atlanta, Georgia

Zeda F. Rosenberg ScD, Assistant to the Director, National Institute of Allergy and Infectious Diseases, National Institutes of Health, Bethesda, Maryland

Andrea Ruff MD, Assistant Professor, Department of International Health, Department of Pediatrics, Johns Hopkins University, Baltimore, Maryland

Sheila J. Santacroce, RM, MSN, CPNP, Doctoral Student, School of Nursing, University of North Carolina, Chapel Hill, North Carolina

Gerald Schochetman PhD, Chief, Laboratory Investigations Branch, Division of HIV/AIDS, National Center for Infectious Disease, Centers for Disease Control and Prevention, Atlanta, Georgia

Daniel D. Sedmak MD, Associate Professor of Pathology, Department of Pathology, College of Medicine, Ohio State University, Columbus, Ohio

Anita Septimus MSW, CSW, Director of Social Services, Department of Immunology and Allergy, Albert Einstein College of Medicine, Bronx, New York

Aziza T. Shad MD, Visiting Scientist, Lymphoma Biology Section, Department of Pediatric Branch, National Cancer Institute, National Institutes of Health, Bethesda, Maryland

R. J. Simonds MD, Medical Epidemiologist, Epidemiology Branch, Division of HIV/AIDS, National Center for Infectious Disease, Centers for Disease Control and Prevention, Atlanta, Georgia

Stephen A. Spector MD, Professor of Pediatrics and Center for Genetics Chief, Division of Infectious Diseases, Department of Pediatrics, University of California at San Diego, La Jolla, California

Reed Tuckson MD, President, Charles R. Drew University of Medicine and Science, Los Angeles, California

John G. Twomey Jr. MD, Assistant Professor, College of Nursing, University of Rhode Island, Kingston, Rhode Island

Richard R. Viscarello MD, Director of Maternal-Fetal Medicine, Department of Obstetrics and Gynecology, Stanford Hospital, Stanford, Connecticut

Ellen R. Wald MD, Department of Pediatrics, University of Pittsburgh School of Medicine, Pittsburgh, Pennsylvania

Thomas J. Walsh MD, Senior Investigator, Infectious Diseases Section, Pediatric Branch, National Cancer Institute, National Institutes of Health, Bethesda, Maryland

Richard J. Whitley MD, Loeb Eminent Scholar Chair in Pediatrics, Professor of Pediatrics, Microbiology, and Medicine, Department of Pediatrics, University of Alabama, Birmingham, Alabama

Lori Wiener PhD, Coordinator, Pediatric HIV Psychosocial Support Program, National Cancer Institute, National Institutes of Health, Bethesda, Maryland

Delbert R. Wigfall MD, Acting Chief, Assistant Professor of Pediatrics, Division of Nephrology, Department of Pediatrics, Duke University Medical Center, Durham, North Carolina

Catherine M. Wilfert MD, Professor of Pediatrics and Microbiology, Chief, Pediatric Infectious Diseases, Department of Pediatrics, Duke University Medical Center, Durham, North Carolina

Christopher B. Wilson MD, Professor of Pediatrics and Immunology, Head, Division of Immunology/Rheumatology, University of Washington, Seattle, Washington

Harland S. Winter MD, Chief, Pediatric Gastro-enterology and Nutrition, Boston University School of Medicine, Boston, Massachusetts

Paul H. Wise MD, MPH, Director, Harvard Institute for Reproductive and Child Health, Harvard Medical School, Associate in Medicine, Children's Hospital, Boston, Massachusetts

Constance Wofsy MD, Professor of Medicine, Department of Medicine, AIDS Activities Program, University of California, San Francisco General Hospital, San Francisco, California

Steven M. Wolinsky MD, BA, Assistant Professor of Medicine, Infectious Diseases, Northwestern University Medical School, Chicago, Illinois

Contents

Vertically Acquired HIV Infection in the United States

Margaret J. Oxtoby

Since the first persons with AIDS were described in 1981, the global impact of this epidemic has been dramatic. The World Health Organization estimated that by the end of 1992 ~2.5 million AIDS cases in men, women, and children had occurred and that 13 million persons had been infected with the human immunodeficiency virus (HIV); 1 million of these were children (1).

In 1983 HIV was established as the cause of the new syndrome, and by early 1985 an antibody assay to detect infection became commercially available. Over the next few years the effect of HIV on its primary target cell, the CD4+ T lymphocyte, was elucidated. The first cases of AIDS in children were described in 1982 (2–5), 1 year after the initial description of AIDS in adults, and the connection with mothers who had AIDS or were at risk for the disease became evident. HIV-infected children manifested similar derangements of their immune systems, with resulting inability to fight infection, as did adults with the syndrome.

In the first decade of the pandemic, much has been learned about vertically acquired HIV infection. This chapter reviews our current understanding of the epidemiology of HIV infection in children and their mothers by using data from AIDS surveillance, HIV surveillance, HIV seroprevalence surveys, and studies of HIV transmission and disease progression (see also Chapters 2–6). Surveillance data delineating the scope of the epidemic will focus on the United States, whereas data from Europe and Africa as well as the United States will be discussed in the sections on transmission and disease progression. This chapter particularly emphasizes information that has emerged since early 1990.

SCOPE OF EPIDEMIC IN UNITED STATES

Epidemiology of AIDS in Women and Children

Historically in the epidemic, AIDS case reporting has helped characterize cases, delineate modes of transmission, and monitor trends. In the United States, surveillance is based on the reporting of AIDS cases to local and state health departments, which in turn report these cases to the Centers for Disease Control and Prevention (CDC). Before the identification of HIV, the AIDS case definition included a list of highly specific opportunistic infections and malignancies, diagnosed by definitive methods such as biopsy or culture, that were due to profound cell-mediated immunodeficiency without other causes. Revision of the case definition in 1987 (6) (Table 1.1) broadened the conditions reportable as AIDS, included diseases diagnosed presumptively, and placed more emphasis on HIV testing as a component of diagnosis. In children as well as adults, these changes reflected increasing understanding of the spectrum of disease attributable to HIV infection and changes in diagnostic practices. In 1993, the AIDS case definition for adults and ado-

Table 1.1.   Diagnoses that Indicate AIDS in 1993 CDC Revised Surveillance Definition for AIDS

Multiple or recurrent bacterial infections[c]
Candidiasis of the trachea, bronchi, or lungs[a]
Candidiasis of the esophagus[a, b]
Invasive cervical cancer[d]
Coccidioidomycosis, disseminated or extrapulmonary[c]
Cryptococcosis, extrapulmonary[a]
Cryptosporidiosis, chronic intestinal[a]
Cytomegalovirus disease (other than liver, spleen, nodes) onset at age >1month[a]
Cytomegalovirus retinitis (with loss of vision)[a, b]
HIV encephalopathy[c]
Chronic herpes simplex ulcer (>1 month duration) or pneumonitis or esophagitis onset at >1 month of age[a]
Histoplasmosis, disseminated or extrapulmonary[a]
Isosporiasis, chronic intestinal (>1 month duration)[c]
Kaposi's sarcoma[a, b]
Lymphoid interstitial pneumonitis[a, b]
Lymphoma, primary brain[a]
Lymphoma (Burkitt's or immunoblastic sarcoma)[c]
Mycobacterium avium complex or *M. kansasii*, disseminated or extrapulmonary[a]
M. tuberculosis or acid-fast infection (species not identified), disseminated or extrapulmonary[c] or pulmonary[d]
Pneumonia, recurrent[d]
P. carinii pneumonia[a, b]
Progressive multifocal leukoencephalopathy[a]
Toxoplasmosis of brain, onset at age >1 month[a, b]
Wasting syndrome caused by HIV[c]

---

[a]If indicator disease is diagnosed definitively (e.g., biopsy, culture) and there is no other cause of immunodeficiency, laboratory documentation of HIV infection is not required.
[b]Presumptive diagnosis of indicator disease is accepted, if there is laboratory evidence of HIV infection (1987 addition).
[c]Requires laboratory evidence of HIV infection (1987 addition).
[d]Requires laboratory evidence of HIV infection (1993 addition; adults and adolescents).

lescents was again expanded to include three new clinical diagnoses: pulmonary tuberculosis, recurrent pneumonia, and invasive cervical cancer, as well as persons with fewer than 200 CD4+ T lymphocytes per microliter (7). Surveillance approaches for children with HIV/AIDS are under review.

Although the AIDS case definition serves as a guide for AIDS reporting, the CDC HIV classification system (8) (Table 1.2), published in 1987, was intended as a structure for describing the entire spectrum of HIV in children, including infants with maternal antibody whose infection status was not yet

determined and asymptomatic infected persons as well as infants and children with overt disease manifestations. A staging classification system for HIV-infected children that incorporates age-specific CD4 levels and mild, moderate, and severe clinical categories is being developed.

It is helpful to examine children with perinatal HIV infection in the context of the whole epidemic, since each of these infections is the result of earlier HIV infections among adults (see also Chapter 6) (9, 10). Overall, women constitute 12% of adult and adolescent AIDS cases in the United States (Table 1.3). The predominant mode of transmission for women has been the sharing of needles during parenteral use of illicit drugs. Sexual contact with an HIV-infected man is also a major mode of transmission for women, accounting for 36% of cases in the United States. Most of these heterosexual contact cases are in turn related to intravenous drug use in the partner. However, increasing trends, particularly evident in the South and Northeast, point to the role of crack, an inexpensive form of smokable cocaine, in relation to heterosexual transmission (11–13). There are also AIDS cases reported among women who have emigrated from countries in the Caribbean and sub-Saharan Africa where heterosexual contact unrelated to drug use is the major mode of transmission. Increasingly, heterosexual transmission unrelated to drug use is becoming an important part of the epidemic within the United States as well. Among vertically infected children with AIDS, their mothers are increasingly less likely to be intravenous drug users and more likely to have been infected heterosexually (Fig. 1.1).

Cases in women and children have continued to increase. In the United States, 6255 new cases in women and 697 cases in children who acquired infection perinatally were reported to CDC in 1992 (Tables 1.3 and 1.4). When examined by month of diagnosis adjusted for reporting delay, AIDS cases in women continued to increase steadily, whereas cases in children appeared to begin to level (Fig. 1.2). However, in the face of increasing numbers of children born each year to infected women, this leveling is most likely attributable to delay in develop-

Table 1.2.   CDC Classification System for HIV in Children

CLASS P-0. INDETERMINATE INFECTION
   Infants <15 months born to infected mothers but without definitive evidence of HIV infection or
      AIDS
CLASS P-1. ASYMPTOMATIC INFECTION
   Subclass A. Normal immune function
   Subclass B. Abnormal immune function
      Hypergammaglobulinemia, T4 lymphopenia, decreased T4-to-T8 ratio, or absolute lymphopenia
   Subclass C. Immune function not tested
CLASS P-2. SYMPTOMATIC INFECTION
   Subclass A. Nonspecific findings (at least two for ≥2 months)
      Fever, failure to thrive, generalized lymphadenopathy, hepatomegaly, splenomegaly, enlarged
         parotid glands, persistent or recurrent diarrhea
   Subclass B. Progressive neurologic disease
      Loss of developmental milestones or intellectual ability, impaired brain growth, or progressive
         symmetrical motor deficits
   Subclass C. Lymphoid interstitial pneumonitis
   Subclass D. Secondary infectious diseases
      Category D-1. Opportunistic infections in CDC case definition
         Bacterial: mycobacterial infection (noncutaneous, extrapulmonary, or disseminated);
            nocardiosis
         Fungal: candidiasis (esophageal, bronchial, or pulmonary), coccidioidomycosis, disseminated
            histoplasmosis, extrapulmonary cryptococcosis
         Parasitic: P. carinii pneumonia, disseminated toxoplasmosis with onset ≥1 month of age,
            chronic crytosporidiosis or isosporiasis, extraintestinal strongyloidiasis
         Viral: cytomegalovirus disease (onset ≥1 month of age), chronic mucocutaneous/disseminated
            herpes (onset ≥1 month age), progressive multifocal leukoencephalopathy
      Category D-2. Unexplained, recurrent, serious bacterial infections (two or more in 2 years)
         Sepsis, meningitis, pneumonia, abscess of an internal organ, bone/joint infections
      Category D-3. Other infectious diseases
         Includes persistent oral candidiasis, recurrent herpes stomatitis (at least two episodes in 1
            year), multidermatomal or disseminated herpes zoster
   Subclass E. Secondary cancers
      Category E-1. Cancers in AIDS case definition
         Kaposi's sarcoma, B cell non-Hodgkin's lymphoma, or primary lymphoma of brain
      Category E-2. Other malignancies possibly associated with HIV
   Subclass F. Other conditions possibly caused by HIV
      Includes hepatitis, cardiopathy, nephropathy, hematologic disorders, dermatologic diseases

ment of AIDS owing to treatment or changes in completeness of reporting. (14).

Projections of the number of persons diagnosed with AIDS suggest that whereas AIDS cases diagnosed annually among homosexual or bisexual men have begun to level (though at a very high rate) and rates among men and women with a history of intravenous drug use are expected to increase not more than 10% per year, the rate of increase among persons infected heterosexually is continuing to increase. Corrected for reporting delay, from 1990 to 1991 AIDS cases in individuals with heterosexually acquired HIV increased by 28%. (15) In addition, some persons who present with no identified risk may have been infected het-

erosexually by persons they did not recognize to be infected or at risk for AIDS.

Of all cases in children reported in the United States in 1992, 90% were attributable to vertical transmission (Table 1.4). Vertically acquired infections account for almost all new infections, because HIV screening of the blood supply has been in place since 1985 and heat treatment of clotting factor/donor screening since 1983 (see Chapters 4 and 39) (16). Recent outbreaks of HIV infection in children in the former Soviet Union and Romania, however, attest to the possibility of nosocomial transmission and the continued need for vigilance in blood screening and sterilization of medical equipment (17). Some children have

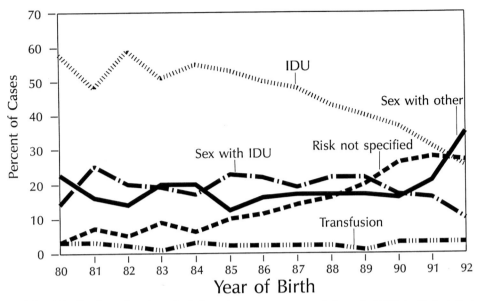

Figure 1.1. Distribution of perinatally infected cases by exposure category of mother for AIDS cases reported through 1992 in United States by child's year of birth. *IDU,* injection drug use.

Table 1.3. Adult and Adolescent AIDS Cases by Exposure Category and Sex Reported in 1992 and Cumulatively (1981–1992) in the United States

	Males				Females			
	1992		1981–1992		1992		1981–1992	
	N	%	*N*	%	*N*	%	*N*	%
Men who have sex with men	23,936	60	142,626	64				
Injection drug use	8,610	21	43,786	20	2,815	45	13,626	50
Men who have sex with men and inject drugs	2,429	6	15,899	7				
Hemophilia/coagulation disorder	313	1	1,983	1	3	0	43	0
Heterosexual contact	1,677	4	6,419	3	2,437	39	9,835	36
Receipt of blood transfusion, blood components, or tissue	397	1	3,036	1	276	4	1,944	7
Other/undetermined	2,718	7	7,965	4	724	12	2,037	7
Total	40,080	100	221,714	100	6,255	100	27,485	100

Table 1.4. AIDS Cases in Children (Age <13 Years) by Exposure Category Reported in 1992 and Cumulative Total Reported in 1981–1992, United States

	1992		1981–1992	
	N	%	*N*	%
Mother with or at risk for HIV infection	697	90	3665	87
Injection drug use	246		1698	
Heterosexual contact	240		1345	
Transfusion or transplant recipient	24		80	
Other/undetermined	187		542	
Hemophilia/coagulation disorder	21	3	188	4
Transfusion recipient	19	2	306	7
Other/undetermined	34	4	90	2
Total	771	100	4249	100

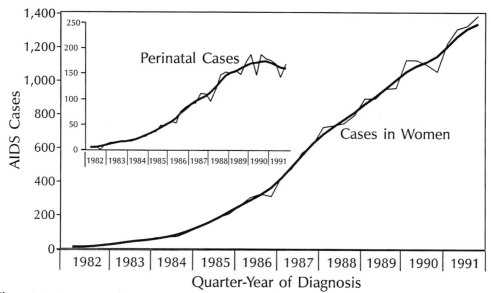

Figure 1.2. Women and perinatally infected children with AIDS by quarter year of diagnosis, adjusted for reporting delays, in United States, 1982–1991.

also been infected through sexual abuse (18, 19).

The demographic characteristics of AIDS cases in women and children with perinatally acquired infection primarily reflect the characteristics of groups at risk for infection, particularly intravenous drug users. Overall, 59% of perinatally acquired AIDS cases in the United States are among African-American children and 26% among Hispanic children; African-American and Hispanic children have cumulative AIDS incidence rates 17 and 7 times the incidence rates in white children. In parts of New York City and northern New Jersey, most intravenous drug users in treatment are black or Hispanic and live in poor inner city communities where the prevalence of HIV infection among these drug users is nearly 50%. Although intravenous drug use is also common in other cities, HIV seropositivity rates in drug users outside the Northeast average under 5%. Fifteen metropolitan areas, most along the East coast, include only one-fifth of the pediatric population of the United States and territories but account for two-thirds of the perinatal cases of HIV infection.

Although the highest number of pediatric AIDS deaths occur in the first year of life, the relative impact of AIDS as a cause of death has been most striking in the 1- to 4-year age group. By 1990, AIDS was the seventh leading cause of death in the United States for this age group. The impact is even greater in some subpopulations; by 1988 in New York State, AIDS was the first leading cause of death among Hispanic children aged 1–4 years and the second leading cause of death (after unintentional injuries) among black children aged 1–4 years (accounting for 15 and 16%, respectively, of all deaths in that age group) (20).

A mathematical model looking at mortality under age 5 years suggests that vertical HIV infection could become the most common cause of death in children in the developed world if maternal infection rates reach 2–3%; rates of 25–30% would be needed to produce a similar effect in the developing world (21).

Prevalence and Incidence of HIV Infection in Women and Infants

AIDS surveillance data have been very useful in characterizing the severe end of the HIV disease spectrum. HIV seroprevalence surveys have complemented data from AIDS surveillance and more accurately present the current situation. Clearly, the highest seroprevalence rates in women are among those who are intravenous drug users or who are sex partners of an HIV-infected man (see Chapter 6). However, several studies have shown that many seropositive women do not acknowledge or know they are at risk for infection. For instance, one early survey among women delivering babies at a New York City hospital that linked blinded HIV results with a questionnaire on behavior related to an increased risk for HIV showed that half the HIV-seropositive women had no reported risk for HIV infection (22); i.e., they were likely infected through heterosexual contact with a partner they did not recognize to be HIV infected or to be at increased risk for infection. Studies in other clinical settings have corroborated this finding.

Various settings in which women are routinely tested for HIV have provided additional estimates of the prevalence in certain populations. Female applicants for military service have been tested since 1985 and have shown a fairly stable seroprevalence rate nationally of 0.06%. Rates are much higher in certain inner city areas in the Northeast: rates are ~0.5% in northern New Jersey and New York City and 0.3% in San Juan, Puerto Rico. Seroprevalence rates in black and Hispanic female military applicants are seven and four times, respectively, those among white applicants (23). Seroprevalence among first-time female blood donors is ~0.01% (24).

Beginning in 1988 the CDC has coordinated many blinded HIV serosurveys in various clinical settings (25). The largest and most nearly population-based sample is the national survey of childbearing women (26–28). This survey measures the prevalence of maternal HIV antibody but is actually conducted through blinded HIV testing of newborn heelstick blood samples collected for routine metabolic testing. The technique for testing filter paper samples was developed in the Massachusetts State Laboratory; in that state the prevalence from December 1986 to June 1987 was 0.21% and from January to December 1988 was 0.25%. This survey is ongoing in 44 states, Puerto Rico, and the District of Columbia. Highest seroprevalence rates have been in the District of Columbia (0.9%), New York (0.61%, with a rate of 1.25% in New York City and 0.16% in upstate New York), New Jersey (0.55%), and Florida (0.54%); most other states have overall rates under 0.1%. (Fig. 1.3 and Table 1.5) The estimated national rate in 1991 was 0.17%; this corresponds to ~7130

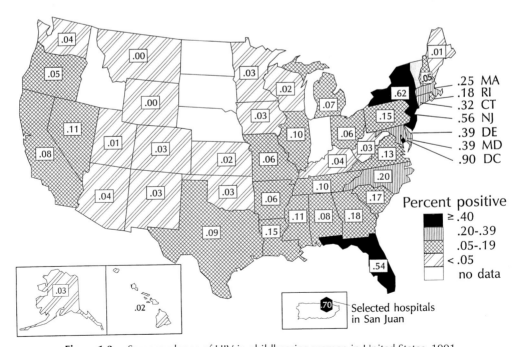

Figure 1.3. Seroprevalence of HIV in childbearing women in United States, 1991.

Table 1.5. Perinatal AIDS Cases Reported 1982–1992 and HIV Prevalence/1000 Childbearing women in 1990[a]

State	Number	%	HIV Prevalence
New York	1066	29	6.2
Florida	578	16	5.4
New Jersey	379	10	5.6
California	201	5	0.8
Texas	123	4	0.9
Puerto Rico	196	5	[b]
Maryland	107	3	3.9
Illinois	100	3	1.0
Pennsylvania	97	3	1.5
Massachusetts	93	3	2.5
Connecticut	80	2	3.2
Georgia	68	2	1.9
Virginia	57	2	1.3
Washington DC	54	1	9.0
North Carolina	51	1	2.0
Louisiana	50	1	1.5
Other	365	10	
Total	3665	100	1.6

[a]Values from states or territories with at least 50 reported perinatal AIDS cases.
[b]Not available island wide.

HIV-infected women delivering live-born infants per year (29). By using 20–30% as an estimate for the rate of perinatal transmission, an estimated 1750 (1400–2200) of these children were infected as a result of maternal infection in 1991. This number is three times the number of children reported with perinatally acquired AIDS in 1991, suggesting that the future number of pediatric cases will be even higher than that experienced to date. Overall, it is estimated that in the United States in 1991 there were 10,000–15,000 HIV-infected children.

Most states that have conducted the survey for multiple years have stable prevalence rates. However, a few areas, particularly in the South, report rising seroprevalence. Among southern states, prevalence per 1000 has increased from 1.7 in 1989 to 2.0 in 1991 (29). Some of this increase has occurred in small towns and rural areas; in Georgia, for instance, the prevalence of infection among childbearing women in Atlanta is similar to that for the rest of the state (30).

Note that the states with the highest syphilis rates in 1991 were also in the southeast. The similarity of distribution between county rates of primary and secondary syphilis of more than 10/100,000 population and counties with HIV rates of more than 100/100,000 among childbearing women is striking (31). Syphilis and other genital ulcer diseases have been associated with an increased risk of acquiring HIV infection. Presumably this is because of risky sexual behavior and the potential enhancement of transmission because of disrupted local mucosal surfaces and the local inflammation that brings increased numbers of potential target cells (CD4+ lymphocytes or macrophages) to the area of contact. Prevention of HIV infection in areas with high rates of syphilis will need to address both these infections. The use of crack cocaine has also been linked to exchange of sex for money and may further fuel the dual epidemics of syphilis and HIV.

Other anonymous HIV seroprevalence surveys have been conducted in various medical clinics in 40 metropolitan areas of the United States. For example, in 1988 and 1989, surveys of women attending sexually transmitted disease clinics showed a median prevalence of 0.8%, but rates in some clinics have been greater than 5% (32). Median seroprevalence rates by clinic type for women attending prenatal, family planning, and abortion clinics were 0.8%, 0.2%, and 0.1%, respectively, but some clinics had much higher rates (33).

In New York City during 1987–1989, parallel studies in 15 abortion facilities showed a prevalence of 1.19% (70/5889), similar to prevalence among childbearing women in New York City during the same time (34).

Newer Surveillance Initiatives

Increasingly, states are moving toward broader forms of HIV/AIDS surveillance. By 1992, more than 30 states had adopted some form of HIV infection reporting, with 26 states requiring reporting by name. This approach can aid HIV-related prevention activities and medical and social support programs. Rather than estimating the actual prevalence of HIV infection or the extent of severe HIV morbidity, HIV infection reporting documents the numbers and characteristics of persons whose infection is detected and who are in need of appropriate follow-up. Surveillance for HIV infection can be particularly helpful for children with perinatal infection by improving the ability to monitor trends and contributing to the development of an appropriate framework for delivering and financing medical and social services to this particularly needy group (see Chapters 52 and 53).

Data from the CDC Pediatric Spectrum of Disease study, conducted in six states or metropolitan areas that report 23% of all United States children with AIDS, help connect the data from AIDS surveillance and HIV seroprevalence. Among children in the Spectrum of Disease study who were receiving medical care for HIV during 1991, the median age for known vertically infected children (class P-1 or P-2) was 3 years, with a range from 0 to 13 years; 32% had AIDS, 55% had symptomatic infection not yet meeting the case definition, and only 13% were considered asymptomatic, with most of these showing immune abnormalities. In addition to these 1000 children, another 600 class P-0 children were under evaluation for possible HIV infection, and many of these children had significant illness as well. Thus, for every child with AIDS in medical care, there were two children with other HIV-related illnesses and two children with indeterminate infection.

HIV infection surveillance can also help determine the number of children in each birth cohort who are detected as HIV infected as a proportion of all those who are estimated to be infected from the neonatal survey and can help ensure that these children are tied into the available community resources. Based on data from Massachusetts, by the time they reached age 3 years, only 35% of HIV-exposed children born in 1988 had been evaluated by the medical system for HIV (35). Although earlier diagnosis and broader recommendations for testing are gradually increasing this proportion, it is clear that many HIV-infected children still lack appropriate early interventions such as early PCP prophylaxis (36, 37).

Impact of AIDS on Family

Children with HIV infection frequently live with other infected or uninfected siblings in families where at least one other adult is HIV infected. Uninfected children share many of the same difficulties as their infected siblings: a high risk of being orphaned at a young age by one or both parents and the heavy medical and social burden of HIV illness on the family. In addition, these children are at increased risk of certain infections, particularly tuberculosis. All children born to HIV-infected women share the "HIV-positive" label and require close follow-up to determine infection status, especially during the first year of life. In certain subpopulations, such as black women aged 15–44 years in New York State and New Jersey, for whom HIV/AIDS is the leading cause of death, the impact on both infected and uninfected children in these communities is already very great (38).

It is estimated that ~20,000 children have already been orphaned by their mother's death to AIDS, with over 80,000 children orphaned by the end of the 1990s (39, 40) (see also Chapter 43).

A high proportion of children born to HIV-infected parents are living in foster care or other alternative family settings because of parental illness or family stresses related to drug use. Of ~1700 children followed in the Pediatric Spectrum of Disease study through 1990, 55% were living with a biologic parent, 10% were with another relative, 28% were in foster care, 3% had been adopted, and 4% lived in group settings or with other caretakers (41).

MOTHER TO INFANT TRANSMISSION
Overall Transmission Rates

Transmission from mother to infant is a relatively efficient mode of transmission of the virus, in contrast to transmission through sexual contact. Calculation of transmission rates is complicated by several factors, in particular the difficulty of establishing a reliable diagnosis of HIV in infancy. Thus, for instance, children who die in their first year of life cannot easily be counted as infected or uninfected unless they have a clinical and immunologic picture characteristic of AIDS or a positive virus test. Various prospective studies have been conducted or are underway in several different countries, and although the rate in individual studies ranges from 10 to 50%, most of the larger studies in the United States and Europe with sufficient follow-up of infants have described rates between 15 and 30%, following the convention of the CDC classification system to determine HIV infection status (see also Chapters 2, 3, and 10C) (42–50). Studies in Africa and Haiti have calculated rates different from those in more industrialized countries, since diagnosis of secondary conditions is more difficult and more children die in infancy (51–56). Minimum rates of transmission in these studies can be calculated by including only children with accepted laboratory documentation of infection—usually, persistence of antibody to the second year of life—whereas a maximum rate can be calculated by adding deaths during the first year to this figure. Because most of these studies have comparison groups of children born to uninfected women, excess mortality above the mortality in this comparison group can be considered related to maternal HIV infection; however, some of these children who die in infancy may not actually be HIV infected. The range of transmission rates of HIV-1 in these studies from Africa and Haiti has been from 25 to 40%. HIV-2, mainly found in West Africa, appears to be much less efficiently transmitted, with one prospective study in Côte d'Ivoire showing only 1 of 34 children of HIV-2-infected mothers becoming infected themselves (57).

It is now clear that rather than thinking in terms of overall rates of transmission, it is important to consider maternal characteristics that might increase or decrease risk of transmission and factors related to an individual pregnancy that could affect transmission at particular times during gestation, parturition, or postpartum. These will be briefly reviewed in this chapter but are discussed in more detail in Chapter 10.

Maternal Characteristics Affecting Risk of Transmission

Many studies suggest that advanced HIV disease in the mother, as represented by increased viral burden (p24 antigenemia (56, 58, 59), higher viral titers (60), altered immune status, particularly low CD4 count, or CD4-to-CD8 ratio (46, 47, 50, 51, 56), or clinical AIDS (47, 51, 53, 56, 59)), are predictive of increased risk of transmission of HIV to the infant. Recent studies have also suggested a high risk of transmission early in the disease among women who seroconvert during pregnancy. A recent study in Zaire suggested that HIV-infected women with normal CD4 counts but high CD8 counts (>1800) were also at increased risk of transmitting HIV, and some of these women may be at an early stage of infection with the virus less well in check (56).

Examination of the relationship between maternal neutralizing antibodies or other HIV-specific humoral and cellular immune responses and risk of HIV transmission to the infant has produced inconsistent results in different studies, and no clear protective or risk factors have emerged. This remains an important area of study. Recent work has focused on maternal and infant immunologic responses to autologous and heterologous viral strains; it remains plausible that a virus which "escapes" maternal immune mechanisms may be involved in selective HIV-1 transmission to the infant (see Chapter 10C).

Timing and Mechanisms of Mother to Infant Transmission

The mechanisms of transmission from mother to infant and the risk of transmission by each route remain a complex puzzle (61). Several promising research approaches are underway, including virologic and immunologic assays of fetuses and infants at different stages of development and comparison of overall transmission rates in cohorts of children born to infected mothers who have different exposures (type of delivery, breast feeding vs. bottle feeding).

It remains unclear when most maternal to infant transmission occurs: early in pregnancy, later in pregnancy, or around delivery. Although case reports have established the presence of virus in fetal tissue as early as 15 weeks, it would seem unlikely that most transmission occurs this early since most infected children are clinically and immunologically normal at birth, and no conclusive evidence of a congenital HIV syndrome has been established. However, from 30 to 50% of children are HIV positive by polymerase chain reaction or culture soon after birth suggesting in utero transmission at some point during gestation (62–64).

For children first showing virologic or immunologic signs of infection after 4–12 weeks, infection in late gestation or intrapartum appears more likely (49, 64). Other recent evidence, although largely indirect, suggests that intrapartum transmission may be more frequent than in utero transmission. The analogy with hepatitis B virus, which is transmitted to the infant mainly through contact with blood and secretions at delivery, suggests this period may be one of high risk for HIV transmission as well. Some studies have suggested a borderline protective effect of cesarean section (47, 50, 65), and most have shown no difference by mode of delivery. Of 1840 HIV-exposed children followed in the Pediatric Spectrum of Disease study with known mode of delivery and HIV infection status, 21% of infected children had been delivered by cesarean section compared with 20% of uninfected children. Among twin sets reported to the International Registry of Twins, 50% of firstborn twins delivered vaginally and 38% of firstborn twins delivered by cesarean were infected compared with 19% of second born twins delivered by either route; the implications of these striking findings and their applicability to singleton births is uncertain (44). A study of prospectively followed sibling pairs found that infection in the older child was not predictive of infection in the subsequent child, and no relationship was found with mode of delivery (66). An important role of chorioamnionitis with funisitis (inflammation of the cord) in transmission of HIV has been found in both prospective studies in Zaire (51, 56), and untreated syphilis was found to increase transmission rate in a United States study (67). Together, these data suggest important transmission factors related to contact with maternal blood or secretions and to placental integrity, which could vary from between pregnancies and even between twins (see Chapter 10A).

Recent studies have also suggested a more important role of breast feeding in transmission of HIV than had been thought initially. Many case reports have established that postpartum transmission in infants who were breast fed has occurred in situations where the mother was transfused with HIV-contaminated blood after the child's delivery or seroconverted during the year after delivery through heterosexual contact, and the risk of transmission to the infant in this circumstance may be 25% or more (68–72). However, this period of acute infection in the mother, before development of an antibody response, may be a time at which she is particularly likely to transmit and may not be generalizable to the more common situation where the mother is infected throughout pregnancy. A meta-analysis of studies of women with prevalent HIV infection estimated a 14% additional risk of transmission related to breast feeding (72).

These findings have clear policy implications, because the risks of breast feeding must be balanced against the risks of not breast feeding, particularly in areas with high infant mortality where the primary causes of infant death are infectious diseases and malnutrition. In areas where there are safe alternatives to breast feeding, such as the United States, HIV-infected women are recommended not to breast feed to avoid risk of transmission to an infant not yet infected (76). Decision analyses evaluating the risk of mortality from other causes associated with not breast feeding, compared with the risk of transmitting HIV through breast feeding, support the current World Health Organization and CDC recommendations for breast feeding in infected mothers (73–77). These recommendations emphasize that in most areas of the world, breast feeding is the best option on a population basis for women. Individual recommendations to known HIV-infected women will vary according to the setting.

Although much remains to be learned about mother to infant transmission, there is a clear need to initiate well-designed collaborative studies of different intervention strategies for prevention of transmission (78). Studies of many interventions, including antiviral agents, passive or active immunization, cleansing of the vaginal canal, and provision of infant feeding alternatives, are underway or being designed (see also Chapters 10C, 41, and 45).

MORBIDITY AND MORTALITY
Clinical Presentations

The full spectrum of HIV disease in children is now becoming evident. To describe the course of HIV disease, estimate average life spans in infected children, and elucidate prognostic factors related to disease progression, prospective studies of children identified at birth will eventually provide the most useful data; but these studies are difficult, and the number of children enrolled is still relatively small. Moreover, such studies can be confounded by changes in supportive care and primary antiviral therapies (see also Chapter 35).

Series of AIDS cases have provided data on the most severely ill children and can be used indirectly to model incubation periods from infection to onset of AIDS. More recently, series of HIV-infected children in clinical settings where HIV antibody testing is frequently recommended in the course of clinical care have provided valuable data on a broader spectrum of clinical manifestations. However, even in these settings, most children are not diagnosed until they have become ill with HIV-related disease.

AIDS case surveillance reports provide data on the most common AIDS indicator diseases (Table 1.6). Among children reported from 1988 through 1992, 35% had *Pneumocystis carinii* pneumonia (PCP), 24% had lymphoid interstitial pneumonitis, 19% had recurrent serious bacterial infections, and 13% had *Candida* esophagitis. Wasting

Table 1.6. Most Commonly Reported AIDS Indicator Diseases[a]

	Number	%[b]
P. carinii pneumonia	1374	37
Lymphoid interstitial pneumonitis	926	25
Recurrent bacterial infections	708	19
HIV wasting syndrome	510	14
Candida esophagitis	506	13
HIV encephalopathy	457	12
Cytomegalovirus disease	308	8
Pulmonary candidiasis	155	4
M. avium infection	156	4
Cryptosporidiosis	106	3
Herpes simplex disease	117	3

[a]Values from 3665 perinatally acquired AIDS cases reported 1982–1992.
[b]Some children had more than one reported disease.

syndrome was reported in 16% and HIV encephalopathy in 14% of the children; various other conditions were reported in less than 10%. Cancers, such as non-Hodgkin's lymphoma, are also seen in ~2% of children with advanced HIV disease but are not as common a sign of HIV disease compared with adults.

Among children diagnosed with AIDS in the first 12 months of life in the national reporting system, 62% have had PCP, whereas only 20% of children diagnosed with AIDS older than 12 months had PCP. PCP most frequently occurs between age 3 and 6 months. In the areas covered by the Spectrum of Disease Study, of the 105 children diagnosed with PCP younger than 6 months only 35% had been evaluated for HIV infection before PCP diagnosis. As one of the most severe opportunistic infections, PCP is associated with shorter survival (median 13 months) compared with overall survival after AIDS of 3 years (37). An analysis of AIDS cases in New York City demonstrated that even among children diagnosed with PCP, survival after AIDS has improved since early in the epidemic; for children reported before mid-1987, 12-month survival was 42% compared with a 62% 12-month survival for children reported from mid-1987 to 1989 (79).

Distinct patterns of disease presentation have emerged. A group of children present early and often suddenly between age 3 and 8 months with symptoms often including PCP, cytomegalovirus, wasting syndrome, and encephalopathy. Older children present later, frequently with a more indolent course and often with a clinical picture including lymphoid interstitial pneumonitis and other evidence of lymphoproliferative processes (lymphadenopathy, hepatosplenomegaly, parotid gland enlargement). Recurrent bacterial infections ranging from persistent otitis media to overwhelming bacterial meningitis or pneumonia are common in children presenting both early and late.

In clinical series as well as the AIDS case reports, PCP is a major cause of sudden early mortality. In one series of 172 children, 9% had PCP at a median age of 5 months, and these children survived a median of only 1 month after diagnosis (80).

In a second study of 111 children, 11 of 16 who had PCP as their presenting infection died during their first episode (81). In studies of children with PCP in Newark and Los Angeles, 50% of the patients first came to medical attention for HIV at the time of their initial PCP evaluation (82, 83). This combination of sudden presentation and high mortality is one reason for encouraging early identification of potentially HIV-infected neonates so that they can be carefully observed and given prophylactic medications as indicated.

Other conditions such as measles can be more severe in these children (84, 85). In fact in 1987 the first deaths in several years attributed to measles were reported, all occurring in HIV-infected children (see also Chapter 19). Measles may have an atypical presentation in children with advanced HIV disease, occurring without the characteristic rash, making diagnosis difficult and enhancing the opportunity for the child with measles to continue to spread it to contacts in community or medical settings. Because measles and HIV infection are both increasing in the United States, particularly in inner cities, the risk of this disease for HIV-infected children is increasing, and both vaccination and postexposure prophylaxis become even more important.

The risk of tuberculosus disease in these children may also be increased because of increased risk of exposure and of disease once infected; however, the impact of tuberculosis at this point in the United States is less among HIV-infected children compared with adults (86–88) (see also Chapter 16).

Rates of Disease Progression

The period from HIV infection to AIDS onset has been called the incubation or clinical latency period. In reality, the interaction of the virus with the host immune system is complex, and recent studies suggest that true latent infection does not occur. In the crude sense, HIV-infected infants usually appear well for the first few months of life, although some immune abnormalities can sometimes be detected. Several infected children can remain well, or present with only mild symptoms, for more than 5 years.

Although among reported perinatal AIDS cases the median age at AIDS diagnosis is 12 months, with a long tail toward the older ages, a few children have been diagnosed as late as age 13 years (Fig. 1.4). Because recently born children have not yet had time to develop AIDS, this observed time underestimates the actual incubation. Of note, more than 50 children reported with AIDS through 1992 did not develop manifestations of AIDS until they were 10 years or older, and perinatal HIV infection was their only reported risk. Studies of these children are important to elucidate factors that may be related to longer survival.

Modeling of data from 838 infected children in the Pediatric Spectrum of Disease study and 2910 children reported with AIDS support the clinical impression, and earlier models, of two distinct populations of children with different rates of survival (89–91). Parametric and nonparametric survival models suggest that an estimated 11–16% of children have a high probability of death before age 4 years (99%; median age at death 5–11 months), whereas the second group had many children surviving beyond 4 years (88%; median age at death over 60 months). Importantly, the difference between the groups was not related to any difference in PCP prophylaxis, specific AIDS-defining conditions, antiviral therapy, or birth weight. These different rates of disease progression may relate to the timing of perinatal infection (those with intragestational infection appear to have a more accelerated disease course), the virus load, or the phenotype of the infecting virus. Description of these two groups is important because of the use of survival analyses in evaluating interventions.

HIV-infected infants clearly progress faster than adults in developing immunodeficiency and related illnesses. Prospective studies as well as case modeling document that the highest incidence of AIDS is during the first year of life. In adults, the median incubation is probably nearer 10 years, and very few adults develop AIDS in the first 3 years after infection.

Prognostic Factors

Except for age at diagnosis and type of clinical presentation (the latter perhaps re-

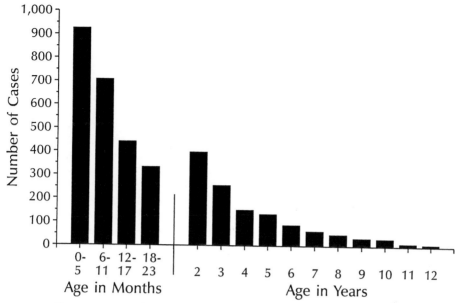

Figure 1.4. Distribution of age at AIDS diagnosis for children with vertically acquired HIV infection through 1992.

flecting only a more advanced immune dysfunction), no demographic or clinical factors have been related to prognosis (89). In several studies, prematurity appears to be a risk factor for more rapid disease progression, but it has been difficult to determine whether it is an independent or dependent prognostic factor. Sex, race or ethnicity, and route of infection of the mother (intravenous drug users compared with mothers who acquired HIV through another route) do not appear to influence the child's age at AIDS presentation or survival after AIDS diagnosis. Therapeutic interventions, particularly administration of zidovudine, appear to have marked benefits in delaying disease progression in some children, and as these therapies are further studied and more widely applied, the course of the disease will likely change.

Low CD4 counts for age are the best markers of immune deficiency and indicators of risk of developing opportunistic infections, although more must be learned about CD4 counts particularly in the first year of life in both infected and uninfected children (see also Chapter 9) (82, 83, 92). Among 147 children followed at the National Cancer Institute, the presence of a very low CD4+ count (<21% of the lower limit of normal values for age, equivalent to

50 cells/μl in an adult) was associated with a significantly increased risk of death within 2 years (93).

Among 94 children followed longitudinally in Paris, a bimodal expression of clinical and biological symptoms was described, with one group experiencing early opportunistic infections or severe encephalopathy and a rate of survival at 3 years of 48%; among children without this early presentation, survival at 3 years was 97%. Laboratory findings of low CD4 counts (<500), negative slope of subsequent CD4 counts, or poor lymphoproliferative response were associated with presence of these early severe clinical syndromes (91, 94).

Among 529 HIV-infected children in the Italian Register for HIV Infection in children (112 infected children followed prospectively from birth), 82% of children developed HIV-1 associated signs at a median age of 5 months, and early symptoms were predictive of shorter survival. Secondary infectious diseases, severe bacterial infections, progressive neurological disease, anemia, and fever were significant and independent predictors of survival. Median survival was 96 months, with ~70% surviving to 6 years (95, 96).

It now appears clear that identification of HIV infection early in the disease process, and regular supportive care, are important in improving survival. Specific prophylactic regimens, such as widespread use of trimethoprim-sulfamethoxazole to prevent PCP or regular infusions of intravenous immunoglobulin, have decreased the risk for certain opportunistic infections and changed the disease course for many children (97). Specific antiretroviral therapy appears to have marked benefits in delaying disease progression in some children, and as these therapies are further studied and more widely applied, the course of the disease will likely change further (98, 99). In the United States, there has been increasing use of PCP prophylaxis and antiretroviral therapy, with over two-thirds of symptomatic children receiving these treatments and nearly one-third receiving intravenous immunoglobulin (100).

EPIDEMIOLOGIC ISSUES FOR THE FUTURE
HIV and AIDS Surveillance Needs

There will be a continuing need to monitor trends in the epidemic through HIV seroprevalence and seroincidence studies and through HIV/AIDS surveillance to track HIV morbidity and mortality. Surveillance must become simplified and more streamlined to accommodate the increasing numbers of cases and to more accurately reflect the full extent of HIV morbidity. Special surveillance studies will be needed to further evaluate certain findings or trends. Increasingly, surveillance data are being used not only to follow the epidemic and target prevention and intervention activities but also to evaluate their impact. Also, flexible mathematical models and projections are increasingly addressing not only national overall trends but also trends in individual transmission categories (such as intravenous drug use, heterosexual acquisition, and perinatal acquisition) and different geographic areas.

As the clinical and immunologic spectrum of disease is more fully understood, and diagnostic tests sensitive and specific for HIV infection in infants become more widely available, it will be possible to design a classification system more indicative of HIV disease stage, which can be used for surveillance as well as clinical needs. A classification system is under consideration that categorizes children by disease severity and degree of CD4+ count suppression.

Biomedical Research

To develop more effective therapies, there is a compelling need to further clarify maternal factors related to transmissibility and the timing and mechanisms of transmission of virus to the infant. Intervention studies will need to go ahead in parallel with these observational studies.

Development of more sensitive and simpler tests for establishing the diagnosis of HIV infection in early infancy has greatly aided medical care; but more work must be done in this area, and tests will need to be more widely available. Nevertheless, it should be recognized that the knowledge that a child was born to an infected mother is a major tool in medical management, and the limitations of currently available diagnostic tests should not discourage clinicians from recommending antibody testing in settings where HIV is a possibility.

Prevention and Early Intervention

Effective strategies for prevention of HIV transmission, through behavioral change and biologic interventions, are closely tied to issues of effective care for HIV-infected persons. As problematic as some diagnostic and therapeutic issues are in children, much has been learned over the first years of the epidemic. These issues deserve further attention and study, but in equal need of emphasis is social science research to better understand the persons at high risk for infections and the factors related to behavior change. More widespread offering of HIV testing in various medical settings will be critical for bringing HIV-infected adults and their children into early care. Practical strategies for delivering, financing, and evaluating care for HIV-exposed children and their families must be pursued.

References
1. World Health Organization Global Programme on AIDS. HIV/AIDS Summary, Jan 1993.
2. Centers for Disease Control. Unexplained immunodeficiency and opportunistic infections in

infants: New York, New Jersey, California. MMWR 1982;31:665–667.

3. Oleske J, Minnefor A, Cooper R, et al. Immune deficiency in children. JAMA 1983;249:2345–2349.

4. Rubinstein A, Sicklick M, Gupta A, et al. Acquired immunodeficiency with reversed T4/T8 ratios in infants born to promiscuous and drug-addicted mothers. JAMA 1983;249:2350–2356.

5. Scott GB, Buck BE, Leterman JG, Bloom FL, Parks WP. Acquired immunodeficiency syndrome in infants. N Engl J Med 1984;310:76–81.

6. Centers for Disease Control. Revision of the CDC surveillance case definition for acquired immunodeficiency syndrome. MMWR 1987;36(suppl 1S):1S–13S.

7. Centers for Disease Control and Prevention. 1993 revised classification system for HIV infection and expanded surveillance case definition for AIDS among adolescents and adults. MMWR 1992;41(RR-17):1–19.

8. Centers for Disease Control. Classification system for human immunodeficiency virus (HIV) infection in children under 13 years of age. MMWR 1987;36:225–230, 235.

9. Centers for Disease Control and Prevention. HIV/AIDS Surveillance Rep 1993;Feb:1–23.

10. Centers for Disease Control. Update: Acquired immunodeficiency syndrome—United States, 1991. MMWR 1992;41:463–468.

11. Ellerbrock TV, Bush TJ, Chamberland ME, Oxtoby MJ. Epidemiology of women with AIDS in the United States: A comparison with heterosexual men with AIDS. JAMA 1992;265:2971–2975.

12. Ellerbrock TV, Lieb S, Harrington P, et al. Heterosexually transmitted human immunodeficiency virus infection among pregnant women in a rural Florida community. N Engl J Med 1992;327:1704–1709.

13. Chaisson MA, Stoneburner RL, Hildebrandt DS, Ewing WE, Telzak EE, Jaffe HW. Heterosexual transmission of HIV-1 associated with the use of smokable freebase cocaine (crack). AIDS 1991;5:1121–1126.

14. Lindegren ML, Simonds RJ, Gwinn M, Fleming P. Why are perinatal AIDS cases in the United States (US) not increasing? [Abstract PoC16-2988]. Ninth International Conference on AIDS, Berlin, Jun 1993.

15. Centers for Disease Control and Prevention. Projections of the number of persons diagnosed with AIDS and the number of immunosuppressed HIV-infected persons, United States, 1992–1994. MMWR 1992;41(RR-18):1–29.

16. Jones DS, Byers RH, Bush TJ, Oxtoby MJ, Rogers MF. Epidemiology of transfusion-associated acquired immunodeficiency syndrome in children in the United States, 1981 through 1989. Pediatrics 1992;89:123–127.

17. Hersh BS, Popovici L, Apetrei RC, et al. Acquired immunodeficiency syndrome in Romania. Lancet 1991;338:645–649.

18. Gutman LT, St. Claire KK, Weedy C, et al. Human immunodeficiency virus transmission by child sexual abuse. Am J Dis Child 1991;145:137–141.

19. Gellert GA, Durfee MJ, Berkowitz CD, Higgins KV, Tubiolo VC. Situational and sociodemographic characteristics of children infected with human immunodeficiency virus from pediatric sexual abuse. Pediatrics 1993;91:39–44.

20. Chu SY, Buehler JW, Oxtoby MJ, Kilbourne BW. Impact of the human immunodeficiency virus epidemic on mortality in children, United States. Pediatrics 1991;87:806–810.

21. Bennett JV, Rogers MF. Child survival and perinatal infections with human immunodeficiency virus. Am J Dis Child 1991;145:1242–1247.

22. Landesman S, Minkoff H, Holman S, McCalla S, Sijn O. Serosurvey of human immunodeficiency virus infection in parturients. JAMA 1987;258:2701–2703.

23. Division of HIV/AIDS, Centers for Disease Control. Prevalence of HIV-1 antibody in civilian applicants for military service, October 1985–December 1992. Department of Defense.

24. Centers for Disease Control. National HIV serosurveillance summary, vol 2. Results through 1990. US Department of Health and Human Services Publication HIV/NCID/11-91/011, 1991.

25. Dondero TJ, Pappaioanou M, Curran JC. Monitoring the levels and trends of HIV infection: The Public Health Service's HIV surveillance program. Public Health Rep 1988;103:213–220.

26. Hoff R, Beradi VP, Weiblen BJ, et al. Seroprevalence of human immunodeficiency virus among childbearing women. N Engl J Med 1988;318:525–530.

27. Novick LF, Berns D, Stricof R, Stevens R, Pass K, Wethers J. HIV seroprevalence in newborns in New York State. JAMA 1989;261:1745–1750.

28. Gwinn M, Pappaioanou M, George JR, et al. Prevalence of HIV infection in childbearing women in the United States. JAMA 1991;265:1704–1708.

29. Gwinn M, Wasser S, Fleming P, Karon J, Petersen L. Increasing prevalence of HIV infection among childbearing women, United States, 1989–1991 [Abstract PoC16-2990]. Ninth International Conference on AIDS, Berlin, Jun 1993.

30. Centers for Disease Control. HIV infection and AIDS—Georgia, 1991. MMWR 1992;41:876–878.

31. Rolfs RT, Nakashima AK. Epidemiology of primary and secondary syphilis in the United States, 1981 through 1989. JAMA 1990;264:1432–1437.

32. McCray E, Onorato IM, Field Services Branch. Sentinel surveillance of human immunodeficiency virus infection in sexually transmitted disease clinics in the United States. Sex Transm Dis 1992;19:235–241.

33. Sweeney PA, Onorato IM, Allen DM, Byers RH, Field Services Branch. Sentinel surveillance of human immunodeficiency virus infection in women seeking reproductive health services in the United States, 1988–1989. Obstet Gynecol 1992;79:503–510.

34. Araneta MRG, Weisfuse IB, Greenberg B, Schultz S, Thomas PA. Abortions and HIV-1 infection in New York City, 1987–1989. AIDS 1992;6:1195–1201.

35. Hsu HW, Moye J, Kunches L, et al. Perinatally acquired human immunodeficiency virus infection:

Extent of clinical recognition in a population-based cohort. Pediatr Infect Dis J 1992;11:941–945.

36. Centers for Disease Control. Guidelines for prophylaxis against *Pneumocystis carinii* pneumonia for children infected with human immunodeficiency virus. MMWR 1991;40:1–13.

37. Simonds RJ, Oxtoby MJ, Caldwell MB, Gwinn ML, Rogers MF. *Pneumocystis carinii* pneumonia among U.S. children with perinatally acquired HIV infection. JAMA 1993;270:470–473.

38. Chu SY, Buehler JW, Berkelman RL. Impact of the human immunodeficiency virus epidemic on mortality in women of reproductive age, United States. JAMA 1990;264:225–229.

39. Caldwell MB, Fleming PL, Oxtoby MJ. Estimated number of AIDS orphans in the United States [Letter]. Pediatrics 1992;90:482.

40. Michaels D, Levine C. Estimates of the number of motherless youth orphaned by AIDS in the United States. JAMA 1992;268:3456–3461.

41. Caldwell MB, Mascola L, Smith W, et al. Biologic, foster, and adoptive parents: Care givers of children exposed perinatally to human immunodeficiency virus in the United States. Pediatrics 1992;90:603–607.

42. Blanche S, Rouzioux C, Moscato MG, et al. A prospective study of infants born to women seropositive for HIV type 1. N Engl J Med 1989;320:1643–1648.

43. Goedert JJ, Mendez H, Drummond JR, et al. Mother-to-infant transmission of human immunodeficiency virus type 1: Association with prematurity or low anti gp-120. Lancet 1989;2:1351–1354.

44. Goedert JJ, Duliege AM, Amos CI, et al. High risk of HIV-1 infection for first-born twins. Lancet 1991;338:1471–1475.

45. Hutto C, Parks WP, Lai S. A hospital-based prospective study of perinatal infection with human immunodeficiency virus type 1. J Pediatr 1991;118:347–353.

46. Burns D, Muenz L, Walsh J, et al. Correlation of perinatal transmission of HIV-1 with mother's lowest prepartum CD4 level [Abstract 463]. 31st Interscience Conference on Antimicrobial Agents and Chemotherapy, Chicago, 1991.

47. European Collaborative Study. Risk factors for mother-to-child transmission of HIV-1. Lancet 1992;339:1007–1012.

48. Gabiano C, Tovo PA, de Martino M, et al. Mother-to-child transmission of human immunodeficiency virus type 1: Risk of infection and correlates of transmission. Pediatrics 1992;90:369–374.

49. Anonymous. Factors involved in mother-to-child transmission of HIV. Consensus Workshop, Siena, Jan 1992. J Acquir Immune Defic Syndr 1992;5:1019–29.

50. Thomas PA, Weedon J, New York City Perinatal HIV Transmission Collaborative Study Group. Maternal predictors of perinatal HIV transmission [Abstract WeC 1059]. Eighth International Conference on AIDS, Amsterdam, Jul 1992.

51. Ryder RW, Nsa W, Hassig S, et al. Perinatal transmission of the human immunodeficiency virus type 1 to infants of seropositive women in Zaire. N Engl J Med 1989;320:1637–1642.

52. Lallemant M, Lallemant-Le-Coeur S, Cheynier D, et al. Mother-child transmission of HIV-1 and infant survival in Brazzavile, Congo. AIDS 1989;3:643–646.

53. Hira SK, Kamange J, Bhat GJ, et al. Perinatal transmission of HIV-1 in Zambia. Br Med J 1989;299:1250–1252.

54. Halsey N, Boulos R, Holt E, et al. Transmission of HIV-1 infections from mothers to infants in Haiti: Impact on childhood mortality and malnutrition. JAMA 1990;264:2088–2092.

55. Workshop on mother-to-child transmission of HIV: Ghent, Belgium, 17–20 February 1992. Brussels: European Economic Community AIDS Task Force, 1992.

56. St Louis ME, Kamenga M, Brown C, et al. Risk factors for perinatal transmission of human immunodeficiency virus type 1: Independent effects of high maternal CD8+ lymphocytes, low CD4+ lymphocytes, and placental inflammation. JAMA 1993;269:2853–2859.

57. Sibailly TS, Adjorlolo G, Gayle H, et al. Prospective study to compare HIV-1 and HIV-2 perinatal transmission in Abidjan, Cote d'Ivoire [Abstract WeC 1065]. Eighth International Conference on AIDS, Amsterdam, Jul 1992.

58. European Collaborative Study. Children born to women with HIV-1 infection: Natural history and risk of transmission. Lancet 1991;337:253–260.

59. d'Arminio Monforte A, Ravizza M, Muggiasca ML, et al. Maternal predictors of HIV vertical transmission. Eur J Obstet Gynecol 1991;42:131–136.

60. Krasinski K, Cao Y, Borkowsky W, Ho DD. Maternal viral load as a risk factor for perinatal HIV-1 transmission. J Cell Biochem 1992;(suppl 16E):109.

61. Douglas GC, King BF. Maternal-fetal transmission of human immunodeficiency virus: A review of possible routes and cellular mechanisms of infection. Clin Infect Dis 1992;15:678–691.

62. Shaffer N, Ou CY, Abrams E, et al. PCR and HIV IgA for early infant diagnosis of perinatal HIV infection [Abstract ThC1580]. Seventh International Conference on AIDS, Amsterdam, Jul 1992.

63. Krivine A, Firtion G, Cao L, et al. HIV replication during the first weeks of life. Lancet 1992;339:1187–1189.

64. Anonymous. Early diagnosis of HIV infection in infants. Consensus Workshop, Siena, Jan 1992. J Acquir Immune Defic Syndr 1992;5:1169–1178.

65. Italian Multicentre Study. Epidemiology, clinical features, and prognostic factors of paediatric HIV infection. Lancet 1988;2:1043–1045.

66. Perinatal AIDS Collaborative Transmission Study. Lack of increased risk of HIV perinatal transmission to subsequent siblings born to an HIV-infected mother [Abstract WeC 1057]. Eighth International Conference on AIDS, Amsterdam, Jul 1992.

67. Pollack H, Borkowsky W, Krasinski K. Maternal syphilis is associated with enhanced perinatal HIV transmission [Abstract 1274A]. 30th Interscience Conference on Antimicrobial Agents and Chemotherapy, Atlanta, 1990.

68. Oxtoby MJ. Human immunodeficiency virus and other viruses in human milk: Placing the issues in broader perspective. Pediatr Infect Dis J 1988;7: 825–835.

69. Hira SK, Mangrola UG, Mwale C, et al. Apparent vertical transmission of human immunodeficiency virus type 1 by breast-feeding in Zambia. J Pediatr 1990;117:421–424.

70. Van de Perre P, Simonon A, Msellati P, et al. Postnatal transmission of human immunodeficiency virus type 1 from mother to infant: A prospective cohort study in Kigali, Rwanda. N Engl J Med 1991;325:593–598.

71. Ruff AJ, Halsey NA, Coberly J, Boulos R. Breast-feeding and maternal-infant transmission of human immunodeficiency virus type 1. J Pediatr 1992;121:325–329.

72. Dunn DT, Newell ML, Ades AE, Peckham CS. Risk of human immunodeficiency virus type 1 transmission through breastfeeding. Lancet 1992; 340:585–588.

73. Heymann SJ. Modeling the impact of breast-feeding by HIV-infected women on child survival. Am J Public Health 1990;80:1305–1309.

74. Hu DJ, Heyward WL, Byers RH, et al. HIV infection and breastfeeding: Policy implications through a decision analysis model. AIDS 1992;6:1505–1513.

75. Lederman SA. Estimating infant mortality from human immunodeficiency virus and other causes in breast-feeding and bottle-feeding populations. Pediatrics 1992;89:290–296.

76. Centers for Disease Control. Recommendations for assisting in the prevention of perinatal transmission of HTLV-III/LAV and acquired immunodeficiency syndrome. MMWR 1985;34:721–731.

77. HIV transmission and breastfeeding. Bull World Health Organ 1992;70:667–669.

78. Mofenson LM, Wright PF, Fast PE. Summary of the working group on perinatal intervention. AIDS Res Hum Retroviruses 1992;8:1435–1438.

79. Thomas P, Singh T, Williams R, Blum S. Trends in survival for children reported with maternally transmitted acquired immunodeficiency syndrome in New York City, 1982–1989. Pediatr Infect Dis J 1992;11:34–39.

80. Scott GB, Hutto C, Makuch RW, et al. Survival in children with perinatally acquired human immunodeficiency virus type 1 infection. N Engl J Med 1989;321:1791–1796.

81. Krasinski K, Borkowsky W, Holzman RS. Prognosis of human immunodeficiency virus infection in children and adolescents. Pediatr Infect Dis J 1989;8:216–220.

82. Connor E, Bagarazzi M, McSherry G, et al. Clinical and laboratory correlates of *Pneumocystis carinii* pneumonia in children infected with HIV. JAMA 1991;265:1693–1697.

83. Kovacs A, Frederick T, Church J, Eller A, Oxtoby M, Mascola L. CD4 T-lymphocyte counts and *Pneumocystis carinii* pneumonia in pediatric HIV infection. JAMA 1991;265:1698–1703.

84. Krasinski K, Borkowsky W. Measles and measles immunity in children infected with HIV. JAMA 1989;261:2512–2516.

85. Palumbo P, Hoyt L, Demasio K, Oleske J, Connor E. Population-based study of measles and measles immunization in human immunodeficiency virus-infected children. Pediatr Infect Dis J 1992;11: 1008–1014.

86. Jones DJ, Malecki JM, Bigler WJ, Witte JJ, Oxtoby MJ. Pediatric tuberculosis and human immunodeficiency virus infection in Palm Beach County, Florida. MJ Dis Child 1992;146:1166–1170.

87. Khouri YF, Mastrucci MT, Hutto C, Mitchell CD, Scott GB. Mycobacterium tuberculosis in children with human immunodeficiency virus type 1 infection. Pediatr Infect Dis J 1992;11:950–955.

88. Moss WJ, Dedyo T, Suarez M, et al. Tuberculosis in children infected with human immunodeficiency virus: A report of five cases. Pediatr Infect Dis J 1992;11:114–120.

89. Byers B, Caldwell B, Oxtoby M, Pediatric Spectrum of Disease Project. Survival of children with perinatal HIV infection: Evidence for two distinct populations [Abstract WS-C10-6]. Ninth International Conference on AIDS, Berlin, Jun 1993.

90. Auger I, Thomas P, De Guttola V, et al. Incubation periods for pediatric AIDS patients. Nature 1988;336:575–577.

91. Blanche S, Tardieu M, Duliege AM, et al. Longitudinal study of 94 symptomatic infants with perinatally acquired human immunodeficiency virus infection: Evidence for a bimodal expression of clinical and biological symptoms. Am J Dis Child 1990;144:1210–1215.

92. McKinney RE, Wilfert CM. Lymphocyte subsets in children younger than 2 years old: Normal values in a population at risk for human immunodeficiency virus infection and diagnostic and prognostic application to infected children. Pediatr Infect Dis J 1992;11:639–644.

93. Butler KM, Husson RN, Lewis LL, Mueler BU, Venzon D, Pizzo PA. CD4 status and p24 antigenemia. Am J Dis Child 1992;146:932–936.

94. Duliege AM, Messiah A, Blanche S, Tardieu M, Griscelli C, Spira A. Natural history of human immunodeficiency virus type 1 infection in children: Prognostic value of laboratory tests on the bimodal progression of the disease. Pediatr Infect Dis J 1992;11:630–635.

95. de Martino M, Tovo PA, Galli L, et al. Prognostic significance of immunologic changes in 675 infants perinatally exposed to human immunodeficiency virus. J Pediatr 1991;119:702–706.

96. Tovo PA, de Martino M, Gabiano C, et al. Prognostic factors and survival in children with perinatal HIV-1 infection. Lancet 1992;339: 1249–1253.

97. Mofenson LM, Moye J, Bethel J, et al. Prophylactic intravenous immunoglobulin in HIV-infected children with CD4+ counts of 0.20×10^9/L or more: Effect on viral, opportunistic, and bacterial infections. JAMA 1992;268:483–488.

98. McKinney RE, Maha MA, Connor EM, et al. A multicenter trial or oral zidovudine in children with advanced human immunodeficiency virus disease. N Engl J Med 1991;324:1018–1025.

99. Working Group on Antiretroviral Therapy: National Pediatric HIV Resource Center. Antiretroviral therapy and medical management

of the human immunodeficiency virus-infected child. Pediatr Infect Dis J 1993;12:513–522.

100. Caldwell MB, Mascola L, Lyons L, et al. Increasing PCP prophylaxis, antiretroviral use and CD4 monitoring in human immunodeficiency virus-infected children [Abstract 907]. 32nd Interscience Conference on Antimicrobial Agents and Chemotherapy, Anaheim, Oct 1992.

2
HIV Infection in Europe

Marie-Louise Newell and Catherine S. Peckham

In Europe, as elsewhere, the AIDS epidemic has emerged as a major health problem. Its impact across regions and subpopulations within Europe is variable and reflected in the number of children with human immunodeficiency virus (HIV) reported from each country or indeed regions within a country.

REPORTS OF AIDS CASES

Cases of AIDS in Europe are reported to the World Health Organization/European Community Collaborating Centre in Paris by 31 countries and are published quarterly. Reporting of cases of AIDS (1, 2) is mandatory in 23 countries of the World Health Organization Europe region and voluntary in eight. In some countries the reports are named, but in most they are coded; in three (Luxembourg, Switzerland (mandatory), and the Netherlands (voluntary) no identifiers are required.

By the middle of 1992, a cumulative total of more than 76,000 cases of AIDS among adults and children had been reported from the 31 countries of the World Health Organization European region (3), and allowing for delays between diagnosis and reporting, a more realistic estimate would be 84,000 AIDS cases. In 1991 the highest annual incidence rates per million population were in France (82.7), Italy (58.6), Spain (104.3), and Switzerland (90.1). Incidence of AIDS cases continues to increase in Europe and also in most individual countries. The proportion of females among total cases reported rose from 15.0% in

1989 to 16.8% in 1990 and 1991 and 17.4% in the first 6 months of 1992, and this has implications for pediatric AIDS reports. In countries, such as Italy and Spain, where the prevalence of HIV infection among intravenous drug users is high, the proportion of female AIDS cases is greater than in northern European countries, such as Sweden, Denmark, and Germany, where there is a preponderance of AIDS cases among homosexual men. It is predicted that in Europe over the next 2 years more cases of AIDS will be diagnosed among intravenous drug users than among homo- or bisexual men. The previously noted (4) leveling off of AIDS cases in the group with a history of intravenous drug use has not continued through 1991. The wide between-country variation in terms of the relative distribution of cases by transmission group is expected to persist (3, 5).

Most women with AIDS are of childbearing age. This has implications for the number of children at risk of HIV infection, because vertical transmission is the main mode of acquisition of infection for children. By the middle of 1992, nearly 3400 children with AIDS had been reported from the WHO Europe region (3), most from Romania (1846), France (400), Spain (419), and Italy (298). For Europe, the proportion of pediatric AIDS cases is constant at 4% of the total AIDS cases. Most children with AIDS reported from Romania had acquired infection through the use of contaminated needles and syringes (6), which highlights the need for continued vigilance in the prevention of infection through this route. If children from Romania are excluded, mother to child transmission accounted for 78% of infection in the remaining 1546 children. This proportion is similar to that reported cumulatively from the United States. About half the mothers of the vertically infected children gave a history of intravenous drug use, and nearly half had acquired infection through heterosexual contact (Fig. 2.1*A*). The relative proportion in each of these categories varied by country (Table 2.1). Of the 1546 children with AIDS, 130 had hemophilia and 121 became HIV infected through a contaminated blood transfusion (Fig. 2.1*B*).

HIV INFECTION

Although AIDS surveillance is important, it is limited as an indicator of trends in HIV infection in adults because of the long latent period and underreporting of AIDS (7). In the future comparisons of trends in adult AIDS will be increasingly difficult to interpret with the widening of the case definition of AIDS to include CD4 counts in the United States (8) (see Chapter 1). The case definition for pediatric AIDS may change pending the outcome of discussions about whether CD4 counts should be included and the possible exclusion of lymphoid interstitial pneumonitis as an indicator disease. To predict the spread of the epidemic, monitoring of HIV prevalence is essential. In eight countries of Europe there is no reporting system for HIV infection. In countries where systems exist, reporting of HIV infection is mandatory in 13 and voluntary in 12, either named, coded, or without identifiers. It has been estimated from available information that there are around 500,000 HIV-seropositive individuals in Europe (3). Laboratory reports of first HIV-positive antibody tests are used in the United Kingdom to monitor the spread of HIV infection (9). However, both laboratory and clinical reporting schemes are likely to underestimate the extent of the problem because of the bias inherent in any reporting system that relies on individuals presenting with symptoms or who come to be tested.

A more reliable approach for estimating the prevalence of HIV infection in a population is unlinked anonymous testing of blood taken for other purposes, although even this is limited to people who have blood taken. Increasingly this approach is being used to monitor the epidemic (10–13). Since the main mode of acquisition of infection in children is vertical transmission from mother to child, the prevalence of HIV infection in the pregnant population is of particular relevance to children. In parallel with AIDS reports, there are marked differences in the seroprevalence of HIV infection among European countries and among areas within one country (11–13). However, the results of unlinked anonymous testing are limited in that they provide no information on maternal risk factors, such as intravenous drug use. Although they are restricted to sample populations in accessible groups, their strength is that they do not suffer from bias resulting from refusal to be tested or failure to identify people at risk. The problem of lack of identifiers has been addressed by relating the results to population characteristics of women delivering in given areas (14).

In England, unlinked anonymous testing among pregnant women has been continuous in selected sites since the beginning of 1990 (10). Residual specimens from antenatal samples collected for rubella serology are tested for HIV antibody. In France (15), a cross-sectional antenatal study that was undertaken in 1990 over 4 months in the Paris region included all women, regardless of pregnancy outcome. In this study blood samples were collected from women or their newborn babies according to availability, and this survey is being extended to the French regions and will be repeated every 2 years.

The first results of these studies from 1990 showed the HIV seroprevalence rate among pregnant women in the Paris area to be 4.14/1000 (Table 2.2) and higher than the overall rate in England (1.14/1000). In inner London the rate was 1.94/1000. However, differences in the population tested make it difficult to compare the two capitals. In Paris all women were tested, irrespective of pregnancy outcome, and the estimate therefore included women whose pregnancies were terminated. This group is

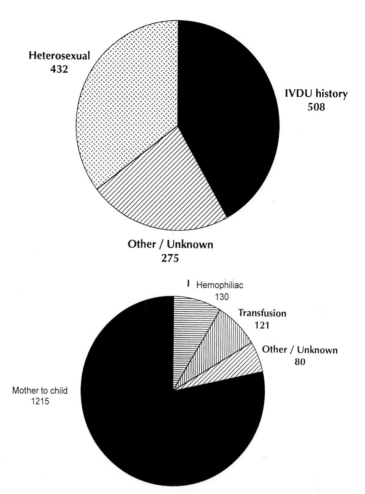

Figure 2.1. *Upper*, maternal transmission group: 1215 vertically infected children from Europe, excluding Romania, by June 30, 1992. *Lower*, pedi-atric AIDS by transmission group: Europe, excluding Romania, June 30, 1992; 1546 cases.

Table 2.1. AIDS in Children Younger Than 13 Years by Risk in Selected Countries by June 30, 1992 (3)

| | Mother to Child | | | | | | |
	IV Drug User	Heterosexual	Other/ unknown	Hemophiliac	Transfusion	Other	Total
Romania	0	34	70	7	573	1162[a]	1846
France	119	174	26	24	54	3	400
Spain	153	37	163	49	11	6	419
Italy	162	85	25	14	7	5	298
UK	9	42	9	13	8	0	81
Germany	21	9	16	8	11	0	65
Commonweatlh of Independent States	0	3	1	0	0	62[a]	66
Switzerland	17	12	6	1	1	0	37
Portugal	0	2	9	6	4	1	22
Netherlands	3	4	4	1	7	0	19
Austria	11	2	3	1	2	0	19

[a]Most were thought to be infected through the use of contaminated needles.

Table 2.2. Results of Anonymous Unlinked Antenatal or Neonatal Screening Programs

Country or City	Year	Prevalence per 1000
Antenatal		
England	1990	1.14
London	1990	1.94
Paris	1990	4.14
Sweden	Mar 1991	0.10
Norway	Aug 1988	0.11
Neonatal		
Italy	1988–1989	1.30
Paris	1990	2.75
Scotland	1990	0.29
Edinburgh	1990	2.46
Rome	1988–1989	4.05
Inner London	1990	1.28
	1991	2.00
Outer London	1990	0.48
	1991	0.33

known to have a higher HIV prevalence than women whose pregnancies continue to term. In England, women who had terminations are less likely to have been tested. Further results will make it possible to examine changes over time.

HIV seroprevalence rates for women with live births are available for Italy, southeast England, and Scotland, based on unlinked anonymous testing of neonatal blood samples taken routinely from all newborns for metabolic screening. In the United Kingdom, continuous unlinked anonymous testing of neonatal blood samples collected onto absorbent filter paper began in three regions in southeast England in 1988 (11) and Scotland in 1990 (13), and this approach is now being extended to other regions. In Italy, cross-sectional surveys using all neonatal blood samples collected over 4 months were set up in nine regions in 1988, repeated in eight regions in 1989, and extended to all 20 Italian regions on an annual basis in 1990 (12).

In Italy during June 1988–April 1989, 39,102 newborns in 92 hospitals were screened, and 51, or 1.3/1000 (95% confidence interval 0.97–1.7), were found to be HIV seropositive. The prevalence was higher in urban and industrialized areas than in rural areas, reflecting the reported cumulative AIDS incidence rate pattern. The HIV seroprevalence rate in the Paris

area (2.75/1000) (16) was close to that reported in Edinburgh, Scotland (2.46/1000) but lower than the rate found in Rome (4.05/1000). Although the rate reported in inner London was low (1.28/1000), an increasing trend in HIV prevalence was observed between 1988 and 1990. Only one-fifth of infected pregnant women in London had been identified through clinical reporting schemes (11), where most infected pregnant women in Scotland were already known by the health services (13) because of the comprehensive voluntary testing program in Edinburgh.

In Sweden, routine confidential antenatal HIV testing is supplemental with anonymous unlinked testing of the 3% of women who refuse named testing (16). By the end of March 1991, 35 HIV infections had been detected among 439,376 pregnant women (0.1/1000) who had a named test, and there were no infections in the samples tested anonymously; 31 of the 35 infected women were considered to have contracted infection through sexual intercourse, over half in Africa, and two-thirds of the 25 women identified as positive early in pregnancy had the pregnancy terminated. During 1988 and 1990, between 89,000 and 98,000 pregnant women were tested each year, and the prevalence of infection remained stable at one in 10,500.

Routine testing of 36,053 sera from pregnant women in southeastern Norway yielded four (0.11/1000) positive results (17). Three of these were already known to be HIV infected before pregnancy. Anonymous testing of sera from 50 women who refused the test yielded one positive result (2%).

OBSTETRIC AND PEDIATRIC SURVEILLANCE

Confidential surveillance schemes where HIV-seropositive pregnant women or HIV-seropositive children are reported centrally can provide useful information. However, these programs are relatively costly, and results are only valuable if they include a substantial proportion of all infected women or children.

In a nationwide, multicenter study in France, 2346 HIV-seropositive pregnant women were reported to a central register over 3 years from 1987 to 1989 (18). Most

HIV-positive women had a history of intravenous drug use, although an increase was observed among women with no such history. The trend toward heterosexual transmission among pregnant women was more marked in the Paris region than in the rest of France.This could have been due in part to changes in population, such as an increase in women from sub-Saharan Africa in the Paris region and an overall increase in testing of intravenous drug users and pregnant women.

In Britain in 1989 a national study of HIV in pregnancy was established through the Royal College of Obstetricians and Gynaecologists to review antenatal screening policies and to establish a confidential register of known HIV-positive pregnancies (19). Results of this surveillance program can be compared with results from the unlinked anonymous neonatal screening program in some regions to provide an estimate of the extent to which HIV infection is not recognized in pregnant women (20).

In Spain, the Spanish pediatric association conducted a survey in public hospitals of children born to HIV-positive mothers between 1981 and 1989 (21). A total of 1938 HIV-positive children were identified, with Madrid, Catalonia, Valencia, Basque, and Andalusia reporting 85% of all cases; 93% of mothers were intravenous drug users.

In the Swiss perinatal HIV study (22), prospective data are collected on children of HIV-infected mothers throughout the country. This allows the combined approach of a population-based case reporting scheme with a prospective cohort study. By July 1991, 286 children had been registered, of whom 201 were identified at birth. Based on these data, the prevalence of HIV infection in women at the time of delivery is estimated to be 0.1% and has remained stable between 1986 and 1989. This agrees with the estimates of 0.11% for Lausanne and 0.2% for Geneva, based on screening programs of pregnant women.

In Italy the register of pediatric HIV infection and AIDS (23, 24) has provided valuable information on children with infection and their presenting symptoms, the natural history of AIDS, and survival. By April 1991, 1887 children had been reported, of whom 1045 were identified at birth and 842 at a median age of 5 months (range: 2 weeks–72 months) (23). In the United Kingdom, a similar pediatric surveillance scheme exists, whereby pediatricians report on a monthly basis any child with HIV infection or born to an HIV-seropositive mother (25). Nil returns are included, and response rates are over 90%. This pediatric surveillance is linked to the obstetrical surveillance scheme to give a comprehensive picture of vertically acquired infection in Britain (20). In both the Italian and British registers, follow-up information is also obtained on the children reported.

VERTICAL TRANSMISSION STUDIES IN EUROPE

Most children in Europe acquire HIV infection through vertical transmission. An estimate of the risk of infection in a child born to an HIV-infected woman and knowledge of the natural history in an infected child are therefore important for both counseling and prediction of future trends in pediatric HIV infection.

There is little variation in the reported rates of vertical transmission from prospective European studies following children born to women known to be HIV infected at the time of delivery. These studies include the French collaborative study (26), the European Collaborative Study (27), and the Swiss perinatal study (22). In the European Collaborative Study (27) (ECS) the rate of transmission was 14.4% (95% confidence interval: 12.0–17.1%), based on 721 children, most (86%) of whose mothers had a history of intravenous drug use. With increasing numbers confidence intervals have narrowed, and the current ECS estimate is more reliable than those previously quoted (28, 29) There was no significant variation between the centers in different parts of Europe. The French collaborative study reported an 18.3% (95% confidence interval: 11.8–24.8%) vertical transmission rate, based on 590 children (S. Blanche, personal communication, 1992), and the Swiss perinatal study (22) reported a 20% (95% confidence interval: 12–30%) transmission rate, based on 201 children.

Vertical transmission rate can only be estimated from prospective studies that identify children at risk at or before birth, and registers of AIDS and HIV infection in children are not designed for this purpose. Vertical transmission rates from the Italian multicenter study (30) must be interpreted with caution, therefore, because this study is essentially a register. Similar caution must be used when interpreting the rates published from the Catalonian register (31). Unless all women who are identified as HIV infected at delivery and their children are followed from birth, bias can be introduced. Several centers participating in the ECS also contribute to the Italian multicenter study. A low rate of vertical transmission has been reported in Edinburgh (32), which is also a ECS participating center; numbers of children enrolled were small, and the confidence interval was therefore wide, overlapping with the rate form the ECS. Further, the possibility that women seeking prenatal care and HIV testing select for a subpopulation of HIV-infected mothers must be considered.

In neither the French study nor the ECS was there an excess of congenital malformations or a dysmorphic syndrome in infected children nor was there an increase in the rate of prematurity (22, 26, 29). Birth weight was related to the mother's intravenous drug use during pregnancy and not to the infection status of the infant; children with drug withdrawal symptoms were lighter than children of mothers who had not used intravenous drugs during pregnancy.

In Edinburgh HIV-infected intravenous drug users had rates of pregnancy termination similar to non-HIV-infected intravenous drug users, and there was no increase in adverse pregnancy outcome nor was there a pregnancy-induced acceleration of HIV infection (33, 34).

In the ECS (27) transmission of infection from mother to child was not associated with maternal intravenous drug use, age, race, or parity. Similarly, in the Swiss perinatal study (22), transmission was not associated with year of birth, sex, race, maternal age, parity, maternal clinical status at time of delivery, mode of delivery, breast feeding, gestational age, or birth weight. In the French collaborative study, there was no significant difference in transmission rates between African women and women with a history of intravenous drug use.

Mother to child transmission was associated with maternal AIDS (but not with less severe HIV-related manifestations), maternal p24-antigenemia, and a CD4 count of $<700/mm^3$ in the ECS (27). Also, children born before 34 weeks gestation were four times more likely to be infected than children born after this time. The rate of infection in children who were breast fed was twice the rate of bottle fed children. Based on data available from several prospective studies, the additional risk of transmission from mother to child in established HIV infection has now been estimated to be about 15% (95% confidence interval: 7–22%) (35). It will be important to monitor vertical transmission rates in Europe because it is anticipated that these rates may increase as the epidemic progresses and a higher proportion of infected women in their childbearing years have more advanced disease.

HIV-2 infection is still uncommon in Europe. However, in the French collaborative study (S. Blanche, personal communication, 1992), there were 40 infants born to mothers who were HIV-2 positive. None of the 15 who had been followed for ≥18 months were infected (95% confidence interval: 0–22%), supporting the evidence from the Ivory Coast that the vertical transmission rate of HIV-2 is likely to be low.

There is increasing evidence to suggest that infection can occur around the time of delivery (27, 36–38). In vaginal deliveries transmission was higher in the ECS (27) when episiotomy, scalp electrodes, forceps, or vacuum extractors were used, but these results were found only in centers where these procedures were not routine, suggesting that it was not these procedures per se that carried a higher risk. In two prospective studies (22, 27), with an overall cesarean section rate of ~25%, there has been some evidence of a protective effect of cesarean section, although in both cases the difference in infection rates by mode of delivery did not reach statistical significance. Based on available evidence, there is no justification for delivery by elective cesarean section for women with HIV infection.

NATURAL HISTORY

Prospective studies based on cohorts of children followed from birth are required to establish the natural history of vertically acquired HIV infection. Information from registers and surveillance provides information on the natural history of specific conditions, usually after diagnosis of AIDS or HIV-related symptoms. In the ECS (29) the most common manifestation of HIV infection was a combination of persistent generalized lymphadenopathy, hepatomegaly, and splenomegaly. Persistent hypergammaglobulinemia occurred early and frequently predated the onset of clinical symptoms or signs. About one-third of infected children developed AIDS within the first year of life, and 17% died of an HIV-related death (Figs. 2.2 and 2.3). Although 90% of infected children showed some manifestation of HIV infection before 12 months, more children improved than deteriorated over the second and third year of life. Few children in this study received prophylactic or antiretroviral treatment before the onset of serious HIV-related symptoms, and it will be important to monitor changes in natural history because in the future children may be treated earlier in the disease. Long-term prognosis for infected children remains to be determined, and follow-up of this cohort is continuing.

Prognosis after AIDS has been diagnosed depends on the age at diagnosis and the AIDS indicator disease. In a longitudinal study in France, Blanche et al. (39) studied 94 symptomatic children with vertically acquired HIV infection. One-third presented with an opportunistic infection early in life, often associated with encephalopathy. Lymphocytic interstitial pneumonitis occurred at a mean age of 29 months, significantly later than opportunistic infections or severe encephalopathy. The children with CD4 cell counts of $<500/mm^3$ or with p24 antigenemia suffered more frequently from life-threatening illness. The presenting clinical manifestions were similar for children born to African mothers and those born to mothers with a history of intravenous drug use. The probability of survival at 3 years was 97% for children without opportunistic infections or severe encephalopathy.

In the Swiss perinatal study (22) the probability for infected children remaining asymptomatic was 29% (95% confidence interval: 14–48%) at 12 months and 12% (95% confidence interval: 3–29%) at 31 months. Although these values are higher than the 10% reported in the ECS (29), they merely reflect the stricter definition of HIV-related symptoms and signs in the ECS. Survival at 12 months was 80% (95% confidence interval: 62–92%) and similar

Age at onset AIDS or age at last visit
103 antibody positive, infected children ECS, Autumn 1992

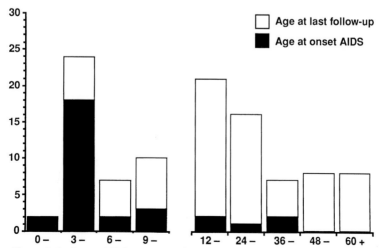

Figure 2.2. Age at AIDS onset or at last visit: 103 antibody-positive infected (27).

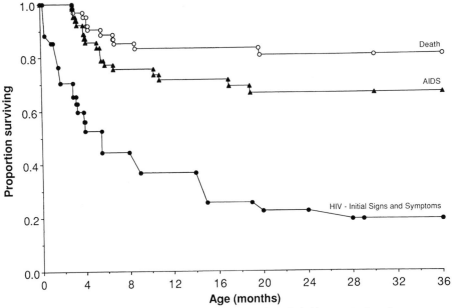

Figure 2.3. Time to death, time to AIDS, and time to HIV-related clinical symptoms and/or signs, based on survival curves, for 64 antibody-positive infected children (29). Based on nonparametric survival analysis, proportion without AIDS or proportion without HIV-related signs and symptoms.

to that reported in the ECS. The overall infant mortality rate in children born to HIV-infected mothers was 4.6%, which compares with 0.7% in the general Swiss population, and the postneonatal mortality rate was 4.0 and 0.3%, respectively. However, it is well-established that infant mortality in children of intravenous drug users is higher than that in the general population.

The Italian register has provided useful information on the clinical presentation of HIV infection and the identification of prognostic factors for survival in children (23). This has contributed to discussions on the clinical staging of pediatric HIV infection. The cumulative proportion of children surviving at age 9 years was 49.5% (95% confidence interval: 27–65%), and the median survival time was 96.2 months. Separate analysis of the 112 seropositive-infected children in the Italian register who had been followed from birth gave similar results to that for the total cohort. However, comparison with the ECS (29) and Swiss perinatal study (22) would suggest that the very early deaths had not been included in this register, possibly they had not been diagnosed as HIV related. The

findings from these European studies suggest that the outlook for children with perinatal HIV infection is better than previously reported.

PEDIATRIC EUROPEAN NETWORK OF TRIALS IN AIDS

Through a European network, pediatricians in several countries are collaborating in a multicenter trial of azidothymidine in children. There have been no placebo-controlled trials of azidothymidine in children, but phase I and II studies in symptomatic children in the United States and Europe have suggested an increase in weight and well-being and an improvement in HIV encephalopathy (C. Giaquinto, personal communication, 1992) (40). Criteria for commencement of treatment with azidothymidine and its duration and dose remain unclear, and practice in Europe varies widely. This European multicenter trial addresses these issues and sets up a network for further trials that may include a comparison of monotherapy with combinations of antiretroviral drugs and trials of prophylactic treatment (D. Gibb, personal communication, 1992).

FAMILY CIRCUMSTANCES

As the number of infected women and children increases, more attention is being given to issues relating to the care of HIV-infected children and their families. Uninfected children born to infected mothers are also affected by their parents' disease. Many are born into socially disadvantaged families in which one or both parents may be an intravenous drug user. In Padova, Italy, 177 children born to HIV-positive mothers were followed from birth (41). About 80% of their mothers had a history of intravenous drug use, and an additional 12% were sexual partners of drug users. Most parents were free of symptoms at the time of the child's birth. Thirty-four (19%) children were abandoned at birth; and by the time they were 6 years old a further 20% were not living with their parent(s). There was no difference in the family situation between HIV-infected and uninfected children. Most (90%) of the orphaned children were living with other relatives, usually grandparents. In Switzerland(22), 20% of children of HIV-infected mothers were placed in foster care by 1 year of life and 50% by 3 years.

IDENTIFICATION OF CHILDREN AT RISK

As early diagnosis of vertically acquired HIV infection (37, 42, 43) and management of HIV-infected children improves, there is increasing awareness of the need to recognize the child at risk of infection. However, evidence from anonymous unlinked antenatal and neonatal screening programs has shown that many children at risk are not being identified. Consequently, as increased efforts are now being made to identify HIV-infected women during pregnancy. If voluntary antenatal testing is to be successful the provision of counseling and satisfactory levels of uptake are an essential. Benefits and risks to mother and child, are well as cost implications, must be carefully considered and the ethical issues addressed.

CONCLUSION

In this chapter we have demonstrated from available information the variation in HIV seroprevalence among women and children in different European countries.

These differences can largely be explained by the prevalence of HIV infection in intravenous drug users and patterns of immigration, and the prevalence of infection in women and children must continue to be monitored. There is, however, a striking similarity in verical transmission rates throughout Europe and in the natural history of pediatric HIV infection. Rates of mother to child transmission are lower than the 30–35% reported from Africa. This could in part be explained by the different distribution of factors associated with increased transmission, such as breast feeding, a higher prevalence of primary infection in pregnancy, and immunological impairment in the mothers. Similarly, the variation in transmission rates reported from the United States may reflect differences in population characteristics. Attention is now being given to possible interventions to reduce vertical transmission. As the children in the current studies age, continued follow-up of the original cohort will be necessary to establish the long-term natural history of pediatric HIV infection. Increasingly widespread treatment may alter the natural history and the age-specific mortality rates.

References

1. Centers for Disease Control. Classification system for human immunodeficiency virus (HIV) infection in children under 13 years of age. MMWR 1987;15:255–236.
2. Centers for Disease Control. Revision of the CDC surveillance case definition for acquired immunodeficiency syndrome. MMWR 1987;36:3s–15s.
3. World Health Organization/EC Collaborating Centre on AIDS. AIDS surveillance in Europe. WHO Q R 1992;34:4–22.
4. World Health Organization/EC Collaborating Centre on AIDS. AIDS surveillance in Europe. WHO Q R 1991;30:1–29.
5. Downs AM, Ancelle-Park RA, Brunet J. Surveillance of AIDS in the European Community: Recent trends and predictions to 1991. AIDS 1990;4:1117–1124.
6. Hersh BS, Popovici F, Zolotusca L, Beldescu N, Oxtoby MJ, Gayle HD. The epidemiology of HIV and AIDS in Romania. AIDS 1991;6(suppl 1):S87–S92.
7. McCormick A. Unrecognised HIV related deaths. Br Med J 1991;302:1365–1367.
8. van Griensven GJP, Boucher EC, Roos M, Coutinho RA. Expansion of AIDS case definition. Lancet 1991;338:1012–1013.
9. Waight PA, Rush AM, Miller E. Surveillance of HIV infection by voluntary testing in England. Commun Dis Rep Rev 1992;2:R85–R90.

10. PHLS Communicable Disease Surveillance Centre, PHLS Virus Reference Laboratory, Academic Department of Genito-urinary Medicine, and Collaborators. The unlinked anonymous HIV prevalence monitoring programme in England and Wales: Preliminary results. Commun Dis Rep 1991;1:R69–R75.

11. Ades AE, Parker S, Berry T, et al. Prevalence of maternal HIV-1 infection in Thames regions: Results from anonymous unlinked neonatal testing. Lancet 1991;337:1562–1564.

12. Ippolito G, Costa F, Stegagno M, Angeloni P, Angeloni U, Guzzanti E. Blind serosurvey of HIV antibodies in newborns in 92 Italian hospitals: A method for monitoring the infection rate in women at time of delivery. J Acquir Immune Defic Syndr 1991;4:402–407.

13. Tappin DM, Girdwood RWA, Follett EAC, Kennedy R, Brown AJ, Cockburn F. Prevalance of maternal HIV infection in Scotland based on unlinked anonymous testing of newborn babies. Lancet 1991;337:1565–1567.

14. Ades AE, Parker S, Cubitt D, et al. Two methods for assessing the risk factor composition of the HIV-1 epidemic in heterosexual women: Southeast England, 1988–1991. AIDS 1992;6:1031–1036.

15. Couturier E, Brossard Y, Larsen C, et al. Prevalence de l'infection VIH chez les femmes enceintes de la region parisienne. Une enquete anonyme non correlee. PREVAGEST Bull Epidemiol Hebdomadaire 1991;33:139.

16. Lindgren S, Bohlin A, Ottenblad C, et al. Swedish national antenatal screening program for HIV-1. Three years experience [Abstract WC 3278]. Seventh International Conference on AIDS, Florence, Jun 1991.

17. Jennum PH. Anti-HIV screening of pregnant women in south-eastern Norway. Natl Inst Public Health Ann 1988;11:54–58.

18. Henrion R, Henrion-Geant E, Mandelbrot L. Evolution du mode de contamination par le VIH des femmes enceintes en France metropolitaine. Presse Med 1991;20:1365–1368.

19. Davison CF, Ades AE, Hudson CN, Peckham CS. Antenatal testing for human immunodeficiency virus. Lancet 1989;2:1442–1444.

20. Davison C, Holland FJ, Newell ML, Hudson CN, Peckham CS. Screening for HIV infection in pregnancy. AIDS Care 1993;5:135–140.

21. Canosa CA, Delgado A, Martin FG, Llorens J, Omenaca F, Contreras JR. Infeccion por el virus de la inmunodeficiencia humana. Encuesta multicentrica espanola. An Esp Pediatr 1991;34:425–435.

22. Kind C, Brandle B, Wyler C-A, et al. Epidemiology of vertically transmitted HIV-1 infection in Switzerland: Results of a nationwide prospective study. Eur J Pediatr 1992;151:442–448.

23. Tovo PA, De Martino M, Gabiano C, et al. Prognostic factors and survival in children with perinatal HIV-1 infection. Lancet 1992;339:1249–1253.

24. de Martino M, Tovo P, Galli L, et al. Prognostic significance of immunologic changes in 675 infants perinatally exposed to human immunodeficiency virus. J Pediatr 1991;119:702–709.

25. Hall S, Glickman M. The British paediatric surveillance unit. Arch Dis Child 1988;63:344–346.

26. Blanche S, Rouzioux C, Guihard Moscato M-L, Veber F, Mayaux M-J, Jacomet C. A prospective study of infants born to women seropositive for human immunodeficiency virus type 1. New Engl J Med 1989;320:1643–1648.

27. European Collaborative Study. Risk factors for mother-to-child transmission of HIV-1. Lancet 1992;339:1007–1012.

28. European Collaborative Study. Mother-to-child transmission of HIV infection. Lancet 1988;2:1039–1042.

29. European Collaborative Study. Children born to women with HIV-1 infection: Natural history and risk of transmission. Lancet 1991;337:253–260.

30. Italian Multicentre Study. Epidemiology, clinical features, and prognostic factors of paediatric HIV infection. Lancet 1988;2:1043–1045.

31. Casabona J, Sanchez E, Salas T. Monitoring vertically acquired AIDS cases [Letter]. AIDS 1991;5:340.

32. Mok JYQ, Hague RA, Yap PL, et al. Vertical transmission of HIV: A prospective study. Arch Dis Child 1989;64:1140–1145.

33. Johnstone FD, Brettle RP, MacCallum LR, Mok J, Peutherer JF, Burns S. Women's knowledge of their HIV antibody state: Its effect on their decision whether to continue the pregnancy. Br Med J 1990;300:23–24.

34. Johnstone FD, MacCallum L, Brettle R, Inglis JM, Peutherer JF. Does infection with HIV affect the outcome of pregnancy? Br Med J 1988;296:467.

35. Dunn D, Newell M, Ades A, Peckham C. Risk of human immunodefiency virus type 1 transmission through breastfeeding. Lancet 1992;340:585–588.

36. Goedert JJ, Duliege A-M, Amos CI, Felton S, Biggar RJ, International Registry of HIV-Exposed Twins. High risk of infection with human immunodeficiency virus type I for first-born, vaginally delivered twins. Lancet 1991;338:1471–1475.

37. Krivine A, Firtion G, Cao L, Francoual C, Henrion R, Lebon P. HIV replication during the first few weeks of life. Lancet 1992;339:1187–1189.

38. Ehrnst A, Lindgren S, Dictor M, et al. HIV in pregnant women and their offspring: Evidence for late transmission. Lancet 1991;2:203–207.

39. Blanche S, Tardieu M, Duliege A, et al. Longitudinal study of 94 symptomatic infants with perinataly acquired human immunodeficiency virus infection. Am J Dis Child 1990;144:1210–1215.

40. Pizzo PA, Wilfert CM. Treatment considerations for children with human immunodeficiency virus infection. Pediatr Infect Dis J 1990;9:690–699.

41. Giaquinto C, Giacomet V, Pagliaro A, et al. Social care of children born to HIV-infected parents. Lancet 1992;339:189–190.

42. De Rossi A, Ades AE, Mammano F, et al. Antigen detection, virus culture, polymerase chain reaction, and in vitro antibody production in the diagnosis of vertically transmitted HIV-1 infection. AIDS 1991;5:15–20.

43. Consensus Workshop on Early Diagnosis of HIV Infection Early diagnosis of HIV infection in infants: Report of a consensus workshop held in Siena, Italy, January 1992. J Acquir Immune Defic Syndr 1992;5:1169–1178.

3
Special Considerations for Developing Nations

Thomas C. Quinn, Andrea Ruff, and Neal Halsey

During the past decade the epidemic of AIDS became a global pandemic with over 500,000 cases officially reported from 165 countries. Because of underreporting in many areas, the World Health Organization (WHO) estimates that 1.7 million cases of AIDS have occurred with over 500,000 deaths during the past 10 years (1, 2). From selected seroprevalence studies and mathematical models, the WHO further estimates that more than 11 million people are infected with human immunodeficiency virus (HIV)-1. Of these individuals, 3 million are women, mostly of reproductive age, and 500,000 are infants and children (3); 80% of these infected women and children reside in sub-Saharan Africa where the estimated prevalence of HIV-1 infection is 2500/100,000 women aged 15–49. Approximately 85% of all children with HIV-1 infection acquired their infection from birth to an HIV-1 infected mother, whereas the remaining 15% acquired their infection parenterally from unscreened blood transfusions or through exposure to blood-contaminated needles and syringes. In developed countries, pediatric AIDS comprises 2% of all reported AIDS cases; however, in developing countries, pediatric AIDS may comprise as much as 15–20% of all AIDS cases (4).

With increasing evidence of heterosexual transmission, the number of infected women and consequently their children is increasing. During the next decade it is estimated that by the year 2000, the cumulative number of adults and children infected with HIV will rise to 30–40 million and that the number of AIDS cases will increase 10-fold to 12–18 million. The HIV-1 pandemic will kill 3 million or more women and 2.7 million children worldwide (3). AIDS will become the leading cause of death for men and women aged 15–49 in major cities throughout the Americas, western Europe, and sub-Saharan Africa. An additional 5.5 million children under age 15 may be orphaned because of the premature death of HIV-1-infected mothers and fathers from AIDS (3, 5). Infant and child mortality rates will also increase as much as 30% greater than previously projected as a direct consequence of perinatal HIV-1 infection. Consequently, pediatric AIDS is now threatening much of the progress that has been made in child survival in developing countries over the past 20 years (3, 6, 7). Unless HIV-1 infection can be controlled among young adults, perinatal transmission of HIV-1 will inevitably continue, further potentiating the spread of HIV-1 infection in children. The greatest tragedy, besides medical and health care costs, will be the loss of thousands of lives, particularly among young adults in their most productive age and the infants born to HIV-infected mothers, which directly affect child survival rates. These will undoubtedly result in a major impact on the economy of all countries throughout the region—in terms of direct medical and patient care costs and indirect costs in the form of absenteeism and de-

31

creased productivity. In many developing countries, the pandemic is likely to overstretch an already fragile health and economic infrastructure.

MAGNITUDE OF HIV-1 INFECTION AND AIDS

As of July 1992, 268,445 cases were reported from all 45 countries in the Americas (Table 3.1). In Africa, 209,805 cases were reported from 53 countries with a sharp increase in reporting since 1986. In Europe, 81,091 cases were reported from 28 of 29 countries. With late introduction of HIV-1 into Asian and Pacific countries, the number of AIDS cases remains low in those areas, with 4846 cases reported from 11 of 19 countries in Oceania and 2764 cases reported in 28 of 40 Asian countries. Thailand and India have reported the largest numbers of cases, 946 and 238, respectively, accounting for over 95% of the cases from the region to date. The relatively small number of AIDS cases reported so far in this region reflects factors such as late introduction of the virus, long average latency period of 10 years, and, to a lesser extent, underrecognition and underreporting. However, data on HIV-1 infection show that although the pandemic in this region is still at an early state, the virus may be spreading at a pace similar to sub-Saharan Africa in the early 1980s.

In Thailand, HIV-1 rates have increased sharply among intravenous drug users from 1% at the start of 1988 to 40% by the end of the same year (8). Seroconversion rates were as high as 3–5%/month. This wave of the HIV-1 epidemic in intravenous drug users was followed by a similar pattern

among female prostitutes (9). A national sentinel survey demonstrated that 44% of lower class prostitutes in Chiang Mai, Thailand were infected with HIV-1, a remarkable rise from <1% in the previous year. Nationally, the HIV-1 seroprevalence among prostitutes increased from 3.5 to 15% over 2 years. Similar patterns were also demonstrated in India and Myanmar. Seroprevalence rates rose from 0% among intravenous drug users to 54% between 1989 and 1990 (10). In Bombay, HIV-1 seropositivity rates among prostitutes increased from 2% in 1989 to 40% in 1991. In Vellore, HIV-1 seroprevalence increased among prostitutes from 0.5 to 34.5% in 1990 (11). Although there is evidence of an increase in HIV-1 prevalence among blood donors and women attending antenatal clinics, the rates are still <0.5%. It is estimated that presently there are 1 million people infected with HIV-1 in India and approximately 500,000 people infected in Thailand. Since heterosexual contact is becoming the predominant mode of HIV-1 transmission in the region, the continued transmission of HIV-1 in the general population appears inevitable. Consequently, WHO estimates that although the annual number of HIV-1 infections will peak in Africa by 1995, infections in Asia will continue to increase well into the early next century and are unlikely to peak before 2015. The annual number of HIV-1 infections by the year 2000 may far exceed that seen in sub-Saharan Africa.

In all regions of the world there are three major modes of HIV-1 transmission: sexual transmission, which may be homosexual, bisexual, or heterosexual; parenteral transmission, including transfusion

Table 3.1. Cumulative Number of AIDS Cases by Continent as of December 22, 1992[a]

Continent	Countries Reporting at Least One Case	Cases Reported	Estimated HIV-1 Infected
Africa	53	209,805	6.0 million
Americas	45	313,083	2.5 million
Asia	28	2,764	1.5 million
Europe	28	81,091	0.5 million
Oceania	11	4,846	<30,000
Total	165	611,589	10.5 million

[a]Data from the WHO Global Programme on AIDS.

of infected blood products or injection with blood-contaminated needles or syringes; and maternal-infant transmission, which may occur in utero during delivery, or postnatally (12, 13). In most developing countries, heterosexual transmission is the major mode of spread of HIV-1 infection, responsible for over 75% of infections (14–16). The virus was probably introduced into these populations in the 1960s, and recent serologic surveys demonstrate that 10–20% of 20- to 40-year old individuals in some urban areas are infected (14, 16–19). Maternal to infant transmission has become a major problem in developing countries since half of the infected individuals are women of reproductive age. In some African and Caribbean cities, 5–30% of pregnant women are HIV-1 seropositive (Table 3.2) (20–33). Because of the rapid spread of HIV-1 among heterosexuals, these areas tend to have the highest rates of HIV-1 infection among the general populations that have been surveyed and represent the most difficult areas for control of the epidemic.

Less is known regarding the extent of HIV-1 infection among children in developing countries. Partially because of the high infant mortality from multiple causes, the full impact of HIV-1 infection in the pediatric population is poorly defined. In several studies, seropositive women in Caribbean and African countries have reported having lost at least twice as many infants before their current pregnancy as had seronegative women (34–37). One-third of children with diarrhea who died after discharge from a rehydration unit in Port-au-Prince had antibody to HIV-1 (34); 45% of children 2–29 months old who were hospitalized consecutively for severe malnutrition in pediatric wards in Bujumbura, Burundi, were HIV-1 seropositive (38). Thus, it appears that most children in developing countries who are infected with HIV-1 may not live long enough to develop clinical AIDS because of the higher mortality rate associated with common childhood diseases in immunocompromised children with HIV-1 infection.

MODES OF TRANSMISSION
Maternal to Infant Transmission

As with other viral infections in pregnant women, maternal HIV-1 infections adversely affect pregnancy outcome and survival of offspring. Mean birth weight for infants born to HIV-1-seropositive women has been lower than the birth weight for infants born to HIV-1-seronegative women (6, 7, 39–46). However, many studies in industrialized countries have been confounded by the

Table 3.2.   Seroprevalence Rates for HIV-1 Infection in Pregnant Women in Selected Countries

Country	City	Year	No. Tested	% Infected	Ref.
Bahamas	National	1991	4825	2.9	20
Brazil	Sao Paulo	1990	3047	1.3	20
Burundi	Bujumbura	1990	1255	17.5	21
Congo	Brazzaville	1991	300	9.0	22
Dominican Republic	Santo Domingo	1991	1056	0.9	20
Haiti	Port-au-Prince	1990	1156	8.0	20
Honduras	San Pedro Sula	1991	416	3.6	20
Ivory Coast	Abidjan	1991	9635	10.5	23
Kenya	Nairobi	1991	5674	15.8	24
Malawi	Blantyre	1990	6482	22.8	25
Rwanda	Kigali	1989	900	30.3	26
Tanzania	Dar Es Salaam	1989	3001	8.9	27
Thailand	Central Regions	1991	4042	1.1	28
Uganda	Kampala	1990	3601	28.1	29
USA	New York City	1988	1192	2.3	30
Zaire	Kinshasa	1989	1491	6.0	31
Zambia	Lusaka	1990	1954	24.5	32
Zimbabwe	Mutebeland	1989	289	11.1	33

high rate of drug abuse in HIV-1-seropositive women. Infants born to cocaine- or heroin-abusing women have significantly lower birth weights and increased mortality rates (38–41). Studies in developing countries have been free of the potentially confounding effects of drug abuse (6, 7, 26, 34–37, 44, 45). When large numbers of infants have been studied in settings without drug abuse, significantly lower birth weights have been observed for infants born to HIV-1-seropositive women compared with -seronegative women in developing nations (Table 3.3).

The lower birth weight for infants born to HIV-1-seropositive women could have been due to in utero infection and decreased fetal growth, or maternal HIV-1 illness could have contributed to shorter duration of pregnancy and decreased weight gain regardless of infection status of the infants. In Zaire and in Kenya, birth weights of infants born to symptomatic HIV-1-seropositive women were lower than for infants born to asymptomatic HIV-1-seropositive women (7, 36). In France, Zaire, and Italy, no significant differences were found in the birth weight for infants subsequently found to be infected compared with uninfected infants (7, 41, 47).

The rate of maternal to infant transmission has ranged from 14 to 40% in recent large series (42, 45–48). The time when most infected infants acquired the HIV-1 infection is unknown. Intrauterine transmission definitely occurs, because HIV-1 has been isolated from fetal tissue and amniotic fluid as early as 13–20 weeks gestation (49–52). However, recent evidence indicates that the most infections probably occur around the time of delivery (53). IgM anti-body responses have been observed 1–2 months after delivery (54). Anti-HIV-1 IgA antibody was present in the first month of life in only 17% of infants who were subsequently shown to have acquired HIV-1 by vertical transmission (55, 56). Also, virus cultures and polymerase chain reaction for HIV-1 DNA at birth have been negative in most infants who were subsequently shown to be infected (7, 57, 58). Maternal to infant HIV-1 transmission may be analogous to hepatitis B transmission from women to their offspring. Although 10% of hepatitis B infections in infants are acquired in utero, the highest risk to the infant occurs at the time of delivery when there is mixing of maternal and fetal circulations (59), and the infant is exposed to infected blood and secretions (see Chapter 10C). Approximately 90% of maternal to infant hepatitis B transmission can be prevented by combined active and passive immunization of infants beginning at birth (60). Therefore interventions just before or shortly after delivery might effectively reduce the rates of maternal to infant HIV-1 transmission.

It is unclear why most infants born to HIV-1-seropositive women do not acquire the infection, and factors associated with maternal to infant HIV-1 transmission have not been fully described. Women with symptomatic HIV-1 infection or low CD4 counts and those who had a previous child with AIDS may be more likely to transmit HIV-1 to their offspring (7, 61). These findings are consistent with the hypothesis that the maternal virus load is an important factor in predicting the risk to offspring (see Chapter 10C). Rossi et al. (62), Goedert et al. (63), and Devash et al. (64) observed that a higher proportion of HIV-1-seropositive

Table 3.3.   Birth Weight of Infants Born to HIV-1-Seropositive and -Seronegative Women in Developing Countries

Ref.	Country	HIV-1 Positive		HIV-1 Negative		P
		No.	Mean birth weight	No.	Mean birth weight	
			g		g	
7	Zaire	85	2698[a]	606	3107	<0.01
		381	2491[b]			
45	Rwanda	174	2800	435	3000	<0.001
6	Haiti	199	2944	1944	3111	<0.001
46	Congo	64	2919	135	3092	?
36	Kenya	180	3090	335	3220	<0.005

[a] Mothers with AIDS.
[b] Mothers without AIDS.

women whose infants did not become infected were more likely to have antibodies to specific HIV-1 proteins or more avid antibody than mothers of infants who did not acquire infections. However, other investigators could not replicate these observations (65, 66). Ugen et al. (67) subsequently compared antibody assays in several different laboratories. They found considerable variability in the levels of antibody directed against different envelope peptides. For some peptides, women who transmitted HIV-1 to their offspring had higher levels of antibody than women who did not transmit HIV-1 to their offspring. However, for other peptides, women who transmitted HIV-1 had lower levels of antibody, and for other peptides, no differences were noted for transmitting or nontransmitting women. The significance of these findings is not yet clear, but the above results may help explain the apparently conflicting results of earlier studies. If the maternal immune response to HIV-1 can be associated with lower rates of vertical transmission, the data would provide the basis for trials of immunotherapy of pregnant women with specific HIV-1 vaccines and possibly other interventions such as passive antibodies administered at birth to infants born of HIV-1-seropositive women (see Chapters 45 and 47).

Higher rates of transmission have been reported for infants delivered vaginally than by cesarean section in some studies (39, 68, 89). However, the differences have been marginally significant, and follow-up of larger numbers in the Italian cohort resulted in a loss of significant differences by type of delivery (41). Goedert et al. (69) reported that the firstborn twin is at higher risk of acquiring HIV-1 infection than the second born. These data suggest that prolonged exposure to the cervical opening during labor or trauma from manipulation of the first twin could be important factors contributing to the risk of maternal to infant HIV-1 transmission. The use of forceps or scalp electrodes during delivery theoretically could predispose to increased risk to the infant if maternal blood is in the birth canal or HIV-1 is present in amniotic fluid. In some areas, obstetricians have initiated the practice of performing cesarean sections on HIV-1-seropositive women to reduce the risk to infants. However, the available data are insufficient to determine whether this practice will have an appreciable impact on the risk to infants.

Precise calculations of maternal to infant HIV-1 transmission in developing countries is confounded by high infant mortality rates. Excess mortality has been observed for infants born to seropositive women as early as 1 or 2 months (6, 7, 68). In Haiti, the infant mortality rate was 24% for infants born to HIV-1-seropositive women and 11% for those born to -seronegative women (6). In Zaire the rates were 21 and 6%, respectively (7). The reasons for higher mortality rates for infants born to HIV-1-seropositive women in underdeveloped countries compared with developed countries are not entirely clear. Infants born in underdeveloped countries are exposed to a larger number of infectious agents that either accelerate the HIV-1 disease process or produce more severe disease and high rates of mortality. Contributing factors probably include the decreased availability of timely medical care for management of bacterial infections and underlying malnutrition. Because 5–12% of infants born to HIV-1-seronegative women in developing countries die before reaching 12 months, all infant deaths cannot be assumed to be due to HIV-1 infections.

In the absence of precise diagnostic tests, several assumptions have been necessary to calculate maternal to infant HIV-1 transmission in developing countries. By assuming that the excess mortality in Haitian infants born to seropositive women was due to HIV-1 infection, adding the excess mortality (13%) to the 11% of surviving infants with persistent HIV-1 antibody provided an estimated 24% rate of HIV-1 transmission from mothers to infants (6). Maternal to infant transmission rates that were also calculated by subtracting infants who lost maternal HIV-1 antibody within the first 12 months of life from the total number of infants born to seropositive women resulted in a similar (25%) estimated rate of maternal to infant HIV-1 transmission. Ryder and coworkers (7) estimated the maternal to infant transmission rate to be 39% based on study of 92 Zairian infants on whom blood cultures and serologic tests were available.

Similar rates were noted in Rwanda (70). Thus, the rate of maternal to infant HIV-1 transmission studied in a few centers of developing countries have been similar to the 25–40% rates observed in some industrialized countries, and higher than the 14% rate reported for the European Collaborative Study (42, 68).

Breast Feeding

The apparent transmission of HIV-1 from mothers to infants by breast feeding was first reported by Ziegler and coworkers (71). Several other instances of possible or probable transmission via breast feeding were summarized by Oxtoby in 1988 (72). With additional reports, 23 infants have now been reported who appear to have been infected via breast feeding (71–74). In several instances, the mothers were not tested for HIV-1 infection before delivery, but the mothers did not have known risk factors for HIV-1 infections, and their sexual partners were seronegative when tested. Van de Perre et al. (73) provided the most convincing data on HIV-1 transmission via breast feeding. The group identified HIV-1 seronegative women at delivery who subsequently seroconverted while breast feeding their infants. Of the 10 infants born to women seroconverted 4 or more months after delivery, four of their infants acquired HIV-1 infection. These women almost certainly were not infected at the time of delivery, and breast feeding was the most likely means of transmission to the infants.

Although the rate of HIV-1 transmission via breast feeding is unknown, the available evidence suggests that breast feeding has resulted in some transmission when women acquired HIV-1 infection after delivery. HIV-1 has been identified in breast milk by electron microscopy, culture, and polymerase chain reaction (74–76). However, the viability of HIV-1 in breast milk has not been determined, and the likelihood of successful transmission via the oral mucous membranes are unknown. The circumstances in the above reports may be unique in that women who recently seroconverted may be more infectious than individuals with longstanding HIV-1 infection. Recent seroconverters have high levels of viremia

(77, 78), which could correlate with higher rates or higher titers of HIV-1 excretion in breast milk, resulting in an increased risk of transmission to infants.

The available data regarding the impact of breast feeding on the risk of HIV-1 acquisition for infants born to women who are seropositive throughout pregnancy are somewhat contradictory (74). In the Italian and European cohort studies, the rate of transmission for breast-fed infants was significantly higher than for non-breast-fed infants (41, 68). In these industrialized countries, the overall rates of transmission were relatively low (18 and 14%). Ryder and coworkers (79) observed no difference in rates of maternal to infant transmission for bottle-fed vs. breast-fed infants in Zaire. Also, the maternal to infant transmission rate of non-breast-fed Haitian infants in Florida was similar to the rate for breast-fed infants in Haiti (6, 80). Thus, the overall rate of maternal to infant transmission for breast-fed infants in developing countries may not appear to be different from the rate for bottle-fed infants or from the rate for non-breast-fed infants in the United States. Randomized, controlled trials in developing countries are indicated to resolve this important question.

In several industrialized countries, advisory bodies have recommended that HIV-1-seropositive women should not breast feed their infants. However, breast feeding is essential for optimal nutrition and survival of infants in underdeveloped countries. Bottle feeding is associated with increased rates and severity of gastroenteritis caused by contamination of other sources of food by enteric pathogens and failure to provide protective factors in human milk (72). The mortality for non-breast-fed infants in developing countries is two to five times higher than for breast-fed infants (76). If breast feeding was withheld from all infants born to HIV-1-seropositive women, the overall mortality in these infants born in areas with poor sanitation would undoubtedly increase (81). Heymann (82) modeled the survival outcomes of children born to HIV-infected women in developing countries who were breast-fed, bottle-fed or wet-nursed. It was estimated that the rate of HIV-1 transmission via breast milk would need to be at least 12% before alternative feeding practices should be recommended. Kennedy et al. (83) used a different model and estimated that a 5–10% increased risk of HIV-1 transmission by breast feeding could be more than offset by overall increased infant mortality caused by a decline in breast feeding rates depending upon the baseline infant mortality. Therefore, the WHO has recommended that biologic mothers should breast feed their infants regardless of maternal HIV-1 status where infectious diseases are the predominant causes of infant mortality (84). Where infectious diseases are not the primary cause of infant death, HIV-infected women should be advised not to breast feed. For women of unknown HIV status, Lederman (85) has noted that the benefits from breast feeding can outweigh theoretical risks of HIV transmission even in some areas of industrialized countries where infant morbidity and mortality are higher than average.

Blood Transfusion

With the implementation of HIV-1 screening of donated blood in 1985, the incidence of new HIV-1 infections among blood transfusion recipients has decreased in most developed countries (86). However, in some developing countries, HIV-1 blood screening has been incompletely introduced because of economic or technical constraints. The potential importance of blood transfusion in HIV-1 transmission is exemplified by the 2–18% seroprevalence rate of HIV-1 infection rate among blood donors in central Africa (8, 15, 18, 19, 87). Previous studies have also shown that transfusion is a frequent occurrence in children from Zaire. Among hospitalized children younger than 24 months in Kinshasa, five of 16 (31%) seropositive infants born to seronegative mothers had been transfused, compared with 15 of 220 (7%) seronegative children in the same age group who had a history of blood transfusion (88). In Kigali, seven of 18 (39%) pediatric cases with AIDS born to seronegative mothers had received a transfusion (89). For hospitalized children aged 2–14 years in Kinshasa, 60% of the seropositive group ($N = 40$), 33% of the seronegative

group ($N = 328$), and 14% of the healthy siblings ($N = 92$), respectively, had received a blood transfusion (90).

In a study that examined the role of blood transfusions in the transmission of HIV-1 among African children, 147 of 1046 (14.1%) pediatric patients in Kinshasa, Zaire, had a history of previous blood transfusion (91). Forty of these 1046 (3.8%) pediatric were HIV-1 seropositive, and there was a strong dose-response association between blood transfusion and HIV-1 seropositivity. The odds ratio of being HIV-1 seropositive increased to 43 in children who had received three or more blood transfusions. In a subsequent study of 167 hospitalized children with acute malaria, 21 (12.6%) were HIV-1 seropositive (92). Ten of the 11 HIV-1-seropositive patients with acute malaria had received blood transfusions during the index hospitalization, and at least four of these children were documented to have been seronegative before transfusion. Follow-up of these four children demonstrated the development of IgM antibodies and the persistence of IgG antibodies to HIV-1 6 months after receiving these blood transfusions.

Efforts to exclude high-risk donors in developing countries on epidemiologic or clinical grounds have thus far been unsuccessful (93), and blood screening for HIV-1 has been limited by the lack of financial resources necessary for routine testing and for adequate facilities for blood banking. A recent report from Zaire clearly underscores the problem with blood transfusions in Africa (94). Of 733 hospitals and medical centers surveyed, 62 (8.5%) transfused blood. Of 3741 units of blood transfused in February 1990, 1045 (27.9%) were not screened for HIV-1 infection. Eighteen of 62 centers (29%) received HIV-1 test kits on a regular basis. Major blood group crossmatching was performed in only 9.7% of the centers. Bacteriologic results indicated contamination in 17% of stocked blood units, 6.4% of solutions used for disinfection, and 22% of sterilized instruments. The authors concluded that transfusion practices in Kinshasa were associated with considerable health risk and that the establishment and appropriate supervision of HIV-1 screening facilities must be integrated into primary health care programs. Muller et al. (95) more recently demonstrated that with the development of transfusion guidelines and continuous education of health workers in at least one hospital in Kinshasa, unnecessary blood transfusion can be reduced further, decreasing the risk of blood-borne HIV-1 transmission.

With the implementation of rapid, inexpensive HIV-1 screening tests, some screening could be implemented in areas where blood facilities do not allow for the storage of blood. Recent technological advances using recombinant antigens have resulted in the development of rapid and inexpensive diagnostic assays that are as sensitive and specific as the standard enzyme-linked immunosorbent assay and Western blot assay (96). In a recent comparative trial, the sensitivity and specificity of five rapid assays ranged from 98 to 99.8 and 99 to 100%, respectively, compared with enzyme-linked immunosorbent assay and Western blot results (96). The use of these and other assays hopefully should allow for the immediate implementation of serologic screening for HIV-1 in developing areas of the world where screening procedures are impractical and unavailable.

CLINICAL ISSUES

Diagnosis

The diagnosis of HIV-1 infection in infants born to HIV-1-seropositive mothers is complicated by the transfer of maternal IgG antibodies in utero. Although newer techniques such as the polymerase chain reaction and HIV-1-specific IgA antibody assay may provide a means of early diagnosis of HIV-1 in infected infants, the assays are being standardized and are not readily available (see also Chapter 12). The diffi-

culty in diagnosing HIV-1 infection in infants and young children is compounded in developing countries where diagnostic resources are limited. Thus, the WHO has developed a provisional clinical case definition of pediatric AIDS for use in areas with limited resources (97). According to WHO criteria, a child is suspected of having AIDS if at least two major signs and at least two minor signs are present in the absence of known immunodeficiency from other causes (Table 3.4).

However, evaluation of the WHO definition in several settings has suggested that it lacks sensitivity and positive predictive value (98–102). Clinical signs are poorly defined, do not include pulmonary disease that is common in children with AIDS, and overlap with endemic disease common in uninfected children. With an emphasis on chronic signs and symptoms, the WHO definition will miss children who die acutely with an overwhelming infection. A WHO working group that addressed these issues in February 1989 recommended that the diagnosis of AIDS be based on serologic testing whenever possible and that the WHO definition, with the addition of "persistent or severe lower respiratory tract infection" as a major sign, continue to be used. Additional clinical studies of pediatric AIDS in developing countries evaluating both the natural history of the disease and the WHO definition are urgently needed.

Clinical Features

Among the more common clinical findings in symptomatic children are failure to thrive, recurrent fever, chronic diarrhea, generalized lymphadenopathy, chronic thrush, hepatosplenomegaly, and recurrent bacterial infections (41, 103, 104). Fewer

Table 3.4.   Provisional WHO Pediatric Clinical Case Definitions of AIDS

Major Signs	Minor Signs
Weight loss or failure to thrive	Generalized lymphadenopathy
Chronic diarrhea for >1 month	Oral thrush
Chronic fever for >1 month	Repeated common infection (otitis media, pharyngitis, etc.)
	Persistent cough
	Generalized dermatitis
	Confirmed maternal infection

Table 3.5.   Clinical Findings in HIV-1-infected African Children

Finding	% of Children with Sign or Symptom by Study			
	Rwanda (N=107)	Zaire (N=201)	Zimbabwe (N=190)	Uganda (N=755)
Weight loss or FTT[a]	88.8	97	53.6	80
Chronic diarrhea	83.2	62	25.4	66
Respiratory involvement[b]	70.1	61	41.4	66
Chronic fever	57.9	61	41.4	49
Persistent generalized lymphadenopathy	90.7	85	NA	71
Hepatomegaly ± splenomegaly	66.4	24	64.6	31
Oral thrush	40.2	52	31.5	NA
Chronic dermatitis	33.6	NA	18.2	55
Chronic parotitis	30.8	NA	NA	35
Neurological complications	NA	NA	4.4	NA
Recurrent infections	NA	18	NA	3
Kaposi sarcoma	NA	NA	40.9	17
	NA	NA	1.1	<1

[a] Failure to thrive.
[b] Chronic cough in Rwanda and Uganda; respiratory infection in Zaire; pneumonia in Zimbabwe.

data are available regarding the presentation of HIV-1-infected children in developing countries where the clinical findings might be expected to differ (Table 3.5). The presence of endemic tropical diseases, ready availability and use of antimicrobials, and limited access to health care and follow-up may affect clinical presentation of HIV-1 infection in developing countries (105). Similarly, the common occurrence of malnutrition and increased frequency and severity of infections among children in those countries, which can adversely affect the immune response, may confound diagnosis and presentation of HIV-1 infection.

Several studies have indicated that infected children in Africa present with many of the same signs and symptoms seem in industrialized countries (99, 100–102). However, the common development of severe protein-energy malnutrition and the more frequent finding of nontyphoid salmonella as a frequent cause of sepsis in African children reflects diseases that occur in most populations and differs somewhat from the clinical presentation of HIV-1 infection in other countries (99). The prevalence of the more commonly reported signs and symptoms such as weight loss, failure to thrive, diarrhea, fever, dermatitis, and respiratory infections vary from country to country and are easily mistaken for the clinical findings of other endemic pediatric diseases. Although there is no pathognomonic symptom or set of clinical findings that readily identifies a child with HIV-1 in-

fection, some investigators have indicated that the failure of children to respond to appropriate medical therapy is a strong indicator of associated HIV-1 infection (106).

Because of the limited availability of diagnostic techniques and the infrequency of autopsies, few data are available regarding the occurrence of opportunistic infections in HIV-1-infected children in developing countries. Although *Pneumocystis carinii* pneumonia is one of the most common opportunistic infections among HIV-1-infected adults and children in industrialized countries, it appears to occur far less frequently in African and Caribbean patients (109–114). Whether the apparent differences in the occurrence of *P. carinii* pneumonia reflect difficulties in establishing the diagnosis, differences in disease susceptibility, or geographic variation in the prevalence of the organism is unknown. However, one recent study showing that 70% of Gambian children have antibodies to *P. carinii* by the time they are 8 years old suggests that although *P. carinii* pneumonia is uncommon, the organism is prevalent (115). Other opportunistic infections such as candidiasis, cryptococcosis, herpes simplex, cryptosporidiosis, and toxoplasmosis have been reported in African children (108). However, as with *P. carinii* pneumonia, the difficulty in diagnosing many of these diseases has undoubtedly resulted in underreporting of opportunistic infections.

In developing countries, tuberculosis has emerged as a major infectious complication of HIV-1 infection. High rates of coinfection with HIV-1 and *Mycobacterium tuberculosis* in adult and, to a lesser extent, pediatric populations have been reported from several countries (116–123). In Port-au-Prince, Haiti, 40% of adult patients with active tuberculosis have been infected with HIV-1. HIV-1 seroprevalence rates of 17 and 55% have been reported among adults with tuberculosis in Zaire and the Central African Republic, respectively (121). Survey of tuberculous children younger than 5 years in Zimbabwe and Ivory Coast have detected HIV-1 seroprevalence rates ranging from 20 to 37.6% (122, 123). The high prevalence of tuberculosis in HIV-1-infected patients has led many physicians in developing countries to empirically treat AIDS patients with antituberculosis therapy. Although response to tuberculosis therapy in adults is generally favorable, relapses have been reported and the duration of antituberculosis therapy for HIV-1-infected adults and children has not been established (120, 121). In contrast to the high prevalence of *M. tuberculosis*, infections caused by *M. avium-intracellulare* and other atypical mycobacteria have been reported much less frequently (111, 121, 124).

Although initially an interaction between malaria and HIV-1 infection was suspected, several cross-sectional studies conducted in Zaire and Zambia indicated similar HIV-1 seroprevalence rates in individuals with and without *Plasmodium falciparum* infections (91, 92, 125). Despite several case reports of severe malaria occurring in HIV-1-infected patients and one study showing a higher prevalence and geometric mean density of parasitemia in HIV-1-seropositive pregnant women, other studies have not indicated a consistent increase in the severity of malaria in seropositive individuals (126, 127). Although malaria is not directly associated with HIV-1 infection, the severe anemia it often causes in young children may result in their receiving HIV-1-contaminated blood transfusions. This has produced a significant dilemma for clinicians in locations where screening of blood is unavailable and has resulted in the modification of criteria for transfusion therapy (128, 129).

Medical Management

Because diagnosis of HIV-1 infection can be difficult to establish in developing countries, practitioners are often required to empirically treat patients based on the presence of characteristic signs and symptoms. Suspect the diagnosis of HIV-1 infection as early as possible to institute more intensive clinical care and follow-up. Although antiretroviral therapy is generally unavailable in developing countries, pediatric patients with known HIV-1 infection can be offered aggressive supportive care including treatment of associated illnesses, nutritional support, and appropriate immunization.

As previously noted, tuberculosis is common among HIV-1-infected individuals in developing countries. The United States Public Health Service has recommended that HIV-1-infected adults with active tuberculosis be treated with isoniazid, rifampin, and pyrazinamide for 2 months followed by isoniazid and rifampin (130) (see Chapter 16A). The WHO has recommended four drugs (isoniazid, rifampin, pyrazinamide, and ethambutol) for 2 months followed by 4 months of isoniazid and rifampin. Few data regarding the optimal antituberculosis therapy for HIV-1-infected children are available, and most practitioners are empirically using at least three drugs, (isoniazid, rifampin, and pyrazinamide) with the addition of ethambutol for patients with disseminated or resistant disease (121). Although studies are being conducted in many developing countries to determine the efficacy and toxicity of several antituberculous regimens in HIV-1-infected adults, it is unlikely that similar data will be available from large numbers of children in the near future. Prospective studies of purified protein derivative-positive HIV-1-infected adults have indicated that they have a high risk of developing active tuberculosis. Advisory groups in the United States recommend that these patients receive prophylactic treatment with isoniazid (130). Although prophylactic antituberculosis therapy is not used in many developing countries, it should be considered for HIV-1-infected individuals (119). Determining the need for prophylactic therapy in children is complicated by the persistence of positive purified protein de-

Table 3.6.   WHO Recommendations for Routine Immunizations of Asymptomatic and Symptomatic HIV-1-infected Children

Vaccine	Asymptomatic	Symptomatic
BCG	Yes[a]	No
DTP[b]	Yes	Yes
OPV	Yes	Yes
IPV[c]	Yes	Yes
Measles	Yes	Yes

[a]Where risk of tuberculosis is high, WHO recommends BCG at birth for asymptomatic HIV-1 infected children; where risk of tuberculosis is low BCG may be withheld.
[b] Diphtheria, pertussis, tetanus.
[c] Inactivated polio vaccine.

rivative skin tests after Calmette-Guérin bacillus (BCG) vaccination during infancy. Alternatives to isoniazid chemoprophylaxis are being evaluated in ongoing clinical trials, and the results should be available by 1994.

Malnutrition is a major contributor to morbidity and mortality of HIV-1-infected children in all countries (105, 131–133). Aggressive nutritional support helps prolong survival of HIV-1-infected children. Nutritional counseling should begin as soon as HIV-1 infection is diagnosed and should emphasize prevention of malnutrition. Parents should be taught to recognize signs of inadequate growth in their children and should know how to appropriately supplement their children's diets with locally available foods. The use of oral rehydration fluids for dehydration and continued provision of appropriate foods during acute and chronic diarrhea episodes should be emphasized (130). Inexpensive food supplements developed as part of diarrhea control programs may prove useful in the management of HIV-1-infected children in developing countries. Unfortunately, limited local resources, poverty, and maternal illness are often major constraints in prevention of malnutrition among HIV-1-infected children in developing countries.

Data from the United States and Africa indicate that measles may be very severe in HIV-1-infected children (134, 135). Two studies in Zaire have provided additional data suggesting that measles is more virulent in HIV-1-infected children. The first study compared mortality rates in HIV-1-seropositive and seronegative children hos-

pitalized with measles (136). Although there was no overall difference in the case fatality ratio between the two groups, there was a trend among children older than 9 months toward a higher case fatality ratio in seropositive children (50 vs. 29%). In a prospective cohort study of infants born to HIV-1-infected mothers in Zaire, the measles case fatality rate in seropositive children was significantly higher than in seronegative children (137). Although HIV-1-infected children may have somewhat lower serologic response rates than HIV-positive seronegative infants after vaccination, most vaccinated infants will be protected against measles, and no serious adverse reactions have been reported (138). The available data support the WHO recommendation to immunize all children with the measles vaccine regardless of known or suspected HIV-1 infections. Current WHO recommendations for immunization of asymptomatic and symptomatic HIV-1-infected children are shown in Table 3.6. Although concerns regarding the safety and efficacy of live vaccines in HIV-1-infected children have been raised, the fears have been largely unjustified.

Disseminated BCG infections have been reported in immunodeficient individuals (132–134). BCG is routinely administered at birth to children in countries where tuberculosis is endemic and local reactions and disseminated disease have been described in HIV-1-infected individuals (132–136). However, the overall rate of complications in HIV-1-seropositive infants appears to be low. In Zaire, Zimbabwe, Rwanda, and Haiti similar rates of regional lymphadenitis were found after BCG vaccination of seropositive and seronegative children (134–138, unpublished data).

The WHO recommends that BCG not be given to symptomatic HIV-1-infected children or adults (138). In countries where the risk of tuberculosis is low, the use of BCG for either HIV-infected or uninfected infants is not recommended. However, in many developing countries the risk of tuberculosis in HIV-1-infected children is greater than the potential risk from the vaccine. Also, BCG is generally given shortly after birth, at which time HIV-1 will generally not have caused significant immunosuppression of infected infants. Moreover, most infants born to seropositive women do not acquire HIV-1 infections. Given the difficulty in identifying HIV-1-infected infants, the probability that most are uninfected and the high incidence of tuberculosis in developing countries, the WHO recommends that BCG continue to be given to asymptomatic HIV-1-infected children.

Although there have been no reports of wild-type poliomyelitis in HIV-1-infected individuals, polio is endemic in most developing countries outside of the Americas, and the risk of infection for young children is significant. In the United States and in almost all of Central and South America where circulation of wild poliovirus has been interrupted through immunization programs and >90% of school age children are adequately immunized against polio, the risk is far less (134). Vaccine-associated poliomyelitis has been reported in normal and immunocompromised hosts and is a theoretical concern in symptomatic HIV-1-infected individuals (146, 147). However, a retrospective review of 180 HIV-1-infected children who had received a total of 468 doses of oral polio vaccine (OPV) revealed no cases of vaccine-associated polio in the children or their contacts (148). Similarly, in prospective studies of infants born to HIV-1-infected mothers in Kenya, Zaire, and Haiti no serious adverse reactions after the use of OPV have been observed (137, 148–150, unpublished data). Advisory groups in the United States recommend that inactivated polio vaccine rather than OPV be given to children born to HIV-infected mothers and their household contacts regardless of clinical status (151). In developing countries the advantages of OPV include ease of administration, lower cost, induction of antibodies into the intestinal tract, and indirect immunization of other individuals through contact with the vaccine virus shed in immunized children's stools.

With HIV-1 seroprevalence continuing to increase among pregnant women in many developing countries, practitioners will encounter increasing numbers of HIV-1-infected children. They will face complex medical and social problems with limited resources. The development of algorithms for the diagnosis and treatment of HIV-1-infected children could assist practitioners in developing countries. However, appropriate algorithms need to be devised on a country-by-country basis taking into account available diagnostic and therapeutic resources and the presence of other endemic diseases. Collaboration with traditional healers, who can identify and assist in the care of HIV-1-infected patients, should also be considered in the development of algorithms. In devising such an algorithm for the care of HIV-1-infected individuals, practitioners and public health planners will confront a major dilemma faced by all developing countries where HIV-1 is endemic. Until antiretroviral therapy becomes available in developing countries, the decision regarding allocation of scarce resources for the medical management of HIV-1-infected patients will plague health personnel. Regardless of the scarcity of resources, every attempt should be made to provide AIDS patients with humane supportive care.

Impact on Child Survival

During the past several decades many developing countries had made substantial progress in the protection of child health. With successful implementation of immunization programs and the use of oral rehydration therapy, mortality rates among infants and children began to decrease. The HIV-1 epidemic is now threatening to nullify many previous gains. In developing countries where heterosexual transmission is common, high rates of maternal HIV-1 infection are resulting in large numbers of perinatally infected infants. The high mortality rates among HIV-1-infected children are due not only to the direct effects of HIV-1 but also to the profound disruption of the family unit associated with the infection. In many cases the parents themselves are incapacitated by HIV-1 infections, becoming progressively less capable of caring for their families. Parental loss and worsening socioeconomic status affect the survival of all children in the family regardless of their HIV-1 serologic status. Previous commitments made by families to ensure appropriate immunization and health care of their children are forgotten in the wake of the disruption caused by HIV-1 infections. In addition, the failure to respond to therapy seen in HIV-1-infected children may create further distrust in health care providers. Resources previously allocated to child health problems may also diminish as governments find it increasingly necessary to allocate funds to the prevention and therapy of AIDS.

In countries with large numbers of HIV-1-seropositive women, the impact of AIDS on child survival is already being felt. Ryder and coworkers (7) have reported a 15% increase in the infant mortality rate in Zaire from perinatal HIV-1 infections. Using available HIV-1 seroprevalence data from women living in several African countries, Valleroy and coworkers (145) estimated that infant and child mortality rates would increase by 6–38% in Kampala and 1–6% in Nairobi because of HIV-1 infections. In Haiti, a 12% increase in infant mortality rates could be directly attributed to HIV-1 infections (6). After evaluating data from 10 central and east African countries, Preble (5) estimated that HIV and/or AIDS will cause between 250,000 and 500,000 deaths annually among children under age five by 2000.

The implications of AIDS in mothers and children in African countries is just beginning to be explored from the perspective of demography, economics, and national policy (3, 5, 152–155). Of particular concern is the increasing number of children orphaned because of maternal AIDS. In some areas, the rising number of AIDS orphans is changing the demographic pattern of society. Half the population in one district in Tanzania consists of children needing food, clothing, and education and who depend on people unable to provide the basic needs. This pattern is repeated throughout the Kagari region, in which 5,000 children have already been orphaned by AIDS (5). In one study in 1989, the number of AIDS orphans in one district of Uganda with a total population of 300,000 was nearly 20,000 (153). Supplementing and supporting the traditional fostering system in some African countries provide a way for meeting the needs of orphans. Although the systems vary ethnically, in general they mediate and offer support to the many orphaned children in the community.

Some children most vulnerable to HIV-1 infection are those who are homeless and living on the streets of major urban centers. An estimated 7–10 million youth struggle to survive on the streets of major Latin American cities, and many more live on the streets of Asia and Africa. These youths live independent of their families and range in age from 6 to 18 years. They are at high risk for HIV-1 infection because of early onset of sexual activity and drug use (154). Studies in North America, Africa, and Latin America have revealed rather high seroprevalence rates of HIV-1 infection among homeless youth. One survey in New York City estimated that almost 7% of more than 1100 16- to 21-year-olds of both sexes living on the street were HIV-1 seropositive (22). Exchange of sex for money or food and child prostitution fuels the epidemic of sexually transmitted diseases and HIV-1 in street children throughout the world. Most of these children have almost no access to health care and have little knowledge about what condoms are or how to use them. Special efforts must be made to reach these high-risk children and change behavior because the usual channels of communication through families or educational institutions are unavailable.

CONTROL AND PREVENTION

HIV-1 infections among infants will undoubtedly continue to increase rapidly since an estimated 3 million women are HIV-1-infected, many of whom will transmit HIV-1 to their offspring (3, 153), and the WHO has projected that 10 million women will be infected by 2000. Most African infants born with HIV-1 infection will not survive beyond their fifth year of life, and AIDS-related increases in child mortality will seriously affect child survival efforts. Given the high fatality rates in this region, the number of AIDS orphans (both infected and noninfected) will increase dramatically as HIV-1-infected women progress to clinical AIDS and death. Clearly, child survival programs in these areas will have to be designed to reach this group of children to ensure coverage and effectiveness.

In the absence of vaccine, public health education about risky behavior is the most important preventive strategy. The stigmatization and psychological effects of HIV-1 infection on individuals have been profound in both developed and developing countries. Although there has been an outreach program to many affected groups in industrialized countries, there has been very little support for HIV-1-infected individuals in developing countries, which leads to further despair and in some countries lack of concerted effort to control AIDS. Thus, for the control of HIV-1 infection in young women, screening women who are anticipating a pregnancy and encouraging them not to become pregnant if they are HIV-1 positive is an important tenet of HIV-1 prevention. However, the cost of laboratory screening on a routine basis in these areas is highly prohibitive, and attempts to identify high-risk individuals by history have proven unsuccessful (156, 157). In these studies most seropositive women who were detected in the screening program became pregnant again after learning their results and elected to carry that pregnancy to term. Strong cultural norms for childbearing have been expressed by women in many developing countries; thus, it is unlikely that HIV-1 control programs will be successful in preventing young women of reproductive age who are found to be HIV-1 seropositive to avoid pregnancy or to contemplate termination of pregnancy, especially when the risk of maternal to infant transmission remains uncertain.

In many developing countries, an HIV-1-seropositive woman must balance the chance she might infect her infant against the possibility that her husband might leave her if she refuses to give him children. The risk of mother to child transmission must also be weighed against the child's survival chances in an environment where many children die from preventable diseases during their first year of life. In these circumstances, particularly for many women who have previously lost a child, the odds of infecting a newborn infant might not seem so great (158, 159). Interruption of maternal to infant transmission will be based on fundamental social-psychological concerns such as sexual behavior, illness behavior, and procreation, which will vary among sub-cultures. On this level, the challenges for AIDS prevention in the developed and developing worlds are similar. The major differences are economic. No individual nation in Africa has the resources required to build and sustain the epidemiologic, laboratory, clinical, and preventive activities required to control AIDS. Thus, a concerted international effort to control AIDS with financial, scientific, educational, and technical support will be required in all countries but most importantly in the developing nations.

References

1. Chin J, Mann J. Global surveillance and forecasting of AIDS. Bull WHO 1989;67:1–7.
2. Chin J. Global estimates of AIDS cases and HIV infection. AIDS 1990;4:S277–S283.
3. Chin J. Current and future dimensions of the HIV epidemic. Lancet 1990;336:221–224.
4. Quinn TC. AIDS in the Americas: A public health priority for the region. AIDS 1990;4:709–724.
5. Preble EA. Impact of HIV/AIDS on African children. Soc Sci Med 1990;31:671–804.
6. Halsey NA, Boulos R, Holt E, et al. Maternal-infant HIV-1 infection in Haiti: Impact on childhood mortaliy and malnutrition. JAMA 1990; 264:2088–2092.
7. Ryder RW, Nsa W, Hassig SE, et al. Perinatal transmission of the human immunodeficiency virus types 1 to infants of seropositive women in Zaire. N Engl J Med 1989;320:1637–1642.
8. Sirivichalyakul S, Phanuphak P, Hanvanich M, Ruxrungtham K, Panmoung W, Thanyanon W. Clinical correlation of the immunological markers of HIV infection in individuals from Thailand. AIDS 1991;6:393–397.
9. Siraprapasiri T, Thanprasertsuk S, Rodklay A, et al. Risk factors for HIV among prostitutes in Chiangmai, Thailand. AIDS 1991;5:579–582.
10. Naik TN, Sarker S, Singh HL, et al. Intravenous drug users: A new high-risk group for HIV infection in India. AIDS 1991;5:117–118.
11. Kaur A, Babu PG, Jacob M, et al. Clinical and laboratory profile of AIDS in India. J Acquir Immune Defic Syndr 1992;5:883–889.
12. Friedland GH, Klein RS. Transmission of the human immunodeficiency virus. N Engl J Med 1987;317:1125–1134.
13. Curran JW, Jaffe HW, Hardy AM, Morgan WM, Selilc RM, Dondero TJ. Epidemiology of HIV infection and AIDS in the United States. Science 1988;239:610–616.
14. Quinn TC, Mann JM, Curran JW, Piot P. AIDS in Africa: An epidemiologic paradigm. Science 1986;234:955–963.
15. Piot P, Plummer FS, Mhalu JL, Chin J, Mann JM. AIDS: An international perspective. Science 1988;239:573–579.
16. Piot P, Kreiss JK, Ndinya-Achola JO, Ngugi E, Plummer FA. Heterosexual transmission of HIV. AIDS 1988;2:1–10.

17. Rwandan HIV Seroprevalence Study Group. Nationwide community-based serological survey of HIV-1 and other human retrovirus infections in a central African country. Lancet 1989;1:941–943.
18. N'Galy B, Ryder RW. Epidemiology of HIV infection in Africa. J Acquir Immune Defic Syndr 1988;1:551–558.
19. Ronald AR, Nydinya-Achola JO, Plummer FA, et al. A review of HIV-1 in Africa. Bull NY Acad Med 1988;64:480–490.
20. Pan American Health Organization. 1991 AIDS/HIV/STD Annu Surveillance Rep 1992:1–50.
21. Sindayirwanya JB. Les implications cliniques de l'infection par VIH pour la mere et l'enfant (a propos de 206 cas) [Abstract WPD5]. Fifth International Conference: AIDS in Africa, Kinshasa, Zaire, Nov 1990.
22. Bazabana M, Loukaka JC, M'Pele P, et al. Tendance de l'infection a VIH chez les femmes encientes au Congo [Abstract MA 268]. Sixth International Conference: AIDS in Africa, Dakar, Senegal, Dec 1991.
23. Ekpini RA, Adjorlolo G, Sibailly T, et al. Prospective study of HIV-1 and HIV-2 mother-to-child transmission [Abstract 1017]. Fourth International Conference on AIDS, Stockholm, Jun 1988.
24. Mungai JN, Maitha GM, Kitabu MZ, et al. Prevalence of HIV and other STD's in three populations in Nairobi for year 1991 [Abstract PoC 4714]. Eighth International Conference on AIDS, Amsterdam, Jul 1992.
25. Liomba, Prevalence of sexually transmitted diseases (STD) and symptomatology in urban pregnant women in Malawi [Abstract A188]. Seventh Meeting of the Africa Union Against Venereal Disease and Treponematoses, Lusaka, Zambia, Mar 1991.
26. LePage P, Dabis F, Serfilira A, et al. Transmission of HIV-1 virus from mother to children in Central Africa: A study of cohort in Kigali, Rwanda [Abstract 243]. Fourth International Conference: AIDS and Associated Cancers in Africa, Marseille, October 1989.
27. Urassa E, Mhalu FS, Mbena E, et al. Prevalence of HIV-1 infection among pregnant women in Dar es Salaam, Tanzania [Abstract TPE 22]. Fifth International Conference: AIDS in Africa, Kinshasa, Zaire, Nov 1990.
28. Thailand Ministry of Public Health. National Sentinel Seroprevalence 1991; Feb 21: 1–20.
29. Hom D, Guay L, Mmiro F, et al. HIV-1 seroprevalence rate in women attending a prenatal clinic in Kampala, Uganda [Abstract WC 3262]. Seventh International Conference on AIDS, Florence, Jun 1991.
30. Centers for Disease Control. Human-immunodeficiency virus infection in the United States: A review of current knowledge. MMWR 1987;36:1–48.
31. Behets F, Bishagara K, Mama A, et al. Diagnosis of HIV infection with a dual rapid assay system as an alternative to ELISA and Western blot testing [Abstract SC 605]. Sixth International Conference on AIDS, San Francisco, Jun 1990.
32. Tembo G, Van Praag E, Mutambo H, et al. Sentinel surveillance of HIV infection in Zambia [Abstract TPE 28]. Fifth International Conference: AIDS in Africa, Kinshasa, Zaire, Oct 1990.
33. Whiteside A. HIV infection and AIDS in Zimbabwe: An assessment. Southern Africa Foundation for Economic Research, Economic Research Unit, University of Natal, 1991: 1–50.
34. Ryder RW, Hassig SE. The epidemiology of perinatal transmission of HIV. AIDS 1988;2(suppl 1): S83–S89.
35. Pape JW, Johnson W. Perinatal transmission of the human immunodeficiency virus. In: AIDS. Profile of an epidemic. Washington, DC: Sci Publ no 514. Pan American Health Organization, 1989: 73–79.
36. Braddick MR, Kreiss JK, Embree JE, et al. Impact of maternal HIV infection on obstetrical and early neonatal outcome. AIDS 1990;4:1001–1005.
37. Miotti PG, Dallabetta G, Ndovi E, et al. HIV-1 and pregnant women: Associated factors, prevalence, estimate of incidence and role in fetal wastage in central Africa. AIDS 1990;4:733–736.
38. Excler JL, Standaert B, Ngendandumwe E, Piot P. Malnutrition et infection of a HIV chez l'enfant en milieu hospitalier au Burundi. Pediatrics 1987; 42:715–718.
39. Italian Multicentre Study: Mother-to-child features, and prognostic factors of paediatric HIV infection. Lancet 1988;2:1043–1046.
40. Selwyn PA, Schoenbaum EE, Davenny K, et al. Prospective study of human immunodeficiency virus infection and pregnancy outcomes in intravenous drug users. JAMA 1989;261:1289–1294.
41. Gabriano C, Tovo PA, de Martino M, et al. Mother-to-child transmission of human immunodeficiency virus Type 1: Risk of infection and correlates of transmission. Pediatrics 1992;90: 359–374.
42. The European Collaborative Study. Children born to women with HIV-1 infection: Natural history and risk of transmission. Lancet 1991;337:253–260.
43. Newell ML, Peckham CS, LePage P. HIV-1 infection in pregnancy: Implications for women and children. AIDS 1990;4(suppl):S111–S118.
44. LePage P, Dabis F, Hitimana D-G, et al. Perinatal transmission of HIV-1: Lack of impact of maternal HIV infection on characteristics of livebirths and on neonatal mortality in Kigali, Rwanda. AIDS 1991;5:295–300.
45. Dabis F, Lepage P, Serufilira A, et al. Transmission du virus VIH-1 de la mere a l'enfant en Afrique Centrale: Une etude de chohorte a Kigali, Rwanda—characteristiques epidemiologiques a l'inclusion [Abstract B12]. The Implications of AIDS for Mothers and Infants. Paris, Nov 1989.
46. Lallemant M, Lall-mant-LeCoeur S, Cheyinier D, et al. Etude prospective de la transmission mere-enfant d-HIV1 + et HIV-1 [Abstract B11]. The Implications of AIDS for Mothers and Infants. Paris, Nov 1989.
47. Blanche S, Rouzioux C, Moscato ML, et al. A prospective study of infants born to women seropositive for human immunodeficiency virus type 1. HIV infection in newborns. French Collaborative Study Group. N Engl J Med 1989; 320:1643–1648.

48. Oxtoby MJ. Perinatally acquired human immunod eficiency virus infection. Pediatr Infect Dis J 1990;9:609–619.

49. Lapointe N, Michaud J, Pekovic D, Chausseau JP, Dupuy J-M. Transplacental transmission of HTLV-III virus. N Engl J Med 1985;312:1325–1326.

50. Sprecher S, Soumenkoff G, Puissant F, Degueldre M. Vertical transmission of HIV in 15-week fetus. Lancet 1986;2:288–289.

51. Mano H, Chermann J-C. Fetal human immunodeficiency virus type 1 infection of different organs in the second trimester. AIDS Res Hum Retroviruses 1991;7:83–88.

52. Courgnaud V, Lauré F, Brossard A, et al. Frequent and early in utero HIV-1 infection. AIDS Res Hum Retroviruses 1991;7:337–341.

53. Ehrnst A, Lindgren S, Dictor S, et al. HIV in pregnant women and their offspring. Evidence for late transmission. Lancet 1991;338:203–207.

54. Schupbach J, Wunderli W, Kind C, et al. Frequent detection of HIV- and IgG specific IgM and IgA antibodies in HIV positive cord blood sera: Fine analysis by Western blot. AIDS 1989;3:583–589.

55. Quinn TC, Kline RL, Halsey, N, et al. Early diagnosis of perinatal HIV infection by detection of viral-specific IgA antibodies. JAMA 1991;266:3439–3442.

56. Landesman S, Weiblen B, Mendez H, et al. Clinical utility of HIV-IgA immunoblot assay in the early diagnosis of perinatal HIV infection. JAMA 1991;266:3442-3446.

57. Rogers MF, Ou CY, Rayfield M, Thomas PA, et al. Use of the polymerase chain reaction for early detection of the proviral sequences of human immunodeficiency virus in infants born to seropositive mothers. N Engl J Med 1989;320:1649–1654.

58. Edwards JR, Utrich PP, Weintrub PS, Cowan MJ, et al. Polymerase chain reaction compared with concurrent viral cultures for rapid identification of human immunodeficiency virus infection among high-risk infants and children. J Pediatr 1989;115:200–203.

59. Smego RA, Halsey NA. The case of routine hepatitis B immunization in infancy for populations at increased risk. Pediatr Infects Dis J 1987;6:11–19.

60. Stevens CE, Toy PT, Taylor PE, Lee T, Yip HY. Prospects for control of hepatitis B virus infection: Implications of childhood vaccination and long-term protection. Pediatrics 1992;90:170–173.

61. Nicholas SW, Sondheimer DL, Wiloughby AD, Yaffe SJ, Katz SL, Human immunodeficiency virus infection in childhood, adolescence, and pregnancy: A status report and national research agenda. Pediatrics 1989;83:293–308.

62. Rossi P, Moschese V, Broliden PA, et al. Presence of maternal antibodies to human immunodeficiency virus 1 envelope glycoprotein gpl20 epitopes correlates with the uninfected status of children born to seropositive mothers. Proc Natl Acad Sci USA 1989;86:8055–8058.

63. Goedert JJ, Mendez H, Drummond JE, et al. Mother-to-infant transmission of human immunodeficiency virus type 1: Association with prematurity or low anti-gpl20. Lancet 1989;1351–1354

64. Devash Y, Calvelli TA, Wood DG, et al. Vertical transmission of the human immunodeficiency virus is correlated with the absence of high-affinity maternal antibodies to gp120 principal neutralizing domain. Proc Natl Acad Sci USA 1990;87:3445–3449.

65. Parekh BS, Shaffer N, Pau CP, et al. Lack of association between maternal antibodies to V3 loop peptides of gpl120 and perinatal HIV-1 transmission. The NYC Perinatal HIV Transmission Collaborative Study. AIDS 1991;5:1179–1184.

66. Halsey NA, Markham R, Wahren B, Boulos R, Rossi P, et al. Lack of association between maternal antibodies to V3 loop peptides and maternal-infant HIV-1 transmission. J Acquir Immune Defic Syndr 1992;5:153–157.

67. Ugen KE, Goedert JJ, Boyer J, et al. Vertical transmission of human immunodeficiency virus (HIV) infection. Reactivity of maternal sera with glycoprotein 120 and 41 peptides from HIV type 1. J Clin Invest 1992;89:1923–1930.

68. European Collaborative Study. Risk factors for mother-to-child transmission of HIV. Lancet 1992;339:1007–1012.

69. Goedert JJ, Duliege A-M, Amos CI, et al. High risk of HIV-1 infection for first-born twins. Lancet 1991;338:1471–1475.

70. Van de Perre P, Simonon A, Hitimana DG, et al. Mother-to-child transmission of HIV: First immunologic and serologic features from an ongoing cohort study in Kigali, Rwanda. Sixth International Conference on AIDS, San Francisco Jun Kigali 1990.

71. Ziegler JB, Cooper DA, Johnson RO, Gold J. Postnatal transmission of AIDS-associated retrovirus from mother to infant. Lancet 1985;1:896–898.

72. Oxtoby M. Human immunodeficiency virus and other viruses in human milk: placing the issues in broader perspective. Pediatr Infect Dis J 1988;7:825–835.

73. Van de Perre P, Simonon A, Msellati P, et al. Postnatal tranmsission of human immunodeficiency virus type 1 from mother to infant. A prospective cohort study in Kigali, Rwanda. N Engl J Med 1991;325:593–598.

74. Ruff AJ, Halsey NA, Coberly J, Boulos R. Breastfeeding and maternal-infant transmission of human immunodeficiency virus type 1. J Pediatr 1992;121:325–329.

75. Ruff A, Coberly J, Farzadegan H, et al. Detection of HIV-1 by PCR in breast milk [Abstract MC 3009]. Seventh International Conference on AIDS, Florence, Jun 1991.

76. Thiry L, Sprecher-Goldberger S, Jonckheer T, et al. Isolation of AIDS virus from cell-free breast milk of three healthy virus carriers. Lancet 1985;1:881–892.

77. Clark SJ, Saag MS, Decker D, et al. High titers of cytopathic virus in plasma of patients with symptomatic primary HIV-1 infection. N Engl J Med 1991;324:954–960.

78. Daar ES, Moudgil T, Meyer RD, Ho, DD. Transient high levels of viremia in patients with primary human immunodefiency virus type 1 infection. N Engl J Med 1991;324:961–964.

79. Ryder RW, Manzila T, Baenda E, et al. Evidence from Zaire that breast-feeding by HIV-1-seroposi-

tive mothers is not a major route for perinatal HIV-1 tranmission but does decrease morbidity. AIDS 1991;5:709–714.

80. Hutto C, Parks WP, Shenghan L, et al. A hospital-based prospective study of perinatal infection with human immunodeficiency virus type 1. J Pediatr 1991;118:347–353.

81. Feachem R, Koblinsky M. Strategies for the reduction of diarrhea disesases among young children: Promotion of breast feeding. Bull WHO 1984;62:271–292.

82. Heymann SJ. Modeling the impact of breast-feeding by HIV-infected women on child survival. Am J Public Health 1990;80:1305–1309.

83. Kennedy KI, Visness CM, Rogan WJ. Breastfeeding and AIDS: A health policy analysis. AIDS Public Policy J 1992;7:18–27.

84. World Health Organization. Consensus statement from the WHO/UNICEF consulation on HIV transmission and breastfeeding. Wkly Epidemiol Rec 1992;67:177–179.

85. Lederman SA. Estimating infant mortality from human immunodeficiency virus and other causes in breast-feeding and bottle-feeding populations. Pediatrics 1992;89:290–296.

86. Centers for Disease Control. Provisional public health service interagency recommendations for screening and donated blood and plasma for antibody to the virus causing acquired immunodeficiency syndrome. MMWR 1985;345:1–5.

87. Mann JM, Francis H, Quinn TC, et al. HTLV-III/LAV seroprevalence among hospital workers in Kinshasa, Zaire: Lack of association with occupational exposure. JAMA 1986;256:3099–3102.

88. Mann JM, Francis H, Davachi F, et al. Risk factors for human immunodeficiency virus seropositivity among children 1 to 24 months old in Kinshasa, Ziare. Lancet 1986;2:654–657.

89. Lepage P, Van de Perre P. Nosocomial tranmission of HIV in Africa: What tribute is paid to contaminated blood transfusion and medical injection. Infect Control Hosp Epidemiol 1988;9:200–203.

90. Mann JM, Francis H, Pavachi F, et al. HTLV-III/LAV seroprevalence in pediatric inpatients 2–14 years old in Kinshasa, Zaire. J Pediatr 1986;78:673–677.

91. Greenberg AE, Nguyen-Dinh P, Mann JM, Kabote N, et al. The association between malaria, blood transfusion, and HIV seropositivity in a pediatric population in Kinshasa, Zaire. JAMA 1988;259:545–549.

92. Nguyen Dinh P, Greenberg AE, Mann JM, et al. Absence of association between malaria, blood transfusion, and HIV seropositivity in a pediatric population in Kinshasa, Zaire. Bull WHO 1987;65:607–611.

93. Nzilambi N, Colebunders RL, Mann JM, et al. HIV blood screening in Afirca: Are there no alternatives? Fourth International Conference on AIDS, Stockholm, Jun 1988.

94. N'tita I, Mulanga K, Dulat C, et al. Risk of transfusion-associated HIV transmission in Kinshasa, Zaire. AIDS 1991;5:437–439.

95. Muller O, N'tila I, Nyst M, et al. Application of blood transfusion guidelines in a major hospital in Kinshasa, Zaire. AIDS 1992;6:431–432.

96. Speilberg F, Kabeya CM, Ryder RW, Kifuani NK, et al. Field testing and comparative evaluation of rapid, visually read screening assays for antibody to human immunodeficiency virus. Lancet 1989;1:580–583.

97. World Health Organization. Acquired immunodeficiency syndrome (AIDS). Wkly Epidemiol Rec 1986;61:69–73.

98. Colebunders RI, Greenberg A, Nguyen-Dinh P et al. Evaluation of a clinical case definition of AIDS in African children. AIDS 1987;1:151–153.

99. Lepage P, Van de Perre P, Dabis F, et al. Evaluation and simplification of the World Health Organization clinical case definition for paediatric AIDS. AIDS 1989;3:221–225.

100. Jonckheer T, Levy J, Ninane J, Allmenti A, Francois A. AIDS case definitions for African children. Lancet 1988;2:690–692.

101. Nsa W, Manzila T, Kabagado U; Mvula M, Ryder R. Validation of a case definition for perinatally acquired AIDS in Africa [Abstract ThGO 34]. Fifth International Conference on AIDS, Montreal, Jun 1989.

102. Mgone CS, Mhalu FS, Shao JF, et al. Prevalence of HIV-1 infection and symptomatology of AIDS in severely malnourished children in Dar Es Salaam, Tanzania. J Acquir Immune Defic Syndr 1991;4:910–913.

103. Scott GB, Hutto C, Makuch RW, et al. Survival in children with perinatally acquired human immunodeficiency virus type 1 infection. N Engl J Med 1989;321:1791–1796.

104. Prober CG, Gershon AA. Medical management of newborns and infants born to human immunodeficiency virus-seropositive mothers. Pediatr Infect Dis J 1991;10:684–695.

105. Conlon CP. Clinical aspects of HIV infection in developing countries. Br Med J 1988;44:101–114.

106. Lambert HJ, Friesen H. Clinical features of pediatric AIDS in Uganda. Ann Trop Paediatr 1989;9:1–5.

107. Clumeck N, Sonnet J, Taelman H, et al. Acquired immunodeficiency syndrome in African patients. N Engl J Med 1984;310:492–497.

108. Viera J, Frank E, Spira TJ, Landesman SH. Acquired immunodeficiency in Haitians. Opportunistic infections in previously healthy Haitian immigrants. N Engl J Med 1983;308:125–129.

109. Elvin KM, Lumbwe CM, Luo NP, Bjorkman A, Kallenius G, Lindner E. *Pneumocystis carinii* is not a major cause of pneumonia in Lusaka, Zambia. Trans R Soc Trop Med Hyg 1989;83:553–555.

110. N'Galy B, Vertozi S, Ryder RW. Obstacles in the optimal management of HIV infection/AIDS in Africa. J Acquir Immune Defic Syndr 1990;3:430–437.

111. Blaser MJ, Cohn DL. Opportunistic infections in patients with AIDS: Clues to the epidemiology of AIDS and the relative virulence of pathogens. Rev Infect Dis 1986;8:21–30.

112. Lucas S, Goodgame R, Kocjan G, Serwadda D. Absence of pneumocystosis in Ugandan AIDS patients. AIDS 1989;3:47–48.

113. Davachi F, Kabongo L, Mayemba N, Ndoko K, Ngoie K, N'Galy B. Clinical findings in 102 symp-

tomatic children with AIDS [Abstract TBP 108]. Fifth International Conference on AIDS, Montreal, Jun 1989.

114. Abouya YL, Beaumel A, Lucas S, et al. Pneumocystis carinii pneumonia. An uncommon cause of death in African patients with acquired immunodeficiency syndrome. Am Rev Respir Dis 1992;145:617–620.

115. Wakefield AE, Stewart TJ, Moxon ER, Marsh K, Hopkin JM. Infection wtih *Pneumocystis carinii* pneumonia in Ugandan African children. Trans R Soc Trop Med Hyg 1990;84:800–802.

116. Meeran K. Prevalence of HIV infection among patients with leprosy and tuberculosis in rural Zambia. Br Med J 1989;298:364–365.

117. Standaert B, Niragira F, Kadenda P, Piot P. The association of tuberculosis and HIV infection in Burundi. AIDS Res Hum Retroviruses 1989;5:247–251.

118. Gilks CF, Brindle RJ, Otieno LS, Bhatt SM, et al. Pulmonary and disseminated tuberculosis in HIV-1 seropostive patients presenting to the acute medical services in Nairobi. AIDS 1990;4:981–985.

119. Morrow RH, Colebunders RL, Chin J. Interactions of HIV infection with endemic tropical diseases. AIDS 1989;3(suppl 1):S79–S87.

120. Nunn PP, McAdam KPWJ. Mycobacterial infections in AIDS. Br Med Bull 1988;44:801–813.

121. Dumois JA. Tuberculosis in children with HIV infection. Pediatr AIDS HIV Infect Fetus Adolesc 1992;3:177–182.

122. Maxwell M, Legg W, Houston S, et al. Association of tuberculosis and HIV infection in Zimbabwe [Abstract ThB 494]. Sixth International Conference on AIDS, San Francisco, Jun 1990.

123. Sassan Morokro M, Gnaore E, Yesso G, et al. HIV-1 infection in children with tuberculosis in Abidjan, Côte d'Ivoire [Abstract MB 2440]. Seventh International Conference on AIDS, Florence, Jun 1991.

124. Okello DO, Sewankambo N, Goodgame R, Aisu T, et al. Absence of bacteremia with Mycobacterium avium-intracellulare in Ugandan patients with AIDS. J Infect Dis 1990;162:208–210.

125. Greenberg E, Nsa W, Ryder RW, et al. *Plasmodium falciparum* malaria and perinatally acquired human immunodeficiency virus type 1 infection in Kinshasa, Zaire. A prospective, longitudinal cohort study of 587 children. N Engl J Med 1991;325:105–109.

126. Katongole-Mbiddle E, Banura C, Kizito A. Blackwater fever caused by Plasmodium vivax infection in the acquired immune deficiency syndrome. Br Med J 1988;296:829–831.

127. Steketee RW, Wirima JJ, Bloland PB, Chelima B, Mermin JH. *Plasmodium falciparum* and HIV infection in pregnant women, Malawi [Abstract 140]. 41st Annual Meeting of the American Society of Tropical Medicine and Hygiene, Seattle, 1992.

128. Schutzhard E, Rainer J, Rwechungura RI. Treatment of severe malarial anaemia in East Africa's underfives—an unsolvable problem since the advent of AIDS? Trans R Soc Trop Hyg 1988;82:220–224.

129. Davachi F, Nseka M, N'Galy B, Mann JM. Effects of an educational campaign to reduce blood transfusions in children in Kinshasa, Zaire [Abstract E 666]. Fifth Interntional Conference on AIDS, Montreal, Jun 1989.

130. CDC. Tuberculosis and human immunodeficiency virus infection: Recommendations of the Advisory Committee for the Elimination of Tuberculosis (ACET). MMWR 1989;38:236–250.

131. Mugo JW, Wafula E, Ngacha DM, et al. HIV seropositivity in paediatrics at Kenyatta National Hospital (KNH), Nairobi, Kenya [Abstract PoC 4276]. Eighth International Conference on AIDS, Amsterdam, Jul 1992.

132. Zadi F, Vetter KM, Diaby L, et al. HIV seroprevalence and AIDS case definitions among hospitalized children, Abidjan, Côte d'Ivoire [Abstract 4465]. Eighth International Conference on AIDS, Amsterdam, Jul 1992.

133. Gayle HD, Gnaore E, Adjorlolo G, et al. HIV-1 and HIV-2 infection in children in Abidjan, Côte d'Ivoire. J Acquir Immune Defic Syndr 1992;5:513–517.

134. Markowitz LE, Chandler FW, Roldan EO, et al. Fatal measles pneumonia without rash in a child with AIDS. J Infect Dis 1988;158:480–483.

135. Centers for Disease Control. Measles in HIV-infected children—United States. MMWR 1988;37:183–186.

136. Sension MG, Quinn TC, Markowitz LE, et al. Measles in hospitalized African children with human immunodeficiency virus. Am J Dis Child 1988;142:1271–1272.

137. Mvula M, Ryder R, Manzila T, et al. Response to childhood vaccinations in African children with HIV infection [Abstract 5107]. Fourth International Conference on AIDS, Stockholm, Jun 1988.

138. Halsey NA, Boulos R, Mode F, et al. Response to measles vaccine in Haitian infants 6 to 12 months old: Influence of maternal antibodies, malnutrition, and concurrent illnesses. N Engl J Med 1985;313:544–549.

139. Lotte A, Wasz-Hockert O, Poisson N, et al. BCG complications. Adv Tuberc Res 1984;21:107–193.

140. Clements CJ, Von Reyn CF, Mann JM. HIV infection and routine childhood immunization: Review. Bull WHO 1987;65:905–911.

141. Nousbaum JB, Garre M, Boles JM, Garo B, Lanul JJ. Deux manifestations inhabituelles d'une infection par le virus LAV-HTLV ~ BCGite et varicelle pulmonaire. Rev Pneumol Clin 1986;42:310–311.

142. Braun MM, Cauthen G. Relationship of the human immunodeficiency virus epidemic to pediatric tuberculosis and *Bacillus Calmette-Guerin* immunization. Pediatr Infect Dis J 1992;11:220–227.

143. Colebunder RL, Ryder RW, Nzilambi N, et al. HIV infection in patients with tuberculosis in Kinshasa, Zaire. Am Rev Respir Dis 1989;139:1082–1085.

144. Centers for Disease Control. BCG vaccination and pediaric HIV infection—Rwanda, 1988–1990. MMWR 1991;40:833–836.

145. Tarantola D, Mann JM. Acquired immunodeficiency syndrome (AIDS) and expanded programmes on immunization. Special Programme on AIDS. Geneva: World Health Organization, 1987.

146. Onorato IM, Markowitz LE, Oxtoby MJ. Childhood immunization, vaccine-preventable diseases and

infection with human immunodeficiency virus. Pediatr Infect Dis J 1988;6:588–595.

147. Nkowane BM, Wassilak SGF, Orenstein WA, et al. Vaccine-associated paralytic poliomyelitis. JAMA 1987;257:1335–1340.

148. McLaughlin M, Thomas P, Onorato I, et al. Use of live virus vaccines in HIV-infected children: A retrospective survey. Pediatrics 1988;82:229–233.

149. Embree J, Datta P, Braddick M, et al. Vaccination of infants of HIV seropositive mothers. Fourth International Conference on AIDS, Stockholm, Jun 1988.

150. Mvula M, Ryder R, Oxtoby M, et al. Measles and measles immunization in African children with human immunodeficiency virus. Fourth International Conference on AIDS, Stockholm, Jun 1988.

151. Centers for Disease Control. General recommendations on immunization. MMWR 1989;38:205–227.

152. Valleroy LA, Harris JR, Way PO. The impact of HIV infection on child survival. AIDS 1990;4:667–672.

153. Chin J, Sankaran G, Mann J. Mother to infant transmission of HIV: An increasing global problem. In: Maternal and child care in developing countries. Geneva: Ott, 1989.

154. Paiva J, Pinto JA, Ruff A, et al. Underprivileged children in Belo Horizonte Brazil: HIV positivity, knowledge and risk behavior [Abstract PoD 5046]. Eighth International Conference on AIDS, Amsterdam, Jul 1992.

155. Hunter S. Demographic and policy implications of the growing orphan burden of AIDS in African countries. Conference on Implications of AIDS in Mothers and Infants, Paris, 1989.

156. Dalglish P. Action for children. UNICEF 1988;3:1–20.

157. Carballo M, Carael M. Impact of AIDS on social organization. In: Fleming AF, Carballo M, Fitzsimmons DW, Bailey MR, Mann J. The global impact of AIDS. New York: Alan R. Liss, 1988: 81–94.

158. Sutherland A, Moroso G, Berthaud M, et al. Influence of HIV infection on pregnancy decisions [Abstract 6607]. Fourth International Conference on AIDS, Stockholm, Jun 1988.

159. Lalleman M. Knowledge and attitude: Mother to child transmission of HIV-1 and prenatal screening in Brazzaville (Congo). First International Conference of AIDS Information, Education and Communication, Ixtapa, Mexico, 1988.

4

Continuing Issues Regarding Transfusion and Coagulation Factor Acquired HIV Infection in Children

M. Elaine Eyster

EPIDEMIOLOGY AND NATURAL HISTORY OF HIV INFECTION

Historical Perspectives and AIDS Surveillance Data

The first cases of hemophilia-associated AIDS were recognized in 1982 (1), at least 2–3 years after the onset of the epidemic in homosexual men and intravenous drug users (2–4). Concerns about a transfusion-acquired infectious agent mounted in 1982, when an infant developed an unexplained cellular immunodeficiency and opportunistic infection after a transfusion of platelets derived from blood of a male donor who subsequently developed AIDS (5). These concerns prompted the Public Health Service to recommend in March 1983 that members of groups at increased risk for AIDS refrain from donating blood or plasma.

By November 1983, the number of cases of AIDS in homosexual men and intravenous drug users had risen exponentially, and additional cases had been reported in hemophiliacs and recipients of blood from donors who subsequently developed AIDS (6). Most cases in transfusion recipients were over age 50 and more closely resembled those from all transfusion recipients than other patients with AIDS. They were observed in states and cities where AIDS was most commonly reported and were linked to donors who were members of high-risk groups (7). This clus-

tering of cases linked by sexual contact and blood transfusions strengthened the evidence that AIDS was caused by an infectious agent, and the search for a putative agent focused on retroviruses known to exhibit a tropism for human CD4 cells, which were consistently depleted in patients with AIDS (8–10).

The codiscovery of the etiologic agent by Montagnier et al. (11) and Gallo et al. (12) accompanied by the finding of a cell line that was permissive to the growth of this virus (13), now termed the human immunodeficiency virus (HIV), soon permitted mass production of viral antigens and the development of a blood test to detect antibodies to HIV. By late 1984, virologic studies provided conclusive evidence that HIV was transmissible through blood cells or plasma and was associated with an asymptomatic but contagious carrier state (14). As culture techniques improved, HIV was frequently isolated from the peripheral blood mononuclear cells of seropositive recipients of blood or blood products and their seropositive high-risk donors (15).

In 1985, with the widespread availability of the enzyme-linked serum immunosorbent assay HIV antibody test, most hemophiliacs who had received clotting factor concentrates were found to be seropositive (see Chapter 12) (16–19). These separate studies showed that ~90% of hemophiliacs intensively treated with factor VIII concentrates were seropositive in 1984 (16–18).

51

Table 4.1. HIV Prevalence and Age-related AIDS Incidence

Mode of Acquisition	Prevalence of HIV Infection[a]	Relation of Age to Incubation and/or Cumulative AIDS Incidence
Vertical	Industrialized countries: 13–32%; unindustrialized countries: 25–48%[b]	Incubation uncertain. Probably two populations: one 4–8 months; one more comparable with adults.
Transfusion	8% of patients wtih congenital anemia and leukemia transfused from 1978 to 1984	Adults (median age 55 yr): 49% cumulative AIDS incidence after 7 yr (95% confidence interval 36–62%). Children: incubation uncertain. Estimated 41 months median for children under age 13 when infected compared with 51 months in adults.[c]
Coagulation factor	Factor VIII deficiency: 70–80%; severe factor IX deficiency: 40–50%	Cumulative 10-yr AIDS incidence: 30 ± 7% when infected between ages 1 and 17; 44 ± 7% when infected between ages 18 and 34; 56 ± 7% when infected between ages 35 and 70.

[a]Transmission rates in infants born to seropositive mothers.
[b]Ref. 149.
[c]With other methods, a mean 8-yr incubation has been calculated, based mainly on adult data.

When stored serum specimens were tested retrospectively, over 50% of seroconversions were found to have occurred during 1981 and 1982 (19). The first seroconversion occurred in late 1978 (20).

By December 1992, 2214 cases of AIDS had been reported in persons with hemophilia, accounting for 1% of the 253,448 reported cases in adults and children. Cases of AIDS in other transfusion recipients numbered 5286, representing 2% of the total. Of the 4249 cases of AIDS in children younger than 13 years, 188 (5%) were in persons with hemophilia and 306 (8%) were in other transfusion recipients (21).

Prevalence of HIV Infections

Hemophilia

Of the estimated 20,000 persons with hemophilia residing in the United States, more than 10,000 are followed regularly at treatment facilities (22). By 1985, about three-fourths of these individuals had received infusions of non-heat-treated clotting factor concentrates that were commercially prepared from large pools of plasma obtained from thousands of donors (22). In a recent survey of over 7000 persons with hemophilia followed at 100 treatment centers throughout the United States from 1985 to 1989, 70% of persons with severe factor VIII deficiency and nearly 50% of persons with se-

vere factor IX deficiency were reported to be seropositive (23). In the largest cohort study reported, the prevalence of HIV antibodies in 908 persons with classic hemophilia (factor VIII deficiency) was 76.5% of those with severe disease, 46.3% of those with moderate disease, and 25.4% of those with mild disease. In 148 persons with Christmas disease (factor IX deficiency), the prevalence was 41.9% of those with severe disease, 26.9% of those with moderate disease, and 8.3% of those with mild disease (24) (Table 4.1).

For reasons not well understood, ~10% of persons with hemophilia repeatedly exposed to non-heat-treated concentrates have not developed HIV antibodies. A similar percentage of recipients of transfusions from HIV-infected donors remain seronegative (25). Because many of these seronegative recipients shared components from donors who subsequently were found to be infected at the time of donation, host factors as well as virulence and size of the inoculum are suspected to be involved in susceptibility to infection. Age at time of first exposure to HIV appears to be unrelated to risk of HIV infection from blood or blood products (P. S. Rosenberg and J. J. Goedert, personal communication, 1993), although age at time of first infection is related to risk of progression to AIDS (24, 26).

In four separate reports involving 227 seronegative hemophiliacs who received virus-inactivated clotting factor concentrates, none were found to be infected using the highly sensitive polymerase chain reaction (PCR) (27–30). Furthermore, except for one child who was infected by a contaminated needle used by his brother, there have been no documented seroconversions associated solely with virus-inactivated screened products in the United States since 1987 (31, 32). However, Nagao and colleagues (33) have reported a 17-year hemophilia B patient in Japan who became seropositive more than 3 years after switching to heat-treated prothrombin complex concentrates.

Transfusion Recipients

In a preliminary report from the Transfusion Safety Study sponsored by the National Heart, Lung, and Blood Institute, 15 of 197 (8%) multitransfused individuals with congenital anemias were found to be infected before self-deferral and HIV-1 antibody screening of donors (34). In a retrospective study from Memorial Sloan Kettering Cancer Center in New York, 18 of 211 (8.5%) patients with leukemia treated from 1978 through 1984 were seropositive (35). Infection with HIV-2 appears to be rare in the United States and has been largely limited to West African immigrants. As of 1991, there were only 18 reported cases. One of these was an American who had traveled to West Africa (36).

AIDS INCIDENCE
Prospective Cohort Studies in Hemophiliacs

Incidence is the measure of risk made by dividing the number of cases that occur in a unit of time by the number of people in the population who are at risk. With AIDS, cumulative rather than annual incidence rates are most informative because few or no symptoms occur early in infection, which in most persons spans many years. The number at risk is determined by testing the study population for HIV antibodies. Those positive at the time of entry are termed *prevalent seropositives*. Those who seroconvert during the study are termed *incident seropositives*. Because the rates of progression to AIDS increase with duration of infection, the more reliable assessment of the natural history of HIV infection is obtained from studies of incident seroconverters.

In the Multicenter Hemophilia Cohort Study, the largest study of incident seroconverters reported, cumulative AIDS incidence for 327 persons with stored sera tested retrospectively was $42 \pm 4.7\%$ (SE) 11 years after HIV seroconversion (J. J. Goedert, personal communication, 1993). Higher values in the range of 50–55% at 10–11 years have been reported in homosexual men (Table 4.2). However, the faster rates in homosexual men are largely due to the increased risk of Kaposi's sarcoma (37) and the rates of

Table 4.2.   Estimated Cumulative AIDS Incidence in Different HIV-infected Populations

Ref.	No. of Incident Seroconverters in Cohort	Time from Known or Estimated Time to Seroconversion or Infection										
		2-yr	3-yr	4-yr	5-yr	6-yr	7-yr	8-yr	9-yr	10-yr	11-yr	12-yr
Hemophiliacs						% of cohort						
Eyster et al. (26)[a]	87					18		26				
Ragni and Kingsley (47)	84									45		
Giesecke et al. (39)	98				5	9						
Lee et al. (88)	111			1							42	
Goedert[b]	327	1	2	7	11	18	22	25	30	37	42	
Transfusion recipients												
Giesecke et al. (39)	48		16	23	29							
Ward et al. (38)	116	5	8	18	33	46	49					
Donegan et al. (111)	111		13									
Homosexual men												
Rutherford et al. (49)	489					13				51	54	
Phair et al. (87)	345	1	3	10								

[a]Included in Goedert Multicenter Cohort Study.
[b]Unpublished update of Ref. 24.

AIDS-defining opportunistic infections in persons with hemophilia, and homosexual men with HIV infections do not differ when the confounding effect of age is excluded.

AIDS Incidence in Transfusion Recipients

Patients infected by HIV as a result of blood transfusions are unique in that their dates of infection are well-defined. Two studies have suggested that the rate at which adult transfusion recipients develop AIDS after HIV infection is more rapid than in persons with hemophilia (38, 39). However, transfusion recipients are generally older and may have other underlying medical conditions that may influence development of HIV-related illnesses. In a longitudinal study in which 694 adult HIV-infected recipients were retrospectively identified after a donor was found to be HIV antibody positive, 49% developed AIDS within 7 years of transfusion. The median age of the recipients with AIDS was 55 years (38). In a Swedish study, 29% of 48 HIV-infected transfusion recipients developed AIDS after 5 years, compared with only 5% of 98 HIV-infected hemophiliacs (39). However, certain assumptions were made in the seroconversion dates for some hemophiliacs, and the average age for the hemophiliacs was lower than for the transfusion recipients.

Incubation Period

The incubation period of AIDS is defined as the time from first infection with HIV to development of AIDS. Because periods of observation have been limited to ≤ 12 years, the distribution of AIDS incubation periods in populations at risk can only be estimated by mathematical modeling.

Most attempts to estimate AIDS incubation periods in transfusion recipients depend on the assumption that AIDS will develop eventually in all infected persons. Furthermore, the denominator, which is the number of people infected by blood transfusions who have not yet developed AIDS, is unknown. Because the period of observation is limited, the exclusion of these individuals leads to an underestimate of the average incubation period. Not surprisingly, estimates vary widely from a mean of 4.5 to 18 years for adults. For example, in 1985–1986, Centers for Disease Control (CDC) estimated the transfusion-associated AIDS incubation to be 4.5–5 years (15, 40), but there was extreme uncertainty in these estimates with a range of 2.6–14.2 years (40). In 1987, Medley et al. (41) used later data and calculated a mean incubation of 8 years for those aged 5–59 years at infection. In an analysis by Andersen et al. in 1988 (42), only 7.4% of cases were diagnosed during the first 3 years of infection. By 7 years, 56.5% were diagnosed, with a long tail beyond the 15th year after which 2.3% of the cases were detected. In the most recent report based on surveillance data from 3518 cases of transfusion-related AIDS reported to the CDC through 1990, the mean incubation was estimated to be 18 years (43).

Age as a Risk Factor for Progression

In persons with hemophilia as well as other risk groups, older age at seroconversion has been clearly shown to be associated with a significantly higher incidence of AIDS (24, 26, 44–47), as well as other HIV-related conditions (oral candidiasis, persistent fever, and weight loss) (48). Cases of AIDS or other HIV-related conditions almost never appear during the first 2 years of infection but occur with increasing frequency thereafter, with cumulative rates by 8 years four times higher in adults than in children and adolescents (24, 26, 48).

In a cohort study of 87 incident seroconverters from a hemophilia center in Pennsylvania, cumulative AIDS incidence was four times higher at 6 years in persons with hemophilia who seroconverted after age 21 than among those who seroconverted between ages 2 and 21 years (26). In a larger study of 1200 HIV-seropositive persons with hemophilia from the United Kingdom, cumulative AIDS incidence 5 years after seroconversion was 4% among patients younger than 25 years after first testing positive for HIV antibodies, 6% among those aged 25–44 years, and 19% among those over age 45 (44). Older age at seroconversion was also associated with an increased risk of AIDS in an Italian study of 499 HIV-positive hemophiliacs (45). However, certain assumptions were made concerning the probability of seroconversion in the periods under study in both the British and the Italian studies.

A more accurate assessment of the risk of AIDS in relation to age was obtained from a multicenter cohort study by Goedert and colleagues (24) of 1219 persons with hemophilia, focusing on 319 subjects with documented dates of seroconversion to HIV (Fig. 4.1). In this study, the incidence rate of AIDS after seroconversion was 2.67/100 person-years and was directly related to age (from 0.83 in persons aged 1–11 years up to 5.66 in persons aged 35–70 years). The annual incidence of AIDS ranged from 0 during the first year after seroconversion to 7% during the eighth year, with 8-year cumulative rates (±SE) of 13.3 ± 5.3% for ages 1–17, 26.8 ± 6.4% for ages 18–34, and 43.7 ± 16.4% for ages 35–70. Similar results were reported by Phillips and colleagues (46) who found a 1.45 relative risk of developing

AIDS for each year of increase in age. More recent data from the multicenter hemophilia cohort study (J. J. Goedert, personal communication, 1993) show 10-year cumulative rates of 30 ± 7% for ages 1–17, 44 ± 7% for ages 18–34, and 56 ± 7% for ages 35–70 (Fig. 4.1). Thus older persons with hemophilia have an incidence of AIDS similar to the cumulative incidence of 54% at 11 years among the cohort of homosexual men in San Francisco (49) and at 7 years in adult recipients (median age 55) of infected blood transfusions (38), whereas children older than 1 year and adolescents clearly have a lower rate of progression to AIDS. This lower rate of HIV progression in children may be partly associated with differences in lymphocyte populations, but functional properties of immune cells may be

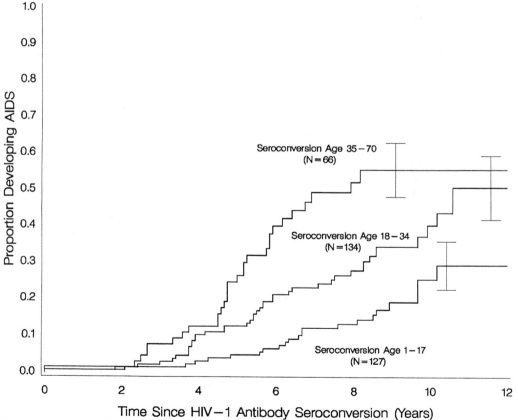

Figure 4.1. Cumulative incidence of AIDS among 327 subjects with hemophilia. Time is measured from the midpoint of each subject's HIV-1 seroconversion date. Number of subjects in follow-up 10 years after seroconversion is in parentheses. *Vertical bars,* ±1 SE. Incidence of AIDS was strongly related to age at seroconversion, with cumulative rates of 30 ± 7% in children and adolescents, 44 ± 7% in younger adults, and 56 ± 7% in adults who seroconverted over age 34. From Goedert JJ, Kessler CM, Aledort LM, et al. A prospective study of human immunodeficiency virus type I infection and the development of AIDS in subjects with hemophilia. N Engl J Med 1989;321:1141–1148.

equally or more important (50). Other possibilities may include age-dependent colonization with microbial agents capable of causing AIDS-defining opportunistic infections (26).

There is also a relationship to age at the time of transfusion-acquired infection. Analysis of CDC AIDS surveillance data as of January 1, 1990, indicated a median incubation of 41 months for children under age 13 and 51 months for adults (D. Ward, personal communication). Medley et al. (41) reported a mean of 1.97 years for children aged 0–4 years at infection compared with 7.97 years for those aged 5–59 years at infection. In an analysis by Lagokos and De Gruttola (51) of 844 transfusion-associated AIDS cases, the median latency was 6.7 years for all cases compared with 3.7 years for those infected under 1 year. Blaxhult et al. (52) also found that age influenced the latency period to AIDS in 58 transfusion recipients from 15 to 60 years of age, with a cumulative AIDS rate of $20 \pm 8\%$ in the younger compared with $39 \pm 9\%$ in older age groups. Thus, the time from transfusion-acquired infection to onset of AIDS is shortest in young infants and older adults, with children, adolescents, and young adults having longer latency periods.

Estimates of AIDS incubation periods of infants infected perinatally and by neonatal transfusion are even more uncertain. In a study by Kraskinski et al. (53), 12 children infected by transfusion had an incubation of 4 months to 5.7 years (median 3.6 years) compared with a shorter incubation of 6 weeks to 7.3 years (median 0.75 years) in 93 with maternally transmitted infection. The median incubation period for nine cases among children in whom the infected transfusion could be accurately dated to within 1 month was 2 years (mean 2.1 years, range 4 months to 5.7 years). In another report by Mundy and coworkers (54) of a cohort of 39 children who were infected with HIV through transfusions as neonates, 26 (67%) were alive at a mean age of 84 months. At a mean of 7 years follow-up, 44% remained asymptomatic, 15% had HIV-related symptoms, and 8% had developed AIDS. This long latency is in marked contrast to that seen in infected infants born to seropositive mothers, most of whom develop symptoms before 1 year of age (55–57). However,

Auger et al. (58) have reported that there is an abrupt knee in the incubation distribution of pediatric patients with AIDS whose only known route of infection is maternal, suggesting the existence of two risk populations, one very short with a median of 4.1 months and the second much longer with a median of 6.1 years, which is comparable with that of 8 years reported for adults. Likewise, Lagakos and De Gruttola (51) estimated that less than 40% of infants infected by their mothers may develop AIDS within 3 years.

Thus, limited data suggest those infants infected perinatally by their mothers have a bimodal distribution for the expression of HIV-related symptoms and that those infected by transfusion may have a more chronic course than most of those infected vertically. This could be due in part to the timing of transmission (see also Chapter 10). HIV transmission can occur during gestation, as supported by identification of HIV in placental and fetal tissue as early as the eighth week of gestation (59–61) and by the finding of a positive culture or PCR during the neonatal period in approximately one-third of infected newborns (62). Conversely, the presence of HIV by culture or PCR cannot be demonstrated at birth in most infected children, suggesting that mother to child transmission occurs late in pregnancy or during delivery in most vertical infections (63, 64). Intrapartum infection is also suggested by the report of discordant infections in twins, with the firstborn being at higher risk (65). Thus, one might speculate that infants infected early in gestation might have a worse prognosis because they have been infected longer and at a time when their developing immune systems are less capable of controlling HIV replication. Other factors, including the size or strain of viral inoculum, the presence of maternal neutralizing antibody, and host factors such as human leukocyte antigen type, may also be involved in the rate of progression to AIDS among HIV-infected neonates, irrespective of the time or mode of acquisition.

Predictive AIDS Markers

The most commonly established laboratory markers used to predict progression to

Table 4.3.   Markers of HIV Infection Commonly Associated with Progression to AIDS

Marker	Abnormality	Diagnostic Value
Serologic		
p24 antigen[a]	Persistence	High positive predictive value in adults; lower in children and adolescents. Poor negative predictive value in all age groups.
Anti-p24	Negativity	With absence of marker, predictive value is high in adults but lower in children and adolescents.
Anti-gp120	Abnormally low level	High in older adults. Uncommon and poor in children and adolescents.
β_2 Microglobulin,[a, b] (μg/liter) (normal: 1.31 ± 2.8)	>4	β_2 Microglobulin and neopterin are strongly correlated and are highly predictive in adults, especially when used in combination with CD4 counts. Both are useful in children.
Neopterin[b] (nmol/liter) (normal: 6.62 ± 1.99)	>17	
α-Interferon[b] (IU) (normal: ≤8)	≥20	Useful in children, adolescents, and adults; less sensitive than CD4 counts. Use not firmly established.
IgA[a,b] (mg/dl) (normal: 251 ± 116)	>300	Least useful. Values applicable only to adults.
Cellular		
CD4 cells/μl (normal: 800 ± 150 or 30–60% of total lymphocytes)	<200 or <20% of total lymphocytes[c]	Most prominent finding in HIV infection. Best single early predictor to identify those progressing to AIDS in 2–3 years in all age groups except infants with persistent infection.
CD4-to-CD8 ratio[a] (normal: 1.57 ± 0.67)	<0.5	Less reliable than CD4 counts because of variability of CD8 counts that show early activation and late decrease.

[a]Widely available clinical tests; independent predictive value.
[b]Soluble products of immune activation.
[c]CD4 counts are age dependent.

AIDS from asymptomatic HIV infection are listed in Table 4.3 (see also Chapter 35). Studies in homosexual men (66–68) and persons with hemophilia (69–71) have shown that low CD4 lymphocyte counts and the appearance of p24 core antigen (69, 70) independently predict progression to AIDS, with CD4 counts being more sensitive and p24 core antigen being more specific (70). These findings are age-related with the incidence of AIDS being higher in adults than in children with falling CD4 counts and detectable p24 antigen (Table 4.2) (24). The appearance of p24 antigen may be preceded by the loss of p24 antibody (69), probably because of the formation of antigen-antibody complexes (72). Both the loss of p24 core and gp120 envelope antibody correlate with progression to AIDS (24; J. J. Goedert et al., unpublished data, 1993).

Plasma viremia has been shown to be a more sensitive marker of the clinical stage of HIV infection and virus replication than either the presence of p24 antigen or antibody in plasma (73). In adults, there is good correlation among the presence of viremia, CD4+ lymphocyte counts, development of symptoms, and duration of infection. However, children infected in the perinatal period are often found to have plasma viremia with CD4 counts within the normal range for age-matched controls (74). Direct quantitation of HIV in peripheral blood mononuclear cells (75) and determination of the frequency of HIV DNA in CD4 cells (76) have also been shown to correlate with disease progression. However, these tests are only available on a research basis.

Serum β_2 microglobulin (β_2M) predicts progression to AIDS both independently of and in addition to CD4 lymphocyte counts in adults (77) as well as infants infected perinatally (78) and in HIV-infected hemophiliacs across a wide age spectrum (J. J. Goedert et al., personal communication). This protein, which is a subunit of the class I histocompatibility antigens, is present on the surface of all nucleated cells. Elevated levels reflecting increased production or cell turnover are found in those patients who progress to AIDS. In the San Francisco General Hospital Cohort Study, β_2M was a better predictor of progression to AIDS than CD4 lymphocyte counts, presence of HIV p24 core antigen, or neopterin (77).

Elevated neopterin levels are found with HIV infection, and progressive infection is associated with a further increase in all age groups (78, J. J. Goedert et al., personal communication, 1993). Neopterin is a product of macrophages stimulated by interferon-γ from activated T cells. High neopterin levels independently predict AIDS up to 3 years before diagnosis (79). In the Los Angeles cohort of the multicenter AIDS cohort study, neopterin was a better predictor of AIDS than β_2M (80). Other products of immune activation that have been found to be markers for progression to AIDS are IgA, increased levels of soluble interleukin-α receptors, and increased levels of soluble CD8 (80).

An unusual form of acid labile interferon-α has been shown to be persistently elevated in some persons with HIV infections (81). In persons with hemophilia, moderate or high serum levels of interferon were predictive of AIDS up to 36 months diagnosis, with relative hazards (standardized for duration of infection) comparable with that of the CD4 counts (24).

It is clear that laboratory markers singly and in combination can be used effectively to predict progression to AIDS over months to years in HIV-infected individuals. In persons with hemophilia, the risk of AIDS at 2 years was 67% among persons who were positive for p24 core antigen compared with only 22% among those who remained antigen negative at the time the CD4 count first fell below 200 cells/μl (70). In the San Francisco study of asymptomatic HIV-seropositive homosexual men, a combination of five variables, including number and proportion of CD4 lymphocytes and serum β_2M and presence of p24 antigen and hematocrit, identified two-thirds of those progressing to AIDS at either 2 or 3 years (77). In the Los Angeles multicenter AIDS cohort, AIDS was predicted most accurately by the level of CD4 cells in combination with either β_2M or neopterin levels (80).

Clinical markers also have predictive value for AIDS. Oral candidiasis, persistent fever, weight loss, and pneumonia not classified as AIDS have all been shown to be associated with an increased risk of AIDS after adjustment for CD4 counts in HIV-infected adults (48, 68, 82, 83), although this association was true only for oral candidiasis in HIV-infected children with hemophilia (48). Surprisingly, herpes zoster has no predictive value in persons with hemophilia, regardless of age (48).

Possible Cofactors That Affect Progression to AIDS

Various exogenous cofactors, including size of inoculum, strain variation, coinfection with other blood-borne viruses, and host factors have been suggested to accelerate progression to AIDS. A familial tendency to serious complications of HIV infection was noted in a study of HIV-infected sibling pairs with hemophilia (84), and an increase in the frequency of certain HLA haplotypes has been associated with development of AIDS in homosexual men (85), and hemophiliacs (86), suggesting that host or immunogenetic factors may act as endogenous cofactors. Sexually transmitted cofactors may also be involved in progression (87). However, except for age (24, 26), and possibly cytomegalovirus (88) and human T cell lymphotrophic virus type I (89), no unequivocal cofactors have been reported in American or European studies.

Future Projections

Back-calculation methods estimate that 8100 persons with hemophilia were infected with contaminated blood products before March 1985 and project a cumulative AIDS incidence of 3475 ± 700 (SD) through January 1, 1993 (90). Estimates of the number of eventual transfusion-associated AIDS cases are more imprecise because of greater uncertainties about the incubation distribution. One analysis estimates from 12,300 to 16,800 eventual cases of AIDS in the age group 13–69 years attributable to infection before July 1985 (91).

Survival

In the Multicenter Hemophilia Cohort Study, 10-year cumulative survivals were 79 ± 2% for adults who seroconverted at age 18 or over and 93 ± 3% for children who seroconverted below 18 years of age (92). These figures are similar to those reported in homosexual men but are considerably longer than the 49.5% (95% confidence interval: 27–65%) cumulative survival at age 9 years for children infected perinatally (57). Survival is related to age at HIV seroconversion, duration of infection, and CD4 lymphocyte counts as well as to therapy. In the Multicenter Hemophilia Cohort Study, actuarial survival at 4 years was 90% (confidence interval: 28–92%) for those with CD4 counts greater than 200 and less than 500 and 31% (confidence interval: 23–39%) with a median of 24 months for those with CD4 counts of <50 cells μl (92).

Effect of Therapy

As with other risk groups (93) therapy with zidovudine in asymptomatic hemophiliacs with CD4 counts of <500 delays progression in AIDS (94). Zidovudine also appears to prolong survival in HIV-infected persons with hemophilia whether given before or after AIDS diagnosis (95) (see also Chapter 35).

TRANSMISSION OF HIV BY BLOOD AND BLOOD PRODUCTS

United States

Seroprevalence of Donors—HIV-1

When nationwide screening was implemented in 1985, 0.04% of donations were found to be positive for HIV-1 by both the enzyme-linked immunosorbent assay and Western blot tests (96). During 1985–1987, with donor education, confidential self-exclusion, and more selective recruitment

of donors, the average prevalence of HIV-positive donors declined by about half (97). In 1987, the average rates of positive Western blot tests were 133 per million donations to the American Red Cross (97). The highest rates of 589 per million were found in males donating for the first time. Intermediate rates of 123 and 154 per million were found in repeat male and new female donors, respectively, with the lowest rates of 36 per million being found in repeat female donors. By 1989, median seroprevalence rates among 4 million donors at 50 American Red Cross Blood Banks had declined to 84 per million overall and 415 per million for first-time donors (98).

Seroprevalence of Donors—HIV-2

The prevalence of HIV-2 is not yet calculble in United States blood donors, but no instances were discovered after screening over 28,140 samples derived from at least 20,000,000 blood donors who were repeatedly reactive on anti-HIV-1 testing (99). Although as of 1992, no transfusion transmission had been found (100), one case of HIV-2 infection has been reported in an American who attempted to donate blood (36). In September 1991 the Food and Drug Administration licensed an anti-HIV-1 and -2 combination test, and in June 1992 blood banks began screening for HIV-2. It is anticipated that future testing will uncover a few HIV-2-infected donors who would not have been detected by cross reactions with anti-HIV-1 test systems.

Risk of Transfusion-acquired HIV Infection

Prescreening

Little information is available regarding the risk of HIV infection for patients transfused before routine screening procedures were adopted. However, in a retrospective study of HIV serology in leukemia patients transfused in New York City in the 6 years before screening, the overall estimated risk based on an average of 133 components per recipient was 0.02–0.11% per component between 1978 and 1985 when antibody screening was implemented (35). In San Francisco, the incidence of transfusion-associated HIV infection is estimated to have risen rapidly from that first described in 1978 to 1.1% per transfused unit in 1982 (101).

Postscreening

Each year, about 3 million persons in the United States are transfused with blood or blood products that are collected from nearly 18 million donations. Calculations that include the "worst case estimates" suggest that as many as 460 recipients of screened blood may have become infected from May 1986 to May 1987, considerably less than the 7200 estimated to have become infected in 1984, the year before routine screening was implemented (102). In another analysis, estimated total infected units entering the blood supply in 1987 were lower, ranging from a low of 67 to a high of 227 (97). Education, donor recruitment, and self-screening in combination with testing is estimated to be 99.83–99.95% effective in eliminating HIV-infected units from transfusion. In 1991, overall risk in the United States was estimated to be 1 in 225,000 per unit transfused (103). In high prevalence areas, estimates were as high as 1 in 60,000 from a review of AIDS cases caused by screened blood transfused between 1985 and 1990 (103) and from testing of 1530 pools of mononuclear cells prepared from 76,500 blood donations that were cultured and evaluated by the PCR (104). In another study of 61,000 units of screened HIV-negative blood, only one unit was found positive by HIV culture and PCR (101). Furthermore, in a large cohort of patients who were transfused with 110,000 units of screened blood during cardiac surgery, only two HIV-1 seroconversions occurred in patients without other identifiable risk factors (105).

Tests Employed

Like all laboratory tests, HIV antibody tests used to screen asymptomatic HIV-infected blood donors are imperfect. However, most nonspecific results caused by cross-reacting proteins or directed against the cell substrate used to grow the virus (106) were seen with first generation tests. The use of so-called "second generation" tests using purified viral proteins rather than whole viral lysates has achieved a sensitivity of >99.99% with a specificity of 99.8% (107, 108). Although the risk of a false negative test is on the order of 1 in 36,000 to 1 in 300,000 (97, 108), both the sensitivity and specificity of the tests depend on the quality of testing in the laboratory. However, most false negative test results are observed among persons who have recently become infected with HIV and who have not yet developed detectable antibody (102, 109).

Acquisition of Transfusion-associated Infection from Donors Later Found to Be Infected with HIV

Most high-risk blood donors implicated in the transmission of HIV are chronic carriers of the virus who have minimal or no symptoms (110). The vast majority, but not all of these, can be shown retrospectively by "look back" studies to have been HIV infectious at the time of donation, and the rate of infection in recipients of blood from donors later found to be infected with HIV is very high (97, 111).

In the Transfusion Safety Study, 90% of the 124 recipients of anti–HIV-positive blood have tested positive (111). In a study from San Francisco that investigated recipients of blood from 92 donors who subsequently developed AIDS, infection in the recipient was apparent in 90% of the cases where the donor developed AIDS within 1 year, in 62% when the donor's AIDS was recognized between 1 and 4 years, and in 20% of those with an interval between 4 and 5 years (25). In a larger longitudinal study of recipients of blood from donors later found to be infected, which included the group mentioned above, 59% of those exposed became infected. Of recipients who received blood from donors who earlier donated to recipients who became seropositive, 95% became infected (38). Different blood components were equally likely to transmit infection. Ho and colleagues (75) have shown that one 250-ml unit of contaminated blood could contain 1.5×10^4 tissue culture infective doses of HIV-1 if it were obtained from an asymptomatic person or 1.75×10^6 if obtained from a symptomatic person. These values explain why transfusion of contaminated blood results in such a high rate of HIV infection among recipients.

Silent Infections

An insensitive test accounts for failure to detect an HIV-infected donor in a few cases. Human error in testing or releasing HIV-positive blood for transfusion also occurs and has been estimated to be <0.1% based on studies of the frequency of such errors in more than 6,000,000 units transfused (96). However, because the antibody test is an indirect test that measures a host immune response rather than some direct property of the virus itself, donor screening for HIV antibodies will never detect all infected donors.

For transfusion recipients, the greatest risk of HIV infection is in the "window period" between the time the donor is infected with HIV and the time the donor develops antibodies (102, 112). Most seroconversions occur within 2–3 months after infection, with few if any donors remaining infectious and seronegative for longer than 6 months (29, 112). In a study from the CDC of 27 homosexual and 12 hemophilic men, stored samples from before and after seroconversion were tested for p24 antigen and for HIV DNA by PCR. Modeling techniques estimated the median time from infection with HIV to be 2.4 ± 2.1 (SE) months. Modeling of cases of HIV infection in published reports suggested that 95% of cases would be expected to seroconvert within 5.8 ± 0.6 months (28). In a recent look back CDC study of the recipients of 179 seronegative donations from blood donors who subsequently developed HIV antibody, the calculated average window was 45 days. It was estimated with 95% certainty that at least 90% of donors had a window of <141 days (112).

Although antigenemia has been detected within 4 weeks of seroconversion (72), screening of blood donors for HIV antigen has not been found useful. Two separate studies that tested more than 700,000 volunteer donors failed to detect any cases that were not detected by routine HIV-1 antibody testing (113, 114). Although there is one recent case of a blood sample that tested positive for HIV antigen but negative for antibody (115), this is such a rare phenomenon that as of August 1992, the Food and Drug Administration has not recommended antigen testing for routine blood donor screening. This conclusion may need to be reversed if more sensitive tests for antigen detection are developed (113). Other methods for direct detection of virus rather than the immune response include viral culture and PCR. However, neither is yet suitable for screening blood donors.

Risk of Transfusion-acquired Idiopathic CD4+ T Lymphocytopenia

The newly reported AIDS-like illness called idiopathic CD4+ T lymphocytopenia (ICL) has no known link to HIV-1, HIV-2, or any other virus. ICL does not occur in clusters of patients linked by sexual activity, injection drug use, or blood transfusion and does not appear to be increasing in frequency. The initial 30 cases of ICL were reported to the CDC from 1985 to 1992, with no apparent increase in frequency over the 7 years. They occurred in persons aged 18–70 years living in 15 different states. Because there is no evidence that associates ICL with blood transfusions or an infectious agent, there is no reason to implement additional screening measures to detect ICL in blood donors.

Worldwide

HIV-1

In an international survey of 33 countries performed by the Canadian Red Cross between 1985 and 1988, the proportion of AIDS cases attributed to blood transfusion-associated AIDS cases increased from 1.8 to 3.6% (116) (see also Chapter 3). Current estimates attribute 10% of the reported cases of AIDS to blood transfusions in some eastern European and developing countries (117).

By 1988, 31 of 33 countries were screening blood routinely with an enzyme immunoassay test. Most showed a decreasing or stable trend in the confirmed positive HIV-1 antibody prevalence rate, which varied from 0 to 0.64%, with most reporting prevalence rates below 0.005%. By 1985, most countries surveyed had already implemented self-exclusion programs and provided alternate test sites (116). By 1988, seroprevalence data were reported to be 0.03% among blood donors in Rome (118), 0.002% in Germany (119), and 0.004% among repeat donors in Switzerland (120) compared with 0.01% in the United States (21). More recent studies have shown a rate of 0.09% in France and Mexico (122, 123) and 0.02% in Greece (124). In marked contrast to these low rates, studies in Zaire in 1986 showed a seroprevalence rate of 6.5% among male blood donors and 8.4% of women attending an antenatal clinic (125). Likewise, studies in Zambia showed a seroprevalence rate of 0–3% in rural areas, compared to 6–10% in urban areas, and 11% in the largest cities (126). In Nigeria, seroprevalence rates in 1991 were 2.8% for the general population and 0–0.25% for blood donors (127).

Preliminary findings from a worldwide survey of blood safety in relation to HIV/AIDS being conducted by the Norwegian Red Cross and the McGill Center for Medicine indicate that only in developed market economy countries are 100% of blood donations screened. About 88% of donations are screened in eastern European countries, 55% in developing countries, and about one-third in the least developed countries (117). Reasons for lack of access to HIV testing include insufficient funds, political instability, lack of organizational services, and infrastructural problems. Compounding these difficulties are a high prevalence of HIV in many urban areas, a high incidence of paid donors, inappropriate utilization of blood, and lack of quality assurance programs.

HIV-2

HIV-2 infection was first described in 1985 in asymptomatic West African prostitutes where the infection appears to be most prevalent. In a study of 5720 Nigerian blood donors, two persons were found to be positive confirmed by Western blot. In the Canadian survey, 16 of 33 countries surveyed were already screening or planning to screen for HIV-2 (116).

Methods to Reduce Transmission
Donor Screening, Education, and Exclusion

Donor education defining persons at high risk who should not give blood, predonation medical screening, confidential unit exclusion (allowing donors to designate their blood for laboratory studies rather than for transfusion), and notification of anti-HIV-positive donors have been accompanied by a significant fall in prevalence of HIV-antibody-positive donors. However, studies have shown that current measures for donor education and screening are not uniformly effective (128). Therefore, future strategies must focus on improved methods of education and screening to eliminate people at high risk from the donor pool and on the development of more effective programs to recruit low-risk donors.

Use of Autologous Blood

It has long been recognized that the safest blood for transfusion is the patient's own blood. Autologous blood donation before elective surgery and intraoperative cell salvage have been widely endorsed as good transfusion practices (129, 130). Use of recombinant human erythropoietin with supplemental iron has been shown to increase red cell production, thereby allowing the safe preoperative collection of more units of autologous blood (131). However, this procedure, when approved for general use, will not be an option for most patients who require homologous transfusions of red cells and will not provide platelet support.

Directed Donations

Some who feel that a relative or a friend would be a safer donor than an unknown anonymous volunteer believe that directed donations designed for a particular patient might reduce the risk of HIV transmission. There is no evidence, however, that directed donors are safer than volunteer donors, and questions arise about whether the directed donor who may feel pressured into giving is as truthful about his or her risk status as the volunteer who donates without obligation. Furthermore, the practice of seeking directed donors leads to the collection of blood from many new donors, and the risk of HIV-infected units from new donors is between two and three times that from previously tested donors, depending on whether the directed donor is female or male (121).

Virus Inactivation of Plasma Products

Unlike red cells and platelets, plasma derivatives can be subjected to virus inactivation procedures to markedly reduce the risk of hepatitis transmission and eliminate the risk of HIV transmission (132–134). Methods of clotting factor virus inactivation include heating in the dry state or aqueous phase, heating in solvent suspension, steam treatment, and treatment with other solvents and detergents, with or without purification by affinity-column chromatography (135, 136). There were a few earlier reports of seroconversions in persons with hemophilia who received donor deferred, but usually not donor tested, concentrates heated in the dry state at lower temperatures and for shorter periods (142). However, as mentioned previously, CDC surveillance data through December 1990 have shown no seroconversions from donor screened, virus-inactivated, donor tested factor concentrates since 1986 (31). In a recent study from Germany of 155 patients exclusively treated with more than 15 million units of pasteurized factor VIII concentrate, no HIV seroconversions were found (134). This study included sufficient patients receiving concentrate that was manufactured before 1985 from plasma presumably contaminated with HIV to prove that pasteurized factor VIII concentrate that is heat-treated at 60° C for 10 hr in aqueous solution is safe and does not carry the risk of HIV transmission.

Alternatives to Blood Products

Desmopressin, a synthetic analogue of vasopressin, has been shown to increase factor VIII levels in persons with mild classic hemophilia and von Willebrand's disease and should be used in preference to plasma-derived products whenever possible (138). With recombinant DNA technology, it is now possible to produce recombinant factor VIII, which is structurally and functionally comparable with plasma factor VIII (139). Recombinant factor VIII has been shown to be effective and well-tolerated in early clinical trials of persons with classic hemophilia without the risk of hepatitis and other transfusion-associated viruses inherent in the use of blood products (141). The technology to produce recombinant factor IX remains underdeveloped.

Physician and Patient Education

Attempts to decrease the risk of HIV by transfusion must also include physician education to carefully evaluate the risk-benefit ratio with each transfusion episode and to consider alternatives to homologous transfusions. Use of components from as few donors as possible for any one procedure must be stressed, because the risk of infection is related linearly to the number of blood units to which one is exposed. Synthetic products such as desmopressin and hematopoietic growth factors should be used when appropriate. Also of importance is the continuing need to educate patients in the risks of transfusion, especially before elective surgical procedures are planned, and in the alternatives to transfusion.

Future
Impact of Current Methods to Reduce Transmission

From April 1985 through March 1990, 158 patients with AIDS (4.8% of all patients with transfusion-associated AIDS) whose cases were reported to the CDC had purportedly acquired their infections from blood that was negative on screening for HIV (141). Upon further investigation, only one case was confirmed HIV positive from screened blood donations. Considering that an estimated 85 million units of blood and blood products were transfused during these 5 yr, HIV infection from screened blood is very rare in the United States.

New Technologies

Future strategies must focus on ways to reduce the risk of HIV transmission during the window of early infection and on the development of methods to inactivate virus from cellular products. The technology for the direct detection of virus markers is rapidly evolving, but a dedicated effort will be needed to perfect and automate techniques such as PCR. These tests may need to be used in combination with indirect antibody tests to achieve maximum sensitivity and specificity. Although virus inactivation methods have substantially improved the safety of plasma derivatives, absolute safety will not be possible unless these methods can be adapted for treatment of cellular components.

TRANSMISSION OF HIV TO FEMALE SEXUAL PARTNERS AND OFFSPRING

Prevalence in Female Sexual Partners of HIV-infected Hemophiliacs

The reported prevalence of HIV seropositivity in female sexual partners of HIV-infected persons with hemophilia in the United States ranges from 7 to 22% (142, 143). In a review of CDC surveillance data through December 31, 1991, 86 female sexual partners were reported to be HIV seropositive, and 14 of their children were reported to have developed AIDS in the first year of life (143). These estimates are similar to those for female heterosexual partners of infected transfusion recipients, but better data are needed regarding the number at risk. The rate of increase in female sexual partners was not as rapid as was observed in the early years of the epidemic, but this could reflect random variation in reporting or a disruptive effect of HIV infection on sexual relationships rather than a change in sexual practices.

Timing of Transmission

Conflicting data are available concerning the temporal relationship of the infection to the duration of sexual contact and the degree of immune deficiency of the male partner (142, 144, 145). Two studies found an association with more severe HIV disease as measured by HIV antigenemia and/or low CD4 counts, whereas another found that transmission occurred early and was unrelated to the clinical or immunologic status of the hemophiliac. These differences may relate in part to high level plasma viremia that has been shown to occur around the time of seroconversion and to reoccur years later when CD4 counts are markedly depressed (146).

Impact on Reproductive Choices and Sexual Partners

During the past decade, an intensive effort has been undertaken by health care providers at hemophilia treatment centers to educate and counsel their patients regarding risk reduction measures. However, data from two studies suggest that these efforts have not been as effective as had been hoped (147, 148). In a survey reporting on 2276 spouses or sex partners of a comparable number of known HIV-seropositive hemophiliacs, 280 couples reported pregnancies between January 1985 and March 1987, representing a fertility rate of 54.7/1000 women/yr. This rate was comparable with the United States fertility rate for this same time, despite recommendations against unprotected intercourse by HIV-seropositive men (147). In a longitudinal study that assessed 217 HIV-negative female sex partners of HIV-positive hemophilic men entered into an open cohort study from March 1985 through January 1991, compliance with the use of a condom for vaginal sex improved in over two-thirds of the patients. However, almost one-third of the women in the cohort continued to have unprotected vaginal sex with their HIV-positive partner, at least occasionally, and one-fourth of the women reported a mean of 2.2 condom failures during 12 months. Furthermore 20% of the women had sex with one or more outside partners while remaining sexually active with their HIV-positive partner. Unprotected sex was more common among women with lower education, and relapse rates to high-risk behavior were significantly higher among women with high-risk behavior at enrollment (148). Thus, an alarming number of women in fairly stable relationships continue to knowingly put themselves, their children, and other outside partners at risk for HIV infection. Future studies should focus on the identification of those most likely to continue high-risk behavior while attempting to develop new strategies and vaccines for prevention.

References

1. Centers for Disease Control. Pneumocystis carinii pneumonia among persons with hemophilia A. MMWR 1982;31:365–367.
2. Gottlieb MS, Schroff R, Schanker HM, et al. Pneumocystis carinii pneumonia and mucosal candidiasis in previously healthy homosexual men: Evidence of a new acquired cellular immunodeficiency. N Engl J Med 1981; 305:1425–1431.
3. Masur H, Michelis MA, Greene JB, et al. An outbreak of community-acquired *Pneumocystis carinii* pneumonia: Initial manifestations of cellular immune dysfunctions. N Engl J Med 1981; 305:1431–1438.
4. Centers for Disease Control. Update on acquired immune deficiency syndrome (AIDS)—United States. MMWR 1982;31:507–508, 513–514.
5. Ammann AK, Cowan MJ, Wara DW, et al. Acquired immunodeficiency in an infant: Possible transmission by means of blood products. Lancet 1983;1:956–958.
6. Centers for Disease Control. Update: Acquired immunodeficiency syndrome (AIDS) among patients with hemophilia—United States. MMWR 1983;32:613–615.
7. Curran JW, Lawrence DN, Jaffe H, et al. Acquired immunodeficiency syndrome (AIDS) associated with transfusions. N Engl J Med 1984;310:69–75.
8. Klatzmann D, Barre-Sinoussi F, Nugeyre MT, et al. Selective tropism of lymphadenopathy-associated virus (LAV) for helper-inducer T lymphocytes. Science 1984;225:59–63.
9. Goedert JJ, Sarngadharan MG, Biggar RJ, et al. Determinants of retrovirus (HTLV-III) antibody and immunodeficiency conditions in homosexual men. Lancet 1984;2:711–716.
10. Fahey JL, Prince H, Weaver M, et al. Quantitative changes in T helper or T suppressor/cytotoxic lymphocyte subsets that distinguish acquired immune deficiency syndrome from other subset disorders. Am J Med 1984;76:95–100.
11. Barré-Sinoussi F, Chermann JC, Rey F, et al. Isolation of a T-lymphotropic retrovirus from a patient at risk for acquired immunodeficiency syndrome (AIDS). Science 1983;220:868–870.
12. Gallo RC, Salahuddin SZ, Popovic M, et al. Frequent detection and isolation of cytopathic retroviruses (HTLV-III) from patients with AIDS and at risk for AIDS. Science 1984;224:500–503.
13. Popovic M, Sarngadharan MG, Read E, Gallo RC. Detection, isolation, and continuous production of cytopathic retroviruses (HTLV-III) from patients with AIDS and pre-AIDS. Science 1984;224:497–500.
14. Groopman JE, Salahuddin SZ, Sarngadharan MG, et al. Virologic studies in a case of transfusion-associated AIDS. N Engl J Med 1984;311:1419–1422.
15. Peterman TA, Jaffe HW, Feorino PM, et al. Transfusion-associated acquired immunodeficiency syndrome in the United States. JAMA 1985;254: 2913–2917.
16. Kitchen LW, Barin F, Sullivan JL, et al. Aetiology of AIDS: Antibodies to human T-cell leukaemia virus (type III) in haemophiliacs. Nature 1984; 312:367–368.
17. Goedert JJ, Sarngadharan MG, Eyster ME, et al. Antibodies reactive with human T-cell leukemia viruses (HTLV-III) in the sera of hemophiliacs receiving factor VIII concentrate. Blood 1985;65: 492–495.
18. Evatt BL, Gomperts ED, McDougal JS, et al. Coincidental appearance of LAV1 HTLV-III antibodies in hemophiliacs and the onset of the AIDS epidemic. N Engl J Med 1985;312:483–486.
19. Eyster ME, Goedert JJ, Sarngadharan MG, et al. Development and early natural history of HTLV-III antibodies in persons with hemophilia. JAMA 1985;253:2219–2223.
20. Ragni MV, Tegtmeier GE, Levy JA, et al. AIDS retrovirus antibodies in hemophiliacs treated with factor VIII or factor IX concentrates, cryoprecipitate or fresh frozen plasma: Prevalence, seroconversion rate, and clinical correlations. Blood 1986;67:592–595.
21. Centers for Disease Control. HIV/AIDS Surveillance Report, Apr 1992.
22. Care of Hemophilia in the USA. National Hemophilia Foundation Report, 1985.
23. National Hemophilia Foundation Information Exchange Medical Bulletin 137, Jul 1991.
24. Goedert JJ, Kessler CM, Aledort LM, et al. A prospective study of human immunodeficiency virus type I infection and the development of AIDS in subjects with hemophilia. N Engl J Med 1989;321:1141–1148.
25. Perkins HA, Samson S, Garner J, et al. Risk of AIDS for recipients of blood components from donors who subsequently developed AIDS. Blood 1987;70:1604–1610.
26. Eyster ME, Gail MH, Ballard JO, Al-Mondhiry H, Goedert JJ. Natural history of human immunodeficiency virus infections in hemophiliacs. Effects of T-cell subsets, platelet counts, and age. Ann Intern Med 1987;107:1–6.
27. Jackson JB, Sannerud KJ, Hopsicker JS, et al. Hemophiliacs with antibody against human immunodeficiency virus are actively infected. Transfusion 1989;29:265–267.
28. Gibbons J, Cory JM, Hewlett IK, Epstein JS, Eyster ME. Silent infections with human immunodeficiency virus type 1 are highly unlikely in multitransfused seronegative hemophiliacs. Blood 1990;76:1924–1926.
29. Bailly E, Kleim JP, Schneweis KE, van Loo B, Hammerstein U, Brackman HH. Absence of human immunodeficiency virus (HIV) proviral sequences in seronegative hemophilic men and sexual partners of HIV-seropositive hemophiliacs. Transfusion 1992;32:104–108.
30. Lefrére JJ, Mariotti M, Vittecoq D, et al. No evidence of frequent human immunodeficiency virus type 1 infection in seronegative at risk individuals. Transfusion 1991;31:205–211.
31. National Hemophilia Foundation Information Exchange Medical Bulletin 155. Reported cases of

AIDS-like or immunodeficiency symptoms among individuals testing HIV antibody negative: Implications for hemophilia. Jul 31, 1992.

32. Centers for Disease Control. HIV infection in two brothers receiving intravenous therapy for hemophilia. MMWR 1992;41:228–231.

33. Nagao T, Honda K, Yoshihara N, Nakanaga K. Delayed human immunodeficiency virus-1 seroconversion in a hemophilia B patient in Japan. Blood 1991;78:1983–1984.

34. Hilgartner M, DeSousa M, Giardina B, Aldelsberg B, Transfusion Safety Study Group. Effect of transfusion and HIV infection on the immune response of patients with congenital hemolytic anemia. Blood 1986;68(suppl 1):128a.

35. Minamoto GY, Scheinberg DA, Dietz K, et al. Human immunodeficiency virus infection in patients with leukemia. Blood 1988;71:1147–1149.

36. O'Brien TR, Polon C, Schable CA, et al. HIV-2 infection in an American. AIDS 1991;5:85–88.

37. Biggar RJ, International Registry of Seroconverters. AIDS incubation in 1891 HIV seroconverters from different exposure groups. AIDS 1990; 4:1059–1066.

38. Ward JW, Bush TJ, Perkins HA, et al. The natural history of transfusion-associated infection with human immunodeficiency virus. Factors influencing the rate of progression to disease. N Engl J Med 1989;321:947–952.

39. Giesecke J, Tomba GS, Berglund O, Berntorp E, Schulman S, Stigendal L. Incidence of symptoms and AIDS in 146 Swedish haemophiliacs and blood transfusion recipients infected with human immunodeficiency virus. Br Med J 1988; 297:99–102.

40. Lui KJ, Lawrence DN, Morgan WM, Peterman TA, Haverkos HW, Bregman DJ. A model-based approach for estimating the mean incubation period of transfusion-associated acquired immunodeficiency syndrome. Proc Natl Acad Sci USA 1986;83:3051–3055.

41. Medley GF, Anderson RM, Cox DR, Billard L. Incubation period of AIDS in patients infected via blood transfusion. Nature 1987;328:719–721.

42. Anderson RM, Medley GF. Epidemiology of HIV infection and AIDS: Incubation and infectious periods, survival and vertical transmission. AIDS 1988;2(suppl 1):S57–S63.

43. Wilson G, Holmes W. Additional supporting evidence from 3518 cases of TA-AIDS that the incubation time to AIDS is greater than 12 years [Abstract WC 3003]. Seventh International Conference on AIDS, Florence, Jun 1991.

44. Darby SC, Rizza CR, Doll R, Spooner RJD, Stratton IM, Thakrar B. Incidence of AIDS and excess of mortality associated with HIV in haemophiliacs in the United Kingdom: Report on behalf of the directors of haemophilia centres in the United Kingdom. Br Med J 1989;298:1064–1068.

45. Schinaia N, Ghirardini A, Chiarotti F, et al. Progression to AIDS among Italian HIV-seropositive haemophiliacs. AIDS 1991;5:385–391.

46. Phillips AN, Lee CA, Elford J, et al. More rapid progression to AIDS in older HIV-infected people: The role of CD4+ T-cell counts. J Acquir Immune Defic Syndr 1991;4:970–975.

47. Ragni MV, Kingsley LA. Cumulative risk for AIDS and other HIV outcomes in a cohort of hemophiliacs in western Pennsylvania. J Acquir Immune Defic Syndr 1990;3:708–713.

48. Eyster ME, Rabkin CS, Hilgartner MW, et al. AIDS-related conditions in children and adults with hemophilia: Rates, relationship to CD4 counts and predictive value. Blood 1993;3: 828–834.

49. Rutherford GW, Lifson AR, Hessol NA, et al. Course of HIV-1 infection in a cohort and bisexual men: An 11 year follow up study. Br Med J 1990;301:1183–1188.

50. Fletcher MA, Mosley JW, Hassett J, et al. Effect of age on human immunodeficiency virus type 1-induced changes in lymphocyte populations among persons with congenital clotting disorders. Blood 80;1992:831–840.

51. Lagakos SW, De Gruttola V. The conditional latency distribution of AIDS for persons infected by blood transfusion. J Acquir Immune Defic Syndr 1989;2:84–87.

52. Blaxhult A, Granath F, Lidman K, Giesecke J. The influence of age on the latency period to AIDS in people infected by HIV through blood transfusion. AIDS 1990;4:125–129.

53. Kraskinski K, Borkowsky W, Holzman RS. Prognosis of human immunodeficiency virus infection in children and adolescents. Pediatr Infect Dis J 1989;8:216–220.

54. Mundy TM, Lieb L, Ward J, et al. Seven year follow-up of HIV infection in neonatal transfusion recipients [Abstract TBP 167]. Fifth International Conference on AIDS, Montreal, Jun 1989.

55. Willoughby A, Mendez H, Goedert J, Berthaud M, Moroso G, Sunderland A. Natural history of infants born to HIV positive women [Abstract MBO 2]. Fifth International Conference on AIDS, Montreal, Jun 1989.

56. Scott GB, Hutto C, Makuch RW, et al. Survival in children with perinatally acquired human immunodeficiency virus type I infection. N Engl J Med 1989;321:1791–1796.

57. Tovo PA, DeMartino M, Gabiano C, et al. Prognostic factors and survival in children with perinatal HIV-1 infection. Lancet 1992;339:1249–1253.

58. Auger I, Thomas P, De Gruttola V, et al. Incubation periods for paediatric AIDS patients. Nature 1988;336:575–577.

59. Maury W, Potts BJ, Rabson AB. HIV-1 infection of first-trimester and term human placental tissue. A possible mode of maternal-fetal transmission. J Infect Dis 1989;160:583–588.

60. Chandwani S, Greco MA, Mittal K, et al. Pathology and human immunodeficiency virus expression in placentas of seropositive women. J Infect Dis 1991;163:1134–1138.

61. Courgnand V, Laure F, Brossard A, et al. Frequent and early in utero HIV-1 infection. AIDS Res Hum Retroviruses 1991;7:337–341.

62. Mofensen LM. Preventing mother to infant HIV transmission: What we know so far. AIDS Reader 1992; Mar/Apr:42–51.

63. Ehrnst A, Lindgren S, Dictor M, et al. HIV in pregnant women and their offspring: Evidence for late transmission. Lancet 1991;338:203–207.

64. De Rossi A, Ometto L, Mammano F, Zanotto C, Giaquinto C, Chieco-Bianchi L. Perinatal transmission of HIV-1: Lack of detectable virus in peripheral blood cells at birth, and prognostic values of polymerase chain reaction results in infants [Abstract WeC 1060]. Eighth International Conference on AIDS, Amsterdam, Jul 1992.

65. Goedert JJ, Duliège AM, Amos CI, et al. High risk of HIV-1 infection for first born twins. Lancet 1991;338:1471–1475.

66. Goedert JJ, Biggar RJ, Melbye M, et al. Effect of T4 count and cofactors on the incidence of AIDS in homosexual men infected with human immunodeficiency virus. JAMA 1987;257:331–334.

67. Polk BF, Fox R, Brookmeyer R, et al. Predictors of the acquired immunodeficiency syndrome developing in a cohort of seropositive homosexual men. N Engl J Med 1987;316:61–66.

68. Moss AR, Bacchetti P, Osmond D, et al. Seropositivity for HIV and the development of AIDS or AIDS related condition: Three year follow up of the San Francisco General Hospital cohort. Br Med J 1988;296:745–750.

69. Allain JP, Laurian Y, Paul DA, et al. Long term evaluation of HIV antigen and antibodies to p24 and gp41 in patients with hemophilia: Potential clinical importance. N Engl J Med 1987;317:1114–1121.

70. Eyster ME, Ballard JO, Gail MH, Drummond JE, Goedert JJ. Predictive markers for the acquired immunodeficiency syndrome (AIDS) in hemophiliacs: Persistence of p24 antigen and low T_4 cell count. Ann Intern Med 1989;110:963–969.

71. Aldeort LM, Hilgartner MW, Pike MC, et al. Variability in serial CD4 counts and relation to progression of HIV-1 infection to AIDS in haemophilic patients. Br Med J 1992;304:212–216.

72. Stramer SL, Heller JS, Coombs RW, Parry JV, Ho DD, Allain JP. Markers of HIV infection prior to IgG antibody seropositivity. JAMA 1989;262:64–69.

73. Coombs RW, Collier AC, Allain JP, et al. Plasma viremia in human immunodeficiency virus infection. N Engl J Med 1989;321:1626–1631.

74. Saag MS, Crain MJ, Decker WD, et al. High-level viremia in adults and children infected with human immunodeficiency virus: Relation to disease state and CD4+ lymphocyte levels. J Infect Dis 1991;164:72–80.

75. Ho DD, Mougdel MS, Alam M. Quantitation of human immunodeficiency virus type I in the blood of infected persons. N Engl J Med 1989;321:1621–1625.

76. Schnittman SM, Greenhouse JJ, Psallidopoulos MC, et al. Increasing viral burden in CD4+ T cells from patients with human immunodeficiency virus (HIV) infection reflects rapidly progressive immunosuppression and clinical disease. Ann Intern Med 1990;113:438–443.

77. Moss AR, Bacchetti P. Natural history of HIV infection. AIDS 1989;3:55–61.

78. Ellaurie M, Rubinstein A. B2 microglobulin concentration in pediatric human immunodeficiency virus infection. Pediatr Infect Dis J 1990;9:807–809.

79. Fuchs D, Hausen A, Reibnegger G, Werner ER, Dierich MP, Wachter H. Neopterin as a marker for activated cell-mediated immunity: Application in HIV infection. Immunology Today 1988;9:150–155.

80. Fahey JL, Taylor JMG, Detels R, et al. The prognostic value of cellular and seriologic markers in infection with human immunodeficiency virus type I. N Engl J Med 1990;322:166–172.

81. Eyster ME, Goedert JJ, Poon M-C, Preble OT. Acid-labile alpha interferon: A possible preclinical marker for the acquired immunodeficiency syndrome in hemophilia. N Engl J Med 1983;309:583–586.

82. Phair J, Munoz A, Detels R, et al. The risk of Pneumocystis carinii pneumonia among men infected with human immunodeficiency virus type 1. N Engl J Med 1990;322:161–165.

83. Dodd CL, Greenspan D, Katz MH, Westenhouse JL, Feigel DW, Greenspan JS. Oral candidiasis in HIV infection; pseudomembraneous and erythematous candidiasis show similar rates of progression to AIDS. AIDS 1991;5:1339–1343.

84. Meropol NJ, Krause PR, Ratnoff OD, et al. Tendency to serious sequelae of infection with the human immunodeficiency virus in sibships with hemophilia. Arch Intern Med 1989;149:885–888.

85. Mann DL, Murray C, Yarchoan R, Blattner WA, Goedert JJ. HLA antigen frequencies in HIV-1 seropositive disease-free individuals and patients with AIDS. J Acquir Immune Defic Syndr 1988;1:13–17.

86. Steel CM, Ludlam CA, Beatson D, et al. HLA haplotype A1B8DR3 as a risk factor for HIV-related disease. Lancet 1988;1:1185–1188.

87. Phair J, Jacobson L, Detels R. Acquired immune deficiency syndrome occurring within 5 years of infection. J Acquir Immune Defic Syndr 1992;5:490–496.

88. Lee CA, Phillips AN, Elford J, Janossy G, Griffiths P, Kernoff P. Progression of HIV disease in a haemophiliac cohort followed for 11 years and the effect of treatment. Br Med J 1991;303:1093–1096.

89. Bartholomew C, Blattner W, Cleghorn F. Progression to AIDS in homosexual men coinfected with HIV and HTLV-1 in Trinidad. Lancet 1987;2:1469.

90. Rosenberg PS, Gail MH, Biggar RJ, Goedert JJ. Simplified back-calculations for the AIDS epidemic [Abstract TAO 35]. Fifth International Conference on AIDS Montreal, Jun 1989.

91. Kalbfleisch JD, Lawless JF. Estimating the incubation time, distribution and expected number of cases of transfusion-associated acquired immune deficiency syndrome. Transfusion 1989;29:672–676.

92. Ehmann WC, Goedert JJ, Eyster ME, Multicenter Hemophilia Cohort Study. Relationship of CD4 counts and zidovudine therapy to survival in a cohort of HIV positive hemophiliacs [Abstract PoC 4199]. Eighth International Conference on AIDS, Amsterdam, Jul 1992.

93. Volberding PA, Lagakos SW, Koch MA, et al. Zidovudine in asymptomatic human immunodeficiency virus infection: A controlled trial in persons with fewer than 500 CD4 positive cells per cubic millimeter. N Engl J Med 1990;322:941–949.

94. Merigan T, Amato DA, Balsley J. Placebo-controlled trial to evaluate zidovudine in treatment of

human immunodeficiency virus infection in asymptomatic patients with hemophilia. Blood 1991;78:900–906.

95. Ragni MV, Kingsley LA, Zhou SJ. The effect of antiviral therapy on the natural history of human immunodeficiency virus infection in a cohort of hemophiliacs. J Acquir Immune Defic Syndr 1992;5:120–126.

96. Schorr JB, Berkowitz A, Cumming PD, Katz AJ, Sandler SG. Prevalence of HTLV-III antibody in American blood donors. N Engl J Med 1985;313:384–385.

97. Cumming PD, Wallage EL, Schorr JB, Dodd RY. Exposure of patients to human immunodeficiency virus through the transfusion of blood components that test antibody-negative. N Engl J Med 1989;321:941–946.

98. Vermund SH. Commentary: Changing estimates of HIV-1 seroprevalence in the United States. J NIH Res 1991;3:77–81.

99. Surveillance for HIV-2 infection in blood donors—United States, 1987–1989. MMWR 1990;39:829–831.

100. Sazama K, Kuramoto IK, Holland PV, Couroucé A-M, Gallo D, Hanson CV. Detection of antibodies to human immunodeficiency virus type 2 (HIV-2) in blood donor sera using United States assay methods for anti HIV type 1. Transfusion 1992;32:398–401.

101. Busch MP, Young MJ, Samson SM, et al. Risk of human immunodeficiency virus (HIV) transmission by blood transfusions before the implementation of HIV-1 antibody screening. Transfusion 1991;31:4–11.

102. Ward JW, Holmberg SD, Allen JR. Transmission of human immunodeficiency virus (HIV) by blood transfusions screened as negative for HIV antibody. N Engl J Med 1988;318:473–478.

103. Holmberg S, Conley LJ, Rogers MF. AIDS from blood transfusions screened negative for HIV antibody, United States [Abstract MoC 0092]. Eighth International Conference on AIDS, Amsterdam, Jul 1992.

104. Busch MP, Eble BE, Khayam-Bashi H, et al. Evaluation of screened blood donations for human immunodeficiency virus type 1 infection by culture and DNA amplification of pooled cells. N Engl J Med 1991;325:1–5.

105. Donahue JG, Nelson KE, Munoz A, et al. Transmission of human immunodeficiency virus (HIV) by transfusion of screened blood [Letter]. N Engl J Med 1990;323:1709.

106. Fang CT, Dare F, Kleinman S, Wehling RH, Dodd RY. Relative specificity of enzyme-linked immunosorbent assays for antibodies to human T-cell lymphotrophic virus, type III, and their relationship to Western blotting. Transfusion 1986;26:208–209.

107. Centers for Disease Control. Update: Serologic testing for antibody to human immunodeficiency virus. MMWR 1988;36:833–845.

108. Zuck TF. Silent sequences and the safety of blood transfusion. Ann Intern Med 1988;108:895–897.

109. Kessler HA, Blaauw B, Spear J, Paul DA, Falk LA, Landay A. Diagnosis of human immunodeficiency virus infection in seronegative homosexu-als presenting with an acute viral syndrome. JAMA 1987;258:1196–1199.

110. Feorino PM, Jaffe HW, Palmer E. Transfusion-associated acquired immunodeficiency syndrome. Evidence for persistent infection in blood donors. N Engl J Med 1985;312:1293–1296.

111. Donegan E, Stuart M, Niland JC, et al. Infection with human immunodeficiency virus type 1 (HIV-1) among recipients of antibody-positive blood donations. Ann Intern Med 1990;113:733–739.

112. Petersen L, Satten G, Dodd R, HIV Lookback Study Group. Time period from infectiousness as blood donor to development of detectable antibody and the risk of HIV transmission from transfusion of screened blood [Abstract MoC 0091]. Eighth International Conference on AIDS, Amsterdam, Jul 1992.

113. Alter HJ, Epstein JS, Swenson SG, et al. Prevalence of human immunodeficiency virus type 1 p24 antigen in U.S. blood donors—an assessment of the efficacy of testing in donor screening. N Engl J Med 1990;323:1312–1317.

114. Busch MP, Taylor PE, Lenes BA, et al. Screening of selected male blood donors for p24 antigen of human immunodeficiency virus type 1. N Engl J Med 1990;323:1308–1312.

115. Irani MS, Dudley AW, Lucco LJ. Case of HIV-1 transmission by antigen-positive antibody-negative blood. N Engl J Med 1991;325:1174–1175.

116. Perrault R, Mankikan S, Adatia A. Human immunodeficiency virus antibody screening of blood donors. An international survey. The Canadian Red Cross, Ottawa, Canada [Abstract TBP 350]. Fifth International Conference on AIDS, Montreal, Jun 1989.

117. Tsoukos C. Risk of HIV infection through blood products, session 18. Eighth International Conference on AIDS, Amsterdam, Jul 1992.

118. Mannella E, Ippolito G, Miceli M, Angeloni P. Seroprevalence of HIV infection among blood donors in Rome [Abstract MAP36]. Fifth International Conference on AIDS, Montreal, Jun 1989.

119. Gluck D, Koerner K, Kubanek B, et al. Prevalence of HIV-antibodies in blood donors in the FRG [Abstract MAP 40]. Fifth International Conference on AIDS, Montreal, Jun 1989.

120. Burckhardt JJ, Butler-Brunner E, Perrin LH, Bachmann P. Anti-HIV seroprevalence in blood donations from July 85 until December 88 in Switzerland [Abstract MAP43]. Fifth International Conference on AIDS, Montreal, Jun 1989.

121. Starkey JM, MacPherson MS, Bolgiano DC, Simon ER, Zuck TF, Sayers MH. Markers of transmission-transmitted disease in different groups of blood donors. JAMA 1989;269:3452–3454.

122. Couroucé AM, Retrovirus Study Group of French Society of Blood Transfusion. [Abstract PoC 4003]. Eighth International Conference on AIDS, Amsterdam, Jul 1992.

123. Herrera F, Gallardo ME, Centro Nacional de la Transfusion Sanguinea (CNTS). Nation-wide HIV 1 seroprevalence in Mexican blood donors. Third report [Abstract PoC 4065]. Eighth International Conference on AIDS, Amsterdam, Jul 1992.

124. Politis C, Fragatou S, Vrettou H, Economidou J. HTLV-1 infection in low and risk groups in Greece [Abstract PoC 4678]. Eighth International Conference on AIDS, Amsterdam, Jul 1992.

125. N'Galy B, Ryder RW, Bila K, et al. Human immunodeficiency virus infection among employees in an African hospital. N Engl J Med 1988;319: 1123–1127.

126. Luo NP, Dallas ABC, Chipuka L, Nshimbi R, Tedder R. HIV seroprevalences amongst health blood donors in 31 hospitals in Zambia [Abstract MBP149]. Fifth International Conference on AIDS, Montreal, Jun 1989.

127. Tekena H, Moses AE, Ola TO, Obi SO, Bajani MD. Increasing risk of transfusion-associated AIDS as the pandemic spreads: Experience in Maiduguri, Nigeria [Abstract PoC 4673]. Eighth International Conference on AIDS, Amsterdam, Jul 1992.

128. Leitman SF, Klein HG, Melpolder JJ. Clinical implications of positive tests for antibodies to human immunodeficiency virus type I in asymptomatic blood donors. N Engl J Med 1989;321: 917–924.

129. Council on Scientific Affairs. Autologous blood transfusion. JAMA 1986;256:2378–2380.

130. Menitove JE. The decreasing risk of transfusion-associated AIDS. N Engl J Med 1989;321:966–968.

131. Goodnough LT, Rudnick S, Price TH, et al. Increased preoperative collection of autologous blood with recombinant human erythropoietin therapy. N Engl J Med 1989;321:1163–1168.

132. McDougal JS, Martin LS, Cort SP, Mozen M, Heldebrant CM, Evatt BL. Thermal inactivation of the acquired immunodeficiency syndrome virus, human T lymphotropic virus-III/lymphadenopathy-associated virus, with special reference antihemophilic factor. J Clin Invest 1985;76: 875–877.

133. Levy JA, Mitra G, Mozen MM. Recovery and inactivation of infectious retroviruses from factor VIII concentrates. Lancet 1984;2:722–723.

134. Schimpf K, Brackmann HH, Kreuz W, et al. Absence of anti-human immunodeficiency virus types 1 and 2 seroconversion after the treatment of hemophilia A or von Willebrand's disease with pasteurized factor VIII concentrate. N Engl J Med 1989;321:1148–1152.

135. Safety of therapeutic products used for hemophilia patients. MMWR 1988;37:441–450.

136. Pierce GF, Lusher JM, Brownstein AP, Goldsmith JC, Kessler CM. The use of purified clotting factor concentrates in hemophilia. Influence of viral safety, cost, and supply on therapy. JAMA 1989; 261:3434–3438.

137. Survey of non-U.S. hemophilia treatment centers for HIV seroconversions following therapy with heat-treated factor concentrates. MMWR 1987; 36:121–124.

138. Mannucci PM. Desmopressin (DDAVP) for treatment of disorders of hemostasis. Prog Hemost Thromb 1986;8:19–45.

139. White GC, Shoemaker CB. Factor VIII gene and hemophilia. Blood 1989;73:1–12.

140. Schwartz RS, Abildgaard CF, Aledort LM, et al. Human recombinant DNA-derived antihemophilic factor (Factor VIII) in the treatment of hemophilia. N Engl J Med 1990;323:1800–1805.

141. Conley LJ, Holmberg SD. Transmission of AIDS from blood screened negative for antibody to the human immunodeficiency virus. N Engl J Med 1992;326:1499.

142. Smiley ML, White GC, Becherer P, et al. Transmission of human immunodeficiency virus to sexual partners of hemophiliacs. Am J Hematol 1988;28:27–32.

143. Chorba TL, Holman RC, Evatt BL. Heterosexual and vertical transmission of AIDS in the hemophilia community. Public Health Rep 1993;108: 99–105.

144. Goedert JJ, Eyster ME, Biggar RJ, Blattner WA. Heterosexual transmission of human immunodeficiency virus (HIV): Association with severe depletion of T helper lymphocytes in men with hemophilia. AIDS Res Hum Retroviruses 1987;3: 355–361.

145. Ragni MV, Kingsley LA, Nimorwicz P. HIV heterosexual transmission in hemophilia couples: Lack of relation to T4 number, clinical diagnosis, or duration of HIV exposure. J Acquir Immune Defic Syndr 1989;2:557–563.

146. Clark SJ, Saag MS, Decker WD, et al. High titers of cytopathic virus in plasma of patients with symptomatic primary HIV-1 infection. N Engl J Med 1991;324:954–960.

147. Jason J, Evatt B, Hemophilia-AIDS Collaborative Study Group. Pregnancies in human immunodeficiency virus-infected sex partners of hemophilic men. Am J Dis Child 1990;144:485–490.

148. Dublin S, Rosenberg PS, Goedert JJ. Patterns and predictors of high-risk sexual behavior in female partners of HIV-infected men with hemophilia. AIDS 1992;6:475–482.

149. Peckham C. Mother to infant transmission, session 87. Eighth International Conference on AIDS, Amsterdam, Jul 1992.

HIV Infection and AIDS in Adolescents

Lawrence J. D'Angelo

Beginning in 1987, increasing concern and attention has focused on adolescents and their involvement in the continued increase in cases of AIDS and the spread of human immunodeficiency virus (HIV) infection (1–5). This growing interest culminated in a special congressional report in the spring of 1992 (6). Although cases of AIDS in adolescents remain less than 0.5% of all those reported, comparisons with adult and pediatric case counts underestimate the contribution that adolescents make to the total number of cases. Given the prolonged incubation of this infection, it is safe to assume that many cases of AIDS diagnosed in young adults aged 20–34 are the result of HIV infection acquired during adolescence. In addition, sexual behaviors and drug and alcohol use patterns established during adolescence will affect an individual's risk of HIV infection for years to come.

Although knowledge of the specific behaviors that put adolescents at risk of HIV infection has increased (7–11), many gaps remain. These gaps impede our ability to provide appropriate medical care and social services that might decrease the risk of acquiring HIV infection in certain adolescents. In addition, the problem of increasing rates of infection in adolescents in the United States and other developed countries is small compared with that faced by youth in many developing countries. High seroprevalence rates in teenagers in sub-Saharan African countries reflects high rates in older adults and promises to sustain the problem of AIDS in all age groups.

EPIDEMIOLOGY OF AIDS IN ADOLESCENTS

As of June 30, 1993, 913 cases of AIDS among adolescents 13–19 years old had been reported to the Centers for Disease Control and Prevention (Table 5.1), which represents 0.4% of the 315,390 total reported AIDS cases. Another 9446 cases have been reported in young adults 20–24 years old, most of whom were presumably infected with HIV during adolescence. Since the first case was reported in an adolescent in 1981, there has been a steady increase in the number of cases that has paralleled the increase in adults and children. From July 1, 1992, until June 30, 1993, there were 420 newly reported cases in adolescents compared with 171 new cases between July 1, 1991, and June 30, 1992. This compares with an overall increase of 25.9% in other nonadolescent age groups. In 13–19-year-olds, cases have been reported from 30 states and the District of Columbia; 19 other states have reported cases in individuals aged 20–24 years. Only North Dakota has not reported a case of AIDS in an adolescent or young adult. Over 70% of cases have been reported from Metropolitan Statistical Areas with populations of 1 million or greater. New York alone accounts for 13% of all reported cases in this age group (12).

Of the 872 cases in 13–19-year-olds, 630 have occurred in males (72.2%) and 242 are reported in females (27.8%). The male-to-female ratio of 2.6:1.0 is remarkably different from the ratio of 8.36:1 for all cases.

The rate of new case reporting is highest in African-American females (averaging almost 30% increase annually) and lowest in Caucasian females (13%/year). By comparison, in the 20–24-year age group, of the 8911 cases reported as of June 30, 1992, 1597 are cases in females (17.9%) and 6765 are cases in males (88.1%). In this age group the male-to-female ratio is 4.24:1.0.

Minority adolescents are disproportionately represented in the reported case count, with 325 (37.3%) cases being reported in African-Americans and 174 (19.9%) in Hispanics. These case counts, when compared with the 358 (41.1%) cases reported in Caucasians and 15 (1.7%) in individuals classified as "other" race (Table 5.2), illustrate the fact that most cases of AIDS in adolescents are now occurring among minority youths. The single largest gender and racial group are Caucasian males, who overall represent 33.6% of all reported cases in adolescents. The cumulative incidence rate (cases/1,000,000 population), however, is still much higher in minority youth, having reached 87.3 in African-American teenagers and 60.8 in Hispanics.

MODES OF TRANSMISSION

The distribution of reported cases of AIDS in adolescents by transmission category is illustrated in Figure 5.1. The largest single transmission category is that representing adolescents who have been infected via transfusion of blood products to correct coagulation defects (30.6% of all adolescent cases). When combined with that group who has acquired their infection via blood transfusion or as a result of tissue transplantation, 36.9% of all cases are accounted for by these medical interventions to alter other underlying chronic or acute illnesses. Given the advances made in screening for the presence of HIV antibody in blood of tissue specimens, it is anticipated that the percentage of all cases that this group represents will continue to fall.

The second largest single category is "men who have had sex with men" (24.4%). When this group is combined with the other groups representing a behaviorally related mode of transmission (injection drug use, heterosexual contact, and the combination category of those who use injection drugs and have had sex with men) 54.1% of cases are represented.

Within the 13–19-year age group, the mode of transmission of HIV infection changes with age. Younger adolescents have acquired their infections as a result of the receipt of blood products, whereas older adolescents and young adults acquired their

Table 5.1. Persons with AIDS by Age and Gender Reported in the United States through June 30, 1992

	<13 yr	13–19 yr	20–24 yr	25–29 yr	All Ages
Males	2,080	630	7,314	30,912	204,038
Females	1,818	242	1,597	4,672	26,141
Total	3,898	872	8,911	35,584	230,179
Percentage of all reported cases	1.7	0.4	3.9	15.5	

Table 5.2. AIDS Cases in Adolescents, Ages 13–19, by Gender and Ethnicity Reported in the United States June 30, 1992

Ethnicity	Male		Female		Total		Cumulative Index (per 1,000,000 population)
	No.	%	No.	%	No.	%	
Caucasian	293	33.6	65	7.5	358	41.1	18.2
African-American	190	21.8	135	15.5	325	37.3	87.3
Hispanic	134	15.4	40	4.6	174	20.0	60.8
Other	13	1.5	2	0.2	15	1.7	32.1
Total	630	72.2	242	27.8	872	100	

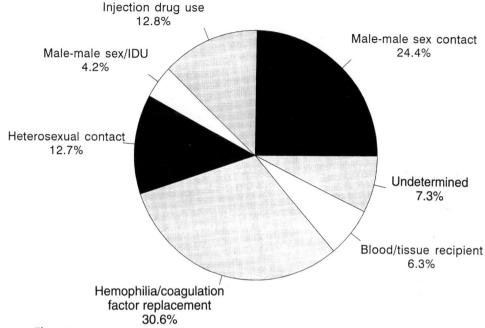

Figure 5.1.   AIDS cases in adolescents by transmission category through June 30, 1992. *IDU,* injection drug use.

infections through behavioral exposures (Table 5.3). A similar difference is also evident between males and females. Male adolescents appear about equally likely to acquire their infection via blood products or via behavioral exposures, whereas over 80% females have been infected through either injection drug use or sexual contact. Finally, analyzing the available mode of transmission data by race reveals that nearly 60% of cases in Caucasians occur as a result of blood or blood component transfusion, whereas over 86% of cases in African-Americans and 67% of cases in Hispanics occur as a result of behavioral exposures (Table 5.4).

INDICATOR DISEASES, NATURAL HISTORY, AND MORTALITY

The percentage distribution of AIDS indicator diseases (diseases that defined AIDS before 1993) is shown in Figure 5.2. Adolescents are more similar to adults than to children in their manner of presentation and nature of their AIDS defining event. *Pneumocystis carinii* pneumonia is the leading diagnosis (32.9%). Other common infectious diseases include *Candida* esophagitis (11.8%), cryptococcosis (8.8%), and chronic herpes simplex infection (7.6%). The leading noninfectious defining events have been wasting syndrome (18.4%) and HIV-related malignancies (Kaposi's, Burkitt's lymphoma, immunoblastic lymphoma, and so forth) (6.1%) and dementia (5.4%). It will be interesting to see how the number of AIDS cases in adolescents changes with the new diagnostic surveillance criteria.

Little is known about the natural history of HIV infection in adolescents. Goedert's report of the natural history of HIV infection in patients with hemophilia suggested that the illness was more slowly progressive in this age group (13). However, this finding may not be substantiated when a broader cross section of adolescents who have acquired their infection through exposures other than transfusions are studied. In fact, given the potential that adolescents who acquire HIV may have had exposures that could result in other types of sexually transmitted infections, others predict that we will find that most infected adolescents have a more aggressive course than adults.

AIDS is the sixth leading cause of death in individuals 15–24 years old. As of December

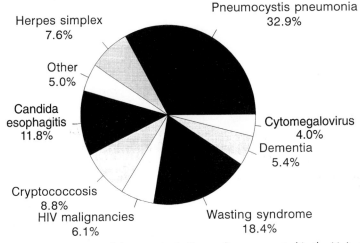

Figure 5.2. AIDS cases in adolescents by indicator disease reported in the United States through June 30, 1992.

Table 5.3. Adolescent and Young Adult AIDS by Age of Diagnosis and Transmission Category Reported in the United States through December 31, 1991

Transmission Category	13–15 yr	16–17 yr	18–19 yr	20–24 yr
		% cases		
Sexual transmission[a]	10	29	66	78
Injection drug use	2	5	16	17
Blood/tissue/clotting factor receipt	86	60	18	5

[a]"Undetermined" case classified as sexually transmitted.

Table 5.4. AIDS Cases in Adolescents, Ages 13–19, by Race or Ethnicity and Transmission Category Reported in the United States through June 30, 1992

Transmission Category	White		Black		Hispanic		Other	
	No.	%	No.	%	No.	%	No.	%
Homosexual or heterosexual contact	102	28.5	187	57.5	69	39.7	3	20.0
Injection drug use	26	7.3	49	15.1	35	20.1	2	13.3
Clotting factor/blood recipient	212	59.2	43	13.2	58	33.3	9	60.0
Other/undetermined	18	5.0	46	14.2	12	6.9	1	6.7
Total	358	100.0	25	100.0	174	100.0	15	100.0

31, 1991, 334 of the 789 cases of AIDS reported by that date had died (42.5%). As with the overall infection rate, the death rate is higher in minority male youth, even though Caucasian males have the highest number of recorded deaths (14).

PREVALENCE OF INFECTION

Although enumerating cases of AIDS is necessary and useful, such an undertaking gives little information about the current situation with regard to transmission of infection. The long latency from acquisition to clinical expression of infection results in most infected adolescents not being diagnosed until they are in their twenties or thirties. Given the accepted median incubation of 8–12 years, it is probably fair to estimate that 20% of all reported cases of AIDS were acquired during ages 13–19 years (15).

Estimates of HIV infection in adolescents exist from multiple sources. There is no one estimate, however, that summarizes the national seroprevalence rate in adolescents. This is even more true in other countries where only the occasional seroprevalence study has been stratified by age to a sufficient degree to allow for analysis of the rates of infection in adolescents.

The most efficacious studies for estimating rate of infection are those that include an entire population of adolescents or at least test specimens without regard to any characteristic that might make it more or less likely for patients to be HIV positive. An example of such a study is the family of serosurveys run under the auspices of the Centers for Disease Control and Prevention (16). Rather than a single study, this is really a group of studies run out of various health care services throughout the country, but focused primarily in family planning and sexually transmitted disease (STD) clinics. All are conducted in a blinded manner by testing discarded blood samples collected for other routine medical purposes. Test results are linked to limited, nonidentifying demographic information. This method provides an unbiased estimation of seroprevalence while preserving anonymity.

Although overall rates in adolescents in family planning clinics involved in these surveys routinely have run less than 0.5%, certain geographic areas have regularly had rates in teenagers that were in the 1.0–1.5% range (17). Data from STD clinics show that the infection rate is higher in this group of adolescents with rates of >2.0% frequently documented. Even as early as 1987, data from STD clinics in Baltimore showed that the overall rate of infection was 2.2% in 15–19-year-olds. Even more significant, the rate in adolescent women attending these clinics was *higher* than the rates in adolescent men, 2.5 vs. 2.2% (18). Data from a rural geographic area, STD clinics in Mississippi, demonstrate a lower overall rate in adolescents (0.40%) but also support the finding of similar rates of infection in males and females (0.41% males, 0.38% females) (19).

Data acquired from the required military and Job Corps (a federally funded training program for disadvantaged youth) screening programs have the advantage of characterizing the universe of adolescents who apply to these programs. However, although surveys are comprehensive in nature, they do not represent a true national cross section of adolescents since they are confined to only adolescents who seek out enrollment in these programs. Adolescents at highest risk might decide not to apply to either of these programs because they know they will be tested.

Military data specific to adolescents analyzed for 4 years (October 1985–September 1989) showed an overall cumulative prevalence of 0.34/1000 specimens tested (20). Rates were similar in males and females (0.35/1000 males and 0.32/1000 females) but varied dramatically by geographic area. Seven regions had rates of 2.0 or greater (Table 5.5), with the rate being the highest in Washington DC (5.32/1000).

Similar data from applicants to the Job Corps collected from October 1987–February 1990 showed an overall seroprevalence rate of 3.6/1000 and also showed that rates in females (3.2/1000) were similar to rates in males (3.7/1000) (21). In younger adolescents, the rate in females actually was higher than the rate in males (2.3/1000 vs. 1.5/1000). Rates were higher in African-Americans (5.3/1000) than in Hispanics (2.6/1000) or Caucasians (1.2/1000). Higher rates were also seen in individuals from the Northeast or South and in those who came from larger metropolitan areas (Fig. 5.3).

Other data on seroprevalence in adolescents and young adults come from various studies, many of which focus on individuals in a particular geographic area or individuals in special social or living situations. For instance, a survey of self-referred students at 19 universities revealed that 0.84/1000 of 18–24-year-olds were positive (22) while a

Table 5.5. Prevalence of Antibodies to HIV in United States Military Applicants, 1985–1989, from Selected Regions

County or City	Prevalence (per 1000)
Total	0.34
Cook County (Chicago)	0.70
Los Angeles	0.85
Dade County (Miami)	1.25
Queens (New York)	1.56
Baltimore	2.19
Washington DC	5.32

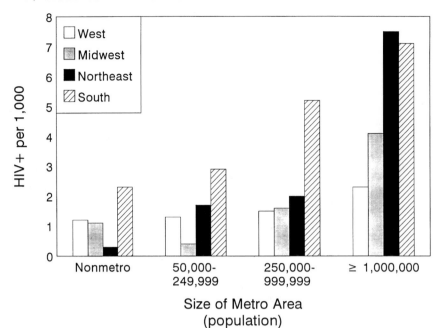

Figure 5.3.   HIV seroprevalence in Job Corps students by regions of the United States and by size of metropolitan area reported from October 1987 to February 1990.

similar survey in a facility for runaway youth showed a prevalence of 5.3% (53.0/1000) (23)! National data obtained from adolescents aged 13–19 who are tested with knowledge and informed consent at publicly funded counseling and testing centers show an overall prevalence of 0.47% (4.74/1000) (24). Finally, an annual seroprevalence survey in an adolescent health clinic in Washington DC has shown an increase in the seroprevalence rate from 4.1/1000 specimens tested in 1987 to 19.34/1000 in 1992 (25). This rapid increase in infected adolescents has recently been commented on by Quinn et al. in their ongoing studies of the prevalence of HIV infection in patients at STD clinic in metropolitan Baltimore (26). Despite the varying methods in these surveys, they indicate heterogeneity in the adolescent population with regard to the risk of HIV infection with certain adolescents in this country being at very high risk of infection but many others still having a measurable albeit lower risk.

Age stratified seroprevalence data from other countries are much harder to access than data from this country. Nonetheless, data that are available indicate that the rate of infection in teenagers is often a reflec-

tion of the overall rate in the community. For instance, data from sexually transmitted disease clinics in the Central African Republic show prevalence rates of 16 and 9% in females and males, respectively. Although extraordinarily high, it is still lower than the rates in other age groups up to 40 years. General seroprevalence in Uganda had reached 16% for women and 7% for men aged 15–20 years. In the western hemisphere, 7.5% of pregnant women aged 15–19 years in Port-au-Prince, Haiti, are HIV positive, but only 1.0% of women and 3.0% of men presenting to STD clinics on Martinique are HIV positive (27).

These national and international data show that a substantial number of adolescents worldwide are already HIV infected. As is true in both the developed and underdeveloped countries, many adolescents are continually at risk of HIV infection on the basis of sexual practices, medical status, or drug use. These risks are reviewed in the next section.

RISK OF HIV TRANSMISSION IN ADOLESCENTS

With over 50% of reported cases of AIDS in adolescents already linked to a mode of transmission that is determined by some behavior in which these individuals have engaged, it is clear that reduction in the acquisition of HIV infection will necessitate an understanding of risk behavior among adolescents. Although participation in risk behaviors traditionally linked to the transmission of HIV infection in adults certainly will place adolescents at risk of infection, a recent study utilizing solely homosexual or bisexual classification, intravenous drug use, sex with either of these "group members" as criteria for screening adolescents missed 62% of seropositive teenagers (10). For this reason, we must be alert to behaviors that might put adolescents into high-risk contact with older individuals who may have a more regularly established profile of risk behaviors even though an adolescent might not classify him or herself as a member of a particular risk group.

Sexual intercourse, either vaginal, anal, or oral-genital, would appear to be the most likely way that adolescents have and will continue to put themselves at risk of HIV infection. Median age of first intercourse has declined to less than 17 years compared with 1970 when it was slightly more than 20 years (28, 29). Although this decrease is dramatic, more troublesome is the fact that an increasing number of sexually active adolescents have had sex with multiple partners. Results from the nationally school-based Youth Risk Behavior indicate that by 12th grade, 17.0% of females and 38.5% of males will have had four or more lifetime sexual partners (30). This was particularly true of males who identified themselves as being "Black"; regardless of grade level, 60.4% had four or more lifetime partners.

For those individuals who are sexually experienced and who do not choose abstinence, barrier protection in the form of a condom appears to be effective in reducing the chances of being infected with any STD pathogen. Condom use by teens in general and individuals who appear to be at increased risk of STDs in specific is poor. For instance, data from the Youth Risk Behavior Survey has shown that adolescents who have had multiple lifetime partners are also less likely to use condoms. Of "highly experienced" males, 45.6% had used a condom at the time of their last intercourse, compared

with 54.2% of those with fewer than four lifetime partners. This difference was even more pronounced in young women where only 29.2% of those with four or more partners used condoms at their last intercourse compared with 44.3% of those with fewer than four partners. Although the relationship of other variables to condom use in young women is complex, a recent study by Orr et al. (31) showed that only the presence of other risk behaviors (drug use, delinquency, school problems) predicted adolescents who were less likely to use condoms. In this study and others previously mentioned (8, 9), a reliable link between use of oral contraceptives and poor attitudes or behaviors with regard to condom use could not be established, although women who use condoms for contraception as well as for protection from sexually transmitted diseases were more likely to have used condoms at last coitus.

An accurate history of male-male sexual contact is often difficult to obtain from adolescent males. Although it is estimated that between 17 and 35% of men have had a sexual experience with another man and that these experiences frequently occur in adolescence, no good studies on the epidemiology and nature of these experiences exist, and adolescents are often unwilling to discuss this aspect of their sexuality (32). It is disturbing, however, that in those young men who relate a history of same sex behavior, behavior changes capable of lessening the risk of HIV infection are less likely to have been adopted (33).

Although anal intercourse is a risk behavior most often associated with male-male sex, in certain surveys between 15 and 20% of women have also experienced this form of sexual intercourse (8, 9, 34). As is true with male-male contact, little is known of the frequency and circumstances of this behavior, other than that in women it appears to be related to total number of sexual partners (8). It is postulated that in some groups of females this form of intercourse is utilized as a method of birth control and is less likely to be associated with condom use (35).

Estimates of injection drug use by adolescents is similarly difficult to obtain. Several studies from the Centers for Disease

Control and Prevention estimate that between 2.3 and 3.7% of male and 0.7 and 1.8% of female adolescents have ever used injection drugs and that an even smaller percentage have shared needles (36, 37). Other forms of drug use are more common, however, and it is less clear how they may influence an adolescent's risk of HIV. Crack cocaine use has been linked to an overall increase in the rate of STDs in adolescents (38), and a history of substance abuse is more commonly reported in adolescents who have syphilis (39). Other drugs such as alcohol and marijuana can lead to impaired judgment and inappropriate choices concerning sex and other potentially risky behaviors (40–42).

PREVENTION OF HIV INFECTION IN ADOLESCENTS

Despite the progress that has been made in the treatment of HIV infection and the hope that a vaccine will emerge as a practical preventive measure, the most immediate hope for influencing a change in the growing number of HIV-infected adolescents is a successful prevention program. Such a program should be national and aimed at changing the behaviors that put adolescents at risk of HIV infection.

Key to effecting such a change in behavior is ensuring that adolescents have an adequate knowledge base about HIV infection and AIDS and what behaviors might put them at risk of infection. In the mid-1980s, it was clear that many adolescents had much incorrect information about HIV infection and AIDS (43, 44). These misconceptions appeared to be greatest in minority youth, many of whom were already engaged in potentially risky behaviors (45, 46). With initiation of the first AIDS education projects, the knowledge of many adolescents concerning HIV infection improved (47, 48). Most studies to date confirm that adolescents are now aware that sexual intercourse and injection drug use are behaviors that can result in the transmission of HIV infection. Misconceptions about the risk of HIV infection and casual contact are still prevalent, however (49).

More controversial is the information surrounding how, if at all, adolescents translate this increased knowledge into behavior change (50). Kegeles et al. (51) followed 151 female and 53 male adolescents for 12–18 months to see if their attitudes or behaviors concerning condom use changed over this time. Unfortunately, the study showed that in this cohort, despite displaying knowledge of the role of condoms in preventing sexually transmitted diseases, neither women nor men increased their use nor their intention to use condoms. This study was conducted just as information on the effectiveness of condoms in preventing the spread of HIV infection was beginning to be accepted. Subsequent studies have shown that an increase in knowledge can be followed by the expected adoption of certain preventive health behaviors; these sorts of changes have often been more successful in men than in women and at times have been offset by the initiation of other behaviors that increasingly contribute to risk of infection (52, 53). When knowledge and attitudes have appeared to influence behavioral change, this change has not usually been assessed over time (54, 55).

More optimistic findings have been reported from a 1988 national survey of adolescent males, where an increase in condom use appeared to have occurred over a 3-year period. This increase appeared to relate to having received formal AIDS education (56). Countering this national survey data is a more focused study on several cohorts of potentially at risk adolescents followed over 4–6 years. A demonstrated overall increase in knowledge was not reflected in the adoption of more positive behavior (57).

Any meaningful attempt to influence behavior will have to target hard-to-reach adolescents, many of whom live in unstable situations (58). The hope that such adolescents might be amenable to changing their behaviors has recently been increased by a study that utilized an intensive educational and behavioral intervention with runaway adolescents in New York City. Rotheram-Borus et al. (59) demonstrated that behavioral changes that were sustained over time could be brought about in a subset of teens who experienced between 15 and 30 1- to 2-hour focused and in-depth AIDS intervention programs that teach practical social skills and basic AIDS information. These programs were distinguished by their rigor and repetitive nature. The implication for other similar programs targeting such youth is that much more intensive efforts may be necessary and that the potential for success should not be overlooked, despite the work entailed.

Preventing HIV infection in adolescents will clearly take more than teaching a few basic facts about the infection. A coordinated effort between schools, families, religious groups, and health professionals is necessary. Despite the existence of comprehensive school-based education programs created at both local and national levels (60), we must remember that many adolescents do not attend school regularly. These adolescents will need to receive their information through other sources. Health professionals have a unique opportunity and responsibility in this regard (61). Out-of-school youth still interact with the health care system and often seek care for behaviors that could put them at risk of HIV infection. This is an appropriate and opportune time to provide guidance as well as care. It is crucial to remember, however, that all counseling must be straightforward and nonjudgmental.

Most adolescents seen by health professionals will not be easily identifiable as being members of an at risk group. They still need, however, to hear a consistent message of concern in the setting where they receive their health care. This message should consist of the following simple facts: 1) any adolescent, particularly one who is sexually active, may now or in the future be at risk of HIV infection; 2) sexual abstinence and avoiding the use of injection drugs will reduce this risk to very low levels; 3) for those adolescents who are sexually active, limiting their number of sexual partners, avoiding high risk practices such as anal intercourse, and using barrier protection particularly in the form of condoms will reduce, but not eliminate, their risk of infection.

Health professionals must also be willing to advocate for comprehensive and truthful teaching in school-based education programs (62), encourage parents to speak with their children and adolescents (63), and actively reach out to groups of adolescents who may be at increased risk of infection. These include gay and bisexual youth, youth in detention, runaway and homeless youth, and youth with coagulation disorders. Adolescents who are infected deserve special services and attention to help them avoid transmitting this infection to others (see Chapter 40).

RESEARCH NEEDS

The fact that adolescents comprise the smallest percentage of cases of AIDS for any age group is probably part of why we know considerably less about HIV infection in adolescents than we do in children and adults. Although it is assumed that adolescents will be similar to adults in the natural history of their infection and their response to therapy, they have been omitted from many studies that would have allowed a scientific basis for this assumption (5). Adolescents are similarly poorly represented in clinical trials (64), although a special initiative on the part of the AIDS Clinical Trials Group will hopefully soon correct this lack of enrollment. We need to know more about the course of HIV infection in adolescents and how medications will affect this course.

With regard to epidemiology of AIDS and HIV infection in adolescents, there is a need to continue to explore what specific behaviors and what additional factors put adolescents at risk of HIV infection. For instance, the role of noninjection drug use in adolescent HIV infection may well be unique given that teenagers often engage in various risk behaviors simultaneously. It is assumed, without appropriate data, that this information will mirror that found in adults. Additional information is necessary concerning adolescents' abilities to access care and services. This access may be blocked by financial and insurance barriers as well as legal barriers to an adolescent's requesting care or participating in research studies.

Finally, we need to know more about how to provide an adequate prevention message to adolescents. Most adolescents feel that they have heard enough about HIV and AIDS despite their acknowledged knowledge deficits. We need better techniques for providing information that will improve knowledge and attitudes and that will allow this to be translated into meaningful behavioral change.

References

1. Hein K. AIDS in adolescents: A rationale for concern. NY State J Med 1987;87:290–295.
2. Hein K, Hurst M. Human immunodeficiency virus infection in adolescence: A rationale for action. Adolesc Pediatr Gynecol 1988;1:73–82.
3. Vermund SH, Hein K, Gayle HD, Cary JC, Thomas PA, Drucker E. Acquired immunodeficiency syndrome among adolescents: Case surveillance profiles in New York City and the rest of the United States. Am J Dis Child 1989;143:1220–1225.
4. Manoff SB, Gayle HD, Mays MA, Rogers MF. Acquired immunodeficiency syndrome in adolescents: Epidemiology, prevention, and public health issues. Pediatr Infect Dis J 1989;8:309–314.
5. D'Angelo LJ, Sondheimer DL. Adolescents and HIV infection: Struggling not to be forgotten. Pediatr AIDS HIV Infect 1990;1:75–77.
6. Select Committee on Children, Youth, and Families. House of Representatives, 102nd Congress. A decade of denial: Teens and AIDS in America. Washington DC: US Government Printing Office, 1992:55–439.
7. Centers for Disease Control. HIV-related beliefs, knowledge, and behaviors among high school students. MMWR 1988;37:717–721.
8. MacDonald NE, Wells GA, Fisher WA, et al. High-risk STD/HIV behavior among college students. JAMA 1990;263:3155–3159.
9. Kotloff KL, Tacket CO, Clemens JO, et al. Assessment of the prevalence and risk factors for human immunodeficiency virus type 1 (HIV-1) infection among college students using three survey methods. Am J Epidemiol 1991;133:2–8.
10. D'Angelo LJ, Getson PR, Luban NLC, Gayle HD. Human immunodeficiency virus infection in urban adolescents: Can we predict who is at risk? Pediatrics 1991;88:982–986.
11. Centers for Disease Control. Selected behaviors that increase risk for HIV infection among high school students—United States, 1990. MMWR 1992;41:231–240.
12. Centers for Disease Control. HIV/AIDS Surveillance Report, Jul 1992:1–18.
13. Goedart JJ, Kessler CM, Aledort LM, et al. A prospective study of human immunodeficiency virus type I infection and the development of AIDS in subjects with hemophilia. N Engl J Med 1989; 321:1141–1148.
14. National Center for Health Statistics. Advance report on final mortality statistics, 1989. Monthly Vital Stat Rep 1992;40(suppl 2):no 8.
15. Bacchetti P, Moss AR. Incubation period of AIDS in San Francisco. Nature 1989;338:251–253.
16. Pappaioanou M, Dondero TJ, Petersen LR, et al. The family of HIV seroprevalence surveys: Objectives, methods, and uses of sentinel surveillance for HIV in the United States. Public Health Rep 1990;105:113–119.
17. Wondell DA, Onorato IM, McCray E, Allen DM, Sweeney PA. Youth at risk: Sex, drugs and human-immunodeficiency virus. Am J Dis Child 1992;146:77–81.
18. Quinn TC, Glaser D, Cannon RO, et al. Human immunodeficiency virus infection among patients attending clinics for sexually transmitted diseases. N Engl J Med 1988;318:197–203.
19. Young R, Feldman S, Brackin BT, Thompson E. Seroprevalence of human immunodeficiency virus among adolescent attendees of Mississippi sexually transmitted disease clinics: A rural epidemic. South Med J 1992;85:460–463.
20. Burke DS, Brundage JD, Goldenbaum MS, et al. Human immunodeficiency virus infections in teenagers: Seroprevalence among applicants for U.S. military service. JAMA 1990;263:2074–2077.
21. St. Louis M, Conway GA, Hayman CR, et al. Human immunodeficiency virus infection in disadvantaged adolescents: Findings from the US Job Corps. JAMA 1991;266:2387–2391.
22. Gayle HD, Keeling RP, Garcia-Tunon M, et al. Prevalence of the human immunodeficiency virus among university students. N Engl J Med 1990;323:1538–1541.
23. Stricof RL, Kennedy JT, Nattell TC, Weisfuse IB, Nouick LF. HIV seroprevalence in a facility for runaway and homeless adolescents. Am J Public Health 1991;81(suppl):50–53.
24. Centers for Disease Control. Publicly funded HIV counseling and testing—United States, 1991. MMWR 1992;41:613–617.
25. D'Angelo LJ, Getson PR, Brasseux CO, Guagliardo MF, Shafer N. A longitudinal study of HIV infection in urban adolescents [Abstract]. 31st Intersciences Conference on Antimicrobial Agents and Chemotherapy, Chicago, Oct 1991.
26. Quinn TC, Groseclose SL, Spense M, Provost V, Hook EW. Evolution of the human immunodeficiency virus epidemic among patients attending sexually transmitted disease clinics: A decade of experience. J Infect Dis 1992;165:541–544.
27. Center for International Research. Trends and patterns of HIV/AIDS infection in selected developing countries: Country profiles. Research Note 5. Washington DC: Bureau of the Census, Feb 1992.
28. Hoffert SL, Kahn JR, Baldwin W. Premarital sexual activity among U.S. teenage women over the past three decades. Fam Plann Perspect 1987;19:46–53.
29. Centers for Disease Control. Premarital sexual experience among adolescent women—United States, 1970-1988. MMWR 1991;39:930–935.
30. Centers for Disease Control. Sexual behavior among high school students—United States 1990. MMWR 1992;40:385–397.
31. Orr DP, Langefeld CD, Katz BP, et al. Factors associated with condom use among sexually active female adolescents. J Pediatr 1992;120:311–317.
32. Remafedi G. Adolescent homosexuality: Psychosocial and medical implications. Pediatrics 1987;79:331–337.
33. Stall R, Barrett D, Bye L, et al. A comparison of younger and older gay men's HIV risk taking behaviors: The communication technologies 1989 cross-sectional survey. J Acquir Immune Defic Syndr 1992;5:682–687.

34. Reinisch JM, Sanders SA, Hill CA, Ziemba-Davis, M. High-risk sexual behavior among heterosexual undergraduates at a midwestern university. Fam Plann Perspect 1992;24:116–121.

35. Jaffe LR, Seehaus M, Wagner C, Leadbeater BJ. Anal intercourse and knowledge of acquired immunodeficiency syndrome among minority-group female adolescents. J Pediatr 1988;112:1005–1007.

36. Centers for Disease Control. HIV related knowledge and behaviors among high school students—selected U.S. sites, 1989. MMWR 1990;39:385–397.

37. Holtzman D, Anderson JE, Kann L, et al. HIV instruction, HIV knowledge, and drug injection among high school students in the United States. Am J Public Health 1991;81:1596–1601.

38. Fullilove RE, Fullilove MT, Bowser BP, Gross SA. Risk of sexually transmitted disease among black adolescent crack users in Oakland and San Francisco. JAMA 1990;263:851–855.

39. Cox JM, D'Angelo LJ, Silber TJ. Substance abuse and syphilis in urban adolescents: A new risk factor for an old disease. J Adolesc Health 1992;13:483–486.

40. Zabin LS, Hardy JB, Smith EA, Hirsch MB. Substance use and its relation to sexual activity among inner-city adolescents. J Adolesc Health Care 1986;7:320–331.

41. Stall R, McKusick L, Wiley L, Coates T, Ostrow D. Alcohol and compliance with safe sex. Health Educ Q 1986;13:359–371.

42. Hingson RW, Strunin L, Berlin BM, Heeren T. Beliefs about AIDS, use of alcohol and drugs, and unprotected sex among Massachusetts adolescents. Am J Public Health 1990;80:295–299.

43. DiClemente RJ, Zorn J, Temoshok L. Adolescents and AIDS: A survey of knowledge, attitudes, and beliefs about AIDS in San Francisco. Am J Public Health 1986;76:1443–1445.

44. Strunin L, Hingson R. Acquired immunodeficiency syndrome and adolescents: Knowledge, beliefs, attitudes, and behaviors. Pediatrics 1987;79:825–828.

45. DiClemente RJ, Boyers CB, Morales ES. Minorities and AIDS: Knowledge, attitudes, and misconceptions among Black and Latino adolescents. Am J Public Health 1988;78:55–57.

46. Goodman E, Cohall AT. Acquired immunodeficiency syndrome and adolescents: Knowledge, beliefs and behaviors in a New York City adolescent minority population. Pediatrics 1989;84:36–42.

47. Hingson R, Strunin L, Berlin B, Acquired immunodeficiency transmission: Changes in knowledge and behaviors among teenagers, Massachusetts statewide surveys, 1986 to 1988. Pediatrics 1990; 85:24–29.

48. Steiner JD, Sorokin G, Schiedermayer DL, Vanstrusteren TJ. Are adolescents getting smarter about acquired immunodeficiency syndrome? Change in knowledge and attitude over the past 5 years. Am J Dis Child 1990;144:302–306.

49. Koopman C, Rotheram-Borus MJ, Henderson R, Bradley JS, Hunter J. Assessment of knowledge of AIDS and beliefs about AIDS prevention among adolescents. AIDS Educ Prev 1990;2:58–70.

50. Zabin LS, Hirsch MB, Smith EA, Hardy JB. Adolescent sexual attitudes and behaviors: Are they consistent? Fam Plann Perspect 1984;16:181–185.

51. Kegeles SM, Adler NE, Irwin CE. Sexually active adolescents and condoms: Changes over the year in knowledge, attitudes and use. Am J Public Health 1988;78:460–461.

52. Zimet GD, Bunch DL, Anglin TM, et al. Relationship of AIDS-related attitudes to sexual behavior changes in adolescents. J Adolesc Health 1992;13:493–498.

53. Ku LC, Sonenstein FL, Pleck JH. The association of AIDS education and sex education with sexual behavior and condom use among teenage men. Fam Plann Perspec 1992;24:100–106.

54. Rickert VI, Gottlieb A, Jay MS. A comparison of three clinic-based AIDS education programs on female adolescents' knowledge, attitudes, and behavior. J Adolesc Health Care 1990;11:298–303.

55. Jemmott JB, Jemmott LS, Fong GT. Reductions in HIV risk-associated sexual behaviors among black male adolescents: Effects of AIDS prevention intervention. Am J Public Health 1992;82:372–376.

56. Sonenstein FL, Pleck JH, Ku LC. Sexual activity, condom use and AIDS awareness among adolescent males. Fam Plann Perspect 1989;21:152–158.

57. Stiffman AR, Earls F, Dore P, Cunningham R. Changes in acquired immunodeficiency syndrome-related risk behavior after adolescence: Relationships to knowledge and experience concerning human immunodeficiency virus infection. Pediatrics 1992;89:950–956.

58. DiClemente RJ, Lanier MM, Horan PF, Lodico M. Comparison of AIDS knowledge, attitudes, and behaviors among incarcerated adolescents and a public school sample in San Francisco. Am J Public Health 1991;81:628–630.

59. Rotheram-Borus MJ, Koopman C, Haignere C, Davies M. Reducing HIV sexual risk behaviors among runaway adolescents. JAMA 1991;266:1237–1241.

60. Centers for Disease Control. Guidelines for school health education to prevent the spread of AIDS. MMWR 1988;37(suppl):S–2.

61. Stiffman AR, Earls F. Behavioral risks for human immunodeficiency virus infection in adolescent medical patients. Pediatrics 1990;85:303–310.

62. DiClemente RJ. Prevention of human immunodeficiency virus infection among adolescents: The interplay of health education and public policy in the development and implementation of school-based AIDS education programs. AIDS Educ Prev 1989;1:70–78.

63. Centers for Disease Control. Characteristics of parents who discuss AIDS with their children—United States, 1989. MMWR 1991;40:789–791.

64. D'Angelo LJ. The participation of adolescents in AIDS clinical trails [Abstract]. J Adolesc Health 1992;13:49.

6

Information for Caretakers of Children about Women Infected with HIV[a]

Deborah Cotton, Judith S. Currier, and Constance Wofsy

The diagnosis of AIDS in a child often is tantamount to the identification of an entire family at risk for human immunodeficiency virus (HIV) infection. The perinatally infected child by definition has a seropositive mother. She may in turn have acquired the infection sexually from the father of the child or another male partner. The family may include siblings who were infected perinatally themselves and others who were not. In addition, because the epidemic of intravenous drug use, a major contributor to the occurrence of AIDS, plagues many communities, extended family members including aunts, uncles, and cousins may be HIV seropositive as well.

Pediatricians caring for children with HIV infection may by interest or default become involved in the counseling, referral, or even direct care of adult family members. In addition, the pediatrician often holds a special place of trust for such families and may be sought for advice and support during the entire family's interaction with the health care system. Thus, pediatricians must be aware of differences in the natural history of HIV infection in adults compared with children, knowledgeable concerning state-of-the art-therapies for adult AIDS, and well-versed in methods to prevent further spread of the disease to other family members.

Because an infected mother is most often the primary caretaker of the child with HIV

infection, the pediatrician must especially understand the unique ramifications of the infection in this population. The intent of this chapter is to provide a practical overview of knowledge concerning the optimal management and prevention of HIV infection in adults, especially in women of childbearing age.

EPIDEMIOLOGY OF HIV INFECTION IN WOMEN

Risk factors for HIV infection in women have been reasonably well delineated. Worldwide the predominant mode of HIV transmission for women is vaginal intercourse with an infected man. Genital ulceration in women, caused by several sexually transmitted diseases, appears to increase the risk of infection as it does in men (1). Intercourse during menses may similarly increase risk to women as may the use of oral contraceptives, perhaps by producing cervical erosion (2). Rectal intercourse is significantly more likely to result in infection in women than vaginal intercourse, probably because of trauma to the rectal mucosa (3).

Although HIV can be recovered from cervical secretions its infectivity is likely less than that of semen. However, the virus can be transmitted from infected women to their male sexual partners during vaginal intercourse (4), and, in addition, several cases of female to female transmission have been reported (5–7).

In the United States, transmission of HIV through intravenous drug abuse is a major contributor to infection in women (8), and

[a]Portions of this chapter also appear in Broder S, et al., eds. *Textbook of AIDS medicine.* Baltimore: Williams & Wilkins, 1994; Sachs B, et al., eds. *Reproductive health care for women.* London: Oxford University Press, 1994.

just over half of all cases of AIDS in women nationally are due to this risk behavior (9). Moreover, such women are also at risk of sexual transmission from partners who use intravenous drugs (10). Drug use, including alcohol intoxication, may indirectly contribute to infection through its disinhibiting effects that may lead to unprotected sex or to exchange of sex for drug money (11). Thus, the dual epidemics of drug abuse and AIDS are closely linked with major ramifications for families of children with HIV infection.

To date, more than 20,000 women in the United States, most of whom are of childbearing age, have been diagnosed with AIDS (9), and it is now the sixth leading cause of death nationally in women between the ages of 15 and 45 (12). Moreover, data suggest that the epidemic started later in women than in men in this country and that as a result a larger proportion of women with HIV are in earlier stages of infection. These women may be entirely well and thus unaware of their infection. Women of color are disproportionately infected with HIV compared with their representation in the general population. A substantial percentage of women with AIDS are immigrants from countries in which heterosexual transmission of HIV is tragically quite common (9). In addition to the above risk factors, many women may have become infected through transfusion. Since testing of the donor blood supply began in 1985 the number infected in this manner has rapidly decreased. However, because of the long incubation cases of AIDS will continue to occur for many years. Finally, although acquisition of HIV infection through accidental percutaneous exposure such as occurs in the medical setting is unusual (9), note that most health care workers are women of childbearing age and comprise a group at risk of acquiring HIV infection.

Thus, women with AIDS have become infected because of various risk factors, and, unlike men, a large percentage of infections have been indirect and caused by high-risk behavior of sexual partners. Therefore, women may be less aware of the possibility that they have been infected with HIV.

In the United States, largely because of the link to drug abuse, AIDS in women is highly concentrated in poor neighborhoods in major urban areas of the Atlantic seaboard (9). In these areas, HIV infection is only one of many threats to family health and safety. Drug abuse, domestic violence, gang warfare, and lack of provision of basic social services are major problems. Besides the rising incidence of HIV infection in cities, certain rural areas in the southeastern United States are also showing a rapid increase in the incidence of AIDS in women. Heterosexual acquisition of HIV infection by women is increasing more rapidly in the South than in other areas of the United States. Economic and geographic barriers to health care access and a relative lack of awareness concerning AIDS in women on the part of many practitioners in the South prevent many women and children from receiving appropriate testing, counseling, and treatment.

Many women with HIV infection are single parents with little or no support available for caring for themselves or their ill children. Paradoxically, diagnosis of HIV infection in a child of such severely disadvantaged families can lead to an improved social situation because of specific services provided to the family that would otherwise be unavailable.

NATURAL HISTORY OF HIV INFECTION IN WOMEN

Unlike perinatally infected infants, most of those infected with HIV as adults have a prolonged asymptomatic phase of illness. It has been estimated from an ongoing study of gay men with the disease that on average frank AIDS does not develop for ten or perhaps more years after infection (13). However, despite the fact that patients may remain well for many years, risk continues to increase with time, and progression to AIDS is expected to ultimately be very high if not universal (14).

Acute infection with HIV can be accompanied by a distinct clinical syndrome consisting of fever, adenopathy, malaise, myalgia, pharyngitis, skin rashes, and in some cases aseptic meningitis (15). However, in many cases the infection is apparently silent and is identified only through HIV testing or after presentation with an opportunistic infection or tumor.

For many years, the development of certain clinical signs such as weight loss, oral thrush, prolonged fever, and disseminated herpes zoster have been recognized as predictive of the subsequent development of AIDS in the HIV-infected man (14). More recently, it has been shown that monitoring of the absolute number or percentage of CD4 cells in such patients is the most sensitive predictor of short-term development of frank AIDS (16, 17). In addition, controlled clinical trials have demonstrated the benefit of specific therapies when the CD4 count has fallen below certain critical levels (18). This finding has led to recommendations for periodic testing of adults with HIV infection by CD4 monitoring (19). The value of additional serologic markers of disease progression in adults such as β_2 microglobulin, neopterin, p24 antigen testing, and quantitative viral culture are unclear but are subject to ongoing research.

Once an adult's CD4 count has fallen below 200 cells/mm^3, the risk of development of opportunistic infections increases markedly (14). In adults, *Pneumocystis carinii* pneumonia remains the most common initial opportunistic infection, although with widespread PCP prophylaxis its incidence may decrease or at least be delayed. Other common opportunistic infections occurring early in frank AIDS include cryptococcal meningitis, cerebral toxoplasmosis, recurrent salmonellosis, and severe herpes simplex infection late in the disease include disseminated cytomegalovirus infection, *Mycobacterium avium intracellulare* infection, and high-grade B cell lymphoma. Recurrent bacterial pneumonia and sepsis and tuberculosis are now included in the Centers for Disease Control AIDS definition and can occur relatively early in the disease, often when the CD4 count is >200 cells/mm^3.

For several years, possible gender-specific differences have been considered in the timing, occurrence, and patterns of HIV complications. Research into these issues has been hampered by a lack of large cohort studies of women with HIV. In part, the emphasis on the role of women in transmitting infection to their fetuses and male sexual partners rather than attention to the impact of the disease on the woman herself was due to the fact that women sought care for their children but were frequently unaware of their own illness until their child was diagnosed with HIV. In addition, as discussed earlier, a greater proportion of women with HIV infection may be in the asymptomatic stage. Thus information on late-stage complications of HIV infection in women is extremely limited. As a result, inferences regarding the natural history of HIV in women, as well as health policy, have often been based on small case series and anecdotal reports. Although there is now increasing interest in recruiting and following larger groups of women, such studies, even if initiated today, would require many years to accumulate definitive data given the long incubation of the infection.

Early studies suggested that women with HIV infection had a more rapid rate of disease progression and a shortened survival after diagnosis compared with men (20, 21). However, several of these studies did not include the striking difference between men and women in the occurrence of Kaposi's sarcoma. Kaposi's, which is far more common in HIV-infected men than women, is associated with longer survival after diagnosis than other HIV-related complications. Recent studies have attributed survival differences between men and women to stage of disease, use of health care resources, and differential use of antiviral therapy (22–24), although others have not found a gender difference in survival (25).

Except for the known dramatic gender difference in the occurrence of Kaposi's sarcoma and several reports suggesting that esophageal candidiasis may be more common in HIV-infected women than men, the incidence of other HIV-related complications appears to be the same (26, 27). There is no indication that women have a different course once opportunistic infections have occurred or that women respond differently to commonly used therapies such as zidovudine, trimethoprim-sulfamethoxazole, or fluconazole. Thus in the absence of data to the contrary, women should be treated in the same manner as men.

The initiation of certain therapies for AIDS is currently based on CD4 cell level. For example, zidovudine is recommended in asymptomatic individuals once the CD4 count is <500 cells/mm³ (18), and PCP prophylaxis is generally initiated at a level of 200 CD4 cells/mm³ based on data from longitudinal cohort studies in males that demonstrated a dramatic rise in the risk of PCP once the CD4 count dropped below this level (28). There are no similar longitudinal data on CD4 counts in women, and thus it is unclear if these cutoffs are appropriate for this population. Uncertainty is compounded if the patient is pregnant when these therapeutic decisions are being made. Normal pregnancy has been demonstrated to result in transient decreases in CD4 cell number that return to normal postpartum (29). Whether a decrease in CD4 cell number from 300 to 200 cells/mm³ occurring during pregnancy has the same, better, or worse prognosis than in the nonpregnant woman is unknown and is subject to ongoing investigation. Again, while waiting for more definitive studies, we recommend using the same criteria as those established in male cohorts for the initiation of HIV therapies.

The possible occurrence of female-specific manifestations of HIV infection is a matter of much current research interest as well as widespread debate among advocates of women with HIV, the medical community, and government agencies. Small studies have concluded that vaginal candidiasis as well as cervical dysplasia, carcinoma in situ, and overt cervical carcinoma are more common and more aggressive in women with HIV infection (26, 30–33). In addition, there are anecdotal reports that HIV-infected women have more frequent or severe pelvic inflammatory disease (34, 35). However, in the absence of large cohort studies, especially ones that include both HIV-infected and demographically matched noninfected women it is difficult to demonstrate a causal relation between HIV and these conditions (36). However, invasive cervical carcinoma has now been added to the list of AIDS-defining conditions by the Center for Disease Control.

Oral thrush has been known for many years to indicate progressive immune destruction in men with HIV infection, and it is plausible that vaginal infection with candida, an extremely common affliction in normal women, may indeed be more severe and more refractory to treatment in women who are HIV infected. In addition, some authors have suggested that vaginal candidiasis may occur earlier than oral candidiasis and might serve as a sensitive marker of disease progression in women (37). In a recent study vaginal candidiasis was not only the most common initial clinical manifestation of HIV infection but also the most common opportunistic infection observed during HIV infection among a prospectively followed cohort of women (26).

Cervical carcinoma has been linked to human papilloma virus (38–40) and epidemiologically is more likely to occur in women who begin sexual intercourse at an early age and who are more likely to have multiple partners (41), supporting the view that cervical carcinoma may be due to the acquisition of an infectious agent. Women who have early sex and multiple partners are also more likely to acquire HIV infection, and thus the occurrence and progression of cervical disease in an individual woman may simply indicate dual infection with both agents rather than a causal role of HIV (42). Despite this, female renal transplant recipients and those immunosuppressed from cancer therapy have been reported to have a greater incidence of, and a more aggressive course with, cervical carcinoma (43, 44). Moreover, the occurrence of cervical dysplasia in HIV-infected women is inversely correlated with CD4 cell number (39, 42), lending biological plausibility to HIV acting either as a potentiator of human papilloma virus or independently to cause cervical carcinoma.

The precise role if any of HIV in the occurrence and virulence of pelvic inflammatory disease is based entirely on uncontrolled studies (35, 45). Pelvic inflammatory disease is linked with early and multiple sex partners and caused by many different infectious agents, making determination of a causal role of HIV in the occurrence of pelvic inflammatory disease even more difficult.

The scientific debate over female-specific manifestations of HIV infection has been hampered not only by inadequate cohort studies but also by the fact that in the United States the provision of medical and social benefits for persons with HIV infection is linked to standardized definitions of AIDS (46). Until recently these definitions have not included possible female-specific conditions, and advocates of women with HIV argue that many such women have significant morbidity and even may die without ever fulfilling the Centers for Disease Control AIDS definition (47). Thus several groups actively lobbied for an expanded definition of AIDS to include cervical dysplasia and carcinoma, pelvic inflammatory disease, and vaginal candidiasis. The Centers for Disease Control has now added invasive cervical carcinoma, only, to the list of AIDS-defining conditions.

Although the causal role of HIV in these gynecological conditions is a critical issue to resolve, the situation is somewhat more straightforward for the clinician than for the policymaker. Women infected with HIV are clearly at greater risk for having cervical dysplasia, whatever the reason. Most practitioners who care for such women favor Pap smear every 6 months with referral to a gynecologist experienced in colposcopy for any question of an abnormality. One recent study (42) has suggested that in this population Pap smears may not be sufficiently sensitive to detect dysplasia, and some have recommended colposcopy for all women with HIV infection. However, the risk-benefit of this approach is unknown, and routine colposcopy in lieu of PAP smear screening is not recommended (36). Conversely, women presenting with cervical dysplasia, with pelvic inflammatory disease, or with recurrent refractory vaginal candidiasis in the absence of other risk factors (such as diabetes or recent antibiotic use) should certainly be advised to have HIV antibody testing.

PROVISION OF MEDICAL CARE FOR WOMEN AND OTHER ADULT FAMILY MEMBERS

When a pediatrician has diagnosed HIV infection in a child there are obviously many issues to be discussed immediately with the child's family. If it is likely that the parents of the child did not suspect or know the diagnosis before, then the pediatrician must decide how much information should be given during this initial discussion regarding the risk to other family members.

The situation is made vastly easier if there is already a system in place for counseling and referral concerning these issues. Early discussions of safe sex are crucial if it is likely that the mother or other family adults are currently sexually active. Appropriate information must also be given as soon as possible regarding the risk of perinatal transmission in future or current pregnancies.

HIV antibody testing to confirm infection and CD4 testing to stage disease progression should be arranged as soon as possible for all family members who are likely to be at risk. Appropriate medical and counseling services should be available to respond to the results of these tests. Once a mother or other adult is identified as HIV infected further care will be determined by initial CD4 results, medical interview, and examination. All adults with confirmed HIV infection regardless of CD4 count should receive pneumococcal vaccine and yearly influenza vaccine, and some experts also recommend Hemophilus influenzae vaccine (49). PPD testing with appropriate controls is important since between 30 and 50% of HIV-infected adults coinfected with tuberculosis may develop active disease during immunosuppression (50). Tuberculosis in a household with any child poses a problem and the risk for disseminated infection. HIV-infected children may be even less able to contain their infection (see Chapter 16). Screening for IgG to toxoplamosis is useful to assess likely risk of cerebral toxoplasmosis and, if the patient is negative, to ensure that precautions are taken to avoid primary infection with *Toxoplasma gondii*.

HIV-infected adults with <500 CD4 cells/mm^3 are in general offered 100 mg zidovudine five times per day or 200 mg TID although the benefit of this therapy in delaying progression to AIDS in this population is now somewhat controversial (18, 19). If the CD4 cell count is <200 cells/mm^3 in an asymptomatic individual or <300 when accompanied by nonspecific AIDS-related complex symptoms (weight loss, fever), PCP prophylaxis with oral trimethoprim-sulfamethoxazole should be initiated (51). If patients cannot tolerate trimethoprim-sulfamethoxazole aerosolized pentamidine or dapsone may be used; however, trimethoprim-sulfamethoxazole has clearly been demonstrated to be the superior agent for the secondary prevention of PCP pneumonia in adults (52).

In general, pediatricians should refer adult patients identified with HIV infection to an experienced general internist, infectious diseases specialist, or family practitioner (in some areas oncologists and a few pulmonologists also provide primary care to HIV-infected adults). The organization of the care is, in many ways, more important than the prior training of those who deliver it. Clinics or private practices that can ensure continuity of providers, have ancillary personnel such as social workers experienced in caring for HIV-infected patients, and have access to clinical trials of promising agents provide ideal settings for the care of the HIV-infected adult. Unfortunately, because many of these women only have coverage by Medicaid, access to such care can be compromised in some areas.

INTEGRATED CARE OF FAMILIES

The HIV-infected women presents unique challenges for care. Unlike most women with life-threatening disease she cannot necessarily rely on the support of those around her. Indeed she is very often caring for other sick family members, despite her own illness.

HIV infection is a disease of a whole family, but care is frequently fragmented for each member. Women with HIV infection may have poor access to appropriate medical care because they are members of a socioeconomic group with reduced access to basic health care (53). When pregnant, they may receive late or even no prenatal care (54). Thus programs that link preventive counseling, disease detection, and medical intervention solely to settings such as family planning or prenatal clinics may miss many women at risk for or actually infected with HIV. Wherever women present for care, HIV testing should be offered.

The time it takes to access appropriate care for herself often is more than an HIV-infected woman can manage while caring for her children. Therefore, care for HIV-infected women and their children (and sometimes other family members as well) should ideally be integrated at one site.

There are several pragmatic obstacles, however. In some cities, tertiary care children's hospitals provide the bulk of care for HIV-infected children, and these are often separate and geographically distant from adult hospitals and clinics specializing in HIV. Neither type of hospital is likely to be equipped to handle all situations occurring in the other patient-age population, and few sites could afford or attract full-time HIV doctors specializing in such care. Thus adult practitioners would need to be brought for sessions at a children's hospital or vice versa. Even if this were successful for routine outpatient visits referral would still have to be made for specialized testing and for inpatient care. An alternative is to have a partnership between adult and pediatric sites with good communication but separate systems of care, but this still has the disadvantage of requiring a woman to make separate appointments and travel to two sites. It is the experience of many pediatric providers that many women seek care for their children but ignore themselves, making it important that these mothers be counseled and guided to appropriate care providers. Many models of integrated care now exist, and they must be evaluated and adapted for other cities (55–57).

Additional problems are raised in trying to provide women with access to experimental therapies. As of the end of 1990, <7% of participants in federally sponsored HIV clinical trials sponsored by the AIDS Clinical Trials Group (ACTG) had been women. Early on, women were in some cases categorically barred from such protocols (as has traditionally been the case in other diseases) largely because of concerns over possible teratogenic effects of experimental drugs. Although all ACTG trials now permit the entry of nonpregnant women, accrual of women for these trials is still poor. Women entering ACTG trials are more likely to be white and less likely to have ever used intravenous drugs than the population of women with AIDS in the United States. However, with time, the demographic characteristics of women participating in these trials has come closer to that of all women with the disease (58). A separate Women's Health Committee has been established within the ACTG to improve accrual of women to trials that will study possible female-specific manifestations of the disease such as cervical carcinoma and pelvic inflammatory disease.

Often sites providing experimental drug protocols require that patients have a separate primary care provider. For a woman with HIV who is already bringing in a child to a pediatric clinic (and perhaps separate pediatric clinical trials site) it is extremely burdensome to obtain her own care at two additional locations. Moreover, few experimental sites are equipped with the kinds of support services needed by mothers to participate successfully in drug trials. The need for transportation and child care are additional needs beyond the mother's own, which are rarely included in budgets of such programs and can create barriers to female participation.

The problems encountered in the area of HIV infection have not been experienced to the same degree in providing care for women of who have life-threatening diseases. In part this is because women with HIV tend to be poorer and have fewer social supports than women with other diseases such as breast cancer or end-stage renal disease. Women with those diseases may often rely on informal networks of support such as family, neighbors, or church volunteers to care for their children and themselves during a life-threatening illness. The unique nature of HIV infection, as a sexually acquired and vertically transmitted infection creating whole families with disease, is especially challenging. Modern western societies are poorly equipped to respond to such a crisis, especially in impoverished areas where HIV infection in women is most prevalent.

PREVENTION OF INFECTION IN WOMEN OF CHILDBEARING AGE

The tragedy of perinatally acquired HIV infection makes imperative the prevention of infection in women of childbearing age. Unfortunately, beyond the issue of prenatal testing there has been little attention to innovative prevention programs for women.

The programs that exist have for the most part been male-oriented and have focused on the use of condoms and voluntary change of sexual behaviors. However, women face a more complex set of challenges in AIDS prevention than can be addressed by these measures. First, HIV may be transmitted more efficiently from men to women (59), and thus the use of a condom for each act of intercourse is essential. Unfortunately, a woman often does not control the decision to use a condom because she is often the less powerful partner in the relationship and may suffer many negative consequences if she demands condom use. For example, her partner may leave her, question her own background, or accuse her of questioning his, may force her to have sex without a condom anyway, or may physically abuse her in other ways.

The development and recent licensure of the "female condom," a vaginal sheath designed to serve both as a contraceptive and safer sex device that a woman controls is a promising development; however, it was licensed without proof of efficacy for either indication because of the urgency of the epidemic so it remains to be seen if it will be useful (60). Some innovative programs to increase the empowerment of women at risk for HIV have also been described, and further efforts in this area seem essential (61, 62).

HIV TESTING OF WOMEN AT RISK

Screening for HIV antibody as a preventive strategy has been suggested as especially critical for women, who may be unaware of being placed at risk for infection through the behaviors of their partners. Much discussion has focussed on prenatal testing. Proponents have argued that such information is so vital to the reproductive decision-making of women that testing should be mandatory. In addition, pediatricians have argued that in the absence of definitive tests of infection in young infants, all children at risk of HIV infection should be identified as soon as possible and have thus argued for prenatal or routine neonatal testing. Because all mothers with AIDS passively transfer antibody to their infants this suggestion is tantamount to suggesting prenatal screening of their mothers. Recently, a workshop was convened under the auspices of the National Pediatric HIV

Resource Center that included more than 60 national experts (including pediatricians, obstetricians, parents, nurses, social workers) and developed recommendations regarding testing and screening (see Table 6.1) as part of their review of the medical management of infants and children with HIV infection.

Opponents of prenatal testing have argued that, overall, the population of pregnant women in the United States is at very low risk for HIV and that the benefits of testing in this population are outweighed by its potential negative consequences, e.g., a false-positive test leading to pregnancy termination and avoidance of future pregnancy and possible discrimination in housing, employment, and even health care. In addition, opponents of prenatal testing indicate that the women at highest risk are also most likely to receive poor, late, or even no prenatal care, which severely limits the benefits of a prenatal testing program.

One difficulty in crafting appropriate policies regarding prenatal testing and counseling has been that the scientific basis for estimates of the risk of perinatal transmission and survival of children with AIDS has been based on incomplete data and has in fact changed dramatically over the past few years. Early in the epidemic a pregnant woman would have been advised that the chance of giving birth to an infected child was close to 50% (63) and that death before the age of 2 would be almost certain. Today, she would likely be given an estimate of no more than 10-30% risk of vertical transmission and informed that the child might well live into school age or beyond (a long time in a disease where new therapies are constantly being introduced). That there is no prenatal test to predict which infants are truly infected also limits the usefulness of prenatal testing.

In 1991 an Institute of Medicine Committee concluded that at that time mandatory prenatal testing was inadvisable (64). Since then, however, the use of HIV testing in the prenatal setting has increased and is now used widely in a voluntary but "routine" manner. Although it is difficult to predict future use, the recent demonstration of a benefit of prophylactic therapy for PCP in infants at risk for HIV makes more likely the adoption of a policy of mandatory or at least aggressive routine testing of those pregnant women perceived to be at increased risk. Such considerations have spawned the recommendations by the National Pediatric HIV Resource Center listed in Table 6.1

Table 6.1.   Recommendations Regarding Prenatal Screening and Testing Developed by National Pediatric HIV Resource Center Workshop[a]

Women of reproductive age should receive HIV counseling, and HIV testing should be routinely offered by all medical providers.

HIV antibody testing accompanied by appropriate counseling should be standard of care in all prenatal settings. HIV testing should be recommended as early as possible during prenatal period. If women are not tested during pregnancy, counseling and testing should be recommended to women during postnatal period.

HIV antibody testing, accompanied by appropriate counseling to mother, should be standard of care for neonates born to mothers who have not received HIV antibody testing or for whom antibody test results are unknown to pediatrician.

Positive maternal or infant HIV tests must be linked to appropriate health care services for mother and infant. This requires that obstetric and/or prenatal medical providers cooperatively develop plans with the child's pediatrician for ongoing care of all infants of seropositive women. Obstetric and/or prenatal medical providers must work collaboratively with woman's ongoing care provider to assure future HIV directed care of mother.

After confirmation of HIV infection in a woman, all children born to that woman since 1980 should be tested for antibody to HIV. Counseling should be provided to woman concerning risk of HIV infection to all partners since 1980. HIV antibody testing after appropriate counseling should be standard of care for all partners who can be located.

[a]Proceedings are available through National Pediatric HIV Resource Center (1-800-362-0071) and have been published (Pediatr Infect Dis J 1993;12:513–522).

CONCLUSIONS

HIV in women differs from the disease in men in virtually all respects. Women have a more diverse set of risk factors than men and are more likely to be unaware of the source of their infection. They are more likely to be poor, young, and of color. Women who have HIV infection are often members of families where others, including their own children, have AIDS. As a group, they have less knowledge concerning AIDS and far less access to health care and experimental drug trials. Women with HIV infection may have additional manifestations of the infection and may have a different pattern and incidence of some opportunistic diseases than men with HIV. Drugs women may be given may not have been previously tested in women. If these women become pregnant, the information available to guide choices about pregnancy termination and future family planning is still incomplete and subject to varying interpretations. There is little published literature to guide their treatment. Perhaps most importantly, the ability of many women to avoid infection or seek appropriate treatment is severely limited because of their low societal status.

For all these reasons HIV infection in women can be best approached in a targeted and gender-specific fashion. The delay in recognizing the enormity of the problem of HIV infection in women is tragic. However, it is heartening that in the last year increasing interest in this problem has culminated in the inclusion of many sessions on HIV infection in women at the last two International Conferences on AIDS, increasing hope that this challenge can yet be met.

References

1. Holmberg SD, Horsburgh CR, Ward JW, Jaffee HW. Biologic factors in the sexual transmission of human immunodeficiency virus. J Infect Dis 1989; 160:116–125.
2. Plummer F, Simonses J, Cameron D, et al. Cofactors in male-female sexual transmission of human immunodeficiency virus type 1. J Infect Dis 1991;163:233–239.
3. Padian N, Marquis L, Francis DP, et al. Male-to-female transmission of human immunodeficiency virus. JAMA 1987;258:780–790.
4. Padian NS, Shiboski SC, Jewell NP. Female-to-male transmission of human immunodeficiency virus. JAMA 1991;25:1664–1667.
5. Monzon OT, Capellan JMB. Female-to-female transmission of HIV [Letter]. Lancet 1987;2:40–41.
6. Marmor M, Weiss LR, Lyden M, et al. Possible female-to-female transmission of human immunodeficiency virus [Letter]. Ann Int Med 1986; 105:969.
7. Chu SY, Buehler JW, Fleming PL, Berkleman RL. Epidemiology of reported cases of AIDS in lesbians, United States 1980–89. Am J Pub Health 1990;80:1380–1381.
8. Guinan ME, Thomas PA, Pinsky PF, et al. Heterosexual and homosexual patients with the acquired immunodeficiency syndrome: A comparison of surveillance, interview, and laboratory data. Ann Intern Med 1984;100:213–218.
9. Centers for Disease Control. HIV/AIDS Surveillance Rep 1992;April 1992:1–18.
10. Brown LS, Primm BJ. Sexual contacts of intravenous drug abusers: Implications for the next spread of the AIDS epidemic. J Natl Med Assoc 1988;80:651–656.
11. DesJarlais DC, Friedman SR. Intravenous cocaine, crack, and AIDS risk reduction. JAMA 1988; 259:1945–1946.
12. Chu SY, Buehler JW, Berkleman RL. Impact of the human immunodeficiency virus epidemic on mortality of women of reproductive age, United States. JAMA 1990;264:225–229.
13. Munoz A, Wang MC, Bass S, et al. Acquired immunodeficiency syndrome (AIDS)-free time after human immunodeficiency virus type 1 (HIV-1) seroconversion in homosexual men. Am J Epidemiol 1989;130:530–539.
14. Lifson AR, Rutherford GW, Jaffee HW. The natural history of human immunodeficiency virus infection. J Infect Dis 1988;158:1360–1367.
15. Cooper DA, Gold J, Maclean P, et al. Acute AIDS retrovirus infection. Definition of a clinical illness associated with seroconversion. Lancet 1985; 1:537–540.
16. Fahey J, Taylor J, Detels R, et al. The prognostic value of cellular and serologic markers in infection with human immunodeficiency virus type 1. N Engl J Med 1990;332:166–172.
17. Polk B, Fox R, Brookmeyer R, et al. Predictors of the acquired immunodeficiency syndrome developing in a cohort of seropositive homosexual men. N Engl J Med 1987;316:61–66.
18. National Institute of Allergy and Infectious Diseases. Recommendations for zidovudine; early infection. JAMA 1990;263:1606–1609.
19. Aboulker JP, Swart AM. Preliminary analysis of the Concorde trial. Lancet 1993;341:889–890.
20. Rothenberg R, Woefel M, Stoneburner R, Milberg J, Parker R, Truman B. Survival with the acquired immunodeficiency syndrome. N Engl J Med 1987;317:1297–1302.
21. Whyte B, Swanson C, Cooper D. Survival of patients with the acquired immunodeficiency syndrome in Australia. Med J Aust 1989;150:358–362.
22. Moore RJH, Sugland B, Chaisson R. Zidovudine and the natural history of the acquired immunodeficiency syndrome. N Engl J Med 1991;324:1412–1416.

23. Stein M, Piette J, Mor V, et al. Differences on access to zidovudine among symptomatic HIV-infected persons. J Gen Intern Med 1991;6:35–40.

24. Lemp G, Hirozawa A, Cohen J, Derish P, McKinney K, Hernandez S. Survival for women and men with AIDS. J Infect Dis 1992;166:74–79.

25. Ellerbrock T, Bush T, Chamberland M, Oxtoby M. Epidemiology of women with AIDS in the United States, 1981 through 1990: A comparison with heterosexual men with AIDS. JAMA 1991;265:2971–2975.

26. Carpenter C, Mayer K, Stein M, Leibman B, Fisher A. HIV infection in Northern American women: Experience with 200 cases and a review of the literature. Medicine 1991;70:307–325.

27. Fleming PC, Ciesielski CA, Berkelman RC. Sex-specific differences, United States, 1988–1989 [Abstract MC 3210]. Seventh International Conference on AIDS, Florence, Jun 1991.

28. Phair J, Munoz A, Detels R, et al. The risk of *Pneumocystis carinii* pneumonia among men infected with human immunodeficiency virus type 1. N Engl J Med 1990;322:769–775.

29. Biggar R, Pahava S, Minkoff H, et al. Immunosuppression in pregnant women infected with human immunodeficiency virus. Am J Obstet Gynecol 1989;161:1239–1244.

30. Henry M, Stanley M, Cruikshank S, Carson L. Association of human immunodeficiency virus-induced immunosuppression with human papillomavirus infection and cervical intraepithelial neoplasia. Am J Obstet Gynecol 1989;160:52–53.

31. Maiman M, Fruchter R, Serur E, et al. Human immunodeficiency virus and cervical neoplasia. Gynecol Obstet 1990;38:377–382.

32. Vermund SH, Kelley KF, Klein RS, et al. High risk of human papillomavirus infection and cervical squamous intraepithelial lesions among women with symptomatic human immunodeficiency virus infection. Am J Obstet Gynecol 1991;165:392–400.

33. Safrin S, Dattel BJ, Hauer L, Sweet RL. High frequency of latent and clinical human papillomavirus cervical infections in immunocompromised human immunodeficiency virus-infected women. Obstet Gynecol 1992;79:321–327.

34. Schrager LK, Friedland GH, Maude D, et al. Cervical and vaginal squamous cell abnormalities in women infected with human immunodeficiency virus. J Acquir Immune Defic Syndr 1989;2:570–575.

35. Safrin S, Dattel B, Haver L, Sweet R. Seroprevalence and epidemiologic correlates of infection in women with acute pelvic inflammatory disease. Obstet Gynecol 1990;75:666–670.

36. Minkoff H, DeHovitz J. Care of women infected with the human immunodeficiency virus. JAMA 1991;266:2253–2258.

37. Rhoads JL, Wright DC, Redfield RR, Burke DS. Chronic vaginal candidiasis in women with HIV infection. JAMA 1987;257:3105–3107.

38. Zur Hausen H. Human papillomavirus and their possible role in squamous cell carcinomas. Curr Top Microbiol Immunol 1977;78:1–30.

39. Vermund SH, Kelley KF. Human papilomavirus in women: Methodologic issues and role of immuno-suppression. In: Kiely M, ed. Reproductive and perinatal epidemiology. Boca Raton: CRC Press, 1991:144–162.

40. Durst M, Gissmann L, Ikenberg H, Zur Hansen M. A papillomavirus DNA from a cervical carcinoma and its prevalence in cancer biopsies from different geographic regions. Proc Natl Acad Sci USA 1983;80:3812.

41. Munoz N, Bosch FX, Jensen OM. Epidemiology of cervical cancer. IARC Sci Publ 1989;94:9–39.

42. Maiman M, Tarricons N, Viera J, et al. Colposcopic evaluation of human immunodeficiency virus seropositive women. Obstet Gynecol 1991;78:84–88.

43. Katz R, Veanattukalathil S, Weiss K. Human papillomavirus infection and neoplasia of the cervix and anogenital region of women with Hodgkin's disease. Acta Cytol 1987;31:845–854.

44. Halpert R, Fruchter R, Sedlis A, Butt K, Boyce J, Sillman F. Human papillomavirus and lower genital neoplasia in renal transplant patients. Obstet Gynecol 1986;68:251–258.

45. Hoegsberg B, Abulafia O, Sedlis A, et al. Sexually transmitted diseases and human immunodeficiency virus infection among women with pelvic inflammatory disease. Am J Obstet Gynecol 1990;163:1135–1139.

46. Levine C, Stein G. What's in a name? The policy implications of the CDC definition of AIDS. Law Med Healthcare 1991;19:278–290.

47. Office of Technology Assessment. The CDC's case definition of AIDS: Implications of the proposed revisions. Background paper OTA-BP-H-89. Washington, DC: Government Printing Office, Aug 1992.

48. 1993 Revised classification system for HIV infection and expanded surveillance case definition for adolescents and adults. MMWR 1993;41:1–19.

49. Hollander H. Care of the individual with early HIV infection. In: Sande MA, Volberding PA, ed. Medical management of AIDS. Philadelphia: Saunders, 1991:93–102.

50. Pitchenik AE, Fertel D, Bloch AB. Mycobacterial disease: Epidemiology, diagnosis, treatment, and prevention. Clin Chest Med 1988;9:425–441.

51. Centers for Disease Control. Recommendations for prophylaxis against *Pneumocystis carinii* pneumonia for adults and adolescents infected with human immunodeficiency virus. MMWR 1992;41:1–11.

52. Hardy WD, Feinberg J, Finkelstein D, et al. A controlled trial of trinethoprim-sulfamethoxazole or aerosolized pentamidine for secondary prophylaxis of *Pneumocytis carinii* pneumonia in patients with the acquired immunodeficiency syndrome. N Engl J Med 1992;327:1842–1848.

53. Muller C. Medicaid: The lower tier of health care for women. Women Health 1988;14:81–103.

54. Anonymous. Blessed events and the bottom line: The financing of maternity care in the United States. New York: Alan Guttmacher Institute, 1987.

55. Kloser P, Pinto RC, Lombardo J, Bais P, Lyunch A, Gibson C. Women's Clinic: A full service clinic for women with HIV disease [Abstract SD 816]. Sixth International Conference on AIDS, San Francisco, Jun 1990.

56. Gregonis S, Tedaldi E, Treston C. Providing health care to families in a pediatric hospital [Abstract PoD 5539]. Eighth International Conference on AIDS, Amsterdam, Jul 1992.

57. Muther J, Keen P, Klein E, Nesbein S, Sawyer M, Pratt-Palmore M. Family clinic: A model for delivery of comprehensive services to HIV positive children and their parents [Abstract PoB 2431]. Eighth International Conference on AIDS, Amsterdam, Jul 1992.

58. Cotton DJ, Feinberg J, Finklestein D. Participation of women in a large multicenter HIV/AIDS clinical trials program in the United States [Abstract TuD 114]. Seventh International Conference on AIDS, Florence, Jun 1991.

59. European Study of the Heterosexual Transmission of HIV. Comparison of female to male and male to female transmission of HIV in 563 stable couples. Br Med J 1992;304:809–813.

60. Guinan M. HIV, heterosexual transmission, and women. JAMA 1992;268:520–521.

61. Norwood C, Cordova R. Health force: Three years successful experience empowering women affected by AIDS as educators, advocates and leaders in a poor urban area [Abstract PoD 5447]. Eighth International Conference on AIDS, Amsterdam, Jul 1992.

62. Lundgren R, Bezmalinovic B, Hirschmann A, Arathoon E. Guatemala City women: Empowering a vulnerable group to prevent HIV transmission [Abstract PoD 5445]. Eighth International Conference on AIDS, Amsterdam, Jul 1992.

63. Friedland GH, Klein RS. Transmission of human immunodeficiency virus. N Engl J Med 1987;317:1125–1135.

64. Institute of Medicine. HIV screening of pregnant women and newborns. Washington, DC: National Academy Press, 1991.

SECTION II

Etiology, Pathogenesis, and Transmission

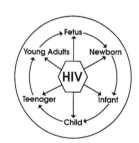

Biology and Molecular Biology of HIV

Ruth I. Connor and David D. Ho

Human immunodeficiency virus (HIV), previously known as lymphadenopathy-associated virus, human T cell lymphotropic virus type III, or AIDS-related virus, is an RNA virus that belongs to the lentivirus family of nononcogenic, cytopathic retroviruses (1). HIV shares morphologic, biologic, and molecular properties with prototypic animal lentiviruses, including visna virus, caprine arthritis encephalitis virus, and equine infectious anemia virus (Fig. 7.1) (2–4). Like HIV in humans, these viruses cause slow progressive wasting disorders, including neurodegeneration, that are often fatal (5, 6). On the basis of viral protein cross-reactivity and sequence similarity, HIV-1 is very closely related to the primate retrovirus, simian immunodeficiency virus (SIV) (7–10). HIV-1 also shares sequence homology and serologic reactivity with another group of human T cell lymphotropic retroviruses referred to as HIV-2, which were first isolated from West Africans (11–13). HIV-2 is clearly associated with immunodeficiency and a clinical syndrome similar to AIDS (14, 15); however, its pathogenicity may be lower than that of HIV-1.

The mature HIV-1 virion is slightly more than 100 nm in diameter and by electron microscopy appears as a dense cylindrical core surrounded by a lipid envelope (Fig. 7.1*A*). The virion core is comprised of structural proteins encoded by the HIV-1 *gag* gene, as well as the RNA genome and virally encoded enzymes, including reverse transcriptase and integrase, that are required for efficient viral replication (Fig. 7.1*B*).

The RNA genome of HIV-1 is ~10 kilobase (kb) pairs long and is characterized by the presence of two flanking long terminal repeat (LTR) sequences and *gag, pol,* and *env* genes characteristic of most retroviruses (Fig. 7.2). Unlike other nonprimate retroviruses, the genome of HIV-1 contains at least six additional genes (*tat, rev, nef, vpu, vpr, vif*) that function in the complex coordination of viral gene expression and replication (Table 7.1).

LIFE CYCLE

CD4 Binding

Early observations of a selective depletion of CD4+ T lymphocytes in patients with AIDS implied a specific tropism of the virus for cells bearing the CD4 surface antigen and suggested that CD4 may serve as the cellular receptor for HIV-1 (16). Subsequent studies have confirmed these observations and further characterized the interaction between HIV-1 and CD4. Binding of HIV-1 to CD4 and initiation of the virus life cycle is mediated by the HIV-1 envelope glycoprotein, gp120. As with other retroviruses, the envelope glycoproteins of HIV-1 are synthesized as a precursor polypeptide (gp160) that is subsequently cleaved to yield the external protein, gp120, and the transmembrane protein, gp41 (17). These envelope proteins are incorporated into the outer lipid bilayer of the virion as either a trimer or tetramer of gp120/gp41, with an estimated total of 72 protrusions per virion (18). Based on mapping studies, several dis-

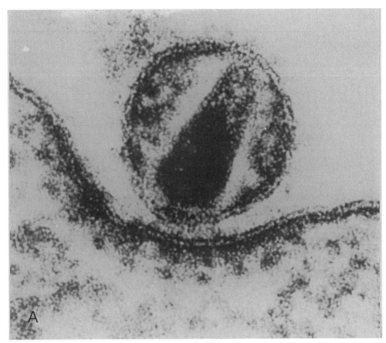

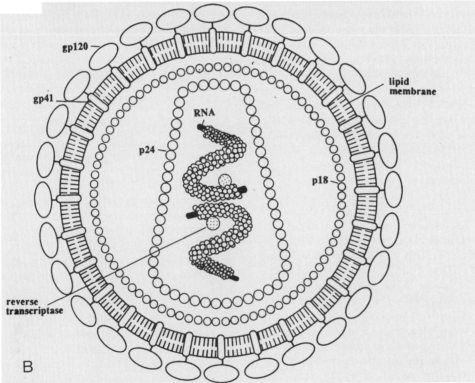

Figure 7.1. **A**, electron micrograph of HIV-1 virion. Characteristic dark cylindrical core is surrounded by a lipid envelope acquired as virion buds from surface of an infected cell (courtesy of H. Gelderblom). **B**, components of HIV-1 virion, including envelope glycoproteins (gp120 and gp41), nucleocapsid proteins, genome, and associated reverse transcriptase. Modified from Gallo RC, Montagnier L. AIDS in 1988. Sci Am 1988;4:41.

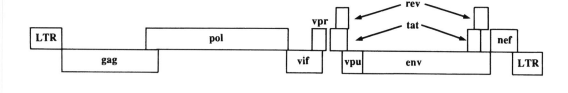

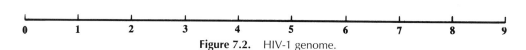

Figure 7.2.   HIV-1 genome.

Table 7.1.   HIV-1 Structural and Regulatory Proteins

Name	Size	Function
Structural proteins		
Gag	p55/p17/p24/p7	Group-specific antigens or capsid proteins
Pol	p66/p51/p32	Viral enzymes; protease, reverse transcriptase, integrase
Env	gp160/gp120/gp41	External and transmembrane envelope glycoproteins
Regulatory proteins		
Tat	p16/p14	Transactivator of viral transcription (38–46)
Rev	p19	Promotes nuclear export and stabilization of viral mRNA (47–51)
Nef	p25	Increases viral burden in vivo (52)
Vif	p23	Increases virion infectivity (53–58)
Vpu	p16	Increases efficiency of virus release; effects processing of envelope glycoproteins (59–64)
Vpr	p10-15	Enhances viral transcription (65, 66)

crete sites on gp120 have been implicated in CD4 binding (19, 20). Although spatially distinct, these regions may be brought together by proper tertiary folding of the molecule to form a conformationally dependent binding site. Antibody mapping studies (21, 22), mutagenesis analysis (22–24), and X-ray crystallography (25) have contributed significantly to defining specific sites on the CD4 molecule that participate in high affinity (10^{-9} M) binding of gp120. Based on these studies, the gp120 binding site has been localized within the first immunoglobulin-like domain (D1) of the CD4 molecule (25).

Fusion and Entry

Binding of gp120 to CD4 triggers a series of events leading to fusion of the virus and host cell membranes. Although poorly understood, the mechanism of virus fusion is believed to involve specific molecular con-

formational changes induced by CD4 binding that allow interaction of the amino-terminal fusion domain of gp41 with the host cell membrane (reviewed in Ref. 26) (Fig. 7.3). Mutations within the first 31 residues of this hydrophobic region (amino acids 511–542) have been shown to disrupt membrane fusion, altering not only virus entry but also affecting the fusion of HIV-1-infected cells with uninfected CD4+ cells (27, 28). Additional sites within the V3 domain of gp120 (29, 30) and the transmembrane region of gp41 (amino acids 661–710) (31) have been identified and appear to be important for virus fusion and infectivity; however, the precise nature of their involvement remains undefined.

Entry of HIV-1 into susceptible cells is dependent on introduction of the virus nucleocapsid core into the host cell cytoplasm. Based on the appearance of virus particles within endosomal compartments, initial studies suggested that HIV-1 was internal-

cytopathicity have been mapped to broader regions within *env* and *tat* (104). The significance of the V3 region in determining cell tropism is unknown, but this domain (amino acids 298–327) is clearly distinct from the CD4 binding site as defined by Lasky et al. (19) (amino acids 397–439) and Olshevsky et al. (20). Mutations within this region have been shown to significantly reduce infectivity without affecting virus binding, suggesting that efficient entry of HIV-1 may be determined by postbinding events and may involve interaction with sites contained within the V3 domain (reviewed in Ref. 106).

One hallmark of HIV-1 infection is selected tropism of the virus for cells bearing the CD4 molecule; however, accumulating evidence suggests that HIV-1 may also infect in vitro cells that express no detectable CD4, including neuronal cells, glial cells, endothelial cells, oligodendricytes, astrocytes, muscle cells, colorectal cells, B cells, and bone marrow progenitor cells (107–112). Entry and replication of the HIV-1 in these cells are frequently inefficient, and the mechanisms that govern infection of CD4− cells are currently unknown. In vivo, there is also evidence of expanded tropism in tissues and cells that are not known to be CD4+. HIV-1 infection has been documented in many nonlymphoid tissues, including colon, rectum, duodenum, cervix, retina, and brain (113–117). Cumulatively, these studies raise the possibility that HIV-1 infection in certain cell types may occur through pathways independent of CD4, perhaps by interaction with a second, as yet unidentified, receptor.

INFECTION OF MONONUCLEAR PHAGOCYTES

Within the peripheral blood, infected CD4+ T lymphocytes form a primary reservoir for HIV-1 (118, 119). Evidence that HIV-1 may also infect cells of macrophage lineage was provided in early studies by Ho et al. (120) in which HIV-1 was directly recovered from peripheral blood monocyte/macrophages of infected patients. Since that time, cells having morphologic and growth properties characteristic of monocyte/macrophages have been associated with virus expression in the brain, lung, lymph nodes, and skin (121–127). The possibility that monocyte/macrophages may be productively infected was further substantiated by the finding that monocytes could support HIV-1 replication in vitro (120) and that infection could be blocked by antibodies to the CD4 receptor (128).

The ability to replicate efficiently in monocyte/macrophages is characteristic of lentivirus infections (129, 130). Prototypical animal lentiviruses, including visna virus and caprine arthritis-encephalitis virus, establish a persistent infection within the host that is characterized by slow but progressive development of immunosuppressive, inflammatory, and/or degenerative diseases. These viruses exhibit a strong tropism for cells of macrophage lineage, although virus replication is restricted by the state of cellular differentiation (130). Levels of virus production are initially low within circulating monocytes; however, as cells enter the tissues and begin to differentiate, the rate of virus replication dramatically increases. By controlling the rate of virus replication, infected monocyte/macrophages serve as reservoirs for the dissemination of infection to target tissues such as the lung and central nervous system (CNS).

Control of HIV-1 replication within infected mononuclear phagocytes is similarly influenced by factors that govern the state of cellular differentiation and/or activation. Cytokines, such as granulocyte macrophage-colony stimulating factor, interferon, tumor necrosis factor-α, interleukin c-1, and interleukin c-6, which are critical in regulation of immune responses in vivo, have been shown in vitro to alter the level of HIV-1 gene expression in infected monocyte/macrophages (131–134). In chronically infected macrophages, HIV-1 replication is predominantly intravacuolar, leading to large accumulations of intracytoplasmic virus particles (135, 136). Paradoxically, these chronically infected cells release only low levels of mature virus progeny, despite the relatively high frequency of infected cells detected in vitro. Moreover, infected macrophages in culture are relatively resistant to HIV-1-induced cytopathic effects and, unlike T lymphocytes, are rarely associated with formation of multinucleated giant cells. The ability to sustain low-level persistent infection while harboring large numbers of virus particles has led many to suggest that infected macrophages may serve as reservoirs for the persistence and dissemination of HIV in vivo.

Examination of tissue samples from AIDS patients has shown virus present in infected cells of macrophage lineage in the skin, lymphatic tissues, lungs, spinal cord, and brain. Within the skin, epidermal Langerhans' cells appear to be a predominant target for infection with HIV-1 (125–127). The presence of these cells in the skin and mucous membranes suggests they may serve as early targets for HIV-1 infection and may subsequently disseminate the virus to regional lymph nodes (126). The first isolate of HIV-1 (then termed lymphadenopathy-associated virus) was derived in 1983 from the lymph node tissue of a patient suffering from persistent generalized lymphadenopathy (137). HIV-1 particles have since been directly demonstrated in the lymph nodes of HIV-1-seropositive patients (138, 139) and have been associated in these tissues with CD4-bearing follicular dendritic cells (140).

Within the lungs, pulmonary macrophages from both AIDS patients and normal donors are susceptible to HIV-1 infection in vitro (124). Spontaneous production of HIV-1 in primary pulmonary macrophage cultures from AIDS patients suggests that these cells may also be targets for infection in vivo (124). Although infected macrophages do not appear to undergo significant cytopathology in vitro, HIV-1-induced defects in functional activity, in particular defense against intracellular pathogens, may increase the likelihood of opportunistic infections. Moreover, infected pulmonary macrophages expressing virus antigens have been shown to be targets for lysis by HIV-specific cytotoxic T lymphocytes and may be responsible for induction of inflammatory reactions in the lungs of HIV-1-infected individuals (141).

CENTRAL NERVOUS SYSTEM INVOLVEMENT

Involvement of the CNS in HIV-1 infection is characterized by several distinct neurologic syndromes, including subacute encephalitis, vacuolar myelopathy, aseptic meningitis, and peripheral neuropathy (reviewed in Ref. 142). Children can also have significant neurodevelopmental changes (see Chapter 23). Considerable evidence now indicates that macrophages within the brain and CNS are a primary target for HIV-1 infection. Detection of HIV-1 DNA in brain tissue by ultrastructural analysis (143), in situ hybridization (122), and immunochemical staining (117, 122, 144–146), as well as the recovery of infectious virus from the brain and cerebrospinal fluid (147, 148) strongly suggests that HIV-1 may have a causal role in the subacute encephalitis associated with AIDS.

The precise mechanism for HIV-1-mediated pathology in the CNS is not well understood; however, several possibilities have been raised by recent studies (Fig. 7.5). HIV-1 isolates derived from the brain and CNS have been shown to replicate efficiently in macrophage and glioma cell cultures in vitro. Although with low frequency, infection of endothelial cells, oligodendrocytes, and astrocytes has also been reported (149, 150). Conceivably, direct cytotoxicity of these cells may arise as a result of infection and replication of the virus. Alternatively, expression of virus antigens on the surface of infected cells may indirectly make them targets for cytotoxic T cells (151). Coinfection with other viruses, in particular cytomegalovirus and JC virus, has also been suggested to be involved in the pathogenesis of AIDS dementia complex (152, 153). These viruses are found with high frequency in immunocompromised patients, including those with AIDS, and may have direct or indirect effects on the neurologic disease induced by HIV-1.

Despite the relatively low cytopathic effects of HIV-1 infection in peripheral blood monocytes and other tissue macrophages, infected macrophages in the brain are frequently associated with the formation of multinucleated giant cells. In patients with AIDS dementia complex, the amount of HIV-1 detected in the CNS has been found in some cases to exceed that detected in the blood or other tissues (147, 148). Moreover, certain isolates of HIV-1, particularly those recovered from brain tissue and cerebrospinal fluid, appear to display preferen-

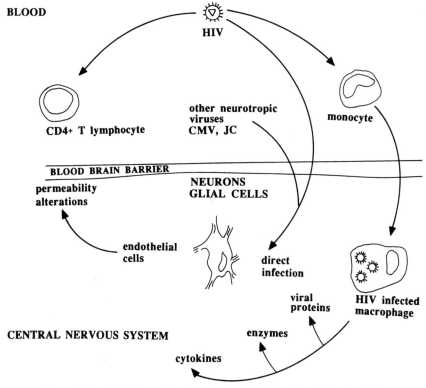

Figure 7.5.   Possible mechanisms for HIV-1-induced pathology in CNS.

tial tropism for cells of macrophage lineage (154). Such neurotropic strains of HIV-1 may be more prone to attack cells of the CNS, which may have implications for development of neurologic dysfunction within the host.

QUANTITATION OF HIV-1

The relationship between virus burden and immunologic status in HIV-1-infected individuals has been studied by several groups (155–157). In early studies, in situ hybridization and immunofluorescent staining were used to determine frequency of cells expressing viral mRNA and surface proteins, respectively (155). Based on these studies it was suggested that the frequency of circulating peripheral blood mononuclear cells (PBMC) infected with HIV-1 in vivo was low (roughly 1 in 10^5 PBMC). However, these techniques may underestimate the virus burden in vivo, since a proportion of latently infected cells may contain HIV-1 DNA yet express no detectable viral RNA or proteins. Indeed, recent studies now

indicate that the levels of HIV-1 in the blood and plasma of infected individuals are much higher than previously estimated (156). Using polymerase chain reaction techniques capable of detecting one molecule of HIV-1 proviral DNA, Simmonds et al. (157) determined the average frequency of PBMC carrying HIV-1 provirus to be 1 in 8000 cells. The frequency was lower in asymptomatic patients (1 in 6000 to 1 in 80,000 cells) but increased in AIDS patients (1 in 770 to 1 in 3300 cells). In a high proportion of peripheral blood leukocytes, HIV-1 proviral DNA has been shown to be replication competent (158), consistent with the high recovery rate of infectious virus from plasma and PBMC of infected patients at all stages of disease (156). Considering that only a small percentage of PBMC are CD4+ cells, the frequency of HIV-1 in these cells may be even higher. Moreover, the high rate of virus recovery from the plasma of HIV-1-seropositive individuals indicates that HIV-1 replication within the host is not completely latent and that circulating antibodies are insufficient to neutralize HIV-1 in vivo.

PATHOGENESIS OF HIV-1 IN MATURE AND IMMATURE HOST

In vivo, the course of infection with HIV-1 is governed by complex interactions between the virus and host immune system. Although little is known of the dynamics of HIV-1 replication within an infected individual, it is reasonable to suggest that immune mechanisms may be elicited in a mature host that contribute to restriction of viral replication and establishment of low-level infection. In adults, initial infection with HIV-1 is characterized by the onset of acute illness, and in the short period before seroconversion, virus may be detected in the cerebrospinal fluid, PBMC and plasma (159, 160). High levels of infectious HIV-1 have recently been demonstrated in both the plasma and PBMC of infected individuals during primary infection, suggesting that the initial viral burden may be rather explosive in an immunologically naive individual. A rapid decrease in the amount of cell-free and cell-associated virus occurs at seroconversion, indicating development within the host of an effective immune response capable of limiting viral replication (160). After primary infection and seroconversion, many individuals enter an asymptomatic period of variable duration characterized by low levels of viral replication and relatively few clinical manifestations. This period of stability may extend for many years, although CD4+ T cell counts usually show a continuous gradual decline during this time. Onset of disease progression in adults is often marked by rapidly decreasing CD4+ T cell counts, clinical deterioration, and increased virus burden in both plasma and PBMC.

In contrast, children infected with HIV-1 in utero or during the perinatal period have a relatively short latency before development of symptomatic disease. Lower levels of HIV-1 are found in the plasma and PBMC of asymptomatic or mildly symptomatic children, whereas severely symptomatic children may have a virus burden comparable with that found in adults (161–163). In studies by Saag et al. (164), HIV-1 was detected in the plasma of each of five infected children regardless of their CD4+ lymphocyte counts or duration of infection. This is in marked contrast to findings in adult patients, where levels of plasma viremia decrease rapidly after seroconversion and remain relatively low throughout the asymptomatic phase of infection. Moreover, those children infected during the perinatal period had a higher incidence of plasma viremia than those infected after the age of 3 months by blood product transfusion (164). Cumulatively, these findings suggest that rapid disease progression in children may occur and may reflect the degree of development of immune function in the host. Infection of immature target cells, such as noncirculating thymocytes or hematopoietic progenitor cells, may initially restrict levels of HIV-1 in tissues and peripheral circulation (165). However, exposure of immunologically naive cells to antigens or immune cytokines in the first few months of life may increase virus replication in infected cells, thereby adding to the virus burden in plasma and PBMC (166). It is unknown whether the overall virus burden in the peripheral blood reflects the level and compartmentalization of HIV-1 in the tissues, and and whether differences in the relative tissue distribution of HIV-1 may contribute to differences in the clinical outcome of infection in adults and children. It is believed, however, that HIV-1 infection may be transmitted at different stages of gestation and the subsequent disease course may be determined in part by the tissue distribution and maturity of CD4+ T cells and bone marrow-derived myelomonocytic cells in the immature host (165). Additional factors, including differential timing of infection and the strain of virus passed from mother to infant, may also contribute to viral pathogenesis and disease progression in infected neonates and children.

CONCLUSIONS

It is clear that protective immunity is not persistent after primary infection with HIV-1, and evidence of increasing virus burden appears coincident with disease progression in infected individuals. Progression to AIDS is marked by an increasing frequency of infected cells and elevated levels of plasma viremia. Mechanisms that govern the persistence of

HIV within the host and ultimately the transition from low level to fulminant infection are unknown. Factors including the virus inoculum, site of infection, and immune status of the host may have bearing on the course of disease (165). Based on our knowledge to date, several additional factors may contribute to this process. Increased sequence diversity coupled with the high mutation rate of specific HIV-1 genes may allow the virus to evade immune surveillance and persist within the host. The emergence of genotypic variants with altered biologic activities, including increased replication rates, cytopathicity, and expanded tropism may increase the overall pathogenicity of the virus. In addition, infection of cells of the macrophage lineage, which appear relatively resistant to HIV-1-mediated cytopathology, may provide a reservoir for dissemination of the HIV-1 to multiple sites in the body, including the brain and CNS. Other factors, including concomitant infection with other viruses, disruption of cytokine regulatory networks, and infection of hematopoietic progenitor cells, may contribute to eventual immune dysfunction. In the face of increasing virus burden, decreases in CD4+ T cells may result directly from HIV-1-mediated cytopathicity or indirectly through autoimmune mechanisms. The profound immunosuppression and opportunistic disease characteristic of HIV-1 infection and AIDS is consistent with the central role these cells play in the induction of immune responsiveness and regulation of immune function in vivo.

References

1. Chiu I-M, Yaniv A, Dahlberg JE, et al. Nucleotide sequence evidence for the relationship of AIDS retrovirus to lentiviruses. Nature 1985;317:366–368.
2. Gonda MA, Wong-Staal F, Galo RC, Clements JE, Narayan O, Gilden RV. Sequence homology and morphologic similarity of HTLV-III and visna virus, a pathogenic lentivirus. Science 1985;227:173–177.
3. Sonigo P, Alizon M, Staskus K, et al. Nucleotide sequence of the visna lentivirus: Relationship to the AIDS virus. Cell 1985;42:369–382.
4. Stephens RM, Casey JW, Rice NR. Equine infectious anemia virus *gag* and *pol* genes: Relatedness to visna and AIDS virus. Science 1986;231:589–594.
5. Narayan O, Cork LC. Lentiviral diseases of sheep and goats: Chronic pneumonia leukoen-cephalomyelitis and arthritis. Rev Infect Dis 1985;7:89–98.
6. Cheevers WP, McGuire TC. Equine infectious anemia virus: Immunopathogenesis and persistence. Rev Infect Dis 1985;7:83–88.
7. Daniel MD, Letvin NL, King NW, et al. Isolation of T-cell tropic HTLV-III-like retrovirus from macaques. Science 1985;228:1201–1204.
8. Kanki PJ, McLane MF, King NW Jr, et al. Serologic identification and characterization of a macaque T-lymphotropic retrovirus closely related to HTLV-III. Science 1985;228:1199–1201.
9. Chakrabarti L, Guyader M, Alizon M, et al. Sequence of simian immunodeficiency virus from macaque and its relationship to other human and simian retroviruses. Nature 1987;328:543–547.
10. Fukasawa M, Miura T, Hasegawa A, et al. Sequence of simian immunodeficiency virus from African green monkey, a new member of HIV/SIV group. Nature 1988;333:457–461.
11. Clavel F, Guetard D, Brun-Vezinet F, et al. Isolation of a new human retrovirus from West African patients with AIDS. Science 1986;233:343–346.
12. Clavel F, Guyader M, Guetard D, Salle M, Montagnier L, Alizon M. Molecular cloning and polymorphism of the human immunodeficiency virus type 2. Nature 1986;324:691–695.
13. Guyader M, Emerman M, Sonigo P, Clavel F, Montagnier L, Alizon M. Genome organization and transactivation of the human immunodeficiency virus type 2. Nature 1987;326:662–669.
14. Clavel F, Mansinho K, Chamaret S, et al. Human immunodeficiency virus type 2 infection associated with AIDS in West Africa. N Engl J Med 1987;316:1180–1185.
15. Brun-Vezinet F, Rey MA, Katlama C, et al. Lymphadenopathy-associated virus type 2 in AIDS and AIDS-related complex: Clinical and virological features in four patients. Lancet 1987;1:128–132.
16. Klatzmann D, Barre-Sinoussi F, Nugeyre MT, et al. Selective tropism of lymphadenopathy associated virus (LAV) for helper-inducer T lymphocytes. Science 1984;225:59–63.
17. Willey RL, Bonifacino JS, Potts BJ, Martin MA, Klausner RD. Biosynthesis, cleavage, and degradation of the human immunodeficiency virus type 1 envelope glycoprotein gp160. Proc Natl Acad Sci USA 1988;85:9580–9584.
18. Özel M, Pauli G, Gelderblom HR. The organization of the envelope projections on the surface of HIV. Arch Virol 1988;100:255–266.
19. Lasky LA, Nakamura G, Smith DH, et al. Delineation of a region of the human immunodeficiency virus type 1 gp120 glycoprotein critical for interaction with the CD4 receptor. Cell 1987;50:975–985.
20. Olshevsky U, Helseth E, Furman C, Li J, Haseltine W, Sodroski J. Identification of individual human immunodeficiency virus type 1 gp120 amino acids important for CD4 receptor binding. J Virol 1990;64:5701–5707.
21. Sattentau QJ, Dalgleish AG, Weiss RA. Epitopes of the CD4 antigen and HIV infection. Science 1986;234:1120–1123.

22. Peterson A, Seed B. Genetic analysis of monoclonal antibody and HIV binding sites on the human lymphocyte antigen CD4. Cell 1988;54:65–72.
23. Mizukami T, Fuerst TR, Berger EA, Moss B. Binding region for human immunodeficiency virus (HIV) and epitopes for HIV-blocking monoclonal antibodies of the CD4 molecule defined by site-directed mutagenesis. Proc Natl Acad Sci USA 1988;85:9273–9277.
24. Brodsky MH, Warton M, Myers RM, Littman D. Analysis of the site in CD4 that binds to the HIV envelope glycoprotein. J Immunol 1990;144:3078–3086.
25. Ryu S-E, Kwong PD, Trunch A, et al. Crystal structure of an HIV-binding recombinant fragment of human CD4. Nature 1990;348:419–425.
26. Moore JP, Jameson BA, Weiss RA, Sattentau QJ. The HIV-cell fusion reaction. In: Bentz J, ed. Viral fusion mechanisms. Boca Raton: CRC Press, 1993:233–289.
27. Kowalski M, Potz J, Basiripour L, et al. Functional regions of the envelope glycoprotein of human immunodeficiency virus type 1. Science 1987;237:1351–1355.
28. Freed EO, Myers DJ, Risser R. Characterization of the fusion domain of the human immunodeficiency virus type 1 envelope glycoprotein gp41. Proc Natl Acad Sci USA 1990;87:4650–4654.
29. Freed EO, Myers DJ, Risser R. Identification of the principal neutralizing determinant of human immunodeficiency virus type 1 as a fusion domain. J Virol 1991;65:190–194.
30. Page KA, Streans SM, Littman DR. Analysis of mutations in the V3 domain of gp160 that affect fusion and infectivity. J Virol 1992;66:524–533.
31. Helseth E, Olshevsky U, Gabuzda D, Ardman B, Haseltine W, Sodroski J. Changes in the transmembrane region of the human immunodeficiency virus type 1 gp41 envelope glycoprotein affect membrane fusion. J Virol 1990;64:6314–6318.
32. Pauza CD, Price TM. Human immunodeficiency virus infection of T cells and monocytes proceeds via receptor-mediated endocytosis. J Cell Biol 1988;107:959–968.
33. Stein BS, Gowda SD, Lifson JD, Penhallow RC, Bensch KG, Engleman EG. pH-independent entry into CD4-positive T cells via virus envelope fusion to the plasma membrane. Cell 1987;49:659–668.
34. Bushman FD, Fujiwara T, Craigie R. Retroviral DNA integration directed by HIV integration protein in vitro. Science 1990;249:1555–1558.
35. Kim S, Byrn R, Groopman J, Baltimore D. Temporal aspects of DNA and RNA synthesis during human immunodeficiency virus infection: Evidence for differential gene expression. J Virol 1989;63:3708–3713.
36. Sodroski J, Patarca R, Rosen C, Wong-Staal F, Haseltine W. Location of the trans activating region on the genome of human T-cell lymphotropic virus type III. Science 1985;229:74–77.
37. Ayra SK, Guo C, Josephs SF, Wong-Staal F. Transactivator gene of human T-lymphotropic virus type III (HTLV-III). Science 1985;229:69–73.

38. Sadaie MR, Benter T, Wong-Staal F. Site-directed mutagenesis of two trans-regulatory genes (tat-III, trs) of HIV-1. Science 1988;239:910–913.
39. Garcia JA, Harrich D, Pearson L, Mitsuyasu R, Gaynor RB. Functional domains required for tat-induced transcriptional activation of the HIV-1 long terminal repeat. EMBO J 1988;7:3143–3147.
40. Dingwall C, Ernberg I, Gait MJ, et al. Human immunodeficiency virus 1 tat protein binds trans-activation-responsive region (TAR) RNA in vitro. Proc Natl Acad Sci USA 1989;86:6925–6929.
41. Gatignol A, Kumar A, Rabson A, Jeang K-T. Identification of cellular proteins that bind to the human immunodeficiency virus type 1 trans-activation-responsive TAR element RNA. Proc Natl Acad Sci USA 1989;86:7828–7832.
42. Cullen BR. Trans-activation of human immunodeficiency virus occurs via a bimodal mechanism. Cell 1986;46:973–982.
43. Laspia MF, Rice AP, Mathews MB. HIV-1 Tat protein increases transcriptional initiation and stabilizes elongation. Cell 1989;59:283–292.
44. Kao S-Y, Calman AF, Luciw PA, Peterlin BM. Anti-termination of transcription within the long-terminal repeat of HIV-1 by tat gene product. Nature 1987;330:489–493.
45. Sodroski J, Goh WC, Rosen C, Dayton A, Terwilliger E, Haseltine W. A second post-transcriptional trans-activator gene required for HTLV-III replication. Nature 1986;321:412–417.
46. Malim MH, Hauber J, Fenrick R, Cullen BR. Immunodeficiency virus rev trans-activator modulates expression of the viral regulatory genes. Nature 1988;335:181–183.
47. Malim MH, Hauber J, Le S-Y, Maizel JV, Cullen BR. The HIV-1 rev trans-activator works through a structured target sequence to activate the nuclear export of unspliced viral mRNA. Nature 1989;338:254–257.
48. Malim MH, Tiley LS, McCarn DF, Rusche JR, Hauber J, Cullen BR. HIV-1 structural gene expression requires binding of the Rev trans-activator to its RNA target sequence. Cell 1990;60:675–683.
49. Chang DD, Sharp PA. Regulation of HIV Rev depends upon recognition of splice sites. Cell 1989;59:789–795.
50. Kestler HW, Ringler DJ, Mori K, et al. Importance of the nef gene for maintenance of high virus loads and for the development of AIDS. Cell 1991;65:651–662.
51. Fisher AG, Ensoli B, Ivanoff L, et al. The sor gene of HIV-1 is required for efficient virus transmission in vitro. Science 1987;237:888–893.
52. Strebel K, Daugherty D, Clouse K, Cohen D, Kolks T, Martin MA. The HIV 'A' (sor) gene product is essential for virus infectivity. Nature 1987;328:728–730.
53. Gabuzda DH, Lawrence K, Langhoff E, et al. Role of vif in replication of human immunodeficiency virus type 1 in CD4+ T lymphocytes. J Virol 1992;66:6489–6495.
54. Sakai K, Ma X, Gordienko I, Volsky DJ. Recombinational analysis of a natural noncytopathic human immunodeficiency virus type 1 (HIV-1) isolate: Role of the vif gene in HIV-1 in-

fection kinetics and cytopathicity. J Virol 1991; 65:5765–5773.

55. Arya SK, Gallo RC. Three novel genes of human T-lymphotropic virus type III: Immune reactivity of their products with sera from acquired immune deficiency syndrome patients. Proc Natl Acad Sci USA 1986;83:2209–2213.

56. Kan NC, Franchini G, Wong-Staal F, et al. Identification of HTLV-III/LAV *sor* gene product and detection of antibodies in human sera. Science 1986;231:1553–1555.

57. Strebel K, Klimkait T, Martin MA. A novel gene of HIV-1, *vpu*, and its 16-kilodalton product. Science 1988;241:1221–1223.

58. Strebel K, Klimkait T, Maldarelli F, Martin MA. Molecular and biochemical analyses of human immunodeficiency virus type 1 *vpu* protein. J Virol 1989;63:3784–3791.

59. Terwilliger EF, Cohen EA, Lu Y, Sodroski JG, Haseltine WA. Functional role of human immunodeficiency virus type 1 *vpu*. Proc Natl Acad Sci USA 1989;86:5163–5167.

60. Klimkait T, Strebel K, Hoggan MD, Martin MA, Orenstein JM. The human immunodeficiency virus type 1-specific protein *vpu* is required for efficient virus maturation and release. J Virol 1990;64:621–629.

61. Schwartz S, Felber BK, Fenyö E-M, Pavlakis GN. Env and Vpu proteins of human immunodeficiency virus type 1 are produced from multiple bicistronic mRNAs. J Virol 1990;64:5448–5456.

62. Willey RL, Maldarelli F, Martin MA, Strebel K. Human immunodeficiency virus type 1 Vpu protein regulates the formation of intracellular gp160-CD4 complexes. J Virol 1992;66:226–234.

63. Willey RL, Maldarelli F, Martin MA, Strebel K. Human immunodeficiency virus type 1 Vpu protein induces rapid degradation of CD4. J Virol 1992;66:7193–7200.

64. Cohen EA, Terwilliger EF, Jalinoos, Proulx J, Sodroski JG, Haseltine WA. Identification of HIV-1 *vpr* product and function. J Acquir Immune Defic Syndr 1990;3:11–18.

65. Cohen EA, Dehni G, Sodroski JG, Haseltine WA. Human immunodeficiency virus *vpr* product is a virion-associated regulatory protein. J Virol 1990;64:3097–3099.

66. Zack JA, Arrigo SJ, Weitsman SR, Go AS, Haislip A, Chen ISY. HIV-1 entry into quiescent primary lymphocytes: Molecular analysis reveals a labile, latent viral structure. Cell 1990;61:213–222.

67. Stevenson M, Stanwick TL, Dempsey MP, Lamonica CA. HIV-1 replication is controlled at the level of T-cell activation and proviral integration. EMBO J 1990;9:1551–1560.

68. Bukrinsky MI, Stanwick TL, Dempsey MP, Stevenson M. Quiescent T lymphocytes as an inducible reservoir in HIV-1 infection. Science 1991;254:423–427.

69. Dougherty JP, Temin HM. Determination of the rate of base-pair substitution and insertion mutations in retrovirus replication. J Virol 1988; 62:2817–2822.

70. Leider JM, Palese P, Smith FI. Determination of the mutation rate of a retrovirus. J Virol 1988; 62:3084–3091.

71. Alizon M, Wain-Hobson S, Montagnier L, Sonigo P. Genetic variability of the AIDS virus: Nucleotide sequence analysis of two isolates from African patients. Cell 1986; 46:63–74.

72. Starich BR, Hahn BH, Shaw GM, et al. Identification and characterization of conserved and variable regions in the envelope gene of HTLV III/LAV, the retrovirus of AIDS. Cell 1986;45:637–648.

73. Willey RL, Rutledge RA, Dias S, Folks T, Theodore T, Buckler CE, Martin M. Identification of conserved and divergent domains within the envelope gene of the acquired immune deficiency syndrome retrovirus. Proc Natl Acad Sci USA 1986;83:5038–5042.

74. Hahn BH, Gonda MA, Shaw GM, et al. Genomic diversity of the AIDS virus HTLV-III: Different viruses exhibit greatest divergence in their envelope genes. Proc Natl Acad Sci USA 1985;82: 4813–4817.

75. Holmes EC, Zhang LQ, Simmonds P, Ludlam CA, Leigh Brown AJ. Convergent and divergent sequence evolution in the surface envelope glycoprotein of human immunodeficiency virus type 1 within a single infected patient. Proc Natl Acad Sci USA 1992;89:4835–4839.

76. Clements JE, Pederson FS, Narayan O, Haseltine WA. Genomic changes associated with antigenic variation of visna virus during persistent infection. Proc Natl Acad Sci USA 1980;77:4454–4458.

77. Montelaro RC, Parekh B, Orrego A, Issel CJ. Antigenic variation during persistent infection by equine infectious anemia virus, a retrovirus. J Biol Chem 1984;259:10539–10544.

78. Salinovich O, Payne SL, Montelaro RC, Hussain KA, Issel CJ, Schnorr KL. Rapid emergence of novel antigenic and genetic variants during persistent infection. J Virol 1986;57:71–80.

79. La Rosa GJ, Davide JP, Weinhold K, et al. Conserved sequence and structural elements in the HIV-1 principal neutralizing determinant. Science 1990;249:932–935.

80. Simmonds P, Balfe P, Ludham CA, Bishop JO, Brown AJL. Analysis of sequence diversity in hypervariable regions of the external glycoprotein of human immunodeficiency virus type I. J Virol 1990;64:5840–5850.

81. Hahn BH, Shaw GM, Taylor ME, et al. Genetic variation in HTLV-III/LAV over time in patients with AIDS or at risk for AIDS. Science 1986;231: 1548–1553.

82. Saag MS, Hahn BH, Gibbons J, et al. Extensive variation of human immunodeficiency virus type-1 *in vivo*. Nature 1988;334:440–444.

83. Meyerhans A, Cheynier R, Albert J, et al. Temporal fluctuations in HIV quasispecies *in vivo* are not reflected by sequential HIV isolations. Cell 1988;58:901–910.

84. Cichutek K, Merget H, Norley S, et al. Development of a quasispecies of human immunodeficiency virus type 1 *in vivo*. Proc Natl Acad Sci USA 1992;89:7365–7369.

85. Pang S, Schlesinger Y, Daar ES, Moudgil T, Ho DD, Chen ISY. Rapid generation of sequence variation during primary HIV-1 infection. AIDS 1992;6:453–460.

86. Fisher AG, Ensoli B, Looney D, et al. Biologically diverse molecular variants within a single HIV-1 isolate. Nature 1988;334:444–447.

87. Sakai K, Dewhurst S, Ma X, Volsky D. Differences in cytopathicity and host cell range among infectious molecular clones of human immunodeficiency virus type 1 simultaneously isolated from an infected individual. J Virol 1988;62:4078–4085.

88. Fenyö EM, Morfeldt-Månson L, Chiodi F, et al. Distinct replicative and cytopathic characteristics of human immunodeficiency virus isolates. J Virol 1988;62:4414–4419.

89. Fouchier RAM, Groenink M, Kootstra NA, et al. Phenotype-associated sequence variation in the third variable domain of human immunodeficiency virus type 1 gp120 molecule. J Virol 1992; 66:3183–3187.

90. Andeweg AC, Groenink M, Leeflang P, et al. Genetic and functional analysis of a set of HIV-1 envelope genes obtained from biological clones with varying syncytium-inducing capacities. AIDS Res Hum Retroviruses 1992;8:1803–1813.

91. DeJong J-J, Goudsmit J, Keulen W, et al. Human immunodeficiency virus type 1 clones chimeric for the envelope V3 domain differ in syncytium formation and replication capacity. J Virol 1992; 66:757–765.

92. Tersmette M, De Goede REY, Al BJM, et al. Differential syncytium-inducing capacity of human immunodeficiency virus isolates: Frequent detection of syncytium-inducing isolates in patients with acquired immunodeficiency syndrome (AIDS) and AIDS-related complex. J Virol 1988; 62:2026–2032.

93. Tersmette M, Gruters RA, DeWolf F, et al. Evidence for a role of virulent human immunodeficiency virus (HIV) variants in the pathogenesis of acquired immunodeficiency syndrome: Studies on sequential HIV isolates. J Virol 1989;63:2118–2125.

94. Schuitemaker H, Koot M, Kootstra NA, et al. Biological phenotype of human immunodeficiency virus type 1 clones at different stages of infection: Progression of disease is associated with a shift from monocytotropic to T-cell-tropic virus populations. J Virol 1992;66:1354–1360.

95. Fujita K, Silver J, Peden K. Changes in both gp120 and gp41 can account for increased growth potential and expanded host range of human immunodeficiency virus type 1. J Virol 1992;66: 4445–4451.

96. Groenink M, Andeweg AC, Fouchier RAM, et al. Phenotype-associated env gene variation among eight related human immunodeficiency virus type 1 clones: Evidence for in vivo recombination and determinants of cytotropism outside the V3 domain. J Virol 1992;66:6175–6180.

97. Cheng-Meyer C, Shioda T, Levy JA. Host range, replicative, and cytopathic properties of human immunodeficiency virus type 1 are determined by very few amino acid changes in tat and gp120. J Virol 1991;65:6931–6941.

98. Kim S, Ikeuchi K, Groopman J, Baltimore D. Factors affecting cellular tropism of human immunodeficiency virus. J Virol 1990;64:5600–5604.

99. Cann AJ, Zack JA, Go AS, et al. Human immunodeficiency virus type 1 T-cell tropism is determined by events prior to provirus formation. J Virol 1990;64:4735–4742.

100. Cheng-Meyer C, Quiroga M, Tung JW, Dina D, Levy JA. Viral determinants of human immunodeficiency virus type 1 T-cell or macrophage tropism, cytopathicity and CD4 antigen modulation. J Virol 1990;64:4390–4398.

101. York-Higgins D, Cheng-Meyer C, Bauer D, Levy JA, Dina D. Human immunodeficiency virus type 1 cellular host range, replication, and cytopathicity are linked to the envelope region of the viral genome. J Virol 1990;64:4016–4020.

102. Liu ZQ, Wood C, Levy JA, Cheng-Meyer C. The viral envelope gene is involved in macrophage tropism of a human immunodeficiency virus type 1 strain isolated from brain tissue. J Virol 1990; 64:6148–6153.

103. O'Brien WA, Koyanagi Y, Namazie A, et al. HIV-1 tropism for mononuclear phagocytes can be determined by regions of gp120 outside the CD4-binding domain. Nature 1990;348:69–73.

104. Shioda T, Levy JA, Cheng-Meyer C. Macrophage and T cell-line tropism of HIV-1 are determined by specific regions of the envelope gp120 gene. Nature 1991;349:167–169.

105. Westervelt P, Trowbridge DB, Epstein LG, et al. Macrophage tropism determinants of human immunodeficiency virus type 1 in vivo. J Virol 1992; 66:2577–2582.

106. Moore JP, Nara PL. The role of the V3 loop og gp120 in HIV infection. AIDS 1991;5(suppl 2): S21–S33.

107. Adachi A, Koenig S, Gendelman HE, et al. Productive, persistent infection of human colorectal cell lines with human immunodeficiency virus. J Virol 1987;61:209–213.

108. Cheng-Meyer C, Rutka JT, Rosenblum ML, McHugh T, Stites Dp, Levy JA. Human immunodeficiency virus can productively infect cultured human glial cells. Proc Natl Acad Sci USA 1987;84:3526–3530.

109. Clapham PR, Weber JN, Whitby D, el al. Soluble CD4 blocks the infectivity of diverse strains of HIV and SIV for T cells and monocytes but not for brain and muscle cells. Nature 1989;337: 368–370.

110. Folks TM, Kessler SW, Orenstein JM, Justement JS, Jaffe ES, Fauci AS. Infection and replication of HIV-1 in purified progenitor cells of normal human bone marrow. Science 1988;242:919–922.

111. Harouse JM, Kunsch C, Hartle HT, et al. CD4-independent infection of human neural cells by human immunodeficiency virus type 1. J Virol 1989;63:2527–2533.

112. Monroe JE, Calender A, Mulder C. Epstein-Barr virus-positive and -negative B cell lines can be infected with human immunodeficiency virus types 1 and 2. J Virol 1988;62:3497–3500.

113. Nelson JA, Wiley CA, Reynolds-Kohler C, Reese CE, Margaretten W, Levy JA. Human immunodeficiency virus detected in bowel epithelium from patients with gastrointestinal symptoms. Lancet 1988;1:259–262.

114. Moyer MP, Huot RI, Ramirez A, Joe S, Meltzer MS, Gendelman HE. Infection of human gastrointestinal cells by HIV-1. AIDS Res Hum Retroviruses 1990;6:1409–1415.

115. Pomerantz RJ, Kuritzkes DR, de la Monte SM, et al. Infection of the retina by human immunodeficiency virus type 1. New Engl J Med 1987;317:1643–1647.

116. Pomerantz RJ, de la Monte SM, Donegan SP, et al. Human immunodeficiency virus (HIV) infection of the uterine cervix. Ann Intern Med 1988;108:321–327.

117. Wiley CA, Schrier RD, Nelson JA, Lampert PW, Oldstone MBA. Cellular localization of human immunodeficiency virus infection within the brains of acquired immune deficiency syndrome patients. Proc Natl Acad Sci USA 1986;83:7089–7093.

118. Schnittman SM, Psallidopoulos MC, Lane HC, et al. The reservoir for HIV-1 in human peripheral blood is a T cell that maintains expression of CD4. Science 1989;245:305–308.

119. McElrath MJ, Pruett JE, Cohn ZA. Mononuclear phagocytes of blood and bone marrow: Comparative roles as viral reservoirs in human immunodeficiency virus type 1 infections. Proc Natl Acad Sci USA 1989;86:675–679.

120. Ho DD, Rota TR, Hirsch MS. Infection of monocyte/macrophages by human T lymphotropic virus type III. J Clin Invest 1986;77:1712–1714.

121. Tenner-Racz K, Racz P, Dietrich M, Kern P. Altered follicular dendritic cells and virus-like particles in AIDS and AIDS-related lymphadenopathy. Lancet 1985;1:105–106.

122. Koenig S, Gendelman H, Orenstein J, et al. Detection of AIDS virus in macrophages in brain tissue from AIDS patients with encephalopathy. Science 1986;233:1089–1093.

123. Gartner S, Markovits P, Markovitz DM, Betts RF, Popovic M. Virus isolation from and identification of HTLV-III/LAV-producing cells in brain tissue from a patient with AIDS. JAMA 1986;256:2365–2371.

124. Salahuddin SZ, Rose RM, Groopman JE, Markham PD, Gallo RC. Human T lymphotropic virus type III infection of human alveolar macrophages. Blood 1986;68:281–284.

125. Braathen LR, Ramirez G, Kunze ROF, Gelderblom H. Langerhans' cells as primary target cells for HIV infection. Lancet 1987;2:1094.

126. Niedecken H, Lutz G, Bauer R, Kreysel HW. Langerhans' cell as primary target and vehicle for transmission of HIV. Lancet 1987;2:519–520.

127. Rappersberger K, Gartner S, Schenk P, et al. Langerhans' cells are an actual site of HIV-1 replication. Intervirology 1988;29:185–194.

128. Collman R, Godfrey B, Cutilli J, et al. Macrophage-tropic strains of human immunodeficiency virus type 1 utilize the CD4 receptor. J Virol 1990;64:4468–4476.

129. Narayan O, Wolinsky JS, Clements JE, Strandberg JD, Griffin DE, Cork LC. Slow virus replication: The role of macrophages in the persistence and expression of visna viruses of sheep and goats. J Gen Virol 1982;59:345–356.

130. Gendelman HE, Narayan O, Kennedy-Stoskopf S, et al. Tropism of sheep lentiviruses for monocytes: Susceptibility to infection and virus gene expression increase during maturation of monocytes to macrophages. J Virol 1986;58:67–74.

131. Koyanagi Y, O'Brien WA, Zhao JQ, Golde DW, Gasson JC, Chen ISY. Cytokines alter production of HIV-1 from primary mononuclear phagocytes. Science 1988;241:1673–1675.

132. Perno C-F, Yarochan R, Cooney DA, et al. Replication of human immunodeficiency virus in monocytes. Granulocyte/macrophage colony stimulating factor (GM-CSF) potentiates virus production yet enhances the antviral effect mediated by 3'-azido-2'3'-dideoxythymidine (AZT) and other dideoxynucleoside congeners of thymidine. J Exp Med 1989;169:933–951.

133. Kornbluth RS, Oh PS, Munis JR, Cleveland PH, Richman DD. The role of interferons in the control of HIV replication in macrophages. Clin Immunol Immunopathol 1990;54:200–219.

134. Poli G, Bressler P, Kinter A, et al. Interleukin 6 induces human immunodeficiency virus expression in infected monocytic cells alone and in synergy with tumor necrosis factor α by transcriptional and post-transcriptional mechanisms. J Exp Med 1990;172:151–158.

135. Gendelman HE, Orenstein JM, Baca LM, et al. The macrophage in the persistence and pathogenesis of HIV infection. AIDS 1989;3:475–495.

136. Orenstein JM, Meltzer MS, Phipps T, Gendelman HE. Cytoplasmic assembly and accumulation of human immunodeficiency virus types 1 and 2 in recombinant human colony-stimulating factor-1-treated human monocytes: An ultrastructural study. J Virol 1988;62:2578–2586.

137. Barre-Sinoussi F, Chermann JC, Rey F, et al. Isolation of a T-lymphotropic retrovirus from a patient at risk for acquired immune deficiency syndrome (AIDS). Science 1983;220:868–871.

138. Baroni CD, Pezzella F, Mirolo M, Ruco LP, Rossi GB. Immunohistochemical demonstration of p24 HTLV-III major core protein in different cell types within lymph nodes from patients with lymphadenopathy syndrome (LAS). Histopathology 1986;10:5–13.

139. Le Tourneau A, Audouin J, Diebold J, Marche C, Tricottet V, Reynes M. LAV-like viral particles in lymph node germinal centers in patients with the persistent lymphadenopathy syndrome and the acquired immunodeficiency syndrome-related complex: An ultrastructural study of 30 cases. Hum Pathol 1986;17:1047–1053.

140. Armstrong JA, Horne R. Follicular dendritic cells and virus-like particles in AIDS-related lymphadenopathy. Lancet 1984;2:370–372.

141. Plata, F, Autran B, Martins LP, et al. AIDS virus-specific cytotoxic T lymphocytes in lung disorders. Nature 1987;328:348–351.

142. Price RW, Brew B, Sidtis J, Rosenblum M, Scheck AC, Cleary P. The brain in AIDS: Central nervous system HIV-1 infection and AIDS dementia complex. Science 1988;239:586–592.

143. Orenstein JM, Janotta F. Human immunodeficiency virus and papova virus infections in acquired immunodeficiency syndrome: An ultrastructural study of three cases. Hum Pathol 1988;19:350–361.

144. Gabuzda DH, Ho DD, de la Monte SM, Hirsch MS, Rota TR, Sobel RA. Immunohistochemical identification of HTLV-III antigen in the brains of patients infected with AIDS. Ann Neurol 1986;20:289–295.

145. Vazeux R, Brousse N, Jarry A, et al. AIDS subacute encephalitis. Identification of HIV-infected cells. Am J Pathol 1987;126:403–410.

146. Pumarola-Sune T, Navia BA, Cordon-Cardo C, Cho ES, Price RW. HIV antigen in the brains of patients with the AIDS dementia complex. Ann Neurol 1987;21:490–496.

147. Levy JA, Shimabukuro J, Hollander H, Mills J, Kaminsky L. Isolation of AIDS-associated retroviruses from cerebrospinal fluid and brains of patients with neurological symptoms. Lancet 1985;2:586–588.

148. Ho DD, Rota TR, Schooley RT, et al. Isolation of HLTV-III from cerebrospinal fluid and neural tissues of patients with neurologic syndromes related to the acquired immunodeficiency syndrome. N Engl J Med 1985;313:1493–1497.

149. Stoler MH, Eskin TA, Benn S, Angerer RC, Angerer LM. Human T-cell lymphotropic virus type III infection of the central nervous system. A preliminary in situ analysis. JAMA 1986;256:2360–2364.

150. Gyorkey F, Melnick JL, Gyorkey P. Human immunodeficiency virus in brain biopsies of patients with AIDS and progressive encephalopathy. J Infect Dis 1987;155:870–876.

151. Sethi KK, Naher H, Stroehmann I. Phenotypic heterogeneity of cerebrospinal fluid-derived HIV-specific and HLA-restricted cytotoxic T-cell clones. Nature 1988;335:178–181.

152. Wiley CA, Nelson JA. Role of human immunodeficiency virus and cytomegalovirus in AIDS encephalitis. Am J Pathol 1988;133:73–81.

153. Nelson JA, Reynolds-Kohler C, Oldstone MB, Wiley CA. HIV and HCMV coinfect brain cells in patients with AIDS. Virology 1988;165:286–290.

154. Koyanagi Y, Miles S, Mitsuyasu RT, Merrill JE, Vinters HV, Chen ISY. Dual infection of the central nervous system by AIDS viruses with distinct cellular tropisms. Science 1987;236:819–822.

155. Harper ME, Marselle LM, Gallo RC, Wong-Staal F. Detection of lymphocytes expressing human T-lymphotropic virus type III in lymph nodes and peripheral blood from infected individual by in situ hybridization. Proc Natl Acad Sci USA 1986; 83:772–776.

156. Ho DD, Moudgil T, Alam M. Quantitation of human immunodeficiency virus type 1 in the blood of infected persons. N Engl J Med 1989; 321:1621–1625.

157. Simmonds P, Balfe P, Peutherer JF, Ludlam CA, Bishop JO, Leigh Brown AJ. Human immunodeficiency virus-infected individuals contain provirus in small numbers of peripheral mononuclear cells and at low copy numbers. J Virol 1990;64:864–872.

158. Brinchmann JE, Albert J, Vartdal F. Few infected CD4+ T cells but a high proportion of replication-competent provirus copies in asymptomatic human immunodeficiency virus type 1 infection. J Virol 1991;65:2019–2023.

159. Goudsmit J, de Wolf F, Paul DA, et al. Expression of human immunodeficiency virus antigen (HIV-Ag) in serum and cerebrospinal fluid during acute and chronic infection. Lancet 1986;2:177–180.

160. Daar ES, Moudgil T, Meyer RD, Ho DD. Transient high levels of viremia in patients with primary human immunodeficiency virus type 1 infection. N Engl J Med 1991;324:961–964.

161. Srugo I, Brunell PA, Chelyapov NV, Ho DD, Alam M, Israele V. Virus burden in human immunodeficiency virus type 1-infected children: Relationship to disease status and effect of antiviral therapy. Pediatrics 1991;87:921–925.

162. Alimenti A, Luzuriaga K, Stechenberg B, Sullivan JL. Quantitation of human immunodeficiency virus in vertically infected infants and children. J Pediatr 1991;119:225–229.

163. Alimenti A, O'Neill M, Sullivan JL, Luzuriaga K. Diagnosis of vertical human immunodeficiency virus type 1 infection by whole blood culture. J Infect Dis 1992;166:1146–1148.

164. Saag MS, Crain MJ, Decker WD, et al. High-level viremia in adults and children infected with human immunodeficiency virus: Relation to disease stage and CD4+ lymphocyte levels. J Infect Dis 1991;164:72–80.

165. McCune JM. HIV-1: The infective process in vivo. Cell 1991;64:351–363.

166. Krivine A, Firtion G, Cao L, Francoual C, Henvion R, Lebon P. HIV replication during the first few weeks of life. Lancet 1992;339:1187–1189.

8
Immunopathology and Pathogenesis of HIV Infection

Zeda F. Rosenberg and Anthony S. Fauci

The common denominator of infection with human immunodeficiency virus (HIV) in children and adults is a profound immunosuppression, rendering the host susceptible to the development of various opportunistic infections and neoplasms. The virus also exerts other direct and indirect effects on the host that may be particularly dramatic in infants and children because of the ongoing developmental stages of different organ systems such as the central nervous system. This chapter focuses on the immunopathogenesis of HIV infection.

Initial infection with HIV in older children and adults can be either asymptomatic or result in an acute, self-limiting mononucleosis-like syndrome occurring 2–4 weeks after initial infection and resolving within 1–2 weeks (1, 2). Both the acute HIV syndrome and asymptomatic infection are followed by production of anti-HIV antibodies, which usually appear 6–12 weeks after infection. After seroconversion, an asymptomatic phase exists that, in adults, may span from several months to years, with a median clinical latency estimated at ~11 years (3). Some perinatally infected infants may fail to produce significant levels of anti-HIV antibody after the loss of maternal antibodies and may be at higher risk for developing AIDS (4). Retrospective studies of children with AIDS who were infected perinatally with HIV suggested that the median time to the onset of clinical symptoms was between 5 and 10 months (5–7). The longest asymptomatic period reported in these studies was

7.3 years. As the time since HIV first appeared in the pediatric population has lengthened, prospective natural history studies have suggested that ~80% of children develop symptoms by the time they are 2 years old. The duration of survival has increased with the introduction of therapy and supportive care.

Much is known about the cells that HIV infects and the mechanism of virus entry into the cell. Relatively little is known, however, about how HIV exerts its pathogenic effect. This chapter discusses the current hypotheses of how infection with HIV ultimately causes destruction of a specific population of T lymphocytes, the CD4+ T helper/inducer subset of cells. In addition, the chapter presents several potential mechanisms whereby HIV causes a functional impairment of otherwise healthy cells. One major unresolved area in the immunopathogenesis of HIV infection is progression of disease from an asymptomatic infection to full-blown immunosuppression and AIDS. This chapter will, therefore, review the current understanding of how factors that can activate immune cells may also activate HIV expression in these cells.

TARGET CELLS FOR HIV
Infection of CD4-positive T Cells

It was observed early in the AIDS epidemic that adult AIDS patients experienced a dramatic decline in the absolute number of circulating CD4+ T cells and in the ratio

115

of CD4+ T to CD8+ T cells (8, 9). This observation, in combination with isolation of HIV from the blood of patients with AIDS (10–12), focussed attention on the CD4+ T cell as the principal target of HIV infection in vivo. HIV was subsequently shown to infect and replicate in CD4+ T cells in culture and to cause a rapid and profound cytopathic effect in these cells (13, 14). Not all cells that are infected with HIV, however, are killed by the virus. Some cells survive acute infection in vitro and have been shown to sustain a low-level chronic infection (15, 16). Factors involved in the conversion of a latent or chronic infection to an active one are discussed below.

The preferential infection of CD4+ T cells by HIV in culture is due to the presence of the CD4 molecule on the surface of the CD4+ T cells (17–19). During normal immune responses, the CD4 molecule binds to its natural ligand, the class II major histocompatibility complex (MHC) molecule, on the surface of antigen-presenting cells (20, 21). The CD4 molecule also functions as a high-affinity receptor for HIV by binding tightly to the external envelope glycoprotein (gp120) of HIV (Fig. 8.1). The affinity of gp120 for CD4 is greater than that of the MHC class II molecule (17–19). Although various cells other than CD4+ T cells may express CD4 and be infected by

HIV (see below), it is the destruction of the CD4+ T cell by HIV that results in the profound immunosuppression characteristic of AIDS. Because of the critical role of CD4+ T cells in induction of the intricate network of immune responses in vivo, the elimination of this one specific subset of cells has devastating consequences. The mechanisms by which HIV can destroy CD4+ T cells are discussed below.

HIV Infection of Monocytes and Macrophages

As a member of the lentivirus subgroup of retroviruses, HIV maintains the ability to infect cells of monocytic lineage that have been shown to express CD4 on their surface (22). In vitro, HIV has been shown to infect monocytic and promyelocytic cell lines, peripheral blood monocytes, and alveolar macrophages. In HIV-infected individuals, HIV has been found in peripheral blood monocytes and in macrophages from both the lung and brain (reviewed in Ref. 23). In comparison with the decline in CD4+ T cells that occurs during HIV infection, the number of monocytes and macrophages does not appear to be affected. Several factors may explain this apparent paradox. First, relatively few HIV-infected monocytes can be detected in the peripheral blood of HIV-infected indi-

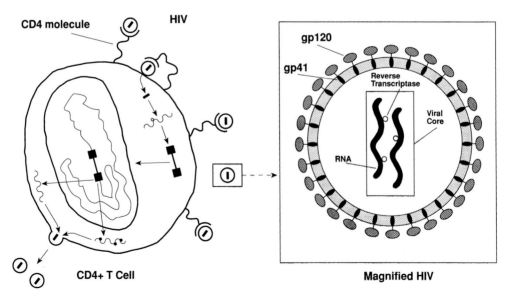

Figure 8.1.   Binding of HIV envelope glycoprotein (gp120) to CD4 receptor that is present on surface of CD4+ T lymphocytes. Adapted from Ref. 23.

viduals (24, 25). In addition, HIV-infected peripheral blood monocytes have been identified in only a small proportion of HIV-infected individuals (24, 26). Second, HIV-infected monocytes and macrophages are not necessarily killed by the virus. It has been demonstrated that HIV-infection of monocytes and macrophages in vitro is associated with a much reduced cytopathic effect when compared with HIV infection of CD4+ T cells (reviewed in Ref. 23).

The role of monocyte and macrophage in immunopathogenesis of HIV infection is unclear. However, it is thought that the HIV-infected monocyte and macrophage may function as a reservoir of virus infection in various organs of the body (27). Depending on the level of cellular differentiation of the monocyte and macrophage, HIV may replicate predominantly intracellularly, within cytoplasmic vacuoles (28, 29). As a result, the virus may be shielded from the immune system and be carried by the infected monocyte and macrophage to different organs of the body, particularly the brain and lung. HIV-infected monocytes and macrophages may also be involved in the spread of HIV to CD4+ T cells. Since cell to cell transmission of HIV from intracellular HIV particles in an infected monocytoid line to T cells has been demonstrated (30), HIV may be transmitted in vivo from HIV-infected macrophages to CD4+ T cells during cellular interactions that normally occur during immune responses.

Infection of Other Cell Types

Owing to the high affinity of HIV gp120 for CD4, any cell in the body that expresses CD4 can potentially be infected by HIV. In vivo, HIV has been detected in epidermal Langerhans' cells, dendritic cells, megakaryocytes, microglia, astrocytes and oligodendroglia, cardiac myocytes, and cells from the retina, renal epithelium, cervix, and rectal mucosa (reviewed in Refs. 23, 31–34). The list of human cells that have been reported to be infected with HIV in vitro is extensive and ranges from B cell lines and colorectal cells to cervical cells and choroid plexus cells (reviewed in Ref. 35). In most of these studies cell lines and not primary cells were infected, bringing into question the physiologic relevance of these observations. The

presence of CD4 protein on the surface of cells that can be infected by HIV has been demonstrated in most cases. However, there have been several reports of HIV infection of cells that do not express detectable levels of CD4, including glial and muscle tumor cells, fibroblastoid cell lines, and primary fetal neural cells (reviewed in Refs. 35, 36). Recent studies have found that galactosyl ceramide is important for HIV infection of CD4– neural and colon epithelial cells (37–39). Although these data suggest that another receptor may be involved in HIV infection of a minor population of cells, the preponderance of evidence establishes CD4 as the principal receptor for HIV and the CD4+ T cell as the primary target cell for HIV infection in vivo.

Infection of Placental and Fetal Tissues

Maury et al. (40) have reported that placental tissue from both first trimester and term placentas expresses CD4 and can be infected by HIV in vitro. Unfortunately, most studies have used placental preparations with a mixture of cell types, making it less certain precisely which cells express CD4 (see Chapter 10A). CD4-negative human transformed trophoblast-derived cells and primary trophoblast cultures can also be infected by HIV or HIV-infected cells in vitro (41–43). Additional studies are at variance because some have determined that placental trophoblasts express CD4 and are susceptible to HIV infection (44, 45), whereas others have found that syncytiotrophoblasts were negative for CD4 (45a). Studies of tissues from 8-week aborted fetuses from HIV-infected women show that HIV could be cultured from trophoblastic and villous Hofbauer cells and hematological precursor cells (46). HIV antigens and nucleic acids are present in the trophoblasts of a few placentas from HIV-infected women (47). However, in another report, HIV antigens were detected solely in placental cells with macrophage-like morphology (48).

The precise timing of maternal to fetal transmission of HIV is not known. The ability to culture HIV or detect HIV DNA in fetal tissue from fetuses during the first and second trimesters of pregnancy suggests that HIV transmission from mother to fetus may occur early in gestation (46, 49). However, other studies have failed to detect either HIV or HIV DNA in fetuses or in most infected infants at birth, suggesting that mother to infant transmission also may occur at or near the time of delivery (50). Twin studies that show a greater chance of the firstborn twin of an HIV-infected mother becoming infected compared with the second born twin suggest that transmission of HIV infection may occur perinatally (51). The precise route(s) of infection of the fetus during maternal to fetal transmission is unknown. The absence of CD4 on syncytiotrophoblasts suggests that binding of HIV to non-CD4 molecules might also be involved in transplacental infection (see Chapter 10A) (40, 43).

Infection of Lymphoid Tissue and Lymphoid Precursor Cells

High levels of HIV have been detected in lymphoid organs from HIV-infected individuals (52). Levels of HIV expression in lymphoid tissue are significantly higher than that observed in the peripheral blood at all stages of infection. Most HIV in lymphoid tissue is not found within infected lymphocytes but is trapped extracellularly within the network of follicular dendritic cells (reviewed in Ref. 53). Since HIV infection of CD4+ T cells may occur within lymphoid tissue, lymphoid organs may serve as the principal reservoir of HIV in the body.

HIV infection of lymphoid precursor cells in the bone marrow and the thymus has been proposed to explain the lack of CD4+ T cell replacement over the course of HIV infection and the presence of hematologic abnormalities in HIV-infected patients (reviewed in Ref. 23) (Fig. 8.2). Although HIV infection of normal human bone marrow progenitor cells has been observed in vitro (reviewed in Ref. 54), in vivo studies have not generated consistently positive findings (54, 55). HIV infection of immature CD4+/CD8+ thymic lymphocytes as well as CD3–/CD4–/CD8– intrathymic T cell precursors has been reported (56, 57). In addition, human fetal thymocytes and mature thymocytes from infants and children can be productively infected with HIV (58–60). However, similar to the in vivo bone marrow studies, in vivo HIV infection of thymuses from aborted fetuses of pregnant HIV-seropositive women has not been consistently observed (49, 61).

MECHANISMS OF CD4+ T CELL DEPLETION
Direct Virus-induced Cytopathicity

Several observations in vivo have led to the assumption that HIV is directly responsible for the loss of CD4+ T cells that invari-

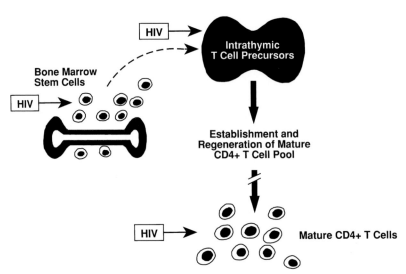

Figure 8.2. HIV infection of lymphoid precursor cells in bone marrow and thymus may explain lack of regeneration of mature CD4+ T cells that are also targets for HIV.

ably occurs over the course of HIV disease. During primary HIV infection, there is a direct association between the level of HIV replication in the peripheral blood and a decline in the number of circulating CD4+ T cells (62–64). In addition, the level of HIV in the plasma as well as the proportion of HIV-infected circulating CD4+ cells is higher in individuals who are symptomatic compared with asymptomatic individuals (reviewed in Refs. 54, 65–71). Similar findings have also been found in prospective studies of HIV-infected individuals (72, 73).

HIV can rapidly kill CD4+ T cells in vitro via several potential mechanisms (reviewed in Ref. 23). The first is through production of large numbers of HIV particles that bud from the external cell membrane. The presence of HIV proteins and budding virus particles may result in the disruption of the cell membrane, leading to osmotic disequilibrium and cell death. Second, the process of HIV replication can result in the accumulation of high levels of unintegrated viral DNA and heterodisperse RNAs and the production of large amounts of virus core protein. The presence of these foreign products in the cell may interfere with normal cellular functions and lead to cell death.

Several researchers have demonstrated that both gp120 and CD4 may be important in cell death (reviewed in Ref. 23). It has been hypothesized that production of HIV envelope glycoprotein within the cell may result in the complexing of gp120 to intracellular CD4 molecules that could interfere with cell function. It is unclear whether any of these mechanisms are involved in cell death in vivo.

Indirect Cell Killing

The potential mechanisms of direct HIV-induced cytopathicity described above are based on the premise that significant levels of virus replication must occur within a cell before a cytopathic effect will be manifested. However, there are several indirect ways in which uninfected CD4+ T cells or cells that are expressing only low levels of HIV may be killed. The formation of multinucleated giant cells, or syncytia, between HIV-infected CD4+ T cells and uninfected CD4+ T cells has been observed during cy-topathic infections in vitro (reviewed in Ref. 23). These short-lived syncytia form through binding of CD4 molecules on the surface of uninfected CD4+ T cells to the gp120 molecules that are expressed on the surface of HIV-infected CD4+ T cells. The role of syncytia formation in the loss of CD4+ T cells in vivo is unclear. Syncytia are rarely seen in vivo; CD4+ T cells can be killed by HIV in vitro without syncytia formation, and syncytia formation can occur in the absence of cell death (reviewed in Ref. 23).

Uninfected CD4+ T cells may be destroyed through a process in which these cells are mistakenly identified as being infected and are killed as a result of antibody-dependent cellular cytotoxicity. "Innocent" bystander CD4+ T cells may become targets for antibody-dependent cellular cytotoxicity by the passive binding of free gp120 to their surface CD4 molecules (74). It has also been shown that uninfected CD4+ T cells can capture and process soluble gp120 and function as class II MHC restricted antigen-presenting cells. These CD4+ T cells that express the processed gp120 peptides have been shown in vitro to be susceptible to killing by CD4+ gp120-specific cytotoxic T cells (75, 76).

Binding of gp120 to CD4 may also be the basis for the generation of autoimmune reactions that can destroy CD4+ T cells. Since the natural ligand for CD4 is the class II MHC molecule, the binding of both class II MHC and gp120 to CD4 must be due to the presence of shared antigenic determinants (reviewed in Ref. 23). The HIV transmembrane glycoprotein, gp41, has also been shown to possess a region of homology with class II MHC. Anti-HIV antibodies from AIDS patients can react with class II MHC antigens and may be involved in antibody-dependent cellular cytotoxicity or complement-mediated cell killing.

Superantigens have recently been invoked as a potential mechanism for CD4+ T cell depletion. In a mouse retroviral model, it has been shown that a virally encoded superantigen can stimulate proliferation and expansion of subsets of T cells bearing specific T cell receptor ß-chain variable (Vß) regions (77). Recently, it has been shown that HIV replicates up to 100-fold more efficiently in T cell lines that express specific ß-chain variables and that cells in vivo that expressed these same ß-chain variables were more likely to express HIV proteins (78). It is more likely that superantigens in HIV-infected individuals are not directly responsible for deletion of T cell subsets but rather activate T cells, rendering them more susceptible to HIV infection (Fig. 8.3). Evidence for the deletion of CD4+ T cells bearing specific ß-chain variables is uncertain (78–80).

Apoptosis or programmed cell death has recently been introduced as a potential mechanism to explain the death of CD4+ T cells that may not directly be infected with HIV (81). It has been hypothesized that apoptosis, which is the normal pathway for elimination of autoreactive T cell clones from the immature thymocyte population (82, 83), is inappropriately initiated in CD4+ T cells in HIV-infected individuals. Initiation of apoptosis may be caused by cross-linking of the CD4 receptor via the binding of gp120 alone or complexes of gp120 bound to anti-gp120 anti-bodies. Apoptosis may then be triggered by subsequent antigenic stimulation of the T cell receptor as has been shown in CD4+ T cells from asymptomatic HIV-infected individuals (81, 84). In addition, acute HIV infection of lymphoblastoid cells or activated peripheral blood mononuclear cells results in apoptosis in vitro (85, 86). Because it has been reported that both CD4+ and CD8+ T cells from asymptomatic HIV-infected individuals spontaneously undergo apoptosis in vitro (84, 87, 88), additional studies are needed to delineate the mechanism of apoptosis and its relevance to CD4+ T cell depletion in HIV infection.

QUALITATIVE ABNORMALITIES OF IMMUNE CELLS IN HIV INFECTION

Infection with HIV not only causes a depletion of CD4+ T cells but can interfere with immune cell function in adults and children before CD4+ T cell loss. Note that median CD4+ T cell counts in infants and children are considerably higher (ranging from 1.8 to 2.95×10^9/liter depending on age of child) than the corresponding levels in adults (89). As a result, children with AIDS frequently present with CD4+ T lymphocyte counts that are substantially higher than those observed in adult AIDS patients (89a). Before recognition of higher levels of CD4+ T cells in healthy children, it was felt that HIV-induced functional abnormalities of immunocompetent cells were more important in HIV-induced immunosuppression in children vs. adults. Qualitative defects in immunologic function may occur to the same degree in children and adults.

Investigators have reported a wide range of functional abnormalities of CD4+ T cells that are present in various stages of HIV infection. Because HIV has been shown to be present in only a small percentage of circulating CD4+ T cells, mechanisms other than direct infection must be operative to explain the existence of a generalized HIV-induced functional defect. In this regard, numerous investigators have shown that exposure of T cells to HIV proteins, in the form of killed virus-infected cells, killed virus, or soluble envelope glycoproteins, can result in an inhibition of prolif-

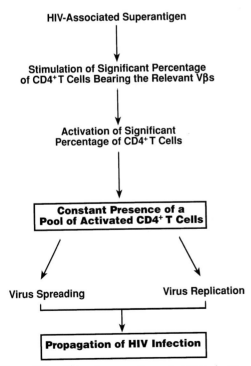

Figure 8.3. Role of superantigens in HIV infection in establishment of a pool of activated CD4+ T cells that are highly susceptible to HIV infection and viral replication. *Vß*, ß-chain variable.

erative responses to T cell activation factors such as mitogens and antigens (reviewed in Ref. 23).

The high-affinity binding of HIV gp120 to CD4 may be responsible for the generation of impaired T cell responses during HIV infection. For example, binding of gp120 to CD4 on the surface of CD4+ T cells may interfere with the interaction of class II MHC molecules with CD4 that occurs in antigen presentation during normal immune responses. Alternatively, the binding of HIV gp120 to CD4 may interfere with transduction of signals that occur after binding of ligands to either the CD4 or antigen receptor complex (27). It has also been suggested that HIV gp120 may interfere with the binding of interleukin (IL)-2 to the IL-2 receptor because of the fact that a region of homology exists between gp120 and IL-2 (90). In these three potential mechanisms, infection of T cells is not necessary for induction of impaired responses since defective HIV virions or soluble gp120 may also bind to CD4.

Infection with HIV may also result in a decreased level of expression of CD4 on the surface of the infected CD4+ T cell that would prohibit effective CD4-class II MHC interactions. It has been observed in vitro that HIV-infected CD4+ T cells exhibit decreased levels of CD4 on their surfaces. Infection with HIV has also been associated with decreased expression of other cell surface molecules, including CD3, CD8, IL-2 receptor, IL-2, class II MHC, and class I MHC (reviewed in Ref. 23). Because these molecules are important during typical T cell responses, HIV-induced suppression of their expression may result in an impairment of CD4+ T cell function.

Like HIV-infected adults, the immunological function of HIV-infected children also is significantly impaired and may contribute to the cause of disease progression. It has been hypothesized that the timing of HIV infection of infants in utero may impact the normal ontogenic development of T cells, thus causing a greater impairment of immunity than infection in the adult (91). This may be due at least in part to a tolerance and/or deletion of HIV-reactive clones of immune competent cells.

ACTIVATION OF LATENT HIV INFECTION

Infection with HIV in vivo is characterized by an asymptomatic state that can last for many years in adults. Although HIV can be cultured from peripheral blood cells from individuals during this period, virus replication, as measured by the presence of HIV core p24 antigen in the peripheral blood or plasma viremia, occurs at significantly lower levels than during the symptomatic stage of disease. In children and adults, persistence of HIV p24 is highly prognostic of disease progression (92, 93). These data suggest that, for variable periods after infection with HIV, virus replication is restricted to chronic, low-level expression (see also Chapter 7). A shift from restricted to active replication presumably occurs after an indeterminate time. Although very little is known about the events that occur in vivo to initiate changes in the level of viral expression, a substantial body of in vitro data suggests that activation of CD4+ T cells by various factors may be key in the induction of HIV expression (Fig. 8.4). In this regard, HIV infection of resting T cells results in incomplete reverse transcription of viral RNA and the accumulation of labile, partial DNA transcripts. The reverse transcriptase process is completed, and virus replication occurs upon activation of these infected resting cells (94).

Infants infected perinatally with HIV generally experience a relatively shorter latent period between infection and disease than adults. The reason for this difference in the rate of disease progression is unknown. It has been hypothesized that HIV infection may progress more rapidly in infants if the timing of transmission in utero coincides with the period of rapid expansion of CD4+ immunocompetent cells in the fetus (91). Such an expansion would allow for the spread of HIV into most immunocompetent cells, whose normal migration between the marrow, spleen, and thymus could result in the spread of HIV throughout the body. The absence of a mature immune system in the infant may augment the unchecked spread of the virus. Thus, activation of HIV infection in the perinatally infected infant could result in a much more rapid and severe abrogation of immune function.

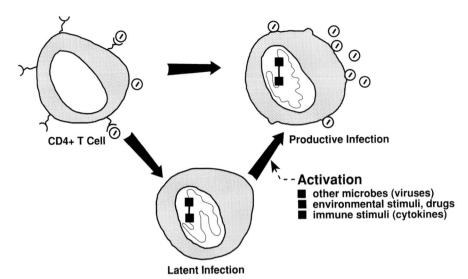

CD4+ T Cell

Productive Infection

`---` **Activation**
  ■ other microbes (viruses)
  ■ environmental stimuli, drugs
  ■ immune stimuli (cytokines)

Latent Infection

Figure 8.4. Activation of CD4+ T cells by exposure to various factors, including heterologous viruses, environmental stimuli, and cytokines, may be key in induction of HIV expression in latently infected cells.

In this regard, it is highly likely that, in any given HIV-infected individual, universal microbiologic latency does not exist. However, individual cells within an infected individual may be latently infected with HIV.

T Cell Activation and HIV Expression in Vitro

The importance of T cell activators in the amplification of HIV expression has been demonstrated by experiments which showed that HIV replicated to higher levels in cells that had been stimulated, before infection, with mitogens or antigens. In addition, mitogen stimulation of cells that exhibited chronic, low-level HIV replication resulted in a marked upregulation of HIV expression. Investigators have found that the molecular mechanisms of mitogen induction of HIV expression involve production of cellular DNA-binding factors that bind to a specific region of the HIV long terminal repeat (LTR) and result in stimulation of virus mRNA transcription (95; reviewed in Ref. 96). These specific sequences of the HIV DNA, known as the NFkB-binding sites, are also found in the genes for both IL-2 and the IL-2 receptor (97).

Virus gene products from heterologous DNA viruses represent another class of factors that have been shown to induce HIV expression in vitro (reviewed in Ref. 96). By using genes from various different DNA viruses, it was initially shown that cotransfection of these genes with HIV LTR constructs resulted in upregulation of an indicator gene (CAT) that was under the

control of the HIV LTR. Similarly, transfection of heterologous virus genes into cells transfected with intact HIV resulted in increased HIV replication. Conversely, infection of HIV LTR-CAT transfected cells with intact heterologous viruses can cause an upregulation of CAT activity. It has subsequently been shown that heterologous virus genes affect HIV transcription via induction of cellular DNA-binding proteins that bind to a multiplicity of sites on the HIV LTR.

Although immunization with common childhood vaccines may be considered a potential activating factor for HIV expression, studies of HIV-infected children have shown that vaccination histories for infants who progressed to AIDS were similar to those who remained asymptomatic. In addition, it has been shown that p24 antigen levels in adults did not increase after influenza vaccination (reviewed in Ref. 98). In HIV-infected children, the risks of developing severe vaccine-preventable diseases far outweighs the hypothetical risk of vaccine-induced HIV expression (see also Chapter 46).

Cytokine Regulation of HIV Expression

Cytokines represent another class of T cell activation factors that may be involved in induction of HIV expression (reviewed in Ref. 99). Tumor necrosis factor (TNF)-α, granulocyte macrophage-colony stimulating factor, and IL-6 have been shown to upregulate HIV expression in chronically infected cell lines. In addition, both TNF-α and granulocyte macrophage-colony stimulating factor could enhance HIV replication during acute HIV infection. By combining TNF-α with either GM-CSF or IL-6, a synergistic activation of HIV expression was detected in chronically infected cell lines. In parallel with results obtained with mitogen-induced activation of HIV expression, it has been demonstrated that TNF-α exposure results in production of cellular factors that bind to the NFkB sequences in the HIV LTR, which, in turn, induces new mRNA transcription and virion production (reviewed in Ref. 100). The mechanisms of IL-6-induced upregulation of HIV expression either alone or in combination with TNF-α appear to involve both post-transcriptional and transcriptional events (101).

A common theme that emerges from these studies is that activation of HIV and activation of the immune system are intricately connected. Thus mechanisms that the immune system uses to generate protective responses against a host of immunological insults may contribute to progression of HIV disease. For example, TNF-α, a normal immunoregulatory cytokine that is produced in humans in response to naturally occurring infections, is found in elevated levels in the sera of AIDS patients and is produced in substantial amounts by the monocytes of HIV-1-infected individuals (reviewed in Ref. 100). In addition, elevated

levels of IL-6 and TNF-α have been found in children with HIV infection (102). It has been shown that phorbol 12-myristate 13-acetate-induced activation of chronically HIV-infected cells results in induction and secretion of TNF-α and HIV and that induction of HIV expression can be suppressed by antibodies to TNF-α. In addition, phorbol 12-myristate 13-acetate exposure of chronically HIV-infected cells results in an increase in the level of TNF receptors (reviewed in Ref. 100). Along with evidence that binding of HIV to monocytes and macrophages causes secretion of TNF-α and IL-6 (103, 104), these data suggest that HIV, TNF-α, and IL-6 may be involved in an autocrine/paracrine loop in which the net result is the unrestricted replication of HIV and the gradual destruction of the immune system. Recent studies which demonstrate that spontaneous production of TNF-α and IL-6 by B cells from HIV-infected individuals results in induction of HIV expression in vitro lend further support for the role of these cytokines in HIV immunopathogenesis (105, 106) (Fig. 8.5).

In addition to the identification of soluble factors that enhance HIV expression, cytokines such as interferon-α, interferon-β, and TGF-β have been shown to suppress HIV expression (reviewed in Ref. 100). Interferon-α acts at the cell membrane level to prevent release of HIV virions from the cell surface. Interferon-γ was originally thought to inhibit HIV expression because extracellular virion formation was significantly reduced. However, the appearance of

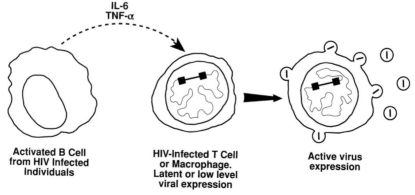

Figure 8.5. Activated B cells from HIV-infected individuals spontaneously secrete cytokines that can induce expression of HIV in latently or chronically infected T cells or macrophages. Adapted from Fauci AS. Immunopathogenic mechanisms in human immunodeficiency virus (HIV) infection. Ann Intern Med 1991;114:678–693.)

reduced HIV production is actually due to the redirection of virion formation from the plasma membrane to intracytoplasmic vacuoles (107). Similar to its pleiotropic effect on immune function, TGF-β exerts a bifunctional effect on HIV replication in that pretreatment of cells with TGF-β before HIV infection results in enhanced HIV expression, whereas exposure of chronically infected cells to TGF-β suppresses HIV expression after mitogen or IL-6 stimulation (reviewed in Ref. 100).

CONCLUSION

Since the recognition of AIDS in the early 1980s, researchers have identified and isolated the etiologic agent, extensively characterized its molecular structure, and delineated the mechanisms by which HIV infects cells. It became widely appreciated that HIV caused the destruction of a specific subset of T lymphocytes, the CD4+ T cells. Because of its pivotal role in immune function, the elimination of CD+4 T cells results in a global immunosuppression that renders the host susceptible to fatal infections and neoplasms. Although it is well-known that CD4+ T cells of HIV-infected individuals are qualitatively and quantitatively impaired, the precise mechanisms of HIV-induced immune destruction are less well understood. This chapter has reviewed the potential mechanisms whereby HIV can directly and indirectly destroy CD4+ T cells, and cause functional impairment of CD4+ T cells, as well as B cells and antigen-presenting cells.

One major area of investigation in the immunopathogenesis of HIV infection is the activation of HIV expression that is thought to occur in vivo after a long and variable asymptomatic phase. In vitro, numerous studies have shown that factors, such as mitogens, antigens, heterologous viruses, and cytokines, can induce HIV expression. Other soluble factors, including the interferons and TGF-β, can exert either suppressive or bifunctional effects on HIV expression. The knowledge generated through these studies is instrumental to the control of HIV expression and the prolongation of the disease-free state.

References

1. Ho DD, Sarngadharan MG, Resnick L, et al. Primary human T-lymphotropic virus type III infection. Ann Intern Med 1985;103:880–883.
2. Cooper DA, Gold J, MacLean P, et al. Acute AIDS retrovirus infection: Definitioin of a clinical illness associated with seroconversion. Lancet 1985;1: 537–540.
3. Lemp GF, Payne SF, Rutherford GW, et al. Projections of AIDS morbidity and mortality in San Francisco. JAMA 1990;263:1497–1501.
4. Andiman WA. Virologic and serologic aspects of human immunodeficiency virus infection in infants and children. Semin Perinatol 1989;13:16–26.
5. Krasinski K, Borkowsky W, Holzman RS. Prognosis of human immunodeficiency virus infection in children and adolescents. Pediatr Infect Dis J 1989;8: 216–220.
6. Rogers MF, Thomas PA, Starcher ET, et al. Acquired immunodeficiency syndrome in children: Report of the Centers for Disease Control National Surveillance, 1982 to 1985. Pediatrics 1987;79:1008–1014.
7. Tovo PA, de Martino M, Gabiano C, et al. Prognostic factors and survival in children with perinatal HIV-1 infection. Lancet 1992;339: 1249–1253.
8. Masur H, Michelis MA, Greene JB, et al. An outbreak of community-acquired *Pneumocystis carinii* pneumonia: Initial manifestation of cellular immune dysfunction. N Engl J Med 1981; 305:1431–1438.
9. Gottlieb MS, Schroff R, Schanker HM, et al: Pneumocystic carinii pneumonia and mucosal candidiasis in previously healthy homosexual men: Evidence of a new acquired cellular immunodeficiency. N Engl J Med 1981;305:1425–1431.
10. Barre-Sinoussi F, Chermann JC, Rey F, et al. Isolation of a T-lymphotropic retrovirus from a patient at risk for acquired immune deficiency syndrome (AIDS). Science 1983;220:868–871.
11. Levy JA, Hoffman AD, Kramer SM, et al. Isolation of lymphocytopathic retroviruses from San Francisco patients with AIDS. Science 1984;225:840–842.
12. Gallo RC, Salahuddin SZ, Popovic M, et al: Frequent detection and isolation of cytopathic retroviruses (HTLV-III) from patients with AIDS and at risk for AIDS. Science 1984;224:500–503.
13. Klatzmann D, Barre-Sinoussi F, Nugeyre MT, et al. Selective tropism of lymphadenopathy associated virus (LAV) for helper-inducer T lymphocytes. Science 1984;225:59–63.
14. Popovic M, Sarngadharan MG, Read E, et al. Detection, isolation, and continuous production of cytopathic retroviruses (HTLV-III) from patients with AIDS and pre-AIDS. Science 1984; 224:497–500.
15. Zagury D, Bernard J, Leonard R, et al. Long-term cultures of HTLV-III–infected T cells: A model of cytopathology of T-cell depletion in AIDS. Science 1986;231:850–853.
16. Folks TM, Powell D, Lightfoote M, et al. Biological and biochemical characterization of a cloned Leu-3-cell surviving infection with the ac-

quired immune deficiency syndrome retrovirus. J Exp Med 1986;164:280–290.

17. Dalgleish AG, Beverley PC, Clapham PR, et al. The CD4 (T4) antigen is an essential component of the receptor for the AIDS retrovirus. Nature 1984;312:763-767.

18. Klatzmann D, Champagne E, Chamaret S, et al. T-lymphocyte T4 molecule behaves as the receptor for human retrovirus LAV. Nature 1984;312:767–768.

19. McDougal JS, Kennedy MS, Sligh JM, et al. Binding of HTLV-III/LAV to T4+ T cells by a complex of the 110K viral protein and the T4 molecule. Science 1986;231:382–385.

20. Gay D, Maddon P, Sekaly R, et al. Functional interaction between human T-cell protein CD4 and the major histocompatibility complex HLA-DR antigen. Nature 1987;328:626–629.

21. Doyle C, Strominger JL. Interaction between CD4 and class II MHC molecules mediates cell adhesion. Nature 1987;330:256-259.

22. Talle MA, Rao PE, Westberg E, et al. Patterns of antigenic expression on human monocytes as defined by monoclonal antibodies. Cell Immunol 1983;78:83-99.

23. Rosenberg ZF, Fauci AS. The immunopathogenesis of HIV infection. Adv Immunol 1989;47:377-431.

24. Schnittman SM, Psallidopoulos MC, Lane HC, et al. The reservoir for HIV-1 in human peripheral blood is a T cell that maintains expression of CD4. Science 1989;245:305–308.

25. Spear GT, Ou Cy, Kessler HA, et al. Analysis of lymphocytes, monocytes, and neutrophils from human immunodeficiency virus (HIV)-infected persons for HIV DNA. J Infect Dis 1990;162:1239–1244.

26. McElrath MJ, Pruett JE, Cohn ZA. Mononuclear phagocytes of blood and bone marrow: Comparative roles as viral reservoirs in human immunodeficiency virus type 1 infections. Proc Natl Acad Sci USA 1989;86:675–679.

27. Fauci AS: The human immunodeficiency virus: Infectivity and mechanisms of pathogenesis. Science 1988;239:617–622.

28. Orenstein JM, Meltzer MS, Phipps T, et al: Cytoplasmic assembly and accumulation of human immunodeficiency virus types 1 and 2 in recombinant human colony-stimulating factor-1-treated human monocytes: An ultrastructural study. J Virol 1988;62:2578–2586.

29. Gendelman HE, Orenstein JM, Baca LM, et al. The macrophage in the persistence and pathogenesis of HIV infection. AIDS 1989;3:475–495.

30. Mikovits JA, Raziuddins S, Gonda M, et al. Negative regulation of human immune deficiency virus replication in monocytes. Distinctions between restricted and latent expression in cells. J Exp Med 1990;171:1705–1720.

31. Rosenberg ZF, Fauci AS. Immunopathogenesis of HIV infection. FASEB J 1991;5:2382–2390.

32. Zucker-Franklin D, Cao Y. Megakaryocytes of human immunodeficiency virus-infected individuals express viral RNA. Proc Natl Acad Sci USA 1989;86:5595–5599.

33. Louache F, Bettaieb A, Henri A, et al. Infection of megakaryocytes by human immunodeficiency virus in seropostitive patients with immune thrombocytopenic purpura. Blood 1991;78:1697–1705.

34. Rodriguez ER, Nasim S, Hsia J, et al. Cardiac myocytes and dendritic cells harbor human immunodeficiency virus in infected patients with and without cardiac dysfunction: Detection by multiplex, nested, polymerase chain reaction in individually microdissected cells from right ventricular endomyocardial biopsy tissue. Am J Cardiol 1991;68:1511–1520.

35. Rosenberg ZF, Fauci AS. Immunopathologic mechanisms of HIV infection. In: Gallo RC, Jay G, eds. The human retroviruses. San Diego: Academic, 1991:141–161.

36. Tsubota H, Ringler DJ, Kannagi M, et al. CD8+ CD4- lymphocyte lines can harbor the AIDS virus in vitro. J Immunol 1989;143:858–863.

37. Harouse JM, Bhat S, Spitalnik SL, et al. Inhibition of entry of HIV-1 in neural cell lines by antibodies against galactosyl ceramide. Science 1991;253:320–323.

38. Bhat S, Spitalnik SL, Gonzalez-Scarano F, et al. Galactosyl ceramide or a derivative is an essential component of the neural receptor for human immunodeficiency virus type 1 envelope glycoprotein gp120. Proc Natl Acad Sci USA 1991;88:7131–7134.

39. Yahi N, Baghdiguian S, Moreau H, et al. Galactosyl ceramide (or a closely related molecule) is the receptor for human immunodeficiency virus type 1 on human colon epithelial HT29 cells. J Virol 1992;66:4848–4854.

40. Maury W, Potts BJ, Rabson AB. HIV-1 infection of first-trimester and term human placental tissue: A possible mode of maternal-fetal transmission. J Infect Dis 1989;160:583–588.

41. Zachar V, Spire B, Hirsch I, et al. Human transformed trophoblast-derived cells lacking CD4 receptor exhibit restricted permissiveness for human immunodeficiency virus type 1. J Virol 1991;65:2102–2107.

42. Zachar V, Nrskov-Lauritsen N, Juhl C, et al. Susceptibility of cultured human trophoblasts to infection with human immunodeficiency virus type 1. J Gen Virol 1991;72:1253–1260.

43. Douglas GC, Fry GN, Thirkill T, et al. Cell-mediated infection of human placental trophoblast with HIV in vitro. AIDS Res Hum Retroviruses 1991;7:735–740.

44. Amirhessami-Aghili N, Spector SA. Human immunodeficiency virus type 1 infection of human placenta: Potential route for fetal infection. J Virol 1991;65:2231–2236.

45. David FJ, Autran B, Tran HC, et al. Human trophoblast cells express CD4 and are permissive for productive infection with HIV-1. Clin Exp Immunol 1992;88:10–16.

45a. Lairmore M, Cuthbert C, Morgan C, Dessatti C, Anderson CL, Sedmak D. Lack of CD4 antigen or RNA expression on syncytiotrophoblasts. [Abstract]. Keystone Conference on HIV Pathogenesis, Albuquerque, Mar 1993.

46. Lewis SH, Reynolds-Kohler C, Fox HE, et al. HIV-1 in trophoblastic and villous Hofbauer cells, and haematological precursors in eight-week fetuses. Lancet 1990;335:565–568.

47. Chandwani S, Greco MA, Mittal K, et al. Pathology and human immunodeficiency virus expression in placentas of seropositive women. J Infect Dis 1991;163:1134–1138.

48. Mattern CF, Murray K, Jesen A, et al. Localization of human immunodeficiency virus core antigen in term human placentas. Pediatrics 1992;89:207-209.

49. Courgnaud V, Laure F, Brossard A, et al. Frequent and early in utero HIV-1 infection. AIDS Res Hum Retroviruses 1991;7:337–341.

50. Ehrnst A, Lindgren S, Dictor M, et al. HIV in pregnant women and their offspring: Evidence for late transmission. Lancet 1991;338:203–207.

51. Goedert JJ, Duliège Am, Amos CI, et al: High risk of HIV-1 infection for first-born twins. The International Registry of HIV-exposed Twins. Lancet 1991;338:1471–1475.

52. Pantaleo G, Graziosi C, Butini L, et al. Lymphoid organs function as major reservoirs for human immunodeficiency virus. Proc Natl Acad Sci USA 1991;88:9839–9842.

53. Pantaleo G, Graziosi C, Fauci AS. New concepts in the immunopathogenesis of human immunodeficiency virus (HIV) infection. N Engl J Med, 1993;328:327–335.

54. Connor RI, Ho DD. Etiology of AIDS: Biology of human retroviruses. In: DeVita VT Jr, Hellman S, Rosenberg SA, eds. AIDS: Etiology, diagnosis, treatment, and prevention. Philadelphia: Lippincott, 1992:13–38.

55. Stanley SK, Kessler SW, Justement JS, et al. CD34+ bone marrow cells are infected with HIV in a subset of seropositive individuals. J Immunol 1992;149:689–697.

56. De Rossi A, Calabro ML, Panozzo M, et al. In vitro studies of HIV-1 infection in thymic lymphocytes: A putative role of the thymus in AIDS pathogenesis. AIDS Res Hum Retroviruses 1990;6:287–298.

57. Schnittman SM, Denning SM, Greenhouse JJ, et al. Evidence for susceptibility of intrathymic T-cell precursors and their progeny carrying T-cell antigen receptor phenotypes TCR -αβ+ and TCR γδ+ to human immunodeficiency virus infection: A mechanism for CD4+ (T4) lymphocyte depletion. Proc Natl Acad Sci USA 1990;87:7727–7731.

58. Tanaka KE, Hatch WC, Kress Y, et al. HIV-1 infection of human fetal thymocytes. J Acquir Immune Defic Syndr 1992;5:94–101.

59. Hatch WC, Tanaka KE, Calvelli T, et al. Persistent productive HIV-1 infection of a CD4- human fetal thymocyte line. J Immunol 1992;148:3055–3061.

60. Hays EF, Uittenbogaart CH, Brewer JC, et al. In vitro studies of HIV-1 expression in thymocytes from infants and children. AIDS 1992;6:265–272.

61. Papiernik M, Brossard Y, Mulliez N, et al. Thymic abnormalities in fetuses aborted from human immunodeficiency virus type 1 seropositive women. Pediatrics 1992;89:297–301.

62. Tindall B, Cooper DA. Primary HIV infection: Host responses and intervention strategies. AIDS 1991;5:1–14.

63. Daar ES, Moudgil T, Meyer RD, et al. Transient high levels of viremia in patients with primary human immunodeficiency virus type 1 infection. N Engl J Med 1991;324:961–964.

64. Clark SJ, Saag MS, Decker WD, et al. High titers of cytopathic virus in plasma of patients with symptomatic primary HIV-1 infection. N Engl J Med 1991;324:954–960.

65. Rosenberg ZF, Fauci AS. Immunopathogenesis of HIV infection. In: DeVita VT Jr, Hellman S, Rosenberg SA, eds. AIDS: Etiology, diagnosis, treatment and prevention. Philadelphia: Lippincott, 1992:61–76.

66. Venet A, Lu W, Beldjord K, et al. Correlation between CD4 cell counts and cellular and plasma viral load in HIV-1-seropositive individuals. AIDS 1991;5:283–288.

67. Saag MS, Crain MJ, Decker WD, et al. High-level viremia in adults and children infected with human immunodeficiency virus: Relation to disease stage and CD4+ lymphocyte levels. J Infect Dis 1991;164:72–80.

68. Srugo I, Brunell PA, Chelyapov NV, et al. Virus burden in human immunodeficiency virus type 1-infected children: Relationship to disease status and effect of antiviral therapy. Pediatrics 1991;87:921–925.

69. Katzenstein DA, Holodniy M, Israelski DM, et al. Plasma viremia in human immunodeficiency virus infection: Relationship to stage of disease and antiviral treatment. J Acquir Immune Defic Syndr 1992;5:107–112.

70. Escaich S, Ritter J, Rougier P, et al. Plasma viraemia as a marker of viral replication of HIV-infected individuals. AIDS 1991;5:1189–1194.

71. Hsia K, Spector SA. Human immunodeficiency virus DNA is present in a high percentage of CD4+ lymphocytes of seropositive individuals. J Infect Dis 1991;164:470–475.

72. Schnittman SM, Greenhouse JJ, Psallidopoulos MC, et al. Increasing viral burden in CD4+ T cells from patients with human immunodeficiency virus (HIV) infection reflects rapidly progressive immunosuppression and clinical disease. Ann Intern Med 1990;113:438–443.

73. Hufert FT, von Laer D, Fenner TE, et al. Progression of HIV-1 infection. Monitoring of HIV-1 DNA in peripheral blood mononuclear cells by PCR. Arch Virol 1991;120:233–240.

74. Lyerly HK, Reed DL, Matthews TJ, et al. Anti-GP 120 antibodies from HIV seropositive individuals mediate broadly reactive anti-HIV ADCC. AIDS Res Hum Retroviruses 1987;3:409–422.

75. Lanzavecchia A, Roosnek E, Gregory T, et al. T cells can present antigens such as HIV gp120 targeted to their own surface molecules. Nature 1988;334:530–532.

76. Siliciano RF, Lawton T, Knall C, et al. Analysis of host-virus interactions in AIDS with anti-gp120 T cell clones: Effect of HIV sequence variation and a mechanism for CD4+ cell depletion. Cell 1988;54:561–575.

77. Hugin AW, Vacchio MS, Morse HC 3rd. A virus-encoded "superantigen:" In a retrovirus-induced immunodeficiency syndrome of mice. Science 1991;252:424–427.

78. Laurence J, Hodtsev AS, Posnett DN. Superantigen implicated in dependence of HIV-1 replication in T cells on TCR VB expression. Nature 1992;358:255–259.

79. Imberti L, Sottini A, Bettinardi A, et al. Selective depletion of HIV infection of T cells that bear specific T cell receptor V beta sequences. Science 1991;254:860–862.

80. Dalgleish AG, Wilson S, Gompels M, et al. T-cell receptor variable gene products and early HIV-1 infection. Lancet 1992;339:824–828.

81. Ameisen JC, Capron A. Cell dysfunction and depletion in AIDS: The programmed cell death hypothesis. Immunol Today 1991;12:102–105.

82. Duvall E, Wylie AH. Death and the cell. Immunol Today 1986;7:115–119.

83. Jenkinson EJ, Kingston R, Smith CA, et al. Antigen-induced apoptosis in developing T cells: A mechanism for negative selection of the TCR repertoire. Eur J Immunol 1989;19:2175–2177.

84. Groux H, Torpier G, Montë D, et al. Activation-induced death by apoptosis in CD4+ T cells from human immunodeficiency virus-infected asymptomatic individuals. J Exp Med 1992;175:331–340.

85. Terai C, Kornbluth RS, Pauza CD, et al: Apoptosis as a mechanism of cell death in cultured T lymphoblasts acutely infected with HIV-1. J Clin Invest 1991;87:1710–1715.

86. Laurent-Crawford AG, Krust B, Muller S, et al. The cytopathic effect of HIV is associated with apoptosis. Virology 1991;185:829–839.

87. Gougeon ML, Olivier R, Garcia S, et al. Evidence for an engagement process towards apoptosis in lymphocytes of HIV-infected patients. C R Acad Sci III 1991;312:529–537.

88. Meyaard L, Otto SA, Jonker RR, et al. Programmed death of T cells in HIV-1 infection. Science 1992;257:217–219.

89. Denny T, Yogev R, Gelman R, et al. Lymphocyte subsets in healthy children during the first 5 years of life. JAMA 1992;267:1484–1488.

89a. Connor E, Bagarazzi M, McSherry G, et al. Clinical and laboratory correlates of *Pneumocystic carinii* pneumonia in children infected with HIV. JAMA 1991;265:1693–1697.

90. Reiher WE 3rd, Blalock JE, Brunck TK. Sequence homology between acquired immunodeficiency syndrome virus envelope protein and interleukin 2. Proc Natl Acad Sci USA 1986;83:9188–9192.

91. Ammann AJ: Immunopathogenesis of pediatric acquired immunodeficiency syndrome. J Perinatol 1988;8:154–159.

92. Goudsmit J, Lange JM, Paul DA, et al. Antigenemia and antibody titers to core and envelope antigens in AIDS, AIDS-related complex, and subclinical human immunodeficiency virus infection. J Infect Dis 1987;155:558–560.

93. Epstein LG, Boucher CA, Morrison SH, et al. Persistent human immunodeficiency virus type 1 antigenemia in children correlates with disease progression. Pediatrics 1988;82:919–924.

94. Zack JA, Arrigo SJ, Weitsman SR, et al. HIV-1 entry into quiescent primary lymphocytes: Molecular analysis reveals a labile, latent viral structure. Cell 1990;61:213–222.

95. Nabel G, Baltimore D. An inducible transcription factor activates expression of human immunodeficiency virus in T cells. Nature 1987;326:711–713.

96. Rosenberg ZF, Fauci AS. Induction of expression of HIV in latently or chronically infected cells. AIDS Res Hum Retroviruses 1989;5:1–4.

97. Hoyos B, Ballard DW, Bohnlein E, et al. Kappa B-specific DNA binding proteins: Role in the regulation of human interleukin-2 gene expression. Science 1989;244:457–460.

98. Onorato IM, Markowitz LE, Oxtoby MJ. Childhood immunization, vaccine-preventable diseases and infection with human immunodeficency virus. Pediatr Infect Dis J 1988;7:588–595.

99. Rosenberg ZF, Fauci AS. Immunopathogenic mechanisms of HIV infection: Cytokine induction of HIV expression. Immunol Today 1990;11:176–180.

100. Poli G, Fauci AS. The effect of cytokines and pharmacologic agents on chronic HIV infection. AIDS Res Hum Retroviruses 1992;8:191–197.

101. Poli G, Bressler P, Kinter A, et al. Interleukin 6 induces human immunodeficiency virus expression in monocytic cells alone and in synergy with tumor necrosis factor alpha by transcriptional and post-transcriptional mechanisms. J Exp Med 1990;172:151–158.

102. Rautonen J, Rautonen N, Martin NL, et al. Serum interleukin-6 concentrations are elevated and associated with elevated tumor necrosis factor-alpha and immunoglobulin G and A concentrations in children with HIV infection. AIDS 1991;5:1319–1325.

103. Merrill JE, Koyanagi Y, Chen IS. Interleukin-1 and tumor necrosis factor alpha can be induced from mononuclear phagocytes by human immunodeficiency virus type 1 binding to the CD4 receptor. J Virol 1989;63:4404–4408.

104. Nakajima K, Martinez-Maza O, Hirano T, et al. Induction of IL-6 (B cell stimulatory factor-2/IFN-beta 2) production by HIV. J Immunol 1989;142:531–536.

105. Rieckmann P, Poli G, Kehrl JH, et al. Activated B lymphocytes from human immunodeficiency virus-infected individuals induce virus expression in infected T cells and a promonocytic cell line, U1. J Exp Med 1991;173:1–5.

106. Boue F, Wallon C, Goujard C, et al. HIV induces IL-6 production by human B lymphocytes. Role of IL-4. J Immunol 1992;148:3761–3767.

107. Biswas P, Poli G, Kinter AL, et al. Interferon-gamma induces the expression of human immunodeficiency virus in persistently infected promonocytic cells (U1) and redirects the production of virions to intracytoplasmic in PMA-differentiated U1 cells. J Exp Med 1992;176:739–750.

Clinical Immunology of HIV-infected Children

Richard A. Koup and Christopher B. Wilson

Because the immune system is both the substrate for replication of the human immunodeficiency virus (HIV) and the defense mechanism against the HIV, differences in the immune system between the mature and the developing host may lead to complex differences in the pathogenesis of infection and disease. Children who acquire HIV infection perinatally have, in many cases, a more rapid progression from latent to symptomatic infection and from onset of symptomatic infection to death. The basis for these differences is unknown. It is likely that there are multiple factors among which may be differences in the capacity of cells from the fetus and neonate to be infected or to support viral replication once infected. Alternatively, the neonate's immunologic response may be less able to restrict viral replication or spread. This chapter will provide background of the ontogeny of the immune system, particularly as it relates to aspects that may influence the pathogenesis of HIV infection. This is followed by a discussion of the immunologic and clinical consequences of HIV infection in the developing host. The approach to characterize the immunologic function of patients and to differentiate between immunodeficiency caused by HIV and from other causes follows.

DEVELOPMENT OF IMMUNE SYSTEM

Cells of the immune system are derived from hematopoietic precursors and include T and B lymphocytes, NK cells, granulocytes, and monocytes/macrophages. These cells, their secreted products (e.g., immunoglobulins, cytokines) and other factors secreted by various hematopoietic and nonhematopoietic cells, such as complement, make up the immune system. All hematopoietic cells derive from pluripotent stem cells. During development these cells are initially derived from the yolk sac; this is supplanted as the principal source of hematopoiesis by the liver at 8 weeks gestation and the bone marrow by ~5 months gestation. Unlike adults, the peripheral blood of neonates contains substantial numbers of hematopoietic precursors (1), as does fetal blood as early as 12 weeks gestation (1). These cells serve as precursors for each lymphocyte lineage: T cells, NK cells, and B cells.

The specific immune system is composed of T cells and B cells, which express on their surface antigen-specific receptors. In the case of T cells this is known as the T cell antigen receptor (TCR) and in the case of B cells it is the membrane bound form of immunoglobulin (Ig). There are two types of TCR, which are composed of $\alpha\beta$ or $\gamma\delta$ heterodimers; the predominant population of T cells (95%) express the $\alpha\beta$ receptor. Studies in transgenic mice strongly suggest that these cell types are derived from distinct lineages (2). For Ig, the heterodimer is composed of a κ or λ light chain paired with a heavy chain. Both T cell and B cell receptors are heterodimeric proteins, the variable region of which determines antigen specificity. Both receptors are derived by controlled genetic rearrangement events, which lead to the juxtaposition of gene segments that will encode the variable region of the molecule important for specific antigen recognition to the gene segment encoding the constant region of the molecule. This process of rearrangement results in the joining of the segments in such a way that additional diversity in the portions of the molecule which serve to engage antigen is achieved by addition or deletion of nucleotides at the junctions of the segments (3). Overall, for Ig a potential repertoire of $\sim 10^{11}$ and for the TCR of $\sim 10^{15-18}$ has been estimated (3).

T cells through their TCR and B cells through surface Ig see antigen in a fundamentally different way. B cells and Ig engage antigen directly, recognizing in many cases secondary or tertiary structure or other complex determinants. In contrast, T cells recognize antigen as short peptides in association with a major histocompatibility (MHC, which is known as HLA in humans) molecule (reviewed in Ref. 4). The peptides are derived by degradation of intact proteins by specific antigen processing and become associated with the MHC molecule within the cell, after which the peptide-MHC complex is transported to the cell surface. In general proteins that are synthesized within the cell (host cell proteins and proteins produced by pathogens, such as viruses, that replicate within cells) associate preferentially with class I MHC molecules (human leukocyte antigen (HLA A, B, and C in humans). In contrast, specific antigen presenting cells (monocytes/macrophages and B cells) internalize and process extracellular proteins (e.g., those derived from bacteria and other pathogens that replicate extracellularly) into peptides that then associate with class II MHC molecules (HLA-D in humans) the expression of which is largely restricted to these cells.

CD8 T cells recognize antigen in association with class I MHC, and CD4 T cells recognize antigen in association with class II MHC. This is due to the fact that the CD4 or CD8 molecule functions as a coreceptor with the antigen-specific TCR by binding to the MHC class II or class I molecule, respectively. The recognition by CD4 T cells of antigen in association with class II MHC endows these cells with the capacity to respond to antigens secreted or released from injured, effete, or infected host cells or from extracellular pathogens. This capacity to survey their environment for antigenic proteins is important in allowing these helper T cells to regulate responses by other cells of the immune system. Conversely, the recognition by CD8 T cells of antigen in association with class I MHC tends to focus their recognition to cells in which the antigenic or foreign proteins are being synthesized. This is a teleologically desirable property for CD8 T cells, since one major function is to mediate cytotoxic destruction of foreign or infected cells.

DEVELOPMENT AND FUNCTION OF T CELL LINEAGE

T cells develop in the thymus from hematopoietic precursors. These precursors first colonize the thymus in the human at ~8 weeks gestation where they (thymocytes) undergo a series of differentiative events, including de novo expression of CD4, CD8, and the TCR (5, 6). Cells that fail to productively rearrange their TCR do not mature and die. Concomitant with expression of their TCR, those thymocytes of the predominant TCR αβ lineage express simultaneously both CD4 and CD8. Based on studies in the mouse, these double-positive (CD4+ and CD8+) thymocytes undergo a dual-selection process, which tests suitability of the TCR on the surface of each T cell. Negative selection removes cells that react strongly with self-antigens, whereas positive selection retains cells that can respond best to foreign antigens in the context of host MHC. During positive selection the thymocyte matures such that expression of the TCR, CD3, and associated signaling molecules increases. Also those cells that recognize antigen in association with class II MHC selectively maintain CD4 and lose CD8 expression, whereas the reverse is true for cells which possess a TCR that recognizes antigen in association with class I MHC. Only ~5% of cells entering the thymus productively rearrange their TCR and successfully undergo positive without negative selection; accordingly ~95% of all thymocytes never mature and reach the periphery as T cells.

By 12 weeks of gestation each major developmental stage of thymocyte is detectable and by 18–20 weeks of gestation the representation of each subset is similar to that observed postnatally (7). Nevertheless, there appear to be differences in the nature and diversity of the TCR in the fetus from that in more mature individuals. In the first half of gestation in the human and in the fetal and neonatal mouse, a very limited range of receptor gene segments is used both by thymocytes expressing the γδ TCR and those expressing the αβ TCR (8, 9). Furthermore, generation of diversity by the addition of extra nucleotides at the junction of the different TCR gene segments is minimal. Although the data set is limited, in the human these differences appear to be most pronounced before midgestation and are much less apparent at term. The net effect of these differences would be to limit the repertoire and perhaps the nature of antigens that may be recognized by T cells in the fetus. Direct evidence in favor of selective differences in repertoire is the diminished frequency of T cells capable of responding to some antigens but not others (10, 11). Whether such differences in repertoire contribute to the age-related limitation in capacity of the fetus and infant to respond to certain antigens is not yet clear.

Mature thymocytes are the immediate precursors of peripheral T cells and have acquired many functional attributes of T cells. They can produce interleukin (IL)-2, express high-affinity IL-2 receptors, and proliferate in response to mitogens (reviewed in Ref. 12). However, there are phenotypic and functional differences that distinguish these cells from T cells of the adult. For example, mature thymocytes express the CD38 antigen, whereas resting T cells from adults do not; the capacity of mature thymocytes to produce certain cytokines, such as interferon-γ and interleukin (IL)-4, is markedly less than that of mature T cells.

ONTOGENY OF T CELL FUNCTION AND PHENOTYPE IN NEONATES

Phenotype

By midgestation ~80% of circulating leukocytes are lymphocytes, and the absolute number is ~3500 cells/mm³ through-out the latter part of gestation (13). Values at term are somewhat higher with mean values of 5500/mm³ (14, 15). Although a slightly lower percentage of circulating lymphocytes in neonates are T cells, neonates actually have increased absolute numbers of T cells (~2500–4000/mm³) compared with adults. However, there are several phenotypic and functional differences between T cells from adults and neonates.

An example is the increased absolute and relative numbers of CD4+ T cells in neonates, a differences of obvious importance in management of the infant and neonate with potential HIV infection. The greater numbers of CD4 than CD8 T cells is established in utero, with ratios declining from ~4–5:1 at 28 weeks gestation to values of ~3:1 at term (16). Unfortunately, no truly definitive study of T cell subpopulations in normal infants and children has been published. The two most complete studies are shown in Table 9.1. Neither study performed the analysis with the reagents and parameters now recommended by the Centers for Disease Control (17). Collectively, the values reported by these investigators (14, 15) appear to encompass the range reported in more limited studies by other groups in various ethnic populations, e.g., an at risk population of American children of <2 years age (18). A more definitive study in which the Centers for Disease Control parameters are followed and in which the population is racially heterogenous is needed to provide definitive data.

Other phenotypic differences in neonatal T cells are consistent with recent derivation from thymic precursors, lack of previous antigenic exposure, or both. Nearly all T cells from neonates express CD38, and those from premature or stressed neonates may express additional thymocyte surface antigens, e.g., CD1. Like mature thymocytes, nearly all neonatal T cells express the high molecular weight isoforms of the CD45 molecule, as identified by antibodies to CD45RA, and do not express the low molecular weight isoform CD45R0 (19, 20). In contrast, 50–60% of circulating T cells in adults express CD45R0, and the remainder express CD45RA in a mutually exclusive fashion. The CD45R0 subset of T cells appears to contain virtually all T cells capable

Table 9.1.   Age-related Changes in T Lymphocyte Populations in Normal Children

Cell Population	Age Groups[a]			
	2–11 mo	1–2 yr	3–4 yr	5–13 yr
Japanese[b]				
PBMC ($\times 10^3$/mm^3)	7.5 (5.1–9.8)	5.1 (3.3–6.9)	4.3 (3.3–5.3)	3.3 (2.7–3.9)
T cells ($\times 10^3$/mm^3) – total (CD3)	5.0 (3.5–6.5)	3.0 (1.9–4.1)	2.6 (1.7–3.5)	1.9 (1.5–2.3)
CD4	3.8 (2.5–5.1)	2.1 (1.3–2.9)	1.8 (1.1–2.5)	1.1 (0.8–1.4)
CD8	1.6 (0.9–2.2)	1.1 (0.6–1.5)	1.0 (0.6–1.4)	0.9 (0.6–1.1)
	2 d–11 mo	1–6 yr	7–17 yr	18–70 yr
European[c]				
Lymphocytes ($\times 10^3$/mm^3)	4.1 (2.7–5.4)	3.6 (2.9–5.1)	2.4 (2.0–2.7)	2.1 (1.6–2.4)
T cells ($\times 10^3$/mm^3) – total (CD3)	2.5 (1.7–3.6)	2.5 (1.8–3.0)	1.8 (1.4–2.0)	1.4 (1.1–1.7)
CD4	2.2 (1.7–2.8)	1.6 (1.1–1.8)	0.8 (0.7–1.1)	0.8 (0.7–1.1)
CD8	0.9 (0.8–1.2)	0.9 (0.8–1.5)	0.8 (0.6–0.9)	0.7 (0.5–0.9)

[a]Values are means (European) or median (Japanese); range in parentheses is from the 25–75 percentile.
[b]Data from Yanase Y, Tomogo T, Okumura K, et al. Lymphocyte subsets identified by monoclonal antibodies in healthy children. Pediatr Res 1986;20:1147–1151.
[c]Data from Erkeller-Yuksel FM, Deneys V, Yuksel B, et al. Age-related changes in human blood lymphocyte subpopulations. J Pediatr 1992;120:216–222.

of response to specific recall antigens. Hence these cells are often referred to as memory T cells. Evidence suggests that the CD45RA subset of T cells are antigenically naive, and most convert to the CD45R0 phenotype after activation. These phenotypic differences in expression of CD45 isoforms are paralleled in part by differences in expression of β1 integrins identified by the CD29 antibody (21) and by a series of functional differences.

Proliferation

Lectin mitogens such as phytohemagglutinin (PHA) and concanavalin A (ConA) induce blastogenesis in fetal thymocytes as early as 10 weeks gestation. By 20 weeks gestation T cells proliferate as well as those of adults in response to PHA, ConA, and alloantigens (reviewed in Ref. 12). Although an allogeneic response is detectable by 14 weeks gestation in blood and splenic lymphocytes, the rare development of graft vs. host disease in the fetus or preterm neonate after intrauterine or postnatal exchange transfusion indicates that all aspects of this response may not be intact, perhaps because of defects in lymphokine production or cytotoxicity described below. In contrast to these findings, neonatal T cells proliferate less well in response to many agents that activate signaling directly through the T cell antigen receptor complex, including anti-CD3, certain bacterial superantigens, and mitogenic antibodies to CD2 (22, 23). This appears to reflect the lack of the putative memory T cell population in the neonate, because in the adult it is the memory T cells that proliferate well in response to these stimuli.

Regulatory and Cytotoxic Functions

Provision of help for B cell Ig production by T cells from neonates appears to vary depending on the assay conditions. Compared with adult T cells, neonatal T cells support B cell Ig production ~50% as well as do T cells from adults in response to stimuli other than pokeweed mitogen and anti-CD3 (23, 24; reviewed in Ref. 12). However, in response to the latter stimuli neonatal T cells do not support and can inhibit B cell Ig production. The lack of help for B cell Ig production can be partly accounted for by deficient production of specific lymphokines (24) and can be overcome by previous activation of neonatal T cells, which is associated with a phenotypic conversion from CD45RA+ to CD45R0+ cells and alteration in lymphokines produced (see below).

T cells, principally the CD8+ subset, mediate antigen-specific, MHC-restricted cytolytic activity. The cytotoxic response generated by neonatal T cells is 30–60% less than that of adult cells in most studies (reviewed in Ref. 12); cytotoxicity of fetal blood mononuclear cells is absent before

~20–23 weeks gestation. Those studies in which the most profound deficits were observed used purified T cells as effectors, suggesting that the studies in which better developed cytotoxicity was observed with neonatal mixed mononuclear cells may not have been as specific for CTL function.

Lymphokine Production and Its Consequences

Because neonatal T cell proliferation is critically dependent on production of IL-2 and on expression of high-affinity IL-2 receptors in response to activation, it can be inferred that these functions would parallel the results of proliferation (reviewed in Ref. 12). This is the case. IL-2 production in response to mitogens and allogeneic stimulation is normal, whereas production of IL-2 in response to anti-CD3 is diminished. The response to mitogens and alloantigen is mature by 20 weeks gestation.

In addition to IL-2, neonatal T cells appear to produce lymphotoxin in amounts at least as great as adult T cells (Table 9.2). However, production of several other lymphokines is diminished to a modest or marked degree, even in response to stimuli that induce proliferation and IL-2 production that equals or exceeds that by adult T cells (reviewed in Refs. 12 and 25). T cells from healthy neonates produce on average 10-fold less interferon-γ and >10-fold less IL-4 than adult T cells and 20–50% as much tumor necrosis factor (TNF), IL-3, and granulocyte macrophage-colony stimulating factor (GM-CSF). In each case mRNA transcription and accumulation parallel differences in lymphokine secretion. Additional studies using RNA analysis only, suggest that production of IL-5 is also diminished (26), a finding supported by unpublished data from our laboratory. This difference may reflect in large part the absence of memory T cells in neonates (27). After short or long-term propagation in vitro, by stimulation with mitogens and IL-2, neonatal T cells or adult naive T cells lose expression of CD45RA, acquire expression of CD45R0, and in parallel acquire the capacity to secrete large amounts of each lymphokine produced in diminished amounts by naive and neonatal T cells (19, 26, 28).

The relevance of this to T cell function in response to specific infectious pathogens is suggested by studies in neonates with herpes simplex virus infection (29). In the first month after infection blood mononuclear cells of the neonates make little interferon-γ in response to specific antigen in comparison to adults with primary herpes simplex virus infection. However, 2 months after onset of infection, and shortly after specific antigen responsive memory T cells are first detectable by proliferation assays, interferon-γ production in response to specific antigen is similar in infected neonates and adults. Together, these data are consistent with the notion that the primary basis for deficient production of many if not all lymphokines by neonatal T cells is the lack of prior experience with foreign antigens rather than an intrinsic, ontogenetically determined immaturity in function.

The lymphokines referred to above have various functions in host defense (reviewed in Refs. 12 and 25). Thus, deficient production of these lymphokines, at least until memory T cells develop in response to antigens of the infecting pathogen, may initially attenuate the response to infection. For example, a combined deficiency in interferon-γ and IL-4 production may impede the efficient induction of specific immune responses by T cells and B cells, impair the generation of antigen-specific cytotoxic T cells, and interfere with the normal effector phase of the immune response. As described below, many of these features are characteristic of the neonate's immune response.

DEVELOPMENT AND FUNCTION OF NK CELLS

Natural killer (NK) cells are a lymphocyte subset that can be identified in the human by expression of the CD16 and/or CD56 surface antigens (30). Many NK cells in the adult also express surface CD57. NK cells are nonadherent and have the morphological appearance of large, granular lymphocytes. NK cells express surface CD2 and the ζ-chain of the CD3 complex in association with CD16. Unlike cytotoxic T cells, NK cells produce MHC-*non*restricted cytotoxicity directed against virus-infected cells and tumor cells. Studies in experimental animals suggest an important role for NK cells in modulating in vivo resistance to tumors and viruses, especially those of the herpes group. Similarly, the report of recurrent, severe infection with herpes group viruses in a patient lacking NK cells supports a role for NK cells in virus defense (31). The cytolytic mechanisms of NK cells are similar to those documented in cytotoxic T cells, and NK cytotoxicity is generally enhanced by in-terferon-γ and IL-2 (32). NK cells also produce certain lymphokines (see Table 9.2), replicate in response to IL-2, augment cytolytic T cell responses, inhibit T and B cell growth and differentiation, and inhibit hematopoietic cell growth and maturation. NK cells are also one mediator of antibody-dependent cell-mediated cytotoxicity (ADCC), a process that is significantly more efficient than nonantibody dependent cell lysis by NK cells.

Table 9.2.   Lymphokines/Cytokines: Partial List Including Source and Major Known Functions

Name	Principal Cell Sources	Functions	Production by Neonatal Cells
Interferon-γ	T cells, NK cells	Pleiotropic effects; activates macrophages; enhances HLA antigen expression; enhances release of IL-1 and TNF; modulates B cell growth and differentiation; augments NK cell cytotoxicity; inhibits HIV infection in macrophages	Markedly diminished
IL-2	T cells, NK cells	Major T cell growth factor; enhances B cell proliferation and differentiation; augments NK cell cytotoxicity	Normal
IL-3	T cells	Stimulates growth of bone marrow stem cells; mast cells	Moderately diminished
IL-4	T cells, mast cells	Stimulates growth and differentiation of and T cells; impedes macrophage activation	Markedly diminished
IL-5	T cells	Regulates B cell growth and differentiation; stimulates growth of eosinophil colonies from myeloid stem cells; augments eosinophil functions	Markedly diminished (mRNA analysis only)
GM-CSF	T cells, monocyte/ macrophages	Stimulates growth of granulocyte-macrophage colonies from myeloid stem cells; modulates macrophage and granulocyte function; may enhance HIV replication	Moderately diminished
Lymphotoxin	T cells, ?NK cells	Lyses or inhibits growth of tumor cells or virus-infected cells	Normal or increased
TNF-α	Macrophages, T cells, NK cells	Same as lymphotoxin; mediates many aspects of acute-phase response; partly mediates septic shock; enhances HIV replication in cell lines	Slightly decreased
IL-1	Monocyte/macrophages; T and B cells; fibroblasts, endothelial cells, etc.	Pleiotropic effects; facilitates T cell activation; regulates B cell and neutrophil function; mediates many aspects of acute-phase response	Normal
IL-6	Monocytes/macrophages; T and B cells; fibroblasts, endothelial cells, other	B cell differentiation and Ig secretion; acute-phase response mediator; hematopoietic stem cell growth; T cell growth and differentiation; may enhance HIV replication	Normal or moderately diminished (see text)
G-CSF	Monocyte/macrophages; fibroblasts, endothelial cells	Stimulates growth of granulocyte colonies from myeloid stem cells; modulates neutrophil function	Normal
M-CSF, CSF-1	Monocyte/macrophages; fibroblasts, endothelial cells	Stimulates growth of macrophage colonies from stem cells; modulates macrophage function	Normal to increased

NK cells make up ~10–15% of circulating lymphocytes in the adult and neonate (Table 9.3). As defined by expression of the CD16 surface antigen, the number of circulating NK cells in the blood of term neonates and adults is similar (30, 32). However, the fraction of NK cells that expresses another NK cell marker, CD57 (HNK-1), is markedly diminished, and the fraction that expresses CD56 (NKH-1) is reduced by ~50% (30, 32, 33). Because the total lymphocyte count in the blood of neonates is greater than in adults, the absolute numbers of NK cells in the neonate exceeds that in adults. However, the cytotoxic activity of neonatal NK cells is reduced to 15–60% of the activity of adults' NK cells in most studies. This may be due to the relative paucity of neonatal NK cells that express CD56. Virtually all adult NK cells that express CD16 also express CD56, whereas a substantial number of neonatal NK cells do not. NK cells that do not express CD56 have poor cytolytic capacity; when only those neonatal NK cells that express CD56 are studied, their cytolytic potential is similar to that of adult cells (30, 32).

Cells with an NK phenotype appear to make up a considerable percentage of mononuclear cells in the fetal liver where they can be detected as early as 6 weeks gestation (30). Cytolytic function increases progressively during fetal and postnatal life with lysis ~50% of that obtained with adult cells at term and comparable with those observed in adult cells by 4–5 years of age in one study and by ~6 months in another (33, 34). The increase in cytolytic activity appears to roughly parallel the increase in percentage of CD56 expressing cells.

As with adult cells, neonatal NK cell activity is augmented by the interferons and IL-2. However, IL-2 improves neonatal NK cell activity relatively more than it does adult NK cell activity, such that IL-2-treated neonatal and adult NK cells have nearly identical cytotoxicity (30, 32, 34). However, interferon-α or -γ enhances the cytotoxic activity of neonatal NK cells minimally, except for those neonates who have normal numbers of CD56-expressing NK cells. ADCC by neonatal lymphocytes is also diminished at birth, averaging ~50% of adult values; ADCC is present at adult levels by ~1 year of age (reviewed in Ref. 12).

In a series of studies employing a murine model of herpes simplex virus infection, Kohl (35) has demonstrated that the age-related maturation of NK cell function parallels the development of resistance to herpes simplex virus infection and that NK-deficient mice could be protected from herpes simplex virus infection by human lymphocytes plus human interferon-α or -γ. Human cord blood cytotoxic activity against herpes simplex virus-infected cells is consistently diminished, even after stimulation with IL-2. ADCC vs. herpes simplex virus is also diminished in the neonatal mouse model as well as in human cord blood cells. NK activity vs. cytomegalovirus-infected targets is also diminished in neonates but matures rapidly postnatally as described for general NK activity (36). NK cell activity and ADCC (if passively acquired maternal antibody is present) are likely important in the initial containment phase of herpes simplex virus and cytomegalovirus infection; diminished NK cytotoxicity may be an important factor allowing the wide dissemination

Table 9.3.   Age-related Changes in NK Cells and NK Cell Function[a]

Age	n	Phenotypic Markers							
		CD16		CD56		CD57		K562 cytotoxic cells	
		%	No.	%	No.	%	No.	%	No.
Birth	11	13.8 ± 4.3	709 ± 316	9.1 ± 4.3	481 ± 198	1.2 ± 0.7	60 ± 40	1.1 ± 0.2	54 ± 24
1–5 mo	6	12.7 ± 4.6	790 ± 352	10.6 ± 5.4	627 ± 308	1.4 ± 0.8	80 ± 40	1.8 ± 0.5	113 ± 48
6–12 mo	7	12.5 ± 4.9	714 ± 300	12.2 ± 6.0	676 ± 295	1.7 ± 1.5	120 ± 110	2.0 ± 0.4	121 ± 42
1–4 yr	8	12.9 ± 4.6	573 ± 264	13.1 ± 5.6	586 ± 310	2.6 ± 1.9	120 ± 90	2.1 ± 0.3	136 ± 37
5–8 yr	6	14.4 ± 5.2	418 ± 134	15.0 ± 6.7	431 ± 181	12.5 ± 6.7	360 ± 170	2.1 ± 0.3	92 ± 23
9–13 yr	7	15.2 ± 4.2	408 ± 196	16.5 ± 5.9	438 ± 181	15.8 ± 6.9	410 ± 190	2.1 ± 0.4	81 ± 26
Adult	12	15.5 ± 5.4	318 ± 191	16.4 ± 6.5	343 ± 214	20.5 ± 5.5	400 ± 150	2.1 ± 0.3	60 ± 23

[a]Data adapted from Ref. 33. Values are means ± SD.

of infection that is characteristic of over-whelming neonatal or intrauterine infection with herpes simplex virus and cytomegalovirus respectively.

PHENOTYPE AND FUNCTION OF B CELLS DURING DEVELOPMENT

B Cells and Immunoglobulin

Pre-B cells are first detected in human fetal liver at ~8 weeks gestation and in fetal bone marrow by 12 weeks gestation; after 30 weeks gestation they are found only in bone marrow (reviewed in Ref. 12). B cells expressing surface IgM can be detected by 10 weeks gestation; B cells expressing surface Ig of the other isotypes are present by 15 weeks gestation. Although adult B cells initially express IgM plus IgD, fetal B cells appear to express IgM without IgD. B cells expressing IgM in the absence of IgD may easily become tolerant to the antigens that they bind, perhaps allowing the fetus to become tolerant to antigens to which it is exposed in utero. Later in gestation, fetal B cells that coexpress IgM and IgD appear. Another major difference in the fetal B cell repertoire is the relative preponderance of B cells expressing CD5 (also known as Ly-1$^+$- or B1-B cells) (37–39). These cells make up to 50% of the B cell and B cell progenitor populations in the fetal spleen and lymph nodes by midgestation but are less abundant in fetal liver and bone marrow. CD5+ or B1-B cells may represent a separate lineage, precursors for which are found only early during development. Unlike conventional (B2) B cells, B1-B cells are capable of self-renewal, commonly produce antibodies of limited diversity that are directed against self-antigens (autoantibodies), and are susceptible to long-term tolerance. It has been suggested that they are involved in regulation and development of the immune system through idiotypic networks.

The preponderance of B1 or CD5+ B cells noted in the fetus, is also observed in neonates. Like adults, neonates have circulating B cells, most of which express IgM and IgD and a smaller fraction of which express IgG or IgA. However, the coexpression of IgM and IgD with IgG or IgA or the coexpression of activation markers and IgD is unique to neonatal B cells. It is unknown

whether the observed differences are accounted for by lineage differences, developmental differences, or recent activation (presumably by self-antigens).

The repertoire for specific antigen recognition, which is dictated by the variable region of the Ig expressed by a particular B cell, appears also to differ and to be more limited in the fetus than in the adult. In the early to midgestation human fetus, the numbers of different gene segments used to generate the Ig variable regions and the potential diversity at the third complementarity determining region of the Ig heavy chain is limited. The B cell repertoire increases during gestation, such that by birth it is considerably more diverse (40, 41). Differences in repertoire, along with functional differences, may be involved in limiting the capacity of the fetus and neonate for production of antibodies to certain antigens. It is unknown if this affects the capacity of the fetus and neonate to produce antibodies to different antigens of the HIV, although the variety of HIV antigens recognized by serum from infected neonates is often more limited than that of adults.

Immunoglobulin Production and Concentrations in Fetus and Neonate

Ig-secreting plasma cells appear later in gestation than B cells; plasma cells secreting IgM have been detected by week 15 of gestation, whereas those secreting IgG and IgA are first detected by weeks 20 and 30, respectively. IgM is first detectable in the blood of the fetus near the end of the second trimester, but only minimal levels of IgM and IgA are detectable at birth (reviewed in Ref. 12). IgM levels increase from a mean of 6 mg/dl in premature neonates at <28 weeks gestation to 11 mg/dl at term. Serum concentrations of IgA in umbilical cord blood are usually 0.1–5.0 mg/dl (levels undetectable by conventional methods) and are similar in term and preterm neonates. Passively derived maternal IgG is the source of virtually all IgG detected in the normal fetus (10). Ig levels do not reach adult norms until ~1 year (IgM), 5–6 years (IgG), and adolescence (IgA), respectively (Table 9.4). IgG subclass production matures in the order IgG_3, IgG_1, IgG_4, IgG_2. In addition to

**Table 9.4.   Serum Ig and T Cell Subsets in Exposed but Uninfected Infants
and in Infants Infected Perinatally with HIV[a]**

Age	Children		
	Uninfected	P-1	P-2
IgG (mg/dl)			
0–1 mo	544 ± 757	836 ± 1091	952 ± 1122
1–6 mo	437 ± 630	551 ± 657	1360 ± 1514
7–12 mo	565 ± 711	615 ± 918	1893 ± 2422
13–42 mo	725 ± 998	774 ± 1120	2125 ± 2855
IgA (mg/dl)			
0–1 mo	16 ± 30	16 ± 27	54 ± 69
1–6 mo	24 ± 32	27 ± 39	74 ± 98
7–12 mo	27 ± 68	26 ± 42	141 ± 191
13–24 mo	42 ± 69	45 ± 89	149 ± 188
IgM (mg/dl)			
0–1 mo	47 ± 78	47 ± 77	103 ± 152
1–6 mo	59 ± 89	85 ± 109	134 ± 159
7–12 mo	79 ± 104	108 ± 134	167 ± 183
13–24 mo	105 ± 130	120 ± 177	149 ± 191
CD3+ lymphocytes (cells/mm³)			
0–1 mo	4050 ± 2073	3809 ± 2760	3984 ± 2553
1–6 mo	5030 ± 2344	4721 ± 1508	3438 ± 2747
7–12 mo	4782 ± 1918	4577 ± 1888	4369 ± 2449
13–24 mo	4116 ± 1643	4144 ± 2011	4016 ± 2025
CD4+ lymphocytes (cells/mm³)			
0–1 mo	2900 ± 1541	2580 ± 1501	2317 ± 1317
1–6 mo	3278 ± 1401	3482 ± 1234	1706 ± 1215
7–12 mo	3051 ± 1285	2769 ± 1326	1951 ± 882
13–24 mo	2584 ± 1105	2030 ± 1481	1680 ± 1089
CD8+ lymphocytes (cells/mm³)			
0–1 mo	1418 ± 791	1404 ± 974	1499 ± 1046
1–6 mo	1626 ± 985	1457 ± 709	1613 ± 958
7–12 mo	514 ± 300	394 ± 334	523 ± 266
13–24 mo	1374 ± 663	1902 ± 844	2242 ± 1290

[a]Data adapted from Ref. 67. Values are means ± SD.

quantitative differences, there are qualitative differences in Ig synthesis by the newborn as well. Some circulating IgM in the neonate may be nonfunctional monomeric instead of pentameric IgM. However, IgM is relatively more abundant in secretions of neonates than in those of adults, and secretory IgA, while absent at birth, is detectable by 1–2 weeks of age in tears, nasopharyngeal secretions, and saliva (42); these may provide partial compensation for the overall diminution in Ig production in the neonate.

In general, neonatal B cells can differentiate into IgM-secreting plasma cells as efficiently as adult cells. However, the ability of neonatal T cells to produce B cell help for IgM production is variable, as noted above. Unlike adult B cells, neonatal B cells do not differentiate into plasma cells that secrete IgG or IgA in most assay systems (43); these functions are not mature until ~2 (IgG) and

5 years (IgA) of age, respectively. However, recent results suggest that under certain conditions, neonatal B cells produce IgG, each of the IgG isotypes, IgA and IgE, in amounts comparable with adult B cells (24, 44). Similar results have been obtained in more limited studies with fetal B cells from as early as 12 weeks gestation, although IgA production was not detected (39). To achieve these results either an artificial form of T cell help was provided (normal adult T cells do not suffice as they do when adult B cells are studied) and/or exogenous lymphokines not produced adequately by neonatal T cells were required. These results suggest that limitation in the capacity of neonatal B cells to produce these Ig isotypes is not absolute, but their limited response under most conditions in vitro is paralleled by their relative inability in these functions in vivo.

Specific Antibody Responses
by Fetus and Neonate

Antibody responses by the fetus have been documented in response to maternal immunization with tetanus toxoid; although the response was primarily IgM, it did appear to prime for a secondary antibody response later (reviewed in Ref. 12). In addition, specific antibody production has been documented in response to various intrauterine infections. However, not all fetuses mount a detectable antibody response to intrauterine infection: specific IgM antibody was absent in 34% of infants with congenital rubella, 19% of infants with congenital *Toxoplasma* infection, and 11% of infants with congenital cytomegalovirus infection. Similar results have been obtained by measuring IgA antibodies. IgA antibodies are detectable in a somewhat greater fraction of infants with congenital *Toxoplasma* infection (89%) than are IgM antibodies, indicating that fetal infection can lead to antibody production and to class switching from IgM to IgA antibodies in the fetus (45). Note that these results were obtained at term or in early infancy and that fetal antibody production as detected by IgM or IgA antibodies to the infecting pathogens is detected in <25–50% of those with established congenital *Toxoplasma* infection at 20–30 weeks gestation. This suggests that production of antibodies by the fetus may be absent or delayed in development relative to adults. As described in more detail below, similar findings have been made in the fetus and infant with HIV infection.

The neonate can mount an antibody response to most protein antigens after either immunization (e.g., tetanus and diphtheria toxoids) or infection (e.g., enteroviruses) (reviewed in Ref. 12). However, the response may be less marked than that of older children or adults, and the switch from IgM to IgG production may be delayed. In contrast, the response to many polysaccharide antigens is absent or severely blunted, as demonstrated by the inability of neonates to mount a response to *Hemophilus influenzae* type B polyribose-ribitol phosphate vaccine or to group B streptococcus type-specific capsular antigens after infec-

tion. In humans the response to some polysaccharide antigens can be demonstrated by 6 months of age, but the response to vaccination with pneumococcal or *H. influenzae* polysaccharides remains poor until ~18–24 months. The basis for the inability of infants to respond to polysaccharides may be multifactorial but does not appear to be due to a lack of the appropriate antibody repertoire, at least for *H. influenzae* (46). In fact, coupling of the *H. influenzae* capsular polysaccharide to protein carriers converts it from type 2 thymus/T cell independent antigen to a T cell dependent antigen and renders it immunogenic in infants as young as 2–6 months. This is not due to a change in the repertoire of the antibodies produced in response to the conjugate compared with the free polysaccharide (46). It is yet unknown whether this is also true for other polysaccharide antigens that are poorly immunogenic in infants.

Preterm neonates of >24 weeks gestation produce antibody in response to protein antigens such as diphtheria toxoid as well as term neonates or infants and respond appropriately to the diphtheria-pertussis-tetanus and oral and inactivated poliovirus (41) vaccines when these are administered at the usual intervals of 2, 4, and 6 months. B cells from preterm infants also synthesize antibody in vitro as well as B cells from term infants. As in term infants, the ability to respond to polysaccharide antigens remains diminished during the first two years of life.

TRANSPLACENTAL PASSAGE OF IgG

Only antibody of the IgG isotype crosses the placenta (reviewed in Ref. 12). IgG transport across the placenta can be detected as early as 8 weeks gestation, but circulating fetal concentrations of IgG remain below 100 mg/dl until ~17–20 weeks. After this time, the levels rise steadily, reaching half of the term serum concentration by ~30 weeks; the term neonate's IgG level usually exceeds the maternal level by 5–10%. All IgG subclasses cross the placenta well, because the relative amounts of IgG_1, IgG_2, IgG_3, and IgG_4 in cord serum are generally comparable with those in maternal serum; however, data from one group suggested that IgG_1 may be preferentially transported. By approximately 2 months of life, the amount of circulating IgG synthesized by the infant equals the amount derived from transplacental transfer; by 10–12 months of age the IgG is nearly all derived from synthesis by the infant. As a consequence of the fall in passively derived IgG and increased synthesis of IgG, values reach a nadir of ~400 mg/dl in term infants at 3–4 months and rise thereafter. The premature infant has proportionally lower IgG concentrations at birth, and values reach a lower nadir: at 3 months values of 82 and 104 mg/dl, are observed in infants born at 25–28 and 29–32 weeks gestation, respectively. This passively transferred maternal antibody is important in protection but confounds the use of antibody tests that measure IgG or total antibody for the diagnosis of infection in the fetus, neonate, and infant.

MONONUCLEAR PHAGOCYTES

Blood monocytes are derived from bone marrow myeloid precursors and themselves are precursors of tissue macrophages; together these cells make up the mononuclear phagocytes system. Under steady-state conditions, >95% of the total mononuclear phagocytes are tissue macrophages, and <2% are monocytes (reviewed in Ref. 12). Differentiation of monocytes into tissue macrophages involves many common maturational changes, but some are seen only in certain tissues (e.g., alveolar macrophages utilize aerobic cytochrome oxidation).

Macrophages are detectable as early as 4 weeks gestation. Initially, macrophages are found in the yolk sac, followed by the fetal liver and then bone marrow. The number of circulating monocytes in the neonate is equal to or greater than that of the adult, and the capacity of fetal marrow to produce monocytes appears to be similar to or greater than that of adult marrow. However, the number of tissue macrophages in the neonate is less well defined. In rodents and monkeys, fetal lung contains very few macrophages until just before term, and this may also be true in humans. In healthy monkeys the number of alveolar macrophages increases rapidly in the first 24–48 hours after birth. Because resident macrophages in the spleen and liver are responsible for removing damaged erythrocytes from the blood, the increased numbers of such erythrocytes circulating in neonates of <36 weeks gestation suggest that these cells are either less abundant or functionally impaired in preterm neonates.

Although monocyte production appears to be normal in the neonate, the delivery of monocytes to the site of infection or inflammation is delayed and attenuated. Macrophages from neonatal rodents are clearly immature in their ability to cooperate with T cells and B cells in the induction of specific response to antigen and express markedly fewer class II MHC molecules. In contrast, human neonatal monocytes express relatively normal amounts of class II MHC molecules and appear to be capable of processing and presenting *Escherichia coli* antigen to T cells. Similarly, neonatal monocytes can support the responses of parental T cells to *E. coli*, tetanus toxoid, purified protein derivative, and other antigens. However, it is uncertain if the response of neonatal monocytes is as efficient as that of adult cells, and the ability of neonatal tissue macrophages to support lymphocyte responses to antigen has not been studied.

Various monocyte/macrophage-derived cytokines, including TNF-α, IL-6, and GM-CSF have been reported to enhance HIV replication (47, 48; see Chapter 8). To the extent that it has been addressed, cytokine production by monocytes from term neonates has been similar to those from adults (reviewed in Ref. 12). In response to endotoxin, monocytes from term neonates secreted as much IL-1, IL-6, and TNF as did adult cells; monocytes derived from preterm neonates produced similar amounts of IL-1 but less TNF. Note that, except for studies on IL-6, the concentrations of endotoxin used may be higher than achieved in the blood even in individuals with Gram-negative sepsis; thus these results must be interpreted with the caveat that they will require replication at more physiologically relevant, lower concentrations of endotoxin. Production of IL-6 by monocytes in response to IL-1 is reduced to ~50 and ~25% of adult values with cells from term and preterm neonates, respectively

lation, but the resultant immune deficiency more closely mimics that observed in adult populations (53–55).

CELLULAR IMMUNE ABNORMALITIES

T Cells

The hallmark of immune deficiency in pediatric HIV infection, as in adult infection, is the loss of lymphocytes bearing a CD4 surface phenotype. As will become evident in this chapter, the simple quantitative loss of CD4 cells does not adequately explain all abnormalities in immune responsiveness described in pediatric HIV infection. In this section, the abnormalities in both the numbers and function of T cells that result from HIV infection will be addressed.

Results in Adults

From the onset of HIV infection in adults, there is a continual loss of CD4 lymphocytes usually in conjunction with a rise in CD8 lymphocytes, resulting in a dramatic reversal of the ratio of CD4 to CD8 T cells in the peripheral blood (53, 54, 56). This pattern has been described in all adult and adolescent HIV-infected populations regardless of route of infection. CD4 T cells with a putative memory function (CD45RO+) are preferentially lost in the early stages of infection, although ultimately all CD4 lymphocytes (CD45RO+) and CD45RA+) are lost (57, 58). There is coexpression on both CD4 and CD8 T cells of the activation marker HLA-DR. Other T cell phenotypes with unresolved function have also been described, such as those coexpressing CD8, CD57, and HLA-DR.

In addition to these quantitative abnormalities in T cell numbers, functional abnormalities have been observed that cannot always be explained by the quantitative decline in CD4 T cells. There are defects in T cell responses to alloantigenic stimulation, soluble antigens, and mitogens (59). In addition, defects in T cell signaling, clonal expansion, IL-2 production, and IL-2 receptor expression have been observed (60–62). Despite the description of these multiple quantitative and qualitative T cell defects, the most reliable predictor of clinically relevant immune deficiency, as manifest by the development of opportunistic infections and malignancies, has been the absolute number of CD4 T cells in the peripheral blood. Although occasional infections, such as oral candidiasis, are seen in adults with CD4 T cell numbers in the 300–500/μl range, most severe infections occur when CD4 T cell numbers drop below the 200–300/μl range. Most opportunistic infections in adult HIV disease are infections classically controlled by the cellular arm of the immune system. This observation reinforces the concept that in adult infection, the loss of CD4 T cells, and the resultant paralysis of the cellular arm of the immune system, are the most pivotal consequences of HIV infection. Not all these observations hold for pediatric HIV infection.

Quantitative Abnormalities in Pediatric Infection

Neonatal HIV infection is characterized by a continual decline in T lymphocytes bearing the CD4 surface phenotype (63–67). As described earlier in this chapter, newborn infants have a much higher percentage of circulating CD4 lymphocytes than adults and that population has a higher percentage of naive (CD45RA+) compared with memory (CD45RO+) T lymphocytes. With age, the percentage and absolute numbers of CD4 T cells in infants begin to approximate those of adults (Table 9.1). The rate of CD4 T cells decline is often much more rapid in neonatal infection than in adults. The mean incubation from HIV infection to AIDS in neonates is difficult to estimate since there appear to be two distinct clinical courses. Some have a rapid decline in CD4 lymphocytes, resulting in an early diagnosis of AIDS and death, whereas others may remain healthy and symptom-free for many years (68). The mean incubation from birth to AIDS has been estimated as 4.1 months for rapid progressors and 6.1 years for slow progressors (69). The exact reason for this bimodal distribution of cases remains controversial, although it has been suggested that the rate of disease progression may be associated with the timing of infection during pregnancy and delivery. In addition to a loss of

CD4 T cells, an increase in CD8 T cells with a resultant reversal in the CD4-to-CD8 ratio is also observed. Other phenotypic abnormalities in T cell populations, such as coexpression of CD57 and HLA-DR in conjunction with CD8, have been noted (K. Luzuriaga, personal communication, 1993). The increased number of T cells that coexpress HLA-DR is suggestive of a loss of immune regulation in HIV infection, which leads to a general state of immune activation. Although this is obviously an oversimplified view of what actually may be occurring, some degree of immune activation is also apparent from the hypergammaglobulinemia and excess levels of circulating lymphokines, which have been described.

As in adult infection, CD4 T cell depletion in neonatal HIV infection correlates with clinical disease as manifest by opportunistic infections and development of tumors. In multiple studies, loss of CD4 T cells or reversal of the CD4-to-CD8 ratio has correlated with p24 antigenemia, virus load, loss of mitogenic responsiveness, and development of opportunistic infections. Note that opportunistic infections, which are the ultimate correlates of clinically relevant immune deficiency, occur in HIV-infected neonates with much higher CD4 T cell counts than in HIV-infected adults. In one study, 8 of 22 infants diagnosed with *Pneumocystis carinii* pneumonia had >450 CD4 T cells/mm^3 at time of infection (70). In addition, P-2 infection status can be associated with near-normal CD4 lymphocyte numbers (Table 9.4). This may result from the fact that functional defects not predicted by CD4 lymphocyte numbers alone can be present in HIV-infected infants (71). Therefore the level of CD4 lymphopenia at which clinically relevant immune deficiency can occur must be adjusted to take into account the high percentage of CD4 lymphocytes in the neonatal circulation, changes in those numbers that normally occur with age (Table 9.1), and functional abnormalities not reflected in CD4 lymphocyte numbers. Current recommendations suggest that prophylaxis is appropriate when CD4 T cell counts fall below values of 1500/μl, 750/μl, 500/μl, or 200/μl, respectively in infants (<1 year old) or children between 1 and 2 years, 2 and 6 years, or over 6 years of age,

respectively (72) (see Chaper 21). Although absolute numbers of memory vs. naive CD4 cells may be what ultimately determines susceptibility to *P. carinii* pneumonia, and explain why infants contract this infection with higher numbers of total CD4 cells, greater functional abnormalities may exist as a result of HIV infection of a developing immune system than occur after infection of a mature adult immune system.

Functional Abnormalities in Pediatric Infection

The most evident manifestation of the functional defects in T cell immunity in neonatal HIV infection is the inability of the host to deal with tumors and infections that rely on cellular immunity for control. Tumors (73–75) or severe clinical syndromes associated with Epstein-Barr virus (EBV) (76–78) and pulmonary infection with *P. carinii* (70) are conditions seen in HIV-infected infants who have only modest decreases in CD4 T cell numbers in their peripheral blood (see Chapters 21 and 33). This has been taken as evidence of a greater functional immune defect in neonatal HIV infection than occurs in adult infection. The implications of these observations on possible pathogenetic mechanisms of HIV infection in neonates were covered in Chapter 8.

The presence of functional T cell abnormalities in neonatal HIV infection is well described. Several studies have documented that near-normal T cell numbers can exist at the time of clinically apparent T cell immunodeficiency (67, 70). In addition, cutaneous anergy is an early manifestation of HIV infection in children (63, 65). To address the basis of the immune nonresponsiveness of infected children with normal T cell numbers, Roilides et al. (79) investigated T helper (CD4) cell function in infected children. In this study, peripheral blood lymphocytes from infants and children at various stages of HIV infection were tested for ability to proliferate in response to soluble antigen (influenza and tetanus antigens), alloantigen, or mitogen. The response to soluble antigen was the first to be lost followed by the alloantigen response and then the mitogenic response. Among the mitogens, the response to pokeweed mitogen (PWM), a T cell-dependent B cell mitogen is often the best predictor of immune deficiency (80), but all mitogenic responses, including those to PHA and ConA, are depressed in HIV-infected infants (63, 64, 66, 79, 81). Loss of these T cell functions often occurs before apparent loss of CD4 T cell numbers and is often the first measurable indication of immune attrition in infants. This pattern of T helper cell dysfunction occurs irrespective of the route or timing of HIV infection.

Less concrete information is available on functional abnormalities of cytotoxic (CD8) T cells in pediatric HIV infection. Since the outgrowth of EBV-related malignancies is felt to be under the control of EBV-specific cytotoxic T lymphocytes (CTL), the common occurrence of such tumors in HIV-infected infants might indicate a functional defect in the EBV-specific CTL response. Indeed, Blumberg et al. (82) in a study of HIV-infected homosexual men found a direct correlation between CD4 T cell numbers and CTL activity against EBV. A similar loss of IL-2 production was noted, indicating that a loss of CD4 help for the CD8 CTL could be the operative defect. This is in agreement with the observation that the cytomegalovirus-specific CTL response of HIV-infected adults could be restored by the addition of IL-2 (83). In contrast to reports of decreases in specific CTL activities, two other studies in adult populations have indicated that CD8 T cells maintain a normal broad cytolytic function (84) or actually exhibit an increase in allogeneic reactivity as a result of HIV infection (85). In a direct attempt to measure the HIV-specific CTL response in HIV-infected children, Luzuriaga et al. (86) found that neonatally infected children were less likely than hemophilic children to have detectable HIV-specific CTL in the peripheral blood. Because as neonatally infected children are known to have levels of replicating HIV in their blood similar to those in adults (51), this lack of detectable HIV-specific CTL did not result from a decrease in antigenic load. Subsequent attempts by Luzuriaga et al. (K. Luzuriaga, personal communication, 1993) to determine precursor frequency of these HIV-specific CTL have also demonstrated a relative deficiency in the number

of functional HIV-specific CTL precursors in neonatally infected children. This deficiency may relate to the decreased clonogenic potential of CD8 lymphocytes in AIDS patients, which has been described in adult populations but has not been adequately investigated in children (51, 87). A lack of CD4 T cell help in providing IL-2 does not explain this defect, since this step was circumvented by the addition of IL-2 to the expanding cultures of CD8 T cells.

In summary, the susceptibility of infants infected by HIV to infections and malignancies routinely controlled by the cellular arm of the immune system can be correlated to specific measurable defects in CD4 and CD8 cell functions. Many of these measurable abnormalities in T cell function are apparent before any quantitative abnormalities in T cell numbers. There still remain many gaps in our understanding of how HIV infection can bring about such broad functional abnormalities in T cells, most which are uninfected.

Monocytes and Macrophages

Monocytes and macrophages are important in the immune response to infection. One key role is to act as antigen-presenting cells to the T and B cells during generation of an immune response. This function is shared with other cells of the immune system, including the Langerhans cells of the skin and the dendritic cells, variants of which are present in the circulation or in the lymphoid organs. In addition, through their phagocytic function, macrophages are responsible for control of pathogens such as mycobacteria. The increased incidence of tuberculous and *Mycobacterium avium* infections in HIV-infected individuals is consistent with functional defects either in these cells or in their activation by T cells or T cell products (see also Chapter 16B).

A direct role for HIV in mediating monocyte and macrophage dysfunction can be hypothesized because HIV can infect these cells directly. Both monocytes and macrophages express low levels of CD4 on their surface, as do Langerhans and dendritic cells. Laboratory and primary isolates of HIV will infect peripheral blood monocytes and transformed cell lines of monocytic origin (88, 89). HIV can also be recovered from relatively pure populations of monocytes isolated from the blood of HIV-infected patients, and studies have indicated that the major reservoir of HIV in the central nervous system resides in multinucleated giant cells of monocytic origin (90, 91). Monocytes and other antigen-presenting cells may serve a further detrimental function to the host by providing a vehicle through which HIV can be spread to other cells. HIV will replicate to high titer in some monocyte lines without causing cell death (92), and recent evidence suggests that follicular dendritic cells, although unable to replicate HIV, can efficiently pass HIV infection to CD4 T cells in the process of HIV antigen presentation (93).

Very little information has been generated in pediatric populations regarding the role of HIV in monocyte/macrophage dysfunction. Most conclusions must therefore be extrapolated from studies performed on adult patients. High levels of MHC-II molecules are expressed by these cells during antigen presentation. It has been suggested that there is less HLA-DR (an MHC-II antigen) expressed on monocytes from HIV-infected than from uninfected individuals (94). The same holds true for Langerhans cells (95). Direct assays of antigen-presenting function have indicated that HIV-infected monocytic cell lines have a decreased capacity to drive a proliferative response to antigen, indicating a direct defect in antigen-presenting function (96). In addition, abnormalities in chemotaxis and Fc receptor function of monocytes have been noted as a result of HIV infection (97, 98).

Natural Killer Cells

As described above, lymphocytes with NK function, which is most commonly assayed by the capacity of these cells to lyse the erythroleukemia cell line K562, are identifiable by the expression of CD16 and commonly also CD56 and CD57. Absolute numbers of circulating CD16 and CD56 cells remain normal in adult and pediatric HIV infection, but expression of CD57 increases, and it is often coexpressed on CD8 T cells. The true function of these CD8/CD57 double-positive cells is controversial, but a similar population of cells has been described in acute cytomegalovirus infection. There are functional abnormalities in the NK cells of HIV-infected children. In a hemophilic population, Sullivan et al. (53) found peripheral blood lymphocytes from HIV-infected individuals lysed K562 cells to a lesser degree than peripheral blood lymphocytes from uninfected controls, although the difference was not striking. Other studies in adult populations have indicated that NK cells from HIV-infected individuals are deficient in the ability to lyse K562 cells but maintain the ability to mediate ADCC activity (99). This specific defect in triggering of K562 lysis may be related to a deficiency in tubulin rearrangement (100). How HIV infection might bring about such a specific defect in NK cell function remains unknown, although some have suggested that NK cells can be infected with, and harbor, HIV.

Granulocytes

Because HIV has such profound effects on lymphocyte populations, little notice is often given to possible effects of HIV on granulocyte function. Bacteria constitute a major fraction of infections encountered in pediatric AIDS. Although this may largely reflect deficits in antibody synthesis, abnormalities in granulocyte function may result from HIV infection and contribute to this susceptibility. In general, granulocyte numbers are normal in both adult and pediatric HIV-infected populations until the later stages of AIDS, when all white blood cells are decreased. Limited studies of granulocyte function in HIV infection have, however, revealed some abnormalities. Several granulocyte functions can be measured in vitro. These include chemotaxis, bacterial phagocytosis, superoxide generation, and bactericidal activity. When each of these activities was measured in granulocytes from HIV-infected individuals, it was found that superoxide generation and bactericidal activities were normal, but bacterial phagocytosis was decreased (101). Of interest was the fact that increased chemotaxis was seen in symptomatic patients, but decreased chemotaxis was observed in patients with asymptomatic HIV infection (101).

Whether these in vitro defects result in clinically relevant deficiency in the ability to control infection remains unknown.

HUMORAL IMMUNE ABNORMALITIES
B Cells

Antibodies that cross the placenta and are present in breast milk are known to provide the infant with some level of protective immunity against multiple pathogens. However, an infant encounters, and must mount primary immune responses, to many bacterial, viral, fungal, and protozoal pathogens early in life. Abnormalities in B cell numbers and function in these individuals can have serious results. B cell dysfunction contributes significantly to the overall morbidity and mortality of pediatric HIV infection, and clinical decisions must be based upon an understanding of the relevant B cell dysfunctions present in these children. B cell abnormalities in adults have less serious repercusions, however, since primary immunity and some level of circulating antibody already exist to most pathogens. B cell dysfunction therefore is minor in the clinically apparent immune deficiency associated with adult HIV infection.

Results in Adults

In the area of B cell deficiencies, most observations and research have been performed in pediatric populations where the abnormalities are more clinically apparent. In adults, increased numbers of circulating B cells, specifically those B cells expressing the CD5 surface phenotype, have been noted (102). Increased levels occur and syndromes associated with immune complexes are not uncommon in HIV-infected adults. Clinically, antibody responses to vaccination with influenza or pneumococcal vaccines are deficient in infected adults, and bacterial infections with encapsulated organisms such as the pneumococcus or *H. influenzae* present a significant health risk to those infected with HIV. B cell abnormalities, however, remain a minor consideration when compared with the devastating consequences of T cell abnormalities present in adult HIV infection.

Quantitative Abnormalities in Pediatric Infection

Whether direct or as a consequence of CD4 T cell dysfunction, B cell abnormalities have a major impact on the clinically relevant immune deficiency of pediatric HIV infection. Increased absolute numbers of circulating B cells including those that coexpress CD5 are present in HIV-infected infants. One of the most common findings among infected infants is hypergammaglobulinemia. This phenomenon is so common among those infants infected with HIV that it is often used as an indicator of infection during the first 12–18 months of life, when HIV serology is of little value in determining infection status. Levels of IgG correlate with the age of the child and also with the stage of HIV infection, the highest levels being present in older children and in P-2 infection rather than in asymptomatic infection (67; Table 9.4). The hypergammaglobulinemia in these patients is polyclonal (103, 104). The most common IgG subclass to be elevated is IgG_1, followed by IgG_3. In one study of 47 infected children, 16 had only elevated IgG_1, 6 had only elevated IgG_3, and 12 had elevations of both subclasses (103). IgG_2 and IgG_4 levels are usually normal or low rather than elevated in these children, but there does not appear to be an increased risk of bacterial infection in those with low levels of these IgG subclasses (103). IgA and IgM levels can also be elevated (67). This is a late manifestation of HIV infection, generally occurring in infants with P-2 infection status (67). Elevated IgE levels have also been seen in some infected infants. Although generally associated with hyperimmunoglobulinemias, sporadic reports of HIV-infected infants with panhypogammaglobulinemia have also surfaced (105). The presence of circulating immune complexes is also common in HIV-infected infants.

Functional Abnormalities in Pediatric Infection

Abnormalities in B cell function are readily apparent in pediatric HIV infection. These abnormalities are manifest clinically by susceptibility to bacterial infections, which are far more prevalent in pediatric HIV disease than in adult HIV disease. Infections with *Streptococcus pneumoniae*, *H. influenzae*, Salmonella species, *Staphylococcus aureus* and *Escherichia coli* are common and constitute a significant proportion of the infections encountered in these children (106). Many studies have been performed to determine the basis of the functional B cell defects. HIV-infected children in general respond poorly to vaccination. This is true of immunization with the T-dependent antigens tetanus toxoid and diphtheria toxin (107). In one study, 6 of 15 HIV-infected infants had poor antibody responses to tetanus toxoid, and 14 of 17 had poor responses to immunization with diphtheria toxoid (107). These poor responses to T-dependent antigens have been confirmed in studies immunizing infants with the bacteriaphage øX 174, a T-dependent antigen that has been classically used to evaluate the ability to generate a primary humoral immune response (108). Further evaluation of the defect in øX 174 responsiveness of these children indicated that there was a poor primary response to immunization and a poor secondary response to boosting and that the IgM to IgG switch was absent (108). Responses to vaccination with T-independent antigens such as pneumococcal polysaccharide have also been poor in HIV-infected children, indicating that a direct defect in B cell responsiveness exists (108).

In vitro assays of B cell function have also demonstrated clear abnormalities. Responsiveness of peripheral blood lymphocytes to the T-dependent B cell mitogen PWM is significantly reduced in infected infants (108). In addition, the in vitro response to the B cell mitogen *Staphylococcus aureus* Cowan strain I (SAC) is diminished (108), although B cell proliferation in response to anti-Ig coated beads is not (53). By using an assay that measures Ig production rather than cellular proliferation as an indicator of immune responsiveness, it has been reported that HIV-infected patients have increased levels of spontaneous Ig secretion from their peripheral B cells and that this level is not augmented by the addition of PWM (109, 110). A similar lack of Ig production has been noted in response to soluble recall antigens (110). As such it is

apparent that HIV-infected infants are deficient in their ability to produce an antibody response to primary and recall antigens and that this defect is multifactorial, involving increased spontaneous Ig secretion and decreased response to new or old antigens. Both B cell and T cell abnormalities probably contribute to this unresponsive state.

Are the B cell abnormalities a direct result of HIV? Amadori et al. (111) have calculated that 20–40% of circulating B cells in HIV-infected children are secreting Ig directed at HIV-specific determinants. This would indicate that a monumental humoral immune response is being directed at HIV in these individuals and that it is this HIV-specific response that constitutes the B cell activation and polyclonal gammopathy of pediatric HIV infection. Schnittman et al. (112) have reported that HIV can stimulate normal B cells to proliferate and differentiate, and Pahwa et al. (113) have determined that sucrose-banded HIV virus particles can stimulate IgG synthesis in peripheral blood lymphocytes. These virus particle preparations would also decrease the differentiation responses of B cells to PWM, SAC, and EBV (113). These results taken together indicate that HIV can indeed stimulate a vigorous B cell response in either an antigen-specific or a mitogenic manner and could therefore be directly responsible for many B cell abnormalities.

CYTOKINES

Cytokines may be both protective and deleterious in HIV infection.

Results in Adults

In adults with HIV infection associated with generalized lymphadenopathy but not AIDS, examination of lymph nodes by in situ hybridization suggests that an ongoing immune reaction to the virus is associated with the production of each cytokine assessed, including IL-1β, IL-2, IL-6, and interferon-γ (114). Compared with non-HIV-infected individuals with reactive lymphadenopathy from other causes, the nodes from the HIV-infected patients had increased numbers of interferon-γ-expressing T cells but similar numbers of T cells and macrophages expressing the other cytokines. These patients did not yet have detectable impairment of their immune response, suggesting that this represents the host's attempt to control HIV infection. It is unknown whether this is altered as infection progresses. In patients with AIDS there is a parallel diminution in the capacity for production of the T cell-derived lymphokines IL-2 and interferon-γ when whole blood mononuclear cells are stimulated with antigens or with mitogens in vitro (115, 116) Interferon-α production is also decreased, but production of TNF-α and lymphotoxin (TNF-β) are increased (116). These changes parallel the decline in CD4 numbers as the disease progresses; the capacity of the remaining CD4 T cells to produce IL-2 and interferon-γ appears to be largely normal (117). In fact, production of IL-2 in response to antigens may be detectable in many HIV-infected individuals when a proliferative response is not, a situation not encountered with cells from normal individuals (118). Nevertheless, there appears to be a perturbation of the capacity of T cells from adults with HIV infection to produce lymphokines (115–119). Overall there appears to be a perturbation in cytokine production in adults with AIDS, such that the lymphokines that act to inhibit viral replication (the interferons) or to enhance the function of cytotoxic cells (IL-2, IL-4, and interferons) are produced in decreasing amounts (as assayed in vitro) as the disease progresses. In contrast, cytokines that may enhance viral replication, induce cachexia, and/or lead to polyclonal B cell activation and hyperglobulinemia (TNF and IL-6) are produced in greater amounts as the disease progresses. There is some additional clinical data supporting this notion. In many adults with AIDS, circulating concentrations of interferon-α, TNF-α, IL-1, and IL-6, increased mRNA for these cytokines, and/or constitutive production of these cytokines by blood mononuclear cells or monocytes ex vivo are observed (120, 121); note that the observation of increased circulating interferon-α contrasts to diminished production by mononuclear cells challenged in vitro. The mechanism for excess production of TNF, IL-1, and IL-6 is less clear than for the loss of production of IL-2 and interferon-γ. Some workers have suggested that infection of monocytes or monocyte cell lines with HIV directly induces or augments production of these cytokines in vitro; in contrast, other studies have shown no impact of HIV infection on production of these cytokines (122).

Results in Children

There is a paucity of data regarding cytokines in children with HIV infection. Two studies have sought to detect circulating cytokines that may lead to cachexia or central nervous system injury. Increased concentrations of circulating TNF-αβ were observed in one study and were strongly associated with a subgroup of children with progressive encephalopathy (123). Concentrations did not correlate with wasting, nor did cerebrospinal fluid concentrations of TNF-α correlate with encephalopathy. Another study examined cerebrospinal fluid for several cytokines, and no consistent observations could be made (124). These results are in part congruent with those in adults, but note that cytokine concentrations may not accurately reflect production in vivo for various reasons. Thus it would be valuable to have parallel data on mRNA content or ex vivo production, as described in adults.

There is little information on lymphokine production by cells from HIV-infected children; most studies have relied on proliferation assays. The data described above (118) and in a recent study (125) suggest that in children as in adults, IL-2 production may detect antigen specific responses, particularly those directed against HIV antigens or peptides, that are not detected by proliferation assays (125). This is all the more surprising, since tetanus antigen and PHA-induced IL-2 production was diminished in HIV-infected children compared with controls. A more complete picture of cytokine production in comparison with normal age-matched controls is needed in HIV-infected children.

CLINICAL CONSEQUENCES OF HIV-INDUCED IMMUNE DEFECTS

The most important clinical consequence of HIV-induced immune dysfunction in infants is susceptibility to opportunistic infections, recurrent infections with capsulated or pyogenic bacteria, and malignancies. There are multiple other clinical consequences of HIV infection, although it is often difficult to determine if these are the result of HIV-induced immune dysfunction, opportunistic infection, or a direct result of virus replication. Laboratory and physical findings common to HIV-infected infants are listed in Table 9.6.

Laboratory Abnormalities

The most common and specific laboratory findings associated with HIV infection in infants are a reduced CD4 T cell count, an inverted CD4-to-CD8 ratio, and polyclonal hypergammaglobulinemia. These findings are not only highly suggestive of HIV infection but indicate associated immune deficiency. Because normal ranges for Ig levels and lymphocyte subset numbers vary with the age of the child, one must be sure that the values reported are outside the limits of normal for a child of that age (Tables 9.1, 9.3, and 9.4). Several other laboratory findings are common and may tip off the physician to the presence of HIV infection. Anemia is often present. This may be a microcytic anemia or, if hemolytic in

Table 9.6. Laboratory and Clinical Findings in HIV-infected Infants and Children

Laboratory findings
    Decreased percentage of CD4 cells
    Increased percentage of CD8 cells
    Inverted CD4:CD8 ratio
    Increased quantitative Ig
    Anemia
    Thrombocytopenia
    Lymphopenia
    Plasmacytosis
    Decreased IGF-1
    Decreased growth hormone
    Decreased thymic hormone
    Increased β_2 microglobulin
Clinical findings
    Diffuse lymphadenopathy
    Hepatosplenomegally
    Failure to thrive
    Recurrent otitis media
    Thrush
    Recurrent diarrhea
    Parotid enlargement
    Neurodevelopmental deficits

nature, a macrocytic anemia. Lymphopenia ($<1500/\mu l$) and thombocytopenia are common, and plasmacytosis may be visible on the differential smear. These hematologic findings, in the correct clinical setting, should warrant further investigation to determine the HIV infection status of the child.

Many tests historically used in the work-up of immune deficiency will be abnormal. These include anergy to skin test antigens, poor proliferative responses to T cell (PHA, ConA), T-dependent B cell (PWM), or pure B cell (SAC) mitogens, decreased proliferative responses to soluble antigens (Tetanus toxoid, Candida), decreased immune responsiveness to primary or secondary immunization with bacteriophage øX 174, and possibly abnormal NK cell function. Although these tests are valuable in the work-up of children with immune deficiency of unknown type, with the availability of testing for HIV, their usefulness in the evaluation of an HIV-infected child is unclear since they will not establish the diagnosis nor will they aid in clinical management of that child.

Other abnormalities, which would not be part of a routine laboratory work-up of a child, include decreased serum levels of neopterin, insulin-like growth factor-1, and growth hormone (126), or increased levels of β_2 microglobulin. The usefulness of any of these tests in either the diagnosis or clinical management of pediatric HIV infection is dubious.

Finally, many nonspecific abnormalities of routine laboratory tests may occur that may not be due to immunologic abnormalities per se but may result from infections or immune complexes related to the HIV infection. These include liver enzyme abnormalities, electrolyte imbalances, acid-base disturbances, and evidence of renal dysfunction. None of these laboratory findings could be considered specific to HIV infection and are mentioned solely for the purpose of completeness.

Physical Findings

Myriad physical findings are associated with the presence and consequences of HIV infection. Most of these result from opportunistic infections and malignancies that afflict the child and are not a direct result of HIV infection itself. One is therefore referred to the chapters of clinical manifestations in infants, children, and adolescents for a more comprehensive description of clinical findings. This section will attempt to describe those findings present in the otherwise asymptomatic HIV-infected patient as yet unaffected by opportunistic infections. A list of common physical findings is presented in Table 9.6.

The most common finding associated with pediatric HIV infection is diffuse lymphadenopathy. This is most likely a direct result of HIV infection, and multiple lymphoid organs can be involved, resulting in hepatosplenomegaly, parotid enlargement, and tonsillar hypertrophy. Developmental abnormalities are also common in HIV-infected infants. These can manifest as growth retardation or failure to reach developmental milestones (126, 127). Even in the absence of immune deficiency, neurologic abnormalities in the growing child may become apparent. These abnormalities, however, are beyond the scope of this chapter and are dealt with more thoroughly in Chapter 23.

Finally, infections common to infants and children may be more recurrent and aggressive in the HIV-infected child than in the normal child. One must therefore be cognizant of unrelenting moniliasis, diarrhea, and recurrent otitis media as possible indicators of a developing immune deficiency in the HIV-infected child.

DIFFERENTIAL DIAGNOSIS

Depending on age and presenting features when the diagnosis of HIV infection is entertained, the differential diagnosis will vary. For the purposes of this chapter, the chief concern is those children in whom hematologic or immunologic evaluation may yield results consistent either with a diagnosis of perinatal HIV infection or another disease process. Children who present in the neonatal period or early infancy with lymphadenopathy, hepatosplenomegaly, thrombocytopenia, anemia, or leukopenia may have another form of congenital or perinatal infection or possibly a hemato-

logic disorder. In congenital or perinatal infection caused by any organism listed in Table 9.7, any or all of these features may be observed. Further, congenital infection with these organisms may be associated with various immunologic abnormalities with similarities to those found in infants infected with HIV perinatally. Each congenital infection is commonly associated with increased concentrations of IgM and sometimes IgA. Increased IgG appears to be relatively uncommon in congenital infections other than HIV but may occur. Congenital rubella infection may be associated with persistent IgA deficiency or panhypogammaglobulinemia, as seen in some children with HIV infection. Abnormalities of cell-mediated immunity or T cell numbers are less common. In congenital toxoplasma (128) and cytomegalovirus (129) infection and in congenital syphilis (130) T cell numbers and subsets are generally normal even in infancy, although activated T cells are sometimes detected in increased numbers. Although these diseases may be associated with relatively poor T cell responses to the infecting pathogen in infancy, proliferative responses to mitogens are generally normal. In contrast, congenital rubella virus infection after maternal infection in the first trimester may be associated with diminished proliferative responses even to mitogens and with a persistent increase in CD8 relative to CD4 T cells (131, 132). This body of findings indicates, that these infections should be specifically considered in children with suspect perinatal HIV infection, and the appropriate testing should be performed as shown in Table 9.7. Other perinatally acquired infections, such as those from herpes simplex virus or hepatitis B, are usually sufficiently different in their clinical features and not associated with obvious immunologic abnormalities that they may be readily distinguished. Acute, post- or perinatally acquired infection with cytomegalovirus, EBV and *Toxoplasma* may also mimic many findings of perinatal HIV infection (lymphadenopathy, hepatosplenomegaly, relative increase in CD8 vs. CD4 T cells) and should be considered.

Primary immunodeficiency disorders may also be confused with HIV infection. These

Table 9.7.   Differential Diagnosis of HIV Infection and Young Children[a]

Illness	Distinguishing Laboratory Feature
Congenital infections	
CMV	CMV in urine, blood, IgM of IgA anti-CMV antibody
Toxoplasmosis	IgM or IgA antitoxoplasma antibody
Rubella	IgM or IgA antirubella antibody
Syphilis	Dark field exam, VRPR antibody titer, IgM-FTA
Acute peri- or postnatal infections	
CMV	CMV isolated + IgM or IgA anti-CMV antibody
Toxoplasmosis	See above
Ebstein-Barr virus	IgM VCA antibody
Primary immunodeficiencies	
X-linked SCID	Low T cells, poor antibody response
Autosomal recessive SCID	Low or absent T and B cells, Ig
Variant SCID	Absent or poor responses to specific antigens, variable T and B cell numbers subset abnormalities
Adenosine deaminase or nucleoside phosphorylase deficiency	Purine pathway enzyme defects
Omenn's syndrome	Lymphadenopathy, activated T cells, eosinophilia, hyper IgE
Bare lymphocyte syndrome	Absent HLA class II and/or class I antigens on lymphocytes
SCID with graft vs. host disease	Lymphoid chimerism
DiGeorge syndrome	Absent thymus on chest X-ray, hypocalcemia
Wiskott-Aldrich syndrome	Microplatelets, thrombocytopenia
X-linked lymphoproliferative syndrome	EBV nuclear antigens in tissue lymphocytes
Mucocutaneous candidiasis	Selective T-cell unresponsiveness to *Candida* skin tests, proliferative assays
Hyperimmunoglobulin M	Lymphadenopathy, increased IgM, decreased IgG and IgA, neutropenia common
Hematologic disorders	
Lymphoma	Positive node biopsy
Reticuloendotheliosis	Positive node or skin biopsy
Idiopathic thrombocytopenic purpura	Antiplatelet antibodies; no other immune abnormalities
Secondary immunodeficiencies	
Malnutrition	Decreased transferrin, prealbumin
Nephrotic syndrome	Kidney biopsy, hypogammaglobulinemia, decreased albumin
Protein-losing enteropathy	Lymphopenia, hypogammaglobulinemia, intestinal biopsy, decreased albumin

[a]CMV, cytomegalovirus; RPR, rapid plasma reagin; FTA, fluorescent treponemal antibody; VCA, viral capsid antigen; SCID, severe combined immunodeficiency disease. Data modified from edition 1, p.105.

can usually be excluded by appropriate history, examination, and immunologic analyses as indicated (Table 9.5). Note that the single most helpful test in differentiating HIV infection from other genetic or acquired conditions leading to abnormalities of the immune system is evidence for HIV infection in the patient or, in the case of perinatally transmitted infection, in the patient's mother. One relatively rare form of

combined immunodeficiency, Omenn's syndrome, may particularly cause confusion. This disease presents in early infancy with severe eczema, lymphadenopathy and hepatosplenomegaly, diarrhea, and increased IgE. Disturbances in other Ig classes, alterations in T cell subsets, increased numbers of activated T cells, and relatively intact T cell proliferative responses to mitogens with absent responses to specific antigens are also common. The other forms of severe combined immunodeficiency vary in their laboratory manifestations and to some extent in their clinical severity. In general responses to specific antigens are invariably absent, numbers of T cells are markedly reduced or absent, and B cells are markedly reduced (autosomal-recessive form) or present in normal numbers (in most cases of the X-linked form); responses to mitogens parallel the overall deficit in T cells. Detailed reviews of combined immunodeficiency and other forms of immunodeficiency, which may be confused with HIV infection, are available (133).

SUGGESTED EVALUATION

The goal of the laboratory evaluation of an infant with possible HIV infection is to establish the presence or absence of that infection and, if present, to determine the degree of resultant immune deficiency. It is necessary to know the degree of immune deficiency so that a prognosis can be established and a decision reached regarding initiation of therapy. In the past, many tests of immunologic function were recommended in the evaluation of HIV-infected children. Many of these are listed above and include delayed type hypersensitivity skin testing, mitogen assays, β_2 microglobulin assays, and bacteriophage øX 174 immunization. Although these tests have been valuable for our understanding of the scope of immune deficiency encountered in pediatric HIV infection, and may remain useful as surrogate markers of immunologic response to experimental therapeutic protocols, they are not useful in management of individual patients and can no longer be recommended except as they apply to clinical research trials.

All current clinical prognostic and therapeutic decisions in HIV-infected children are based upon virologic markers of HIV (p24 antigen or culture results, see Chapter 35) and the degree of CD4 lymphopenia relative to normal values for age. It is often difficult to diagnose HIV infection in infancy (see Chapters 11 and 12). In the absence of other possible exposures (blood or blood product transfusion, sexual exposure) most infants and children acquire HIV infection from their mothers. Thus serologic testing of the mother for HIV will usually establish if the child is at risk. During the first 12–18 months of life, serologic testing of a child born to an HIV-infected mother will not be useful in determining the infection status of that infant because of the presence of maternal antibodies in the infant's circulation. Direct detection of HIV in the infant, through assays of p24, virus culture, or polymerase chain reaction amplification of virus DNA, is the best way to establish the diagnosis of HIV infection at this age. However, these tests may be unreliable in the first months of life, are often not standardized, and are not readily available to all physicians. One is often forced to use other methods to establish if a child is infected with HIV.

Immunologic tests that may establish the existence of HIV infection in a child include HIV-specific Ig production after in vitro stimulation of infant B cells (134), detection of HIV-specific IgM (135), or the presence of HIV-specific IgA (136). None of these tests is as yet clinically reliable. The physician must often use clinical judgment and surrogate immunologic studies until virologic results become available. The most reliable and clinically important tests, which can be performed on infants with indeterminate infection status, are a CD4 lymphocyte count and quantitative Ig. A low CD4 count and high Ig (particularly IgG) level in a child with physical signs of HIV infection (diffuse lymphadenopathy, hepatosplenomegaly) and a possible source of exposure to HIV are very suggestive of HIV infection. Once HIV infection is diagnosed, either through virologic testing or the persistence or re-emergence of HIV-specific antibodies after 12–18 months of age, the CD4 lymphocyte count is the most important immunological parameter on which clinical decisions will be based.

References

1. Christensen RD. Hematopoiesis in the fetus and neonate. Pediatric Res 1989;26:531–535.
2. Philpott KL, Viney JL, Kay G, et al. Lymphoid development in mice congenitally lacking T cell receptor $\alpha\beta$-expressing cells. Science 1992;265:1448–1452.
3. Davis MM, Bjorkman PJ. T-cell antigen receptor genes and T-cell recognition. Nature 1988;334:395–402.

4. Jorgensen JL, Reay PA, Ehrich EW, Davis MM. Molecular components of T-cell recognition. Annu Rev Immunol 1992;10:835–873.

5. Haynes BF, Martin ME, Kay HH, Kurtzberg A. Early events in human T cell ontogeny: Phenotypic characterization and immunohistologic localization of T cell precursors in early human fetal tissue. J Exp Med 1988;168:1061–1080.

6. Schwartz RH. Acquisition of immunologic self-tolerance. Cell 1989;57:1073–1081.

7. Campana D, Janossy G, Coustan-Smith E, et al. The expression of T cell receptor-associated proteins during T cell ontogeny in man. J Immunol 1989;142:57–66.

8. McVay LD, Carding SR, Bottomly K, Hayday AC. Regulated expression and structure of T cell receptor $\gamma\delta$ transcripts in human thymic ontogeny. EMBO J 1991;10:83–91.

9. George JF Jr, Schroeder HW Jr. Developmental regulation of Dβ reading frame and junctional diversity in T cell receptor-β transcripts from human thymus. J Immunol 1992;148:1230–1239.

10. Fischer HP, Sharrock CEM, Panayi GS. High frequency of cord blood lymphocytes against mycobacterial 65-kDa heat-shock protein. Eur J Immunol 1992;22:1667–1669.

11. Hayward AR, Herberger MJ, Groothuis J, Levin MR. Specific immunity after congential or neonatal infection with cytomegalovirus or herpes simplex virus. J Immunol 1984;133:2469–2473.

12. English BK, Wilson CB. Neonate as an immunocompromised host. In: Patrick CC, ed. Infections in immunocompromised infants and children, New York: Churchill Livingstone, 1992:95–118.

13. Forestier F, Daffos F, Galacteros F, Bardakjian J, Rainaut M, Beuzard Y. Hematological values of 163 normal fetuses between 18 and 30 weeks of gestation. Pediatric Res 1986;20:342–346.

14. Yanase Y, Tango T, Okumura K, Tada T, Kawasaki T. Lymphocyte subsets identified by monoclonal antibodies in healthy children. Pediatr Res 1986;20:1147–1151.

15. Erkeller-Yuksel FM, Deneys V, Yuksel B, et al. Age-related changes in human blood lymphocyte subpopulations. J Pediatr 1992;120:216–222.

16. Wilson M, Rosen FS, Schlossman SF, Reinherz EL. Ontogeny of human T and B lymphocytes during stressed and normal gestation: Phenotypic analysis of umbilical cord lymphocytes from term and preterm infants. Clin Immunol Immunopathol 1985;37:1–12.

17. Centers for Disease Control. Guidelines for the performance of CD4+ T-cell determinations in persons with human immunodeficiency virus infection. MMWR 1992;41:1–17.

18. McKinney RE Jr, Wilfert CM. Lymphocyte subsets in children younger than 2 years old: Normal values in a population at risk for human immunodeficiency virus infection and diagnostic and prognostic application to infected children. Pediatr Infect Dis J 1992;11:639–644.

19. Sanders ME, Makgoba MW, Sharrow SO, et al. Human memory T lymphocytes express increased levels of three cell adhesion molecules (LFA-3, CD2, and LFA-1) and three other molecules (UCHLI, CDw29, and Pgp-1) and have enhanced IFN-γ production. J Immunol 1988;140:1401–1407.

20. Lewis DB, Prickett KS, Larsen A, Grabstein K, Weaver M, Wilson CB. Restricted production of interleukin-4 by activated human T cells. Proc Natl Acad Sci USA 1988;85:9743–9747.

21. Pilarski LM, Yacyshyn BR, Jensen GS, Pruski E, Pabst HF. $\beta1$ integrin (CD29) expression on human postnatal T cell subsets defined by selective CD45 isoform expression. J Immunol 1991;147:830–837.

22. Pirenne H, Aujard Y, Eijaafari A, et al. Comparison of T cell functional changes during childhood with the ontogeny of CDw29 and CD45RA expression on CD4+ T cells. Pediatr Res 1992;32:81–86.

23. Clement LT, Vink PE, Bradley GE. Novel immunoregulatory functions of phenotypically distinct subpopulations of CD4+ cells in the human neonate. J Immunol 1990;145:102–108.

24. Splawski JB, Lipsky PE. Cytokine regulation of immunoglobulin secretion by neonatal lymphocytes. J Clin Invest 1991;88:967–977.

25. Wilson CB, Lewis DB, English BK. T cell development in the fetus and neonate. Adv Exp Med Biol 1991;310:17–29.

26. Ehlers S, Smith KA. Differentiation of T cell lymphokine gene expression: The in vitro acquisition of T cell memory. J Exp Med 1991;173:25–36.

27. Lewis DB, Yu CC, Meyer J, English BK, Kahn SJ, Wilson CB. Cellular and molecular mechanisms for reduced interleukin-4 and interferon-gamma production by neonatal T cells. J Clin Invest 1991;87:194–202.

28. Wilson CB, Penix L, Melvin A, Lewis DB. Lymphokine regulation and the role of abnormal regulation in immunodeficiency. Clin Immunol Immunopathol, in press.

29. Burchett SK, Corey L, Mohan KM, Westall J, Ashley R, Wilson CB. Diminished interferon-γ and lymphocyte proliferation in neonatal and postpartum primary herpes simplex virus infection. J Infect Dis 1992;165:813–818.

30. Phillips JH, Hori T, Nagler A, Bhat N, Spits H, Lanier LL. Ontogeny of human natural killer (NK) cells; Fetal NK cells mediate cytolytic function and express cytoplasmic CD3ϵ,δ proteins. J Exp Med 1992;175:1055–1066.

31. Biron CA, Byron KS, Sullivan JL. Severe herpesvirus infections in an adolescent without natural killer cells. N Engl J Med 1989;320:1731–1735.

32. Sancho L, de la Hera A, Casas J, Vaquer S, Martinez-A C, Alvarez-Mon M. Two different maturational stages of natural killer lymphocytes in human newborn infants. J Pediatr 1991;119:446–454.

33. Yabuhara A, Kawai H, Komiyama A. Development of natural killer cytotoxicity during childhood: Marked increases in number of natural killer cells with adequate cytotoxic abilities during infancy to early childhood. Pediatr Res 1990;28:316–322.

34. McDonald T, Sneed J, Valenski WR, Dockter M, Cooke R, Herrod HG. Natural killer cell activity

in very low birth weight infants. Pediatr Res 1992;31:376–380.

35. Kohl S. The neonatal human immune response to herpes simplex virus infection: A critical review. Pediatr Infect Dis J 1989;8:67–74.

36. Harrison CJ, Waner JL. Natural killer cell activity in infants and children excreting cytomegalovirus. J Infect Dis 1985;151:301–307.

37. Bofill M, Janossy G, Janossa M, et al. Human B cell development. II. Subpopulations in the human fetus. J Immunol 1985;134:1531–1538.

38. Antin JH, Emerson SG, Martin P, Gadol N, Ault KA. Leu-1+ (CD5+) B cells. A major lymphoid subpopulation in human fetal spleen: Phenotypic and functional studies. J Immunol 1986;136: 505–510.

39. Punnonen J, Aversa GG, Vanderkerckhove B, Roncarolo M-G, de Vries JE. Induction of isotype switching and Ig production by CD5+ and CD10+ human fetal B cells. J Immunol 1992; 148:3398–3404.

40. Sanz I. Multiple mechanisms participate in the generation of diversity of human H chain CDR3 regions. J Immunol 1991;147:1720–1729.

41. Mortari F, Newton JA, Wang JY, Schroeder HW Jr. The human cord blood antibody repertoire. Frequent usage of the V_H7 gene family. Eur J Immunol 1992;22:241–245.

42. Burgio GR, Lanzavecchia A, Plebani A, Jayakar S, Ugazio AG. Ontogeny of secretory immunity: Levels of secretory IgA and natural antibodies in saliva. Pediatr Res 1980;14:1111–1114.

43. Durandy A, Thuillier L, Forveille M, Fischer A. Phenotypic and functional characteristics of human newborns' B lymphocytes. J Immunol 1990;144:60–65.

44. Tucci A, Mouzaki A, James H, Bonnefoy J-Y, Zubler RH. Are cord blood B cells functionally mature? Clin Exp Immunol 1991;84:389–394.

45. Decoster A, Darcy F, Caron A, et al. Anti-P30 IgA antibodies as prenatal markers of congenital toxoplasma infection. Clin Exp Immunol 1992; 87:310–315.

46. Anderson EE, Shackelford PG, Quinn A, Carroll WL. Restricted Ig H chain V gene usage in the human antibody response to *Haemophilus influenzae* type b capsular polysaccharide. J Immunol 1991;147:1667–1674.

47. Poli G, Kinter A, Justement JS, et al. Tumor necrosis factor α functions in an autocrine manner in the induction of human immunodeficiency virus expression. Proc Natl Acad Sci USA 1990; 87:782–785.

48. Poli G, Bressler P, Kinter A, et al. Interleukin 6 induces human immunodeficiency virus expression in infected monocytic cells alone and in synergy with tumor necrosis factor α by transcriptional and post-transcriptional mechanisms. J Exp Med 1990;172:151–158.

49. Schibler KR, Liechty KW, White WL, Rothstein G, Christensen RD. Defective production of interleukin-6 by monocytes: A possible mechanism underlying several host defense deficiencies of neonates. Pediatr Res 1991;31:18–21.

50. Kornbluth RS, Oh PS, Munis JR, Cleveland PH, Richman DD. Interferons and bacterial lipopolysaccharide protect macrophages from productive infection by human immunodeficiency virus in vitro. J Exp Med 1989;169:1137–1151.

51. Alimenti A, Luzuriaga K, Stechenberg B, Sullivan JL. Quantitation of human immunodeficiency virus in vertically infected infants and children. J Pediatr 1991;119:225–229.

52. Schnittman SM, Denning SM, Greenhouse JJ, et al. Evidence for susceptibility of intrathymic T-cell precursors and their progeny carrying T-cell antigen receptor phenotypes TCRαβ+ and TCRγδ+ to human immunodeficiency virus infection: A mechanism for CD4+ (T4) lymphocyte depletion. Proc Natl Acad Sci USA 1990;87: 7727–7731.

53. Sullivan JL, Brewster MS, Brettler DB, et al. Hemophiliac immunodeficiency: Influence of exposure to factor VIII concentrate, LAV/HTLV-III, and herpesviruses. J Pediatr 1986;108:504–510.

54. Eyster ME, Gail MH, Ballard JO, Al-Mondhiry H, Goedert JJ. Natural history of human immunodeficiency virus infections in hemophiliacs: Effects of T-cell subsets, platelet counts, and age. Ann Intern Med 1987;107:1–6.

55. Goedert JJ, Kessler CM, Aledort LM, et al. A prospective study of human immunodeficiency virus type 1 infection and the development of AIDS in subjects with hemophilia. N Engl J Med 1989;321:1141–1148.

56. Lifson AR, Rutherford GW, Jaffe HW. The natural history of human immunodeficiency virus infection. J Infect Dis 1988;158:1360–1367.

57. van Noesel CJM, Gruters RA, Terpstra G, Schellekens PTA, van Lier RAW, Miedema F. Functional and phenotypic evidence for a selective loss of memory T cells in asymptomatic human immunodeficiency virus-infected men. J Clin Invest 1990;86:293–299.

58. Schittman SM, Lane HC, Greenhouse J, Justement JS, Baseler M, Fauci AS. Preferential infection of CD4+ memory T cells by human immunodeficiency virus type 1: Evidence for a role in the selective T-cell functional defects observed in infected individuals. Proc Natl Acad Sci USA 1990; 87:6058–6062.

59. Clerici M, Stocks NI, Zajac RA, et al. Detection of three distinct patterns of T helper cell dysfunction in asymptomatic human immunodeficiency virus-seropositive patients. J Clin Invest 1989;84:1892–1899.

60. Tsang K, Fundenberg H, Galbraith G. In vitro augmentation of interleukin-2 production and lymphocytes with the tat antigen marker in patients with AIDS [Letter]. N Engl J Med 1984;310:987.

61. Prince H, Kermani-Arab V, Fahey J. Depressed interleukin-2 receptors expression in acquired immune deficiency and lymphadenopathy syndrome. J Immunol 1984;133:1313–1317.

62. Prince H, John J. Abnormalities of interleukin-2 receptor expression associated with decreased antigen-induced lymphocyte proliferation in patients with AIDS and related disorders. Clin Exp Immunol 1987;67:59–65.

63. Oleske J, Minnefor A, Cooper R, et al. Immune deficiency syndrome in children. JAMA 1983; 249:2345–2349.

64. Rubinstein A, Sicklick M, Gupta A, et al. Acquired immunodeficiency with reversed T_4/T_8 ratios in infants born to promiscuous and drug-addicted mothers. JAMA 983;249:2350–2356.

65. Blanche S, Le Deist F, Fischer A, et al. Longitudinal study of 18 children with perinatal LAV/HTLV III infection: Attempt at prognostic evaluation. J Pediatr 1986;109:965–970.

66. Pahwa S, Kaplan M, Fikrig S, et al. Spectrum of human T-cell lymphotropic virus type infection in children. JAMA 1986;255:2299–2305.

67. de Martino M, Tovo P-A, Galli L, et al. Prognostic significance of immunologic changes in 675 infants perinatally exposed to human immunodeficiency virus. J Pediatr 1991;119:702–709.

68. Scott GB, Hutton C, Makuch RW, et al. Survival in children with perinatally acquired human immunodeficiency virus type 1 infection. N Engl J Med 1989;321:1791–1796.

69. Auger I, Thomas P, De Gruttola V, et al. Incubation period for paediatric AIDS patients. Nature 1988;366:575–577.

70. Leibovitz E, Rigaud M, Pollack H, et al. *Pneumocystic carinii* pneumonia in infants infected with the human immunodeficiency virus with more than 450 CD4 T-lymphocytes per cubic millimeter. N Engl J Med 1990;323:531–533.

71. Petersen J, Church J, Gomperts, Parkman R. Lymphocyte phenotype does not predict immune function in pediatric patients infected with human immunodeficiency virus type 1. J Pediatr 1989;115:944–948.

72. Centers for Disease Control. Guidelines for prophylaxis against *Pneumocystis carinii* pneumonia for children with human immunodeficiency virus infection/exposure. MMWR 1991;40:1–13.

73. Groopman JE, Sullivan JL, Mulder C, et al. Pathogenesis of B cell lymphoma in a patient with AIDS. Blood 1986;67:612–615.

74. Rechavi G, Ben-Bassat I, Berkowicz M, et al. Molecular analysis of Burkitt's leukemia in two hemophilic brothers with AIDS. Blood 1987;70: 1713–1717.

75. Kamani N, Kennedy J, Bradsma J. Burkitt lymphoma in children with human immunodeficiency virus infection. J Pediatr 1988;112:241–244.

76. Fackler JC, Nagel JE, Adler WH, Mildvan PT, Ambinder RF. Epstein-Barr virus infection in a child with acquired immunodeficiency syndrome. Am J Dis Child 1985;139:1000–1004.

77. Andiman WA, Martin K, Rubinstein A, et al. Opportunistic lymphoproliferations associated with Epstein-Barr viral DNA in infants and children with AIDS. Lancet 1985;2:1390–1393.

78. Katz BZ, Berkman AB, Shapiro ED. Serologic evidence of active Epstein-Barr virus infection in Epstein-Barr virus-associated lymphoproliferative disorders of children with acquired immunodeficiency syndrome. J Pediatr 1992;120:228–232.

79. Roilides E, Clerici M, De Palma L, Rubin M, Pizzo PA, Shearer GM. Helper T-cell responses in children infected with human immunodeficiency virus type 1. J Pediatr 1991;118:724–730.

80. Andrews CA, Sullivan JL, Brettler DB, et al. Isolation of human immunodeficiency virus from hemophiliacs: Correlation with clinical symptoms and immunologic abnormalities. J Pediatr 1987;111:672–677.

81. Culver KW, Ammann AJ, Partidge C, Wong DF, Wara DW, Cowan MJ. Lymphocyte abnormalities in infants born to drug-abusing mothers. J Pediatr 1987;111:230–235.

82. Blumberg RS, Paradis T, Byington R, Henle W, Hirsch MS, Schooley RT. Effects of human immunodeficiency virus on the cellular immune response to Epstein-Barr virus in homosexual men: Characterization of the cytotoxic response and lymphokine production. J Infect Dis 1987;155: 877–889.

83. Rook AH, Masur H, Lane HC, et al. Interleukin-2 enhances the depressed natural killer and cytomegalovirus-specific cytotoxic activities of lymphocytes from patients with the acquired immune deficiency syndrome. J Clin Invest 1983; 72:380–403.

84. Pantaleo G, De Maria A, Koenig S, et al. CD8+ T lymphocytes of patients with AIDS maintain normal broad cytolytic function despite the loss of human immunodeficiency virus-specific cytotoxicity. Proc Natl Acad Sci USA 1990;87:4818–4822.

85. Tung KSK, Koster F, Bernstein, Kriebel PW, Payne SM, Shearer GM. Elevated allogeneic cytotoxic T lymphocyte activity in peripheral blood leukocytes of homosexual men. J Immunol 1985;135: 3163–3171.

86. Luzuriaga K, Koup RA, Pikora CA, Brettler DB, Sullivan JL. Deficient human immunodeficiency virus type 1-specific cytotoxic T cell responses in vertically infected children. J Pediatr 1991;119: 230–236.

87. Pantaleo G, Koenig S, Baseler M, Lane HC, Fauci AS. Defective clonogenic potential of CD8+ T lymphocytes in patients with AIDS. J Immunol 1990;144:1696–1704.

88. Ho DD, Rota TR, Hirsch MS. Infection of monocyte/macrophages by human T lymphotropic virus type III. J Clin Invest 1986;77:1712–1715.

89. Landay A, Kessler HA, Benson CA, et al. Isolation of HIV-1 from nonocytes of individuals negative by conventional culture. J Infect Dis 1990;161: 706–710.

90. Stoler MH, Eskin TA, Benn S, Andere RC, Angere LM. Human T-cell lymphotropic virus type III infection of the central nervous system. JAMA 1986;256:2360–2364.

91. Gartner S, Markovitz P, Betts RF, Popovic M. Virus isolation from and identification of HTLV III/LAV-producing cells in brain tissue from a patient with AIDS. 1986;256:2365–2371.

92. Gartner S, Markovits P, Markovitz DM, Kaplan MH, Gallo RC, Popovic M. The role of mononuclear phagocytes in HTLV-IIII/Lav infection. Science 1986;233:215–219.

93. Cameron PV, Freudenthal PS, Barker JH, Gazelter S, Inaba K, Steinman RM. Dendritic cells exposed to human immunodeficiency virus type 1 transmit a vigorous cytopathic infection to CD4+ T cells. Science 1992;257:383–387.

94. Heagy W, Kelly VE, Strom TB, et al. Decreased expression of human class II antigens on monocytes from patients with acquired immune deficiency syndrome. J Clin Invest 1984;74:2089–2096.

95. Belsito DV, Sanchez MR, Baer RL, Valentine F, Thorbecke GJ. Reduced Langerhans' cell I$_A$ antigen and ATPase activity in patients with the acquired immunodeficiency syndrome. N Engl J Med 1984;310:1279–1282.

96. Petit AJC, Tersmette M, Terpstra FG, De Goede REY, Van Lier RAW, Miedema F. Decreased accessory cell function by human monocytic cells after infection with HIV. J Immunol 1988;140:1485–1489.

97. Smith PK, O'Hara K, Masur H, Lane HC, Fauci AS, Wahl SM. Monocyte function in the acquired immunodeficiency syndrome: Defective chemotaxis. J Clin Invest 1984;74:2121–2128.

98. Bender BS, Frank MM, Lawley TS, Smith WJ, Brickman CM, Quinn TC. Defective reticuloendothelial system Fc receptor function in patients with acquired immunodeficiency syndrome. J Infect Dis 1985;152:409–412.

99. Katz JD, Mitsuyasu R, Gotlieb MS, Lebow LT, Bonavida B. Mechanism of defective NK cell activity in patients with acquired immunodeficiency syndrome (AIDS) and AIDS-related complex. J Immunol 1987;139:55–60.

100. Sirianni MC, Soddus S, Malorni, Arancia G, Aiuti F. Mechanism of defective natural killer cell activity in patients with AIDS is associated with defective distribution of tubulin. J Immunol 1988; 140:2565–2568.

101. Roilides E, Mertin S, Eddy J, Walsh TJ, Pizzo PA, Rubin M. Impairment of neutrophil chemotactic and bactericidal function in children infected with human immunodeficiency virus type 1 and partial reversal after in vitro exposure to granulocyte-macrophage colony-stimulating factor. J Pediatr 1990;117:531–540.

102. Alberto A, Mion M, Indraccola S, Panozzo M, Francavilla E, Chievo-Bianchi L. CD5+ B cells during HIV infection [Abstract PoA2037]. Eighth International Conference on AIDS, Amsterdam, Jul 1992.

103. Roilides E, Black C. Reimer C, Rubin M, Venzon D, Pizzo PA. Serum immunoglobulin G subclasses in children infected with human immunodeficiency virus type 1. Pediatr Infect Dis J 1991;10:134–139.

104. Church JA, Lewis J, Spotkov JM. IgG subclass deficiencies in children with suspected AIDS. Lancet 1984;1:1279.

105. Maloney MJ, Guill MF, Wray BB, Lobel SA, Ebbeling W. Pediatric acquired immune deficiency syndrome with panhypogammaglobulinemia. J Pediatr 1987;110:266–267.

106. Bernstein LJ, Krieger BZ, Novick B, Sicklick MJ, Rubinstein A. Bacterial infection in the acquired immunodeficiency syndrome of children. Pediatr Infect Dis 1985;4:472–475.

107. Borkowsky W, Steele CJ, Grubman S, Moore T, La Russa, Krasinski K. Antibody responses to bacterial toxoids in children infected with human immunodeficiency virus. J Pediatr 1987;110:563–566.

108. Bernstein LJ, Ochs HD, Wedgewood RJ, Rubinstein A. Defective humoral immunity in pediatric acquired immune deficiency syndrome. J Pediatr 1985;107:352–357.

109. Lane HC, Masur H, Edgar LC, Whalen G, Rook AH, Fauci AS. Abnormalities of B-cell activation and immunoregulation in patients with the acquired immunodeficiency syndrome. N Engl J Med 1983;309:453–458.

110. Teeuwsen VJP, Logtenberg T, Siebelink HJ, et al. Analysis of the antigen- and mitogen-induced differentiation of B-lymphocytes from asymptomatic human immunodeficiency virus-seropositive male homosexuals. J Immunol 1987;139:2929–2935.

111. Amadori A, Zamarchi R, Ciminale V, et al. HIV-1-specific B cell activation: A major constituent of spontaneous B cell activation during HIV-1 infection. J. Immunol 1989;143:2146–2152.

112. Schnittman SM, Lane HC, Higgins SE, Folks T, Fauci AS. Direct polyclonal activation of human B lymphocytes by the acquired immune deficiency syndrome virus. Science 1986;233: 1084–1086.

113. Pahwa S, Pahwa R, Saxinger C, Gallo RC, Good RA. Influence of the human T-lymphotrophic virus/lymphadenopathy-associated virus on functions of human lymphocytes: Evidence for immunosuppressive effects and polyclonal B-cell activation by banded viral preparations. Proc Natl Acad Sci USA 1985;82:8198–8202.

114. Emilie D, Peuchmaur M, Maillot MC, et al. Production of interleukins in human immunodeficiency virus-1-replicating lymph nodes. J Clin Invest 1990;86:148–159.

115. Murray HW, Scavuzzo DA, Kelly CD, Rubin BY, Roberts RB. T4+ cell production of interferon gamma and the clinical spectrum of patients at risk for and with acquired immunodeficiency syndrome. Arch Intern Med 1988;148:1613–1616.

116. Voth R, Rossol S, Klein K, et al. Differential gene expression of IFN-α and tumor necrosis factor-α in peripheral blood mononuclear cells from patients with AIDS related complex and AIDS. J Immunol 1990;144:970–975.

117. Lane HC, Depper JM, Greene WC, Whalen G, Waldmann TA, Fauci AS. Qualitative analysis of immune function in patients with the acquired immunodeficiency syndrome. N Engl J Med 1985;313:79-84.

118. Clerici M, Stocks NI, Zajac RA, et al. Interleukin-2 production used to detect antigenic peptide recognition by T-helper lymphocytes from asymptomatic HIV-seropositive individuals. Nature 1989;339:383–385.

119. Maggi E, Macchia D, Parronchi P, et al. Reduced production of interleukin 2 and interferon-gamma and enhanced helper activity or IgG synthesis by cloned CD4+ T cells from patients with AIDS. Eur J Immunol 1987;17:1685–1690.

120. Grunfeld C, Feingold KR. Metabolic disturbances and wasting in the acquired immunodeficiency syndrome. N Engl J Med 1992;327:329-337.

121. Breen EC, Rezai AR, Nakajima K, et al. Infection with HIV is associated with elevated IL-6 levels and production. J Immunol 1990;144:480–484.

122. Molina J-M, Schindler R, Ferriani R, et al. Production of cytokines by peripheral blood monocytes/macrophages infected with human immunodeficiency virus type 1 (HIV-1). J Infect Dis 1990;161:888–893.

123. Mintz M, Rapaport R, Oleske JM, et al. Elevated serum levels of tumor necrosis factor are associ-

ated with progressive encephalopathy in children with acquired immunodeficiency syndrome. Am J Dis Child 1989;143:771–774.

124. Galo P, Laverda AM, de Rossi A, et al. Immunological markers in the cerebrospinal fluid of HIV-1-infected children. Acta Paediatr Scand 1991;80:659–666.

125. Wiseman G, Rubinstein A, Martinez P, Lambert S, Devash Y, Goldstein H, Cellular and antibody responses directed against the HIV-1 principal neutralizing domain in HIV-1 infected children. AIDS Res Human Retroviruses 1991;7:839–845.

126. Lepage P, Van de Perre P, Van Vlet G, et al. Clinical and endocrinologic manifestations in perinatally human immunodeficiency virus type 1-infected children aged 5 years or older. Am J Dis Child 1991;145:1248–1251.

127. Brettler DB, Forsberg A, Bolivar E, Brewster F, Sullivan J. Growth failure as a prognostic indicator for progression to acquired immunodeficiency syndrome in children with hemophilia. J Pediatr 1990;117:584–588.

128. McLeod R, Mack DG, Boyer K, et al. Phenotypes and functions of lymphocytes in congenital toxoplasmosis. J Lab Clin Med 1990;116:623–635.

129. Alford CA, Stagno S, Pass RF, Britt WJ. Congenital and perinatal cytomegalovirus infections. Rev Infect Dis 1990;12:S745–S753.

130. Samson GR, Beatty DW, Malan AF. Immune studies in infants with congenital syphilis. Clin Exp Immunol 1990;81:315–318.

131. Rabinowe SL, George KL, Loughlin R, Soeldner JS, Eisenbarth GS. Congenital rubella: Monoclonal antibody-defined T cell abnormalities in young adults. Am J Med 1986;81:779–782.

132. Buimovici-Klein E, Lang PB, Ziring PR, Cooper LZ. Impaired cell-mediated immune response in patients with congenital rubella: Correlation with gestational age at time of infection. Pediatrics 1979;64:620–626.

133. Stiehm ER. Immunologic disorders in infants and children. 3rd ed. Philadelphia: WB Saunders, 1989.

134. Pahwa S, Chirmule N, Leombruno C, et al. In vitro synthesis of human immunodeficiency virus-specific antibodies in peripheral blood lymphocytes of infants. Proc Natl Acad Sci USA 1989;86:7532–7536.

135. Pyun KH, Ochs HD, Dufford MTW, Wedgewood RJ. Perinatal infection with human immunodeficiency virus: Specific antibody responses by the neonate. N Engl J Med, 1987;317:611–614.

136. Quinn TC, Kline RL, Halsey N, et al. Early diagnosis of perinatal HIV infection by detection of viral-specific IgA antibodies. JAMA 1991;266:3439–3442.

10
Vertical Transmission of HIV

PART A / PLACENTA AS BARRIER

Clark L. Anderson, Daniel D. Sedmak, and Michael D. Lairmore

The remarkable paradox of the placenta, that it permits the fetus to develop protected from the hazards of its environment yet supplied with all necessary nutrients, is central to an understanding of vertical transmission of HIV from infected mother to fetus. How the placenta protects the fetus from HIV infection, how it might serve as a conduit for infection, what its role might be in the risk and timing of fetal infection are questions that can only be contemplated after a review of the essential features of placental biology and pathology. We will therefore outline relevant characteristics of the structure and function of the placenta at parturition and during development and will discuss what is known about transplacental infections including those caused by human immunodeficiency virus (HIV) and other microorganisms.

PLACENTA BIOLOGY

For purposes of assessing the risks of vertical HIV transmission, four biological aspects of the normal human placenta must be understood: interface of the two circulatory systems, maternal-placental interface, development of the placenta, and placental changes at parturition (1). Comparisons with other animal placentas, which are often significantly different, should be made cautiously.

Circulatory Interface

The blood of the fetus, entering the placenta through two arteries in the umbilical cord and returning through a single umbilical vein (Fig. 10A.1A and B), circulates through an immense capillary network terminating in tiny finger-like villi, displaying a surface area of ~12 m². These villi in turn are bathed in a 140-ml pool of maternal blood, circulating at the rate of 600 ml/min and fed by the vasculature of the uterus. The cellular and structural elements of the villus interface, all derived from fetal tissue, are several (Fig. 10A.1C and D). The syncytiotrophoblast, constituting the true interface with the maternal blood, is a single, seamless layer of cytoplasm, delimited by the basal and apical plasma membranes, that covers the entire surface of the branching villi, like a rubber glove covers a hand. It is responsible for the bulk of the transport function of the placenta and can move nutrients by various mechanisms ranging from simple diffusion to receptor-mediated endocytosis. Out of contact with maternal blood and beneath 20% of the syncytiotrophoblast in the mature placenta lie cytotrophoblasts (Langhans' cells), which are stem cells from which the syncytiotrophoblast is derived and presumably from which in vitro cultures of trophoblasts and syncytium are derived (3, 4). Beneath these two trophoblast layers lies a basement membrane about which little has

159

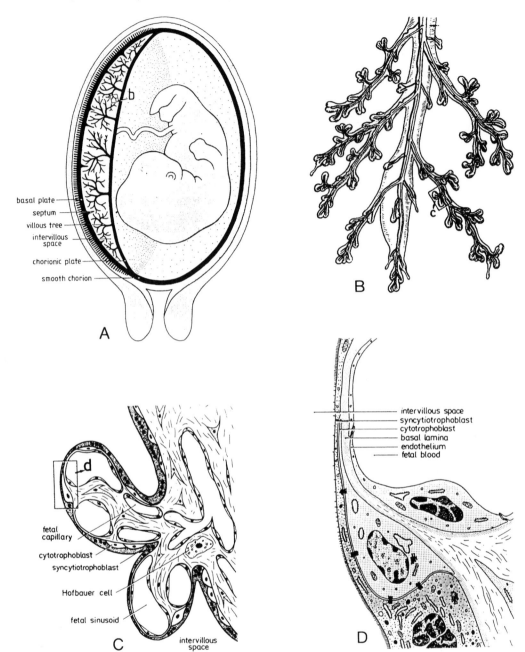

Figure 10A.1. Basic morphology of human placental villi. **B** shows a magnification of *b* in **A**. **C** shows a magnification of *c* in **B**. **D** shows a magnification of *d* in **C**. From Benirschke K, Kaufmann P. Pathology of the human placenta. 2nd ed. New York: Springer-Verlag, 1990.

been written but which appears freely permeable to all elements transported by the surrounding cells. Containing the circulating fetal blood is a monocellular layer of endothelium overlying a basal lamina. The endothelial layer, like the syncytiotrophoblast, allows passage of all relevant nutrients by similar transcellular mechanisms and in addition possibly by an intercellular route through gaps between the endothelial cells. Between the two cellular layers is interspersed connective tissue containing resident macrophages (Hofbauer cells) and occasional fibroblasts and mast cells.

The actual circulation interface in its simplest form in the mature terminal villus of the term placenta consists of just three layers: the syncytiotrophoblast, a fused basal lamina, and an endothelial cell monolayer (Fig. 10A.1*D*). All nutrients, and presumably most infectious agents, must pass this barrier. Maternal antibody of the IgG class, vital for protection of the newborn whose immature immune system is just beginning to synthesize antibody, crosses this barrier by a presumably active process. Specific transport receptors are likely involved although the molecular mechanism is virtually unknown. The route taken by HIV across this barrier is not obvious because the CD4 protein, the HIV receptor, has not been shown to the satisfaction of all to be displayed on the syncytiotrophoblast nor on the endothelial cell nor is it accepted that the syncytiotrophoblast becomes infected with HIV. The CD4 molecule is, however, expressed on the villus Hofbauer cells, which upon infection might serve as a reservoir for the virus just as do macrophages elsewhere in the body. No one seems to dispute the possibility that infected cells of the villus interstitium might traverse the villus connective tissue and diapedese through the endothelial layer to reach fetal circulation, but whether and how and to what extent maternal cells normally pass through the syncytiotrophoblast into the villus connective tissue is a more vexing issue. Maternal cells have frequently been found in newborn circulation, but it cannot be clearly defined that these are prepartum events; they may be intrapartum. Regardless, HIV might pass by this mechanism.

Whether and with what frequency rents are formed in the villus barrier is unclear. All normal placentas show small fibrinoid deposits that appear to fill gaps in the seamless trophoblast layer and are thought to represent the scarred filling of traumatic damage to the integrity of the barrier. These gaps, if present, may serve as conduits for transplacental infection, but data supportive of this notion are scant.

Although the syncytiotrophoblast layer of the placenta is believed to represent an uninterrupted barrier between the maternal circulation and the fetus, recent evidence suggests that transtrophoblastic channels exist in the placentas of animals and perhaps humans. These channels appear capable of transporting water-soluble molecules normally in the range of 1.5 nm; however, during conditions of increased fetal venous pressure or decreased osmotic pressure of the fetal compartment, these channels may dilate and permit the passage of molecules independent of size. They may represent a potential pathway for direct entry of virus from mother to fetus.

Cellular Interface

Although the great bulk of the functional interface between mother and fetus resides in the villus, the point of contact between the two circulatory systems, one must consider as well the barrier capacity of the cellular interface between the placenta with its membranes and the mother, i.e., the extraplacental and the materno-placental interface (Fig. 10A.1*A*). It consists of several elements which all pose barriers, albeit limited ones, to infection. The developing fetus is bathed in somewhat less than 1 liter amniotic fluid that to some extent is exchangeable with the contents of the respiratory and gastrointestinal tracts of the fetus; amniotic fluid is aspirated and swallowed, the fetus contributes urine and often meconium. In turn, the amniotic fluid is contained by the placental membranes, a thin (<1 mm) trilayered envelope that interfaces with the uterine endometrium throughout the internal circumference of the uterine cavity. The inner two layers are derived from fetal tissue and the outermost layer from the mother. Immediately adjacent to the amniotic fluid is the amnion, a single layer of epithelial cells of fetal origin enveloping the cord and continuous with the outermost layer of epithelium of the fetus. It is under-plied with a basement membrane and a connective tissue layer containing fibroblasts and macrophages but no vessels. The amnion appears reasonably permeable and also shows evidence at birth of large defects that would allow cells and macromolecules to pass.

Peripheral to the amnion is the chorion layer, itself a trilamellar tissue consisting first of a layer of connective tissue in which sit fibroblasts and macrophages and, until the sixth month of gestation, through which course chorionic vessels that are contiguous with the umbilical vein. Beneath lies a basement membrane and then a multicellular layer of trophoblasts within which sit remnants of primordial villi. Peripheral to the chorion is the maternal contribution to the placental membranes, the capsular decidua, which is derived from the outermost cells of the endometrium. The decidua contains maternal macrophages and inflammatory cells. Maternal blood vessels course through the deeper elements but are sparse near the chorion. The capsular decidua, enveloping the amnion and chorion, is contiguous with the decidua underlying the placenta proper, called the basal decidua, which is a frequent site of hemorrhage, inflammation, and degeneration. To what extent infections might cross this area is unclear.

Developmental Aspects of Barrier

The placental barrier as described above exists only at term; obviously in considering the prospects for HIV transmission one must consider the placenta as a developing organ, differentiating between the implanting blastocyst of about 250 cells to the mature placenta roughly one-sixth the weight of the term fetus over the course of about 40 weeks. Consider that it is not for several weeks that maternal-fetal circulation is intact. Thus for a considerable period of early gestational life, the fetus develops in close proximity to various maternal cells and fluids that provide ample opportunity for HIV transmission given appropriate circumstances, i.e., infection of the surrounding tissues.

Parturition and Barrier Rents

The process of labor, offering abundant opportunities for infection of the fetus, occurs in three stages. First, as the uterus begins its accelerating course of rhythmic contractions it also changes its shape, becoming longer and slimmer, and it differentiates into two segments, an active, contracting segment at the vertex and a passive, thin birth canal segment at the inferior pole, with the cervix dilating and thinning. Fetal movements and uterine contractions serve to detach the amnio-

chorion from underlying decidua in the lower uterine segment; the membranes often appear to slide through the cervix. After rupture of the membranes and expulsion of amniotic fluid, the fetus is delivered with the aid of increased intra-abdominal pressure exerted by voluntary pushing efforts of the mother. The birth canal in the highly vascular area of the perineum is often torn, resulting in minor hemorrhage that might contaminate an unprotected fetus. Finally, as a result of the intense contractions at the peak of labor the placenta separates from the uterus at its weakest section, the decidua spongiosa, where a hematoma creates a cleavage plane over the course of a few minutes. As the uterus continues to contract, obliterating its lumen, the placenta passes through the birth canal dragging along the membranes as they peel off the uterine decidual surface.

Obviously, many opportunities for infection are present during birth. Furthermore, the risk of fetal infection, both prenatal and intranatal, is enhanced by any number of obstetrical maneuvers including amniocentesis, amnioscopy, scalp blood sampling, cordocentesis, electronic monitoring by scalp electrodes, and episiotomy.

PLACENTAL TRANSMISSION OF NON-HIV INFECTION

Because the mechanisms by which HIV-1 infects the fetus and newborn are poorly understood, we will develop a conceptual framework for understanding how this infection may occur by reviewing what is known about maternal-fetal transmission of other microorganisms.

Intrauterine fetal infections have been classically described as resulting from either ascension of organisms through the endocervical canal and vagina or from hematogenous spread of organisms through the villous placenta (Table 10A.1) (5, 6). This delineation encompasses >95% of all fetal infections. It excludes that small percentage of infections that may result from contiguous spread of a microorganism directly from myometrium into the chorioamnion, descent through the fallopian tubes, and, as yet undescribed, infection of the sperm or oocyte.

Ascending Infections

Ascending infections are caused by organisms that transiently colonize the vagina and endocervix (Fig. 10A.1*A*) such as group B streptococcus, *Hemophilus influenzae*, coliforms, anaerobes, and the fungus *Candida albicans*. Ascending infections initially result in chorioamnionitis, an acute inflammation of the fetal membranes that most commonly affects the membrane region directly opposed to the endocervical canal. Chorioamnionitis occurs in 4–24% of all live births, and its prevalence is increased in the presence of certain microorganisms such as *Neisseria gonorrhea* (7), reviewed in Refs. 1 and 8. Fetal infection secondary to chorioamnionitis results from fetal inhalation or ingestion of contaminated amniotic fluid and from direct invasion of fetal skin or umbilical cord (funisitis) by organisms in the amniotic fluid.

Most microorganisms that cause congenital abnormalities, or are associated with chronic infections of the infant, result from hematogenous spread, i.e., transplacental passage of blood-borne maternal organisms to the fetus. The most common of these microorganisms include the protozoan parasites *Toxoplasma gondii* and *Plasmodium* species; the bacteria *Treponema pallidum*, tuberculosis, and *Listeria monocytogenes;* and viruses such as cytomegalovirus (CMV), rubella, and parvoviruses (Table 10A.1).

Hematogenous Route

The role of the placenta in the hematogenous route of maternal to fetal infection has slowly emerged over the last century. It appears that when maternal infections are characterized by a phase of numerous blood-borne organisms, whether they be cell-free or cell-associated, there is frequent involvement of the placenta. However, a significant percentage of these placental infections never result in fetal infection. This is particularly true for the *Trypanasoma cruzi* and malaria parasites, the tubercle bacillus, and the rubella virus and CMV. As an example, only 30–40% of infants born to mothers with primary CMV infection have evidence of congenital infection (6). In summary, it appears that the placenta is a

Table 10A.1. Pathways of Fetal Infection[a]

| Organism | In Utero | | Intrapartum |
	Transplacental	Ascending	
Bacteria			
Group B streptococci		+++	
Enterococcus		+++	
Chlamydiae		+	+++
T. pallidum	+++		+
L. monocytogenes	++	+	
Tuberculosis	++		
N. gonorrhea		+	+++
Viruses			
Rubella	+++		
CMV	+++		+
Herpes simplex	+		+++
Coxsackie/enteroviruses	++		+
Varicella-zoster	++		
Human papilloma virus	+		++
Hepatitis B	+		+++
Parvovirus B19	++		
HIV	++		+?
Protozoa			
T. cruzi	+++		
T. gondii	+++		
Plasmodium	+++		
Fungi			
Candida		++	++

[a]Adapted from Ref. 5.

barrier, albeit imperfect, to maternal-fetal transmission of microorganisms.

The barrier mechanisms of the placenta are not well-defined. They probably include both physical blockade of access by microorganisms into the placental villi and functional containment of organisms within the villous placenta. Functional containment could include local antimicrobial effects of cytokines, including interferons, released by infected villus cells. They also could include containment by cell-mediated immune responses of the fetal immune system. Known examples of this include granuloma formation in tuberculosis and mononuclear cell villitis in virus infections, as with rubella. Endogenous villus macrophages, the Hofbauer cells, likely contain and prevent the spread of some microorganisms, such as *T. cruzi*. In this aspect, the placenta may function much like the normal spleen in the immune response to systemic infection.

Transplacental infection of the fetus must involve several discrete steps that include 1) attachment to and passage through the syncytiotrophoblast by cell-free or cell-associated organisms, 2) passage through the villus core, in particular the fused basement membranes of the syncytiotrophoblast and endothelium, and 3) migration through the villus endothelial cell layer into the fetal circulation.

Little is known about the expression by the syncytiotrophoblast of receptors for microorganisms. Furthermore, syncytiotrophoblast surface antigens utilized as receptors may be different from those normally utilized by the organism. There is some evidence that CMV infects normal cells as a result of binding surface human lymphocyte antigen class I molecules, particularly the β_2 microglobulin component (9), yet CMV has been shown to infect syncytiotrophoblast that does not express human lymphocyte antigen class I (10). Conversely, the lack of a syncytiotrophoblast receptor for hepatitis B may explain why transplacental infection of this organism is relatively uncommon compared with intrapartum infection.

The first step of invasion, syncytiotrophoblast binding, may be circumvented by placental lesions in which the syncytiotrophoblast layer is focally disrupted and replaced by fibrin or inflammatory cells. Villitis of unknown etiology (VUE), also referred to as chronic villitis, occurs in 6–34% of otherwise normal deliveries (11). It is characterized by a CD4 lymphocyte-rich mononuclear cell infiltrate and fibrinoid necrosis. VUE may result from infection by as yet unknown organisms or may represent a focal maternal-fetal immunologic reaction (12). VUE could provide the required receptors for microbial invasion, i.e., through expression of CD4 on the infiltrating T lymphocytes and monocytes. Conversely, VUE may contain infected maternal leukocytes localized in response to the production of chemoattractant molecules. Furthermore, VUE may result in destruction of the fused syncytiotrophoblast-endothelial cell basement membrane, facilitating entry into the fetal vasculature.

Migration of organisms through the villus vasculature into the fetal circulation may be a crucial component of fetal infection. CMV, which is a common cause of congenital infections, is characterized by prominent virus inclusions in villus endothelial cells (1). Infection of villus endothelial cells could result in induction of leukocyte adhesion molecules either directly by the infecting microorganism or indirectly by cytokines, such as interleukin-1 or tumor necrosis factor. In this setting adhesion molecules could facilitate transfer of microorganisms to circulating fetal leukocytes.

Indirect evidence indicates that some fetal infections are dependent upon placental maturation. Hematogenous spread of *T. gondii* from mother to fetus increases with each trimester, and infection of the placenta with tuberculosis occurs most commonly in the third trimester. Conversely, maternal rubella infections are rarely transmitted to the fetus beyond the second trimester. These timed infections may be secondary to maturational acquisition or loss of expression of normal placental antigens utilized by these microorganisms for adherence and invasion. Thus it is conceivable that fetal HIV infection may be affected by placental maturation.

Several organisms, such as coxsackieviruses and parvovirus B19, are remarkable for the absence of placental histopathology in the presence of fetal infection. This phenomenon suggests that some organisms may cross the placenta without actively infecting, i.e., replicating, within villus cells. This phenomenon may represent the use by microorganisms of one normal placental molecular transport shuttle, a pathway that would avoid the generation of an inflammatory reaction. One possibility yet to be proven is the shuttling of an IgG-coated organism by the placental IgG transport mechanism into the fetal vasculature.

Risks during Parturition

A significant number of newborn infections are acquired during parturition. Most of these are attributed to either direct fetal contact with microorganisms infecting the birth canal or to infected maternal blood released during delivery. Infectious organisms include bacteria, fungi, and viruses (Table 10A.1). Viruses that gain access to the fetus as a result of contact with genital tract lesions include herpes simplex and human papilloma virus. The hepatitis B virus is the classic example of a microorganism that infects the newborn as a result of exposure to infected maternal blood.

ROUTES OF PLACENTAL HIV TRANSMISSION

Several factors potentially affect the transmission of HIV from mother to fetus (Table 10A.2). These include 1) the placental barrier against HIV transmission (e.g., expression of CD4 and other receptors for HIV, 2) transfer of HIV-infected maternal leukocytes during pregnancy or birth, in part influenced by placental pathology associated with AIDS, 3) quantity and strain of virus present in a maternal blood or secretions, and 4) the nature of maternal antibodies against the virus (reviewed in Ref. 13).

Placenta as a Barrier to Cell-free HIV Infection

The primary receptor for HIV cell infection is CD4, although the virus may also gain entry into certain target cells through alternative molecules including Fc receptors, complement receptors, and perhaps certain galactosyl ceramides (reviewed in Ref. 14). The facts regarding CD4 expression in the human placenta are controversial. Unfortunately, most studies have evaluated placental preparations containing a mixture of cell types using methods with limited ability to discriminate which cells contained CD4. These studies have resulted in confusion over which cells of the human placenta express CD4 and what role the receptor may have in fetal transmission of HIV. However, the issue of CD4 expression on the placental syncytiotrophoblast, the primary cellular barrier between maternal blood and fetal tissues, is critical.

Table 10A.2. Potential Factors Affecting in Utero HIV Transmission

Factor	Role in Transmission
Placental barrier to cell-free HIV	
HIV receptor expression in placenta tissue	Determinate of primary cellular route of transmission
CD4 receptor	Trophoblast expression negative expressed by tissue leukocytes
Fc receptor	Alternate antibody-mediated entry
Focal disruption of barrier (e.g., chorioamnionitis)	Inflammatory nidus of infection, enhanced by coinfecting agents
Placental barrier to cell-associated HIV	
Placenta lesions	Site of HIV-infected leukocyte infiltration enhanced by coinfecting agent
Virological factors of HIV transmission	
HIV strain	Selective transmission of specific strains
Maternal virus load	Potential for increased risk of transmission
HIV promoter enhancement	Pregnancy hormonal enhancement of HIV replication
Maternal immune response	
Low maternal gp120 antibodies	Associated with increased risk of transmission
Maternal antibodies to V3 loop	Not conclusively associated with HIV transmission

We have examined both placental sections and cultures of highly purified trophoblasts for the expression of CD4 (15). In placental sections CD4 protein expression was found exclusively in leukocytes of the placental villi. These cells were identified morphologically as Hofbauer cells or lymphocytes. In contrast, the syncytiotrophoblast, clearly identified using cytokeratin monoclonal antibody, was negative for CD4 using three different monoclonal antibodies. These data are consistent with the immunohistochemical findings of several investigators that have failed to detect CD4 protein in trophoblasts from placental sections (16–19) or in purified cytotrophoblast or syncytiotrophoblast cultures (20–22). Similarly, others have demonstrated immunohistochemically that Hofbauer cells of the first and third trimesters of gestation are strongly positive for CD4 protein expression (16). However, our data conflict with those of some who report that cells consistent with trophoblast cells were positive for CD4 by an immunofluorescence method (23) and of others who have described that trophoblasts of explant cultures are CD4 positive (24). The basis for this discordance is likely methodological.

Molecular studies have generally failed to identify CD4 RNA from immunoaffinity-purified trophoblast preparations. Using both Northern blot assay and reverse transcriptase-polymerase chain reaction amplification of RNA we could not identify CD4 RNA in immunoaffinity-purified cytotrophoblast and more mature cultures containing syncytia (15). Similarly, others did not detect CD4 RNA in purified trophoblasts by Northern blot hybridization and have reported only minimal signals from rare contamination by leukocytes in CD4 polymerase chain reaction analysis from these same cell preparations (21). Reports demonstrating CD4 RNA from nonpurified placental tissues or explants are of little value to localize the cell type that expresses the CD4 receptor in the placenta (23, 25). It is our impression that these studies collectively suggest that leukocytes (Hofbauer cells, lymphocytes) are the principal villus cells that express CD4 and that trophoblasts bear neither CD4 protein nor mRNA. This conclusion explains, in part, the difficulty in demonstrating primary HIV infection of purified trophoblast cultures (20–22). Conversely, HIV has been demonstrated by immunohistochemistry or in situ hybridization to infect from 10 to 45% of the placentas from HIV-seropositive women (26). Cells within the placental villi (Hofbauer cells, lymphocytes) appear to be the principal cells that express HIV antigens in infected placentas (17, 26). However, less frequently cells at the periphery of villi consistent with trophoblasts have been demonstrated to express HIV proteins (17). The absence of CD4 on the villus syncytiotrophoblast suggests that alternative mechanisms exist for transplacental HIV infection of the fetus. Alternative to CD4, non-CD4 molecules may be involved in transplacental HIV infection. These molecules include Fc and complement receptors, both of which participate in antibody-mediated enhancement of HIV infection by monocytes at least in vitro (27). Considerable evidence indicates that the maternal surface of the villus syncytiotrophoblast bears an Fc receptor for IgG that functions to transport maternal IgG to the fetus (28, 29). One might postulate that HIV-antibody complexes are transported across the syncytiotrophoblast by the same process, allowing the virus to reach the villus interstitium where it could infect CD4+ Hofbauer cells, thereby gaining access to the fetal circulation. Direct infection of the syncytiotrophoblast, i.e., virus replication within the cell, need not accompany transcellular passage of the virus. Complement receptors have not been found on the syncytiotrophoblast. It is easy to image that disruption of the syncytiotrophoblast barrier would readily lead to fetal infection. Focal villus Hofbauer cells would easily be infected by a CD4-mediated process, and they in turn could serve as the nidus of a more widespread infection of the fetus were they to release their cellular contents or to move from their residence into the fetal circulation. Although most blood-borne infections of the placenta are accompanied by some form of chorionic villitis, this lesion has not been consistently associated with HIV infections of pregnant women (13). In contrast, chorioamnionitis is frequently found in the placentas of HIV-seropositive women and may be the result of concurrent coexisting (non-HIV) infections in these women (30). The isolation of HIV from aborted fetuses as early as 8 weeks gestation (17) and from amniotic fluid (31) supports the fact that transplacental HIV infections may occur early in the fetus. Still it is unclear if a specific morphologic lesion of the placenta is associated with an increased risk for HIV infection of the fetus.

Cell-associated HIV Transmission

Because the exchange of maternal cells with the fetus during gestation is rare, it is unlikely that cell-associated transmission of virus across a normal placenta is the predominant mode of transmission of HIV to the fetus. However, inflammatory lesions may promote the infiltration of infected maternal cells into the villus where they would meet CD4+ fetal inflammatory cells (Hofbauer cells and lymphocytes). During asymptomatic stages of HIV infection the virus is often maintained in a cell-associated state. In cell culture systems, HIV has been clearly demonstrated to be transported from cell to cell without participation of extracellular virus particles (32).

Virological Factors of HIV in Utero Transmission

Additional factors peculiar to the virus may influence in utero transmission of HIV. Recently, it was noted that minor genetically distinct subsets of HIV were selectively transmitted from infected mothers to their fetuses (33). Such observations imply the existence of either selected transmission of specific HIV strains which can cross the placenta or HIV strains with enhanced ability to infect the fetus. The phenomenon of selective cellular tropisms with HIV is well established. Thus it is conceivable that strains with enhanced ability to infect the placenta are more likely to be transmitted to the fetus.

Maternal virus load may influence the risk of HIV infection to the fetus. This is suggested by an initial report that mothers with AIDS are more likely to have virus-positive cord blood cultures than asymptomatic seropositive mothers (34) and by the observation that patients with AIDS often have larger titers of cell-free and cell-associated HIV in their blood and secretions compared with asymptomatic individuals. Thus those mothers with AIDS appear to be at greater risk to transmit the virus to their children.

The virus may also have more insidious ways to enhance its chances for transmission to the fetus. HIV promoter regions, necessary viral genes that enhance virus replication, are induced by glucocorticoids in tissue culture and by pregnancy in HIV-transgenic mice (35). Thus it is theoretically possible that HIV takes advantage of the hormonal microenvironment during pregnancy to enhance transplacental transmission. HIV replication in both monocytes and lymphocytes has been demonstrated to be enhanced by selected cytokines known to be elicited during the inflammatory process. Therefore, just as hormonal influences may enhance the virus replication, cytokines (e.g., tumor necrosis factor) released locally in sites of placental inflammation may serve to increase HIV replication and promote transmission across the placenta.

Maternal Antibodies

The influence of specific anti-HIV immune responses in determining the rate of transmission of the virus to the fetus is not clearly understood. Low maternal anti-gp120 (HIV external envelope) antibody titers have been associated with an increased risk for vertical transmission of HIV (36). Initial studies (37) suggested a role for antibodies to the principal neutralizing epitope (V3) of HIV in the transplacental transmission of the virus, but subsequent work shows no correlation (38). To understand the extent of the role that specific anti-HIV antibodies play in determining the rate of transmission of the virus to the fetus will require more extensively controlled epidemiologic studies or the development of appropriate nonprimate models of the infection (see Chapter 10B).

CONCLUSIONS

The foregoing review makes clear that HIV has many opportunities to pass from an infected mother to her fetus during pregnancy and delivery. Although the placenta is an efficient barrier to infection, it is imperfect, and just as various other mi-

women coupled with a more complete phenotypic characterization of the virus emerging in the neonate should answer this question.

Taken together, these results suggest that, like hepatitis virus, a significant proportion of neonatal infection involving SIV, and by extrapolation HIV, may occur at or near birth. The requirement for active maternal disease and the emergence in the neonate of a subspecies of SIV from the mother further implies a role for virus genes in the transport of virus across the placental barrier.

Similar results were obtained by Mossman and colleagues (57) in a serial sacrifice of pregnant rhesus females infected during the second and third trimesters of pregnancy with the pathogenic molecular clone SIVmac239. SIV was identified in three placentae and one fetus. No significant association between maternal cell-free viremia and fetal infection was observed. Surprisingly, however, the presence of SIV in the infected fetus and the fetal portion of the one placenta correlated with maternal antibody to gag proteins.

The Tulane Primate Center has also initiated studies in a third species of macaque, the cynomolgus monkey (*M. fascicularis*; Davison-Fairburn and Murphey-Corb, unpublished data). Five pregnant females were inoculated intravenously with SIV/DeltaB670 during the first and second trimesters of pregnancy (50–92 days gestation). One aborted 61 days postinoculation, two died in utero shortly after inoculation, one was born premature and died 24 hours after birth, and one died 3 months after birth with pneumonia. Intrauterine growth retardation was noted in several pregnancies. Much fetal material was either too autolyzed or unavailable for further study; however, the premature infant and placental tissue collected from the intrauterine deaths were PCR positive for SIV sequences. The severe consequences of SIV infection seen in this preliminary study of pregnant cynomolgus macaques raises the issue of relevancy as a model for human infection, but further studies are warranted.

Transmission of SIV may also occur via breast feeding, as evidenced by the study of McClure et al. (58, 59), who have shown seroconversion by 9–12 months of age in three of 12 infants born to SIV-infected rhesus monkeys. Two other infants born to infected dams were stillborn, and another died 3 days after birth; the virological status of these three are unknown, but these premature deaths may have occurred as a result of a transplacentally acquired infection.

In summary, 49 pregnant females spanning three species of macaques and involving both cloned and uncloned virus stocks have been utilized in a preliminary examination of maternal-fetal transmission of SIV in the macaque. Of these, seven females (14%) have given birth to infected offspring confirmed by either PCR and/or virus isolation. Nine abortions suspected to be infected were also observed, which may elevate the frequency of transplacental transmission to 33%. Several cases of postnatal transmission via breast milk were also identified. This transmission frequency appears similar to that observed in HIV-infected humans.

Detailed pathological examination of placental and fetal tissues derived from these studies will elucidate the mechanism(s) by which these viruses gain entry into the fetal circulation. The type of placental lesion may reveal the route of entry. For example, inflammation of fetal chorioamnionic membranes or maternal decidua imply an ascending route of infection from the vaginal mucosa, whereas villitis or placentitis suggest entry via the maternal circulation. The inclusion in these studies of specialized techniques such as immunohistochemistry and in situ hybridization, and combinations thereof, should reveal the type of cell responsible for virus transport through placental tissue.

Several investigators have also successfully infected the macaque fetus by direct inoculation of SIV into amnionic fluid. Ruprecht et al. (60) infected seven of eight fetuses when virus was delivered during the second or third trimesters. More recently, Tarantal et al. (61) inoculated the amnionic fluid from four rhesus monkey fetuses each during early (day 26), middle (day 65), and late (day 130) gestation with SIVmac251. All fetuses became infected, and fetal death occurred in three of four, two of four, and one of four fetuses, respectively. Marked intrauterine growth retardation was also observed in those fetuses that survived to term. Ochs et al. (62) also successfully infected pigtailed macaque fetuses by amnionic inoculation during the second trimester with SIVmne. In addition, two of five pigtailed macaque fetuses died as a result of intra-amnionic inoculation with HIV-1.

Studies at the Tulane Primate Center did not result in uniform infection of all fetuses inoculated via amnionic fluid. Only one of three fetuses inoculated during the first trimester and two of five fetuses inoculated during the second trimester showed signs of infection. In contrast, two of two inoculated during the third trimester died in utero 2 weeks postinoculation. This limited study may suggest that the timing of fetal exposure may be critical to the outcome, with a higher incidence of infection expected near term.

Taken together, these data demonstrate that fetal infection can result from exposure to virus-containing amnionic fluid that comes in direct contact with fetal mucosal surfaces. Although artifically created in the macaque system, this condition could arise naturally in the HIV-infected pregnant woman by an ascending infection from the vaginal mucosa. Other viral or bacterial agents could potentially aid HIV in this process by attracting mononuclear cells to the site of inflammation.

SUMMARY

Several animal models are now available to increase our understanding of maternal-fetal transmission of HIV. These models will be vital in identifying the mechanism(s) of viral transport across the placental barrier and cofactors that aid and/or enhance this process. Preliminary studies performed with limited numbers of SIV-infected macaques suggest that HIV, like hepatitis virus, may be transmitted to neonates predominantly perinatally, with some transmission occurring earlier in gestation, perhaps with the aid of opportunistic infections or other cofactors such as cocaine use, that are known to cause changes in placental pathology. Selection of a single genetic species from a swarm of genetically distinct forms of the virus found in the maternal circulation fur-

ther suggests that forms of virus with particular tropisms may also be involved in allowing the virus to enter the fetal circulation. Further studies using more animals, however, must be performed to confirm these observations.

Once the pathobiology of this process is understood, these models can be further utilized to evaluate antiviral drugs and vaccines effective in prevention. The need for nonhuman trials for these experimental strategies must be underscored given the proven potential of drugs to alter fetal development and for vaccines to enhance transmission and/or disease.

References

1. La Pointe N, Michaud J, Pekovic D, Chausseau JP, Dupuy J-M. Transplacental transmission of HTLV-III virus. N Engl J Med 1985;312:1325–1326.
2. Jovias E, Koch MA, Achafer A, Stauber M, Lowenthal D. LAV/HTLV-III in 20-week fetus. Lancet 1985;2:1129.
3. Sprecher S, Soumenkoff G, Puissant F, Degueldre M. Vertical transmission of HIV in 15-week fetus. Lancet 1986;2:288–289.
4. Cournaud V, Laure F, Brossard A, et al. Frequent and early in utero HIV-1 infection. Aids Res Hum Retroviruses 1991;7:337–341.
5. Mano H, Chermann J-C. Fetal human immunodeficiency virus type 1 infection of different organs in the second trimester. Aids Res Hum Retrovirus 1991;7:83–88.
6. Goedert JJ, Duliege A-M, Amos CI, et al. High risk of HIV-1 infection for first-born twins. Lancet 1991;338:1471–1475.
7. Krivine A, Firtion G, Cao L, Francoual C, Henrion R, Lebon P. HIV replication during the first weeks of life. Lancet 1992;339:1187–1189.
8. Ryder RW, Nsa W, Hassig SE, Behets F, Rayfield M, Ekungola B. Perinatal transmission of the human immunodeficiency virus type 1 to infants of seropositive women in Zaire. N Engl J Med 1989;320:1637–1642.
9. Goedert JJ, Drummond JE, Minkoff HL, Stevens R, Blattner WA, Mendez H. Mother-to-infant transmission of human immunodeficiency virus type 1: Association with prematurity or low anti-gp120. Lancet 1989;2:1351–1354.
10. European Collaborative Study. Risk factors for mother-to-child transmission of HIV-1. Lancet 1992;339:1007–1012.
11. Italian Multicentre Study. Epidemiology, clinical features, and prognostic factors of paediatric HIV infection. Lancet 1988;2:1043–1046.
12. Mok JQ, Rossi A, De Ades A, et al. Infants born to mothers seropositive for human immunodeficiency virus: Preliminary findings from a multicenter European study. Lancet 1987;1:1164–1168.
13. Rossi P, Moschese V, Broliden PA, et al. Presence of maternal antibodies to human immunodeficiency virus 1 envelope glycoprotein gp 120 epi-

topes correlates with the uninfected status of children born to seropositive mothers. Proc Natl Acad Sci USA 1989;86:8055–8058.

14. Blanche S, Rouzioux C, Giuhard Moscato M-L, et al. A prospective study of infants born to women seropositive for human immunodeficiency virus type 1. N Engl J Med 1989;320:1643–1648.

15. Kind C, Brandle B, Wyler CA, et al. Epidemiology of vertically transmitted HIV-1 infection in Switzerland: Results of a nationwide prospective study. Eur J Pediatr 1992;151:442–448.

16. Hutto C, Parks W, Lai S, et al. A hospital-based prospective study of perinatal infection with human immunodeficiency virus type 1. J Pediatr 1991;118:347–353.

17. Parekh BS, Shaffer N, Pau C-P, et al. Lack of correlation between maternal antibodies to V3 loop peptides of gp120 and perinatal HIV-1 transmission. AIDS 1991;5:1179–1184.

18. Van de Perre P, Simonon A, Msellati P, et al. Postnatal transmission of human immunodeficiency virus type 1 from mother to infant: A prospective cohort study in Kigali, Rwanda. N Engl J Med 1991;325:593–598.

19. Lewis SH, Reynolds-Kohler C, Fox HE, Nelson JA. HIV-1 in trophoblastic and villous Hofbauer cells, and haematological precursors in eight-week fetuses. Lancet 1990;335:565–568.

20. Douglas GC, Fry GN, Thirkill T, et al. Cell-mediated infection of human placental trophoblast with HIV in vitro. AIDS Res Human Retroviruses 1991; 7:735–740.

21. Mano H, Chermann J-C. Replication of human immunodeficiency virus type 1 in primary cultured placental cells. Res Virol 1991;142:95–104.

22. Zachar V, Norskov-Lauritsen N, Juhl C, et al. Susceptibility of cultured human trophoblasts to infection with human immunodeficiency virus type 1. J Gen Virol 1991;72:1253–1260.

23. Beutler B, Cerami A. The biology of cachectin/TNF—a primary mediator of the host response. Annu Rev Immunol 1989;7:625–655.

24. Reuben JM, Gonik B, Li S, et al. Induction of cytokines in normal placental cells by the human immunodeficiency virus. Lymphokine Cytokine Res 1991;10:195–199.

25. Fitzgerald NA, Shellan GR. Host genetic factors on fetal susceptibility to murine cytomegalovirus after maternal or fetal infection. J Infect Dis 1991;163: 276–281.

26. Abzug MJ, Rotbart HA, Levin MJ. Demonstration of a barrier to transplacental passage of murine enteroviruses in late gestation. J Infect Dis 1989; 159:761–765.

27. Abzug MJ, Rotbart HA, Magliato SA, Levin MJ. Evolution of the placental barrier to fetal infection by murine enteroviruses. J Infect Dis 1991;163: 1336–1341.

28. Mbawuike IN, Six HR, Cate TR, Couch RB. Vaccination with inactivated influenza A virus during pregnancy protects neonatal mice against lethal challenge by influenza A viruses representing three subtypes. J Virol 1990;64:1370–1374.

29. Ruprecht RM, Bernard LD, Chou T-C, et al. Murine models for evaluating antiretroviral therapy. Cancer Res 1990;50:5618s–5627s.

30. Ruprecht RM, O'Brien LG, Rossoni LD, Nusinoff-Lehrman S. Suppression of mouse viremia and retroviral disease by 3'-azido-5'deoxythymidine. Nature 1986;323:467–469.

31. Sharpe AH, Hunter JJ, Ruprecht RM, Jaenisch R. Maternal transmission of retroviral disease and strategies for preventing infection of the neonate. J Virol 1989;63:1049–1053.

32. Gardner MB. Retroviral spongiform polioencephalopathy. Rev Infect Dis 1985;7:99–110.

33. Pederson NC. The feline immunodeficiency virus. In: Levy JA, ed. The retroviridae. Vol 2. New York: Plenum, 1993.

34. Yamamoto J, Hansen H, Ho E, et al. Epidemiologic and clinical aspects of feline immunodeficiency virus infection in cats from the continental United States and Canada and possible mode of transmission. J Am Vet Med Assoc 1989;194:213–220.

35. Hosie MJ, Robertson C, Jarrett O. Prevalence of feline leukemia virus and antibodies to feline immunodeficiency virus in cats in the United Kingdom. Vet Rec 1989;125:293–297.

36. Callanan JJ, Hosie MJ, Jarrett O. Transmission of feline immunodeficiency virus from mother to kitten. Vet Rec 1991;128:332–333.

37. Wasmoen T, Armiger-Luhman S, Egan C, et al. Transmission of feline immunodeficiency virus from infected queens to kittens. Vet Immunol Immunopathol 1992;35:83–93.

38. Martin CB Jr, Ramsey EM. Gross anatomy of the placenta of rhesus monkeys. Am J Obstet Gynecol 1970;36:167–177.

39. Giddens WE, Tsai C-C, Morton WR, Ochs HD, Knitter GH, Blakeley GA. Retroperitoneal fibromatosis and acquired immunodeficiency syndrome in macaques: Pathologic observations and transmission studies. Am J Pathol 985;119: 253–263.

40. Tsai C-C, Follis KE, Snyder K, et al. Maternal transmission of type D simian retrovirus (SRV-2) in pigtail macaques. J Med Primatol 1990;19:203–216.

41. Letvin NL, Daniel MD, Sehgal PK, et al. Induction of AIDS-like disease in macaque monkeys with T-cell tropic retrovirus STLV-III. Science 1985;230: 71–73.

42. Murphey-Corb M, Martin LN, Rangan SRS, et al. Isolation of and HTLV-III related retrovirus from macaques with simian AIDS and its possible origin in asymptomatic mangabeys. Nature 1986;321: 435–437.

43. Zhang J-Y, Martin LM, Watson EA, et al. Simian immunodeficiency virus/delta-induced immunodeficiency disease in rhesus monkeys: Relation of antibody response and antigenemia. J Infect Dis 1988;158:1277–1286.

44. Baskin GB, Murphey-Corb M, Watson EA, Martin LN. Necropsy findings in rhesus monkeys experimentally infected with cultured simian immunodeficiency virus (SIV)/delta. Vet Pathol 1988;25: 456–467.

45. McClure HM, Anderson DC, Ansari AA, Fultz PN, Klumpp SA, Schinazi RF. Nonhuman primate models for evaluation of AIDS therapy. Ann NY Acad Sci 1990;616:287–298.

46. Lundgren B, Bottiger D, Ljungdahl-Stahle E, et al. Antiviral effects of 3'-fluorothymidine and 3'-

azidothymidine in cynomolgus monkeys infected with simian immunodeficiency virus. J Acquir Immune Defic Syndr 1991;4:489–498.

47. Martin LN, Murphey-Corb M, Soike K, Davison-Fairburn B, Baskin GB. Effects of initiation of 3′azido-3′-deoxythymidine treatment at different times after infection of rhesus monkeys with simian immunodeficiency virus. J Infect Dis, in press.

48. Daniel MD, Letvin NL, Sehgal PK, et al. Prevalence of antibodies to 3 retroviruses in a captive colony of macaque monkeys. Int J Cancer 1988;41:601–608.

49. Ochs HD, Morton WR, Tsai CC, et al. Maternal-fetal transmission of SIV in macaques: Disseminated adenovirus infection in an offspring with SIV infection. J Med Primatol 1991;20:193–200.

50. Ochs HD, Morton WR, Kuller LD, et al. Prenatal inoculation of macaque fetuses with SIV and HIV [Abstract]. 10th Annual Symposium on Nonhuman Primate Models for AIDS, San Juan, Nov 1992:32.

51. Davison-Fairburn B, Blanchard B, Hu F-S, et al. Experimental infection of timed-pregnant rhesus monkeys with simian immunodeficiency virus (SIV) during early, middle and late gestation. J Med Primatol 1990;19:381–393.

52. Davison-Fairburn B, Baskin B, Murphey-Corb M. Maternal-fetal transmission of SIV in 2 species of macaques [Abstract]. 10th Annual Symposium on Nonhuman Primate Models for AIDS, San Juan, Nov 1992:29.

53. Hirsch VM, Philip M, Zack A, Vogel P, Johnson PR. Simian immunodeficiency virus infection of macaques: End-stage disease is characterized by widespread distribution of proviral DNA in tissues. J Infect Dis 1991;163:976–988.

54. Hahn BH, Shaw GM, Taylor ME, et al. Genetic variation in HTLV-III/LAV over time in patients with AIDS or at risk for AIDS. Science 1986;232:1548–1553.

55. Burns DPW, Desrosiers RC. Selection of genetic variants of simian immunodeficiency virus in persistently infected rhesus monkeys. J Virol 1991;65:1843–1854.

56. Wolinsky SM, Wike CM, Korber BT, et al. Selective transmission of human immunodeficiency virus type 1 (HIV-1) variants from mother to infants. Science 1992;255:1134–1137.

57. Mossman SP, O'Neil SP, Hoover EA, Maul DH. Vertical transmission of SIVmac239 in rhesus macaques [Abstract]. 10th Annual Symposium on Nonhuman Primate Models for AIDS, San Juan, Nov 1992:32.

58. McClure HN, Anderson DC, Fultz PN, et al. Maternal transmission of SIVsmm in rhesus macaques. J Med Primatol 1991;20:182–187.

59. Klumpp SA, Anderson DC, Novembre FJ, McClure HM. Animal model for pediatric AIDS: Pathology in infant rhesus monkeys infected with SIVsmm [Abstract]. 10th Annual Symposium on Nonhuman Primate Models for AIDS, San Juan, Nov 1992:30.

60. Ruprecht R, Fazely F, Sharma P, et al. Prenatal infection of rhesus monkey fetuses with the simian immunodeficiency virus: A model to study lentiviral pathogenesis during ontogeny. J Cell Biochem 1992;suppl 16E:111.

61. Tarantal AF, Marthas ML, McChesney MB, et al. Prenatal SIV infection in the rhesus macaque (*Macaca mulatta*) [Abstract]. 10th Annual Symposium on Nonhuman Primate Models for AIDS, San Juan, Nov 1992:33.

62. Ochs HD, Morton WR, Kuller LD, et al. Prenatal inoculation of macaque fetuses with SIV and HIV [Abstract]. 10th Annual Symposium on Nonhuman Primate Models for AIDS, San Juan, Nov 1992:32.

PART C / CURRENT INSIGHTS REGARDING VERTICAL TRANSMISSION

Lynne M. Mofenson and Steven M. Wolinsky

The number of children with vertically acquired HIV infection is increasing with the expanding AIDS pandemic. By the end of 1992 the World Health Organization had estimated that 4 million women and 1 million of their children were infected with HIV worldwide. By the year 2000, the World Health Organization projects that 3 million women and children will die from HIV-related disease; cumulatively, 10 million children will be born infected (1).

The spread of HIV by heterosexual contact and intravenous drug use has increased the prevalence of infection among sexually active women of childbearing age. Epidemiologic surveys in Europe and North America indicate that 0.15–0.24% of women delivering infants in 1989–1991 were infected, although seroprevalence as high as 6.6% has been observed in some inner city areas (2–4). In sub-Saharan Africa, as high as 20–30% of pregnant women receiving antenatal care are infected (5).

Many epidemiological surveys, reviewed in detail in Chapter 1, have evaluated the rate of vertical transmission of HIV infection (5, 6). In Africa, reported transmission rates have ranged from 28 to 52% of infants born to infected mothers. In Europe and North America, reported transmission rates have ranged between 10 and 39%. Vertically acquired HIV infection accounts for 85% of reported pediatric AIDS cases in the United States (7) and for the vast majority of pediatric HIV infection worldwide.

Pediatric HIV infection has high morbidity and mortality. It has been estimated that ~20% of HIV-infected infants will develop AIDS during the first year of life (8), and >90% of infected infants can be expected to develop HIV-related symptoms by age 12–18 months (9–11). In the New York City metropolitan area, AIDS is the leading cause of death among black women aged 25–44 years and the second leading cause of death among black children aged 1–4 years (5). Particularly in the developing world, HIV infection may have a substantial impact on infant and child mortality rates, abolishing the gains achieved over the last 30 years through programs such as childhood immunization (12).

Prevention of vertically acquired HIV infection must be a public health priority. Strategies to interrupt mother to child HIV transmission require an understanding of factors influencing viral transmission during pregnancy and the postnatal period. Understanding the pathogenesis of other perinatally acquired viruses provides insight into both the potential timing and mechanisms of HIV transmission. Furthermore, successful prevention strategies used for other viruses may assist in designing appropriate interventions for interrupting perinatal HIV infection.

LESSONS FROM OTHER VERTICALLY TRANSMITTED VIRUS INFECTIONS

Among viruses that can be transmitted before, during, or after birth, rubella, hepatitis B, herpes simplex virus (HSV), human T cell lymphotropic virus type I (HTLV-I), and cytomegalovirus (CMV) each provide unique lessons for HIV transmission (Table 10C.1). The time during gestation when transmission occurs differs among these viruses and is important in influencing transmission rates and disease manifestations in the infant.

Timing of Vertical Virus Transmission

Virus transmission may occur in utero by direct transplacental hematogenous spread, by ascending infection of the amniotic membranes and fluid, or iatrogenically by direct invasive methods for diagnosis. Infections, such as rubella, that are primarily transmitted in utero can result in abortion, stillbirth, prematurity, congenital malformations, intrauterine growth retardation, active disease at birth or neonatal period, or persistent infection with late sequelae.

Infection of the fetus with rubella virus presumably occurs secondary to placental infection from maternal viremia during primary infection and before development of protective maternal antibody. Gestational age at the time of maternal infection is an important determinant of both the rate and pathogenic manifestations of infection. Fetal infection with rubella declines from over 50% when maternal infection occurs during the first 8 weeks of gestation to 34% during 9–12 weeks gestation and a low of 10% between 13 and 24 weeks gestation (13). However, significant teratogenic effects are most common when maternal infection occurs between the 4th and 12th weeks of gestation, the period of most rapid fetal tissue growth and organ differentiation. Among infants infected during the first 8 weeks of gestation, as many as 90% have detectable defects during the first 4 years of life; this decreases to 52% for those infected between 9 and 12 weeks gestation and to 16% for those infected between 13 and 20 weeks (13–14).

In contrast to rubella, hepatitis B and HSV are most commonly transmitted at the time of delivery. Intrapartum transmission occurs by mucocutaneous contact of the infant with maternal blood and cervico-vaginal secretions during passage through the birth canal, by ascending infection from the cervix, or by maternal-fetal transfusion at delivery. Viruses transmitted primarily during the intrapartum period can cause acute systemic illness that can lead to death or, more commonly, persistent infection with late sequelae.

Evidence for late transmission of these viruses included the known presence of infectious virus in blood and/or vaginal fluids, the lack of distinct congenital malformations in infected newborns, the lack of acute disease manifestations at birth, diagnostic laboratory findings arising within a time most consistent with acquisition of infection at birth, and, most importantly, the efficacy of preventive strategies targeted to the newborn period in preventing infection in infants of infected women.

The mechanism of intrapartum transmission may be modified by the site of persistent virus in the mother. For HSV, after an initial short-lived viremic phase, virus remains latent within sensory nerve ganglia. Upon reactivation, HSV spreads via the nerve to locally replicate in epithelial cells; viremia only rarely occurs. Hence, HSV is not typically found in maternal blood but in genital tract cells and secretions. Whereas intrapartum exposure to virus in blood, either through maternal-fetal transfusion or direct contact, is primary in hepatitis B transmission, for HSV, direct contact of the infant with cell-free or cell-associated virus in infectious genital secretions during passage through the birth canal at delivery is critical. Ascending infection is also involved, as demonstrated by the increasing risk of neonatal HSV infection with increasing duration of ruptured membranes (15).

Postpartum virus transmission can occur during the neonatal period by exposure to infectious maternal secretions or ingestion of infected breast milk; such infections may be associated with virus persistence and subsequent late sequelae.

HTLV-I is a highly cell-associated virus infecting lymphocytes that is transmitted primarily during the postpartum period. Virus load in the peripheral blood is relatively low ($\leq$1:100 to 1:10,000 lymphocytes are infected) (16). Exposure of the infant to a sufficiently high infectious dose of virus to establish infection occurs principally by ingestion of infected lymphocytes present in breast milk. This is supported by the high cell-associated virus burden in breast milk

of carrier mothers, the transmission of HTLV-I through breast milk in animal models, and infrequent infection of children born to carrier mothers who are fed only formula (17, 18). The serologic profile observed in infected children is also most consistent with postpartum transmission. HTLV-I antibody titers decrease during the first few months of life, with essentially all becoming seronegative by 6 months of age. In infected children, however, HTLV-I antibody reappears after the age of 12 months. Cord blood surveys of infants born to carrier mothers have failed to detect evidence of infection, such as IgM antibody or virus-bearing cells, except on very rare occasions, making intrauterine transmission unlikely (17, 19).

Vertical transmission of CMV, unlike the previous viruses, does not appear limited to a specific time. After primary infection, asymptomatic intermittent virus excretion can be detected from various body sites, including the cervix, urinary tract, breast milk, and pharynx, although viremia is unusual. Although intrauterine transmission of CMV is most likely to occur during the viremic phase of primary infection, later transmission can also occur through exposure to excreted virus present in maternal genital secretions or breast milk.

Evidence for in utero CMV transmission includes detection of virus within the placenta and in fetal organs from abortuses, ability of the virus to replicate in a wide variety of fetal cells and tissues, virus isolation from amniotic fluid, presence at birth of symptomatic disease affecting multiple organ systems in 10–15% of infants infected after maternal primary infection, and presence of viruria or detection of CMV IgM in the first few days after birth (15, 20).

Ingestion of CMV from infectious maternal genital secretions during passage through the birth canal or in breast milk also can be a significant source for neonatal infection. In contrast to infants infected in utero, infants acquiring infection intra- or postpartum are usually asymptomatic at birth, becoming viruric after age 4–8 weeks. Intrapartum transmission is relatively efficient: ~57% of infants who pass through a genital tract actively shedding CMV become infected (15). Postpartum transmission by

Table 10C.1.   Comparison of HIV-1 with Other Vertically Transmitted Viruses[a]

	Rubella	Hepatitis B	HSV	HTLV-1	CMV	HIV-1
Persistence						
Causes persistent maternal infection	0	+	+	+	+	+
Persistent infection in presence of antibody	0	0	+	+	+	+
Site of maternal infection						
Commonly found in vagina-cervix	0	0	+	0	+	+
Commonly found in blood						
Cell free	+ (primary infection)	+	0	?	+	+
Cell associated	0	0	0	+	+	+
Time of transmission						
Intrauterine	++	± (<5%)	± (rare)	? ± (rare)	+	+
Intrapartum						
From genital site	0	0	++	0	++	?+
From blood	0	++	0	0	?+	?+
Postpartum from breast milk	0	± (rare)	0	++	+	+
Overall transmission rate and modifying factors	*Intrauterine* 10–50% depending on gestational age at time of maternal primary infection	*Intrapartum* 10–90% depending on hepatitis B antigen and antibody status of mother	*Intrapartum* 3–50% depending on primary vs. recurrent infection	*Breast Milk* 20–25%	*Intrauterine* 40–50% if primary infection during pregnancy 1–2% if chronic infection during pregnancy *Intrapartum Breast milk* 50–60% if active viral shedding in cervix at delivery or into breast milk	12% lowest (European Collaborative Study) to 45% highest (Nairobi),

Table 10C.1.—*continued*

	Rubella	Hepatitis B	HSV	HTLV-1	CMV	HIV-1
Infant outcome						
Fetal demise/congenital anomalies	++	0	± (rare)	0	+	?0
Acute symptomatic disease at birth	++	± (rare)	± (<10%)	0	++	± (rare)
Acute symptomatic disease after birth but during neonatal period	0	± (rare)	++	0	±	± (rare)
Persistent infection without symptoms in neonatal period with late sequelae	+	++	±	++	++	++
	Deafness	Liver disease and cancer	Recurrent HSV lesion	ATL, TSP	Deafness; other CNS	AIDS, death
Preventive strategies available	+	+	+	?+	0	0
	Childhood immunization with rubella to ensure immunity before childbearing	Neonatal postexposure immunoprophylaxis immunoglobulin and vaccine	Cesarean section delivery if active lesion present at labor	Formula rather than breast feeding of infants born to carrier mothers		
Availability of curative treatment or adjunctive therapies for infected infants with disease	0	0	+	0	?+	Adjunctive antiretroviral therapy and PCP prophylaxis for infected infants
			Acyclovir for acutely ill infected infant		?Ganciclovir for acutely ill infected infant being evaluated	

[a]ATL, adult T cell leukemia; TSP, tropical spastic paraparesis; CNS, central nervous system; PCP, *Pneumocystis carinii* pneumonia. Modified from Schwartz DA, Nahmias AJ. Human immunodeficiency virus and the placenta. Ann Clin Lab Sci 1991;21:264–274.

breast milk is also relatively efficient; up to 53–63% of infants breast fed with milk containing virus become infected. CMV is more common in mature milk (36–50% of milk specimens from seropositive mothers) than colostrum (8–11% of milk specimens) (21), and infection is more common in infants who breast feed for longer than 1 month (21, 22).

Factors Modifying Vertical Transmission and Neonatal Disease Manifestations

As shown in Table 10C.2, many different factors may influence risk of virus transmission from mother to child. Since the pregnant woman is the source of virus causing fetal or neonatal infection, the pattern of maternal infection and her immune response influences the degree of neonatal protection.

The exact mechanisms for transplacental virus spread have not been identified. For

Table 10C.2. Factors Influencing Mother to Child Virus Transmission

Maternal factors
    Clinical and immunologic status
    Site of persistent virus expression
    Level and duration of viremia
    Virus-specific immune response
Viral factors
    Virus phenotype
    Virus genotype
Placental factors
    Placental cell susceptibility to virus infection
    Developmental stage of placenta
    Integrity of placenta
Fetal factors
    Gestational age at time of virus exposure
    Fetal immune response
    Fetal cell susceptibility to viral infection
    Genetic factors (e.g., HLA type)
Obstetrical factors
    Route of delivery
    Invasive monitoring
    Postdelivery infant handling
Neonatal factors
    Skin and mucus membrane integrity
    Neonatal immune response
    Gastrointestinal maturity
Breast milk factors
    Level and duration of virolactia
    Nonspecific antiviral defenses
    Virus-specific local immunity

both rubella and CMV, isolated infection of the placenta has been observed in the absence of fetal infection, suggesting possible protection of the fetus by the placental barrier in some instances (13, 23). Alternatively, infection of the fetus has been observed without concomitant infection of the placenta.

Maternal virus burden and immune response may be important determinants of virus transmission. Highest rates of hepatitis B transmission, ≥85%, are observed from hepatitis B e antigen positive mothers (serum hepatitis B e antigen significantly correlates with high amount of infectious virions) (24, 25). The risk of neonatal HSV infection is highest when primary maternal infection occurs late in pregnancy, possibly because of neonatal exposure to a high amount of virus in the absence of a maternal immune response; Whitley and colleagues (26) have observed that 51% of neonates with HSV infection lack HSV antibody in initial blood samples. Fifty percent of women delivering vaginally with primary HSV genital lesions transmit infection to their neonates, compared with <10% if the lesion is secondary to HSV reactivation (27, 28).

In utero CMV transmission is most frequent after primary infection in the mother (average transmission rates of 40–50%) and less frequently results from reactivation of latent virus in the presence of maternal immunity (transmission rates between 0.2 and 1.8%) (29), although intra- and postpartum transmission may more often occur in this setting. Although maternal immunity may not completely protect against CMV transmission, it appears to be involved in reducing the virulence of infection in the fetus and infant. Symptomatic neonatal CMV occurs principally after primary maternal infection, and infected infants asymptomatic at birth are more likely to suffer severe late sequelae if born to mothers with primary infection during pregnancy (30, 31). Although greater pathologic impact on the fetus may be seen with transmission during primary maternal infection, less frequently clinically significant CMV disease may occur in infants who acquire disease from mothers with reactivated infection.

Regardless of time of acquisition, the immaturity of the neonatal immune system appears to affect both the severity and chronicity of disease manifestations when compared with infection occurring in older children or adults. Whereas HSV infection outside the perinatal period generally remains a localized epithelial cell infection, HSV infection of the neonate presents acutely after the 1st week of life with disseminated, multiorgan involvement or disease localized to the central nervous system, skin, eyes or mouth; encephalitis is observed in 50–75% of infected infants with disseminated disease. Similarly, primary infection with CMV in nonimmunocompromised individuals outside the perinatal period is generally subclinical with persistent infection manifest only by intermittent asymptomatic virus excretion. In contrast, 10% of infected newborns born to mothers with a primary infection experience severe symptomatic CMV disease at birth, and an additional 5–17% of initially asymptomatic infected infants develop long-term sequelae such as sensorineural hearing loss, chorioretinitis, mental retardation, and other neurologic sequelae (29, 31).

The manifestations of CMV disease in the infant are also affected by developmental maturity of the fetus-newborn at the time of infection; although infection acquired by the infant during the intrapartum or postpartum period can occasionally be associated with self-limited signs of pulmonary or reticuloendothelial involvement, severe neurologic sequelae are confined to infections transmitted in utero (29).

Virus infection of the fetus and newborn often produces persistent infection. Vertically acquired rubella is associated with persistence of viremia and virus excretion for months postnatally, even in the face of specific antibody response (32). Similarly, persistent infection is more common with vertically acquired hepatitis B infection (85-90%) than with infection acquired in adults (5–10%).

Development and Success of Preventive Strategies

The development of modalities to prevent mother to child transmission are highly dependent on the timing and mechanism of virus transmission. For viruses transmitted in utero, such as rubella, intervention strategies aimed at preventing maternal infection or possibly enhancing immune response in infected mothers are indicated. Prevention of congenital rubella syndrome focused on development of a safe and effective vaccine to render women of childbearing age immune before pregnancy. Since the licensure of live, attenuated rubella vaccine in the United States in 1969, the incidence of rubella and congenital rubella syndrome have dramatically declined because of universal childhood immunization and targeted immunization of women of childbearing age. Despite these programs, congenital rubella has not been completely eradicated, and missed opportunities for vaccination occur all too frequently (33).

For viruses primarily transmitted during the intrapartum or postpartum periods, the opportunity exists to interrupt transmission from an infected pregnant woman to her newborn. For hepatitis B, intervention focuses on the window period between exposure of the infant to maternal virus during delivery and the actual development of infection in the infant. Because neutralizing antibody is associated with immunity, this strategy relies upon immunoprophylaxis of the newborn through administration of hyperimmune hepatitis B immunoglobulin at birth followed by active immunization to ensure persistence of protective neutralizing antibody in the infant; this regimen has proven to be over 90% effective. Most infants who become infected despite this regimen have intrauterine infection unlikely to be reversed by immunoprophylaxis provided after birth. Despite a highly effective intervention, implementation has been limited by failure to identify a high proportion of hepatitis B-infected mothers. Universal prenatal screening of pregnant women is now recommended; additionally the Immunization Practices Advisory Committee to the Public Health Service has recently recommended universal childhood immunization for hepatitis B (34), an approach similar to that taken for rubella.

Because intrapartum HSV transmission occurs principally by mucocutaneous contact of the neonate with infectious maternal genital tract secretions during vaginal delivery, cesarean section in mothers with active genital herpes at the time of delivery has been the primary preventive strategy. Maternal case identification may be less than optimal because a large proportion of mothers have asymptomatic or unrecognized infection. Furthermore, serial antepartum vaginal cultures fail to predict virus shedding at delivery, and no rapid and sensitive screening test is available. Prophylactic systemic acyclovir therapy of mothers with active genital herpes late in gestation remains controversial and of uncertain efficacy. However, early diagnosis of infected infants with prompt initiation of antiviral therapy has been demonstrated to decrease mortality and improve long-term outcome (15).

For viruses transmitted primarily by breast feeding, such as HTLV-I, formula feeding by carrier mothers may be an effective measure to dramatically reduce infection and chronic sequelae. This strategy is limited by the availability of alternative forms of infant nutritional supplementation.

Prevention of vertical CMV transmission is much more complex. Significant rates of transmission are observed before, during, and after birth. However, the most damaging neurologic sequelae of vertically acquired CMV infection occur in the infants of immunologically naive women who develop primary maternal CMV infection during the intrauterine period. Therefore prevention of primary CMV infection in pregnant women through a rubella-like universal immunization strategy would be necessary to prevent the most damaging effects of congenital CMV (35). The specific virus epitopes that induce immunity or prevent virus transmission are not defined, however, and there is some concern regarding the oncogenic potential of live vaccines, given the ability of CMV to transform human cells in vitro.

As is evident from Table 10C.1, infant outcome as well as design of preventive strategies are highly dependent on timing and mechanism of viral transmission. For viruses that can be transmitted during all periods of fetal and neonatal development, such as CMV and HIV, preventive strategies will need to be multifaceted, and delineation of factors that enhance or prevent transmission during each of these periods is of great significance.

HIV VERTICAL TRANSMISSION: TIMING OF TRANSMISSION

HIV can be transmitted before, during, or after delivery. Data are limited, however, about the relative proportion and efficiency of transmission during the intrauterine, intrapartum, or postpartum periods (Table 10C.3).

Intrauterine Transmission

The clinical observation that 20–30% of infected infants appear to develop rapid, early onset of AIDS during the first few months of life provided initial indirect evidence for intrauterine transmission. The early manifestation of disease in these infants is consistent with the clinical outcome of infants infected with other viruses transmitted in utero, although some viruses, such as HSV, transmitted intrapartum may also present with acute illness in the neonatal period. The development of easily performed, reliable tests for the detection of HIV proteins and nucleic acids in placental tissue and aborted fetal organs has provided more direct evidence for transmission during gestation.

Apparently, intrauterine transmission can occur during each trimester of gestation. Data documenting transmission during the first trimester, however, are limited. HIV has been identified by culture or polymerase chain reaction (PCR) in fetal tissue obtained from therapeutic abortions as early as 10 weeks gestation (36–42). HIV has also been be detected in placental tissue from HIV-infected women as early as 8 weeks gestation by techniques including ultrastructural examination, virus culture, immunocytochemistry, and in situ hybridization (43–47). Although contamination with maternal blood could potentially confound studies of placental or fetal tissue obtained from abortuses, many investigators have demonstrated the ability of certain placenta-derived cells to support HIV replication in vitro (48–52).

Evidence for an HIV-associated embryopathy similar to that induced by other viruses transmitted during the early intrauterine period of fetal organogenesis must be regarded with great reservation. Although

Table 10C.3.   Timing of Vertical Transmission[a]

Intrauterine Transmission	Intrapartum Transmission	Postpartum Transmission
Early onset symptoms (<6 months) ~30%	Later onset symptoms (>12 months) ~70%	Transmission of other retroviruses by breast milk
Neonatal period virus identification (<1week) ~30–50%	Delayed virus identification (≥1 week) ~50–70%	HIV isolation from breast milk
? Dysmorphic syndrome	Acute primary infection virologic-immunologic pattern	Transmission of HIV from mothers who became infected postpartum and breast fed their infant
HIV identified in placentas (≥8 weeks gestation)	HIV isolation from vaginal-cervical secretions	Possible increased risk of HIV transmission from mothers with established infection who breast fed their infants
In vitro infection of placenta-derived cells	Discordant twins: Increased risk of infection in first born twin	
HIV identified in fetal tissue (≥10 weeks gestation)	Intrapartum blood exposure	
HIV identified in amniotic fluid	? Possible decreased risk transmission with cesarean section	
HIV identified in fetal blood specimens		

[a]Modified from Ref. 6.

some investigators have described a craniofacial dysmorphism associated with perinatal HIV transmission (53–55), subsequent studies have not confirmed this association with the same malformations observed in infants born to HIV-infected and uninfected mothers who used drugs during pregnancy (56, 57). Either HIV is not an embryopathic virus or the virus crosses the placenta so infrequently during the first 8 weeks of pregnancy that congenital malformations are rarely documented. Furthermore, intrauterine growth retardation, a clinical consequence of other intrauterine viral infections, has not been observed in most studies (58). Although low birth weight and adverse fetal outcome have been reported in a few African cohorts of HIV-infected pregnant women (50–61), association with the HIV infection status of the infant was not provided. However, it may be difficult to detect an effect of intrauterine HIV infection on fetal growth if in utero transmission occurs infrequently, because only a small proportion of any infected cohort might then be expected to demonstrate growth retardation.

Several investigators have detected virus in fetal tissue from abortuses obtained during the second trimester. Proviral DNA sequences have been detected by PCR in fetal organs from abortions performed between 16 and 24 weeks gestation (39, 40). Potential maternal blood contamination was assessed by coamplification of a polymorphic genomic DNA sequence adjacent to the cystic fibrosis locus. Although tissue from 33 fetuses between 16 and 24 weeks gestation were analyzed, potential maternal blood contamination could be excluded in only nine (39). HIV proviral DNA sequences were detected in fetal thymus (six of eight), spleen (8 of 9), and peripheral blood (five of nine) sampled from these nine fetuses. Although all nine fetuses had evidence of HIV proviral DNA in one or more sites, all fetal organ samples were negative for HIV by both virus isolation and p24 antigen testing. Lyman et al. (62) used PCR to detect proviral DNA in fetal central nervous system tissue from second trimester abortions. Maternal blood contamination was addressed by wiping the intact fetus with alcohol. Proviral sequences were detected in 8 of 23 (30%) fetal organs.

These studies involved a limited number of fetuses, and the relatively high proportion of infected fetuses detected by either virus isolation or PCR suggests some selection bias. Significantly lower fetal tissue infection rates have been reported. A recent study could not substantiate the presence of HIV in 12 first and second trimester fetuses (63), although two fetuses had nonconfirmable PCR or in situ hybridization positivity in a single organ.

HIV has been isolated from both amniotic fluid cells and amniotic fluid supernatant obtained during the first and second trimester of pregnancy (64, 65). Fetal blood from 13 fetuses of women undergoing elective termination of pregnancy between 16 and 24 weeks gestation was sampled by cor-

docentesis and analyzed for p24 antigen (64). HIV p24 antigen was found in both maternal serum and amniotic fluid samples from five of 13 mothers and in fetal blood from three of their five fetuses.

Indirect evidence for intrauterine transmission is provided by the detection of HIV by virus isolation and/or PCR in samples obtained from cord blood or birth samples in ~30–50% of infants born to infected mothers (67–77). (Table 10C.4). Inadvertent maternal blood contamination of cord blood samples could represent a significant source of potential bias in some of these results.

Comparative analysis of virus sequences in a mother's peripheral blood obtained dur-

Table 10C.4. Detection of HIV by Culture, PCR or p24 Antigen in HIV-infected Infants with Sequential Testing, or Age at Time of Testing[a]

Ref.	Method of HIV Detection	Age of Infected Infant at Testing	No. Positive at Specified Age/Total Infected Infants Sequentially Tested
Rogers et al. (68)	DNA PCR, culture, p24 antigen	Birth (cord blood) to 16 days (PCR)	6/11 (55%)
		2–13 months (culture, p24 antigen)	11/11
Ehrnst et al. (63)	Culture (plasma/PBMC)	First few days of life (peripheral blood)	0/3 (0%)
		Between birth and 6 months	3/3
Burgard et al. (69)	Culture (PBMC)	Birth (peripheral blood)	19/40 (48%)
		Between birth and 3 months	30/40 (75%)
De Rossi et al. (70)	DNA PCR, culture (PBMC)	<2 days	1/7 (14%)
		3–15 days	3/4 (75%)
		30–90 days	7/7
Borkowsky et al. (71)	DNA PCR, culture, p24 antigen	Birth to 2 days	3/6 (50%)
		15–60 days	6/6
Bryson et al. (72)	Culture (PBMC)	Birth (cord blood) to <72 hrs	6/10 (60%)
		2 weeks to 6 months	10/10
Quinn et al. (73)	ICD p24 antigen	<1 week	0/9 (0%)
		1–9 months	9/9
Miles et al. (74)	ICD p24 antigen	Birth (cord blood)	5/9 (55%)
		2 weeks to 9 months	8/9 (89%)
Lee et al. (75)	ICD p24 antigen	<5 days	0/3 (0%)
		6–30 days	3/3
Burchett et al. (76)	RNA PCR, culture (plasma/PBMC)	Birth (cord blood)	1/5 (20%) (PBMC culture only)
		1 month	3/5 (60%) (1 RNA PCR; 2 all tests positive)
		3 months	5/5 (5 PBMC culture positive; 2 also plasma culture positive)
Krivine et al. (77)	DNA PCR, culture (PBMC), p24 antigen	Birth	5/16 (31%)
		4–9 weeks	16/16
	RNA PCR	Birth	1/7 (14%)
		4–9 weeks	7/7

[a]PBMC, peripheral blood mononuclear cells; ICD; immune complex dissociated.

ing gestation with virus from her infant's blood sequences obtained at parturition may be used to estimate timing of vertical transmission. A study of three mother-infant transmission pairs showed that the homogeneous quasi-species population in the infant at 1–3 months most closely resembled a minor genetic variant in the mother's virus swarm (78). In a prospective study of one mother-infant pair, nested PCR was used to amplify the third hypervariable domain (V3) within the envelope coding region from virus RNA sequences in cord blood and maternal blood sampled after each trimester and delivery and 9 months postpartum (79). Virus sequence analysis showed that the infant's V3 consensus sequence represented a minor genotype in the mother at delivery and most closely resembled the genetic variants found in the mother early in pregnancy after the first trimester.

Although current data provide convincing evidence that intrauterine HIV transmission occurs, the relative proportion of transmission that arises in utero, the timing of infection during gestation, and the mechanisms involved are poorly understood.

Intrapartum Transmission

Direct evidence for intrapartum transmission analogous to hepatitis B has been difficult to obtain. Much of the data that indicate HIV transmission from mother to infant occurs during the intrapartum period are indirect.

Among twin sets reported to the International Registry of HIV-exposed Twins, HIV infection was more common in first-born than in second-born twins, particularly with vaginal delivery (80, 81). An updated analysis of 92 twin sets showed that 30 sets were discordant for infection. In 23 of 30 discordant twin sets, the firstborn twin was infected, whereas in seven twin sets the second born was infected ($p = 0.004$). Therefore the presenting twin had a 3-fold greater risk of infection than the second born twin. Although this relationship was not influenced by the mode of delivery, risk of transmission was higher overall in twins delivered vaginally than those delivered operatively. No data were available, however, regarding duration of ruptured membranes, length of labor, or indication for cesarean delivery. These data suggest that the presenting twin would have a prolonged exposure to infected blood and cervical secretions in the genital tract during the later stages of pregnancy and delivery. If direct mucocutaneous exposure to virus during delivery or ascending infection during labor are significant factors in HIV transmission, preventive strategies aimed at reducing virus inoculum by methods such as viricidal lavage of the birth canal or immediate surface decontamination of the newborn might be utilized.

There have been conflicting results from studies of singleton births regarding the influence of mode of delivery on transmission rates. Several investigators have reported similar infection rates regardless of mode of delivery (9, 58, 82). The European Collaborative Study found that cesarean delivery tended to decrease the risk of perinatal infection but only for emergency and not elective cesarean deliveries (83). This trend in relative risk reduction with cesarean delivery has also been reported by others, although reported reductions in transmission are marginal (84). Since only a few infants in these studies were delivered operatively, no study has had sufficient power to eliminate a protective effect. Similar to hepatitis B, significant transmission could also occur by maternal-fetal transfusion during labor or mucocutaneous exposure to maternal blood, which operative delivery would not prevent.

Virus sequences were analyzed in peripheral blood from a mother during gestation and her dizygotic twin pair after birth to estimate timing of perinatal infection (85). Virus was found by isolation and PCR of proviral DNA at 1 and 2 months of age for both twins, but only the second twin had proviral DNA detected by PCR at 16 hr postpartum. The V3 consensus sequence from the first twin most closely resembled the mother's V3 consensus sequences at parturition. The V3 consensus sequence from the second twin, however, most closely resembled the mother's V3 consensus sequences at 25 weeks gestation. Although these limited data indicate both intrauterine and intrapartum transmission in this twin set, the interpretation of infection timing is confounded by the probable multifactorial nature of this transmission. A genetic variant prevalent in the mother during gestation may either infect the infant directly or enter the fetal compartment and infect the fetus at a later time. Additionally, the dichotomy observed between proviral DNA and virus RNA sequences observed during longitudinal infection may be relevant to whether cell-associated or free virus was transmitted and when the transmission occurred (86).

About 30–50% of infants ultimately found to be HIV infected are PCR or culture positive at birth, consistent with virus acquisition in utero. Conversely, as shown in Table 10C.4, 50–70% of infants do not demonstrate detectable virus until later in infancy, consistent with acquisition during the intrapartum period. Some investigators have proposed a laboratory-based definition of early vs. late HIV infection (Table 10C.5) (87). A few investigators using quantitative culture and HIV RNA-PCR have noted peak virus production at age 1–3 months with a subsequent decline in some infants prospectively followed from birth, compatible with primary infection acquired during birth (77, 88, 89).

Collectively, these data imply that both intrauterine and intrapartum transmission occurs. The observed bimodal distribution of HIV-related symptomatic disease expression may reflect differences in the timing of virus transmission (90): infants with in utero infection having a rapid onset of clinical disease, and infants with intrapartum or postpartum infection having a slower onset of clinical disease. The proposed definition

of early vs. late infection in Table 10C.5 may assist in validating this hypothesis. The higher rate of intrapartum transmission suggested by some studies could be attributable to the relative insensitivity of the diagnostic tests used at time of birth. Similarly, latent virus sequestered in a privileged site that was not amenable to sampling could escape detection. After birth, antigenic stimulation of latent virus in these noncirculating cells could stimulate active viral replication, permitting biological amplification and virus detection.

Postpartum Transmission

Analogous to other human (HTLV-I) and animal (bovine leukemia virus and caprine arthritis-encephalitis virus) retroviruses (91), HIV can also be transmitted by breast feeding. Although both free virus and proviral DNA have been found in breast milk (92–94), demonstration of breast milk transmission has been epidemiologically complex.

Several studies have shown an increased risk of postpartum transmission by breast feeding among women with primary HIV infection during the peripartum period (9, 93, 95–100). The infant, therefore, could be potentially exposed to secretions or cells containing a high virus or proviral burden, respectively. These studies, however, are confounded by the limited size of the cohorts, the potential for intrauterine or intrapartum transmission, and the presence of antibodies in the breast milk of healthy HIV-infected women (101, 102).

Prospective studies of HIV transmission in breast fed infants have also been compromised by these variables and have given conflicting results. Evaluation of matched mother-infant populations that only vary by method of infant feeding has not been possible because of the homogeneity of feeding practices in current prospective cohorts, with breast feeding being the norm in developing countries and formula feeding the norm in industrialized countries. Both high (9, 100) and low (82, 103) rates of HIV transmission in breast fed infants have been reported. For example, the European Collaborative Study group reported a 2-fold increase in the risk of infection among

Table 10C.5.   Proposed Laboratory-based Definition of Early vs. Late HIV Infection[a]

Early (in utero) HIV infection
  Positive HIV culture or PCR within 48 hr of birth[b]
Late (intrapartum) HIV infection
  Negative HIV culture, PCR, or p24 antigen within one week of life and
  Positive HIV culture, PCR, or p24 antigen between age 7 and 90 days[c]

[a]Modified from Ref. 87.
[b]Positive cord blood sample must be confirmed with sample from peripheral blood obtained within 48 hrs of birth. Second confirmatory sample obtained outside neonatal period should be positive by HIV culture or PCR.
[c]Infant must not be breast feeding.

breast fed infants (31 vs. 14%), but only 38 of 828 children evaluated were breast fed (83). A meta-analysis of published prospective studies estimated the additional attributable risk of transmission posed by breast feeding from mothers with established HIV infection before pregnancy was 16% (95% confidence interval 8–25%) and was 26% (95% confidence interval 14–39%) from mothers who develop primary HIV infection postpartum (104).

Although HIV can be transmitted by breast milk, infected women in developing countries may not have a reasonable alternative to breast feeding. The potential to reconstitute infant formulas under unsanitized conditions poses significant risk of perinatal morbidity and mortality (105–108). Infant morbidity and mortality can be further reduced by protective maternal antibodies to endemic diseases. Therefore the risk of HIV transmission by breast feeding must be addressed in the context of specific patient populations (109).

FACTORS ASSOCIATED WITH TRANSMISSION AND POTENTIAL INTERVENTION STRATEGIES
Maternal and Virologic Factors

Maternal factors influencing the rate of HIV transmission from mother to child are incompletely defined. Indirect measures of increased virus burden including p24 antigenemia, CD4+ number, mother's disease state, and absence of maternal antibody to specific HIV epitopes have been associated with an increased risk of transmission. Additionally, characteristics of the maternal virus strains may also influence transmissibility.

Clinical and General Immune Status of the Mother

Advanced disease stage (defined as AIDS and Centers for Disease Control class IV disease stage), either during pregnancy or within months of giving birth, has been associated with increased rates of vertical transmission in many studies from different areas of the world, including Italy, Scotland,

Sweden, Africa, and Europe (83, 100, 110–113). Nonspecific symptoms of HIV disease, in the absence of other findings, have not correlated with increased transmission risk (83, 114). However, the presence of HIV-related symptoms combined with CD4+ number <200 µl was associated with transmission (114).

Low CD4+ number has been associated with increased transmission (100, 115, 116). Data from 146 HIV-infected pregnant women in Zaire have shown a relationship between the risk of transmission and low CD4+ number (77% transmission for <10% CD4+ cells vs. 23% for >30% CD4+ cells) (115). Similarly, a study from New York City also demonstrated association of low CD4+ percent with mother to child transmission and also found that transmission correlated highly with the mother's CD4+ numbers enumerated during the last trimester (116).

Although other studies have failed to correlate risk of perinatal transmission with low CD4+ number or advanced disease state, data were confounded by the higher CD4+ numbers and asymptomatic disease state of the enrolled women (9, 117). Studies of larger cohorts of HIV-infected pregnant women that have permitted stratification by both Centers for Disease Control classification of the disease state and CD4+ numbers have validated these initial findings (83, 118). A trend toward higher transmission between women with AIDS (31%) vs. asymptomatic women (14%) was found for the 615 women evaluated by the European Collaborative Study. A significant risk for transmission was found if the women were stratified by CD4+ number (<400/µl (19%), <700/µl (22%), and >700/µl (6%)) or CD4+/CD8+ ratios (>0.6 (12%) and <0.6 (24%)) (83). Similarly, among HIV-infected women enrolled in a large prospective cohort study in Rwanda, women with a CD4+:CD8+ ratio of <0.5 at parturition had a 3.2 times higher risk of perinatal transmission than women with a CD4+/CD8+ ratio of >0.5 (119).

Maternal Virus Characteristics

Several studies have noted a correlation between p24 antigenemia and risk of vertical transmission (10, 110, 120). However, some smaller cohort studies have not affirmed this association (121). High p24 antigen coupled with low CD4+ number or advanced disease stage has been linked with elevated transmission risk in several studies (110, 120, 122).

One prospective study of 47 pregnancies did not find an association between maternal viremia during pregnancy and transmission (63), but virus quantitation was not performed. In one limited study, an increased risk of perinatal transmission was associated with an increased proviral burden in maternal blood as measured by a quantitative PCR DNA assay (123). The rate of transmission has also been correlated with the maternal virus burden as measured by end-point dilution cultures in a small cohort of mother-infant pairs (124).

Several investigators have attempted to define the biologic and genetic features of the virus associated with perinatal transmission. In one study, the biological characteristic of the virus isolated from three transmitting and four nontransmitting mothers and their infants were evaluated (125). The virus isolated from nontransmitting mothers had slow-low growth properties, whereas the viruses isolated from the transmitting mothers and their infants had rapid-high growth characteristics. A previous study did not find a correlation between phenotype and risk of transmission (126).

The HIV genome is characterized by a high degree of genetic variability. Virus variants arise by mutation during replication by error-prone reverse transcription. The complex mixture of variants that exists in an infected individual are the result of competition and selection in response to immunologic pressure for change, and to alterations in cell tropism and replication efficiency among the variants (127).

In an initial study to investigate the role of selection in perinatal HIV transmission, the distribution of distinguishable genotypes transmitted between mother and child were analyzed (78). Comparisons of virus sequences from the three transmission pairs showed that specific sequences were highly conserved between each mother and her infant and that the infant's prevalent virus sequence was derived from a single variant present in its mother. Furthermore,

the infants' virus sequences were less diverse than those of their mothers. A low proportion of synonymous to nonsynonymous substitutions suggested that there was positive selection for change. The lower ratios of synonymous to nonsynonymous substitutions for infants' V3 sequence variation suggested that the infants' V3 region is under greater selective pressure for change than the V4-V5 region.

A conserved N-linked glycosylation site preceding the first cysteine of the V3 loop (the N-X-T sequon) was present in each mother's sequence set and absent in all of the infants' sequence sets (78). This finding has been corroborated by some investigators (125, 128) but not others (79). The absence of this site may be critical for a particular mode of transmission (transplacental transmission) but not relevant to others (direct contact at the time of delivery).

Sequence sets from additional mothers and their infants have confirmed the observation that the infant's virus sequences are less diverse than those of their mothers (79, 125, 128). The relatively narrow distribution of variants in the infant is compatible with random transmission of a limited number of virions during gestation where, because of genetic evolution, these variants may be a minor form in the mother postpartum but represent a prevalent form found during gestation (85); selection of an antigenically distinct variant in the mother that escapes a critical immune surveillance mechanism; or specific biological characteristics of the transmitted virus such as differences in cell tropism or replicative capacity (78).

Maternal HIV-specific Immune Response

HIV-specific humoral and cellular immune response, while ultimately unsuccessful, inhibits virus replication and spread after infection and may be important in determining long-term disease outcome (129). Maternal HIV-specific immune response may be involved in preventing, or possibly enhancing, vertical transmission. Several investigators have proposed the level and specificity of maternal HIV-specific antibody may be important in determining transmission.

Antibodies to the hypervariable domain of gp120, the V3 region, have HIV neutralizing activity in vitro, and a monoclonal chimeric antibody against the V3 domain was recently shown to protect chimpanzees against HIV challenge (130); mutations in this region have been associated with changes in cell tropism and neutralization escape (127). Several early studies have suggested that HIV-infected pregnant women with high antibody titer to conserved portions of the V3 hyper-variable loop and/or high avidity-high affinity antibody against the principal neutralizing domain of the V3 loop may have a lower rate of HIV transmission to their infants (117, 131–133). However, these investigators evaluated antibody to V3 peptides that encompassed different areas of the V3 loop, and more recent investigators could not replicate these associations (134–137). The linear synthetic peptides used for the antibody assays may not reflect the immunogenic epitopes that exist in vivo or the V3 sequence that predominates in the study population. Therefore it is unclear whether conflicting results are due to minor differences in technique, the use of V3 peptides derived from consensus sequences of laboratory isolates rather than from autologous viral isolates, or because important virus neutralizing activity is associated with conformational epitopes of gp120 or antibody to regions other than gp120 (138). A recent study reported antibody to gp41 peptides was lower in transmitting than nontransmitting mothers in a small cohort of mother-infant pairs (139). Additionally, other factors, such as the maternal cytotoxic immune response to HIV, may be important in protection against HIV transmission.

Maternal antibody neutralization activity may need to be evaluated in the context of autologous viral isolates. One study from Sweden evaluated the neutralizing activity of maternal sera to autologous as well as heterologous viral isolates in a small number of mother-child pairs (140). Nontransmitting mothers were found more frequently to have autologous as well as cross-neutralizing antibody. Significantly, none of the mothers who transmitted had neutralizing activity against their child's virus isolate. The emergence of neutralization-resistant or enhancement-sensitive virus variants caused by genetic mutation under selective immune pressure has been demonstrated both in vitro and in vivo (141, 142) and may be involved in mother to child transmission. In a limited study of sera from four transmitting mothers, maternal antibody could not neutralize respective infant isolates in two mother-infant pairs and was found to enhance infection in the remaining pairs (143), corroborating the Swedish study.

These data are consistent with the hypothesis that selective vertical transmission occurs with a neutralization-resistant virus variant that develops under immune pressure in the mother. Further evaluation of this hypothesis will require sequential studies of virus and immunologic parameters in the mother during pregnancy and her infant at and after birth.

The potential protective role of maternal cellular immune response to HIV has had little evaluation to date. Maternal HIV antibodies mediating antibody-dependent cellular cytotoxicity were not associated with protection from vertical transmission, although they correlated with a more favorable clinical stage in infected children (144).

Maternal and virologic data that correlate with protection from transmission suggest that therapy capable of reducing maternal virus burden may reduce incidence of maternal-fetal transmission. Additionally, enhancement of the maternal humoral and/or cellular immune response to HIV through passive or active immunization, or both, may also be involved in prevention of transmission. If protective virus epitopes that induce antibody with broad neutralizing capacity can be identified, passive immunization of the mother and/or infant with one or more monoclonal antibodies or active immunization with a subunit HIV vaccine may provide optimal preventive interventions. If, however, there is selective vertical transmission of a maternal virus neutralization-escape variant, a polyvalent hyperimmune HIV globulin preparation or vaccine will be necessary.

Placental Factors

As discussed in detail in Chapter 10A, a formidable placental barrier separates the infectious maternal circulation from the fetal circulation. Detection of HIV in the placenta has been observed in the absence of fetal infection (47), and conversely no detectable HIV has been reported in placentas from infants subsequently identified as infected (145).

Because placental morphology changes during gestation, if different placental cells have disparate susceptibilities to HIV infection, there may be changing risk of placental infection throughout gestation. Virus transmission to the fetus might also occur without actual placental infection by passage of cell-free virus through the placental barrier by active Fc receptor-mediated transport of HIV immune complexes or mixing of maternal and fetal cells from breaches in the placental barrier. Maternal coinfections associated with chorioamnionitis could perturb the integrity of the placenta. Some reports have noted an increased incidence of chorioamnionitis in placentas from HIV-infected mothers (44, 45), and a recent study from Zaire noted a significant, independent association of placental inflammation with vertical HIV transmission (146). One investigator has reported increased rates of vertical transmission during pregnancy in women with untreated syphilis (121).

If placental cell HIV infection is necessary for fetal transmission, provision of antiretroviral therapy during pregnancy could potentially prevent placental infection or restrict HIV replication within placental cells. If placental disruption is an important cofactor in transmission, measures aimed at identifying and treating known causes of placental dysfunction, such as maternal syphilis and smoking, may assist in reducing HIV transmission.

Fetal Factors

Fetal cell susceptibility to HIV infection could vary by gestational age (possibly because of developmental differences in CD4 expression), and different fetal organ systems could vary in susceptibility to infection. Immature thymic cells have been shown to be readily infected with HIV (147, 148), and neonatal and cord blood macrophages have been found to be more susceptible to infection by HIV isolates than adult macrophages (149).

If certain fetal cells or organ systems were particularly susceptible to HIV infection, virus could infect these tissues (i.e., the thymus or central nervous system), escaping detection in peripheral blood samples obtained during the neonatal period. Infection of fetal stem cells may be more immunologically devastating than infection of more mature cells because of resulting stem cell destruction or dysfunctional cellular maturation, perhaps resulting in the more rapid disease course observed in perinatal HIV infection when compared with HIV infection in adults.

The potential role of the maturing immunologic capabilities of the fetus and fetal response to HIV infection has not yet been evaluated; however, an immature immune system may be less able to restrict HIV replication. A relative deficiency of circulating HIV-1 *gag*-specific cytotoxic T lymphocytes has been described in infants with vertical HIV infection when compared with HIV-infected adults (150). It has been theorized that HIV infection of early precursor thymic cells could lead to immunologic tolerance, inhibiting the ability of the newborn immune system to mount an effective immune response owing to perception of HIV antigen as "self."

A genetic predisposition to infection was suggested by the finding that monozygotic twin sets were more likely to be concordant for HIV status (16 of 19 sets, 84%) than were dizygotic twin sets (40 of 62 sets, 62%) in the International Registry of HIV-exposed Twins (80, 81), although this finding is confounded by the presence of common vs. separate placentas in mono- or dizygotic twins, respectively. A role for genetic susceptibility or resistance to HIV infection has just begun to be explored. A study evaluating infectivity of peripheral blood lymphocytes from uninfected persons showed reproducible differences in peripheral blood lymphocyte susceptibility to infection by various HIV isolates (151). These differences were donor-specific and segregated within members of one family, suggesting that a highly polymorphic gene, such as the human lymphocyte antigen (HLA) locus, may influence susceptibility to infection. Recent reports indicate that a conserved portion of the HIV envelope glycoprotein has striking homology with major histocompatibility complex class II and/or I HLA antigens (152–154). Thus, individuals who have HLA alleles that share determinants with these virus proteins theoretically might be more susceptible to HIV infection and/or disease progression.

Several studies have addressed the role of HLA antigens in HIV disease expression. Some studies have found an association between the HLA-B8-DR3 haplotype with disease progression (155, 156). A recent study from Scotland found this haplotype to be more frequent in HIV-infected compared with HIV-uninfected infants born to HIV-infected mothers (157). Just et al. (158) evaluated susceptibility to HIV infection in 106 African-American perinatally exposed infants from New York City and San Francisco and observed an increased likelihood of infection in infants with the HLA-DQA1 allele 0102 and a lower risk of infection in infants with a critical amino acid sequence of HLA-DPB1. Differences in HLA haplotypes associated with risk of infection between studies may reflect differences in population variation in HLA antigen frequency among different ethnic groups.

Prevention and/or treatment of fetal infection may prove difficult. Indirect therapy to the fetus could be provided by transplacental passage of maternal antiretroviral therapy. However, toxicity to the developing placenta and fetus is a concern. Passive immunization of the fetus with neutralizing antibody could be accomplished through transplacental active transport of antibody exogenously administered to the mother after the second trimester of pregnancy or induced in the mother by active immunization. However, once infection of fetal cells has occurred, the ability to avert infection in the newborn may be lost.

Intrapartum and Birth Canal Factors

Langerhans cells in the skin and certain gastrointestinal cells have been shown to express CD4 and to be productively infected by HIV (159). Intensive exposure of the thin skin or mucosal surfaces of the fetus or newborn to maternal secretions during birth or through swallowing of infected amniotic fluid could provide a significant dose of virus. The importance of HIV-specific mucosal IgA or IgG in maternal genital and cervical secretions in reducing the risk of infection of the infant during birth is unknown, although one study suggests IgA levels correlate with transmission of HIV to the fetus, rather than protection (159a).

Modification of obstetrical practices could influence virus transmission occurring during the intrapartum period. If intrapartum transmission of HIV occurs primarily through direct exposure of the infant to cell-associated or free virus in genital secretions, comparable with vertical transmission of HSV, cesarean section performed before labor might be expected to reduce the risk of transmission. Additionally, virucidal cleansing of the birth canal before vaginal delivery and immediate surface decontamination of the infant by washing may provide less costly strategies to reduce transmission. However, if maternal-fetal blood exchange at the time of delivery is a significant source of virus, analogous to transmission of hepatitis B, such measures might prove less beneficial. In the absence of prospective, controlled evaluations of operative delivery, current obstetric guidelines do not recommend cesarean delivery in HIV-infected pregnant women other than for standard obstetric indications (160).

Provision of antiviral therapy to the infant before intense virus exposure during delivery could reduce risk of infection. Transplacental passage of antiviral therapy provided during late gestation or labor to the mother could provide systemic antiviral activity in the infant at the time of exposure during delivery. Maintenance of antiviral activity in the infant for a period after delivery through short-term administration of an antiretroviral agent might be desirable.

Newborn and Infant Factors

The role of the newborn immune response to HIV exposure in averting transmission is unclear. Although one report noted HIV-specific cytotoxic immune responses were reduced in HIV-infected infants (150), other researchers have noted relatively normal cell-mediated and humoral immune responses in HIV-infected infants during the first 2 years of life, with subsequent attrition (161). The presence of HIV-specific antibodies mediating cellular cytotoxicity, neutralization and syncytium inhibition has correlated with slower disease progression in infected infants in several reports but not with protection from transmission (144, 162).

The strategy of passive-active immunization has been successfully employed to prevent vertical transmission of hepatitis B. If the intrapartum period is the predominant time of HIV transmission, boosting the HIV immune response of the newborn may reduce transmission. Even if such a strategy does not prevent transmission, it may modify the manifestations of HIV disease in infected children.

Breast Milk Factors

Factors associated with infectivity and potential protective effects of breast milk have just begun to be evaluated. A dose-response effect between the amount of breast milk consumed and risk of HIV infection was not observed in one report (163), although a recent study found an association between duration of breast feeding and risk of infection (164). Transmission via breast milk may be less related to the amount of exposure and more related to specific infectivity of the milk itself, specific susceptibility in the infant, or timing of exposure.

The constitution of colostrum and early milk differs from that of mature milk, particularly in cellular content. Studies have shown that the concentration of leukocytes, primarily macrophages, is quite high in colostrum, whereas later milk is relatively acellular (165, 166). If cell-associated virus were crucial in transmission, then ingestion of colostrum and early milk may constitute a greater risk of transmission than ingestion of later milk. HIV has been demonstrated both within the cellular fraction as well as the cell-free fraction of breast milk (92, 94, 168). Recent in vitro HIV infection of human mammary epithelial cells (169) suggests that localized virus production in breast tissue could account for cell-free virus observed in breast milk.

Several investigators have demonstrated proviral DNA as well as cell-free virus are more common in colostrum samples (obtained 0–7 days after delivery) than mature milk samples (169–171). No correlation was observed between clinical stage of maternal disease and detection of HIV in breast milk, although breast milk containing proviral DNA was more common in mothers with p24 antigenemia (170, 171). In a small number of mother-infant pairs, infection rates were slightly higher (25%) in infants who breast fed from mothers with detectable HIV in their breast milk (compared with 10% if HIV was not detected) (169).

The local production and secretion of immunoglobulin could affect infectivity of breast milk; secretory IgA is the major immunoglobulin found in milk and is present in high concentration in colostrum (50 mg/ml) and somewhat lower concentrations in mature milk (1 mg/ml) (172). HIV IgG and IgA have been identified in breast milk of a significant proportion of healthy HIV-infected mothers (101, 102, 108, 173). The association between risk of HIV transmission via breast milk and the presence of HIV-specific antibody in breast milk is unknown.

In addition to organism-specific immunoglobulin, there are nonspecific components of human milk, such as leukocytes, lysozymes, lactoferrin, and macromolecules such as milk glycolipids and oligosaccharides, that could decrease risk of transmission of pathogenic agents (108, 172, 174, 175). A factor that inhibits the binding of HIV envelope glycoproteins to CD4 has been identified in breast milk from HIV-infected and uninfected women (175, 176). This inhibitory activity is confined to the macromolecular fraction of breast milk, is not found in bovine milk or human sera, and is postulated to be a sulfated protein, glycoprotein, mucin, or glycosaminoglycan.

The mechanism of HIV acquisition through breast feeding is unknown. Transmission might occur via skin or mucosal lacerations present in the infant or direct penetration of gastrointestinal mucosa. The neonatal gastrointestinal barrier is immature at birth and must undergo significant changes to adapt to an extrauterine environment. Neonates have diminished gastric acidity, a thinned gastrointestinal mucosa with an immature microvillus membrane, and a transient deficiency in IgA-producing cells in the intestinal wall mucosa (177). It is hypothesized these factors are associated with increased transport of macromolecules, including allergens and pathogens, across the neonatal intestinal epithelium, accounting for the unique susceptibility of the newborn to diseases such as necrotizing enterocolitis, toxigenic diarrhea, and intestinal allergy (174). The mature intestinal mucosa has M cells capable of transporting bacteria and viruses through the epithelium. These cells could provide yet another mechanism for HIV to gain access to lymphoid tissues. Thus the neonatal gastrointestinal tract may be particularly permeable to macromolecules, permitting HIV to come into contact with CD4-bearing monocytes, Langerhans cells, or T helper cells present in the gastric mucosa.

Although the immature gastrointestinal barrier of the neonate may facilitate transmission of HIV via breast feeding, it is not required for transmission. Breast milk HIV transmission has been reported in a child 2 years old at the time of initiation of breast feeding (177). Maternal HIV infection was secondary to transfusion after delivery of a younger sibling; the 2-year child was breast fed by the mother for several months after delivery of the sibling.

If breast feeding poses a significant risk of HIV transmission to the infant, alternative methods of feeding would be recommended. Recommendations about infant feeding must consider the setting in which the mother and infant reside. In areas in which safe and effective alternatives are unavailable, the benefits of breast feeding may outweigh the risk of HIV transmission.

POTENTIAL INTERVENTIONS TO PREVENT VERTICAL HIV TRANSMISSION

As has been indicated, knowledge remains limited regarding relative importance of the multiple factors involved in vertical transmission. It will be years before the intricacies of transmission are unraveled, but the urgency of the problem is so great that development of interventions cannot be postponed. Specific clinical trials are being developed, and some are underway.

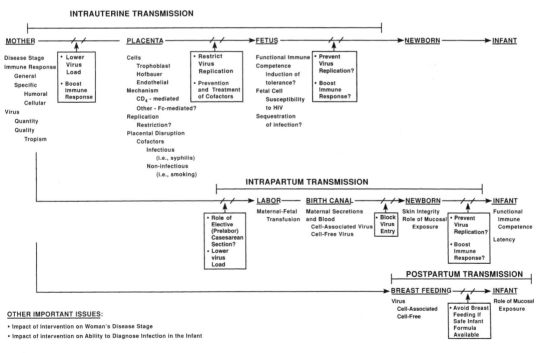

Figure 10C.1. Mediating factors and potential strategies for prevention of vertical transmission of HIV. From Mofenson LM. Preventing mother to infant transmission: What we know so far. AIDS Reader 1992;Mar/Apr: 42–51.

Figure 10C.1 portrays potential points of intervention in the process of vertical transmission. Present clinical trials are targeted to several intervention points to maximize their success. Current and planned strategies to interrupt vertical transmission will be addressed in detail in Chapters 35, 45, and 47.

References

1. Chin J. Current and future dimensions of the HIV/AIDS pandemic in women and children. Lancet 1990;336:221–224.
2. Gwinn M, Pappaioanou M, George JR, et al. Prevalence of HIV infection in childbearing women in the United States. JAMA 1991;265:1704–1708.
3. Peckham CS, Tedder RS, Briggs M, et al. Prevalence of maternal HIV infection based on unlinked anonymous testing of newborn babies. Lancet 1990;335:516–519.
4. Novick LF, Berns D, Stricof R, Stevens R, Pass K, Wethers J. HIV seroprevalence in newborns in New York State. JAMA 1989;261:1745–1750.
5. Oxtoby M. Perinatally acquired human immunodeficiency virus infection. Pediatr Infect Dis J 1990;9:609–619.
6. Mofenson LM. Preventing mother to infant HIV transmission: What we know so far. AIDS Reader 1992;Mar/Apr:42–51.
7. Centers for Disease Control. HIV/AIDS Surveillance. Department of Health and Human Services, Atlanta, Jul 1992.
8. Auger L, Thomas P, DeGruttola V, et al. Incubation periods for pediatric AIDS patients. Nature 1988;336:575–577.
9. Blanche S, Rouzioux C, Moscato MG, et al. A prospective study of infants born to women seropositive for HIV type 1. N Engl J Med 1989;320:1643–1648.
10. European Collaborative Study. Children born to women with HIV infection: Natural history and risk of transmission. Lancet 1991;337:253–260.
11. Tovo PA, de Martino M, Gabiano C, et al. Prognostic factors and survival in children with perinatal HIV infection. Lancet 1992;339:1249–1253.
12. Vermund SH, Sheon AR. The worldwide impact of HIV/AIDS on child survival: A review of the model of Bennett and Rogers. Pediatr AIDS HIV Infect Fetus Adolesc 1992;3:49–52.
13. Alford CA, Neva FA, Weller TH. Virologic and serologic studies on human products of conceptions after maternal rubella. N Engl J Med 1964;272:1275–1281.
14. Assaad F, Ljungars-Esteves K. Rubella—world impact. Rev Infect Dis 1985;7(suppl 1):S29–S36.
15. Stagno S, Whitley RJ. Herpesvirus infection in the neonate and children. In: Homes KK, Mardh PA, Sparling PF, Wiesner PJ, eds. Sexually transmitted diseases. 2nd ed. New York: McGraw-Hill, 1990:863–887.
16. Mofenson LM, Blattner WA. Human retroviruses. In: Feigin RD, Cherry JD, eds. Textbook of pediatric infectious diseases. 3rd ed. Philadelphia: WB Saunders, 1992:1757–1788.
17. Tsuji Y, Doi H, Yamabe T, Ishimaru T, Miyamoto T, Hino S. Prevention of mother-to-child transmission of human T-lymphotropic virus type I. Pediatrics 1990;86:11–17.
18. Sawada T, Iwahara Y, Ishii K, Taguchi H, Hoshino H, Miyoshi I. Immunoglobulin prophylaxis against milkborne transmission of human T cell leukemia virus type I in rabbits. J Infect Dis 1991;164:1193–1196.
19. Narita M, Shibata M, Togashi T, Koga Y. Vertical transmission of human T cell leukemia virus type I [Letter]. J Infect Dis 1991;163:204.
20. Grose C, Meehan T, Weiner CP. Prenatal diagnosis of congenital cytomegalovirus infection by virus isolation after amniocentesis. Pediatr Infect Dis J 1992;11:605–607.
21. Alford C. Breast milk transmission of cytomegalovirus infection. In: Mestecky J, et al. eds. Immunology of milk and the neonate. New York: Plenum, 1991:293–299.
22. Dworsky M, Yow M, Stagno S, Pass RF, Alford C. Cytomegalovirus infection of breast milk and transmission in infancy. Pediatrics 1983;72:295–299.
23. Hayes K, Gibas H. Placental cytomegalovirus infection without fetal involvement following primary infection in pregnancy. J Pediatr 1971;79:401–405.
24. Shikata T, Karasawa T, Abe K, et al. Hepatitis B e antigens and infectivity of hepatitis B virus [Letter]. J Infect Dis 1977;136:571.
25. Hindman SH, Gravelle CR, Murphy BL, et al. "e" Antigen, Dane particles, and serum DNA polymerase activity in HBsAG carriers. Ann Intern Med 1976;85:458–460.
26. Whitley RJ, Nahmias AJ, Visintine AM, Fleming CI, Alford DA. The natural history of herpes simplex virus infection of mother and newborn. Pediatrics 1980;66:489–494.
27. Nahmias AJ, Josey WE, Naib ZM, et al. Perinatal risk associated with maternal genital herpes simplex virus infection. Am J Obstet Gynecol 1971;110:825–836.
28. Brown AZ, Vontver LA, Benedetti J, et al. Effects on infants of first episode of genital herpes during pregnancy. N Engl J Med 1987;317:1246–1251.
29. Demmler GJ. Summary of a workshop on surveillance for congenital cytomegalovirus disease. Rev Infect Dis 1991;13:315–329.
30. Fowler KB, Stagno S, Pass RF, Britt WJ, Boll TJ, Alford DA. The outcome of congenital cytomegalovirus infection in relation to maternal antibody status. N Engl J Med 1992;326:663–666.
31. Stagno S, Pass RF, Dworsky ME, et al. Congenital cytomegalovirus infection: The relative importance of primary and recurrent maternal infection. N Engl J Med 1982;306:945–949.
32. Cooper LZ. The history and medical consequences of rubella. Rev Infect Dis 1985;7(suppl 1):S2–S10.
33. Lee SH, Ewert DP, Frederick PD, Mascola L. Resurgence of congenital rubella syndrome in the 1990's: Report on missed opportunities and failed prevention policies among women of childbearing age. JAMA 1992;267:1616–1620.

34. Centers for Disease Control. Hepatitis b virus: A comprehensive strategy for eliminating transmission in the United States through universal childhood vaccination. MMWR 1991;40(suppl RR-13):1–25.

35. Yow MD, Demmler GJ. Congenital cytomegalovirus disease—20 years is long enough. N Engl J Med 1992;326:702–703.

36. Jovaisas E, Koch MA, Schafer A, Stauber M, Lowenthal D. LAV/HTLV-III in a 20-week fetus [Letter]. Lancet 1985;2:1129.

37. Sprecher S, Soumenkoff G, Puissant F, Degueldre M. Vertical transmission of HIV in a 15-week fetus. Lancet 1986;2:288–289.

38. Peutherer JF, Rebus S, Smith I, et al. Detection of HIV in the fetus: A study of six cases [Abstract 7235]. Fourth International Conference on AIDS, Stockholm, Jun 1988.

39. Courgnaud V, Laure F, Brossard A, et al. Frequent and early *in utero* HIV-1 infection. AIDS Res Hum Retroviruses 1991;7:337–341.

40. Soiero R, Rubenstein A, Rasbaum WK, Lyman WD. Maternal-fetal transmission of AIDS: Frequency of human immunodeficiency virus type 1 nucleic acid sequences in human fetal DNA. J Infect Dis 1992;166:699–703.

41. Mano H, Cherman JC. Fetal human immunodeficiency virus type 1 infection in different organs in the second trimester. AIDS Res Hum Retroviruses 1991;7:83–88.

42. Papiernik M, Brossard Y, Mulliez N, et al. Thymic abnormalities in fetuses aborted from human immunodeficiency virus type 1 seropositive women. Pediatrics 1992;89:297–301.

43. Hill WC, Botlon V, Carlson JR. Isolation of acquired immunodeficiency syndrome virus from the placenta. Am J Obstet Gynecol 1987;157:10–11.

44. Jauniaux E, Nessmann C, Imbert C, et al. Morphological aspects of the placenta in HIV pregnancies. Placenta 1988;9:633–642.

45. Lewis SH, Reynolds-Kohler C, Fox HE, et al. HIV-1 in trophoblastic and villous Hofbauer cells and haematological precursors in eight-week fetuses. Lancet 1990;335:565–568.

46. Chandwani S, Greco MA, Mittal K, et al. Pathology and human immunodeficiency virus expression in placentas of seropositive women. J Infect Dis 1991;163:1134–1138.

47. Mattern CFT, Murray K, Jensen A, Farzadegan H, Pang J, Modlin JF. Localization of human immunodeficiency virus core antigen in term human placentas. Pediatrics 1992;89:207–209.

48. Maury W, Potts BJ, Rabson AB. HIV-1 infection of first-trimester and term human placental tissue: A possible mode of maternal-fetal transmission. J Infect Dis 1989;160:583–588.

49. Zachar V, Spire B, Norskov-Lauritsen N, et al. Cultured trophoblastic choriocarcinoma cells differentially express HIV-1 and cloned provirus. AIDS 1991;5:457–458.

50. David FJ, Tran HC, Autran B, et al. Maternal-fetal HIV transmission: Placental cells CD4 expression and permissivity to infection with HIV [Abstract MA 79]. Seventh International Conference on AIDS, Florence, Jun 1991.

51. Douglas GC, Fry GN, Thirkill T, et al. Cell-mediated infection of human placental trophoblast with HIV *in vitro*. AIDS Res Hum Retroviruses 1991;7:735–740.

52. Mano H, Cherman JC. Replication of human immunodeficiency virus type 1 in primary cultured placental cells. Res Virol 1991;142:95–104.

53. Marion RW, Wiznia AA, Hutcheon G, et al. Human T-cell lymphotrophic virus type III embryopathy: A new dysmorphic syndrome associated with intrauterine HTLV-III infection. Am J Dis Child 1988;140:638–640.

54. Iosub S, Banjii M, Stone RK, Gromisch DS, Wasserman E. More on human immunodeficiency virus embryopathy. Pediatrics 1987;80:512–516.

55. Perro M: Dysmorphism leading to a diagnosis of acquired immunodeficiency syndrome [Letter]. Am J Dis Child 1987;141:474.

56. Embree JE, Braddich M, Datta P, et al. Lack of correlation of maternal human immunodeficiency virus infection with neonatal malformations. Pediatr Infect Dis J 1989;8:700–704.

57. Qazi QH, Sheikh TM, Fikrig S, et al. Lack of evidence for craniofacial dysmorphism in perinatal human immunodeficiency virus infection. J Pediatr 1988;112:7–11.

58. Lingren S, Anzen B, Bohlin AB, Lidman K. HIV and child-bearing: Clinical outcome and aspects of mother-to-infant transmission. AIDS 1991;5:1111–1116.

59. Temmerman M, Plummer FA, Mirza NB, et al. Infection with HIV as a risk factor for adverse obstetrical outcome. AIDS 1990;4:1087–1093.

60. Braddick MR, Kreiss JK, Ebree JE, et al. Impact of maternal HIV infection on obstetrical and early neonatal outcome. AIDS 1990;4:1001–1005.

61. Miotti PG, Dallabetta G, Ndovi E, Liomba G, Saah AJ, Chiphangwi J. HIV-1 and pregnant women: Associated factors, prevalence, and estimate of incidence and role in fetal wastage in central Africa. AIDS 1990;4:733–736.

62. Lyman WD, Kress Y, Kure K, Rashbaum WK, Rubinstein A, Soeiro R: Detection of HIV in fetal central nervous system tissue. AIDS 1990;4:917–920.

63. Ehrnst A, Lindgren S, Dictor M, et al. HIV in pregnant women and their offspring: Evidence for late transmission. Lancet 1991;338:203–207.

64. Viscarello RR, Cullen MT, DeGennaro NJ, Hobbins JC. Fetal blood sampling in HIV-seropositive pregnancies before elective midtrimester termination of pregnancy. Am J Obstet Gynecol 1992;167:1075–1079.

65. Mundy DC, Schinazi RF, Gerver AR, et al. Human immunodeficiency virus isolated from amniotic fluid. Lancet 1987;2:459–460.

66. Rogers MF, Ou CY, Kilbourne B, Schochetman G. Advances and problems in the diagnosis of human immunodeficiency virus infection in infants. Pediatr Infect Dis J 1991;10:523–531.

67. Shaffer N, Ou CY, Abrams E, et al. PCR and HIV IgA for early infant diagnosis of perinatal HIV infection [Abstract ThC 1580]. Eighth International Conference on AIDS, Amsterdam, Jul 1992.

68. Rogers MF, Ou CY, Rayfield M, et al. Use of the polymerase chain reaction for early detection of

the postviral sequences of human immunodeficiency virus in infants born to seropositive mothers. N Engl J Med 1989;320:1649–1654.

69. Burgard M, Mayaux MJ, Blanche S, et al. The use of viral culture and p24 antigen testing to diagnose human immunodeficiency virus infection in neonates. N Engl J Med 1992;327:1192–1197.

70. De Rossi A, Ometto L, Mammano F, Zanotto C, Giaquinto C, Chieco-Bianchi L: Vertical transmission of HIV-1: Lack of detectable virus in peripheral blood cells of infected children at birth. AIDS 1992;6:1117–1120.

71. Borkowsky W, Krasinski K, Pollack H, Hoover W, Kaul A, Ilmet-Moore T. Early diagnosis of human immunodeficiency virus in children <6 months of age: Comparison of polymerase chain reaction, culture, and plasma antigen capture techniques. J Infect Dis 1992;166:616–619.

72. Bryson Y, Chen I, Miles S, et al. A prospective evaluation of HIV coculture for early diagnosis of perinatal HIV infection [Abstract WB 2014]. Seventh International Conference on AIDS, Florence, Jun 1991.

73. Quinn TC, Kline R, Moss M, Livingston RA, Hutton N. Acid dissociation of immune complexes improves the diagnostic utility of p24 antigen detection in perinatally acquired HIV-1 infection [Abstract ThC 1579]. Eighth International Conference on AIDS, Amsterdam, Jul 1992.

74. Miles SA, Baldwin E, Magpantay L, et al. Early detection of HIV-1 infection in infants of seropositive mothers by acid dissociated HIV p24 antigen [Abstract TuB 0512]. Eighth International Conference on AIDS, Amsterdam, Jul 1992.

75. Lee F, Nesheim S, Sawyer M, Slade B, Nahmias A. Early diagnosis of HIV infection in infants by detection of p24 antigen in plasma specimens after acid hydrolysis to dissociate immune complexes [Abstract PoB 3702]. Eighth International Conference on AIDS, Amsterdam, Jul 1992.

76. Burchett SK, Henrard D, Watts DH, et al. Early diagnosis of HIV in infants born to seropositive women [Abstract PoB 3630]. Eighth International Conference on AIDS, Amsterdam, Jul 1992.

77. Krivine A, Firtion G, Cao L, Francoual C, Henrion R, Lebon P. HIV infection in newborns: Evidence for viral replication within the first weeks of life [Abstract ThC 1581]. Eighth International Conference on AIDS, Amsterdam, Jul 1992.

78. Wolinsky SM, Wike CM, Korber BT, et al. Selective transmission of human immunodeficiency virus type-1 variants from mothers to infants. Science 1992;255;1134–1136.

79. Kampinga GA, Boer K, Scherpbier HJ, et al. Homogeneous V3 sequences in newborn closely relates to V3 sequences in mother in first trimester of pregnancy, but less at delivery [Abstract PoA 2083]. Eighth International Conference on AIDS, Amsterdam, Jul 1992.

80. Goedert JJ, Duliege AM, Amos CI, et al. High risk of HIV-1 infection for first-born twins. Lancet 1991;338:1471–1475.

81. Duliege AM, Felton S, Goedert JJ, et al. High risk of HIV-1 infection for the first-born twin: The role of intrapartum transmission [Abstract WeC 1062]. Eighth International Conference on AIDS, Amsterdam, Jul 1992.

82. Hutto C, Parks WP, Lai S, et al. A hospital-based prospective study of perinatal infection with human immunodeficiency virus type 1. J Pediatr 1991;118:347–353.

83. European Collaborative Study. Risk factors for mother-to-child transmission of HIV-1. Lancet 1992;339:1007–1012.

84. Italian Multicentre Study. Epidemiology, clinical features, and prognostic factors of pediatric HIV infection. Lancet 1987;2:1043–1046.

85. Weiser B, Nachman S, Burger H, Hsu YJ, Gibbs R. Serial HIV sequences from a pregnant woman and her vertically infected twins suggest one twin was infected in utero and one at birth. 5th Annual Meeting of the National Cooperative Vaccine Development Groups for AIDS, Chantilly, VA, Aug 30–Sep 3, 1992.

86. Zhanq LQ, Leigh-Brown AJ, Holmes EC, Cleland A, Simmonds P: Selection for specific V3 sequences on transmission of HIV [Abstract PoA 2105]. Eighth International Conference on AIDS, Amsterdam, Jul 1992.

87. Byson YJ, Luzuriaga K, Sullivan JL, Wara DW. Proposed definition for in utero versus intrapartum transmission of HIV-1 [Letter]. N Engl J Med 1992;327:1246–1247.

88. Krivine A, Firtion G, Cao L, et al. HIV replication during the first weeks of life. Lancet 1992;339: 1187–1189.

89. Alimenti A, Luzuriaga K, Stechenberg B, et al. Quantitation of HIV-1 in vertically-infected infants and children. J Pediatr 1991;119:225–229.

90. Blanche S, Tardieu M, Duliege AM, et al. Longitudinal study of 94 symptomatic infants with perinatally acquired human immunodeficiency virus infection: Evidence for a bimodal expression of clinical and biological symptoms. Am J Dis Child 1990;144:1210–1215.

91. Van de Perre P, Lepage P, Homsy J, Dabis F. Mother-to-infant transmission of human immunodeficiency virus by breast milk: Presumed innocent or presumed guilty? Clin Infect Dis 1992; 15:502–507.

92. Thiry L, Sprecher-Goldberger S, Jonckheer T, et al. Isolation of AIDS virus from cell-free breast milk of three healthy carriers. Lancet 1985;2: 891–897.

93. Zeigler JV, Cooper DA, Johnson RO, et al. Postnatal transmission of AIDS-associated retrovirus from mother to infant. Lancet 1985;1: 896–897.

94. Bucens M, Armstrong J, Stuckey M. Virological and electron microscopic evidence for postnatal HIV transmission via breast milk [Abstract 5099]. Fourth International Conference on AIDS, Stockholm, Jun 1988.

95. Van de Perre P, Simonon A, Msellati P, et al. Postnatal transmission of human immunodeficiency virus type 1 from mother to infant: A prospective cohort study in Kigali, Rwanda. N Engl J Med 1991;325:593–598.

96. Colebunders R, Kapita B, Nekwei W, et al. Breastfeeding and transmission of HIV [Letter]. Lancet 1988;1:1487.

97. Weinbreck P, Loustaud V, Denis F, Vidal B, Mounier M, de Lumley L. Postnatal transmission of HIV infection [Letter]. Lancet 1988;1:482.

98. Hira SK, Mangrola UG, Mwale C, et al. Apparent vertical transmission of human immunodeficiency virus type 1 by breast-feeding in Zambia. J Pediatr 1990;117:421–424.

99. Stiehm ER, Vink P. Transmission of human immunodeficiency virus infection by breast feeding. J Pediatr 1991;118:410–412.

100. Ryder RW, Nsa W, Hassig SE, et al. Perinatal transmission of the human immunodeficiency virus type 1 to infants of seropositive women in Zaire. N Engl J Med 1989;320:1637–1642.

101. Belec L, Bouquety JC, Georges AJ, et al. Antibodies to human immunodeficiency virus in the breast milk of healthy, seropositive women. Pediatrics 1990;85:1022–1026.

102. Davis MK. Human milk and HIV infection: Epidemiologic and laboratory data. In: Mestecky J, Blair C, Ogra PL, eds. Immunology of milk and the neonate. New York: Plenum, 1991:271–280.

103. Halsey N, Boulos R, Holt E, et al. Transmission of HIV-1 infections from mothers to infants in Haiti. JAMA 1990;264:2088–2092.

104. Newell ML, European Collaborative Study. Risk factors for vertical transmission of HIV-1 infection [Abstract ThC 1520]. Eighth International Conference on AIDS, Amsterdam, Jul 1992.

105. Bennett JV, Rogers MF. Child survival and perinatal infections with human immunodeficiency virus. Am J Dis Child 1991;145:1242–1247.

106. Heymann SJ. Modeling the impact of breast-feeding by HIV-infected women on child survival. Am J Public Health 1990;80:1305–1309.

107. Lederman SA. Estimating infant mortality from human immunodeficiency virus and other causes in breast-feeding and bottle-feeding populations. Pediatrics 1992;89:290–296.

108. Ruff AJ, Halsey NA, Coberly J, Boulos R. Breast-feeding and maternal-infant transmission of human immunodeficiency virus type 1. J Pediatr 1992;121:325–329.

109. World Health Organization. Consensus statement from the WHO/UNICEF consultation on HIV transmission and breastfeeding, Geneva, Apr 30–May 1, 1992.

110. d'Arminio MA, Ravizza M, Muggiasca ML, et al. HIV-infected pregnant women: Possible predictors of vertical transmission [Abstract WC 49]. Seventh International Conference on AIDS, Florence, Jun 1991.

111. Hague RA, Mok JYQ, MacCallum L et al. Do maternal factors influence the risk of HIV? [Abstract WC 3237]. Seventh International Conference on AIDS, Florence, Jun 1991.

112. Lallemant M, Lallemant LCS, Samba L, et al. Assessing the risk for mother-infant HIV-1 transmission: A challenge in developing countries [Abstract MC 3078]. Seventh International Conference on AIDS, Florence, Jun 1991.

113. Hira SK, Kamanga J, Bhat GJ, et al. Perinatal transmission of HIV-1 in Zambia. Br Med J 1898; 299:1250–1252.

114. Thomas P, Weedon J, New York City Perinatal HIV Transmission Collaborative Study Group.

115. Maternal predictors of perinatal HIV transmission [Abstract WeC 1059]. Eighth International Conference on AIDS, Amsterdam, Jul 1992.

115. St. Louis ME, Kabagabo U, Brown C, et al. Maternal factors associated with perinatal HIV transmission [Abstract MC 3027]. Seventh International Conference on AIDS, Florence, Jun 1991.

116. Burns D, Muenz L, Walsh J, et al. Correlation of perinatal transmission of HIV-1 with mother's lowest prepartum CD4 level [Abstract 463]. 31st Interscience Conference on Antimicrobial Agents and Chemotherapy, Chicago, Oct 1991.

117. Goedert JJ, Mendez H, Drummond JE, et al. Mother-to-infant transmission of human immunodeficiency virus type 1: Association with prematurity or low anti-gp120. Lancet 1989;2:1351–1354.

118. Tibaldi C, Palomba E, Ziarati N, et al. Maternal factors influencing vertical HIV transmission [Abstract WC 3277]. Seventh International Conference on AIDS, Florence, Jun 1991.

119. Gratias HD, Lepage P, Van de Perre P, et al. Perinatal study of HIV-1 in Kigali, Rwanda: Estimation of the mother-to-child transmission rate and analysis of its determinants [Abstract PoC 4226]. Eighth International Conference on AIDS, Amsterdam, Jul 1992.

120. Boue F, Pons JC, Keros L, et al. Risk for HIV-1 perinatal transmission vary with the mother's stage of HIV infection [Abstract ThC 44]. Sixth International Conference on AIDS, Montreal, Jun 1990.

121. Borkowsky W, Krasinski K. Perinatal human immunodeficiency virus infection: Ruminations on mechanisms of transmission and methods of intervention. Pediatrics 1992;90:133–136.

122. Scarlatti G, Lombardi V, Plebani A, et al. Polymerase chain reaction, virus isolation and antigen assay in HIV-1 antibody positive mothers and children. AIDS 1991;5:1173–1178.

123. Kreiss J, Datta P, Willerford D, et al. Vertical transmission of HIV in Nairobi: Correlation with maternal viral burden [Abstract MC 3062]. Seventh International Conference on AIDS, Florence, Jun 1991.

124. Krasinski K, Cao Y, Borkowsky W, Ho D. Maternal viral load as a risk factor for perinatal HIV-1 infection [Abstract WD109]. Critical Research Directions in Pediatric HIV Infection, Keystone, CO, Mar 1992.

125. Rossi P, Siena, Consensus Workshop. Maternal factors involved in mother-to-child transmission of HIV-1. J Acquir Immune Defic Syndr 1992; 5:1019–1029.

126. M-Fontelos P, Mellado MJ, Villota J, et al. Evolution of a series of pediatric AIDS related to different strains of HIV [Abstract WB 2030]. Seventh International Conference on AIDS, Florence, Jun 1991.

127. Johnson MA, Cann AJ. Molecular determination of cell tropism of human immunodeficiency virus. Clin Infect Dis 1992;14:747–755.

128. Wade NA, Rathbun D, Flaherty L. Sequence comparison of the human immunodeficiency virus en-

velope V3 loop and CD4-binding region in infected mother/infant pairs [Abstract WD 124]. Proceedings of Critical Research Directions in Pediatric HIV Infection, Keystone, CO, Mar 1992.

129. Yarchoan R, Mitsuya H, Broder S. The immunology of HIV infection: Implications for therapy. AIDS Res Hum Retroviruses 1992;8:1023–1031.

130. Emini EA, Schleif WA, Nunberg JH, et al. Prevention of HIV-1 infection in chimpanzees by gp120 V3 domain-specific monoclonal antibodies. Nature 1992;355:728–730.

131. Rossi P, Moschese V, Broliden PA, et al. Presence of maternal antibodies to human immunodeficiency virus 1 envelope glycoprotein gp120 epitopes correlates with the noninfective status of children born to seropositive mothers. Proc Natl Acad Sci USA 1989;86:8055–8058.

132. Broliden PA, Moschese V, Ljungren K, et al. Diagnostic implications of specific immunoglobulin G patterns born to HIV infected women. AIDS 1989;3:577–582.

133. Devash Y, Calvelli T, Wood DG, et al. Vertical transmission of HIV is correlated with absence of high affinity/avidity maternal antibodies to the gp120 principal neutralizing domain. Proc Natl Acad Sci USA 1990;87:3445–3449.

134. Parekh BS, Shaffer N, Pau CP, et al. Lack of correlation between maternal antibodies to V3 loop peptides of gp120 and perinatal HIV-1 transmission. AIDS 1991;5:1179–1184.

135. Allain JP, Matthew T, Coombs R, et al. Antibody to V3 loop does not predict vertical transmission of HIV [Abstract WC 2263]. Seventh International Conference on AIDS, Florence, Jun 1991.

136. Halsey N, Markham R, Rossi P, et al. V3 loop peptide antibodies in Haitian women and infant HIV-1 infection [Abstract WA 1311]. Seventh International Conference on AIDS, Florence, Jun 1991.

137. Robertson CA, Mok JYQ, Froebel KS, et al. Maternal antibodies to gp120 V3 sequence do not correlate with protection against vertical transmission of human immunodeficiency virus. J Infect Dis 1992;166:704–709.

138. Mofenson LM, Burns DN. Passive immunization to prevent mother-infant transmission of human immunodeficiency virus: Current issues and future directions. Pediatr Infect Dis J 1991;10:456–462.

139. Ugen KE, Goedert JJ, Boyer J, et al. Vertical transmission of human immunodeficiency virus infection: Reactivity of maternal sera with glycoprotein 120 and 41 peptides from HIV type 1. J Clin Invest 1992;89:1923–1930.

140. Scarlatti G, Albert J, Rossi P, et al. Homologous and heterologous neutralization activity in sera of HIV-1 infected mothers: Correlation to transmission [Abstract WeC 1061]. Eighth International AIDS Conference, Amsterdam, Jul 1992.

141. Tremblay M, Weinberg MA. Neutralization of multiple HIV-1 isolates from a single subject by autologous sequential sera. J Infect Dis 1990;162:735–737.

142. Reitz MS, Wilson C, Naugle C, Gallo RC, Robert-Guroff M. Generation of a neutralization-resistant variant of HIV-1 is due to selection for a point mutation in the envelope gene. Cell 1988;54:57–63.

143. Kliks SC, Fadem MB, Wara DW, Levy JA. Evidence for the maternal transfer of neutralization-escape or enhancement variants into newborn infants [Abstract PoA 2463]. Eighth International Conference on AIDS, Amsterdam, Jul 1992.

144. Ljunggren K, Moschese V, Broliden PA, et al. Antibodies mediating cellular cytotoxicity and neutralization correlate with a better clinical stage in children born to human immunodeficiency virus-infected mothers. J Infect Dis 1990;161:198–202.

145. Peuchmaur M, Delfraissy JF, Pons JC, et al. HIV proteins absent from placentas of 75 HIV-1 positive women studied by immunochemistry. AIDS 1991;5:741–745.

146. St Louis M, Nelson A, Kamenga, et al. Placental inflammation as a risk factor for perinatal HIV-1 transmission independent of maternal immune status [Abstract 601]. Proceedings of 32nd Interscience Conference on Antimicrobial Agents and Chemotherapy, Anaheim, Oct 1992.

147. Schnittman SM, Donnury SM, Greenhouse JJ, et al. Evidence of susceptibility of intrathymic T cell precursors and their progeny carrying T-cell receptor phenotypes TCR alpha/beta+ and TCR gamma/delta+ to human immunodeficiency virus infection: A mechanism for CD4+ (T4) lymphocyte depletion. Proc Natl Acac Sci USA 1990;87:7727–7731.

148. Daye N, Johnson DK, Walker CW, et al. In vitro HIV infection of midgestation human thymocytes [Abstract MC 3026]. Seventh International Conference on AIDS, Florence, Jun 1991.

149. Sperduto AR, Bryson YJ, Chen ISY. Effect of HIV-1 infection of neonatal lymphocytes [Abstract 641]. Proceedings of 31st Interscience Conference on Antimicrobial Agents and Chemotherapy, Chicago, Oct 1991.

150. Luzuriaga K, Koup RA, Pikora CA, et al. Deficient human immunodeficiency virus type 1-specific cytotoxic T cell responses in vertically infected children. J Pediatr 1991;119:230–236.

151. Williams LM, Cloyd MW. Polymorphic human gene(s) determines differential susceptibility of CD4 lymphocytes to infection by certain HIV-1 isolates. Virology 1991;184:723–728.

152. Dalgleish AG, Wilson S, Gompels M, et al. T-cell receptor variable gene products and early HIV-1 infection. Lancet 1992;339:824–828.

153. Editorial. AIDS: How can a pussycat kill? Lancet 1992;339:839–840.

154. Imberti L, Sottini A, Bettinardi A, Puoti M, Primi D. Selective depletion in HIV infection of T cells that bear specific T cell receptor V-beta sequences. Science 1991;254:860–862.

155. Kaslow RA, Duquesnoy R, Van Raden M, et al. Ai, Cw7, B8 HLA antigen combination associated with rapid decline of T-helper lymphocytes in HIV-1 infection. Lancet 1990;335:927–930.

156. Steel CM, Ludlam CA, Beatson D, et al. HLA haplotype A1 B8 DR3 as a risk factor for HIV-related disease. Lancet 1988;1:1185–1188.

157. Kilpatrick DC, Haguera RA, Yap PL, et al. HLA antigen frequencies in children born to HIV-infected mothers. Dis Markers 1991;9:21–26.

158. Just J, Louie L, Abrams E, et al. Genetic risk factors for perinatally acquired HIV-1 infection. Pediatr Perinatal Epidemiol 1991;6:215–224.
159. Moyer M, Huot R, Ramirez A, Joe S, Meltzer M, Gendelman H. Infection of human gastrointestinal cells by HIV-1. AIDS Res Hum Retroviruses 1990;6:1409–1415.
159a. Yolken R, Miott P, Dallabetta G, Chiphangwi J, Clayman B, Viscidi R. Secretory immune response to HIV and perinatal transmission [Abstract 1114]. Pediatr Res 1993;33:189A.
160. Minkoff HL, Feinkind K. Management of pregnancies of HIV-infected women. Clin Obstet Gynecol 1989;32:467–476.
161. Borkowsky W, Rigaud M, Krasinski K, Moore T, Lawrence R, Pollack H. Cell mediated and humoral immune responses in children infected with human immunodeficiency virus during the first four years of life. J Pediatr 1992;120:371–375.
162. Brenner TJ, Dahl KE, Olson B, et al. Relation between HIV-1 syncytium inhibition antibodies and clinical outcome in children. Lancet 1991;337:1001–1005.
163. Ryder RW, Manzila T, Baende E, et al. Evidence from Zaire that breastfeeding by HIV-1 seropositive mothers is not a major route for perinatal HIV-1 transmission but does increase mortality. AIDS 1991;5:709–714.
164. de Martino M, Tovo PA, Tozzi AE, et al. HIV-1 transmission through breast-milk: Appraisal of risk according to duration of feeding. AIDS 1992;6:991–997.
165. Lawton JWM, Shortridge KF. Protective factors in human breast milk and colostrum [Letter]. Lancet 1977;1:253.
166. Goldman AS, Garza C, Nichols BL, Goldblum RM. Immunologic factors in human milk during the first year of lactation. J Pediatr 1982;100:563–567.
167. Vogt MW, Witt DJ, Craven DE, et al. Isolation patterns of human immunodeficiency virus from cervical secretions during the menstrual cycle of women at risk for the acquired immunodeficiency syndrome. Ann Intern Med 1987;106:380–382.
168. Toniolo A, Conaldi PG, Serra C, Dolei A, Basolo F. Susceptibility of human mammary epithelial cells to HIV-1 infection [Abstract PoA 2028]. Eighth International Conference on AIDS, Amsterdam, Jul 1992.
169. Ruff A, Coberly J, Burnley A, et al. Prevalence of HIV in breast milk and correlation with maternal-infant transmission [Abstract ThC 1523]. Eighth International Conference on AIDS, Amsterdam, Jul 1992.
170. Bulterys M, Chao A, Farzadegan H, et al. Detection of HIV-1 in breast milk, multiple sexual partners and mother to child transmission of HIV-1: A cohort study [Abstract ThC 1524]. Eighth International Conference on AIDS, Amsterdam, Jul 1992.
171. Van de Perre P, Simonson A, Hitimana DG, et al. Milk HIV-1 IgG, SIgA, and IgM in a cohort of HIV-1 infected mothers, Kigali, Rwanda (1988–1990) [Abstract ThC 1521]. Eighth International Conference on AIDS, Amsterdam, Jul 1992.
172. Welsh JK, May JT. Anti-infective properties of breast milk. J Pediatr 1979;94:1–9.
173. Van de Perre P, Hitimana DG, Lepage P. Human immunodeficiency virus antibodies of IgG, IgA, and IgM subclasses in milk of seropositive mothers. J Pediatr 1988;113:1039–1041.
174. Bines JE, Walker WA. Growth factors and the development of neonatal host defense. In: Mestecky J, Blair C, Ogra PL, eds. Immunology of milk and the neonate. New York: Plenum, 1991:31–37.
175. Newburg DS, Yolken RH. Characterization of a human milk factor that inhibits binding of HIV gp120 to its CD4 receptor. In: Mestecky J, et al., eds. Immunology of milk and the neonate. New York: Plenum, 1991:281–291.
176. Newburg DS, Viscidi RP, Ruff A, Yolken RH. A human milk factor inhibits binding of human immunodeficiency virus to the CD4 receptor. Pediatr Res 1991;31:22–28.
177. Rubini NPM, Passman LJ. Transmission of human immunodeficiency virus infection from a newly infected mother to her two-year old child by breast feeding. Pediatr Infect Dis J 1992;11:682–683.

SECTION III

Diagnostic Challenges in Fetus and Infant

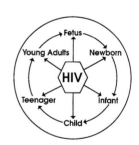

11
Advances in Prenatal Diagnosis of HIV-1 Infection

Richard R. Viscarello and Daniel V. Landers

The prenatal diagnosis of genetic disorders has become routine in many parts of the world. The commonly employed techniques, such as amniocentesis, chorionic villus sampling (CVS), and cordocentesis, are being applied to the prenatal diagnosis of myriad other disorders, in particular congenital infectious diseases. Varying degrees of success in prenatal diagnosis of fetal infection has been achieved for many congenital infections, including toxoplasmosis (1, 2), rubella (3–5), cytomegalovirus (6), and varicella-zoster virus (7).

Considerable attention is now being focused on the applicability of these diagnostic techniques in the prenatal diagnosis of human immunodeficiency virus type-1 (HIV-1) infection (8–10). This chapter discusses the available prenatal diagnostic techniques and their applicability to the diagnosis of fetal HIV-1 infection. The discussion includes a description of these techniques, the maternal and fetal risks of the procedures, the methods of confirming fetal infection, and the prospects in prenatal diagnosis and treatment of intrauterine fetal HIV-1 infection.

SAMPLING TECHNIQUES USED FOR PRENATAL DIAGNOSIS

It is estimated that 13–35% of infants born to seropositive women will be infected with HIV-1, and the remainder will lose their antibody to HIV-1 (11). Currently, the diagnosis of HIV-1 infection in infants can be established in asymptomatic infants by a positive virus culture, polymerase chain reaction (PCR), or p24 antigen. However, these tests may be falsely negative during the first few weeks of life in approximately half of those infants who are subsequently shown to be infected. The presence of AIDS-defining symptoms and a declining CD4 count provides strong evidence for infection during infancy. If a safe and effective method for the prenatal diagnosis of HIV-1 were to exist, counseling regarding the risk of vertical transmission would be possible. The currently available diagnostic techniques are discussed below with reference to their use in the in utero detection of HIV-1 infection. Advantages and disadvantages of these prenatal diagnostic techniques are summarized in Table 11.1.

Ultrasound

Marion and coworkers (12) first suggested the possibility of the existence of an HIV-1-associated embryopathy in 1986. They reported that the constellation of certain craniofacial features associated with growth delay could detect those children who would ultimately develop infection with HIV-1 before the appearance of demonstrable clinical signs or symptoms (13, 19). Other, more recent, studies have failed to confirm the existence of a facial dysmorphism associated with congenital HIV-1 infection (14).

Sonographic measurements of craniofacial morphometrics have been used to de-

207

Table 11.1.   Characteristics of Techniques Available for Prenatal Diagnosis of HIV-1

	Timing	Risk of Fetal Loss	Cost	Comments
Ultrasound	≥5 weeks	None over background rate	$200–$350	Noninvasive; high resolution
Amniocentesis	≥12 weeks	0.25–0.5%	$700–$1000	Lowest risk of invasive procedures, easiest to perform
CVS	≥9–11 weeks	1.0–1.5%	$900–1200	Greatest risk of fetal to maternal transfusion
Fetal blood sampling	≥16 weeks	1.0–2%	$1000–1500	Provides direct access to fetal circulation for diagnosis and therapy; most promising technique.
Embryoscopy	≥5–14 weeks	2–3%	Currently experimental; for research use only in United States	Provides direct visualization and access to fetal circulation for diagnosis and therapy in first trimester
Fetoscopy	≥14 weeks	4–5%	Not currently used	Virtually replaced by cordocentesis

tect other congenital malformations of the head and face. To determine whether high resolution sonography could be used to detect such a dysmorphology associated with in utero HIV-1 infection, measurements from serial ultrasound examinations were reviewed in 171 pregnancies: 57 HIV-1-seropositive women and 114 HIV-1-seronegative matched controls. The two groups did not differ with respect to age, gravidity, stage of maternal HIV-1 infection or tobacco, alcohol, or drug abuse. No significant difference was found in measurements of head circumference, biparietal diameter, occipitofrontal diameter, outer-orbital diameter, inner-orbital diameter, or transcerebellar diameter in fetuses who were subsequently found to be HIV-1 infected compared with noninfected infants (Fig. 11.1). Similar rates of intrauterine growth were observed in the infected and noninfected groups (15).

These findings support the lack of an association between congenital infection with HIV-1 and the existence of a characteristic facies. Additionally, it does not seem that infection with HIV-1 has an adverse effect on fetal growth. These data suggest that the application of other, more invasive methods of prenatal diagnosis such as amniocentesis or cordocentesis must be evaluated if the HIV-1-infected fetus is to be detected in utero.

Amniocentesis

The term amniocentesis refers to the transabdominal insertion of a needle into the amniotic sac. This is the most widely used technique for prenatal diagnosis of genetic disorders. Amniocentesis is used for various purposes, including assessing amniotic fluid for factors predictive of fetal lung maturity during the third trimester and monitoring the severity of isoimmunization. In the past, amniocentesis was performed blindly after palpation of the uterus, but current practice dictates constant sonographic visualization during the procedure, regardless of the indication.

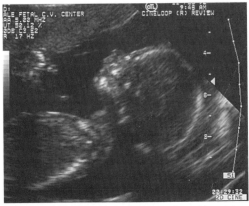

Figure 11.1.   Ultrasound image of profile of face from a 24-week fetus.

The procedure is usually performed after 16 menstrual weeks of gestation, although first trimester amniocentesis is gaining in popularity (16). If pregnancy termination is a consideration, then the procedure must be performed at an early enough gestation to allow time for final results of testing and the subsequent pregnancy termination procedure. Since abortions are not performed electively beyond 24 weeks and some diagnostic testing may take 2–3 weeks, diagnostic procedures usually should be performed by 20 or 21 weeks of gestation; otherwise fetal blood sampling, with its more rapid time to resuls, should be considered as an alternative.

The actual technique for amniocentesis involves inserting a 22-gauge, 3.5-inch spinal needle with stylet transabdominally through the uterine musculature into the amniotic sac under direct sonographic visualization. After the stylet is removed, 10–20 ml amniotic fluid is withdrawn into a sterile syringe. Risks of the procedure to the mother are minimal; however, there is a small risk of fetal loss (0.25–0.5%) caused by spontaneous rupture of membranes, premature contractions, or infection. There may be maternal immunization with fetal red blood cells, so Rh immunoglobulin should be given to Rh-negative mothers to prevent sensitization. The amniotic fluid removed can be cultured, stained with various reagents, and tested for the presence of immunoglobulins, microbial DNA or RNA, or antigen (Fig. 11.2).

There has been limited experience with the prenatal diagnosis of congenital infections from amniotic fluid samples. In 1988, Daffos and coworkers (2) isolated *Toxoplasma gondii* from seven amniotic fluid samples; but toxoplasmosis-specific IgM could not be identified in these fluids. Since viruses require cells for replication they may be more difficult to isolate from amniotic fluid samples than bacteria or parasites. Nevertheless, virus isolation has been achieved via amniocentesis for such viruses as cytomegalovirus (6) and herpes simplex virus (7). In fact, cytomegalovirus has been isolated from the amniotic fluid in numerous cases in which fetal infection was found (7). However, Stagno and coworkers (6) reported three cases with negative amniotic fluid cultures in which cytomegalovirus was isolated from fetal or placental tissue.

There is even less information available on the value of amniocentesis for the prena-

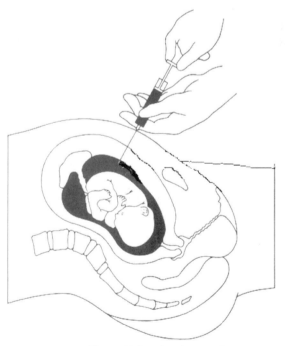

Figure 11.2.   Amniocentesis.

tal diagnosis of fetal HIV-1 infection. Virus antigen and HIV-1 reverse transcriptase activity has been identified in amniocytes and fluid collected at 15 weeks gestation from a pregnant woman with AIDS (17). There has yet to be a report of HIV-1 being isolated from the amniotic fluid of an asymptomatic seropositive woman.

HIV-1 p24 antigen assays were performed in 18 HIV-1 seropositive women between 9 and 24 weeks gestation before elective termination of pregnancy to investigate the transplacental transfer of HIV-1 antibody and p24 antigen and to explore the diagnostic potential of fetal blood sampling in the prenatal diagnosis of intrauterine HIV-1 infection (18). Twelve women were Centers for Disease Control group II (asymptomatic, seropositive), five were group III (symptomatic, seropositive), and one had AIDS (group IV). Amniotic fluid and fetal blood were obtained transabdominally via a single insertion into an anterior cord in 15 cases and transcervically using an embryoscope in three patients. HIV-1 antibody was detected by Western blot analysis in all samples of maternal serum, amniotic fluid, and fetal serum. Each mother-fetus pair displayed identical banding patterns. In contrast, p24 antigen was found in the maternal serum and amniotic fluid from only 5 of 18 patients, three of which also had p24 in the fetal serum. HIV-1 p24 antigen was only found in fetuses of patients with group III disease. Of note, p24 antigen was not detected in the three fetuses sampled in the first-trimester. Detection of HIV-1 or p24 antigen in the amniotic fluid will need to be correlated with fetal or neonatal infection to determine usefulness of this approach for prenatal diagnosis of HIV-1 infection. Fetal cells obtained from amniocentesis could also be studied using PCR and in situ hybridization techniques, although the risk of iatrogenic infection of the fetus remains to be determined.

The risk of infecting the fetus during the procedure is generally regarded as low, since there are no reports of vertical transmission of any congenital infection caused by invasive prenatal diagnosis; however, there is little or no direct information supporting this hypothesis for HIV-1. Thus the risks and benefits must be established be-fore this procedure can be offered clinically for prenatal HIV-1 diagnosis. The sensitivity, specificity, and predictive value of the diagnostic procedure should be established in HIV-1-positive women undergoing elective pregnancy termination before the procedure is offered as an HIV-1 diagnostic tool in women desiring to carry their pregnancies to term. In women electing prenatal diagnosis for genetic risks (i.e., maternal age, prior progeny with trisomy, etc.) the special risk in HIV-1-seropositve women should be discussed in the course of counseling.

Chorionic Villus Sampling

CVS is a technique that allows very early prenatal diagnosis of certain genetic disorders. The approach can be either transcervical or transabdominal and is performed as early as 8 weeks after the last menstrual period. The procedure involves insertion of a narrow catheter into the decidual-chorionic space. A sample of chorionic membrane (fetal tissue) is then removed by suction aspiration using a syringe. Since chorionic villi must be obtained, the tissue is immediatly examined microscopically to determine if the specimen is adequate for diagnostic purposes. CVS offers the advantage of first-trimester prenatal diagnosis but is more subject to procedural failure and ambiguous diagnoses (Fig. 11.3).

There is a paucity of information on the use of CVS in the prenatal diagnosis of congenital virus infection. In one case of rubella infection just before conception, Terry and coworkers (5) reported that the tissue obtained from CVS performed at 12 weeks gestation induced the characteristic effect in culture and produced a positive immunoblot reaction with rubella-specific monoclonal antibody. The virus was subsequently isolated from both fetal and placental tissue following pregnancy termination.

The role of CVS in the prenatal diagnosis of fetal HIV-1 infection is very uncertain. Because of the disruptive nature of the procedure, there is a high risk of exposing fetal tissue to maternal blood. Furthermore, the procedure is performed so early in gestation that the CD4 receptor for HIV-1 may not yet be present on developing T lympho-

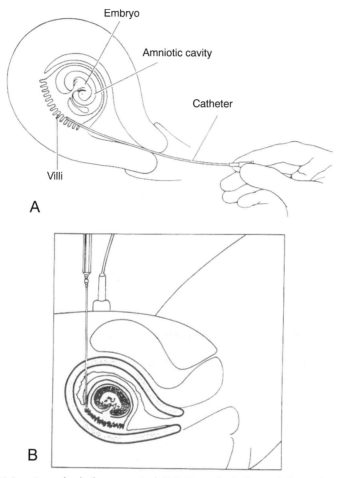

Figure 11.3. **A,** method of transcervical CVS; **B,** method of transabdominal CVS.

cytes. The predominant theory regarding HIV-1 infection suggests that a receptor on the cell surface is necessary for the virus to infect. This receptor has been confirmed to be the CD4 molecule present on certain T lymphocytes and some cells of the monocyte-macrophage line. Other cell types may be infected if they display the CD4 molecule or perhaps a very similar molecule that has enough homology in the region of the HIV-1 binding site.

Cordocentesis

Cordocentesis, also known as percutaneous umbilical blood sampling or fetal blood sampling, is a prenatal diagnostic technique first reported in the early 1980s. It has since gained routine acceptance as a method for prenatal diagnosis when fetal blood samples are necessary. The use of cordocentesis for prenatal diagnosis of HIV-1 infection has many potential problems, and all the risks and benefits must be carefully considered.

If it is shown that HIV-1 transmission occurs early in gestation, cordocentesis may prove useful for identification of infected fetuses early enough for a mother to elect termination of an affected fetus; it may also prove useful in screening HIV-1-infected fetuses for selective in utero treatment. Furthermore, reports of craniofacial dysmorphism among HIV-1-infected infants suggest that HIV-1 infection in early pregnancy may be teratogenic (12, 19). This latter point, however, remains controversial since there is debate about whether a true

HIV-1 or a function of other cofactors such as maternal drug use, race, or even another virus.

Cordocentesis is usually performed after 16 menstrual weeks of gestation. The technique involves the transabdominal insertion of a needle into the umbilical vein at or near its placental origin to remove 1–3 ml fetal blood. The entire procedure is performed under high resolution sonographic guidance using aseptic techniques. The sample can be tested for maternal blood contamination by red blood cell mean corpuscular volume testing, Kleihauer-Betke acid elution testing, or red blood cell anti-agglutination testing for *i* antigen. More recently, investigators have begun using flow cytometry to distinguish maternal cells from fetal cells. Fetal loss has been reported to be <2% (7). The most frequent complications include transient bleeding from the umbilical cord puncture site, usually subsiding within 1 min, occasional transient fetal bradycardia, and, rarely, premature rupture of the amniotic membranes. (Fig. 11.4).

In recent years, cordocentesis has become an extremely important tool in the prenatal diagnosis of intrauterine fetal infection. Daffos and coworkers (1, 2) have reported on 746 pregnancies at risk for congenital toxoplasmosis. The procedure was performed on 278 pregnant women at risk for vertical transmission with the fetal blood being studied for toxoplasmosis-specific

IgM by immunosorbent assay and for isolation of the organism. They isolated the organism from nine samples of fetal blood. Toxoplasmosis-specific IgM was detected in only four of these nine fetuses, possibly because of the lack of fetal IgM production in some fetuses at midgestation. Cordocentesis has also been used with some success to diagnose congenital rubella infection (3, 4).

Daffos and coworkers (8) have performed cordocentesis on two HIV-1-seropositive mothers. Fetal blood samples were obtained just before pregnancy termination at 24 and 27 weeks gestation. The virus was detected from stimulated T lymphocytes by reverse transcriptase activity in one mother. Although anti-HIV-1 IgG antibody was detected in both fetuses as expected (the placenta is permeable to IgG), the virus was not detected in either fetal blood specimen by reverse transcriptase activity assay on the cell-free supernatant of stimulated T lymphocytes. Fetal immune studies, including total lymphocyte counts, CD4+ lymphocyte counts, CD4:CD8 ratios, and total IgM levels were within the ranges found in normal peripheral fetal blood (20). Although both fetuses were pathologically normal, no postmortem virologic studies were performed on the fetal tissue after termination. The absence of detectable HIV-1 in these two isolated cases may relate to the fact that the rate of vertical transmission at term is between 14 and 35% and these fetuses had no evidence of altered immune status.

To date, there has been only one report of the successful prenatal diagnosis of in utero infection with HIV-1 (21). Thirteen HIV-1-infected pregnant women underwent cordocentesis from 23 to 39 weeks gestation. One insertion into an anterior cord was performed in all cases. HIV-1 p24 antigen assay and PCR techniques for HIV-1 were performed on the maternal and fetal samples. Seven fetal blood samples were negative and three were positive using PCR analysis. PCR was unavailable in three cases. Two of the three PCR-positive fetuses have developed AIDS, and one has seroreverted. Both these "infected" fetuses were also HIV-1 p24 antigen positive. One fetus who was PCR negative and two who were p24 antigen negative at the time of sampling

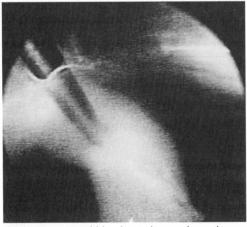

Figure 11.4.   Fetal blood sampling performed transabdominally using a 22-gauge spinal needle as visualized via an embryoscope inserted transcervically.

were later shown to be HIV-1 infected. We concluded that PCR and p24 antigen testing for HIV-1 on samples obtained by cordocentesis during the second and third trimester was predictive of ultimate pediatric infection with HIV-1. We noted, however, that a negative test, while reassuring, is not absolute, suggesting the possibility of intrapartum acquisition of HIV-1 and cautioned that studies into the efficacy and safety of fetal blood sampling must be performed before its acceptance in routine clinical practice for HIV-1-infected women.

It is likely that further attempts will be made to diagnose HIV-1 prenatally using cordocentesis and other prenatal diagnostic techniques, but particular attention must be paid to avoiding the possibility of false-positive results from fetal samples contaminated with maternal blood. This is especially important when using DNA amplifying techniques such as PCR. The likelihood of false negatives can be decreased significantly by combining immunologic, virologic, molecular biologic, and histopathologic techniques for HIV-1 identification.

Embryoscopy

The rapid emergence of prenatal diagnosis has been facilitated by the development of advanced technologies to visualize the fetus and to obtain tissue and fluid for analysis. Embryoscopy is a promising new technique that allows direct visualization of the first trimester conceptus, thus providing true and precise anatomic detail beyond that provided by ultrasound (22). The technique also permits direct access to the developing fetal circulation in the first trimester, providing an opportunity for early fetal diagnosis and therapy.

To determine the feasibility of obtaining fetal blood and amniotic fluid from first trimester pregnancies in seropositive women and to investigate the existence of an embryopathy associated with congenital HIV-1 infection, we studied nine HIV-1-seropositive mother-fetus pairs between 9 and 14 weeks gestation with transvaginal ultrasound, transcervical embryoscopy, and fetal blood sampling before elective termination of pregnancy (23). By using transcervical embryoscopy, a detailed examination

of the gross morphology of nine HIV-1-seropositive conceptuses was performed between 9 and 14 weeks gestation. Access to the fetal circulation was established successfully in all cases. Samples of amniotic fluid and fetal blood were obtained using the embryoscope that were reactive for the presence of antibodies to HIV-1 by enzyme-linked immunosorbent assay (ELISA) and Western blot techniques. HIV-1 p24 antigen was not detected in aliquots from either compartment. No direct evidence of an HIV-1 embryopathy was noted. This method for direct access to the fetal circulation, if proven safe and effective, may permit the prenatal detection and therapy of HIV-1 infection in the first trimester (Fig. 11.5).

PRENATAL PREDICTION OF VERTICAL TRANSMISSION

Maternal factors may be key in predicting the likelihood and timing of fetal infection. The gestational age at which the fetus may become infected has been the subject of considerable speculation, but there remains a paucity of data on the subject. It has been suggested that vertical transmission could occur as early as 12–13 weeks gestation, when CD4 expression first appears on T lymphocytes in the fetal thymus (24). This, of course, would require transplacental passage of the virus. There have been rare reports of documenting HIV-1 infection in fetal tissue from abortus material of HIV-1-seropositive women (25, 26). However, transplacental and intrapartum transmis-

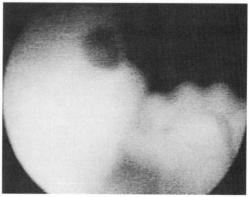

Figure 11.5. Embryoscopic view of fetal face at 9 weeks gestation.

sion may both contribute to the vertical transmission rate. Infected infants have been delivered by cesarean section with intact fetal membranes, making intrapartum transmission highly unlikely in these cases (27). There has also been documentation of vertical transmission via breast milk (28).

The fetus may be vulnerable to infection with HIV-1 throughout gestation, although the timing of transmission has not been ascertained. Fetal lymphocytes undergo progressive phenotypic maturation early in gestation, as evidenced by the appearance of differentiation antigen expression. In fact, specific T cell subsets can be identified as early as the late first trimester. A predictable pattern of antigenic expression associated with fetal immune maturation occurs as the pregnancy progresses (24, 29, 30). Nevertheless, even at birth the fetal immune system remains relatively immature, lacking the functional capacity of the adult immune system. In this regard, studies of the fetal immune system become even more important, particularly in view of recent studies showing detectable immune abnormalities in HIV-1-infected children well before detection of endogenous anti-HIV-1 antibodies. Nadal and coworkers (31) reported immune deficiencies (including hypogammaglobulinemia, IgG subclass deficiency, low serum IgA concentration, antibody deficiency, decreased numbers of CD4+ T cells, and defective cellular response to antigens) in 17 of 33 children born to HIV-1-infected mothers. Seven of these 17 neonates with immune deficiencies were HIV-1 culture positive; another seven had anti-HIV-1 antibody persisting beyond the age of 15 months, and three lost HIV-1 antibodies.

Although the vulnerability of the fetus to infection is important in vertical transmission, maternal status may be even more crucial to the timing of transplacental passage of the virus. Does the risk of vertical transmission increase in pregnancies when maternal disease undergoes rapid progression to symptomatic disease (i.e., AIDS or AIDS-related complex)? Does maternal viremia increase the risk? The stage of maternal disease, the presence or absence of viremia, the maternal antigenic load, maternal immune status, and virulence of the particular

HIV-1 strain may all be involved in determining risk of transmission. Thus maternal factors may provide some keys to prenatal diagnosis of HIV-1 infection. In fact, preliminary studies indicate that HIV-1-infected pregnant women with symptomatic HIV-1 disease are at a higher risk for transmitting the virus to their infants (32, 33). Recent reports indicate that very low absolute CD4+ lymphocyte counts are associated with HIV-1 transmission to the fetus (34, 35). Recently, antibody to HIV-1 gp120 has been negatively correlated with vertical transmission (36).

Maternal serum, amniotic fluid, and cord blood samples, obtained prospectively from 26 HIV-1-infected pregnancies at the time of labor and delivery, were studied to investigate the prognostic significance of HIV-1 p24 antigen as a marker of perinatal transmission (37). Amniotic fluid was obtained by amniocentesis in seven pregnancies and in 13 by needle aspiration before artificial rupture of membranes during labor. Amniotic fluid was not obtained in the six women who presented in labor with premature rupture of the membranes. Cord blood was collected at the time of delivery in 27 newborns (including one set of twins). ELISA and Western blot antibody analyses and p24 antigen determinations were performed on all samples. Sixteen patients had Centers for Disease Control group II, eight had group III, and two had group IV disease. HIV-1 p24 antigen was detected in maternal serum from seven of the 26 women. Amniotic fluid was available in four of these seven patients and was positive in all cases.

HIV-1 p24 antigen was detected in cord blood from only five of the seven infants (71%) whose mothers were noted to have p24 antigen. One premature, antigen-positive infant died 48 hr postpartum. Two newborns, who were symptomatic early in life, have died and the other two remain seropositive and asymptomatic at age 35 and 27 months. The two antigen-negative infants who were born to antigen-positive mothers have seroreverted and remain healthy at 28 and 46 months follow-up. Eighteen of 19 antigen-negative infants born to antigen-negative mothers have seroreverted and are clinically free of disease at a mean follow-up of 33 months. These findings indicate that the presence of

HIV-1 p24 antigen in either cord blood or maternal serum is significantly associated with the development of HIV-1 disease in the infant (Fisher's exact test; $P < 0.01$). We concluded that maternal p24 antigen may identify a subset of women who are at increased risk for the delivery of an HIV-1-infected infant. If confirmed by larger studies, the existence of such a marker of vertical transmission would have considerable utility in the prenatal diagnosis of the HIV-1-infected fetus.

Currently numerous maternal serum factors that have been shown to be predictive of HIV-1 disease progression or response to therapy, such as HIV-1 p24 antigen, β_2-microglobulin, neopterin, interleukin-2 receptor, and plasma viral titers are under investigation to determine their role in predicting vertical transmission. In the future, as these studies continue, we may be able to identify prenatally patterns of maternal factors that are highly predictive of vertical transmission of HIV-1. For a more complete discussion of maternal factors involved in the transmission of HIV-1 from mother to child, refer to Ref. 11 and see Chapter 10C.

RISKS OF PRENATAL DIAGNOSIS OF FETAL HIV-1 INFECTION

The major concern surrounding prenatal diagnosis of fetal HIV-1 infection is the risk that the procedure itself will inoculate the fetus with the virus from maternal sources. Since a deep needle stick is a serious risk factor for HIV-1 infection, cordocentesis may carry some risk of fetal inoculation with maternal HIV-1-infected blood. There are numerous patients in whom cordocentesis has been used for prenatal diagnosis of toxoplasmosis, rubella, and other perinatal infections with no reports of subsequent neonatal infection.

Women with chronic hepatitis B undergoing prenatal diagnostic procedures do not transmit to their neonates at a higher rate than those without prenatal testing. Large numbers of women undergo invasive fetal diagnosis in China, where the prevalence of hepatitis B approaches 20%. There have been no reports, to date, of an increased incidence of vertical transmission of hepatitis B virus from these areas. Whether the pattern of intrauterine (vs. intrapartum) infection, or that associated with e antigen, impact these transmission rates is unresolved. This is quite relevant since HIV-1 is thought to be transmitted in much the same way as hepatitis B but with much less frequency and infectivity. However, the infectious potential of invasive diagnostic methods remains controversial.

There has been one report regarding the risk of mother to fetus transmission of HIV-1 related to invasive diagnostic procedures including amniocentesis, CVS, fetal scalp electrode placement, fetal scalp pH sampling, and fetal blood sampling (38). Neonatal outcome was compared to determine if the risk of HIV-1 transmission is increased after antepartum invasive procedures. Group I consisted of 46 pregnancies in which invasive fetal testing was performed. There were 32 amniocenteses (indications: preterm labor–18; premature rupture of the membranes–9; lung maturity–5), 18 fetal scalp electrode placements, 10 fetal scalp samplings, and three fetal blood samplings (indications: idiopathic thrombocytopenic purpura–2; fetal distress–1). Group II included 93 women who had completed their pregnancies without undergoing an invasive procedure. Both groups were matched for maternal age (27.0 vs. 27.6 years), HIV-1 status, racial breakdown, and HIV-1 risk behavior. The groups did not differ with respect to mean CD4 count (401 vs. 385 cells/ml), HIV-1 p24 antigen status, mean gestational age at delivery (36.2 vs. 36.4 weeks), or mean birth weight (2426 vs. 2754 g). No statistically significant difference was noted between the groups with respect to infant disease status with all invasive procedures ($\chi^2 = 0.99$) or with amniocentesis alone ($\chi^2 = 1.37$). Infant outcome did not differ significantly based on the number of invasive procedures performed during pregnancy ($\chi^2 = 2.26$). The mean time from invasive procedure to delivery was the same in infected infants and those who seroreverted ($t = 0.49$). These data suggest that modern techniques of invasive prenatal diagnosis may predict which fetuses are truly infected with HIV-1 without increasing the risk of iatrogenic infection (38).

Risk of transmission from mother to fetus is probably least with amniocentesis, although the diagnostic capabilities may be equally low, since fetal T cells are not obtained with this procedure. Because of these risks, it will be necessary initially to perform these prenatal diagnostic procedures on seropositive women who have already elected pregnancy termination. It will also be necessary to study some seropositive women who elect to carry their pregnancies so that the risk of transmission can be determined. This will likely be performed for the most part in seropositive women who elect prenatal diagnostic testing for reasons other than HIV-1 status (i.e., maternal age, previous genetic disorder, etc.).

HIV-1 IDENTIFICATION METHODS

The means by which fetal material is studied will be important in determining accuracy of the diagnostic procedure. The state of the art in HIV-1 diagnosis includes various immunologic, virologic, molecular biologic, and histopathologic diagnostic techniques. These techniques are covered in more detail in Ref. 39 and in Chapter 12. The advantages and disadvantages of these techniques are summarized in Tables 11.2 and 11.3.

SUMMARY

Prenatal diagnostic techniques available today may allow physicians to identify fetal HIV-1 infection early in gestation. This would enable HIV-1 seropositive women to make better informed decisions about carrying vs. terminating their pregnancies. Furthermore, as therapeutic agents become

Table 11.2.   Characteristics of Available Laboratory Detection Methods for Prenatal Diagnosis of HIV-1 Infection[a]

Laboratory Method	Specimen Required	Technical Expertise	Relative Cost	Advantages and Disadvantages
HIV-1 IgG antibody testing (ELISA/ Western blot)	Serum/plasma	Low	Low	Not useful for prenatal diagnosis since maternal IgG is present in fetus
HIV-1 IgA antibody testing (ELISA)	Serum/plasma	Low	Moderate	Predictive of ultimate HIV-1 infection in infants 3–6 months
ELISPOT	PBMC	Moderate	Moderate	
IVAP	PBMC	Moderate	Moderate	
HIV-1 p24 antigen	Serum/plasma	Low	Low	May be negative over much of patient's lifetime
In situ hybridization	PBMC/placenta	High	High	Unreliable if maternal contamination
PCR	PBMC	High	High	Unreliable if maternal contamination
Viral culture	PBMC	High	High	Definitive evidence of HIV-1 infection

[a]PBMC peripheral blood mononuclear cells; IVAP, in vitro antibody production; ELISPOT, enzyme-linked immunospot.

Table 11.3.   Sensitivity of Early Diagnostic Tests for HIV-1 Infection in Infants

Laboratory Method[a]	Time to Detection				
	1 week	2–4 weeks	1–2 months	3–6 months	>6 months
			%		
HIV-1 IgA antibody testing (ELISA)	<10	10–30	20–50	50–80	70–90
ELISPOT				>95%	>95%
IVAP				>95%	>95%
HIV-1 p24 antigen	10–25%	20–50%	30–60%	30–50%	20–40%
In situ hybridization					
PCR	30–50	50	70–90	>95%	>95%
Viral culture	30–50	50	70–90	>95%	>95%

[a]HIV-1 IgG antibody testing (ELISA/Western blot) not useful for detection of HIV-1 infection.

available for use in pregnancy, the HIV-1 status of the fetus may be used in deciding if and when to institute therapy and in assessing responses to therapy. There are, however, several important questions that must be answered before prenatal HIV-1 diagnosis will be attempted routinely. It must first be determined that an HIV-1-infected fetus can be detected with a high degree of reliability. The risk of both missing the diagnosis in an infected fetus and making the diagnosis of fetal infection because of maternal contamination of fetal specimens must be dramatically reduced. Finally, it is crucial that the techniques used have virtually no risk of infecting an otherwise healthy fetus. Although the technology may exist to satisfactorily achieve these goals, the state of the art does not provide any safe and reliable prenatal diagnostic methods for HIV-1 infection of the fetus. The techniques discussed in this chapter should be considered research techniques; their utility in clinical practice has yet to be determined. Although the prospect of reliable prenatal diagnosis seems promising, remember that this addresses only part of the perinatal transmission problem. Intrapartum and postpartum transmissions also remain major concerns and are addressed in Chapter 10.

References

1. Desmonts G, Daffos F, Forestier F, et al. Prenatal diagnosis of congenital toxoplasmosis. Lancet 1985;1:500–503.
2. Daffos F, Forestier F, Capella-Pavlovsky M, et al. Prenatal management of 746 pregnancies at risk for congenital toxoplasmosis. N Engl J Med 1988; 318:271–275.
3. Morgan-Capner P, Rodeck C, Nicolaides K, Cradock-Watson J. Prenatal detection of rubella-specific IgM in fetal sera. Prenat Diagn 1985;5: 2126–2129.
4. Enders G, Jonath W. Prenatal diagnosis of intrauterine rubella infection. Infection 1987;15:162–164.
5. Terry G, Ho-Terry L, Warren R, et al. First trimester prenatal diagnosis of congenital rubella: A laboratory investigation. Br Med J 1986;292:930–941.
6. Stagno S, Pass R, Dworsky E, Alford C. Maternal cytomegalovirus infection and perinatal transmission. Clin Obstet Gynecol 1982;25:563–576.
7. Grose C, Itani O, Weiner C. Prenatal diagnosis of fetal infection: Advances from amniocentesis to cordocentesis—congenital toxoplasmosis, rubella, cytomegalovirus, varicella virus, parvovirus and human immunodeficiency virus type-1. Pediatr Infect Dis J 1989;8:459–468.
8. Daffos F, Forestier F, Mandelbrot L, et al. Prenatal diagnosis of HIV-1 infection: Two attempts using fetal blood sampling. J Acquir Immune Defic Syndr 1989;2:205–207.
9. Viscarello RR. In utero detection of human immunodeficiency virus infection: Preliminary studies. Arch AIDS Res 1990;4:232–244.
10. Viscarello RR, Cullen MT, DeGennaro NJ, Hobbins JC. Fetal blood sampling in human immunodeficiency virus-seropositive women prior to elective termination of pregnancy. Am J Obstet Gynecol 1992;167:1075–1079.
11. Ammann A, Bolme P, Borkowsky W, et al. Maternal factors involved in mother-to-child transmission of HIV-1: Report of the Consensus Workshop held in Siena, Italy, Jan 17–18, 1992. J Acquir Immune Defic Syndr 1992;5:1019–1029.
12. Marion R, Wiznia M, Hutcheon R, Rubinstein A. Human T-cell lymphotrophic virus type-III (HTLV-III) embryopathy: A new dysmorphic syndrome associated with intrauterine HTLV-III infection. Am J Dis Child 1986;140:638–640.
13. Marion RW, Wiznia AA, Hutcheon G, Rubinstein A. Fetal AIDS syndrome score: Correlation between severity of dysmorphism and age at diagnosis of immunodeficiency. Am J Dis Child 1987; 141:429–431.
14. Qazi QH, Sheikh TM, Fikrig S, Menikoff H. Lack of evidence for craniofacial dysmorphism in perinatal human immunodeficiency virus infection. J Pediatr 1988;112:7–11.
15. Viscarello R, DeGennaro N, Hobbins J. Sonographic evidence against the existence of a craniofacial dysmorphology associated with congenital infection with human immunodeficiency virus type-1 [Abstract]. 40th Annual Meeting of Society for Gynecologic Investigation, San Antonio, 1991.
16. Viscarello R, Gollin Y, Hobbins JC. Alternative methods of first trimester diagnosis. Obstet Gynecol Clin North Am 1991;18:875–890.
17. Sprecher S, Soumenkoff G, Puissant F, Degueldre M. Vertical transmission of HIV in 15-week fetus. Lancet 1986;2:288–289.
18. Viscarello R, Cullen M, DeGennaro NJ, Hobbins JC. Fetal blood sampling in HIV-1 seropositive pregnancies prior to elective termination of pregnancy [Abstract]. Am J Obstet Gynecol 1992;166: 384.
19. Perro M. Dysmorphism leading to a diagnosis of acquired immunodeficiency syndrome [Letter]. Am J Dis Child 1987;141:474.
20. Rainout M, Pagniez M, Hercend T, Daffos F, Forestier F. Characterization of mononuclear cell subpopulations in normal fetal peripheral blood. Hum Immunol 1987;1B:331–337.
21. Cullen M, Viscarello R, Paryani S, Sanchez-Ramos L. Prenatal diagnosis of HIV-1 infection: The use of cordocentesis, polymerase chain reaction, and p24 antigen assay [Abstract]. Am J Obstet Gynecol 1992;166:386.
22. Cullen MT, Reece EA, Whetham J, Hobbins JC. Embryoscopy: Description and utility of a new technique. Am J Obstet Gynecol 1990;162:82–86.
23. Viscarello R, Cullen M, Whetham J, Hobbins J. Embryoscopy and fetal blood sampling prior to elective first-trimester termination of pregnancy in

human immunodeficiency virus-seropositive women [Abstract]. Annual Meeting of Society of Perinatal Obstetricians, Houston, 1990.

24. Lobach D, Hensley L, Ho W, Haynes B. Human T cell antigen expression during the early stage of fetal thymic maturation. J Immunol 1985;135: 1752–1759.

25. LaPointe N, Michaud J, Pekovic D, et al. Transplacental transmission of HTLV-III virus [Letter]. N Engl J Med 1985;312:1325.

26. Jovais S, Koch M, Schafer L, et al. HTLV-II/HTLV-III in a 20 week fetus [Letter]. Lancet 1985;2:1129.

27. Minkoff H, Nanda D, Menez R, Fikrig S. Pregnancies resulting in infants with acquired immunodeficiency syndrome or AIDS-related complex. Obstet Gynecol 1987;69:285–287.

28. Ziegler J, Johnson R, Cooper D, Gold J. Postnatal transmission of AIDS-associated retrovirus from mother to infant. Lancet 1985;1:896–897.

29. Kamps W, Cooper M. Development of lymphocyte subpopulations identified by monoclonal antibodies in human fetuses. J Clin Immunol 1984;4: 36–39.

30. Holzgreve B, Goldsmith P, Holzgreve W, Golbus M. A monoclonal antibody micromethod for studying fetal lymphocytes—potential for prenatal diagnosis of inherited immunodeficiencies. J Reprod Immunol 1984;6:341–344.

31. Nadal D, Hunziker U, Schupbach J, et al. Immunological evaluation in the early diagnosis of prenatal or perinatal HIV infection. Arch Dis Child 1989;64:662–669.

32. Ryder R, Nsa W, Hassig SE, et al. Perinatal transmission of the human immunodeficiency virus type-1 to infants of seropositive women in Zaire. N Engl J Med 1989;320:1637–1642.

33. Blanche S, Rouzioux C, Moscata M, et al. A prospective study of infants born to women seropositive for human immunodeficiency virus type-1. N Engl J Med 1989;320:1643–1648.

34. Dattel B, Hauer L, Wofsy C, et al. Perinatal transmission of HIV-1: Is a decreased CD4+ cell count predictive? [Abstract TPB 198]. Fifth International Conference on AIDS, Montreal, Jun 1989.

35. Viscarello R, DeGennaro N, Andiman W. Maternal CD4 lymphocyte counts as a predictor of perinatal transmission of HIV-1 [Abstract]. Am J Obstet Gynecol 1993;168:418.

36. Goedert J, Mendez H, Drummond J, et al. Mother-to-infant transmission of human immunodeficiency virus type-1: Association with prematurity or low anti-gp 120. Lancet 1989;2:1351–1354.

37. Viscarello R, DeGennaro N, Gollin YG, Andiman WA, Hobbins JC. Is maternal p24 antigenemia a marker for vertical transmission of human immunodeficiency virus? [Abstract] Annual Meeting of Society for Gynecologic Investigation, San Antonio, 1992.

38. Viscarello R, DeGennaro N, Griffith S, Andiman W, Hobbins JC. Does an antepartum invasive procedure increase the risk of perinatal transmission of HIV-1? [Abstract] Am J Obstet Gynecol 1992;166:384.

39. Albert J, Biberfeld G, Borkowsky W, et al. Early diagnosis of HIV-1 infection in infants: Report of the Consensus Workshop held in Siena, Italy, January 17–18, 1992. J Acquir Immune Defic Syndr 1992;6:1125–1134.

12
Advances in Diagnosis of HIV Infection in Infants

Martha F. Rogers, Gerald Schochetman, and Rod Hoff

Approximately 6000 human immunodeficiency virus-type 1 (HIV-1)-infected women give birth each year in the United States (1). Over three-quarters of all AIDS cases reported to the Centers for Disease Control and Prevention (CDC) in children younger than 13 years are attributed to perinatal (mother to infant) transmission. Some AIDS cases among children who became infected through blood transfusions before donor screening began in 1985 are still being reported, but virtually all current transmission of HIV infection to children in the United States has been through the perinatal route. Studies have shown that 13–40% of infants born to women with HIV infection will have acquired the virus from their mothers (2–6). Differentiating infected from uninfected infants born to these women is clinically difficult in the early stages of the disease and has been hampered by the lack of sensitive, specific, and practical laboratory tests for early detection.

Early diagnosis of HIV infection in infants is needed to identify infants that might benefit from early antiviral therapy, prophylactic treatment for opportunistic infections, and aggressive treatment of bacterial infections, growth and development disorders, and psychosocial problems. Differentiating infected from uninfected infants will eliminate unnecessary procedures and therapy in uninfected infants. Some early diagnostic tests may also provide information that helps establish the timing of transmission

from mother to infant. The effectiveness of possible preventive measures such as prophylactic antiviral therapy, HIV hyperimmune globulin, or future HIV vaccines may depend on timing of transmission. The natural history and prognosis of HIV infection may also be affected by the timing of transmission. Early diagnosis enables parents or caretakers to know the status of these children as soon as possible and, if necessary, to speed the placement of children who cannot be cared for by their parents.

Although tests for antibody to HIV remain the mainstay for laboratory diagnosis in adults and children acquiring HIV through blood products, antibody tests are inadequate for diagnosing infection in infants born to HIV-infected women. Infants passively acquire maternal antibody in utero, which may persist up to age 18 months. In infants younger than 18 months, serum tests for IgG antibody to HIV do not differentiate between infant and maternal antibody; thus a positive HIV antibody test in an infant only indicates exposure and possible infection, and further testing and follow-up is needed to determine infection status.

Significant advances in diagnostic tests for detecting HIV infection in infants born to HIV-infected mothers have been made in the past few years. Care providers for children no longer must wait until age 18 months to diagnose HIV infection in infants. Several diagnostic assays can reliably detect HIV infection by age 6 months with sensitivities and specificities approaching 100%. Problems remain, however, in transferring this technology to community hospital settings in the industrialized world and developing countries. Licensure and standardization will take time, and many tests remain costly.

This chapter discusses the problems of HIV diagnosis encountered by pediatricians and others caring for HIV-infected children and the progress in developing and using new technologies to overcome these problems. It also stresses the need for continued priority research in this area. Accurate and practical diagnostic tests are a key component to optimal management of the infected child and to the development of effective public health programs aimed at preventing morbidity and mortality from HIV infection (see also Chapter 38).

CURRENT LABORATORY TESTS

Antibody to HIV

Serologic tests for HIV-specific antibody are the mainstay of laboratory diagnosis of HIV infection in adults, children suspected of acquiring HIV through nonperinatal routes (i.e., blood or blood products), and children with suspected perinatally acquired infection who are older than 18 months. In most persons, HIV-specific antibody is detectable by currently licensed tests within 4–12 weeks after exposure (7), although an occasional prolonged seroconversion period has been reported. IgG antibody is generally detectable throughout the disease; however, patterns of antibody production to certain viral proteins may change during the disease. A broad antibody response to both envelope and core viral proteins is usually observed in the asymptomatic stage of HIV infection, whereas some symptomatic patients may show a loss of antibody to the core (gag) proteins (8). In addition, some HIV-infected infants will become hypogammaglobulinemic and will not produce antibody including antibody to HIV (9).

The most common antibody tests are enzyme-linked immunosorbent assays (ELISA) used in conjunction with supplemental tests such as the Western blot or an immunofluorescence assay (IFA) to confirm ELISA reactions. The Food and Drug Administration (FDA) has licensed several commercial ELISA kits for detecting antibody to HIV-l, HIV-2, or both viruses (combination tests). Other licensed methods include a latex slide agglutination test and a single use dot-blot method. Commercial Western blot tests and one IFA for confirmatory testing have also been licensed.

For the ELISA, viral antigens derived from either whole disrupted virus produced in culture or from recombinant p24, gp41, or gp120 viral antigens are bound to a solid support (Fig. 12.1), usually in microtiter wells. Patient serum is incubated for a specified time with the immobilized antigen. The wells or beads are washed, removing all but the bound anti-HIV antibody if present. Enzyme-labeled anti-human antibody is then added, followed by substrate. The enzymatic reaction causes a color change proportional to the amount of antibody present in the sample. An optical density reading is obtained, and the result is read as reactive or nonreactive based on the cutoff values established for the kit. If the sample is nonreactive, then the result is reported as negative. If the sample is reactive, a second aliquot of serum is run in duplicate (Fig. 12.2). Only repeatedly reactive specimens are considered ELISA positive.

ELISA is used as the primary screening test. Its sensitivity and specificity are high (>99.8% each); however, the predictive value of a positive test is low in persons at low risk of HIV infection. Therefore repeatedly reactive ELISAs must be confirmed with a supplemental test. Western blot tests are the most common supplemental tests. For the Western blot assay, virus antigens are electrophoresed in a polyacrylamide gel to separate the proteins according to their molecular size. Separated proteins are then transferred onto nitrocellulose membranes and incubated with patient serum to determine the presence of HIV-specific antibodies. As with the ELISA, enzyme-labeled anti-human antibody is added, followed by substrate. A colored antigen band appears at the site of antibody binding, identifying a specific antibody response to the various virus proteins (Fig 12.3).

Standard criteria for interpretation of Western blot tests have been published by

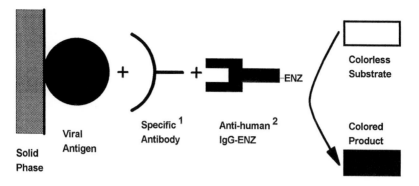

¹ Patient serum

² Horseradish peroxidase, Alkaline phosphatase

β-galactosidase, Glucose oxidase

Figure 12.1. For ELISA, viral antigens derived from whole disrupted virus in culture are bound to a solid support, usually in microtiter wells. Patient serum is incubated with fixed antigen. Wells are washed, removing all but complexed anti-HIV antibodies if present. Enzyme-conjugated antihuman antibody is then added, followed by substrate. Generally used enzymes (*ENZ*) include horseradish peroxidase, al-kaline phosphatase, β-galactosidase, or glucose oxidase. Enzymatic reaction causes a color change that is proportional to amount of antibody present in sample. An optical density reading is obtained, and the result is read as reactive or nonreactive based on cut-off values for positive and negative controls for that run.

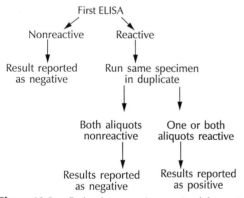

Figure 12.2. Patient's serum is examined for antibody by ELISA. If initial assay is nonreactive, the result is read as negative for anti-HIV. If initial assay is reactive, a second aliquot is assayed in duplicate. If both aliquots are nonreactive, then the result is read as negative for anti-HIV. If one or both assays are reactive, then the result is read as positive for anti-HIV. Only patient specimens that are repeatedly reactive by ELISA are read as positive for anti-HIV. Repeatedly reactive specimens should be confirmed by a supplementary test such as the Western blot or IFA before informing patient of results.

several groups (10, 11). CDC and the Association of State and Territorial Public Health Laboratory Directors (ASTPHLD) have recommended that a positive test be defined by the presence of any two of the following bands: p24, gp41, and gp 120/160 (Table 12.1). These criteria are used by more than 70% of testing laboratories in the United States. Other groups have slightly different criteria for a positive test. All groups agree that a negative test is defined as having no bands. An indeterminate test is one with band(s) not meeting the criteria for a positive test (10, 11). The CDC/AST-PHLD guidelines also stress that no patient be told they are positive until a screening test such as an ELISA has been repeatedly reactive on the same sample and a supplemental test such as Western blot has confirmed the positive ELISA. Persons who test positive by ELISA and are indeterminate by Western blot should be followed clinically and evaluated by other means including an interview for risk factors, a physical exam, immunologic function, and repeat HIV testing. Asymptomatic persons without the usual risk factors for HIV infection who have repeatedly tested positive by ELISA but have remained indeterminate by Western blot for more than 6 months have generally been shown to be uninfected with HIV in studies of blood donors with these results (12).

The current recommendation for HIV testing in the United States is to screen sera with an ELISA and confirm any repeatedly

WESTERN BLOT

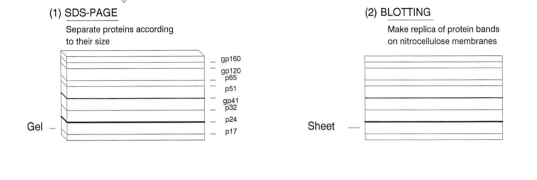

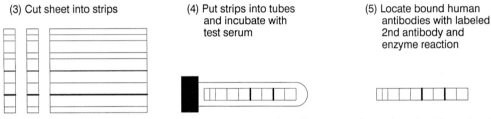

Figure 12.3. For Western blot assay, viral antigens are electrophoresed in a sodium dodecyl sulfate-polyacrylamide gel (*SDS-PAGE*) to separate proteins according to their molecular weight. Separated proteins are transferred onto nitrocellulose, and sheets are cut into strips. A strip is placed into tubes or troughs of a tray and incubated with patient's serum. As with the ELISA, enzyme-conjugated anti-human antibody is added, followed by substrate. A colored band occurs at site of antigen-antibody (from patient serum) complex, identifying specific antibody response to various viral proteins.

Table 12.1. Criteria for Interpretation of Western Blot Tests by Several Organizations[a]

Result	Criteria
Positive	
CDC and ASTPHLD	Any two of these bands: p24, gp41, gp120/gp160
FDA-licensed Du Pont test	p24 and p31 *and* gp41 or gp120/gp160
American Red Cross	At least three bands—one from each gene product group: *gag* and *pol* and *env*
Consortium for retrovirus serology standardization	At least two bands: p24 *or* p31, plus gp41 or gp120/gp160
Negative	No bands present (all groups agree)
Indeterminate	Any pattern other than clearly positive or negative by that group's criteria

[a]From Centers for Disease Control. Interpretation and use of the Western blot assay for serodiagnosis of human immunodeficiency virus type 1 infections. MMWR 1989;38:S3.

reactive tests with either a Western blot assay or IFA. The cost for each positive specimen is about $50 ($3–$5 for (ELISA and $40–$50 for the Western blot). Although this testing algorithm has proven to be highly sensitive and specific, it is not appropriate for use in most developing countries because of its cost, the time needed to complete the testing, the need for sophisticated and costly instruments, and the need for reliable refrigeration of reagents. These problems could be overcome by the use of two rapid HIV tests that would eliminate the use of ELISAs and Western blot tests for testing most sera; the Western blot would only need to be performed on indeterminate sera (positive on one test and negative on the other). The use of a combination of rapid tests could cut testing costs by 50%, save time and labor, and eliminate the need for costly sophisticated instruments.

Several antibody tests for rapid, "on the spot" screening for HIV antibody have been developed. These tests offer several advantages over the standard ELISA tests. They can be performed in a few minutes with materials supplied in the kit or with simple inexpensive equipment. These characteristics make them ideal for blood donation screening in many developing countries that do not have blood storage capabilities. Use of these tests in United States clinic settings, however, offers some advantage in speed and convenience, but a supplemental test is still required to confirm the diagnosis. These rapid tests may be useful in identifying a subset of patients that will likely need further follow-up.

To date, two rapid tests have been licensed by the FDA. One test uses a latex direct agglutination assay and can be performed in fewer than 15 minutes with simple equipment. For this test, serum or whole blood is diluted on a card, mixed with a suspension of antigen-coated latex beads, gently rocked for a few minutes at room temperature, and read with the naked eye for agglutination. Sensitivity and specificity is comparable with licensed ELISA tests (13). However, the end point (agglutination) is a subjective reading, and can be misread by inexperienced technicians.

The second licensed rapid test uses a dot-blot format. This test uses a microfiltration enzyme immunoassay procedure. The solid phase capture reagent is a mixture of latex particles coated with HIV-1 gag (p24) proteins and a purified synthetic peptide representing a conserved and immunodominant sequence of the viral transmembrane protein. The device is a small plastic cartridge designed to filter, concentrate, and absorb all liquid reagents added during the test, including the specimen. The entire test is performed at room temperature. Serum or plasma is mixed with the capture reagent and poured into the plastic cartridge to trap the capture reagent latex beads and any absorbed HIV-1-specific antibodies present in the test specimen. Any bound HIV-1-specific antibodies are detected by addition of anti-human immunoglobulin conjugate and substrate similar to a standard ELISA. A positive or reactive specimen yields a distinct blue in the center circle in the bottom of the cartridge. The entire procedure requires ~10 minutes to perform.

Recent technology for testing dried blood samples collected on filter paper has been developed (14). ELISA, Western blot assay, and IFAs have been adapted for testing for HIV-specific antibody on as little as $5\mu l$ sample. For testing, a 0.25-inch punch from the dried blood spot or collection paper is placed into microtiter plate wells with ELISA diluent buffer, and eluted for several hours. The eluate is then tested by ELISA, and repeatedly reactive specimens are confirmed by Western blot. HIV surveillance with this technique is being used extensively in the United States and other countries for unlinked (no accompanying identifying information) specimens collected from newborns for routine metabolic evaluation (1). Currently, 44 states, Washington DC, and Puerto Rico are participating in a government-sponsored survey to determine the number of infants born to HIV-infected mothers each year. State surveys indicate that prevalence rates are generally stable and that approximately 6000-7000 infants are born each year to HIV-infected women (1). Data from these surveys can also be used to evaluate the effectiveness of HIV counseling and testing programs for pregnant women and their children by comparing the number of HIV-infected women detected through prevention programs with the number that actually gave birth as measured by the unlinked, blinded survey.

Since commercial ELISAs detect IgG, these tests are not sufficient alone to diagnose HIV infection in infants born to HIV-infected mothers because of the persistence of maternal IgG in the infant. Studies have shown that virtually 100% of infants born to HIV-seropositive mothers will test antibody positive at birth, but only about 20–30% will be infected. Those who are uninfected lose maternal antibody usually between 6 and 12 months of age, but a small proportion may retain maternal antibody for up to 18 months (2, 4, 15).

A positive antibody test alone identifies perinatally exposed infant who requires careful follow-up and management (see Chapter 38). Clinical evaluation with repeated testing over at least the first 2 years of life has been the primary means of establishing diagnosis in these infants. Infants who become antibody negative (serorevert) and remain well are generally considered uninfected (16), although there have been a few reports of asymptomatic infants who have seroreverted but have positive virus tests such as culture or PCR (17). In addition, rare reports have described perinatally infected children who had lost maternal antibody and later seroconverted (18, 19). Prospective studies of infants born to HIV-infected women indicate that the frequency of occurrence of antibody-negative/virus-positive children is rare (20, 21).

Repeat Western blot testing over the first year of life and comparison of the band pattern over time can occasionally identify an infected infant. The infant's band pattern at birth is usually identical to the mothers pattern, since most of the detectable antibody is of maternal origin. The appearance of new bands on postneonatal samples that were not present in the birth sample indicates production of antibody by the infant (18, 22).

Rising antibody titers have been used to diagnose other congenital infections in infants, whereas declining titers have been used to indicate noninfection. In the few studies published to date, rising or falling antibody titers have not always correlated with infection status of the infant (18, 23). A more recent study using an IgG capture assay found a rapid decay of maternal antibody in uninfected infants who seroreverted according to the capture assay by age 6 months. HIV-infected infants showed an initial decline followed by a rise at about age 2–3 months (24).

HIV-specific IgA and IgM Assays

Because maternal IgM and IgA antibodies do not cross the placenta, the presence of these HIV-specific antibodies can be used to indicate the presence of HIV infection in infants. Several studies indicate that HIV-specific IgA assays can detect most HIV-infected infants by age 6 months but are generally negative in infected infants younger than 3 months, presumably because HIV-specific IgA antibody is not produced in sufficient quantity to be detected during the first months of life in many infants (25, 26). Less success has been obtained using HIV-specific IgM assays, presumably because production of this antibody type in infants is more transient and at lower serum levels (27). Serum, plasma, and saliva samples have been used for IgA assays (28).

Immunoblot assays for detecting infant HIV-IgA or-IgM antibody require that the more abundant maternal IgG antibody be removed before performing the specific assay for IgA/IgM (29). Failure to remove IgG reduces sensitivity caused by the competing maternal IgG antibody and can cause nonspecific reactions. IgG is generally removed using one or more treatments with recombinant protein G. Samples with high titer IgG may require more than one treatment with protein G for complete removal of maternal IgG, especially samples from African and Haitian infants who tend to have higher concentrations of serum IgG. IgA and IgM antibodies are generally detected using an immunoblot assay, but a recent study found comparable results using an IgA ELISA capture assay (30). This assay does not require removal of IgG and is much less expensive than the immunoblot assay.

p24 Antigen Assay

The standard p24 antigen assay has been a helpful but limited method for diagnosing pediatric HIV infection. Studies of infants born to HIV-infected mothers have found very few infants to be antigen positive early in the course of infection, because of the apparent low levels of antigen in the first month of life and the presence of excess maternal antibody which complexes to any free p24 antigen that is present (15, 3l). The standard p24 antigen assay does not detect p24 that is complexed with antibody, and therefore the test may not be positive unless there are sufficient levels of circulating free p24 antigen.

Despite its limitations for early diagnosis, the antigen test can be helpful in certain settings when virus is likely to be present, but antibody is at low levels or absent. Hypogammaglobulinemic infants with HIV infection can have positive antigen tests (32). Patients (other than infants born to HIV-infected mothers) with recently acquired infection can have detectable antigen levels during the seroconversion between initial infection and before the production of antibody (33).

p24 antigen can be detected in serum from patients in the end stage of their disease process when anti-HIV p24 antibodies may disappear and levels of p24 antigen are high because of increased viral replication. p24 antigen assays have been used to monitor the effect of antiviral therapy in patients with advanced disease (34) and as a prognostic marker for progression to AIDS (35). The antigen assay is also used as the standard method to detect HIV growth in cocultures (36).

Recent studies have shown that modification of the standard p24 antigen assay by acidification of the sample to dissociate the immune complexes can increase sensitivity of the assay to detect HIV infection in infants (37–39). The immune complex dissociation p24 antigen assay has been shown to be highly sensitive and specific for diagnosis of HIV infection in infants, although samples taken in the first week of life have been somewhat problematic in that false-positive and false-negative tests have been observed. Licensed assay kits using this methodology are not yet available in the United States, but ongoing clinical trials in infants of different ages and at different disease stages should establish advantages and limitations of this assay for pediatric diagnosis of HIV infection in the near future.

In the standard p24 antigen assay (Fig. 12.4), patient serum is incubated with anti-HIV-p24 bound to a solid support. Free (non-complexed) HIV antigen, if present, is "captured" by the bound antibody. All other material (including patient HIV antigen-antibody complexes) is washed off. Rabbit anti-HIV antibody is then added along with antirabbit antibody conjugate and substrate, which produces a color change if the test specimen contains HIV p24 antigen. Specimens that are repeatedly reactive should undergo a neutralization assay to ver-

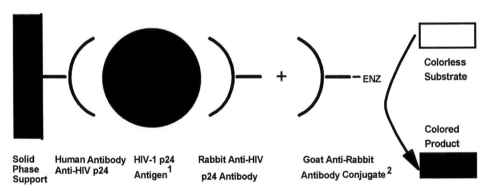

Solid Phase Support   **Human Antibody Anti-HIV p24**   **HIV-1 p24 Antigen**[1]   **Rabbit Anti-HIV p24 Antibody**   **Goat Anti-Rabbit Antibody Conjugate**[2]

[1] Serum specimen from patient

[2] Enzymes include: Horseradish peroxidase
Alkaline phosphatase, β-galactosidase, Glucose oxidase

Figure 12.4. For the HIV p24 antigen assay, anti-HIV antibody is bound to a solid support and is incubated with patient serum. Free (noncomplexed) HIV antigen, if present, reacts with antibody. All other material (including patient HIV antigen-antibody complexes) is washed off. A rabbit anti-HIV p24 antibody and a goat antirabbit antibody enzyme conjugate is then added along with substrate, which produces a color change. Generally used enzymes (*ENZ*) include horseradish peroxidase, alkaline phosphatase, β-galactosidase, or glucose oxidase. Reactive specimens are run in duplicate. Specimens that are repeatedly reactive should undergo an antibody neutralization assay to verify the presence of HIV antigen (not shown). Instructions for neutralization assay are supplied in package insert from manufacturer.

ify the presence of HIV antigen (not shown in Fig. 12.4). The acid dissociation method uses the same methodology except that samples are pretreated with acid to dissociate the immune complexes allowing for the detection of the free HIV p24 antigen (39).

HIV Culture

Virus culture is one of the most sensitive techniques for detecting HIV infection in infants and has been used extensively in research settings. Microcultures in 12-, 24-, and 96-well plates are equally sensitive and specific compared with standard flask methods and require far less blood (40). Virus cultures may be difficult to perform for many laboratories, because they require considerable experience and special facilities to deal with biosafety precautions to prevent exposure of laboratory personnel. HIV culture is not useful as a rapid diagnostic test, because cultures typically take 7–28 days or more to complete.

The standard isolation technique involves coculturing patients' peripheral blood mononuclear cells (PBMC) that have been separated from whole blood with phytohemagglutinin-stimulated PBMC feeder cells from healthy uninfected donors. At least 2×10^6 patient cells should be cocultivated with an equal number of donor cells. The cocultured cells should be stimulated with T cell growth factor (interleukin-2), which appears to enhance viral growth. Cultures must be supplemented every 3–5 days with feeder cells and monitored at least weekly for the presence of virus by antigen or reverse transcriptase production (41, 42).

Ultracentrifugation concentrates viral particles and has been reported to enhance detection of p24 antigen in culture supernatants and shorten the time required for detection of a positive culture (43). This modification reduces the amount of laboratory and technician time required for positive cultures, thus reducing cost and increasing efficiency. One note of caution: investigators recommend use of the confirmatory neutralization assay for p24 antigen assay that is used for detecting virus in the culture, because of possible reduced specificity when using ultracentrifugation.

Polymerase Chain Reaction

PCR is one of the most sensitive diagnostic techniques for detecting HIV infection. HIV is an RNA retrovirus that transcribes its RNA into DNA using the viral enzyme, reverse transcriptase, after entry into the human host cell. These DNA sequences, termed proviral DNA, can then integrate into the human cellular DNA. Because the amount of proviral DNA is very small compared with the amount of human DNA and because the number of infected cells in the blood is small, direct detection of proviral DNA with standard molecular biologic techniques is not feasible. PCR is a method for amplifying proviral DNA up to 1 million times or more to increase the probability of detection.

PCR can be used for diagnosing HIV infection in infants by detection of proviral DNA in PBMCs. Studies evaluating the use of PCR for early diagnosis of HIV infection in infants have shown that ~30–50% of HIV-infected infants will test positive around the time of birth (15, 44). This percentage increases to nearly 100% by age 1–3 months. These sensitivities are comparable with those of virus culture (43). In situ PCR techniques that detect the presence of HIV in specific cells or tissues (45) and quantitative PCR techniques to measure viral load have also been developed.

PCR can also be used to measure active virus replication by detecting viral RNA in plasma (44). Amplification of RNA virus sequences of HIV, as would be found in viral particles in plasma or from messenger RNA in infected cells, can be performed by first making a DNA copy using a commercially available reverse transcriptase enzyme. RNA PCR is most useful for monitoring circulating virus and should not be used in place of DNA PCR for routine diagnostic purposes, because plasma viremia is not always detectable in HIV-infected persons. A recent study used RNA PCR to examine newborn plasma samples and found that 7 of 10 HIV-infected infants had detectable HIV-1 RNA at 4–9 weeks, whereas only 1 of these infants had detectable RNA at birth (44).

In addition to diagnosing infected infants, both PCR and virus culture can also be used to evaluate infants who lose maternal antibody. Several studies indicate that infants who lose maternal antibody and remain healthy are uninfected based on negative virus cultures and PCR (20, 21). Some laboratories have reported rare seroreverting children who will occasionally test positive by PCR on a single specimen, but negative on subsequent specimens (20, 21). The reasons why these infants tested positive on one occasion are unclear. A mix-up in specimens or other laboratory errors is one possible explanation. Alternatively, transient PCR positivity may represent 1) true infection that has cleared, 2) a proviral blood level that is below the level detectable by the test, or 3) maternal blood cell contamination. Continued evaluation of these infants is important.

Because PCR detects the presence of HIV proviral DNA rather than antibody to the virus, it avoids the problem of persistent maternal antibody. PCR requires <1 ml blood, an amount that is feasible to obtain from a newborn. Unlike virus culture that can take up to 4 weeks or longer to complete, PCR testing can be performed in 1–2 days.

For detection of HIV proviral DNA, standard PCR sample preparation requires separation of PBMCs from a blood specimen using a Ficoll-hypaque gradient. After preparation of the PBMCs, the cells are incubated with nonionic detergents followed by treatment with proteinase K to liberate cellular DNA. Proteinase K is then inactivated by heating, and the resulting DNA preparation is ready for PCR; 1 μg DNA (equivalent to the DNA from ~150,000 mononuclear cells) is routinely used per PCR reaction. The PCR technique is a three-step repetitive process (Fig. 12.5): 1) denaturation of cellular double stranded DNA into single strands, 2) annealing of specific primers to the target sequences, and 3) extension of the annealed primers. If a specific RNA sequence is to be amplified, a DNA copy (cDNA) of the RNA sequence is produced using the enzyme reverse transcriptase before PCR amplification of the resulting DNA.

After PCR amplification, many techniques can be used to detect the amplified DNA sequences. Typically, confirmation of amplification of HIV DNA requires hy-bridization of an aliquot of the amplified DNA to a synthetic DNA probe that is complementary to a portion of the amplified-DNA sequence. The probe can be labeled by various means, both isotopic (radioactive) or nonisotopic (colorimetric or chemiluminescent).

A PCR system for qualitative detection of HIV-1 has been developed as a simplified diagnostic kit (46). This kit should provide ease of use through a user-friendly system format while providing the inherent sensitivity and specificity of any research PCR assay. The kit consists of three components: 1) a specimen collection and preparation kit, 2) an amplification kit, and 3) a detection kit. All components are premixed for easy and reliable amplification and detection using the familiar microwell plate colorimetric format. The test specimen is whole blood, and ambient temperature storage allows for convenient shipping of clinical specimens. The whole blood lysis procedure is an easy method that utilizes only 0.5 ml blood. This small sample volume is especially beneficial for testing infants. A modified procedure utilizing 0.1 ml blood has also been developed. In the whole blood lysis procedure, red blood cells are selectively lysed in the procedure while the leukocytes remain intact. Leukocytes are pelleted and washed several times, and the final pellet is extracted for DNA. The entire procedure takes fewer than 2 hrs. A 50-μl aliquot (representing DNA from ~200,000 cells) is used to amplify proviral HIV-1 DNA. Biotinylated primers used to amplify the HIV-1 DNA represent a 142-base pair sequence of the *gag* gene region. These primers have been tested on thousands of samples and amplify all efficiently, detecting virtually 100% of HIV-1 isolates worldwide.

In the early days of PCR, the exquisite sensitivity of the technique and the potential to amplify minute amounts of contaminating material from previous reactions resulted in problems of false positivity. Extremely small amounts of amplified target (patient) DNA (10^{-8} μl) from a previous amplification contaminating a reaction tube may result in a false-positive reaction. To solve this problem, deoxyuridine triphosphate is incorporated into the ampli-

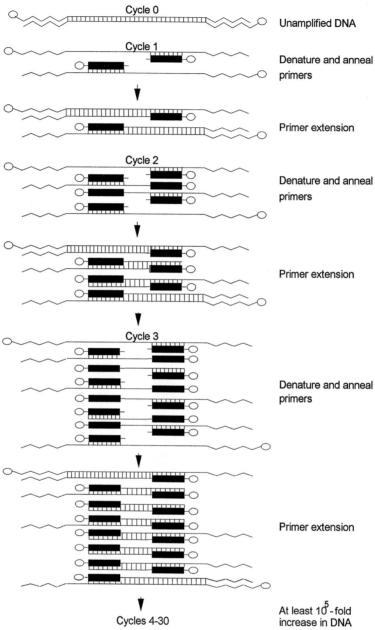

Figure 12.5. PCR involves separating double-stranded DNA from patient's peripheral blood mononuclear cells into two single strands by heating (denaturization). When cooled, DNA strands containing HIV proviral sequences reanneal with complementary nucleotide sequences of primers specific for HIV that have been added in vast excess. A thermostable DNA polymerase catalyzes synthesis of new strands of DNA by adding nucleotides complementary to unpaired DNA strand onto annealed primer (primer extension). At this point (cycle 1), the number of DNA strands containing HIV proviral sequence has doubled. This cycle of heating, cooling, and synthesis of new DNA strands is then repeated multiple times resulting in enormous amplification of targeted sequence. HIV proviral sequences can be detected by hybridization with a synthetic HIV DNA probe labeled with a radioactive phosphate group (^{32}P) or nonisotopically using probes labeled by other means such as with an acridinium ester yielding a chemiluminescent readout (not shown). An ELISA format can also be used for detection of amplified sequences.

fication reaction, making it possible to distinguish amplified DNA from native thymidine-containing DNA found in patient specimen cellular DNA. The active enzyme, uracil-*N*-glycosylase, selectively recognizes and destroys the U-containing amplicons (the contaminating material) while leaving target DNA from the patient specimen unaffected. Because all amplified products are synthesized with deoxyuridine triphosphate rather than deoxythymidine triphosphate (as in the patient specimen), all amplified products will be susceptible to uracil-*N*-glycosylase activity in subsequent reactions. The development of this procedure was critical to the successful transfer of PCR from the research laboratory to the clinical laboratory.

All reagents necessary for amplification are provided in the kit, and it is only necessary to add uracil-*N*-glycosylase to the premixed master mix vial and 50 μl premixed master mix to the appropriate number of amplification tubes. Then 50 μl of prepared specimen are added to the appropriate tube: the tube is capped, and the rack of reaction tubes is placed in the thermal cycler. After the amplification cycle, the reaction tubes should be held at 72°C until the denaturation solution is added.

Detection is based on the ELISA-like colorimetric microwell plate format. Amplified DNA is captured by DNA probes that are specific for HIV and have been coated on the bottom of the well of the microwell plate. Specificity of the detection is given by the bovine serum albumin-conjugated probe that is coated onto the walls of the microplate wells. Denatured amplification reaction is pipetted into the wells that contain the hybridization solution. The plate is covered and incubated for 1 hr at 37°C. After the 1-hr hybridization, the plate is washed; avidin-horseradish peroxidase conjugate is added to the wells and incubated for 15 min at 37°C. The plate is then washed again, and the substrate-chromogen is added. Color development is allowed to proceed for 10 min at room temperature in the dark. Acidic stop solution is added to the wells, and the resulting absorbances are read at 450 nm. The test kit should prove to be rapid, easy to perform, and amenable for use in the clinical labora-

tory. This system should also provide a means to standardize testing among laboratories and is under investigation by many designated clinical trial sites in the United States for FDA licensure. Once the kit is licensed, it will likely become the standard method for diagnosis of HIV infection in infants because of its high sensitivity and specificity and rapid method.

In Vitro Antibody Production Assays

Another promising technique for infant diagnosis is the in vitro antibody production assay (IVAP). This assay detects the presence of HIV-specific antibody-producing B lymphocytes in the infant, which indicates that the infant's immune system has been stimulated by HIV infection. IVAP assays require less time to complete than culture. The standard IVAP assays require 7–10 days to complete and the ELISPOT (described below) can be performed in 1–2 days.

Two methods for this technique have been described. In one method, PBMCs are separated from whole blood, carefully washed to remove plasma, placed in medium, and stimulated to produce antibody with either pokeweed mitogen (47) or Epstein-Barr virus (48). HIV-sensitized B cells will produce antibody that is released into the culture supernatant. HIV-specific antibody in culture supernatants can be detected using standard methods.

In an alternative method, called ELISPOT (49), washed PBMCs are placed in wells with nitrocellulose membrane bottoms coated with HIV antigen (Fig.12.6). Cells are incubated, washed, then treated sequentially with biotinylated antihuman IgG, horseradish-conjugated avidin, and enzyme substrate. The appearance of spots on the nitrocellulose membrane indicates the presence of HIV-specific antibody-producing lymphocytes in the patient.

Both types of assays for detecting antibody-producing cells have been successful in identifying HIV-infected infants, but there are some important limitations. False-positive tests in uninfected infants have been reported in the first 2 months of life. These spurious results might result from the detection of maternal B lymphocytes

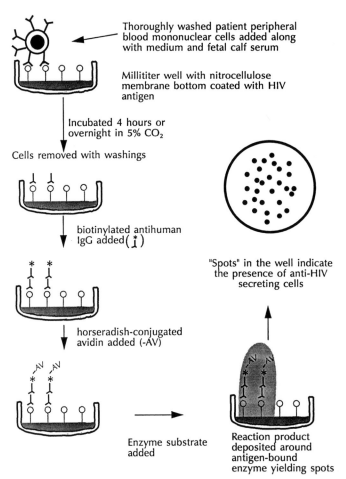

Figure 12.6. For the ELISPOT assay, washed peripheral blood mononuclear cells are placed in wells with nitrocellulose membrane bottoms coated with HIV antigen. Cells are incubated, washed, then treated sequentially with biotinylated antihuman IgG, horseradish-conjugated avidin, and enzyme substrate. Appearance of spots on nitrocellulose membrane indicates presence of HIV-specific antibody-producing lymphocytes.

that are producing antibody but may not harbor the virus, although this has not been carefully studied. Additionally, in the presence of abundant maternal IgG in the infant's serum, false-positive tests may result from maternal anti-HIV antibody that has adhered to infant B cells in the culture. The ELISPOT method may be able to differentiate between this carry-over of maternal antibodies from true HIV antibody-producing cells (50). The adsorbed antibody will yield a diffuse pink background staining that can be readily distinguished from the intense red spots resulting from true antibody-producing cells.

False-negative IVAP tests have been observed in HIV-infected persons with ad-

vanced immunodeficiency who cannot produce antibody. Active virus replication is the stimulus for the replication of antibody-producing cells. Suppression of viral replication by immune mechanisms or by antiviral therapy could suppress production of antibody-producing cells below the level of detection. In one study, 22 (63%) of 34 asymptomatic HIV-seropositive persons, 12 (75%) of 16 symptomatic patients, and 1 (8%) of 13 zidovudine-treated symptomatic patients were ELISPOT positive (49). Another study found that although some zidovudine-treated patients were IVAP negative 3–5 months after starting therapy, most were positive when tested after more than 6 months of treatment (48).

Surrogate Tests—Immunologic Parameters

Tests that measure immunologic abnormalities most commonly associated with HIV infection can also be useful for diagnosis in infants and children. According to the criteria in the CDC classification system for HIV disease in children, the combination of both humoral and cellular immunodeficiency in a symptomatic infant born to an HIV-infected mother is diagnostic of HIV infection in the absence of specific diagnostic tests (16). The classic immunologic abnormalities include low T helper (CD4+) lymphocyte counts for age; elevated T suppressor (CD8+) counts (particularly early on), reversed CD4:CD8 ratio, depressed lymphocyte responses to mitogens, strikingly elevated immunoglobulin levels (most commonly IgG) or rarely hypogammaglobulinemia, and decreased specific antibody responses (9). In adults, decreasing CD4+ cell counts and elevated β_2 microglobulin and neopterin levels frequently herald the development of AIDS (35).

CD4+ cell counts are used to monitor immunosuppression and disease progression in infants. Guidelines based on CD4+ cell counts or percentages for age indicating a need for initiating *Pneumocystis carinii* prophylaxis have been published (51), and guidelines for initiating antiretroviral therapy are under development (see Chapters 21 and 35).

QUANTITATION OF HIV IN BLOOD

Techniques that measure the level of HIV in blood and other tissues have been used to monitor antiviral therapy and to study the pathogenesis of HIV in children. Picograms of p24 antigen per milliliter serum or plasma can be measured, and this assay is often used to monitor the effectiveness of antiretroviral therapy (34). Quantitative cultures can also be performed; the technique involves coculturing serial dilutions of patient PBMCs (separated from whole blood) with a constant number of uninfected donor cells (52). Cultures are then monitored in the same way as described above (see "HIV Culture"). The lowest dilution of cells required to produce a positive culture is the

end point, and the titer of HIV is expressed as the tissue culture infective dose per 10^6 cells. Plasma viral titers can also be measured using serial dilutions of plasma cultured in the same manner as above and results expressed as tissue culture infective dose per milliter plasma (52). By these techniques, studies have found that the mean viral titers in plasma were lowest in asymptomatic HIV-infected patients and higher in symptomatic patients (52). Likewise, the percentage of infected PBMCs was also lowest among asymptomatic patients and higher among symptomatic patients.

PCR can also be used to quantitate virus load with techniques that are less biohazardous and time-consuming compared with the culture techniques (53). DNA lysates of patient PBMCs are serially diluted, amplified, and detected with probes. The signal intensity from each aliquot of serially diluted patient sample are compared with PCR performed on serial dilutions of a plasmid containing a full-length copy of HIV-1 DNA or DNA from a cell line containing one integrated copy of HIV-1 proviral DNA per cell. A rapid, quantitative detection technique has been described that uses a nonisotopic chemiluminescent DNA probe (54). Plasma viremia could also be quantitated by use of RNA PCR on virus concentrated from known volumes of plasma.

HIV-2 INFECTION

In 1986, a second HIV called HIV-2 was isolated from both asymptomatic patients (55) and those with AIDS (56). Most infected persons reside in West African countries or have been exposed sexually or parenterally to residents of these countries. Fewer than 50 cases have been reported in the United States (57). HIV-2 can be transmitted perinatally but appears to be less transmissible compared with HIV-l. In one study, 28% of HIV-1-infected mothers transmitted to their infants compared with 3% of HIV-2-infected mothers (58).

In June 1992, routine screening of the United States blood supply for HIV-2 was initiated. Most blood banks use a combination test that simultaneously detects antibodies to both HIV-l and HIV-2 but does not indicate which virus is present.

The core antigens of HIV-1 and HIV-2 share some common epitopes, but their external gpl20 glycoproteins share fewer epitopes and exhibit minimal cross reactivity (59). Sera from HIV-2-infected persons usually cross reacts with HIV-l ELISA antibody tests using whole virus lysates, and, vice versa, HIV-1 sera will frequently cross react similarly with HIV-2 in the whole viral lysate antibody test. Thus additional testing with specific assays are required to differentiate the two viruses. Whether using a combination test for antibody to both HIV types or separate ELISA tests for each virus, repeatedly positive assays must be confirmed with more specific confirmatory tests to verify infection. HIV-2-specific Western blots, synthetic peptide assays, PCR, and viral cultures may be needed for definitive diagnosis of HIV-2 infection (60). Confirmatory tests for HIV-2 have recently become available, and reference laboratories such as those at CDC can perform such tests when indicated. An algorithm for the laboratory diagnosis of HIV-1 and HIV-2 infection has been recommended by the United States Public Health Service (Fig. 12.7) (60).

FACTORS AFFECTING PERFORMANCE OF DIAGNOSTIC ASSAYS

Several factors must be considered when choosing assays for diagnosis of perinatal HIV infection. Probably the most important is age of the infant at the time of testing. Although the precise kinetics of virus replication and antibody production remain to be defined, several studies indicate that virus load is probably lowest at the time of birth in most infants and increases during the first few months of life (15, 43, 44). IgA antibody production appears to also be low during the first few months of life (25, 26). IVAP assays may yield false-positive results in the first 1–2 months of life (see "In Vitro Antibody Production Assay"). Thus, in the neonatal period, most studies have shown that the greatest percentage of infected infants are detected using sensitive virologic assays such as PCR or virus culture, whereas several assays can detect infection by age 3–6 months (61). Even the most sensitive assays can detect no more than 50% of infected infants around the time of birth; presumably because the viral load is extremely low, virus is suppressed or sequestered in

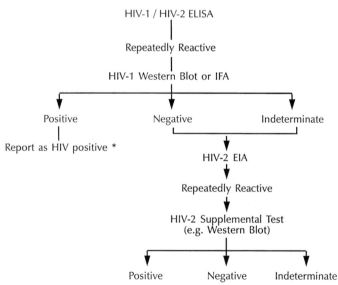

Figure 12.7.   CDC and FDA testing algorithm for use with combination HIV-1/HIV-2 ELISAs. If HIV-1/HIV-2 combination ELISA is repeatedly reactive, an HIV-1 Western blot or IFA is performed. If the HIV-1 Western blot is negative or indeterminate, an HIV-2 ELISA should be performed. Repeatedly reac- tive HIV-2 ELISAs should be confirmed with supplemental tests such as HIV-2 Western blot. * If positive, patient should be told that they are HIV positive. In this case, only patients with identified risk factors for HIV-2 infection should be further tested with HIV-2-specific tests to differentiate virus type.

other tissues, or infection has only recently been transmitted in the case of intrapartum transmission. Figure 12.8 summarizes the sensitivity of the various assays to detect HIV infection by age at time of testing.

The stage of disease also affects the likelihood that a given assay will detect HIV infection in perinatally infected infants and in older children and adults. As disease progresses, the virus load both in the plasma and percentage of infected cells increases (52, 62), and it has been reported that phenotypic properties of the virus swarm change from slowly growing to rapidly growing and syncytia forming (63). Assays that detect the virus, its proteins, or virus genome are more likely to be positive during later stages of the disease compared with earlier, asymptomatic stages in infants. Some severely immunosuppressed adults and children with end-stage disease may lose antibody. Some perinatally infected infants may be hypogammaglobulinemic and will not produce antibody.

Some antiretroviral therapies may affect results of diagnostic tests by lowering virus load. Patients who tested p24 antigen positive before therapy may become negative after therapy. Reducing the virus load decreases the stimulus for antibody production, and IVAP and ELISPOT assays may also become negative (48, 49).

Finally the timing of transmission may also affect the likelihood of early detection of infection in perinatally infected infants.

Theoretically, infants infected in utero should be positive at birth, whereas those infected late in pregnancy and during the intrapartum or postpartum periods may not become positive until sometime after birth.

PRACTICAL ASPECTS OF DIAGNOSTIC ASSAYS

Several practical aspects of the various diagnostic assays must to be considered including costs, technical difficulty of the assay and sample preparation, time required to complete the assay, commercial availability, and FDA licensure (61). The routine use of certain assays may vary depending on sophistication of the laboratory and available technology and resources. Many developing countries have additional considerations such as availability of equipment, consistent electrical power, purified water, and trained laboratory personnel.

Table 12.2 summarizes several of these practical aspects. Unfortunately the most sensitive and specific assays for the earliest diagnosis (e.g., virus culture) are also the most technically difficult and costly. Although availability of PCR is limited, test kits are under development. These kits have greatly simplified sample preparation and require only 0.1–0.5 ml blood, which is critical for testing infants for whom obtaining blood samples is often problematic. The costs of these kits, however, may be prohibitively expensive for most developing coun-

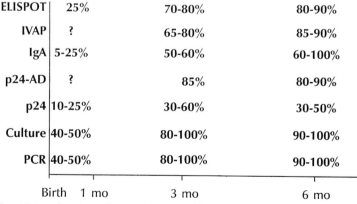

	Birth	1 mo	3 mo	6 mo
ELISPOT	25%		70-80%	80-90%
IVAP	?		65-80%	85-90%
IgA	5-25%		50-60%	60-100%
p24-AD	?		85%	80-90%
p24	10-25%		30-60%	30-50%
Culture	40-50%		80-100%	90-100%
PCR	40-50%		80-100%	90-100%

Figure 12.8. Sensitivity of various diagnostic tests by age of infant at time of testing. Percentages represent sensitivity of diagnostic test to identify HIV-infected infants at a given age. In general, sensitivity is lowest at birth and is increased thereafter. *IgA*, HIV-specific IgA assay; *p24 AD*, acid dissociation p24 antigen assay.

Table 12.2. Practical Aspects to Be Considered When Choosing Diagnostic Tests for Infants Born to HIV-infected Mothers[a]

Assay	Overall Sensitivity/Specificity[b]	Technical Difficulty	Time to Result	Specimen Required	Cost[c]
			days		
Culture	++++/++++	High	15–35	PBMC	$250
PCR	++++/++++	High[d]	1–2	PBMC[d]	$175
p24 Antigen[e]	++/+++[f]	Low	1–2	Serum/plasma	$25
IgA	+++/+++[f]	Low	1–2	Serum/plasma	$10–50
IVAP	+++/++[f]	Moderate	7–10	PBMC	$50–75
ELISPOT	+++/+++	Moderate	1–2	PBMC	$20–30

[a]From Anonymous. Early diagnosis of HIV infection in infants. Consensus Workshop, Siena, Jan 1992. J Acquir Immune Defic Syndr 1992;5:1169–1178.
[b]Sensitivity of assay for detecting HIV-infected infants, specificity of assay in giving negative results for uninfected infants; both consider reliability of the test at different ages. ++++ excellent, +++ good, ++ moderate, + poor.
[c]Approximate commercial costs.
[d]Current methods for PCR are technically difficult and require PBMC. Newer methods under development are of moderate technical difficulty and can be performed using whole blood.
[e]Standard assay that does not use acid hydrolysis.

tries. Other less technically difficult assays such as the serologic tests may prove to be more practical for these settings.

The type of sample and sample preparation must also be considered. Virus culture and currently used methods for PCR, IVAP, and ELISPOT require that mononuclear cells be separated from whole blood, which is more difficult and time consuming than separating serum or plasma for serologic tests such as p24 antigen or antibody ELISA. PCR kits under development offer the advantage of using whole blood samples. Although venipuncture samples are often difficult to obtain and are limited in volume in newborns, cord blood samples are not generally recommended for use in diagnosis unless careful attention is paid to collection to prevent maternal blood contamination (64). This is often not possible in most hospital delivery room settings.

A diagnostic algorithm to be used as a guide for choosing diagnostic tests is shown in Figure 12.9. This algorithm includes age at time of testing, whether the child is symptomatic or asymptomatic, and predictive value of the assay at a given age. The algorithm assumes that the infants are not being breast fed (no ongoing exposure after birth) and that the health care provider would choose the most cost-efficient assay whenever possible. Tests with greater sensitivity (but also greater cost) such as PCR or virus culture would be used to clarify negative or inconclusive results from the less expensive assays.

For children up to 6 months old, PCR and virus culture are recommended because of the greater sensitivity of these tests at this age. HIV IgA or p24 antigen assays are another option particularly in children 3–6 months old, but these tests are less likely to be positive in infected infants younger than 3–6 months as discussed earlier. The IVAP assays should not be used for diagnosis in children younger than 3 months unless technical modifications under study are found to eliminate the problem of maternal antibody adherence.

For children 6–18 months old an initial standard antibody test should be performed to determine whether seroreversion (loss of maternal antibody) has already occurred. If the antibody test is negative on initial and repeat testing, this child should be considered uninfected unless further follow-up reveals other signs or symptoms of HIV disease. Children 6–18 months old with positive antibody tests should be tested with other assays as indicated in the algorithm. Until the reliability of these assays for early diagnosis are firmly established, the tests should be repeated, and when possible another test should be used to confirm the diagnosis.

FUTURE PROSPECTS

Continued development of highly sensitive and specific tests for detecting HIV infection will be necessary to better understand when the virus is transmitted from

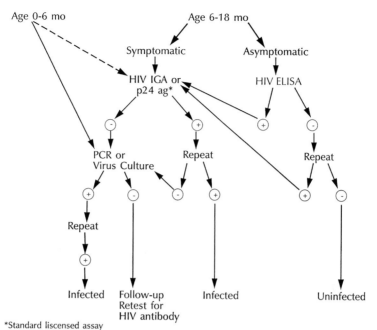

Figure 12.9. Diagnostic testing algorithm for infants born to HIV-infected mothers which assumes that infants are not being breast fed (no ongoing exposure after birth) and that health care provider would choose a less expensive assay whenever possible. Tests with greater sensitivity (but also greater cost) such as PCR or virus culture would be used to clarify negative or inconclusive results from the less expensive assays. For children 0–6 months old, PCR and virus culture is recommended because of the greater sensitivity of these tests at this age. HIV IgA or p24 antigen assays are another option particularly in children 3–6 months old, but these tests are less likely to be positive in infected infants younger than 3–6 months. IVAP assays should not be used for diagnosis in children younger than 3 months unless technical modifications under study are found to eliminate the problem of maternal antibody adherence. For asymptomatic children 6–18 months old an initial standard antibody test should be performed to determine whether seroreversion (loss of maternal antibody) has already occurred. If antibody test is negative on initial and repeat testing, this child should be considered uninfected unless follow-up reveals other signs or symptoms. Children aged 6–18 months with positive antibody tests should be tested with other assays as indicated in algorithm. Repeat testing of children at any age with positive results is recommended to eliminate laboratory or other error.

mother to infant and to detect the virus in infants early in their illness. With this information, more effective approaches to prevention of infection or amelioration of disease in the fetus and newborn can be developed. For example, if most transmission occurs early in gestation, then interventions aimed at treating the infected pregnant woman and fetus would need to be further developed. Trials of antiretrovirals in pregnant women to prevent perinatal transmission are already in place. Early identification of infected pregnant women then becomes critical and further emphasizes the need for prevention programs for pregnant women that include prenatal testing, counseling, and provision of health care services for both mother and infant.

For preventing transmission that occurs near or at the time of birth, additional strategies may be needed. Antiviral treatment of the mother late in gestation or at the time of labor and delivery might still be effective, but greater emphasis should be given to other possible interventions such as HIV hyperimmune globulin and possibly HIV vaccination.

Regardless of the strategy for prevention and treatment, effective intervention for HIV and various other health problems requires adequate provision of primary health care and prenatal and family planning services for indigent, often minority, women and their children. We must address these basic health care needs in our communities in addition to providing specific strategies for eliminating HIV transmission and infection.

References

1. Gwinn M, Pappaioanou M, George R, et al. Prevalence of HIV infection in childbearing women in the United States: Surveillance using newborn blood samples. JAMA 1991;265:1704–1708.
2. European Collaborative Study. Risk factors for mother-to-child transmission of HIV-1. Lancet 1992;339:1007–1012.
3. Mayers MM, Davenny K, Schoenbaum EE, et al. A prospective study of infants of human immunodeficiency virus seropositive and seronegative women with a history of intravenous drug use or of intravenous drug-using sex partners in the Bronx, New York City. Pediatrics 1991;88:1248–1256.
4. Blanche S, Rouzioux C, Moscato MG, et al. A prospective study of infants born to women seropositive for human immunodeficiency virus type 1. N Engl J Med 1989;320:1643–1648.
5. Gabiano C, Tovo P-A, de Martino M, et al. Mother-to-child transmission of human immunodeficiency virus type 1: Risk of infection and correlates of transmission. Pediatrics 1992;90:369–374.
6. Ryder RW, Nsa E, Hassig SE, et al. Perinatal transmission of the human immunodeficiency virus type 1 to infants of seropositive women in Zaire. N Engl J Med 1989;320:1637–1642.
7. Horsburgh CR, Ou C-Y, Jason J, et al. Duration of human immunodeficiency virus infection before detection of antibody. Lancet 1989;2:637–640.
8. Weber JN, Weiss RA, Roberts C, et al. Human immunodeficiency virus infection in two cohorts of homosexual men: Neutralizing sera and association of anti-gag antibody with prognosis. Lancet 1987;1:119–122.
9. Parks WP, Scott GB. An overview of pediatric AIDS: Approaches to diagnosis and outcome assessment. In: Broder S, ed. AIDS—modern concepts and therapeutic challenges. New York: Marcel Dekker, 1987:245–262.
10. Centers for Disease Control. Interpretation and use of the Western blot assay for serodiagnosis of human immunodeficiency virus type 1 infections. MMWR 1989;38:S1–S7.
11. Centers for Disease Control. Interpretive criteria used to report Western blot results for HIV-1-antibody testing—United States. MMWR 1991;40:692–695.
12. Jackson JB, MacDonald K, Cadwell J, et al. Absence of HIV infection in blood donors with indeterminate Western blot tests for antibody to HIV-1. N Engl J Med 1990;322:217–222.
13. Francis HL, Kabeya M, Kafuama N, et al. Comparison of sensitivities and specificities of latex agglutination and an enzyme-linked immunosorbent assay for detection of antibodies to the human immunodeficiency virus in African sera. J Clin Microbiol 1988;26:2462–2464.
14. Hoff R, Berardi VP, Weiblen BJ, Mahoney-Trout L, Mitchell ML, Grady GF. Seroprevalence of human immunodeficiency virus among childbearing women. N Engl J Med 1988;318:525–530.
15. Rogers MF, Ou C-Y, Rayfield M, et al. Use of the polymerase chain reaction for early detection of the proviral sequences of human immunodeficiency virus in infants born to seropositive mothers. N Engl J Med 1989;320:1649–1654.
16. Centers for Disease Control. Classification system for human immunodeficiency virus (HIV) infection in children under 13 years of age. MMWR 1987;36:225–236.
17. European Collaborative Study. Mother to child transmission of HIV infection. Lancet 1988;2:1039–1043.
18. Johnson JP, Nair P, Hines SE, et al. Natural history and serologic diagnosis of infants born to human immunodeficiency virus-infected women. Am J Dis Child 1989;143:1147–1153.
19. Aiuti F, Luzi G, Mezzaroma I, Scano G, Papetti C. Delayed appearance of HIV infection in children [Letter]. Lancet 1987;2:858.
20. Jones DS, Abrams E, Ou C-Y, et al. The lack of detectable human immunodeficiency virus (HIV) infection in antibody-negative children born to HIV-infected mothers. Pediatr Infect Dis J 1993;12:222–227.
21. Wiznia A, Conroy J, Liu HK, Nozyce M. Virus isolation, PCR, and neurodevelopmental delay in children who are HIV seroreverters (P-3) [Abstract ThC 1578]. Eighth International Conference on AIDS, Amsterdam, Jul 1992.
22. Johnson JP, Nair P, Alexander S. Early diagnosis of HIV infection in the neonate [Letter]. N Engl J Med 1987;316:273–274.
23. Scott GB, Hutto C, Parks WP. HIV-1 infection in infants: Practical laboratory diagnosis. In: Hudson CN, Sharp F, eds. AIDS and obstetrics and gynecology. London: Royal College of Obstetricians and Gynecologists, 1988:95–100.
24. Parekh, B, Shaffer N, Schochetman G, et al. Dynamics of maternal IgG antibody decay and HIV-specific antibody synthesis in infants born to seropositive mothers. Eighth International Conference on AIDS, Amsterdam, Jul 1992.
25. Quinn TC, Kline RL, Halsey N, et al. Early diagnosis of perinatal HIV infection by detection of viral-specific IgA antibodies. JAMA 1991;266:3439–3442.
26. Landesman S, Weiblen B, Mendez H, et al. Clinical utility of HIV-IgA immunoblot assay in the early diagnosis of perinatal HIV infection. JAMA 1991;266:3443–3446.
27. Weiblen BJ, Lee FK, Cooper ER, et al. Early diagnosis of HIV infection in infants by detection of IgA HIV antibodies. Lancet 1990;335:988–990.
28. Archibald DW, Johnson JP, Nair P, et al. Detection of salivary immunoglobulin A antibodies to HIV-1 in infants and children. AIDS 1990;4:417–420.
29. Weiblen BJ, Schumacher RT, Hoff R. Detection of IgM and IgA HIV antibodies after removal of IgG with recombinant protein G. J Immunol Methods 1990;126:199–204.
30. Parekh BS, Shaffer N, Coughlin R, et al. HIV-1-specific IgA-capture enzyme immunoassay and IgA-Western blot assay for early diagnosis of HIV-1 infection in infants. Pediatr Infect Dis J, in press
31. Borkowsky W, Krasinski K, Paul D, et al. Human immunodeficiency virus type 1 antigenemia in children. J Pediatr 1989;114:940–945.

32. Borkowsky W, Krasinski K, Paul D, Moore T, Bebenroth D, Chandwani S. Human-immunodeficiency-virus infections in infants negative for anti-HIV by enzyme-linked immunoassay. Lancet 1987;1:1168–1171.

33. Ward JW, Holmberg SD, Allen JR, et al. Transmission of human immunodeficiency virus (HIV) by blood transfusions screened as negative for HIV antibody. N Engl J Med 1988;318:473–478.

34. Chaisson RE, Allain J, Volberding PA. Significant changes in HIV antigen level in the serum of patients treated with azidothymidine. N Engl J Med 1986;315:1610–1611.

35. Fahey JL, Taylor JMG, Detels R, et al. The prognostic value of cellular and serologic markers in infection with human immunodeficiency virus type 1. N Engl J Med 1990;322:166–172.

36. Feorino PM, Forrester B, Schable C, Warfield D, Schochetman G. Comparison of antigen assay and reverse transcriptase assay for detecting human immunodeficiency virus in culture. J Clin Microbiol 1987;25:2344–2346.

37. Palomba E, Gay V, de Martino M, Fundaro C, Perugini L, Tovo P-A. Early diagnosis of human immunodeficiency virus infection in infants by detection of free and complexed p24 antigen. J Infect Dis 1992;165:394–395.

38. Lee F, Nesheim S, Sawyer M, Slade B, Nahmias A. Early diagnosis of HIV infection in infants by detection of p24 antigen in plasma specimens after acid hydrolysis to dissociate immune complexes [Abstract PoB 3702]. Eighth International Conference on AIDS, Amsterdam, Jul 1992.

39. Miles SA, Balden E, Magpantay L, et al. Rapid serologic testing with immune-complex-dissociated HIV p24 antigen for early detection of HIV infection in neonates. N Engl J Med 1993;328:297–302.

40. Alimenti A, Luzuriago K, Stechenberg B, et al. Quantitation of HIV-1 in the blood of vertically infected infants and children. J Pediatr 1991; 266:3443–3446.

41. Rayfield MA. Human immunodeficiency virus culture. In: Schochetman G, George JR, eds. AIDS testing: Methodology and management issues. New York: Springer-Verlag, 1992:111–122.

42. Hollinger FB, ed. ACTG virology manual for HIV laboratories. Bethesda: National Institutes of Health, 1993.

43. Burgard M, Mayaux M-J, Blanche S, et al. The use of viral culture and p24 antigen testing to diagnose human immunodeficiency virus infection in neonates. N Engl J Med 1992;327:1192–1197.

44. Krivine A, Firtion G, Cao L, Francoual C, Henrion R, Lebon P. HIV replication during the first weeks of life. Lancet 1992; 339:1187–1189.

45. Bagasra O, Hauptman SP, Lischner HW, Sachs M, Pomerantz RJ. Detection of human immunodeficiency virus type 1 provirus in mononuclear cells by in situ polymerase chain reaction. N Engl J Med 1992;326:1385–1391.

46. Butcher A, Spadoro J. Using PCR for detection of HIV-1 infection. Clin Immunol Newslett 1992;12:73–76.

47. Amadori A, De Rossi A, Giaquinto C, Faulkner-Valle G, Zacchello F, Chieco-Bianchi L. In-vitro production of HIV-specific antibody in children at risk of AIDS. Lancet 1988;1:852–854.

48. Pahwa S, Chirmule N, Leombruno C, et al. In vitro synthesis of human immunodeficiency virus-specific antibodies in peripheral blood lymphocytes of infants. Proc Natl Acad Sci USA 1989;86:7532–7536.

49. Lee FK, Nahmias AJ, Lowery S, et al. ELISPOT: A new approach to studying the dynamics of virus-immune system interaction for diagnosis and monitoring of HIV infection. AIDS Res Hum Retroviruses 1989;5:517–523.

50. Nesheim S, Lee F, Sawyer M, et al. Diagnosis of human immunodeficiency virus infection by enzyme-linked immunospot assays in a prospectively followed cohort of infants of human immunodeficiency virus-infected women. Pediatr Infect Dis J 1992;11:635–639.

51. Centers for Disease Control. Guidelines for prophylaxis against *Pneumocystis carinii* pneumonia for children infected with human immunodeficiency virus. MMWR 1991;40:1–13.

52. Ho DD, Moudgil T, Alam M. Quantitation of human immunodeficiency virus type 1 in the blood of infected persons. N Engl J Med 1989; 321:1621–1625.

53. Schochetman G, Sninsky JJ. Direct detection of human immunodeficiency virus infection using the polymerase chain reaction. In: Schochetman G, George JR, eds. AIDS testing: Methodology and management issues. New York: Springer-Verlag, 1992:90–110.

54. Ou C-Y, McDonough SH, Cabanas D, et al. Rapid and quantitative detection of enzymatically amplified HIV-1 DNA using chemiluminescent oligonucleotide probes. AIDS Res Hum Retroviruses 1990,6:1323–1329.

55. Kanki PJ, Barin F, M'Boup S, et al. New human T-lymphotropic retrovirus related to simian T-lymphotropic virus type III (STLV III). Science 1986; 232:238–243.

56. Clavel F, Guetard D, Brun-Vezinet F, et al. Isolation of a new human retrovirus from West African patients with AIDS. Science 1986;233:343–346.

57. O'Brien TR, George JR, Holmberg SD. Human immunodeficiency virus type 2 infection in the United States. JAMA 1992;267:2775–2779.

58. Sibailly TS, Adjorlolo G, Gayle H, et al. Prospective study to compare HIV-1 and HIV-2 perinatal transmission in Abidjan, Cote D'Ivoire [Abstract WeC 1065]. Eighth International Conference on AIDS, Amsterdam, Jul 1992.

59. Guyader M, Emerman M, Sonigo P, Clavel F, Montagnier L, Alizon M. Genome organization and transactivation of the human immunodeficiency virus type 2. Nature 1987;326:662–669.

60. Centers for Disease Control. Testing for antibodies to human immunodeficiency virus type 2 in the United States. MMWR 1992;41:1–9.

61. Anonymous. Early diagnosis of HIV infection in infants. Consensus Workshop, Siena, Jan 1992. J Acquir Immune Defic Syndr 1992;5:1169–1178.

62. Alimenti A, O'Neill, Sullivan JL, Luzuriaga K. Diagnosis of vertical human immunodeficiency

virus type 1 infection by whole blood culture. J Infect Dis 1992;166:1146–1148.

63. Tersmette M, Gruters RA, de Wolf F, et al. Evidence for a role of virulent human immunodeficiency virus (HIV) variants in the pathogenesis of acquired immunodeficiency syndrome: Studies on sequential HIV isolates. J Virol 1989;63:2118–2125.

64. Bryson YJ, Luzuriaga K, Wara D. Proposed definitions for in utero versus intrapartum transmission of HIV-1. N Engl J Med 1992;327:1246–1247.

SECTION IV

Clinical Manifestations in Infants, Children, and Adolescents

Problems with Infections

Organ-specific Manifestations

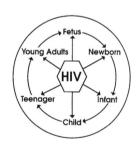

13
Bacterial Infections

Keith Krasinski

Bacterial infections were implicated as significant contributors to morbidity among human immunodeficiency virus (HIV)-infected children from the earliest recognition of the AIDS epidemic even before the etiologic agent had been identified. Bacteremia was detected in 45% of the first 52 patients identified between 1981 and 1983 at the Children's Hospital of New Jersey (1). The importance of bacterial infections was highlighted by their subsequent inclusion in the 1987 revision of the Centers for Disease Control surveillance definition for AIDS as recurrent severe bacterial infections. The P2D2 subclass of pediatric AIDS is now defined as the occurrence of two or more bacteriologically documented, systemic bacterial infections including septicemia or bacteremia, meningitis, pneumonia, osteomyelitis, septic arthritis, or abscesses of body cavity or internal organ (2). In addition to their substantial contribution to morbidity in HIV-infected children, bacterial infections merit significant consideration as potentially preventable and successfully treatable. Furthermore, reducing the frequency and intensity of antigenic stimulation and its associated T lymphocyte activation could potentially modify HIV replication and primary disease progression.

MICROBIAL CONSIDERATIONS

The major bacterial pathogens associated with HIV infection in children comprise those pathogens frequently encountered in routine pediatric practice with immunologically normal children. Table 13.1 indicates pathogens most frequently recovered from blood cultures of febrile HIV-infected children in published studies. The spectrum of bacterial isolates is largely predicted from the clinical site of infection and the association of bacterial pathogens with other clinical infection syndromes (Table 13.2) (3–11).

Table 13.1. Blood Isolates Associated with Disease in HIV-infected Children

Bacterial Isolate	Approximate Frequency[a]
	%
Pneumococcus	30
Salmonella species	14
Enterococcus	8
S. aureus	6
P. aeruginosa	6
Enterobacter cloacae	6
H. influenzae	5
S. viridans	3
Klebsiella pneumoniae	3
E. coli	3
Citrobacter species	<2
P. maltophilia	<2
Acinetobacter species	<2
S. epidermidis	<2
Group A streptococci	<2
Group B streptococci	<2
Group D streptococci, not *Enterococcus*	<2
Lactobacillus species	<2
Diphtheroids	<2
Leuconostoc mesenteroides micrococcus	<2
Neisseria meningitidis	<2
Xanthomonas maltophilia	<2

[a]Values compiled from Ref. 16, 17, and 20. Numbers may not total 100% because of rounding.

241

Table 13.2.   Association of Bacterial Pathogens with Clinical Syndromes in HIV-infected Children[a]

Meningitis
  S. pneumoniae
  H. influenzae
  S. agalactae (GBS)
  Treponema pallidum
Lower respiratory infection
  S. pneumoniae
  H. influenzae
  S. aureus
  Streptococcus viridans
  S. sanguis
  K. pneumoniae
  Proteus mirabilis
  P. aeruginosa enterococcus
  S. enteridis
  N. asteroides
  L. monocytogenes
  Bordetella pertussis
  Moraxella catarrhalis
  Legionella species
  Rhodococcus equi
Gastrointestinal disease
  Salmonella species
  Shigella species
  Campylobacter
  Clostridium difficile toxin
  K. pneumonia
  Aeromonas hydrophilia
Otitis media
  S. epidermidis
  S. pneumoniae
  E. coli
  P. aeruginosa
  Enterococcus
Otitis externa
  Pseudomonas species
Sinusitis
  S. pneumoniae
  S. group G
  S. aureus
  S. epidermidis
	Urinary tract infection
	  E. coli
	  Klebsiella species
	  Enterobacter species
	  Morganella species
	  Enterococcus
	  Pseudomonas species
	Skin and soft tissue
	  S. aureus
	  S. epidermidis
	  Streptococcus viridans
	  Enterobacter species
	  Escherechia coli
	  Acinetobacter species
	  Enterococcus
	  Rochalimaea species
	Intra-abdominal infections
	  Serratia species
	  Pseudomonas species
	  K. pneumoniae
	  Clostridium difficile
	  Salmonella species
	Catheter associated infections
	  S. aureus
	  S. epidermidis
	  P. species
	  S. fecalis
	  K. pneumonia
	  X. maltophilia
	Nosocomial infections
	  S. aureus including MRSA
	  S. epidermidis
	  Enterococcus
	  Pseudomonas species
	  Acinetobacter species
	  Enterobacteriaceae
	Other isolates
	  A. hydrophila
	  Hafnia avei
	  Branhamella catarrhalis
	  Anaerobes

[a]GBS, group B streptococcus; MRSA, methicillin-resistant S. aureus.

Neonatal infections with *Streptococcus agalactiae, Enterobacteriaceae,* and *Listeria monocytogenes* would all be expected to occur in this population but may occur beyond the expected age and be regarded as opportunists (3, 6). Congenital syphilis also occurs in HIV-infected children. Infections with *Nocardia, Actinomyces,* and *Pseudomonas* could also be predicted in individuals with altered cell-mediated immunity, hospitalization, and invasive monitoring and those who are nec-essarily subjected to the selective pressures of antimicrobial chemotherapy resulting in alterations of protective commensal bacteria. Tuberculosis and infections caused by non-tuberculous (atypical) mycobacteria also occur as opportunistic infections in children and adults with HIV infection. Mycobacterial infections are addressed in Chapter 16. Various unusual pathogens associated with lacunar or global defects in host defenses have also been recovered, although less frequently, from HIV-infected children, as they have from other children and adults with immunocompromising conditions. Although infections caused by *Chlamydia* and *Mycoplasma* hae not been systematically addressed among HIV-infected children, they almost certainly occur but may not be suspected, may be difficult to diagnose, or may have the same clinical evolution as these infections in immunologically normal individuals (12). Despite immunization and likely because of the impaired B cell responses from HIV infection, vaccine preventable diseases including pertussis have been recognized in HIV-infected children (7).

EPIDEMIOLOGY
Case Finding and Ascertainment Bias

Most reports of bacterial infections in HIV-infected children are based on retrospective reviews of experience and, as a result, represent a skewed analysis of the true incidence of bacterial disease. Furthermore, the difficulties in establishing bacteriologic diagnoses for clinical syndromes in children are well recognized. For example, the traditional means to document bacterial pneumonia in children is with a positive blood culture; however, if invasive means such as needle biopsy of the lung are employed, many more infections can be substantiated as bacterial. Another familiar example is acute otitis media with effusion, frequently demonstrated to be of bacterial origin but infrequently documented with middle ear cultures in routine clinical practice. Additionally, anaerobic cultures are infrequently employed. Ascertainment bias among the available published data also results from attention to different clinical syndromes, making it difficult to compare among the various studies. Local epidemiology, particularly the medical practices and hospital flora of individual institutions, is likely to contribute significantly to the types of infections that occur and are subsequently documented. At least three medical interventions (*Pneumocystis carinii* pneumonia (PCP) prophylaxis with antimicrobials, antiretroviral therapy, and passive immunization with immunoglobulin products), could be hypothesized to alter bacterial in-

fections and confound interpretation of the various published data. Because HIV case finding is incomplete in several areas of high incidence and utilization of health care by children at risk of HIV is often haphazard, occurrences of bacterial infection may not be attributed to underlying HIV disease.

Recurrent Severe Bacterial Infections (P2D2)

Epidemiologic information based on the surveillance definition of AIDS in children focuses only on the most severe bacterial infections that have occurred in individual patients at least twice. Therefore available information substantially underestimates and distorts the true contribution of bacterial infection to morbidity among HIV-infected children. The CDC reports recurrent severe bacterial infection as an AIDS indicator disease among ~23% of reported cases of AIDS. From 1988 to 1989, the proportion of reported AIDS cases in children with recurrent severe bacterial infection declined 23%, possibly as a result of antimicrobial therapy, immunoprophylaxis, or chemoprophylaxis (13). Changes in diagnostic practices or reporting artifacts could also influence these figures. This decline persisted with recurrent severe bacterial infections accounting for 16 and 18% of reported pediatric AIDS in 1990 and 1991, respectively (Centers for Disease Control unpublished data, 1993). Similarly the New York City AIDS Surveillance Report, which summarizes 563 pediatric AIDS cases from 1981–1989, has found recurrent severe bacterial infections in 103 (18%) (14). There were an additional 46 cases (8%) of *Mycobacterium avium-intracellulare* infections diagnosed. However, this represents only those that meet the CDC pediatric AIDS definition. The Lawrence et al. (15) preliminary report indicates severe, laboratory documented, bacterial infections account for <20% of the presenting clinical syndromes in HIV-infected children.

Retrospective Reviews—North American Experience

More focused reports from New York City groups define bacterial infections among HIV-1-infected children more explicitly. In a review of 46 symptomatic children younger than 6 years, including 17 with AIDS and 29 with what would now be classified as CDC P1 symptomatology, Bernstein et al. (16) reported 27 episodes of sepsis, including five cases of meningitis, two of cellulitis, and one of pneumonia, among 21 of the 46 patients. Additionally, there were five episodes of pneumonia, nine urinary tract infections, two cases of cellulitis, three of lymphadenitis, two of impetigo, three of chronic draining otitis media, two cases of polymicrobial enterocolitis, and one child with a perinephric abscess. Krasinski et al. (17) reported on 71 children including 13 with AIDS, 52 with symptomatic disease not meeting an AIDS definition, and six who were asymptomatic. Over 3.5 years 44 of the 71 children required a bacterial culture with 27 of the children having documented bacterial infections. These children had 125 episodes of infection (most frequently, pneumonia in 24 (19%) and wound infection in 12 (10%) resulting in 35 episodes of bacteremia. The most common clinical syndromes associated with documented bacterial infection are listed in Table 13.3.

Retrospective Reviews—African Experience

The same ascertainment biases are expected to apply to data generated in Africa and to be compounded by sociocultural factors, impaired nutrition, and lack of sophisticated laboratory services. Nevertheless, the report compiled by Lepage and VanDePerre (18) summarizing the experience among 107 HIV-infected children in Rwanda reiterates the importance of bacteremias in 20% of children with AIDS. These were predominantly due to *Salmonella typhimurium* ($n =$ 10) and *S. enteritidis* ($n = 1$) probably from local epidemiologic factors. However, the pneumococcus ($n = 5$), *P. aeruginosa* ($n = 2$), *Escherichia coli,* and *Haemophilus influenzae* ($n = 1$ each) were also represented. Additional syndromes in the Rwandan children included acute pneumonia ($n = 20$), cellulitis and abscesses ($n = 10$), and osteomyelitis ($n = 1$). Chronic otitis media ($n = 29$) was reported more frequently than in the North American experience.

Prospective Experiences

In a prospective study among African children, LePage and VanDePerre (19) determined that bacteremia in children younger than 2 years was significantly associated with HIV infection (odds ratio 3.47, $p = 0.035$); however, this relationship did not hold for children older than two years. A prospectively collected data set is available from the National Institute of Child Health sponsored, multicenter, double-blind study of intravenous immonoglobulin's efficacy in preventing bacterial infection among 372 HIV-1-infected children. The group of 187 children assigned to placebo in this study serve as natural history controls for the development of bacterial infections. In this group 30 bacteremias occurred in 25 children (13% of the population), accounting

Table 13.3.   Site or Clinical Syndrome Associated with Bacterial Infections in HIV-1-infected Children

Site or Clinical Syndrome	Approximate Frequency among Documented Bacterial Infections[a]
	%
Bloodstream	31
Primary bactermia	18
Secondary bacteremia[b]	13
Respiratory tract	29
Pneumonia	15
Other	
Otitis media	4
Otitis externa	1
Sinusitis	1
Rhinitis	2
Conjunctivitis	5
Pharyngitis	1
Genitourinary tract	18
Urinary tract infection	17
Vaginitis	1
Skin and soft tissue	14
Impetigo/other cutaneous	4
Adenitis	3
Wound infection	7
Perirectal abscess	1
Gastrointestinal tract	6
Central nervous system	5
Catheters and devices	2

[a]Compiled from Ref. 16 and 17. Numbers may not total 100% because of rounding.
[b]Most frequently recognized primary sites include lungs, skin, catheter associated infections, gastrointestinal tract, urinary tract, and meninges. Additional sites include perinephric abscesses, subdural empyema

for ~70% of children with laboratory-documented serious bacterial infections. Laboratory proven pneumonias were the next most common and accounted for almost all (20%) the remaining bacteriologically documented infections with single additional cases of acute sinusitis, osteomyelitis, and meningitis. The impact of PCP prophylaxis and antiretroviral therapy cannot be inferred from the data generated in that study. When clinically diagnosed infections that were thought to result from bacterial infection are included, there were 633 episodes in 187 children with 232 bacterial infections/100 patient-years of observation. In the subset of children with CD4 T lymphocyte above 0.2×10^9/liter there were 246 episodes/100 patient-years of observation (20). Minor bacterial infections alone accounted for 159.7 episodes/100 patient-years of observation (21). The distribution of bacterial infection syndromes in this subset of children who were relatively intact immunologically is shown in table 13.4.

Preliminary analysis of the recently concluded National Institute of Allergy and Infectious Disease sponsored prospective study of intravenous immunoglobulin prophylaxis for bacterial infection v. placebo in children with more advanced immunodeficiency who were receiving zidovudine estimated that ~20% of immunocompromised HIV-infected children had at least one serious bacterial infection over a 2-year observation. In this study, the protective effect of intravenous immunoglobulin did not achieve statistical significance. However, when subjects receiving trimethoprim-sulfamethoxazole prophylaxis against PCP, which could also prevent some bacterial infections, were excluded a statistically significant advantage of intravenous immunoglobulin was demonstrated. However, a significant impact on survival was not demonstrated (22).

Effects of Viral Coinfection

Reports summarizing experiences with viral infections in HIV-infected children reveal that bacterial infections are also commonly associated with primary viral syndromes and may contribute to morbidity and mortality. Jura et al. (23) reported five children with bacterial coinfection (including cellulitis, osteomyelitis, and sepsis) among seven with chronic and severe varicella. The bacteria recovered from these infections included *Staphylococcus aureus*, *Salmonella* species, and *L. monocytogenes*. Chandwani et al. (24) noted that respiratory syncytial virus infections frequently were complicated by PCP and bacterial superinfection with such pathogens as pseudomonas, emphasizing the importance of the hospital environment on the type of flora causing nosocomial infections (24). The role of pseudomonas deserves emphasis because infection must be treated vigorously and early. Pseudomonas infections occur in neutropenic and nonneutropenic HIV-infected children, are often catheter related, result in pneumonias or otic infection, and are frequently associated with significant bacteremia (25).

Table 13.4.   Distribution of Minor Bacterial Infection Syndromes in HIV-1-infected Children with Relatively Intact Immune Function (CD4 count >0.20 × 10⁹/liter) Who Were Not Receiving Monthly Intravenous Immunoglobulin[a]

| Infection Syndrome | Episodes | | Rate /100 yr Observation |
	No.	%	
Otitis	225	62	100
Skin/soft tissue	52	14	23
Upper respiratory	36	10	16
Eye	12	3	5
Adenitis	8	2	4
Genitourinary	8	2	4
Lower respiratory	8	2	4
Gastrointestinal	8	2	4
Orodontic	1	<1	<1
Other	3	1	1

[a]Adapted from Ref. 21.

Effect of Clinical Care

Patterns of care also determine to some extent the nature of bacterial infections. In the retrospective study of 204 bacterial infections, other than otitis media, among 105 children referred to the Pediatric Branch of the National Cancer Institute conducted by Roilides and colleagues (26), soft tissue infection (34%), bacteremia (28%), pneumonia (13%), and sinusitis (13%) were the most frequently occurring syndromes. Catheter-related staphylococcal infections followed by enterococcus were the most common infections in children with central venous catheters and were more common in those younger than 6 years. Among patients with 14,250 catheter days of observation (median duration 420 days, range 30–1080 days) there were 80 episodes of central venous catheter-related infections yielding 0.56 bacterial infections/100 catheter days and 0.25 bacteremias/100 catheter days (26). As with other experiences, pneumococcus was the most common isolate in children without catheters. Another effect of the pattern of care was apparent reduction of the frequency of bacterial infections in children receiving antiretroviral therapy; however, the bacterially infected and uninfected groups may not be strictly comparable.

Effect of Survival

Most bacterial infections in children are amenable to therapy, and although they contribute appreciably to morbidity, they do not often cause death of the individual. There is no detailed analysis of actuarial survival among children with bacterial infection who have not met the CDC P2D2 criteria. HIV-infected children with recurrent severe bacterial infections (CDC P2D2) appear to constitute a distinct subclass of children with regard to prognosis, apparently as a result of progressive immunodeficiency, since these children also seldom have bacterial infection as the proximate cause of death. Scott et al. (27) have reported that 29/171 (18%) of children followed in Miami were noted to have recurrent bacterial infections, 16 of these as their presenting manifestation of AIDS. The me-

dian appearance of the first infection was 10 months of age (range 1–39 months). The median survival of children with recurrent bacterial infections was 50 months, an interval much longer than survival of children with PCP (1 month), encephalopathy (11 months), or *Candida* esophagitis (12 months) but substantially shorter than the other major AIDS defining illness in children, lymphocytic interstitial pneumonitis (70 months) (27, 28). Bacterial infections can be identified postmortem in HIV-infected children but are usually comorbidities, such as a mixed enterococcal and fungal infection in a child with varicella pneumonia or *Pseudomonas* infection in a child with PCP (23, 24). One autopsy series identified three bacterial infections, one case each of *Pseudomonas* and *E. coli* sepsis and one case of pneumococcal meningitis among 12 pediatric deaths (29). Although intravenous immunoglobulin administration significantly alters the occurrence of severe and mild bacterial infections in HIV-infected individuals with CD4 counts >200/mm^3, mortality is not apparently affected, suggesting that bacterial infections may not make large contributions to deaths among HIV-infected children (21). Most mortality occurs in children with a CD4 count of <200 and usually in association with an opportunistic infection. Approximately one-third of deaths had a concurrent bacterial infection as the sole identifiable association (30). Alternatively, those bacterial infections contributing to mortality may not be affected by this intervention.

Effect of Antiretroviral Therapy

The beneficial effects of antiretroviral therapy are well recognized clinically in adults and children and are reviewed in Chapter 35. However, clinical improvement is not always associated with manifestly improved immunologic status assessed by CD4 lymphocyte numbers. Recently, therapy with 2' 3'-didioxyinosine has been associated with enhanced elaboration of interlukin-2 by CD4 lymphocytes in vitro in response to stimulation with alloantigens and mitogens (31). The ability to respond in this way was also associated in a decrease in recurrent bacterial infection. Thus with wider experience, antiretroviral therapy may also be recommended as adjunctive therapy to decrease bacterial infections as a result of immune reconstitution in addition to its primary role in treating HIV infection.

PATHOGENESIS AND NATURAL HISTORY

The comparative physiologic immunodeficiency of newborn infants together with antigenic naivete synergize to heighten newborn infants' susceptibility to bacterial infections. As a consequence neonates have particular susceptibility to infections from *S. agalactiae* (group B streptococci), *Enterobacteriaceae*, and *L. monocytogenes.* Furthermore, maternal drug use is often associated with maternal HIV infection, perinatal HIV infection, and prematurity with its attendant inherent risks. Children ultimately determined to have HIV infection are also often exposed to additional risks of invasive monitoring and intensive care. Thus typical nosocomial infections as well as anticipated neonatal infections occur among HIV-infected neonates and appear to have courses similar to those among HIV-uninfected neonates. With immunologic development and antigenic experience, HIV-uninfected neonates acquire immune competence, whereas the immunodeficiency of neonates may persist in HIV-infected infants and result in presentation with these pathogens beyond the neonatal period because of their inability to mount a response against bacteria that normally colonize infants and children. In contrast, although these infections can occur in HIV-infected adults, they are less common, suggesting that when HIV infection occurs after immunologic priming, immunologic responses are not significantly impaired until late in immunosuppression.

Multiple immunologic abnormalities resulting from HIV infection have consequences related to antibacterial host defense (Tables 13.5 and 13.6). Although depletion of CD4-bearing T lymphocytes is considered to be the central determinant of HIV-related immunodeficiency, alterations in function including impaired responses to soluble antigens and impaired secretion of interferon-γ and other lymphokines also occur (32–34). The effects on cell-mediated immunity also occur at the level of the gastrointestinal mucosa and may contribute to the high rate of dissemination and local relapse of enteric pathogens (35). B lymphocyte dysregulation results from altered T lymphocyte help as well as direct B lymphocyte effects and manifests as polyclonal hypergammaglobulinemia, hypogammaglobulinemia, immunoglobulin G subclass deficiency, and impaired primary and secondary antibody responses to T lymphocyte dependent (bacteriophage ϕX 174, tetanus, diphtheria) and independent (pneumococcal and *H. influenzae)* antigens (17, 36–41). As well, immunoglobulin class switching from IgM to IgG antibodies may be absent. CD4-bearing mononuclear phagocytes are also infected and altered by HIV resulting

Table 13.5. Impaired Host Defenses Predisposing to Bacterial Infections

T lymphocytes
Depletion, impaired delayed type hypersensitivity, impaired antigen and mitogen proliferative responses, altered production of interferon-γ
B lymphocytes
Increased or decreased production of immunoglobulins, impaired response to immunization, impaired response to soluble recall antigens, deficient opsonization of bacterial antigens
Monocytes and macrophages
Deficient chemotaxis, impaired phagocytosis, impaired cytokine elaboration
Polymorphonuclear phagocytes
Decreased chemotaxis, decreased phagocytosis, decreased killing, neutropenia
Complement
Deficiency
Integumentary and mucosal barriers
Impaired local cell-mediated responses, impaired secretory antibody responses, breaches in skin from invasive devices and dermatitis, breaches in mucosa because of immunodeficiency, viral infection, reactions to anti-infective chemoprophylaxis or therapy, altered mucosal microflora

Table 13.6.   Association of Host Defense Defects in HIV-infected Children with Bacterial Pathogens

Impaired Host Defense	Associated Bacterial Infection
T lymphocytes, monocytes, macrophages Impaired cell-mediated immunity	Salmonella species, M. tuberculosis, atypical mycobacteria, disseminated Bacille Calmette Guérin infection, Nocardia
B lymphocytes Humoral immune disorders	Encapsulated bacteria S. pneumonia, H. influenzae, N. meningitidis,
Impaired opsonization	Staphylococcal species
Polymorphonuclear leukocytes Neutropenia, functional impairment	Pseudomonads, enteric bacilli (E. coli, Klebsiella species, Enterobacter species) staphylococcal species, α-hemolytic and group D streptococcal species, anaerobes
Complement	Pneumococci, staphylococci, enteric organisms, H. influenzae, Neisseria species
Integumentary and mucosal barriers Skin	Staphylococci, streptococci, cornybacteria, bacillus species
Upper gastrointestinal	α-Hemolytic streptococci, anaerobes, staphylococci
Lower gastrointestinal	Group D streptococci, Enterobacteriaceae, anaerobes
Urinary tract	Group D streptococci, Enterobacteriaceae, Pseudomonads
Reticuloendothelial system	Pneumococcus, H. influenzae, Salmonella species

in depressed interleukin-1 contributing to impaired antigen responses, impaired chemotaxis and killing contributing to abnormal granuloma formation, and decreased expression of complement and Fc receptors resulting in deficient phagocytosis (42–46). Decreased serum levels of the third and to a lesser extent the fourth component of complement also occur in children with AIDS (47). Functional asplenia assessed by elevations in the proportion of circulating pocked red blood cells indicates impairment of tissue macrophages resulting in increased likelihood of bacteremia illness and the propensity for dissemination (48). Neutropenia, resulting from viral or mycobacterial infection or anti-infective chemoprophylaxis or therapy and impaired neutrophil chemotaxis, phagocytosis, superoxide generation, and killing also likely contribute to the enhanced susceptibility of HIV-infected children to bacterial infection (49). Functional impairment of neutrophils could result from direct effects of HIV-1 viral envelope components on polymorphonuclear leukocytes, indirect effects of

circulating immune complexes, alterations in the elaboration of cytokines, or other unknown mechanisms (49–53).

Immunologic abnormalities in HIV-infected children specifically associated with increased risk of bacterial infections include low CD4 T lymphocytes, depressed lymphocyte-proliferative responses to diphtheria and tetanus toxoids, Candida antigen, and pokeweed mitogen (17, 26). However, B lymphocyte dysregulation manifesting only as hypergammaglobulinemia does not appear to significantly heighten risk of bacterial infection. Children with a prior history of opportunistic infections are at great risk for bacterial infections; similarly antecedent recurrences of encapsulated pediatric pathogens such as H. influenzae, pneumococcus, as well as other pyogenic organisms are associated with enhanced risk of bacterial infections. In contrast, children with nonspecific HIV-associated findings such as adenopathy or hepatosplenomegaly only do not appear to be at substantially increased risk of bacterial infections (20).

CLINICAL PRESENTATIONS

There are few data to suggest that clinical presentations of bacterial infections among HIV-infected children differ from the same syndromes in other children. Fever is a common presenting complaint but is nonspecific. Patients with bacteremia frequently have leukocytosis with a left shift; however, this is not invariable. Neutropenia is also a risk factor for and a concomitant of bacterial infections.

In contrast to children with cancer receiving cytotoxic chemotherapy, who develop profound neutropenia and frequently have localized infections without classic signs of inflammation, localized infection in HIV-infected children is usually accompanied by signs of inflammation.

Limited data suggest that pneumococcal bacteremias most often present as otherwise unexplained fever in ~60% of HIV-infected children ultimately demonstrated to have pneumococcal bacteremia; however, pneumonias or other focal infections such as meningitis or stomatitis may coexist (54, 55). Children with bacteria isolated from blood cultures tend to have higher fever (104.4 v. 102°F) and higher white blood cell counts (19,000 v. 11,000) and are more ill appearing than febrile HIV-infected children with negative blood cultures (54). Pneumococcal infections occur in ~6.7/100 children-years of observation, the same frequency as observed in children with sickle cell anemia. Pneumococcal infections can break through active or passive immunization and chemoprophylaxis (55).

The hallmark of pneumonia in children is fever and tachypnea. Although classical presentations for pneumonia of viral, bacterial, and mycoplasma pneumonia are well-known, in individual febrile immunodeficient children it is often impossible to clearly discern the underlying etiologic agent. Since acute diffuse infiltrates, patchy lobar infiltrates, and lobar consolidations all occur in bacterial pneumonias, it is prudent to avoid over-interpretation of the chest roentgenogram in terms of specific etiologic agents. Additionally, since viral, bacterial, parasitic, and fungal infections may coexist it is important to be cautious in withdrawing broad spectrum coverage when a single etiology is suspected, before others can be eliminated.

Gastroenteritis is discussed in greater detail in Chapter 27. The intracellular habitat of *Salmonella* species and the importance of cellular immunity in their eradication are illustrated by the frequency of invasive disease in individuals with HIV infection, in dissemination, and frequent recurrences.

Infection syndromes that have been reported among HIV-infected adults that bear watching among children include bacillary angiomatosis, a dermatologic infection associated with fever, lymphadenopathy, and hepatosplenomegaly caused by *Rochalimaea quintana* or *R. henselae;* pneumonias caused by *Rhodococcus equi;* and pyomyositis caused by staphylococcus or other organisms.

DIAGNOSTIC CONSIDERATIONS

The chief aid to diagnosis is a high index of suspicion. Presenting complaints direct assessment at specific organ systems. Detailed understanding of the individuals' current immune status focuses diagnostic considerations on the likelihood of usual pathogens in individuals who are relatively immunological well and the enhanced possibility of opportunists among those with progressive immunodeficiency. Primary bacteremias and secondary invasion from a recognized or occult site of infection are common. Therefore peripheral venous blood cultures are requisite and should be accompanied by cultures from all lumens of central venous catheters in patients who have them. The frequent occurrence of pneumonias dictates a chest roentgenogram in children with fever, and urine analysis and culture should reveal the presence of urinary tract infections. It is frequently necessary to rely on all diagnostic maneuvers, including sophisticated imaging, that are available to come to the correct determination; however, the needle for obtaining culture material as part of physical diagnosis has not gone out of fashion. Bronchoalveolar lavage and bronchial brush biopsy are useful adjuncts in determining the etiology of pneumonia, with elevations in pulmonary lavage neutrophils and elevations in bacterial counts (>10,000 cfu) obtained by semiquantitative means correlating with bacterial infection. Because of immunosuppressive disease, pulmonary polymorphonuclear responses may not be as exuberant in HIV-infected individuals (56). Additional culture procedures should focus on the organ system involved with specific syndromes. Additionally, antigen detection in blood or body fluids is a useful diagnostic adjunct, but negative results do not eliminate infection with that organism. In the future innovations in gene amplification using the polymerase chain reaction should allow for sensitive and specific detection of organisms in body fluids and tissues.

TREATMENT

Empiric antibiotic therapy is warranted in febrile HIV-infected children because of the unacceptable consequences of missed bacterial infections among immunodeficient individuals. Antimicrobial selection depends on the specific immunologic status of the child, the presenting clinical syndrome, the likelihood that the infection is community acquired v. hospital acquired, the organisms most likely associated with that particular syndrome and anticipated antibiotic susceptibilities, the assessment of the need for oral or parenteral therapy, the expected compliance with any prescribed regimen, and the assurance of follow-up. Antibiotic therapy must be individualized and modified based on culture and sensitivity information and deviations from the expected clinical course.

Patients with community acquired respiratory infections are likely to have encapsulated bacteria typical in children; therefore single daily use of ceftriaxone (50–75 mg/kg) with daily return for reassessment and readministration of the drug is becoming essentially common for outpatient management of infections. For localized community acquired staphylococcal infections oral antistaphylococcal therapy is indicated unless sepsis is suspected. For nosocomial infections, particularly among individuals with central venous catheters, methicillin resistant staphylococcal coagulase positive and negative organisms occur together with Gram negative organisms; thus combination vancomycin with an extended spectrum β-lactam or aminoglycoside is appro-

priate in areas where methicillin resistant *S. aureus* infections are prevalent. In centers where methicillin resistant *S. aureus* are less common, cerftriaxone is appropriate empiric therapy while awaiting culture results.

Once infection is diagnosed, treatment with traditional antibiotic approaches using drugs of appropriate specificity is warranted. Since immune mediated clearance of bacteria is likely to be impaired, it may be useful to extend the duration of therapy for longer than is customary for immunologically normal individuals. Fluoroquinolones are not specifically approved for use in children; however there is increasing evidence of their safety. As a result of their oral bioavailability and broad spectrum they are attractive for some infections caused by resistant organisms and for prolonged therapy needed in individuals.

Recurrences and recrudescence of bacterial infections are common; thus careful search for hidden loci of infection and adequate drainage of sequestered pyogenic foci is indicated. Recurrences are particularly problematic with *Salmonella,* and may be reduced by substituting ceftriaxone for ampicillin or trimethoprim-sulfamethoxazole.

Antibiotics alone have been able to eradicate infection in 89% of catheter related infections. The remainder required catheter removal for success. These infections included six recurrent bacteremias, four tunnel infections, and one recurrent exit site infection from *Pseudomonas* species. There were no deaths related to bacterial infections in this group of patients during observation.

PREVENTION

Pediatricians traditionally approach diseases with an emphasis on prophylaxis. This bias has influenced many individuals to attempt to reduce the incidence of bacterial infections in HIV-infected children as if they had hypogammaglobulinemia, despite the presence of high levels of antibodies. The rationale for this treatment is to provide passively specific antibodies to common agents when the HIV-infected child cannot produce them as a result of their immunosuppression. The use of passive immunization to prevent bacterial and other infections is detailed in Chapter 45. This strategy might be expected to succeed for those pathogens that are common among immunologically normal individuals but might fail for those bacterial pathogens that are uncommon or do not usually elicit exuberant antibody responses. This strategy also fails to explain defective phagocytosis of adequately opsonized bacterial pathogens.

Active immunization against pneumococcal, meningococcal, and *Haemophilus* pathogens is effective for immunologically normal individuals and has enjoyed some success among other immunodeficient populations; however, HIV-infected children have not appeared to benefit, possibly as a result of their impaired β-lymphocyte responses. The availability of conjugated vaccines and the possibility of earlier immunization at a time of relative immunologic integrity may improve the outlook for children. Active immunization is detailed in Chapter 46.

Chemoprophylaxis is another traditional approach for the prevention of bacterial infections. The use of penicillin congeners, cephalosporin congeners, or trimethoprim-sulfamethoxazole might be expected to reduce the incidence of infections with encapsulated bacteria; however, this hypothesis has not been adequately tested in HIV-infected children. Penicillin is a relatively narrow spectrum agent used as pneumococcal prophylaxis for asplenic individuals. Because of the significant occurrence of pneumococcal infections among HIV-infected children it is a logical and inexpensive agent that might be expected to be effective. However, oral prophylaxis requires faithful daily administration. Uncontrolled data using prior pneumococcal infection experience in the same patients suggests that oral or intramuscular penicillin prophylaxis for the prevention of pneumococcal infections in HIV-infected children (57) may be useful. The use of trimethoprimsulfamethoxazole prophylaxis to prevent PCP among leukemic children was also shown to reduce the incidence of bacterial infections, making this an attractive possibility for antibacterial prophylaxis in HIV-infected children. Unfortunately, among leukemic children there was a concomitant increase in fungal infections, which could exacerbate an already difficult problem in immunodeficient HIV-infected children. Because of this problem and the potential for serious allergy, anemia, neutropenia, and thrombocytopenia, recommendations regarding antibacterial prophylaxis must await development of further safety and efficacy data. Preliminary analysis of the data from the placebo controlled trial of intravenous immunoglobulin in zidovudine-treated children appears to demonstrate a beneficial trimethoprim-sulfamethoxazole effect in reducing bacterial infections (22).

Haemophilus and meningococcal diseases are preventable with traditional methods of postexposure chemoprophylaxis. Appropriate and complete vaccination of routine childhood contacts, including day care and school, would also be expected to be valuable in reducing the incidence of bacterial infections in HIV-infected children. Infection control precautions recommended for specific bacterial diseases require no modification in the presence of HIV infection.

The experience at the National Cancer Institute that catheter associated infections in HIV-infected children were very similar to such infections in cancer patients indicates that well recognized principles of catheter care among children with cancer, (including instruction in proper catheter care, Gram stain and culture of exit site and tunnel infections, oral therapy for superficial infections, hospitalization and parenteral therapy for catheter infections per se and associated bacteremias, and catheter removal for tunnel infections) can be generalized to HIV-infected children (26, 58).

AREAS FOR FUTURE RESEARCH

With the advent of antiretroviral therapy there is the possibility that early intervention will be associated with substantial delays in progressive immunodeficiency with consequent shifts in the age and etiologic agent specific patterns of bacterial infections in HIV-infected children. Further advances in immunoglobulin therapy that could prove beneficial include generation of hyperimmune globulins to specific pathogens, production of monoclonal antibodies to pathogens that escape current interventions, and even the mixing of cocktails of monoclonal antibodies to extend their spectrum. Another possible intervention for the prevention or treatment of bacterial infections is the use of specific cytokines to stimulate granulocyte or macrophage production and migration to sites of infection and to enhance their natural function of phagocytosis and killing.

References

1. Siegal FP, Oleske J. Management of the acquired immunodeficiency syndrome: Is there a role for immune globulins? In: Clinical use of intravenous immunoglobulins. London: Academic, 1986:373–383.
2. Centers for Disease Control. Revision of the CDC surveillance case definition for acquired immunodeficiency syndrome. MMWR 1987;36(suppl 1s):1s–15s.
3. DiJohn D, Johnson JP, Lawrence R, et al. Very late onset group B streptococcal sepsis in infants with HIV infection [Abstract TBP 262]. Fifth International Conference on AIDS, Montreal, Jun 1989.
4. Ocana I, DeLuis A, Planes A, et al. Salmonella bacteremia and HIV infection [Abstract MBP 67]. Fifth International Conference on AIDS, Montreal, Jun 1989.
5. Cone L, Polkinghorn G, Woodard D, et al. Nocardia asteroides infections in patients with the acquired immunodeficiency syndrome [Abstract MBP 204]. Fifth International Conference on AIDS, Montreal, Jun 1989.
6. Real FX, Gold JWM, Krown SE, et al. Listeria monocytogenes bacteremia in the acquired immunodeficiency syndrome [Letter]. Ann Intern Med 1984;101:883.
7. Adamson PC, Wu TC, Meade BD, et al. Pertussis in a previously immunized child with human immunodeficiency virus infection. J Pediatr 1989;115:589–592.
8. Kotloff K, Johnson JP, Nair P, et al. Diarrhea and its consequences in HIV infected children [Abstract TBP 263]. Fifth International Conference on AIDS Montreal, Jun 1989.,
9. Peters B, Francis N, Boylston AW, et al. Investigation of HIV positive patients with gastrointestinal symptomatology [Abstract MBP 239]. Fifth International Conference on AIDS, Montreal, Jun 1989.
10. McLaughlin LC, Nord KS, Joshi VV, et al. Severe gastrointestinal involvement in children with the acquired immunodeficiency syndrome. J Pediatr Gastroenterol Nutr 1987;6:517–524.
11. Kales CP, Holzman RS, Krasinski K, et al. Nosocomial infection (NI) in patients with HIV infection [Abstract MBP 70]. Fifth International Conference on AIDS, Montreal, Jun 1989.
12. Cosentini R, Blasi F, Legnani D, et al. Chlamydia [Abstract POB 3158]. Seventh International Conference on AIDS, Florence, Jun 1991.
13. Fleming PL, Simonds RJ, Hansen D, et al. Decline in bacterial infections among US Pediatric AIDS cases. [Abstract 470]. 31st Interscience Conference on Antimicrobial Agents and Chemotherapy, Chicago, Sep 29–Oct 2, 1991.
14. New York City Department of Health. AIDS surveillance update. Dec 28, 1989.
15. Lawrence RM, Rigaud M, Pollack H, et al. Presentations of HTLV-III infections in children [Abstract 937]. Pediatr Res 1986;20:314A.
16. Bernstein LJ, Krieger BZ, Novick B, et al. Bacterial infection in the acquired immunodeficiency syndrome of children. Pediatr Infect Dis J 1985;4:472–475.
17. Krasinski K, Borkowsky W, Bonk S, et al. Bacterial infections in HIV-infected children and adolescents. Pediatr Infect Dis J 1989;8:216–220.
18. Lepage P, VanDePerre P: Clinical manifestations in infants and children. Baillieres Clin Trop Med Commun Dis 1988;3:89–101.
19. LePage P, VanDePerre P, Nsengumuremyi F, et al. Bacteremia as a predictor of HIV infection in African children. Acta Paediatr Scand 1989;78:763–766.
20. National Institute of Child Health and Human Development Intravenous Immunoglobulin Study Group. Intravenous immune globulin for the prevention of bacterial infections in children with symptomatic human immunodeficiency virus infection. N Engl J Med 1991;325:73–80.
21. Mofenson LM, Moye J, Bether J, et al. Prophylactic intravenous immunoglobulin in HIV-infected children with CD4 counts of 0.20 x 10^9/L or more: Effect on viral, opportunistic, and bacterial infections. JAMA 1992;268:483–488.
22. Spector S, Sacks H, Wara D, et al. Pediatric AIDS clinical trials group and the NICHD pediatric HIV treatment centers. Results of the ACTG 051: A double blind placebo controlled trial to evaluate intravenous immunoglobulin in children with symptomatic HIV infection receiving zidovudine. 30th Annual Infectious Diseases Society of America Meeting, Anaheim, Oct 1992.
23. Jura E, Chadwick E, Josephs S, et al. Varicella-zoster virus infections in children infected with HIV. Pediatr Infect Dis J 1989;8:586–590.
24. Chandwani S, Borkowsky W, Krasinski K, et al. Respiratory syncytial virus infection in HIV infected children. J Pediatr 1990;117:251–254.
25. Roilides E, Butler K, Husson RN, et al. Pseudomonas infections in children with human immunodeficiency virus infection. Pediatr Infect Dis J 1992;11:547–553.
26. Roilides E, Marshall D, Venson D, et al. Bacterial infections in human immunodeficiency virus type 1-infected children: The impact of central venous catheters and antiretroviral agents. Pediatr Infect Dis J 1991;10:813–819.
27. Scott GB, Hutto C, Makuch RW, et al. Survival in children with perinatally acquired HIV-1 infection. N Engl J Med 1989;321:1791–1796.
28. Krasinski K, Borkowsky W, Holzman RS. Prognosis of human immunodeficiency virus infection in children and adolescents. Pediatr Infect Dis J 1989;8:216–220.
29. Ross LA, Wong VK, Gomperts ED, et al. Spectrum of infections identified at autopsy in pediatric AIDS [Abstract TBP 267]. Fifth International Conference on AIDS, Montreal, Jun 1989.

30. Mofenson LM, Moye J, Nugent R, et al. Serious infection and mortality in HIV-infected children in a clinical trial of immunoglobulin (IG) [Abstract 908]. 32nd Interscience Conference on Antimicrobial Agents and Chemotherapy, Anaheim, Oct 1992.

31. Clerici M, Roilides E, Butler K, et al. Changes in T helper cell function in human immunodeficiency virus-infected children during didioxyinosine therapy as a measure of antiretroviral activity. Blood 1992;80:2196–202.

32. Giorgi JV, Fahey JL, Smith DC, et al. Early effects of HIV on CD4 lymphocytes in vivo. J Immunol 1987;139:3725–3730.

33. Hoy JF, Lewis DE, Miller GC. Functional versus phenotypic analysis of T cells in subjects seropositive for human immunodeficiency virus: A prospective study of in vitro responses to *Cryptococcus neoformans*. J Infect Dis 1988;158:1071–1078.

34. Murray HW, Rubin BY, Masur H, et al. Impaired production of lymphokines and immune (gamma) interferon in the acquired immunodeficiency syndrome. N Engl J Med 1984;310:883–889.

35. Rogers VD, Kagnoff MF. Gastrointestinal manifestations of the acquired immunodeficiency syndrome. West J Med 1987;146:57–67.

36. Lane HC, Masur H, Edgar LC, et al. Abnormalities of B-cell activation and immunoregulation in patients with the acquired immunodeficiency syndrome. N Engl J Med 1983;309:453–458.

37. Pahwa S, Fikrig S, Menez R, Pahwa R, Pediatric acquired immunodeficiency syndrome: Demonstration of B lymphocyte defects in vitro. Diagn Immunol 1986;4:24–30.

38. Bernstein LJ, Ochs HD, Wedgewood RJ, et al. Defective humoral immunity in pediatric acquired immune deficiency syndrome. J Pediatr 1985;107:352–357.

39. Kamani N, Lightman H, Leiderman I, et al. Pediatric acquired immunodeficiency syndrome-related complex: Clinical and immunologic features. Pediatr Infect Dis J 1988;7:383–388.

40. Borkowsky W, Steele CJ, Grubman S, et al. Antibody responses to bacterial toxoid in children infected with human immunodeficiency virus. J Pediatr 1987;110:563–566.

41. Church JA, Lewis J, Spotkov JM. IgG subclass deficiencies in children with suspected AIDS [Letter]. Lancet 1984;1:279.

42. Lepe-Zuniga JL, Mansell PWA, Hersh EM. Idiopathic production of interleukin-1 in acquired immune deficiency syndrome. J Clin Microbiol 1987;25:1695–1700.

43. Smith PD, Ohura K, Masur H, et al. Monocyte function in the acquired immune deficiency syndrome. J Clin Invest 1984;74:2121–2128.

44. Eales L-J, Moshtael O, Pinching AL. Microbicidal activity of monocyte derived macrophages in AIDS and related disorders. Clin Exp Immunol 1987;67:227–235.

45. Bender BS, Frank MM, Lawley TJ, et al. Defective reticuloendothelial system Fc receptor function in patients with acquired immunodeficiency syndrome. J Infect Dis 1985;152:409–412.

46. Bender BS, Davidson BL, Kline R, et al. Role of the mononuclear phagocyte system in the immunopathogenesis of human immunodeficiency virus infection and the acquired immunodeficiency syndrome. Rev Infect Dis 1988;10:1142–1154.

47. Lin RY, Wildfever O, Franklin MM, et al. Hypocomplementemia and human immunodeficiency virus infection: Clinical correlation and relationships to circulating immune complex and immunoglobulin G levels. Int Arch Allergy Appl Immunol 1988;87:40–46.

48. Pollack H, Noel G, Fikrig S, et al. Ability of RBC pocked counts to identify HIV+ children who are at risk for bacterial sepsis [Abstract p. 19]. First International Conference on AIDS in Children, Adolescents, and Heterosexual Adults, Atlanta, 1987.

49. Rolides E, Mertins S, Eddy J, et al. Impairment of neutrophil chemotaxis and bactericidal function in children with human immunodeficiency virus type 1 and partial reversal after in vitro exposure to granulocyte-macrophage colony stimulating factor. J Pediatr 1990;117:531–540.

50. Ming WJ, Bersani L, Mantovani A. Tumor necrosis factor is chemotactic for monocytes and polymorphonuclear leukocytes. J Immunol 1987;138:1469–1474.

51. Wang JM, Colella S, Allavena P, et al. Chemotactic activity of human recombinant human granulocyte-macrophage colony-stimulating factor. Immunology 1987;60:439–444.

52. Buescher SE, McIleheran SM, Vahan-Raj S. Effects of in vivo administration of recombinant granulocyte-macrophage colony stimulating factor on human neutrophil chemotaxis and oxygen metabolism. J Infect Dis 1988;158:1140–1141.

53. McDougal JS, Hubbard M, Nichobon JK, et al. Immune complexes in the acquired immunodeficiency syndrome (AIDS): Relationship to disease manifestations, risk group, and immunologic defect. Clin Immunol 1985;5:130–138.

54. Arpadi S, Hauger S. Clinical and laboratory findings in HIV infected children with pneumococcal bacteremias [Abstract WB 2207]. Seventh International Conference on AIDS, Florence, Jun 1991.

55. Hsu J, Moye J, Ng P, et al. Pneumococcal bacteremia in children with HIV infection [Abstract WB 2062]. Seventh International Conference on AIDS, Florence, Jun 1991.

56. Dalhoff K, Korber M, Kothe H, et al. Bronchoalveolar lavage in bacterial pneumonia in AIDS patients: Quantitative cultures and assessment of local inflammation [Abstract PWB 7133]. Eighth International Conference on AIDS, Amsterdam, Jul 1992.

57. Peters V, Diamant E, Hodes D. Efficacy of penicillin prophylaxis against invasive pneumococcal infections in HIV-infected children [Abstract 909]. 32nd Interscience Conference on Antimicrobial Agents and Chemotherapy, Anaheim, Oct 1992.

58. Hiemenz J, Skelton J, Pizzo P. Perspective in the management of catheter-related infections in cancer patients. Ped Infect Dis J 1986;5:6–11.

14
Otitis Media and Sinusitis in Patients with HIV Infection

Barry Dashefsky and Ellen R. Wald

Otitis media and sinusitis are among the most common minor bacterial infections affecting children with normal immune function. There is a paucity of systematic study of these infections in immunocompetent hosts in general, but substantial experience and a limited literature suggest that, in their acute, chronic, and recurrent forms, they also occur commonly in children who are infected with human immunodeficiency virus (HIV). Although the causes, manifestations, and clinical course of most episodes of otitis media and sinusitis in HIV-infected children are indistinguishable from those in immunocompetent children, unusually frequent, prolonged, severe, or otherwise problematic episodes, or those caused by unusual or opportunistic pathogens, may be the sentinel expressions of immunodeficiency that should prompt an assessment for HIV infection. Ten of 21 HIV-infected children described by Church (1) exhibited either severe, chronic, or recurrent otitis media (*r* = 8) or chronic sinusitis (*n* = 2) 4–34 months before being diagnosed with HIV infection.

This chapter will review what is known about the causes, pathogenesis, natural history, and clinical features of these two common infections in HIV-infected children, and provide suggestions for their evaluation and management. Given the many similarities of these conditions among both HIV-infected and non-HIV-infected children, the discussion will include selected and summary comments regarding otitis media

and sinusitis in normal children. For more complete discussions of these topics, the reader is referred to comprehensive reviews of otitis media (2–4) and sinusitis (5, 6) and of these conditions in immunocompromised pediatric hosts (7).

OTITIS MEDIA
Microbiologic Considerations

In immunocompetent children, the bacterial organisms responsible for otitis media vary with age of the patient and duration of infection. The pathogens most often isolated from middle ear aspirates obtained from children younger than 6 years with acute otitis media (AOM) are *Streptococcus pneumoniae* (30–40%), nontypable *Haemophilus influenzae* (15–20%, of which up to 30–40% may be amoxicillin resistant on the basis of β-lactamase production), and *Moraxella catarrhalis* (formerly *Branhamella catarrhalis*; 8–12%, of which up to 80% are β-lactamase-positive) (4, 7, 8). *S. pyogenes* (4%), *Staphylococcus aureus* (2%), anaerobic species (up to 5–6%), and other organisms are much less frequently implicated (4, 7). In older children and adults with AOM, *S. pneumoniae* and *H. influenzae* are the predominant pathogens, occurring in similar proportions (8). Respiratory viruses have been isolated from middle ear or nasopharyngeal specimens from 20% of cases of AOM. Their importance in the pathogenesis and etiology of AOM, and as a possible explanation for some apparent

255

antibiotic failures, is newly appreciated. Recurrent episodes of AOM, as well as 20–66% of cases of chronic otitis media, are caused by the same array of organisms (7). Chronic suppurative otitis media (CSOM), characterized by persistent otorrhea through a perforated tympanic membrane, is usually attributable to *Pseudomonas aeruginosa*, staphylococci, or *Proteus* spp; anaerobic organisms have been documented in up to 50% of cases (7). Occasionally fungi, especially *Aspergillus* and *Candida* spp and rarely *Blastomycosis,* have been implicated in CSOM, either alone or in combination with bacterial pathogens (7). *P. aeruginosa,* staphylococci, *P. vulgaris,* and *Escherichia coli* are the pathogens most frequently responsible for acute and chronic bacterial otitis externa. Fungal otitis externa is usually caused by *Aspergillus; Phycomycetes, Rhizopus, Actinomyces, Penicillium,* and *C. albicans* are sometimes implicated.

The microbiology of otitis media in immunoincompetent hosts has not been systematically assessed. Based on limited data and the implication of clinical improvement in response to standard therapy used for AOM in immunocompetent children, it is highly probable that most episodes in HIV-infected children are caused by the same pathogens that are responsible for disease in normal hosts. However, like other immunoincompetent hosts, HIV-infected children occasionally sustain otitis media because of uncommon or opportunistic organisms, and this possibility must be anticipated and clarified. Circumstances that would make this more probable include chronic or repeated episodes of otitis media, prolonged exposure to broad-spectrum antimicrobials, prolonged hospitalization (especially in an intensive care unit), long-standing placement of either gastric or endotracheal tubes, infection caused by uncommon or opportunistic pathogens at another site, and advanced stages of deficient humoral and cell-mediated immunity or neutropenia, whether from HIV infection or treatment. In their report of AOM in HIV-infected children in Italy, the only prospective controlled study to date, Principi and colleagues (9) reported the microbiology to be similar to that associated with AOM in non-HIV-infected Italian children. Cultures of middle ear fluid obtained by tympanocentesis from 17 of 19 HIV-infected children with AOM yielded *S. pneumoniae* (six cases, 35%), nontypable *H. influenzae* (two cases, 12%), *S. pyogenes* (two cases, 12%), *P. mirabilitis* (two cases, 12%), *E. coli* (one case, 6%), and no organism (four cases, 23%). All isolates were susceptible to amoxicillin, with which patients were initially treated. Thirteen episodes of AOM that, by clinical criteria, failed to respond to amoxicillin (including 10 for which tympanocentesis had been performed before initial treatment) were retreated with amoxicillin/clavulanate potassium (without benefit of repeated tympanocentesis). Eleven of these 13 were cured, implying that, at worst, the pathogens responsible for initial treatment failures were similar to those implicated in immunocompetent hosts (for whom amoxicillin/clavulanate potassium is an effective agent) and not unusually resistant or opportunistic pathogens. The two persistent treatment failures resulted in CSOM caused by (amoxicillin-susceptible) *S. pyogenes.*

Other investigators have isolated various other organisms from HIV-infected children with otitis media including staphylococci, *P. aeruginosa,* enterococci, and *Candida* (1, 10, 11).

Reports of middle and external ear canal infection associated with unusual or opportunistic pathogens in adults with HIV infection include two cases of otomastoiditis caused by *A. fumigatus* (12), one case of otitis media caused by *Nocardia asteroides* (13), and seven cases of either aural polyps, otitis media, or both caused by *Pneumocystis carinii* (14–20).

Although not descriptive of HIV-infected patients per se, two reports (21, 22) document the high frequency with which pediatric patients hospitalized in intensive care units, especially those with gastric or tracheal tubes (87% of whom develop otitis media within 4 days of incubation), develop otitis media because of various nosocomially acquired Gram-positive and Gram-negative bacteria and *C. albicans.*

Epidemiology

AOM is a very common occurrence in immunocompetent children with peak frequency during the first 2 years of life (2). In a cohort of children followed prospectively from birth, Teele et al. (23) documented at least one episode of AOM in 83% and at least three episodes in 46% of 698 children followed to 3 years of age; among the cohort of 498 children followed for 7 years, the respective rates were 93 and 74%. Risk factors for AOM, in addition to young age, include male gender, sibling history of severe or recurrent AOM, early age of first AOM, absence of breast feeding, winter season, race, day care attendance, lower socioeconomic status, and craniofacial anomalies (2, 3, 23).

The literature suggests that otitis media is sometimes problematic in HIV-infected adults but gives no sense of its relative frequency (24–26). Many authors have reported that acute, recurrent, or chronic middle-ear infections occur commonly in HIV-infected children (1, 9–11, 27–32).

There are two controlled studies that enable determination of the relative frequency of AOM among HIV-infected children (9, 30). Both clearly indicated that, although this common childhood condition does not affect a greater proportion of HIV-infected children than normal children, it recurs significantly more often among children with symptomatic HIV infection.

Barnett and colleagues (30) retrospectively compared the frequency of AOM in 28 HIV-infected children in Boston with that in 33 children who, born to HIV-infected mothers, had seroreverted by age 18 months. The mean number of episodes of AOM during the first year of life did not differ (1.89 for HIV-infected children vs. 1.33 for those who ultimately seroreverted). However, whereas this annual rate decreased to 0.13 by the third year of life among seroreveters, it increased to 2.4 in the HIV-infected cohort. By 3 years of age, all HIV-infected children had experienced at least one episode of AOM, and 80% had experienced six or more in contrast to the seroreverters, 75% of whom had experienced at least one but none of whom had experienced six or more episodes.

In the comparative cohort study by Principi and colleagues (9), 27 pairs of HIV-infected children and closely matched non-HIV infected controls were followed prospectively for 543 cumulative months

(mean period of observation 19.4 ± 11 months). Data were evaluated for the HIV-infected cohort as a whole and, by HIV classification status (33), as either P-1 (asymptomatic) or P-2 (symptomatic). Forty-six episodes of AOM were diagnosed in 15 HIV-infected subjects and 22 in 16 controls; 27 episodes occurred in 11 P-1 subjects vs. 17 in 13 controls, and 19 episodes occurred in six P-2 subjects vs. five in four controls. The mean number of episodes per child was significantly higher among HIV-infected children than in controls. Recurrent episodes of AOM (three or more within 6 months) also occurred significantly more often, but only among the symptomatic (P2) cohort compared with their controls (four of ten vs. zero of ten). Rates of clinical cure in response to amoxicillin therapy were similar among P1 subjects (89%) and their controls (88%) but were significantly lower among P2 subjects (47%) compared with their controls (100%). These differences were not associated with demonstrated significant differences in microbiology, immunologic parameters, treatment with zidovudine, or IVIG prophylaxis.

Pathogenesis and Natural History

In the immunocompetent host, AOM is attributable to dysfunction of the eustachian tube which is responsible for 1) ventilation of the middle ear cavity, 2) clearance of secretions produced by the mucosa of the middle ear, and 3) protection of the middle ear from nasopharyngeal contents (3).

Virus infection of the upper respiratory tract (URI) is the major pathogenetic factor that, by virtue of the mucosal inflammation it incites, produces both physiologic and anatomic obstruction of the eustachian tube and effusion within the middle ear. When the tube fails to open or is obstructed, negative pressure is established in the middle ear cavity. The absence of ventilation results in further inflammation within the middle ear and production of an effusion. When the eustachian tube next opens, the negative pressure results in aspiration of the heavily colonized nasopharyngeal contents into the middle ear. There, organisms proliferate, leading to a suppurative process manifest as AOM.

A similar pathogenesis probably obtains in the immunoincompetent host. Neutropenia, caused by HIV infection or antiviral therapy, is associated with mucositis, causing eustachian tube dysfunction. Likewise, nasopharyngeal lymphoid hyperplasia, associated with HIV infection, may extrinsically obstruct or infiltrate the eustachian tube.

Abnormal local and systemic immunity, characteristic of advanced HIV infection, would be considered to contribute to the predilection for recurrent and persistent otitis media among children with symptomatic HIV infection. Barnett et al. (30) reported that abnormally low CD4 lymphocyte counts ($<1500/mm^3$) were associated with significantly greater mean numbers of episodes of AOM during the first year of life (2.35 vs. 1.18) as well as an increased risk for recurrent AOM (47 vs. 18%). In contrast, Principi et al. (9) reported the absence of any significant association between neutrophil count, CD4 count, or CD4-to-CD8 ratio and the risk of either recurrent AOM, treatment failure, or persistence of middle ear effusions.

Clinical Presentation

In both immunocompetent and immunoincompetent hosts, AOM usually presents with the abrupt onset of otalgia, fever, or irritability in association with typical otoscopic findings described below. The many patients in whom middle ear effusion persists long after an episode of AOM are usually asymptomatic or mildly symptomatic, although sometimes they have significant complaints of pain, hearing loss, vertigo, or tinnitus.

Nonsuppurative complications of otitis media include hearing loss, adhesive otitis media, tympanosclerosis, and ossicular discontinuity. Suppurative complications include tympanic membrane perforation, sometimes with CSOM, cholesteatoma, mastoiditis, and intracranial suppuration (including meningitis, encephalitis, brain, subdural or extradural abscess, sinus thrombosis, phlebitis, and otitic hydrocephalus) (3).

Diagnostic Considerations

The diagnosis of otitis media is based on otoscopic findings (2). The tympanic membrane is assessed with respect to its contour, color, transparency, architecture, and, most importantly, its mobility. Decreased mobility implies the presence of middle ear effusion that is almost always present in both acute and chronic otitis media. This impression would be supported by the findings of a flattened (type B) curve and/or an absent stapedial reflex if tympanometry is performed. Fullness or bulging of a white or yellow, sometimes hyperemic tympanic membrane are typical findings in AOM. Sometimes purulent fluid can be visualized behind an intact tympanic membrane or as it spills through a perforation. Such signs, coupled with the appropriate symptoms, establish a diagnosis of AOM. Opacity of the tympanic membrane or the presence of clear or mucoid fluid behind it, and decreased mobility suggest a more chronic, nonsuppurative otitis media.

Tympanocentesis should be performed selectively in both immunocompetent and immunoincompetent hosts for diagnostic and therapeutic purposes. According to Bluestone (4), relative indications for tympanocentesis (or myringotomy) for otitis media include the following: 1) severe otalgia, 2) severe illness, 3) poor response to antimicrobial therapy, 4) onset while receiving appropriate antimicrobial therapy, 5) suppurative complications, and 6) immunologically deficient hosts at risk for unusual pathogens. Given the predictability of the microbiology of AOM in the usual HIV-infected child, tympanocentesis should generally be reserved for the severely ill, symptomatic (P2) patient with multiple, recurrent, or otherwise problematic episodes of otitis media.

Radiographs or computerized tomography scanning may be required to confirm the presence of inner ear or mastoid involvement or intracranial complications.

Otitis externa usually presents with a complaint of otalgia. Diagnosis is established by visualizing an erythematous, tender external ear canal that is variably occluded by edema and/or seropurulent debris and may be associated with periauricular edema and pain elicited by movement of the tragus. Bacterial and fungal cultures are helpful, but it is frequently difficult to distinguish pathogens from colonizing flora and invasive from superficial disease. Differential diagnostic considerations include foreign bodies, furunculosis, suppurative and chronic otitis media, mastoiditis, malignant otitis externa, and malignancies.

Treatment

As with immunocompetent hosts, most episodes of AOM in nontoxic HIV-infected children are managed in the absence of specific microbiologic data with an orally administered antimicrobial agent that is predictably active against the most likely pathogens. Candidate antimicrobial agents and dosage recommendations are presented in Table 14.1. In general, amoxicillin, administered for 10–14 days, is the agent of choice for empiric treatment of the first episode of AOM or the occasional recurrence. A broader spectrum, orally administered antimicrobial should be substituted for the following: penicillin allergic patient; when AOM occurs in conjunction with conjunctivitis (a circumstance implicating *H. influenzae*, a pathogen with up to a 40% rate of amoxicillin resistance); frequently recurrent episodes of AOM; episodes that recur shortly after a previous episode; and when symptoms of AOM fail to remit within 48–72 hours of initiation of amoxicillin. Given the observations that children with AOM who have symptomatic HIV infection (P2) are at significantly increased risk for recurrences of AOM, treatment failures with amoxicillin, and prolonged middle ear effusion (9), it should be reasonable to treat recurrent episodes of AOM in this population with a broader spectrum antimicrobial and to extend therapy to ~3 weeks (or for at least 1 week beyond the complete resolution of symptoms). In the case of an HIV-infected child who appears systemically ill or toxic at presentation or during treatment of AOM, tympanocentesis should be performed, aspirated fluid should be cultured, and a parenterally administered broad spectrum antimicrobial (e.g., cefuroxime, cefotaxime, ceftazidime, or ceftriaxone) should be empirically initiated. (If the tympanic membrane has perforated spontaneously, the canal should be suctioned, cleaned, and a sample of middle ear fluid obtained for culture.) Specific treatment is given as dictated by microbiologic data and results of susceptibility testing and as indicated for specific uncommon or opportunistic organisms that may be implicated.

In immunocompetent children, middle ear effusion persists in up to 50% of children with resolution of signs and symptoms after treatment of AOM and gradually resolves in all but 10% over 3 months (3, 4). Because a small percentage of these asymptomatic persistent effusions may be associated with persistent bacterial infection and because subtle or nonspecific symptoms are often difficult to exclude, immediate retreatment with a broader spectrum antimicrobial is often attempted. If not attempted and effusion persists for more than 2–3 months, a second course of treatment with a broader spectrum antimicrobial is recommended, especially before electing a surgical treatment. When middle ear effusion

Table 14.1.   Oral Antimicrobial Therapy for Acute Otitis Media and Acute Sinusitis in Children

Antimicrobial	Daily Dosage	Maximum Daily Dose	No. Daily Doses
	mg/kg	*mg*	
Amoxicillin (many brands)	40	1500	3
Amoxicillin-clavulanate potassium (Augmentin)[a]	40/10	1500	3
Erythromycin-sulfisoxazole (Pediazole, Eryzole)	40–50/120–150	400/1200	4
Trimethoprim-sulfamethoxazole (Bactrim, Septra)	8/40	320/1600	2
Cefaclor (Ceclor)	40	1500	3
Cefuroxime axetil (Ceftin)[b]	30/40	500	2
Cefprozil (Cefzil)	30	1000	2

[a]Amoxicillin-to-clavulanate potassium ratio is 4:1 in all formulations except in Augmentin 250 tablets in which it is 2:1.
[b]Available only as 125- and 250-mg tablets; often prescribed as 125 mg BID for children younger than 2 years and 250 BID for those older than 2 years.

persists unabated for more than 3 months despite treatment with antimicrobials, especially when bilateral, occurring in a young child, or associated with hearing loss, tinnitus, vertigo, or significant changes in the tympanic membrane or middle ear, myringotomy (usually with tympanostomy tube placement) should be considered. These same recommendations apply to HIV-infected children; in symptomatically HIV-infected children (P2), early retreatment of persistent effusion with a broader spectrum antimicrobial is recommended, especially if amoxicillin had been initially used. To date, *P. carinii* has not been reported to cause ear infections in HIV-infected children. The few such adults who have been described appear to have responded to oral trimethoprim-sulfamethoxazole with or without dapsone or to intravenously administered pentamidine. Aural polyps from which *P. carinii* was isolated did not always require excision (14, 17, 19, 20 25).

Chronic suppurative otitis media should be managed in conjunction with an otolaryngologist who will provide a diagnostic specimen from culture, daily aural toilet, and serial examinations. Topical antimicrobial therapy with Cortisporin or Coly-mycin, often in conjunction with gentamicin, is advised despite theoretical concerns for ototoxicity when instilled directly into the middle ear. Parenteral antimicrobials, initially selected empirically for activity against *P. aeruginiosa* and *S. aureus* (e.g., ticarcillin disodium/clavulanate potassium) and subsequently chosen according to culture and antimicrobial susceptibility results, are usually necessary and sufficient to effect a cure. Tympanomastoidectomy is sometimes required.

Although systemic or intranasal decongestants may relieve symptoms of nasal congestion caused by a concurrent viral URI and antihistamines may be effective in relieving symptoms in the allergic patient, neither modality will affect the course of acute otitis media, prevent recurrences of AOM, nor prompt the resolution of subacute or chronic effusions and are therefore not recommended. Results of trials of systemic or intranasal corticosteroids in the treatment of persistent effusion are ambiguous. We would not recommend their use for this indication, although intranasal corticosteroids or sodium cromolyn are efficacious and appropriate for relieving symptoms of allergic rhinitis (4).

Bacterial otitis externa is treated topically with a broad spectrum antimicrobial in conjunction with an anti-inflammatory agent such as Cortisporin solution or suspension (containing polymixin, neomycin, and hydrocortisone in an acid pH medium) four times daily. Local instillation of Burow's solution or acetic acid as well as topically or systemically administered analgesics are frequently indicated. Systemic antibiotics (selected empirically or on the basis or results of cultures) are required for coincidental otitis media or for complicating chondritis, cellulitis, or systemic infection.

Fungal otitis externa is usually satisfactorily treated with cleansing and topical administration of various agents. Cultures may be helpful to direct the selection of a specific agent. For dermatophytes, clotrimazole or tolnaftate are appropriate; nystatin is specific for *Candida* species. amphotericin B is a broad spectrum antifungal. Other useful topical biochemically fungicidal preparations include m-cresyl acetate, nystatin, gentian violet, 1% iodine, and 3% iodochlorhydroxyquin. With more extensive infections, systemic antifungal agents such as amphotericin B may be required.

Prevention

Three effective options exist for preventing or at least reducing episodes of recurrent AOM and middle ear effusion: chemoprophylaxis, myringotomy with tympanostomy tube placement, and adenoidectomy (4, 34–35).

Chemoprophylaxis (4, 34) is the first option that should be utilized. Although in immunocompetent hosts, this modality is usually implemented after the occurrence of more than three episodes with 6 months, a lower threshold is appropriate for initiating chemoprophylaxis in children with symptomatic (P2) HIV infection. Agents with demonstrated efficacy that are recommended include amoxicillin (at 20 mg/kg/day) and sulfisoxazole (at 50–75 mg/kg/day in two divided doses). It is reasonable to assume that any broader spectrum agent listed in Table 14.1 would probably be effective for prophylaxis when given once daily at half the usual therapeutic dose. We recommend considering use of one of these agents for prophylaxis for children with symptomatic (P2) HIV infection. Although concern for its toxicity has led some authorities to caution against the use of trimethoprim-sulfamethoxazle for preventing recurrences of otitis media, it has demonstrated efficacy for this purpose when given daily. Although its ability to prevent otitis media when administered less frequently (as in thrice weekly schedules often used in HIV-infected patients for prophylaxis against *P. carinii* pneumonia) is unknown, daily administration, if tolerated, would provide satisfactory protection for both concerns. Chemoprophylaxis should generally be given throughout the respiratory season for those who experience the usual seasonal pattern of otitis media; it should be given for at least 1 year for those whose disease occurs year-round.

Myringotomy and tube placement is recommended for patients whose frequency of recurrent AOM is not substantially reduced by chemoprophylaxis and for selected patients with chronic effusion (e.g., those with significant hearing loss) (4, 34).

Adenoidectomy (with or without myringotomy and tympanostomy tube placement) has been shown to be modestly efficacious in reducing both middle ear effusion and, to a lesser extent, recurrent middle ear infection in selected populations of children (34–36). It is unclear if tonsillectomy contributes further to a favorable outcome.

Monthly intravenous infusion of immunoglobulin (IVIG) has been demonstrated to reduce the frequency of both serious and minor bacterial infections, including AOM, in HIV-infected children with CD4 lymphocyte counts of ≥200/mm^3 (although the possibility that concomitant trimethroprim-sulfamethoxazole and/or zidovudine therapy confounded the results of the study has not been conclusively excluded). The rates of otitis media per 100 patient-years among IVIG and placebo recipients were 63.5 and 99.5, respectively, representing a 36% decrement in infection frequently (31). A recent study in which children receiving zidovudine were randomized to receive or not receive monthly IVIG demonstrated that IVIG was beneficial in reducing bacterial infections if trimethoprim-sulfamethoxazole was not being administered (See Chapter 45). Although prevention of recurrent otitis media would not typically be a sufficient indication for use of IVIG, it may prove to be a welcome by-product if IVIG therapy is given for other purposes (37).

SINUSITIS
Microbiologic Considerations

Bacterial organisms most commonly responsible for causing acute and chronic sinusitis in immunocompetent adults and children are *S. pneumoniae* (30–40%), nontypable *H. influenzae* (20%), and *M. catarrhalis* (20%) (5–7, 38). Less often, group A streptococcus, group C streptococcus, streptococcus viridans, *Peptostreptococcus, Moraxella* spp and *Eikenella corrodens* are implicated (6). Viruses, such as rhinovirus, parainfluenza, influenza A, and adenovirus, either alone or together with bacterial pathogens, have been identified in ~10% of cases (6). *S. aureus* and anaerobic organisms, as well as streptococcus viridans and *H. influenzae* are most often associated with sinusitis of very prolonged duration. Many fungi, most commonly *A. fumigatus,* are occasionally responsible for chronic sinusitis in immunocompetent hosts (7).

There have been no systematic studies documenting the microbiology of sinusitis in HIV-infected adults or children. It is likely that they become infected with the same organisms that usually infect immunocompetent hosts, as well as the panoply of uncommon and opportunistic bacterial, viral, fungal, mycobacterial, and protozoal pathogens that have been implicated in various compromised hosts (7). The following organisms have been specifically documented to cause sinusitis in HIV-infected patients: *S. aureus* (39, 40), *S. pneumoniae* and *P. aeruginosa* (10, 41–43), *S. epidermidis* (10), group G streptococcus (10), *R. arhizus* (44), *Legionella pneumophila* (in an adult without pneumonia) (45), *C. albicans* (1, 46) *Encephalitozoon cuniculi* (47), *Acanthamoeba castellanii* (48), *A. fumigatus*

(49), *Mycobacterium avium-intracellulare* (in two children with disseminated MAI) (50), and *Cryptococcus neoformans* (51). Patients with HIV infections, like other frequently hospitalized populations, are at increased risk of developing nosocomial sinusitis caused by any of an array of Gram-negative enteric and Gram-positive coccal agents (7).

Epidemiology

Acute sinusitis is an extremely common problem among young children with normal immunity. It has been estimated that 5–10% of viral URIs in young children (which occur six to eight times annually) are complicated by bacterial sinusitis (6). It is probable that, at least, repeated and prolonged episodes of sinusitis occur more frequently among HIV-infected children than among immunologically uncompromised children, although this has not been rigorously documented. The incidence of sinusitis in (mostly adult) AIDS patients has been observed retrospectively to be 10–20% and prospectively 30–68% (41). In a trial of IVIG prophylaxis for serious bacterial infection in HIV-infected children, clinically diagnosed acute sinusitis occurred in 39% of the episodes of "serious" infection and obtained irrespective of CD4 count, HIV classification, and receipt of IVIG (37).

Pathogenesis and Natural History

The paranasal sinuses develop as outpouchings of the nasal cavity (6). Secretions are normally cleared from the sinuses through individual orifices (ostia) that open into a drainage system which empties into the nose by way of meatuses located beneath the nasal turbinates. The frontal, maxillary and anterior ethmoid sinuses drain through an area known as the osteomeatal complex that culminates in the middle meatus; the sphenoid and posterior ethmoid sinuses drain through the superior meatus.

Normal sinus function depends on 1) patency of the sinus ostia and drainage system, 2) a functioning mucociliary apparatus, and 3) a normal quality and quantity of secretions. Retention of secretions within the sinuses occurs when there is 1) anatomic (ex-

trinsic or intrinsic) or physiologic obstruction of normal drainage, 2) reduction in the number or impairment of the function of cilia, or 3) overproduction or increased viscosity of secretions.

In the usual case of sinusitis, either a viral URI or allergy leads to mucositis, resulting in obstruction of drainage. Colonizing nasopharyngeal flora, which have gained access to the formerly sterile sinuses, proliferate, producing a local inflammatory reaction which damages the mucosa and thereby further impairs ciliary function and local phagocytic activity (5, 6). Other less common pathogenetic factors include trauma, polyps, gastric or endotracheal tubes or other foreign bodies, septal deviation, dysmotile cilia syndrome, and cystic fibrosis. Exposure to infected siblings or other young children (e.g., at day care) increases the risk of acquiring a viral URI, the usual prelude to sinusitis. Use of broad spectrum antibiotics also fosters colonization by more resistant bacterial flora and fungi, from which pathology may stem. Likewise, increased susceptibility to colonization by fungi or parasites may occur because of the cellular and humoral immunodeficiency and neutropenia associated with HIV infection and/or its treatment.

Clinical Presentation

There are two patterns of illness with which acute sinusitis presents in immunocompetent children: either persistent or severe symptoms (5, 6). Persistent symptoms are more common. Unlike the usual course of a viral URI, in which symptoms typically improve or resolve within 10 days, acute sinusitis with persistent symptoms is characterized by the presence of unimproving cough and/or rhinorrhea for 10–30 days. Nasal discharge may have any quality (thin, thick, clear, mucoid, or purulent) and cough may be either dry or productive and, although often worse at night, occurs throughout the day. Breath may be malodorous. Affected children do not usually appear very ill. If present, fever is usually low grade. Facial pain and headache are unusual complaints; mild periorbital edema (frequently present upon arising and resolving while upright during the day) may occur. Less commonly, acute sinusitis may present with features of a more severe nature: high fever (>39° C) and purulent nasal discharge. Severe headache (supra- or retroorbital), toxicity, or severe periorbital edema may occur in this presentation.

In immunoincompetent hosts, including children with HIV infection, clinical presentation of sinusitis is most often indistinguishable from that in immunocompetent patients. However, frequent, prolonged, and recurrent episodes, as well as lack of or slow improvement in response to usual management may signify a compromised host. Fever without an apparent source, subtly or belatedly associated with localizing features, such as rhinorrhea, presinus tenderness, facial swelling or erythema, nasal pain or ulceration may characterize the clinical presentation (7).

In the immunocompetent host, physical examination is usually not helpful in differentiating acute sinusitis from a viral URI. Mucopurulent rhinorrhea, edema, and erythema of the nasal mucosa occur in both conditions. Facial tenderness, swelling, or the presence of mucopus emanating directly from a meatus occur rarely in children but, if present, strongly suggest a diagnosis of sinusitis. In sinusitis of chronic duration, hypertrophied nasal turbinates and nasal polyps may be present. Fungal sinusitis is suggested by the presence of nasal mucosa that are focally pale, gray, or black, have decreased or absent pain sensation, increased friability and do not bleed following trauma.

Sinusitis in either the immunocompetent or immunoincompetent host may be complicated by extension of infection to adjacent bone, the orbit, or the central nervous system (in the form of an epidural abscess, brain abscess, meningitis, cavernous sinus thrombosis, optic neuritis, or carotid aneurysm). Orbital involvement is signified by the onset of proptosis, ophthalmoplegia, ocular tenderness, or decreased visual acuity.

Diagnostic Considerations

Often, diagnosis of sinusitis is inferred on the basis of clinical criteria alone. This practice is justified by the strong correlation (88% agreement) between abnormal sinus radiographs and features of persistent sinusitis described above in children younger than 6 years (6).

In acute sinusitis, radiographic findings include diffuse opacification, mucosal thickening of at least 4–5 mm, or, rarely in children, an air-fluid level. The presence of any of these abnormalities in a child with features of sinusitis of either the persistent or severe variety is associated with high-density bacterial maxillary sinusitis in 70% of cases (6).

Sinus radiographs should be used to confirm diagnosis of sinusitis in children younger than 6 years with severe symptoms and in all children older than 6 years suspected of having sinusitis. These recommendations apply to both immunocompetent and immunoincompetent hosts.

Computerized tomography scans with contrast enhancement are more sensitive than radiographs for detecting sinusitis but in general should be reserved for evaluation of recurrent or chronic sinusitis or suspected complications of the orbit or brain. Magnetic resonance imaging is also useful for diagnosing sinusitis but is less helpful than computerized tomography scans. Ultrasonography is not a practical diagnostic technique.

Although not routinely utilized for diagnostic purposes, maxillary sinus aspiration can be safely and effectively performed as an outpatient procedure using a transnasal approach after careful decontamination and adequate local anesthesia of the area below the inferior turbinate which the trocar traverses. Aspirated material should be processed promptly for aerobic and anaerobic bacterial cultures as well as for Gram's stain. Recovery of organisms in a density of at least 10^4 cfu/ml is considered indicative of infection (5, 6).

Indications for sinus aspiration in an immunocompetent host include 1) failure to respond to multiple courses of antibiotics, 2) severe facial pain, and 3) orbital or intracranial complications. The same criteria would apply to an immunoincompetent host. In addition, 1) suspicion for an unusual or opportunistic pathogen or 2) sinusitis in a moderately to severely ill patient should prompt sinus aspiration and biopsy of sinus mucosa. In such cases, in addition to bacterial cultures, aspirated and biopsied material should be processed to facilitate identification of fungi, viruses, mycobacteria, *Legionella*, protozoa, and possibly *P. carinii* and should be submitted for histologic examination. When fungal infection is suspected on the basis of nasal or facial findings, a biopsy of nasal mucosa should be similarly processed (7). Adequacy of platelets and the coagulation profile must be checked before performance of an invasive procedure.

Treatment

In both immunocompetent and immunoincompetent patients who are only mildly ill from sinusitis, outpatient treatment with orally administered antimicrobial therapy empirically aimed at the most likely bacterial pathogens is appropriate (5, 7, 52). Table 14.1 lists candidate antimicrobial agents and dosage schedules. Amoxicillin is recommended for most initial and uncomplicated cases of sinusitis. If improvement does not ensue with amoxicillin within 48–72 hours or in more complicated cases of sinusitis (e.g., episodes associated with development of high fever or periorbital swelling), or if micro-biologic data so indicate, a broader spectrum oral antimicrobial should be substituted. Most comprehensive coverage is afforded by amoxicillin-clavulanate potassium, erythromycin-sulfisoxazole, or cefuroxime axetil. Large comparative studies of these agents in immunocompetent children with sinusitis have not been performed.

No systematic studies have been performed to determine the optimal duration of antimicrobial therapy in either immunocompetent or immunoincompetent hosts. For those who show a prompt clinical response, a 10- to 14-day course appears to be sufficient. For patients who respond slowly or incompletely, we recommend extending treatment for 1 week beyond clinical resolution of symptoms.

When treating patients who have presented with very long-standing symptoms (months rather than weeks) antimicrobial selection should reflect a concern for staphylococci and respiratory anaerobes in addition to *S. pneumoniae*, *H. influenzae*, and *M. catarrhalis*. In this circumstance

amoxicillin-potassium clavulanate, erythromycin-sulfisoxazole, and cefuroxime axetil are suitable. Response to treatment is characteristically slow in these patients. However, as long as continued improvement is noted, treatment should be maintained. Again, it is recommended that therapy be extended for 1 week beyond the resolution of all respiratory symptoms; 4–8 weeks of antimicrobial therapy may be required.

When used as adjunctive treatment of sinusitis, inhaled decongestants appear to provide relief of nasal symptoms, to increase patency of the sinus drainage apparatus, and to decrease nasal airway resistance. However, there is concern that they may cause ciliostasis. The net effect of inhaled decongestants on the course of sinus symptoms has not been systematically studied. Routine use of decongestants is not recommended; however, in selected cases (severe nasal congestion or periorbital swelling) their use for a few days may be helpful. Systemic and local antihistamines, intranasal corticosteroids, and sodium cromolyn appear to help improve symptoms of nasal allergy.

For those patients who present with moderate to severe clinical sinusitis or who, by virtue of being immunoincompetent, are considered at increased risk for unusual or opportunistic organisms or severe courses of illness, hospitalization, diagnostic sinus aspiration, initiation of empiric broad spectrum antimicrobials parenterally, and eventual refinement of antimicrobial selection based on culture and susceptibility testing results are appropriate. Most patients will respond with an impressive diminution of symptoms within 48–72 hours. Rarely, when symptoms do not respond to parenteral therapy, surgical drainage may be necessary to restore physiologic function to a paranasal sinus.

In children with very persistent or recurrent acute sinusitis, antimicrobial prophylaxis should be considered. Although antimicrobial prophylaxis has not been studied in patients with recurrent acute sinusitis, by analogy to its demonstrated effectiveness in reducing episodes of recurrent AOM, it is an attractive preventive modality. Indications should be similar to those used for prophylaxis of recurrent AOM, i.e., three episodes in 6 months or four episodes in 1 year. Similar antimicrobials are recommended as are used in recurrent AOM.

Although there are no data available to help define the specific indications for surgical treatment of sinusitis in HIV-infected children, when maximal medical therapy, including chemoprophylaxis, has failed to reduce chronic symptoms or frequent recurrences, surgical therapy should be considered. In children with chronic sinusitis, creation of a nasoantral window in the maxillary sinus was formerly a therapy which, when critically evaluated, demonstrated little efficacy. Currently, functional endonasal sinus surgery (endoscopic removal of obstructions in the osteomeatal complex, enlargement of the meatus of the maxillary sinus outflow tract, and anterior ethmoidectomy) represents the most promising surgical option. Preliminary reports suggest that this procedure results in substantial improvement in children with chronic sinusitis (6, 53, 54).

When fungal sinusitis is highly suspected or documented, treatment with amphotericin B should be instituted in an accelerated schedule to quickly achieve a daily dose of 1 mg/kg. Addition of 5-fluorocytosine or rifampin should be considered as adjunctive therapy. Liposomal amphotericin has been effective in some cases unresponsive to conventional amphotericin B or when the use of the latter has been complicated by deteriorating renal function. The utility of new antifungal agents such as fluconazole and intraconazole has yet to be defined. Extensive surgical debridement is usually required. Hyperbaric oxygen may be helpful in cases of rhinocerebral mucormycosis (7).

Prevention

Systematic study of antimicrobial prophylaxis for recurrent acute sinusitis in immunocompetent or immunoincompetent patients has not been reported; however, it is an attractive preventive modality which was discussed in "Treatment".

Although in the National Institute of Child Health and Human Development trial, administration of IVIG was associated with a reduction in the overall number of episodes of "severe" bacterial infection, in those HIV-infected patients with CD4 counts of $\geq 200/mm^3$, there was no demonstrated difference in the frequency of clinically diagnosed acute sinusitis incurred by IVIG and placebo recipients (37).

Areas for Future Research in Otitis Media and Sinusitis

Research regarding the following issues pertaining to otitis media and sinusitis in HIV-infected children would have practical applications to management of these common conditions: 1) better definition of the microbiology (especially for sinusitis) including the rolls of antibiotic-resistant and unusual organisms; 2) elucidation of the role of respiratory viruses in the etiology and pathogenesis of otitis media and sinusitis among HIV-infected and uninfected children; 3) determination of optimal antimicrobial agents for treatment and chemoprophylaxis including the possible role of new antifungal triazoles; and 4) development of vaccines that are protective against pathogens commonly responsible for otitis media and sinusitis and immunogenic in children with HIV infection.

References

1. Church JA. Human immunodeficiency virus (HIV) infection at Children's Hospital of Los Angeles: Recurrent otitis media or chronic sinusitis as the presenting process in pediatric AIDS. Immunol Allergy Pract 1987;9:25–32.
2. Paradise JL. Otitis media in infants and children: A current, critical review. Pediatrics 1980;65: 917–943.
3. Bluestone Cd. Recent advances in the pathogenesis, diagnosis, and management of otitis media. Pediatr Clin North Am 1981;28:727–755.
4. Bluestone CD. Modern management of otitis media. Pediatr Clin North Am 1989;36:1371–1387.
5. Wald ER. Acute and chronic sinusitis: Diagnosis and management. Pediatr Rev 1985;7:150–157.
6. Wald ER. Sinusitis in children. N Engl J Med 1992; 326:319–323.
7. Wald ER. Infections of the sinuses, ears, and hypopharynx. In: Shelhamer J, Pizzo PA, Parrillo JE, Masur H, eds. Respiratory disease in the immunosuppressed host. Philadelphia: JB Lippincott, 1991: 450–468.
8. Wald ER. Haemophilus influenzae as a cause of acute otitis media. Pediatr Infect Dis J 1989;8:S28–S30.
9. Principi N, Marchisio P, Tornaghi R, Onorato J, Massironi E, Picco P. Acute otitis media in human immunodeficiency virus-infected children. Pediatrics 1991;88:566–571.

10. Krasinski K, Borkowsky W, Bonk S, Lawrence R, Chandwani S. Bacterial infections in human immunodeficiency virus-infected children. Pediatr Infect Dis J 1988;7:323–328.

11. Williams MA. Head and neck findings in pediatric acquired immune deficiency syndrome. Laryngoscope 1987;97:713–716.

12. Strauss M, Fine E. Asperigillus otomastoiditis in acquired immunodeficiency syndrome. Am J Otol 1991;12:49–53.

13. Forrett-Kaminsky MC, Scherer C, Bemer M, Robert V, Steinbach G, Poussel JF. Otite moyenne à nocardia asteroïdes au cours du SIDA. Presse Méd 1991; 20:1512–1513.

14. Schinella RA, Breda SD, Hammerschlag PE. Otic infection due to *Pneumocystis carinii* in an apparently healthy man with antibody to the human immunodeficiency virus. Ann Intern Med 1987;106: 399–400.

15. Coulman C, Greene I, Archibald R. Cutaneous pneumocystosis. Ann Intern Med 1987;106:396–398.

16. Breda S, Hammerschlag P, Gigliotti F, Schinella R. *Pneumocystis carinii* in the temporal bone as a primary manifestation of the acquired immunodeficiency syndrome. Ann Otol Rhinol Laryngol 1988; 97:427–431.

17. Gherman CR, Ward RR, Bassis ML. *Pneumocystis carinii* otitis media and mastoiditis as the initial manifestation of the acquired immunodeficiency syndrome. Am J Med 1988;85:250–252.

18. Smith M, Hirschfield L, Zahtz G, Siegal F. Pneumocystis carinii otitis media. Am J Med 1988; 85:745–746.

19. Sandler ED, Sandler JM, LeBoit PE, Wenig BM, Mortensen N. *Pneumocystis carinii* otitis media in AIDS: A case report and review of the literature regarding extrapulmonary pneumocystosis. Otolaryngol Head Neck Surg 1990;103:817–821.

20. Park S, Wunderlich H, Goldenberg RA, Marshall M. *Pneumocystis carinii* infection in the middle ear. Arch Otolaryngol Head Neck Surg 1992;118: 269–270.

21. Derkay CS, Bluestone CD, Thompson AE, Kardatske D. Otitis media in the pediatric intensive care unit: A prospective study. Otolaryngol Head Neck Surg 1989;100:292–299.

22. Perisco M, Barker GA, Mitchell DP. Purulent otitis media: A "silent" source of sepsis in the pediatric intensive care unit. Otolaryngol Head Neck Surg 1985;93:330–334.

23. Teele DW, Klein JO, Rosner B, Greater Boston Otitis Media Study Group. Epidemiology of otitis media during the first seven years of life in children in Greater Boston: A prospective cohort study. J Infect Dis 1989;160:83–94.

24. Marcussen DC, Sooy CD. Otolaryngologic and head and neck manifestations of acquired immunodeficiency syndrome (AIDS). Laryngoscope 1985; 95:401–405.

25. Kohan D, Rothstein SG, Cohen HL. Otologic disease in patients with acquired immunodeficiency syndrome. Ann Otol Rhinol Laryngol 1988;97: 636–639.

26. Fairley JW, Dhillon RS, Weller IVD. HIV, glue ear and adenoidal hypertrophy [Letter]. Lancet 1988;2: 1422.

27. Bernstein LJ, Krieger BZ, Novick B, Sicklick MJ, Rubinstein A. Bacterial infection in the acquired immunodeficiency syndrome of children. Pediatr Infect Dis J 1985;4:472–475.

28. Sculerati N, Borkowsky W. Pediatric human immunodeficiency virus infection: An otolaryngologist's perspective. J Otolaryngol 1990;19:182–188.

29. Chanock SJ, McIntosh K. Pediatric infection with the human immunodeficiency virus: Issues for the otorhinolaryngologist. Pediatr Otolaryngol 1989; 22:637–660.

30. Barnett ED, Klein JO, Pelton SI, Luginbuhl LM. Otitis media in children born to human immunodeficiency virus-infected mothers. Pediatr Infect Dis J 1992;11:360–364.

31. Mofenson LM, Moye J, Bethel J, et al. Prophylactic intravenous immunoglobulin in HIV-infected children with CD4+ counts of 0.20 X 10⁹/L or more. JAMA 1992;268:483–488.

32. Chow JH, Stern JC, Kaul A, Pincus RL, Gromisch DS. Head and neck manifestations of the acquired immunodeficiency syndrome in children. Ear Nose Throat J 1990;69:416–423.

33. Centers for Disease Control. Classification system for human immunodeficiency virus (HIV) infection in children under 13 years of age. MMWR 1987;36:225–230, 235.

34. Paradise JL. Antimicrobial drugs and surgical procedures in the prevention of otitis media. Pediatr Infect Dis J 1989;8:S35–S37.

35. Paradise JL, Bluestone CD, Rogers KD, et al. Efficacy of adenoidectomy for recurrent otitis media in children previously treated with tympanostomy-tube placement. JAMA 1990;263:2066–2073.

36. Gates GA, Avery CA, Prihoda TJ, Cooper JC. Effectiveness of adenoidectomy and tympanostomy tubes in the treatment of chronic otitis media with effusion. N Engl J Med 1987;317:1444–1451.

37. National Institute of Child Health and Human Development Intravenous Immunoglobulin Study Group. Intravenous immune globulin for the prevention of bacterial infections in children with symptomatic human immunodeficiency virus infection. N Engl J Med 1991;325:73–80.

38. Wald ER, Milmoe GJ, Bowen AD, Ladesma-Medina J, Salamon N, Bluestone CD. Acute maxillary sinusitis in children. N Engl J Med 1981; 304:749–754.

39. Hadderingh RJ. Recurrent maxillary sinusitis in AIDS patients [Abstract MBP 203]. Fifth International Conference on AIDS, Montreal, Jun 1989.

40. Slavit DH. Chronic sinusitis and dyspnea: Could this be AIDS? Otolaryngol Head Neck Surg 1990; 103:650–652.

41. Rubin JS, Honigberg RH. Sinusitis in patients with the acquired immunodeficiency syndrome. Ear Nose Throat J 1990;69:460–463.

42. Schrager LK. Bacterial infections in AIDS patients. AIDS 1988;S183–S189.

43. Poole MD, Postma D, Cohen MS. Pyogenic otorhinologic infections in acquired immune deficiency syndrome. Arch Otolaryngol 1984;110:130–131.

44. Blatt SP, Lucey DR, Dettoff D, Zellmer RB. Rhinocerebral zygomycosis in a patient with AIDS. J Infect Dis 1991;164:215–216.

45. Schlanger G, Lutwick LI, Kurzman M, Hoch B. Sinusitis caused by *Legionella pneumophila* in a patient with the acquired immune deficiency syndrome. Am J Med 1984;77:957–960.
46. Colmenero C, Monux A, Valencia E, Castro A. Successfully treated candida sinusitis in an AIDS patient. J Craniomaxillofac Surg 1990;18:175–178.
47. Metcalfe TW, Doran RML, Rowlands PL, Curry A, Lacey CJN. Microsporidial keratoconjunctivitis in a patient with AIDS. Br J Ophthalmol 1992;76: 177–178.
48. Gonzalez MM, Gould E, Dickinson G, et al. Acquired immunodeficiency syndrome associated with acanthamoeba infection and other organisms. Arch Pathol Lab Med 1986;110:749–751.
49. Carrazana EJ, Rossitch E, Morris J. Isolated central nervous system aspergillosis in the acquired immunodeficiency syndrome. Clin Neurol Neurosurg 1991;93:227–230.
50. Brady MT, Van Dyke RB. Involvement of the ear, sinuses, oropharynx, parotid, cervical lymph nodes, and ear. In: Yogev R, Connor E, eds. Management of HIV infection in infants and children. Philadelphia: Mosby, 1992:287–322.
51. Grant IH, Armstrong D. Fungal infections in AIDS: Cryptococcus. In: Sande MA, Volberding PA, eds. The management of AIDS. Philadelphia: WB Saunders, 1988;225–233.
52. Lusk RP, Lazar RH, Muntz HR. The diagnosis and treatment of recurrent and chronic sinusitis in children. Pediatr Clin North Am 1989;36:1411–1421.
53. Gross CW, Gurucharri MJ, Lazar RH, Long TE. Functional endonasal sinus surgery (FESS) in the pediatric age group. Laryngoscope 1989;99: 272–275.
54. Lusk RP, Muntz HR. Endoscopic sinus surgery in children with chronic sinusitis: A pilot study. Laryngoscope 1990;100:654–658.

15

Sexually Transmitted Diseases in Children and Adolescents with HIV Infection

Laura T. Gutman

This chapter focuses on the presentation, diagnosis, management, and complications of sexually transmitted diseases (STD) of children who are infected with human immunodeficiency virus (HIV). Because the primary means of transmission of STDs to children, beyond infancy, is through episodes of child sexual abuse, this chapter will also focus on several aspects of the recognition of sexual abuse and evaluation of children who are suspected of having been abused. Policies for HIV testing of children who are being examined for suspected sexual abuse will be discussed.

The term "child sexual abuse" encompasses abusive sexual acts that do not involve sexual contact, such as exposure to sexually explicit acts of others, voyeurism and child pornography; sexual acts during which there is physical contact but the perpetrator is unlikely to exchange body fluids with the child such as digital abuse and external genital rubbing; and sexual acts during which exchange of body fluids between perpetrator and child is possible or likely such as contact between the perpetrator's genitalia and the child's vagina, anus, or mouth.

Several characteristics of the lives of most children who are born into families in which members are HIV infected overlap with social risk factors for child sexual abuse. In later childhood and adolescence, behavioral consequences of earlier abuse may lead to risk-taking behaviors that thereby increase the likelihood that the

child will acquire HIV and other STDs during volitional sexual activity. For adults, the acquisition of STDs has been found to be highly correlated with increased prevalence of HIV infection and predictive of infection with HIV. The ways in which this correlation applies to children are discussed in this chapter.

RECOGNITION OF YOUNGER CHILDREN WHO ARE AT RISK OF BEING SEXUALLY ABUSED

Presentations of children who have been sexually abused are extremely variable. Sexually abused children are often also physically abused, neglected, or emotionally abused. This chapter cannot provide full coverage of the various clinical signs of abuse. However, Appendixes 15.1 and 15.2 include findings and behaviors that commonly characterize normal and abused children or nonabusing and abusing caretakers.

Child sexual abuse occurs in all social classes and may affect children whose families appear to be functioning appropriately. However, there are several social settings that, when present, correlate with significantly increased prevalence of child sexual abuse. They appear to have in common living conditions that bring greater stress to the family, conditions that lead to loss of inhibitions regarding sexual conduct, and conditions that decrease the perceived value of the child to the family. These conditions follow.

269

- The household lives in poverty.
- The child is raised for 3 months or more by persons other than the two biologic parents.
- One or more members of the household is alcoholic.
- One or more members of the household uses illegal substances.
- The child is disabled or has a chronic illness or disability.

Other characteristics of homes in which sexual abuse is more prevalent than in the general population have been less well studied but include families headed by adults who were themselves abused, who have punitive and/or rigid attitudes regarding sexuality, who are socially isolated, in which the mother is disabled, and in which the adults suffer from serious psychiatric illness. Although most sexual abusers are males who are under age 35, abuse by females also occurs, and abusers have included persons of all age ranges.

EVALUATION OF SEXUAL ABUSE

The presence of screening findings may help the clinician to identify those children at risk, to identify social circumstances in which abuse is more likely, and to decide which children require a complete evaluation for suspected child sexual abuse (CSA). An adequate evaluation for child sexual abuse requires participation of skilled professionals from several disciplines formed into a diagnostic team. Child protection teams commonly are composed of a social worker, pediatrician, and nurse or psychologist.

The diagnosis of CSA is imperfect at best. Children who are subsequently confirmed to be abused commonly fail to show physical evidence of abuse, and abused children often initially refrain from disclosing abusive experiences to interviewers. Conversely, children who are probably not abused may present with medical and behavioral symptoms that are similar to those of abused children. Because of these limitations, evaluation of a child for suspected CSA requires that all available diagnostic modalities be used. These include diagnostic interviews with the child, review of medical and behav-

ioral histories, physical examinations, and evaluation for sexually transmitted organisms. The following description is a summary of an evaluation process that would adhere to currently accepted standards and is adapted from the Duke Child Protection Team (Dr. St. Claire, personal communication, 1992).

MEDICAL EXAMINATION
Diagnostic Interview

The process of the evaluation is discussed with the caretaker and the child. An examination often includes more than one interview. The interviewer uses age appropriate techniques such as anatomical dolls, drawings, stories, and writing to help the child express details regarding what may have happened. Affect is important in assessing the reliability of what is being said. Children younger than 3 years usually cannot participate adequately in a diagnostic interview. Leading questions are avoided.

After the diagnostic interviews, an evaluation of the evidence regarding CSA should be made (see Table 15.1A and 1B).

Physical Examination

The physical examination requires understanding of normal prepubertal male and female genital and anal anatomy and characteristics of children who have been sexually assaulted. Rapport must be established with the child since the examinations are not performed if the child cannot cooperate. If the child cannot cooperate and there is a history of genital bleeding and/or persistent discharge the child may need to be examined with generalized anesthesia. Invasive procedures are usually not required to examine a child.

Boys are more difficult to evaluate because physical findings are less well described than for girls.

The examination begins with a medical history from the parents or caretakers and from the child when appropriate, as well as a review of documents and medical records. A physical examination is performed with special attention to the mouth, genital, and anal areas. The Tanner stage for breast and genital development is determined. Details

Table 15.1A.   Interpretation of Findings from Evaluation for Sexual Abuse[a]

Strong evidence of abuse includes a detailed disclosure of a specific act, usually supported by one or more of the following.
Spontaneous descriptions of sexual acts.

Affect: anxious, sad, angry, afraid, guarded demeanor.

Behavior: regressed, avoidant, situational, hyperactive, distractible, eroticized—displayed by humping or imitation of oral sex with dolls.

Detailed sexual knowledge inconsistent with a child's level of development.

Personalized descriptions of sexual behavior.

Knowledge of dynamics of sexually abusive relationships inconsistent with a child's level of development.

Consistency in describing the basic facts of the disclosure to interviewer and others.

Behavioral history consistent with that of a sexually abused child (e.g., sexual acting out, sudden changes in behavior, nightmares).

Probable evidence of child sexual abuse in the absence of detailed disclosure usually include the following.
Child exhibits eroticized behavior.

Child's behavioral history includes sexual acting out with other children, stuffed toys, dolls, animals, or attempted sexual acting out with adults.

Child engages in excessive masturbation in a public manner and/or uses objects to masturbate.

Child has disclosed sexual abuse to another professional or to a parent and does not appear to be vindictive toward the alleged perpetrator.

Ruled Out. No concerns or minimal concerns based upon history and interview with respect to factors outlined above.
Unknown.
Evaluation is incomplete.

Concerns arise from interview but are insufficient to warrant a reasonable suspicion.

Children younger than 3 years are usually preverbal, and results of interviews are consequently limited. Diagnosis is common in children this age.

[a]Compiled from diagnostic interviews.

of the vulva, urethra, posterior forchette, and hymenal tissue are noted. The horizontal diameter of the hymenal opening is measured. Magnification and illumination may be provided by a colposcope or otoscope. The anus is inspected and if gaping is present, the horizontal diameter is measured. Photographs and a detailed written description provide documentation of the findings. Laboratory studies may include urinalysis, vaginal and rectal cultures for chlamydia and gonorrhea, and pharyngeal culture for gonorrhea. A wet preparation of vaginal secretions can be examined for trichomonas and bacterial vaginosis. Other cultures and specimens are collected as warranted by symptoms and history. Some centers obtain serologies for syphilis and HIV when abuse is confirmed or probable.

Results of the diagnostic interviews and physical examinations are considered in reaching the final diagnosis. The final diag-

Table 15.1B.   Final Diagnostic Categories for Evaluation of Child Sexual Abuse[a]

Confirmed
Clear/valid disclosure to professional and/or perpetrator admission and/or one or more grossly abnormal physical finding consisting of the following.
1) Acute trauma: open tears of hymen, vagina, perivaginal tissue, or anal/perianal tissues (when there is not witnessed accidental penetrating trauma which reasonably explains the injury).
2) Presence of culture-proven gonorrhea that is not perinatally acquired or acquired syphilis.
3) Presence of motile sperm or positive acid phosphatase from oral, anal, or vaginal sites.

Probable
No confirmatory data but other medical indicators of abuse present: when a suspect exists who has access to child or when a behavioral or interview history is concerning for inappropriate sexual contact.

Acute trauma: bleeding or significantly friable tissue in vaginal, perivaginal, or anal areas in the absence of infectious etiology or other medical diagnosis such as lichen sclerosis.

Nonacute or healed trauma: age-specified enlargement of hymenal opening plus any combination of the following regardless of opening diameter.
1) Rapid (within 30–45 sec), repeated (on more than one look on the same day or subsequent exams) dilatation of internal and external anal sphincters.
2) Distinct scars, adhesions, or evidence of healed traumas in tissue of posterior fourchette, fossa navicularis, hymen, vagina, or anus.

Confirmed infection with other STDS when not perinatally acquired including *C. trachomatis, T. vaginalis* herpes simplex type II of genital region, condyloma acuminata, and bacterial vaginosis.

Perianal bruising, bleeding, anal gaping in the absence of rectal stool, and scars in perianal areas.

Ruled Out
Based on information available and recognizing that it is not possible to know with certainty that a child has not been abused.

Unknown
Incomplete evaluations and inconclusive evaluations, often because of young age or failure to return for follow-up.

[a]Compiled from diagnostic interviews.

nosis may be categorized according to certainty of findings. For example, Confirmed, Probable, Ruled Out, and Unknown. Bases for the diagnostic categories that incorporate all aspects of the evaluation are found in Table 15.1B. Recognize that most children who have been sexually abused lack specific physical findings. Consequently, the absence of physical findings does not provide evidence against abuse.

Children with the diagnosis of confirmed or probable CSA by law must be reported to the appropriate social agency for further evaluation. Arrangements should be made for a mental health evaluation and treatment.

EPIDEMIOLOGY OF ACQUIRED STD IN OLDER CHILDREN AND ADOLESCENTS

The following behaviors in adolescents put the child at risk for acquiring an STD or suggest that the child may have future behaviors that will incur an increased risk of acquiring an STD, including HIV.

• Initiation of sexual activity at a young age. Studies indicate that younger adolescents (usually defined as age 16 or younger) are less skilled in negotiating and implementing recommended measures designed to decrease transmission of STDs. The approaches of a large proportion of young persons to sexual encounters are characterized by inconsistent use of barrier protection, reluctance to recognize and avoid high-risk partners, difficulty in applying abstinence, and failure to require that a partner be free of a history of STDs or risk factors for STDs. Rates of STDs in adolescent populations are summarized on Table 15.2.

- Use of alcohol in conjunction with sexual activity. The association presumably derives from the decrease in inhibition of risky behavior and suspension of judgment.

- Substance abuse, especially cocaine. The child must finance the purchase of the drug, for which the child may turn to prostitution or the exchange of sex for money or drugs. Furthermore, substances such as cocaine, which stimulate sexual activity, may lead to sexual contact with multiple and anonymous partners.

- Sexual contact with multiple partners. Each contact provides a separate opportunity to become infected, and partners who are also sexually active with multiple other persons are more likely to disseminate one or more infections. Further, multiple partners are often anonymous partners, making impossible effective contact tracing.

- Sexual abuse during childhood or adolescence. The consequences of abuse and violence during childhood and adolescence have been found to include an increase in nonsexual risk-taking behaviors, entry into risky sexual activity at an immature age, prostitution, increased substance abuse, abuse of others, early and unplanned pregnancy, and multiple STDs.

- Homelessness and thrown-away, runaway, and "street child" statuses. Children and adolescents in those desperate circumstances are usually without support or protection and are poorly prepared to build a safe life for themselves. Attempts to support themselves often lead to trading support for sexual favors, prostitution, and drug-related activities.

- A history of a prior STD. These conditions have been primarily identified to be gonorrhea, syphilis, chancroid, chlamydia, genital herpes simplex virus infection, genital warts, and bacterial vaginosis. Current studies are exploring the extent, if any, to which infection with one of these agents facilitates the acquisition of other STDs by reducing the effectiveness

Table 15.2.   Representative Reports of Adolescent Patients in STD and Family Planning Clinics[a]

Report	Population	Infection	Prevalence %	Comments
VA Rahm, 1991, Sweden	301 sexually active teen females	Ct	19	Association between cervical ectopy and Ct infection.
MK Oh, 1988, Alabama	102 sexually active teen females	Ct	26	Mixed infections in 13% of girls
		Tv	13	
		Ng	10	
		HPV	5	
RE Fullilove, 1990, California	222 teen crack cocaine users	Any STD	41	Association of crack cocaine use and STD
TC Quinn, 1992, Maryland	Patients at an STD clinic	HIV	2.1	Greatest rise in prevalence in adolescents
BJ Dattel, 1988, California	127 females adolescents, sexually abused	Ct	14	
		Ng	12	
FM Mulcahey, 1986, England	210 adolescent females, in residential care	Ng	14	Pelvic inflammatory disease common
		Ct	16	
		Tv	16	
DA Frank, 1988, Massachusetts	Pregnant crack users	Any STD	19	
YM Sohn, 1991, Alabama	173 CMV-infected girls in contraceptive clinic	Ng	9	Study of relation of CMV to other STDs
		Ct	21	

[a]Ct, *C. trachomatis;* Ng, *N. gonorrhoeae;* Tv, *T. vaginalis;* CMV, cytomegalovirus.

of physical and immunological barriers. An increase in prevalence of HIV infection has been observed in exposed populations who have preexisting genital ulcer disease compared with those who do not. A prior history of an STD is an indicator of prior risk-taking behavior and may in addition indicate increased susceptibility to infection if exposed.

- Use of oral contraceptives. It is not established whether the increased rates of some STDs (such as chlamydial cervicitis) that are observed in young women using oral contraceptives represent a relative increase in risk-taking behavior, failure of the partner to use condoms or other barrier methods, or increased susceptibility.
- Cigarette smoking. The mechanism of this risk factor is also uncertain. Studies have made this observation in regard to several STDs, including genital human papilloma virus (HPV) infection, but other studies have found no association between smoking history and prevalence of STDs.
- Cervical ectopy. This condition refers to the persistence of columnar lining cells on the ectocervix. This type of mucosal lining cell provides a relatively weak defense to many STDs, and persistence of this type of membrane is believed to increase the susceptibility to infection after exposure. In addition, infections may act to retard the involution of this membrane, which normally decreases or resolves as a child reaches adolescence.

INFECTIONS AND LABORATORY DIAGNOSIS
Treponema pallidum

An important aspect of the microbiology of this organism has been that, with a minor technical exception, it cannot be adequately cultured outside the human body. It is a sobering fact that the means by which the emergence of penicillin-resistant strains would be recognized, should they develop, would be through the clinical recognition of failures of therapy. Diagnostic tests depend in large part upon serologic reactions to infection.

Nontreponemal tests (primarily the Rapid Plasma Reagin test) should be used for screening and to evaluate changes in antibody titer. These tests are less specific than treponemal tests and require that the laboratory perform the test in a manner which allows possible prozone phenomena to be recognized. Treponemal tests (microhemagglutination *T. pallidum*; Fluorescent treponema antibody-absorption tests) should be used to confirm a reactive nontreponemal test.

Human infections caused by *T. pallidum* may be transmitted through vertical transmission from an infected mother (congenital syphilis) or during contact with infected mucosal membranes or secretions (acquired syphilis). The following comments pertain to each form of transmission, again emphasizing only newer developments.

Congenital Syphilis

The epidemic of HIV has been accompanied by a dramatic increase in acquired syphilis in adults and that has led in turn to a concomitant increase in incidence rates of congenital syphilis. The expected ratio of infectious syphilis in women of childbearing age to cases of congenital syphilis is approximately 80:1. Since the populations experiencing most new cases of acquired syphilis are also the populations who are at greatest risk of infection with HIV, the burden of the mortality and morbidity of congenital syphilis now commonly falls on offspring of women who are also HIV infected. Consequently, women and infants infected with either HIV or syphilis should always be fully evaluated for both infections.

A complete statement regarding the evaluation of an infant for congenital syphilis is beyond the scope of this chapter, and the reader is referred to the recent article by Ikeda and Jensen. Several recent developments that merit emphasis include the following.

Since 1988, one criterion for the presumptive diagnosis of congenital syphilis, for which the child requires an adequate course of therapy, is that the infected mother was not treated or was inadequately treated for syphilis. An adequate course of therapy for the mother must include: 1) mother receiving an appropriate course of penicillin; 2) The mother must have serologic follow-up indicating that therapy has been successful and reinfection has not occurred.

Indications that the mother's course of therapy may have been inadequate and the baby therefore requires therapy are raised if 1) the mother was not treated; 2) documentation of the mother's treatment is inexact or unavailable; 3) there is clinical, epidemiologic, or serologic evidence of relapse, reinfection, or failure of therapy in the mother; 4) the mother received a nonpenicillin regimen; 5) an HIV-positive mother received a regimen not recommended for treatment of neurosyphilis; 6) the mother was treated ≤1 month before delivery; 7) the mother was not examined for a decline in antibody titers, or an appropriate decline did not occur. If any of the above pertain, the child's evaluation should be completed, and the child should receive treatment with parenteral penicillin for 10–14 days.

In all instances in which a newborn infant is undergoing a screening serologic evaluation for possible congenital syphilis, the specimen of choice is *maternal* serum, rather than cord blood.

Finally, negative serological results from the mother and/or infant may occur if the mother has primary syphilis at the time of delivery. Only epidemiologic recognition that the mother was exposed will enable these situations to be identified. In instances of documented recent material exposure, even in the absence of positive serologic result, the mother should be evaluated for the possible presence of a chancre, and the infant should receive a course of therapy for presumed congenital syphilis.

Acquired Syphilis

The prevalence of congenital syphilis is greater for infants born to adolescent and teenage women than to women who are ≥21 years old. For these reasons, it is appropriate to give particular attention to the evaluation for syphilis of adolescents who are known or expected to be at increased risk for STDs, who are pregnant, and who are known or suspected of being infected with HIV.

Progression from secondary disease to tertiary disease may be unusually rapid

and common in persons with HIV and is often manifested as early neurosyphilis. Neurosyphilis is now a relatively frequent presenting finding in the initial diagnosis of acquired syphilis. Many HIV-positive adults who have developed neurosyphilis had been treated for primary or secondary syphilis with standard courses of therapy, course that ordinarily would have been highly successful in the treatment of early forms of syphilis. The serologic diagnosis of syphilis in persons who are HIV positive or have AIDS appears to be similar to that of HIV-negative persons, except for a possible tendency late in the course of AIDS to become nonreactive to treponemal and/or nontreponemal antibody tests.

Sexual transmission of syphilis to children may occur as a complication of child sexual abuse. In a recent study of sexually abused children, the prevalence of syphilis was 49/100,000, which is similar to that in adults in high-risk areas and greatly exceeds the national rate of 0.1/100,000 for children aged 0–9 years and 1.4/100,000 for children aged 10–14. Rates of acquired syphilis in adolescents and teenagers who are sexually active are rising rapidly.

The clinical presentations of neurosyphilis in HIV-positive persons have been similar to presentations in the prepenicillin era. Cerebrospinal fluid findings in HIV-infected persons with acquired neurosyphilis are highly variable. The clinician must not rely upon a single parameter in assessing a patient for neurosyphilis.

There are relatively few data regarding the presentations and courses of acquired syphilis in HIV-infected children or adolescents, but there is nothing to suggest that their courses differ significantly from those of adults. Consequently, therapeutic considerations that pertain to HIV-infected adults provide the only guidance to treatment of children and adolescents.

Recommended therapy for early syphilis in the pre-AIDS era has been a single dose of 2.4×10^6 units benzathine penicillin. Musher et al. has suggested an increase of this therapy in HIV-infected persons to three doses at weekly intervals, and a review of the clinical outcomes after three administrations has indicated that failures and relapses are uncommon. An alternative regimen is use of ceftriaxone on a daily basis for 10 days. However, failures have also been reported with this regimen.

These experiences indicate that universally efficacious therapy for early neurosyphilis in HIV-positive persons has not been identified. Consequently repeated and careful evaluations of all HIV-infected syphilitic patients is indicated. An initial examination of the cerebrospinal fluid should be made, and repeated examinations are indicated if the patient has abnormal findings or if there are findings suggesting that the disease has recurred, failed initial therapy, or progressed. Careful and repeated monitoring is strongly advocated.

Neisseria gonorrhoeae

Gonococcal disease is more common in populations at high risk for STDs who reside in the southeastern regions of the United States than in several other areas such as the Midwest and Northwest. The prevalence in high-risk adult groups is usually reflected in populations of abused children, such that some areas commonly recognize gonorrhea in children and in other regions it is rarely recognized. Prevalence data in children also depend upon policies regarding selection of children who will be evaluated for gonorrhea, adequacy of the methods used for collecting specimens, adequacy of the laboratory processes, and prevalence of gonorrhea in the community in which the child resides. Prevalence rates in the 1980s from reported series of children who were being evaluated for child sexual abuse ranged from a high of 19% in North Carolina to 0 in several other states in the United States.

Clinical Management

Reports from some populations indicated that virtually all infected children are clinically symptomatic, and consequently collecting culture samples from asymptomatic children should be discontinued. However, other experiences included children whose vaginal infections were asymptomatic. Consequently we advise that cultures should be taken from both symptomatic and asymptomatic children if the evaluation for STDs is to be complete.

Child sexual abuse may involve mucosal contact between infected adults and the child's anal, pharyngeal, urethral, and vaginal mucosa. In prepubertal children, culture specimens from girls should include anal, pharyngeal, and vaginal specimens. Prepubertal boys should have anal and pharyngeal specimens. For both sexes, urethral specimens should be taken if the child has urethritis or pyuria. A voided urine has been found to be a good specimen for culture of *N. gonorrhoeae* if processed promptly. Samples from conjunctiva should also be taken from children with symptomatic conjunctivitis.

Laboratory Diagnosis

Gonorrhea has been the most prominent of the STDs that cause acute salpingitis and pelvic inflammatory disease in adolescent women, although infection with *Chlamydia trachomatis* has also been shown to be responsible for a more common and chronic presentation. (See pelvic inflammatory disease below). Over 10% of children and adolescents with gonococcal disease are concomitantly infected with *C. trachomatis*. Consequently, children older than 7 years should be treated for both infections whenever gonococcal disease is diagnosed. Younger children may be evaluated for chlamydia and treatment restricted to those who have been shown to be infected.

Good technique in choosing and collecting adequate specimens and initial processing of specimens is vital in the diagnosis of gonorrhea. Swabs should be moistened in nonbacteriostatic saline to cause less irritation to the vagina and anus. Rayon fiber swabs or treated cotton fiber swabs are suitable for collecting samples. Since the organism is highly sensitive to both drying and cooling, clinical samples for *N. gonorrhoeae* are best handled when the clinician plates the specimen at the site of collection onto prewarmed agar media. The inoculated plate should be incubated promptly in CO_2 containing atmosphere at 37°C. Cooling will cause falsely negative results. After overnight incubation, the mature colonies are relatively resistant to cooler temperatures and if necessary can be transported at room temperature. A somewhat less satisfactory alternative is to collect samples in transport media.

Since implications of the diagnosis of gonorrhea in a child are medically as well as socially important, suspected isolates should be securely identified. After the preliminary identification of *Neisseria* species, the result should be confirmed with at least two of the three major confirming techniques. The three available methods are patterns of utilization of carbohydrates, immunofluorescence using monoclonal antibody, and the enzymatic release of certain products from aryl-substituted substrates.

Chlamydia trachomatis

C. trachomatis is a small bacterium that is an obligate intracellular pathogen, requiring tissue culture methods for isolation. Diagnosis of anal-genital chlamydial infection in all ages of children has been impeded by the fact that facilities for culture of *C. trachomatis* are not universally available, are technically difficult, and are expensive. Presenting symptoms have been variable, and some infected children have minimal or no recognized findings. Despite these factors, which have probably led to under-recognition of infections, prevalence rates of genital chlamydial infections in children being evaluated for suspected sexual abuse have been approximately 1–10%. In adolescent females who are sexually active and receiving medical care in urban clinics, prevalence rates have been reported to be 10–26%, and sexually active asymptomatic urban adolescent males have had prevalence rates of 8–14%.

Tissue culture methods for the isolation of *C. trachomatis* are highly specific, and the sensitivity in symptomatic adults has been estimated to be 80% for females and 90% for males. Two other means of identifying *C. trachomatis* are antigen detection systems and a DNA probe method. Antigen detection systems include a commercially available kit using monoclonal antibody (MicroTrak) and enzyme immunoassay (Chlamydiazyme). The diagnostic system based on a chemiluminescent probe for chlamydial DNA is the Pace assay. This is a newly released product, and experience in pediatric populations is minimal. These systems are suitable for screening populations with a high prevalence of disease, and consequently most field trials have been in adolescents and adults. Because of the legal and forensic significance of the diagnosis of an STD, the diagnostic method of choice for children has remained the tissue culture system.

The effect of HIV infection on the presentation or course of genital chlamydial infections of children or adolescents is unknown.

Pelvic Inflammatory Disease

This is a syndrome that involves an inflammatory reaction, usually to an infectious disease, in the female reproductive tract. The condition is usually recognized in adolescents and women, although acute disease has been reported in prepubertal girls infected with gonorrhea. It is a condition with the frequent potential for severe long-term sequelae, including ectopic pregnancy, infertility, and chronic pelvic pain. The condition has increased in prevalence during the past two decades, and it is now estimated that 10–15% of women of reproductive ages have had one or more episodes.

This disease is of particular importance for clinicians who care for children because sexually active adolescents (age 10–14) have the highest prevalence of disease of any group.

A major problem in the control of pelvic inflammatory disease is the difficulty in diagnosis, which is based on clinical findings which may be subtle. Chronic pelvic inflammatory disease is especially likely to be unrecognized and untreated but nevertheless may progress with late complications. The clinical diagnosis is usually based on a combination of systemic findings of fever and leukocytosis with signs of localized inflammatory disease including abdominal pain and pain on examination of cervix and adnexa. Laparoscopic findings may widen the scope of the diagnosis but have not been widely accepted as standards of diagnosis in community settings.

The etiology of the syndrome includes an inciting infection, often caused by *N. gonorrhoeae* or *C. trachomatis*, formation of obstructions and abscesses of the Fallopian tubes, and chronic superinfection with other pelvic anaerobic flora. The condition may be recognized at any time, including during silent periods when the patient is unaware of the evolving condition.

Prevention is usually aimed at preventing the initial infection and focuses on barrier protection, decreasing numbers of sexual partners, avoiding high-risk partners, and seeking medical care for exposures or early symptoms. Abstinence in young adolescent women and postponing entrance into initial sexual activity are the most effective means of prevention.

The effect of infection with HIV on the evolution of pelvic inflammatory disease in children and adolescents is unknown.

Treatment may be provided in an ambulatory setting or parenterally during hospitalization. Because of the poor outcome of pelvic inflammatory disease in adolescents, several investigators recommend hospitalization to ensure adequate therapy. Guidelines for considering hospitalization are shown in Table 15.3. Recommendations for therapy require that treatment be adequate for pelvic anaerobic flora, *C. trachomatis*, and *N. gonorrhoeae*. Several regimens have been approved, and all are designed to treat women who are of an age to receive doxycycline (see Table 15.4).

Trichomonas vaginalis

This organism is a protozoal pathogen and a common cause of urethritis and vaginitis in females. Urethral infection of males is usually clinically silent. This infection has not been systematically studied and is infrequently recognized in populations of sexually abused children. Recent prevalence rates in sexually active adolescent girls have been 8–16%.

Table 15.3. Criteria for Consideration of Hospitalization for Treatment of Pelvic Inflammatory Disease

Young age (<14 years)
Pelvic or tubo-ovarian abscess
Failure to respond to oral antibiotics within 48 hours
Pregnancy

Screening studies for *T. vaginalis* are usually performed by direct observation of a wet mount of vaginal secretion or urine. The sensitivity of this method has been reported to be as low as 50–60%, depending in part on the concentration of trichomonads in the specimen. Since there is a general correlation between the burden of parasites and symptomatology, children and other persons with minimal symptoms or who are asymptomatic have a significant risk of remaining undiagnosed. Diagnosis of infection in males using wet mount techniques is even less reliable. Culture methods are recommended as the most sensitive diagnostic method but are not universally available and are expensive. Other techniques are being developed, such as a direct immunofluorescent assay, but the necessary field studies have not been completed. Therefore, at present, the clinician may employ a wet mount examination for symptomatic patients as a screening study. For patients with mild symptoms, who are asymptomatic or for whom a diagnosis is important, a culture is the method of choice.

Effects of infection with HIV on the presentation or course of infection with genital trichomoniasis, if any, are unknown.

Human Papilloma Virus

Papilloma viruses are a family of small double-stranded DNA viruses. Papilloma viruses are strictly host specific, so HPV infect only humans. Although over 60 genotypes have been identified so far, there are approximately seven genotypes that are commonly implicated in genital infections. HPV infect primarily human keratinocytes. There is no in vitro tissue culture system for the diagnosis of HPV infection.

The epidemiology of genital HPV infection is interesting and complicated. These viruses are the cause of genital warts, laryngeal papillomatosis, and squamous intraepithelial neoplasia. They are highly associated with carcinoma of genital mucosa, but additional cofactors appear to be required, such as smoking, for a lesion to progress to a malignant state. In sexually active adults, infection with HPV is very common. By using the polymerase chain reaction, prevalence rates

Table 15.4.   Treatment of Common STD in Children and Adolescents

Disease	Antimicrobial Agent	Dose	No. Doses/Day	Route[a]	Duration
Syphilis					
Congenital					
Age 0–7 days	Aqueous penicillin G	100,000 μg/kg/day	2	IV	10–14 days
Age 8–28 days	Aqueous penicillin G	150,000 μg/kg/day	3	IV	10–14 days
Acquired					
HIV negative	Benzathine penicillin G	50,000 μg/kg	1	IM	Once
HIV positive	Benzathine penicillin G or	50,000 μg/kg	1	IM	Three doses at weekly intervals
	Aqueous penicillin G	200,000 μg/kg/day	4	IV	10–14 days
Gonorrhea					
Mucosal					
Age <8 years	Ceftriaxone	125 mg	1	IM	Once
Age ≥8 years					
Age ≥45 kg	Ceftriaxone plus	250 mg	1	IM	Once
	doxycycline	100 mg	2	PO	7 days
Disseminated					
<45 kg	Ceftriaxone	50mg/kg	1	IV	7 days
≥45 kg	Ceftriaxone	1 g	1	IV	2 days after asymptomatic
Chlamydia (genital)					
Age ≤7 years	Sulfasoxazole	150 mg/kg/day	4	PO	7–10 days
	or erythromycin ethylsuccinate	40 mg/kg/day	4	PO	7–10 days
Age >7 years	Tetracycline	40 mg/kg/day	4	PO	14 days
Trichomoniasis	Metronidazole	15 mg/kg/day	3	PO	7–10 days
Primary genital herpes simplex	Acyclovir	200 μg	5	PO	7–10 days
Bacterial vaginosis	Metronidazole	15 mg/kg/day	3	PO	7–10 days
Pelvic inflammatory disease					
Ambulatory	Ceftriaxone	250 mg	1	IM	once
	plus doxycycline	100 mg	2	PO	10–14 days
Parenteral (regimen A)	Cefoxitin	2 gm	4	IV	2 days
	plus doxycycline	100 mg	2	PO	10–14 days
Parenteral (regimen B)	Clindamycin	900 mg	3	IV	2 days
	plus gentamicin	2 mg/kg	3	IV	2 days
	plus doxycycline	100 mg	2	PO	10–14 days

[a]Clinician should be aware that changes in treatment recommendations may occur. Good resources are Morbidity and Mortality Weekly Report and the Red Book from the American Academy of Pediatrics.

of over 30% are common, and for STD clinic populations, rates of over 50% pertain. Several factors that influence the prevalence of HPV-related disease include cigarette smoking, several dietary factors, numbers of sexual partners, and HIV infection. Infections may be latent, subclinical, clinical, or progressive. After infection the patient may have a rapid spontaneous cure, remission with subsequent exacerbations, stable infection with dysplastic features on histologic examination, or progression to advanced dysplasia, intraepithelial neoplasia, and localized or metastatic carcinoma.

HPV is one of the most well-studied of the human oncogenic viruses. Several factors appear to influence the progression of an infection to cancer. Several HPV genotypes (16, 18 especially) are associated with most progressive lesions, although even in persons infected with one of these types only a few will progress, with the others remaining unchanged or regressing. Second, age may be a factor, and infection with a high-risk HPV genotype may be more hazardous to younger patients. Third, all medical conditions that decrease the competence of the cellular immune system, including HIV, are associated with increased prevalence of HPV infections and HPV-associated dysplasia, neoplasia, and carcinoma.

Almost all experience with HPV infection in HIV-infected persons has been accrued in adults and has focused on cervical, penile, and intra-anal lesions and carcinoma. In HIV-infected persons, the progression of HPV-associated disease parallels the decline in cellular immunity.

Although relatively few HIV-infected children have been evaluated for HPV infection, there are several case reports indicating that genital warts and laryngeal papillomatosis (usually caused by HPV genotypes 6 or 11) may be unusually severe and refractory to treatment in HIV-infected prepubertal children. In addition, HIV-infected adolescents appear to share with adults the increased risk of progressive cervical, anal, and penile dysplasia if they contract infection with HPV. Consequently, these infections are of great concern to clinicians who care for sexually assaulted children and sexually active adolescents who are also HIV infected.

Diagnosis of HPV infections of the genital tract requires biopsies or cellular specimens from infected areas. Thus, the collaboration with clinicians trained in obstetrics-gynecology and/or dermatology may be required. The following diagnostic methods may be employed.

- Exfoliative cytology (Papanicolaou smear preparations) provides samples of epithelial cells which may be examined for cytologic abnormalities that frequently accompany infections with HPV. These preparations are relatively easy to obtain in sexually active populations, are technically easy to prepare, but require experienced readers to obtain an adequate interpretation. The correlation between cytologic findings and assays for HPV is inexact, and cytologic examinations are relatively insensitive. Sampling errors may account for failures to recognize an infection. Obtaining an appropriate genital specimen from a prepubertal child may be very difficult or require an examination with generalized anaesthesia.

- Histopathological findings of biopsy specimens from involved areas provide information regarding the extent of the lesion and assist in decisions regarding therapy and follow-up.

- Several tests are available for the assay for HPV DNA, RNA, or capsid antigen. These assays vary in sensitivity, specificity, dependence on technical expertise, samples which may be used, and extent to which that technique has been compared with other methods. The reader is cautioned that the results of population studies depend heavily upon the methods used and skills of the laboratory. The clinician should remember that the diagnosis of HPV infection carries particularly important implications for children. Therefore diagnostic methods should be chosen that are not only sensitive but also highly specific.

Treatment of HPV infections is restricted, with few exceptions, to methods that ablate the infected epidermal layer. These methods include laser ablation, cryotherapy, application of locally toxic compounds such as podophylotoxin, and surgical excision. Each method has indications, adverse consequences, and frequent failures with recurrent disease. Nonablative therapy includes investigational use of local and systemic interferon. Recurrences of genital warts or laryngeal papillomatosis in HIV-infected children have been particularly common, and there is no therapy with established and reliable efficacy.

Genital Herpes

Genital herpes virus infections are caused by herpes simplex virus, usually type II.

Genital infections of children with this virus, when acquired beyond the perinatal period, are infrequent, and most data come from individual case reports. Studies of children who are being evaluated for suspected child sexual abuse indicate that the prevalence in that population is about 0.5%. In sexually active adolescent populations the prevalence rises to resemble that of adult STD clinics (1–5%).

Herpes simplex virus infections share the characteristic of all other herpes viruses that primary infections are followed by latency and a potential for periodic reactivation. The primary infection is usually the most clinically severe episode and may include systemic symptoms of fever, malaise, headache, as well as locally severe ulceration. HIV-infected persons appear to be vulnerable to more severe primary herpes simplex virus disease and recurrences that are more frequent and severe. Locally progressive erosive lesions have been reported. Despite this, there are very little data regarding characteristics of genital herpes simplex virus infection in HIV-infected children.

Diagnosis of genital herpes simplex virus infection should rest primarily on viral culture of material taken from the base of a fresh lesion. However, a culture may be negative in a lesion that is not freshly erupted or in recurrent lesions. Additional diagnostic information can be obtained from a biopsy of a lesion. In testing lesional specimens for HSV, labeled monoclonal antibody assays and enzyme immunoassay methods appear to have the best sensitivity and specificity.

During the primary episode of genital herpes, in adults, it is accepted clinical practice to provide a 7–10-day oral course of acyclovir. This therapy hastens healing and decreases acute local and systemic symptoms but has no effect on frequency or severity of recurrences. For patients with frequent recurrences (at least six episodes per year), suppressive daily therapy with acyclovir will diminish the rate of subsequent recurrences. HIV-infected persons have an enhanced rate of recurrences, and some require suppressive therapy. Despite suppressive therapy, immunodeficient persons occasionally continue to exhibit recur-

rent disease, some apparently associated with the development of acyclovir-resistant strains of HSV and others with strains that remain sensitive. The concern that suppressive therapy may lead to emergence of an acyclovir-resistant strain has provided an incentive to some clinicians to restrict the use of suppressive courses.

HIV

There has not been a prospective study of the prevalence of CSA in HIV-infected children in which currently accepted methods of diagnosing CSA were routinely utilized for evaluation of all infected children, but such a study has also not been made of any other population of children in the United States. The only data indicating the prevalence of CSA in an HIV-infected population of children has come from the Duke Pediatric AIDS Clinic. During clinic visits for primary medical care and using case ascertainment methods that are standard for pediatric practices, clinic personnel recognized that many clinic children had demonstrated physical, behavioral, or medical findings which indicated that an evaluation for sexual abuse was warranted. By 1990 14 of the 96 clinic patients had been evaluated by the Duke Child Protection Team and were confirmed to have been sexually abused. Of these 14, the single identified exposure category for HIV for four was sexual abuse. Accordingly, at least 4 of 96 (4.1%) children in the entire clinic population had become HIV infected through abusive sexual contact. Another six patients may have acquired their HIV infection through abuse, although additional possible exposure categories were also present.

The absolute numbers of children who have acquired HIV through sexual abuse is, of course, unknown, but an inquiry conducted by Gellert et al. from major child protection services in the United States yielded 28 cases of HIV-infected children whose only exposure category was CSA (Table 15.5). This number is certainly an underestimation, since there are numerous barriers to diagnosing sexual abuse as a transmission category for pediatric AIDS. These include the general reluctance and difficulty of diagnosis of CSA in all popula-

Table 15.5.   Children and Adolescents Infected with HIV—Prevalence of Other STDs[a]

Report	Population	Infection	Prevalence[a]	Comments
LJ D'Angelo, 1991, Washington DC	At-risk adolescents	HIV	<%M 0.1, F 0.4	Adolescent clinic and ER population
G Gellert, 1991, United States	26 children who acquired HIV through sexual abuse	Ng syphilis Ct HPV	9 9 3 3	National survey of children who acquired HIV through sexual abuse
LT Gutman, 1991, North Carolina	14 children who were HIV-infected and sexually abused	HPV	7	Report of sexually abused children from HIV treatment center
J Oleske, 1990, New Jersey	15 children sexually abused by HIV-infected assailant	HIV	20	Author noted the need for data regarding sexual transmission of HIV

[a]Ng, *N. gonorrhoeae*; Ct, *C. trachomatis*, ER, emergency room.

tions of children, the absence of seroprevalence data for HIV infection in populations of children being evaluated for suspected child sexual abuse, the absence of sexual contact as an exposure category on the national reporting forms for pediatric AIDS, and reluctance to consider sexual abuse as a possible exposure category when there is another possible route of infection for the child.

Because of these impediments to understanding the role of sexual abuse in the transmission of HIV to children, there are neither data regarding the results of HIV testing of abused children nor established policies regarding indications for testing. Gellert et al. reported that the characteristics of a child that 65 child protection services agreed should be tested for HIV included only those children already known or suspected of having AIDS/AIDS-related complex, adolescents with a high risk behavioral profile, or a parent or child who was insistent on HIV testing. Knowledge regarding risk status of assailants that teams agreed would trigger HIV testing of the child generally are not accessible to child protection services.

Recommendations from the Centers for Disease Control in 1989 were that testing of abused children should depend upon local prevalence of infection and exposure risks. This has been interpreted to apply when

the assault was invasive and if the perpetrator was at high risk of being HIV infected.

These recommendations are very difficult to apply because child protection services often cannot know the nature of the abusive act, cannot know the identity of the perpetrator, cannot know whether an identified perpetrator acted alone, and almost never is in a position to evaluate risk factors for HIV on the part of the perpetrator. No data are available regarding the prevalence of HIV infection of sexual assailants of children. Furthermore, the correlation between physical findings and the occurrence of specific invasive sexual acts, even when known, is poor. Abuse is usually chronic, and the type of abuse may change with time. In summary, the child protection service is usually not privy to the information needed to determine if the abusive acts were such that HIV might have been transmitted or if the assailant(s) was at increased risk for being HIV infected.

Because of the major areas in which there are no or only inadequate data, a data-based plan for HIV testing of children suspected of child sexual abuse cannot be and has not been formulated. However, populations of children being evaluated for suspected CSA are probably at greater risk of exposure to HIV than are other children, and certain categories of children who are undergoing an evaluation for abuse are even more likely to have been exposed to HIV. Pending development of data, we suggest that children who are being evaluated for suspected sexual abuse are at highest priority for HIV testing when they meet the following descriptions.

- Child sexual abuse is confirmed or probable.
- Evaluation for abuse was inadequate or incomplete, and diagnosis of abuse therefore unknown. This includes children who are younger than 3 years and therefore cannot participate in an adequate disclosure interview.
- Sexual abuse disclosed by the child or witness included anal, oral, or vaginal contact.
- Child has a vaginal injury or discharge or has proctitis.
- Child is infected at vaginal, anal, urethral, or oral sites with a sexually transmitted organism or is infected with an organism that is associated with sexual contact. These include *N. gonorrhoeae, T. pallidum, T. vaginalis,* genital herpes simplex virus infection, HPV disease (including anal-genital warts), and bacterial vaginosis.
- Child has anal or genital physical findings which suggest that mucosal or dermal injuries may have occurred.
- Perpetrator is not identified.
- It is known or suspected that the child was assaulted by more than one perpetrator.
- Perpetrator is known or suspected to be at increased risk, for any reason, of being HIV infected.
- Child or parents ask to have the child tested.

Children who do not fall under one of the above categories, and for whom HIV testing cannot be specifically urged on the basis of recognizable risks, are children who have been adequately evaluated for child sexual abuse and for whom the results of the evaluation were that abuse was unlikely. Remembering that it is not possible to assure that a child has not been abused with certainty, evaluation of those children for HIV would also be at the discretion of the clinician and/or family.

Repeat serologic evaluation for HIV should be conducted within 6 months after documentation that the child is not subject to reabuse or periodically if the child's safety is in doubt. Since serologic reevaluation for syphilis is also necessary, both test samples can be collected simultaneously.

SEXUALLY ASSOCIATED ORGANISMS

Several microorganisms cause or are associated with symptomatic genital disease and appear to be more prevalent in sexually active persons than in persons who are not (nonabused prepubertal children and virginal adults). However, these infections may not be transmitted solely by sexual contact, and the diagnosis of one of these infections in a child is not usually accepted to be strong or conclusive evidence of sexual abuse.

- *Ureaplasma urealyticum.* Few data regarding *Ureaplasma* infections in children are available. In adults, it is found with greater prevalence in males with urethritis and females with risk factors for STDs. In adolescent males, it is restricted to those who have initiated sexual activity.
- *Mycoplasma hominis.* Studies regarding the prevalence in nonabused children have been controversial and made more so by the paucity of data regarding vaginal flora of prepubertal girls who have undergone a screening process to select nonabused girls. Recent data indicate that this infection is rare in nonabused girls and that approximately 30% of invasively abused girls harbor this organism. In some cases of persistent vaginal discharge, *M. hominis* is the only isolated organism. There are no data regarding the findings of *M. hominis* infected women or children who are also HIV positive.
- *Gardnerella vaginalis* and bacterial vaginosis. *Gardnerella* species are small Gram-negative rods that are anaerobic. They are highly associated, but not always present, in the syndrome "bacterial vaginosis." The pathogenesis of BV is unknown but appears to represent an overgrowth of abnormal vaginal flora. The syndrome has been reported to follow sexual abuse in children. The syndrome includes a thin, grey vaginal discharge that has a particular odor, a raised pH from vaginal secretions, the release of amines from vaginal secre-

tions when in contact with potassium hydroxide, and squamous epithelial cells to which are attached large numbers of small Gram-negative rods. The epithelial cells are frayed at the edges.

- *Candida* sp vaginitis. All adult women are susceptible to overgrowth of *Candida* sp, and *Candida* sp vaginitis is not considered primarily to be an STD. In children infected with HIV, *Candida* sp infections of mucous membranes occur commonly. Children with inflammatory disease of the genital tract should be evaluated for *Candida* sp and the possibility of abusive causes of vaginitis considered. The presence of *Candida* does not eliminate sexual abuse.

ADDITIONAL THERAPEUTIC CONSIDERATIONS

After diagnosis of any STD in a child or adolescent, a major goal is to identify the source of infection. Since an acquired STD in a child is evidence that the child has been the victim of a crime, except in highly unusual circumstances, the identification of perpetrator is usually resisted and denied by the perpetrator. When the perpetrator is a member of the family, which is usually the case, the child's family may also fail to support the child or cooperate in the investigation. However, it is important to attempt to make this identification to ensure a safe environment for the index child and other exposed children.

Another reason to identify the perpetrator is to provide and enforce specific, long-term perpetrator therapy for the assailant in addition to medical treatment of infections. When presented with opportunities, sexual assailants of children characteristically abuse multiple children. In a setting in which HIV infection may be contracted or transmitted, it is even more important that the perpetrator be restrained from further abuse of the index or other children.

When a child is recognized to have been sexually assaulted, the other children who have been exposed to the perpetrator require an evaluation for suspected child sexual abuse. Two recent studies, one of a population of abused HIV-positive children, have documented that the majority of other children who have been exposed to the perpetrator or are in the household of an abused child have also been sexually abused. This includes both siblings of the initially identified child as well as playmates. Again, in a setting in which infection with HIV may accompany child sexual abuse, evaluation and protection of other children is especially important.

The diagnosis of sexual abuse can lead to provision of therapy for the abused child and nonabusing caretakers. Although data regarding the outcomes of therapy are sparse, there are indications that children benefit from therapy and can decrease or eliminate many behavioral disturbances that accompany abuse. Since some late disturbances may include behaviors that are risk factors for acquiring an STD (vulnerability to abuse, early initiation of sexual activity, unprotected sexual intercourse at a young age, multiple partners), it is again particularly important to ensure that children have made a recovery from the abuse if they are HIV infected or living in a setting in which other persons are HIV infected.

Suggested Reading

1. Allers CT, Benjack KJ. Connections between childhood abuse and HIV infection. J Counseling Dev 1991;70:309–313.
2. American Academy of Pediatrics Committee on Child Abuse and Neglect. Guidelines for the evaluation of sexual abuse of children. Pediatrics 1991;87:254–260.
3. Bagley C, McDonald M. Adult mental health sequels of child sexual abuse, physical abuse, and neglect in maternally separated children. Can J Commun Ment Health 1984;3:15–26.
4. Bays J, Chadwick D. The serologic test for syphilis in sexually abused children and adolescents. Adolesc Pediatr Gynecol 1991;4:148–151.
5. Carpenter CCJ, Mayer KH, Stein MD, Leibman BD, Fisher A, Fiore TC. Human immunodeficiency virus infection in North American women: Experience with 200 cases and a review of the literature. Medicine 1991;70:307–325.
6. D'Angelo LJ, Getson PR, Luban NLC, Gayle HD. Human immunodeficiency virus infection in urban adolescents: Can we predict who is at risk? Pediatrics 1991;88:982–986.
7. Centers for Disease Control. Sexually transmitted diseases treatment guidelines. MMWR 1989;38:1–43.
8. Desenclos J-CA, Garrity D, Wroten J. Pediatric gonococcal infection, Florida, 1984 to 1988. Am J Public Health 1992;82:426–428.
9. Faller KC. Child sexual abuse. New York: Columbia University Press, 1988.
10. Friedrich WH, Gramosch P, Broughton D, Kniper J, Beilke R. Normative sexual behavior in children. Pediatrics 1991;88:456–464.

11. Fullilove R, Fullilove M, Bowser BP, Gross SA. Risk of sexually transmitted disease among black adolescent crack users in Oakland and San Francisco, California. JAMA 1990;263:851–856.
12. Gellert GA, Durfee MJ, Berkowitz CD, Higgins KV, Tubiolo VC. Situational and sociodemographic characteristics of children infected with HIV from pediatric sexual abuse. Pediatrics 1993;91:39–44.
13. Gellert GA, Durfee MJ, Berkowitz CD. Developing guidelines for HIV antibody testing among victims of pediatric sexual abuse. Child Abuse Negl 1990;14:9–17.
14. Gershenson HP, Musick JS, Ruch-Ross HS, Magee V, Rubino KK, Rosenberg D. The prevalence of coercive sexual experience among teenage mothers. J Interpersonal Violence 1989;4:204–219.
15. Gutman LT, St Claire KK, Weedy C, et al. Human immunodeficiency virus transmission by child sexual abuse. Am J Dis Child 1991;145:137–141.
16. Gutman LT, St Clair KK, Weedy C, Herman-Giddens M, McKinney RE Jr. Sexual abuse of human immunodeficiency virus-positive children: outcomes for perpetrators and evaluation of other household children. Am J Dis Child 1992;146:1185–1189.
17. Gutman LT, Herman-Giddens M, Phelps WC. Transmission of human genital papillomavirus disease: Comparison of data from adults and children. Pediatrics 1993;91:31–38.
18. Gutman LT, Herman-Giddens ME, McKinney RE Jr. Pediatric AIDS: Barriers to recognizing the role of child sexual abuse. J Dis Child 1993;147:775–780.
19. Hein K, Hurst M. Human immunodeficiency virus infection in adolescents: A rationale for action. Adolesc Pediatr Gynecol 1988;1:173–182.
20. Ikeda MK, Jenson HB. Evaluation and treatment of congenital syphilis. J Pediat 1990;117:843–852.
21. Katz DA, Berger JR. Neurosyphilis in acquired immunodeficiency syndrome. Arch Neurol 1989;46:895–898.
22. Lawson L, Chaffin M. False negatives in sexual abuse disclosure interviews: Incidence and influence of caretaker's belief in abuse in cases of accidental abuse discovery by diagnosis of STD. J Interpersonal Violence 1992;7:532–542.
23. Manoff SB, Gayle HD, Mays MA, Rogers MF. Acquired immunodeficiency syndrome in adolescents: epidemiology, prevention and public health issues. Pediatr Infect Dis J 1989;8:309–314.
24. Moore KA, Nord CW, Peterson JL. Nonvoluntary sexual activity among adolescents. Fam Plann Perspect 1989;21:110–114.
25. Moss GB, Clementson D, D'Costa L, et al. Association of cervical ectopy with heterosexual transmission of human immunodeficiency virus: Results of a study of couples in Nairobi, Kenya. J Infect Dis 1991;164:588–591.
26. Muram D, Speck PM, Gold SS. Genital abnormalities in female siblings and friends of child victims of sexual abuse. Child Abuse Negl. 1991;15:105–110.
27. Musher DM. Syphilis, neurosyphilis, penicillin, and AIDS. J Infect Dis 1991;163:1201–1206.
28. National Institutes of Health Expert Committee on Pelvic Inflammatory Disease. Pelvic inflammatory disease. Research directions in the 1990s. Sex Transm Dis 1991;18:46–64.
29. Oleske J. Human immunodeficiency virus testing of sexually abused children and their assailants. Pediatr Infect Dis J 1990;9:67.
30. Orr DP, Beiter M, Ingersoll G. Premature sexual activity as an indicator of psychosocial risk. Pediatrics 1991;87:141–147.
31. Paradise JE. The medical evaluation of the sexually abused child. Pediatr Clin North Am 1990;37:839–862.
32. Peters JM, Dinsmore J, Toth P. Why prosecute child abuse? South Dakota Law Rev 1989;34:649–659.
33. Remafedi GJ. Preventing the sexual transmission of AIDS during adolescence. J Adolesc Health Care 1988;9:139–143.
34. Smith PB, Weinman M, Mumford DM. Knowledge, beliefs, and behavioral risk factors for human immunodeficiency virus infection in inner city adolescent females. Sex Transm Dis 1992;19:19–24.
35. Vermund SH, Hein K, Gayle H, Cary JM, Thomas PA, Drucker E. AIDS among adolescents: Case surveillance profiles in NYC and the rest of the U.S. Am J Dis Child 1989;143:1220–1225.
36. Wasserheit JN. Epidemiological synergy. Interrelationships between human immunodeficiency virus infection and other sexually transmitted diseases. Sex Transm Dis 1992;19:61–77.
37. Whitaker CJ, Bastian LD. Teenage Victims. A national crime survey report. US Department of Justice, Office of Justice Programs, Bureau of Justice Statistics. May 1991 (NCJ-128129).
38. Wilbur DC, Stoler MH. Testing for papillomavirus: Basic pathobiology of infection, methodologies, and implications for clinical use. Yale J Biol Med 1991;64:113–125.
39. Zierler S, Feingold L, Laufer D, Velentgas P, Kantrowitz-Gordon I, Mayer K. Adult survivors of childhood sexual abuse and subsequent risk of HIV infection. Am J Public Health 1991;81:572–575.

APPENDIX 15.1

Listing of Helpful Findings That Clinician May Use to Identify Children at Risk for Child Sexual Abuse[a]

General Findings During a Clinic Visit
(comparisons between nonabused children-nonabusing parents and
abusecd children-abusing parents)

Nonabused child
- May cling to parents
- May turn to parents for reassurance
- May show by words and actions they want to leave the clinic or hospital
- May find safety in parent and is reassured by their presence

Abused child
- May cry hopelessly during treatment/examination
- May turn to parents for reassurance
- May show no expectation of being comforted
- May be wary of physical contact or may seek physical contact from strangers
- May not be afraid of new ward
- Constantly on alert for danger asking what will happen next, asking for things: food, favors, etc.
- May be excessively compliant or have a "frozen" affect

Nonabusing parent
- Give voluble, spontaneous report and explanation of injury
- May show genuine concern regarding degree of damage, treatment, residual damage
- Often show sense of guilt, especially if child is young and even if not responsible for injury
- Often show warmth, positive relation to child
- May ask many questions
- May be difficult to separate child for admission
- May visit frequently, stay long, discuss progress, bring things

Abusing parent
- Often does not volunteer information regarding injury
- May show little concern regarding injury, treatment, or prognosis
- Little guilt may be shown
- May be critical of child, claim child hurt self, blame child for causing injury
- May avoid looking at, touching child
- May respond to child inappropriately, show little warmth, little sense of how child feels, be indifferent, be constantly criticizing child
- May disappear from hospital before child admitted
- May tend not to visit
- May have little involvement and few questions regarding discharge date
- May show feeling that they and child are worthless
- May show that they were abandoned, punished by parents, unloved, etc.
- May be neglectful of own health, care, etc.

[a]A version of this table has been used for teaching purposes by the Department of Pediatrics, Duke University Medical Center, for many years.

APPENDIX 15.2

Range of Sexual Behavior of Children
(Findings that Clinician May Use to Help to Identify Children at Risk for Child Sexual Abuse)[a]

Probably not indicative of abuse
- Genital or reproduction conversations with peers or similar age siblings
- "Show me yours"/"I'll show you mine" with peers
- Playing "doctor"
- Imitating seduction (i.e., kissing, flirting)
- Dirty words or jokes within cultural or peer group norm

Possibly indicative of abuse
- Preoccupation with sexual themes (especially sexually aggressive)
- Attempting to expose others' genitals (i.e., pulling other's skirt up or pants down)
- Sexually explicit conversation with peers
- Sexual graffiti (especially chronic or affecting individuals)
- Sexual innuendo/teasing/embarrassment of others)
- Precocious sexual knowledge
- Preoccupation with masturbation
- Mutual masturbation/group masturbation
- Simulating foreplay with dolls or peers with clothing on (i.e., petting, French-kissing)

Seriously consider as possibly indicative of abuse or exposure to inappropriate situations
- Sexually explicit conversations with children at a significant age difference
- Touching genitals of others
- Degradation/humiliation of self or others with sexual themes
- Forced exposure of other's genitals
- Inducing fear/threats of force regarding sexual themes
- Sexually explicit proposals/threats including written notes
- Repeated or chronic peeping/exposing/obscenities/pornographic interests/frottage
- Vaginal or anal self-instrumentation
- Simulating intercourse with dolls, peers, animals (i.e., humping)

Further evaluation should be considered
- Oral, vaginal, anal penetration of dolls, children, animals
- Simulating intercourse with peers with clothing off

[a]A version of this table has been used for teaching purposes by the Department of Pediatrics, Duke University Medical Center, for many years.

16
Mycobacterial Infections

PART A / TUBERCULOSIS

Robert N. Husson

Mycobacteria have been major human pathogens from prehistoric times to the present. *Mycobacterium leprae* was the first human bacterial pathogen to be described (1), and Koch's achievement of culturing *M. tuberculosis* and demonstrating it to be the cause of tuberculosis was a major landmark in early bacteriology (2). The extent of human disease caused by tuberculosis in Europe and the United States in the 17th through early 20th centuries led to its being considered "the greatest single cause of disease and death in the Western World" during the period (3).

The mid-20th century saw the rapid decline of tuberculosis in economically developed countries but its continued prominence in less-developed countries of the world. Leprosy, nearly eliminated from much of the developed world, also remains a major health problem in parts of Africa, Asia, and Latin America. Though over 25 species of cultivable mycobacteria have been isolated from clinical specimens, most nontuberculous (atypical) mycobacteria have not been considered to be major human pathogens except in immunocompromised patients.

The AIDS epidemic opened a new chapter on the role of mycobacteria in causing human disease in both the developed and less-developed world. In the United States, the progressive decline in the incidence of tuberculosis initially slowed and then was reversed in 1986, when an increase occurred in the number of cases of tuberculosis reported to the Centers for Disease Control (CDC) (4). From 1985 to 1990 the number of cases of tuberculosis reported to CDC increased by 16% and the number of excess cases during this period relative to prior trends is estimated to be 28,000 (5). The most recent full year data show that this alarming trend has continued, with a total of 26,283 cases reported in 1991, an increase of 582 cases (2.3%) from 1990 (6). This excess of tuberculosis has been attributed to the high incidence of tuberculosis among persons who are infected with the human immunodeficiency virus (HIV) (7–10), as well as to worsening social and economic conditions coupled with decreased resources for prevention and treatment of tuberculosis in the 1970s and 1980s (11, 12).

Perhaps the most ominous development in the resurgence of tuberculosis is the emergence of multidrug-resistant *M. tuberculosis*, with several outbreaks of multiply resistant tuberculosis among HIV-infected individuals documented in the recent literature (13–16). The increasing prevalence of these pathogens that are difficult to treat constitutes a major threat to our ability to combat this infection, even with increased resources.

In the less-developed countries of the world, coinfection with HIV and *M. tubercu-*

289

losis is extremely common. Tuberculosis is a major cause of morbidity and mortality in populations where both infections are endemic (17–21). The interaction between HIV infection and leprosy in areas where the latter is endemic is not as well characterized; however, it appears that an association between HIV infection and leprosy morbidity exists as well (18, 22, 23).

This chapter will focus on clinically important aspects of infection with *M. tuberculosis* in children with HIV infection. Chapter 16B reviews the atypical mycobacterial infections in HIV-infected children. Although much of what is known about this infection derives from the observation and treatment of HIV-infected adults and from the clinical experience of individuals caring for HIV-infected children, recent publications have illuminated specific manifestations of tuberculosis in HIV-infected children.

MICROBIOLOGY

Tuberculosis is caused by *M. tuberculosis* or *M. bovis*, a closely related species that is now a rare cause of infection in the United States. These two organisms can be differentiated on the basis of biochemical tests in the microbiology laboratory but cause essentially identical illness. This section will focus on *M. tuberculosis* as the major cause of tuberculosis (Table 16A.1).

M. tuberculosis is a small (1–4 μm long), slender, rod-shaped bacterium. It is a non-spore-forming, nonencapsulated, slow-growing obligate aerobe, with a generation time of 15–20 hrs. Colonies are rough and characteristically buff colored (nonpigmented). Because of the unusual lipids in their cell walls, *M. tuberculosis* and other mycobacteria retain stain after exposure to acid alcohol. This property is the basis of the acid-fast staining characteristic used in the microscopic examination of clinical specimens.

In the clinical microbiology laboratory, specimens for mycobacterial culture are usually planted on specialized culture media such as Lowenstein-Jensen or Middlebrook 7H10 or 7H11, because *M. tuberculosis* will not grow well on many routine bacterial media. Initial isolation from contaminated clinical specimens such as sputum requires special processing and may involve planting on media containing inhibitors of other bacterial flora. Growth is enhanced in the presence of 5–10% CO_2. Colonies often appear on solid media after 2–3 weeks incubation, but cultures are generally held for 6 weeks before being considered negative.

Once sufficient growth has occurred, *M. tuberculosis* can be identified on the basis of biochemical tests or, more rapidly, with the use of nucleic acid probes. Lack of growth in liquid media containing *p*-nitro-α-acetyl-β-hydroxypropiophenone (NAP test) is often the first test result that indicates that a mycobacterial isolate is a member of the *M. tuberculosis* complex. Newer culture methods, particularly growth in liquid media containing ^{14}C-labeled substrate with radiometric detection of $^{14}CO_2$ (BACTEC system), have decreased the time required to culture, identify, and test for drug suscepti-

Table 16A.1. Clinical Microbiology of *M. tuberculosis*

Gram smear	Weakly Gram-positive beaded rods or invisible (may see negative image of organism)
Acid-fast staining	Positive
Growth rate	Slow (>2 weeks to form colonies; radiometric detection more rapid)
Colony characteristics	Rough, buff colored (nonphotochromogen)
Important biochemical tests in speciation	Niacin positive, nitrate reduction positive
Nucleic acid probes available for rapid speciation	Yes
Isolation from blood	Uncommon except in disseminated disease; more common in AIDS
Isolation from respiratory specimens and gastric aspirates	Common
Isolation from other sites	Variable

bility in laboratories where this system is available. Because of the specialized media and techniques required, difficulty in maintaining proficiency, risk of laboratory exposure, and expense, it has been recommended that clinical microbiology laboratories that do not receive large numbers of specimens for mycobacterial culture refer specimens to reference laboratories (levels II and III) that can better undertake these procedures (24).

EPIDEMIOLOGY

The change in tuberculosis epidemiology associated with the HIV epidemic has been noted above. In the United States, the initial association of active tuberculosis with HIV infection was observed in areas where both infections are highly prevalent such as Florida and New York (8, 25–27). This association between geographic areas and populations with high incidences of both HIV and tuberculosis infection remains valid, with the majority of both infections occurring in urban areas among the poor, racial and ethnic minorities, immigrants from endemic countries, and intravenous drug users. Persons living in group settings, including homeless shelters, correctional facilities, and nursing homes, are additionally at increased risk for tuberculosis because of the higher prevalence of infection in residents of these facilities, as well as the increased likelihood of transmission occurring in these confined settings. (8, 9, 11, 25–28) (Table 16A.2).

Children in the risk groups described for adults, or living with adults in these risk groups, are those who are at risk for exposure to and infection by *M. tuberculosis*. The increased incidence of tuberculosis since the mid-1980s observed in the United States population as a whole has occurred in children as well. The 1991 total of 1662 cases of tuberculosis in children younger than 15 years represents a 4.1% increase over 1990 and a 42% increase over 1987, the last year in which a decline in pediatric tuberculosis occurred (29), (CDC, unpublished data). In addition, the greatest increases in adult tuberculosis have occurred in young adults (5), the age group of most parents and other child care providers, so that further increases in pediatric tuberculosis can be expected in the 1990s. Two recent reports of children with HIV infection and tuberculosis document that the risk categories for coinfection with HIV and tuberculosis for children are the same as for adults (30, 31).

The association of HIV infection with active tuberculosis is not surprising, given the overlap in the groups at greatest risk for these infections and the importance of cell-mediated immunity in controlling tuberculous infection. Early reports of this association were notable for the fact that tuberculosis was often the initial manifestation of HIV-associated illness, thereby serving as a sentinel illness for HIV infection. This finding led to the recommendation that persons with newly diagnosed tuberculosis, particularly those who are in a risk group for HIV infection or who have disseminated or other severe forms of tuberculosis, be screened for HIV infection (9, 32). This association also led to the inclusion of extrapulmonary tuberculosis as an AIDS indicator illness in the 1987 revision of the CDC case definition of AIDS (33), as well as the recommendation that all HIV-infected persons be screened for tuberculous infection and active tuberculosis (34).

Worldwide, areas of high prevalence of tuberculosis, including parts of Africa, Asia, the Caribbean, and South America, overlap substantially with areas of high prevalence of HIV infection. A recent commentary on

Table 16A.2.   Epidemiology of Infection with *M. tuberculosis*

Incidence in AIDS in United States	Few cases reported in children; ~4% in adults; much higher in high risk groups in United States (and in countries where tuberculosis is prevalent)
High risk groups	Urban, poor, some ethnic minorities, some immigrants, intravenous drug users
Environmental source	Adults with pulmonary infection
Transmission	Person to person via respiratory route

the re-emergence of tuberculosis details the scope of the problem of tuberculosis worldwide (12). Among the grim statistics cited are the 8 million new cases of tuberculosis and the 2.9 million deaths from tuberculosis that occur each year. In most of these areas of the less-developed world, where HIV transmission is primarily heterosexual, large numbers of HIV-infected children are at risk for coinfection with *M. tuberculosis*. As expected from this epidemiology, it has become clear that tuberculosis is an important cause of morbidity and mortality among HIV-infected children and adults in these areas and that HIV seroprevalence rates are much higher in patients with tuberculosis than in the general population (17–21).

PATHOGENESIS, CLINICAL PRESENTATION, AND NATURAL HISTORY

Tuberculosis has been a relatively uncommon manifestation of pediatric HIV infection in this country, and few data are available from countries where both tuberculosis and HIV infection are highly prevalent. Two recent reports provide some insight into pathogenesis and manifestations of tuberculosis in HIV-infected children (30, 31) (Table 16A.3).

As is the case in children who are not HIV infected (35), active tuberculosis in HIV-infected infants and young children appears to be a manifestation of primary tuberculous infection rather than reactivation of latent infection. In the older child or adolescent, active tuberculosis may be the result of either primary infection or reactivation, although the former is much more

likely given the higher rates of progression from infection to disease in HIV-uninfected children and adolescents relative to adults (29, 36) and in HIV-infected adults relative to HIV-uninfected adults (13–16, 37).

In contrast, a large proportion of tuberculosis in HIV-infected adults appears to be the result of reactivation of prior infection. HIV infection markedly increases the probability of reactivation of latent tuberculosis infection to active tuberculosis in adults. Indeed, in a study of patients in a methadone maintenance program, the rate of development of active tuberculosis in patients who were both purified protein derivative (PPD) and HIV positive exceeded 7%/year (28). This rate is dramatically higher than both the 0.3%/year observed in the population of PPD-positive and HIV-negative patients in the same study and the ~10% lifetime risk for the development of tuberculosis after PPD conversion in the absence of HIV coinfection (24).

In addition to reactivation of latent tuberculous infection of HIV-infected individuals, however, investigation of outbreaks of tuberculosis among HIV-infected individuals has demonstrated that newly acquired infection with *M. tuberculosis* results in active disease in a high proportion of cases (13–15, 37, 38). In addition, there is much greater overlap in patterns of pulmonary disease in primary and reactivation tuberculosis in HIV-infected individuals. Thus, in the absence of a well-documented source of recent exposure or information from laboratory analysis of the infecting strains, it is difficult to differentiate primary from reactivation disease in an individual case in an older child or adult. Because of the high

Table 16A.3.   Pathogenesis and Clinical Manifestations of *M. tuberculosis* Infection

Initial localization of infection	Respiratory tract
Dissemination	Regional lymph nodes then lymphohematogenous spread throughout body limited by development of immunity in normal host; frequent persistence of disseminated infection in HIV infected
Disease manifestations	Pulmonary most common; extrapulmonary common in HIV infected
Timing in relation to symptomatic HIV disease	Early or late; often first manifestation of HIV infection; may also occur late with rapid disease progression
Treatment	If drug susceptible, generally successful with standard antituberculosis agents. High mortality if multidrug resistant

likelihood of primary infection in children, however, an essential result of any child presenting with tuberculosis should be an active search for an adult source with infectious tuberculosis in the child's environment.

The sequence of events that follow entry of *M. tuberculosis* through the respiratory tract are presumed to be the same in HIV-infected children as in those who are not infected, except that development of immunity is more likely to be inadequate to limit mycobacterial replication in the HIV-infected child. Initial local replication is followed by spread to regional lymph nodes and then lymphohematogenous spread of *M. tuberculosis* to sites throughout the body. In the normal host the development of cell-mediated immunity, thought to correlate with the onset of skin test hypersensitivity that generally occurs between 3 and 12 weeks after infection, limits further spread and results in the elimination of the organism from most sites. In locations where bacteria persist, the infection becomes latent. Reactivation, the result of renewed bacterial replication and/or decreased elimination by the host immune response, may occur in the future and cause active disease.

In patients who do not develop effective immunity to tuberculosis, including those with HIV infection, continued replication may occur in the lung and elsewhere. This uncontrolled infection results in active tuberculosis that may be disseminated or limited to the lung. When limited to the lung, the disease may remain localized or evolve to progressive primary disease, with involvement of increasing areas of the lung and ultimately cavitation if the process is not arrested.

The 14 pediatric patients presented in reports from New York City and Miami provide a limited but important view of the clinical manifestations of tuberculosis in HIV-infected children (30, 31). Respiratory distress and/or cough were present in 12 of the 13 children who had pulmonary tuberculosis, and prolonged fever was noted in seven of the nine patients reported from Miami. Extrapulmonary disease, including meningitis (two patients), mycobacteremia (two patients), mastoiditis (one patient), and lymph node involvement (1 patient)

was observed in five of the 14 reported patients and occurred in association with pulmonary disease in three of these five. Chest radiograph patterns were variable and included focal infiltrates in the upper lobes or hilar regions, multilobar infiltrates, interstitial infiltrates, and hilar adenopathy. Although not observed in these series, a separate case report describes extensive cavitary lesions in a 5-year child with HIV infection and tuberculosis (39). Only two of the 14 patients, one from each report, were reported to have a positive tuberculin test (using the earlier criterion of ≥10 mm induration). Both these children had normal CD4 cell counts, whereas nearly all the others had low CD4 counts. Cultures positive for *M. tuberculosis* were obtained in 13 of 14 patients. Children with pulmonary disease had positive cultures from gastric washings, bronchoalveolar lavage, or tracheal aspirate specimens. Response to therapy was good except in patients with disseminated disease or multidrug-resistant organisms.

Clinical manifestations of tuberculosis in HIV-infected adults have been extensively described. Fever is nearly always present. Chest radiographic findings in HIV-infected persons are often not typical of reactivation disease in HIV-uninfected individuals (apical infiltrates with hilar adenopathy). Cavitation is much less common in tuberculosis in HIV-infected persons than in HIV-uninfected adults. More common are pulmonary infiltrates that may be localized, diffuse, or multiple, with or without hilar adenopathy (20, 40–43). In addition to this nonspecific appearance of pulmonary disease on chest radiographs, the incidence of extrapulmonary disease is much higher in HIV-infected adults than in those who are uninfected, being >50% in several series (26, 41, 42, 44, 45). Meningitis, the most lethal form of extrapulmonary tuberculosis, was found in 10% of HIV-infected adults, compared with 2% in HIV-uninfected individuals, in a large study from Spain (46). Also striking is the occurrence of bacteremia with *M. tuberculosis* in HIV-infected adults (42, 47, 48), a rare finding in patients with tuberculosis who are not HIV-infected.

Taken together, the extensive descriptions of tuberculosis in HIV-infected adults, the manifestations of tuberculosis that have been described in HIV-infected children, and the patterns of tuberculosis that characterize HIV-uninfected children provide a reasonably accurate picture of pediatric tuberculosis in this population. In contrast to adults, most tuberculosis in HIV-infected children is the result of primary infection, as it is in HIV-uninfected children. The probability of disease developing from primary infection is much higher in children without HIV infection than in adults, decreasing gradually from infancy to adolescence, with a second peak in the teenage years (36). The markedly higher rate of active disease observed with primary infection in outbreaks among HIV-infected adults suggests that the likelihood of active disease after primary infection is even higher in HIV-infected children than in those who are uninfected.

Because essentially all pediatric tuberculosis results from initial infection of the lung through inhalation of droplet nuclei, most cases of tuberculosis in HIV-infected children will have evidence of pulmonary disease, as was observed in the two series that have been reported. No typical pattern of pulmonary findings can be discerned, so that any type of infiltrate should be considered to be consistent with a diagnosis of tuberculosis. Hilar adenopathy, a common finding in HIV-uninfected children, may be less common in children with HIV infection. It was present in seven of the 14 cases reported from Miami and New York, however, and may be the only radiographic abnormality present. The admonition that the child with hilar adenopathy in the absence of other pulmonary abnormalities should be treated for active disease (i.e., multidrug therapy and not isoniazid preventive therapy) is especially important for HIV-infected children because of the increased likelihood of disseminated disease. As noted previously, because pediatric tuberculosis results from an exposure to an infected adult, attempts to find the source of infection through cooperation with state and local public health programs are essential in the management of pediatric tuberculosis. It is also of great importance to look for exposed children when an adult is found to be infected.

Although pulmonary disease will be evident in most cases, rapid hematogenous dissemination may result in severe disease, including meningitis, without obvious pulmonary findings. Indeed, in the large series of tuberculous meningitis from Spain, only one-third of patients had pulmonary infiltrates, 22% had adenopathy as the only chest radiographic abnormality, and 46% had a normal chest radiograph (46). HIV infection is certain to be an additional risk for disseminated disease in children, who have a higher baseline risk than adults. Thus, tuberculosis should be considered in the HIV-infected child presenting with meningitis, and evidence of disseminated disease should be sought in the HIV-infected child who is diagnosed with pulmonary tuberculosis.

DIFFERENTIAL DIAGNOSIS

Although it is significantly less common than many other causes of pulmonary disease in HIV-infected children, tuberculosis should be considered as a diagnostic possibility in any child presenting with pulmonary infiltrates. As such, the main differential possibilities include *Pneumocystis carinii* pneumonia, bacterial pneumonia, especially pneumococcal pneumonia, virus pneumonia, and lymphocytic interstitial pneumonitis.

For nonpulmonary lesions, relevant differential diagnostic possibilities depend on the site of involvement. *M. tuberculosis* should be considered in the differential diagnosis of mass lesions in the brain, as well as of meningitis (46, 49). For mass lesions in the brain, the major differential diagnostic possibilities are all relatively uncommon in children and include other infections, particularly toxoplasmosis and cryptococcosis, as well as bacterial abscess and neoplasm, particularly lymphoma. The major differential diagnoses for tuberculosis meningitis are bacterial, viral (including HIV), and fungal (especially *Cryptococcus*) etiologies. For lymphadenitis, the major differential diagnosis would include HIV, cytomegalovirus, other bacteria, and disseminated *M. avium* infection (see also Chapters 8, 13, 16B, and 18).

DIAGNOSIS

The most important aspect of the diagnosis of tuberculosis in HIV-infected patients is for the clinician to consider this diagnosis in the appropriate clinical setting. Preoccupation with more common pulmonary processes such as *P. carinii* pneumonia and bacterial pneumonia may lead to the possibility of tuberculosis being overlooked. Failure to diagnose tuberculosis may lead not only to delay in appropriate therapy but to the spread of tuberculosis in the community or the health care setting (Table 16A.4).

The major modalities available for the diagnosis of tuberculosis include the tuberculin skin test, acid fast stain of clinical material, mycobacterial culture, and histology of biopsy specimens. As noted above, a typical radiographic appearance of pulmonary tuberculosis in the HIV-infected child has not emerged, so tuberculosis should be considered in any child with lung disease and should be diagnosed in any child with lung disease and a positive tuberculin test. The epidemiologic setting, including the mycobacterial culture and sensitivity results of the source case, is an essential part of the diagnostic evaluation and may ultimately provide the only bacteriologic information on which to base treatment decisions for the exposed child. The availability of this information should not, however, be the rationale for curtailing the evaluation of the HIV-infected child with suspected tuberculosis because of the significant risk of multiple exposures and the acquisition of drug-resistant tuberculosis.

Tuberculin skin testing with PPD has been found to be relatively insensitive for documenting tuberculous infection in adults with HIV infection and tuberculosis, with less than half of HIV-infected patients being tuberculin skin test positive at the time of diagnosis of tuberculosis (26, 41, 42, 46, 50). The likelihood of tuberculin positivity, and delayed type hypersensitivity to other antigens, depends on the state of HIV disease, with progressively fewer individuals having a positive test with more advanced HIV disease and/or lower CD4 counts (20, 32, 45, 51). There are no data on the overall frequency of tuberculin-specific skin test anergy among HIV-infected children. Among the 14 children with tuberculosis reported from New York and Miami, only two were reported to have positive tuberculin tests. A tuberculin test is nevertheless highly informative if positive, and therefore should be performed, along with appropriate controls consisting of two additional antigens (*Candida*, mumps, or tetanus toxoid) administered by the Mantoux method, in HIV-infected children in whom tuberculosis is being considered (51).

A recent review of tuberculosis in children provides an extensive discussion of the issues and controversies in tuberculin testing (29). The Mantoux technique of intradermal injection of 5 tuberculin units PPD should be used rather than one of the less sensitive and specific multipuncture tests, both for screening and diagnostic purposes in HIV-infected children. In infants and young children, a positive tuberculin test indicates primary or recent infection even without clinical evidence or radiographic

Table 16A.4.   Diagnosis of Infection with *M. tuberculosis*

Usual clinical presentations	Pulmonary disease, often with extrapulmonary involvement; extrapulmonary without pulmonary findings also occurs
History of contact with infected individual	Useful if positive; drug susceptibility of source case important
PPD skin testing	Useful for screening in asymptomatic child; evidence of active tuberculosis if positive in child with clinical illness; low sensitivity in HIV infected.
Chest radiograph findings	Localized or diffuse infiltrates; hilar adenopathy common
Acid-fast stain of clinical material	Useful if positive, culture required for speciation
Culture of clinical material	Necessary to confirm diagnosis and for antibiotic susceptibility testing
Blood culture	Occasionally positive, especially if extrapulmonary infection

evidence of disease (35). In an HIV-infected child with a consistent clinical illness, a positive tuberculin test is compelling evidence of active tuberculosis.

Tuberculin screening has been recommended for all HIV-positive individuals (9, 24, 34, 52, 53). New guidelines for the interpretation of tuberculin skin tests, based on prevalence among different risk groups for tuberculous infection, were recently developed by the CDC and the American Thoracic Society (24). One of the most important changes in these guidelines is the use of 5 mm induration as the definition of a positive test (vs. the previous 10 mm standard) in persons with HIV infection. False-positive tuberculin reactions, presumed to be caused by infection with nontuberculous mycobacteria, are uncommon in normal adults using current criteria for a positive test. False-positive reactions would be expected to be even less common in HIV-infected individuals because of their typically diminished delayed type hypersensitivity responses (51).

Acid-fast stain and mycobacterial culture are important elements in the evaluation of tuberculosis in HIV-infected children. Stain is relatively insensitive compared with culture, especially for cerebrospinal fluid. Fluorochrome (e.g., auramine-rhodamine) staining is more sensitive than traditional Ziehl-Neelsen or Kinyoun type stains, however, and most clinical microbiology laboratories that receive specimens for mycobacterial diagnosis will perform fluorescent staining. Sites from which samples for stain and culture should be obtained depend on site of disease. Pulmonary samples (sputum, tracheal aspirate, bronchoalveolar lavage fluid, lung biopsy tissue) and gastric aspirates should be obtained when pulmonary disease is present. Samples from blood, bone marrow, lymph node, liver, cerebrospinal fluid, or other sites for histopathology and acid-fast stain may be appropriate depending on the extent and location of disease. Given the high frequency of nontuberculous mycobacterial infection in HIV-infected children (54, 55), a positive acid-fast stain from a nonpulmonary specimen does not provide a definitive diagnosis of tuberculosis. Depending on the clinical setting and the nature of the positive specimen however, it may be an indication for initiating antituberculous therapy pending the results of culture.

The observation of acid-fast organisms on smears of pulmonary samples (sputum, tracheal aspirate or bronchoalveolar lavage specimens) from a child with pulmonary disease should be considered to be tuberculosis until proven otherwise for several reasons. Pneumonia is a relatively uncommon manifestation of *M. avium* infection, and in one study of adults, acid-fast organisms were much less likely to be observed on smear (10% of 40 patients) in patients with *M. avium* infection than in patients with *M. tuberculosis* (48% of 31 patients) (56) (see also Chapter 16B). The rapid course of tuberculosis in HIV-infected individuals indicates that presumptive therapy pending definitive diagnosis is appropriate. In addition, smear positivity is a sign of highly infectious tuberculosis, so this finding should lead to the institution of isolation precautions to protect other patients and health care workers from exposure.

Aggressive efforts to obtain appropriate culture material are often essential not only to document *M. tuberculosis* infection but to be able to determine sensitivities to available antituberculous agents. Morning gastric aspirates are the most readily available samples from children with pulmonary tuberculosis, and multiple samples should be obtained. A recent review of pediatric tuberculous in Houston, however, found the culture sensitivity of these specimens to be only 39% in HIV-uninfected children (57). The use of bronchoalveolar lavage has been shown to increase the yield for smear and culture over sputum samples in HIV-infected adults (56, 58). The incremental yield from bronchial brushings or transbronchial biopsy samples in addition to simple lavage and washings appeared to be minimal in these studies. In contrast the yield for culture from BAL specimens was surprisingly low (13%) in a small study of tuberculosis in HIV-uninfected children, although this study did not directly compare the yields from bronchoscopy and gastric aspirates (59). The results of these studies in HIV-infected adults combined with the difficulty in obtaining sputum from children, the variable sensitivity of culture, and the lack of specificity of acid-fast stain of gastric aspirates indicate that bronchoalveolar lavage to obtain pulmonary specimens should be strongly considered early in the diagnostic evaluation of tuberculosis in the HIV-infected child. In addition to providing specimens for mycobacterial stain and culture, specimens important for the diagnosis of other pulmonary pathogens as well as direct visual information that may support the diagnosis of pulmonary tuberculosis in the absence of positive cultures may be obtained (60).

Indeed, both gastric lavage and bronchoscopy appear to have had higher yields for mycobacterial culture in the small series of tuberculosis in HIV-infected children than the results in HIV-uninfected children. In the report from Miami, gastric aspirates yielded positive culture for *M. tuberculosis* in six of seven cases, and a bronchoalveolar lavage specimen was positive in the one patient with a negative gastric aspirate, as well as in the other four patients in whom bronchoalveolar lavage specimens were obtained (31).

Once samples are obtained, mycobacterial culture is painfully slow because of the long generation time of *M. tuberculosis*. The time required for colonies to appear on solid media is generally at least 2–3 weeks and may be as long as 6 weeks. As noted above, the use of radiometric detection in liquid media (BACTEC system) is now widely used and decreases the time to positive culture to as little as 1 week. Although traditional methods of species identification may take several more weeks, newer methods of speciation using nucleic acid probes or chromatography/mass spectrometry may allow identification within days after initial growth. Commercially available probes that are specific for *M. tuberculosis* and *M. avium* are now widely used in clinical microbiology laboratories for early speciation of mycobacterial cultures.

Additional approaches that remain experimental include use of nucleic acid probes directly on clinical specimens and use of the polymerase chain reaction to amplify mycobacterial DNA directly in clinical samples (61, 62). Reports on the use of polymerase chain reaction in clinical diagnosis of infectious diseases have become extremely numerous in the infectious disease literature, and commercially available kits are beginning to appear to detect pathogens in clincal specimens. Because of the time required for traditional culture, the application of this technology to mycobacterial infections holds great promise to facilitate diagnosis of tuberculosis and *M. avium* infection in ways that will directly affect patient management.

Diagnostic evaluation of an HIV-infected child with a clinical syndrome or epidemiologic history suggestive of tuberculosis or exposure to an adult with tuberculosis is relatively straightforward, although obtaining a definitive diagnosis may be difficult. Tuberculin skin testing should be performed using the Mantoux method, with appropriate controls placed at the same time. Chest radiographs should be obtained, because pulmonary disease will be present in most cases of active tuberculosis in HIV-infected children, regardless of whether extrapulmonary tuberculosis is also present. In the clinically well child, with a normal chest radiograph who has had a potential or documented exposure to a person with infectious tuberculosis, the initial evaluation may stop here and a decision made regarding preventive therapy based on the exposure history (see below). In the clinically ill child with pulmonary disease, additional evaluation would include obtaining morning gastric aspirates for culture and pulmonary samples for acid-fast stain and mycobacterial culture. Specimens from other sites should be obtained for stain and culture depending on the clinical syndrome (e.g., cerebrospinal fluid in the child with meningitis.)

TREATMENT

Approaches to treatment of tuberculosis in HIV-uninfected adults and children have changed markedly over the past decade, with the acceptance of short course (6–9 months) chemotherapy as standard. Although caution is warranted as more patients with advanced HIV disease and tuberculosis are treated, it appears that with timely diagnosis and completion of the prescribed course of therapy, drug susceptible tuberculosis in HIV-infected adults usually responds well to standard therapeutic regimens (26, 41, 42, 44, 45). This favorable experience in adults is supported by the outcomes reported in the limited pediatric literature (30, 31). The qualifiers noted above (timely diagnosis, patient compliance, and absence of drug resistance) may be particularly problematic, however, in HIV-infected patients, so treatment of tuberculosis in this population is rarely a straightforward proposition.

Two recent reviews in the pediatric literature provide excellent discussions of issues in the treatment of pediatric tuberculosis, including detailed recommendations, that are relevant for the treatment of HIV-infected as well as HIV-uninfected children (29, 63). Isoniazid (INH) and rifampin are the backbones of all currently accepted regimens for the treatment of tuberculosis where the organism is sensitive to these agents (63, 64). Although the optimal therapy for tuberculosis in children with HIV infection has not been established, the American Thoracic Society, the CDC Advisory Committee for the Elimination of Tuberculosis, and the American Academy of Pediatrics have recommended daily treatment with three drugs (INH, rifampin, and pyrazinamide) (32, 63, 65) for the first 2 months of therapy, followed by the two-drug regimen of INH and rifampin to complete at least 9 months therapy, for patients with HIV infection. In adults, therapy is also continued for at least 6 months after sputum becomes culture negative. Because of the increased frequency of multidrug-resistant tuberculosis, the CDC Advisory Committee for the Elimination of Tuberculosis is formulating new treatment guidelines that will recommend a four-drug regimen (INH, rifampin, pyrazinamide, and streptomycin or ethambutol) as initial therapy for all new cases of active tuberculosis unless infection with fully susceptible *M. tuberculosis* is essentially certain.

If poor compliance with treatment is anticipated, twice weekly therapy under direct observation is acceptable for the maintenance two-drug portion of standard therapy. Indeed the link between failure to complete therapy and the emergence of drug resistance (see below) has led to new and greatly increased emphasis on the use of directly observed therapy to ensure compliance with antituberculous therapy (66). If disseminated disease with meningitis or bone or joint involvement is present or if INH resistance is suspected, ethambutol or streptomycin is added for the initial 2 months, with two-drug therapy for an additional 10 months. If INH or rifampin is not included in the initial regimen for any form disease, prolonged therapy for a minimum total of 18 months is recommended (65). Considerations in the treatment of multidrug resistant tuberculosis are discussed below.

Pediatric doses and toxicities for the commonly prescribed agents are shown in Table 16A.5. Detailed weight-based doses for these agents may be found in Ref. 63. In general, these medications are well tolerated in children. Particular caution must be exercised with ethambutol, however, because early signs of optic neuritis, the major toxicity of this agent, are difficult to monitor in young children (67). In addition, complications of therapy and drug intolerance may be more common in HIV-infected children. The high incidence of liver function test abnormalities in children with HIV infection together with the high rate of intolerance of other agents such as trimethoprim-sulfamethoxazole, indicates that closer monitoring of HIV-infected children, including monitoring of liver function tests, may be required. Indeed a large review of tuberculosis therapy in HIV-infected adults noted an 18% incidence of adverse reactions requiring a change in therapy compared with 3.7% in HIV-uninfected patients from the same institution (45). For patients who cannot take medications orally, parenteral formulations of isoniazid and rifampin are available in addition to the orally administered products, and streptomycin is available only for intramuscular administration.

Decisions regarding the use of preventive INH therapy in HIV-infected patients without signs of tuberculosis is often extremely difficult because of the low sensitivity of tuberculin testing in this setting. The HIV-infected child with a positive tuberculin test and no evidence of active disease after careful evaluation including a chest radiograph, and in whom INH resistance is not anticipated, should receive 12 months preventive therapy with INH. The efficacy of INH pre-

Table 16A.5.   Recommended Drugs for Initial Treatment of Tuberculosis in Children[a]

Drug	Dosage Forms	Daily Dose[b]	Maximal Daily Dose	Twice Weekly Dose	Major Adverse Reactions
Isoniazid	Tablets: 100 mg, 300 mg Syrup: 50 mg/5 ml[c] Vials: 1 g	10–15 mg/kg PO or IM	300 mg	20–40 mg/kg max. 900 mg	Hepatic enzyme elevation, peripheral neuropathy, hepatitis hypersensitivity
Rifampin	Capsules: 150 mg, 300 mg Syrup: formulated from capsules, 10 mg/ml Vials: 600 mg	10–20 mg/kg PO or IV	600 mg	10–20 mg/kg max. 600 mg	Orange discoloration of secretions and urine; nausea, vomiting, hepatitis, febrile reaction, purpura (rare)
Pyrazinamide	Tablets: 500 mg	20–40 mg/kg PO	2 g	50–70 mg/kg	Hepatotoxicity, hyperuricemia, arthralgias skin rash, gastrointestinal upset
Streptomycin	Vials: 1 g, 4 g	20–40 mg/kg IM	1 g	25–30 mg/kg IM	Ototoxicity, nephrotoxicity
Ethambutol	Tablets: 100 mg, 400 mg	15–25 mg/kg PO	2.5 g	50 mg/kg	Optic neuritis (decreased red-green color discrimination, decreased visual acuity), skin rash

[a]Adapted from Ref. 88, which provides detailed weight-based dosage of isoniazid, rifampin, pyrazinamide, and ethambutol.
[b]Doses based on weight should be adjusted as weight changes
[c]Many experts do not recommend the use of isoniazid syrup because of drug instability and frequent gastrointestinal side effects.

ventive therapy is well documented in immunocompetent individuals, and limited data suggest that it is effective in HIV-infected persons as well (68). Preventive therapy after exposure to drug-resistant tuberculosis is discussed below.

In the case of the child with a negative tuberculin test but a history of exposure, the decision to use preventive therapy requires careful consideration of the likelihood of infection. Algorithms for the assessment of infection risk that were developed to assist in decision making regarding prophylaxis of multidrug-resistant tuberculosis are also applicable in the setting of exposure to susceptible tuberculosis and are described below and in Figure 16A.1. In general, if the risk of infection is moderate to high based on close exposure (household or other enclosed space contact), preventive therapy should be administered. Whether or not preventive therapy is administered, close follow-up of the exposed child is essential because of the high risk of progression to active disease after infection (estimated to be 170 times greater for persons with HIV infection relative to persons without this or other risk factors for progres-

sion) (68). As is the case with therapy of active disease, directly observed preventive treatment should be considered for patients in whom compliance may not be optimal.

MULTIDRUG-RESISTANT TUBERCULOSIS

The increasing prevalence of multidrug-resistant tuberculosis, particularly among HIV-infected individuals, has raised a host of new problems. In 1991, 14.4% of cases reported to the CDC had organisms that were resistant to at least one antituberculous agent. In 1991, 3.1% of new cases and 6.9% of recurrent cases were resistant to INH and rifampin, compared with 0.5% and 3.0% in 1982–1986 (66, 69). In the report of pediatric tuberculosis from Miami, three of nine cases had organisms that were resistant to both isoniazid and rifampin (31).

Beyond the increase in overall prevalence of multidrug-resistant tuberculosis, the phenomenon of institutional outbreaks of multidrug-resistant tuberculosis in hospitals and correctional facilities further threatens the ability of public health and medical systems to manage this problem (13–16, 66, 70). In addition to extensive spread among other

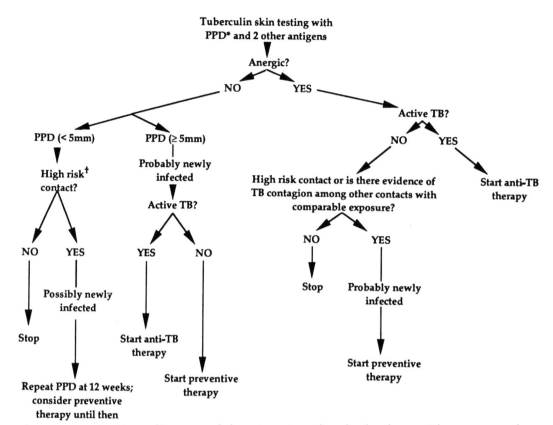

Figure 16A.1. Decision-making approach for estimating likelihood of new infection with *M. tuberculosis* and need for preventive therapy in persons with HIV infection. *TB*, tuberculosis. †Members of immediate family, close social contacts, or others who shared same indoor environment with infectious tuberculosis patient for substantial periods. Adapted from Ref 68.

HIV-infected residents of these facilities, infection of hospital workers and other employees of these institutions has occurred, with 33 and 50% of exposed workers infected in two hospital outbreaks (66). Mortality rates among AIDS patients infected with multidrug-resistant tuberculosis in these outbreaks has been extremely high, ranging from 72 to 89%, and survival from the time of diagnosis has been extremely short (median 4–16 weeks) (69).

The major factor in the de novo emergence of multidrug resistance in an individual is the failure to complete an appropriate course therapy with two or more drugs. In the United States the increased prevalence of multidrug resistance has been linked to several factors including social and economic conditions and diminished federal state and local resources for the public health and case management of tu-

berculosis. A report from one hospital in New York City, an area with a high prevalence of multidrug-resistant tuberculosis and HIV infection, indicated that as many as 80% of patients with tuberculosis did not complete the prescribed treatment (11).

The many problems raised by multidrug-resistant tuberculosis are extensively covered in a series of reports from the CDC (66, 68, 69). Treatment of active multidrug-resistant tuberculosis and the management of exposure to multidrug-resistant tuberculosis in the HIV-infected individual are the two issues most likely to be faced by clinicians treating HIV-infected children.

The treatment of multidrug-resistant (resistant to two or more agents) tuberculosis has been extremely difficult. Whereas INH resistance was a significant but manageable obstacle to effective therapy, HIV-infected individuals infected with multidrug-resistant tuberculosis have responded poorly to treatment, with mortality rates essentially equivalent to those of untreated tuberculosis, as noted above. Coresistance to INH and rifampin, mycobactericidal drugs that form the core of standard therapy, has occurred in most outbreaks of multidrug-resistant tuberculosis and is the most likely reason for this poor response to therapy. Resistance to pyrazinamide, the third component of standard therapy, has been much less frequently reported (13–16, 70, 71). Although resistance to this agent clearly occurs, it may prove to be useful in regimens for treating multidrug-resistant tuberculosis. In addition to older second-line agents that have been incorporated into treatment regimens for multidrug-resistant tuberculosis, increasing attention has been focused on the quinolones, many of which have shown antimycobacterial activity in vitro (72, 73).

The specific therapy of multidrug-resistant tuberculosis depends on the exact pattern of drug susceptibility observed for the infecting organism. Because a high proportion of multidrug-resistant tuberculosis cases have occurred in HIV-infected individuals, drug susceptibility testing should be undertaken for all isolates from HIV-infected children and/or the source case, even if drug resistance is not suspected on an epidemiologic basis. The early use of additional agents (four or more drugs) if drug resistance is suspected or if initial clinical response to standard therapy is poor is appropriate to achieve effective treatment of drug-resistant tuberculosis.

The management of persons, including those with HIV infection, exposed to multidrug-resistant tuberculosis is a complex issue that was the subject of a recent report from the CDC. As noted above, the low sensitivity of the tuberculin test in HIV-infected persons greatly complicates this issue. Figure 16A.1 and Table 16A.6 provide an approach to estimating the likelihood of new infection with tuberculosis in general and multidrug-resistant tuberculosis in particular and to decision making regarding the use of preventive therapy. Intermediate to high likelihood of new infection with multidrug-resistant tuberculosis should lead to consideration of multidrug-preventive therapy, if there is no evidence of active disease. The importance of close follow-up is essential because of the high likelihood of active disease following tuberculosis infection in HIV-infected individuals.

Note that efficacy of preventive regimens for drug-resistant tuberculosis is not established. For INH resistance alone, rifampin may be used. It has been recommended, however, that if INH resistance is partial (<100%), INH should still be the drug of choice for preventive therapy (68). If multidrug resistance is present, alternatives may be tried based on the susceptibility patterns of the source case. If preventive therapy is initiated, more than one drug should be used. Alternatives that have been suggested include pyrazinamide plus ethambutol or pyrazinamide plus a fluoroquinolone or possibly the use of an aminoglycoside or capreomycin with pyrazinamide (68).

Table 16A.6.   Likelihood of Infection with Multidrug-resistant *M. tuberculosis* among Contacts Thought to Be Newly Infected[a]

Infectiousness of the Source MDR TB Case	Closeness and Intensity of MDR TB Exposure	Contact's Risk of Exposure to Drug-susceptible TB	Estimated Likelihood of Infection with MDR *M. tuberculosis*[b]
+	+	−	High
+	−	−	High-intermediate
−	+	−	High-intermediate
−	−	−	Intermediate
+	+	+	Intermediate
+	−	+	Low-intermediate
−	+	+	Low-intermediate
−	−	+	Low

[a]Anergic contacts should be considered likely to be newly infected if there is evidence of contagion among contacts with comparable exposure. MDR TB, multidrug-resistant tuberculosis. + high; − low. From Centers for Disease Control. Management of persons exposed to multidrug-resistant tuberculosis. MMWR 1992;41 (RR-11):65.
[b]Multidrug preventive therapy should be considered for persons in high, high-intermediate, and intermediate categories.

Specific toxicities, particularly of ethambutol and the quinolones, should be considered in addition to the susceptibility pattern of the organism in designing a multidrug-preventive regimen for children exposed to multidrug-resistant tuberculosis.

INFECTION CONTROL

Because tuberculosis is spread by airborne droplet nuclei, attention to established infection control and case management procedures is essential to prevent the spread of tuberculosis in the health care setting and in the community. The emergence of multidrug-resistant tuberculosis and the documented nosocomial outbreaks of multidrug-resistant tuberculosis have added even greater urgency not only to adherence to established procedures but to the need to assess the efficacy of these procedures (66). It is important to note in this context failure to consider the diagnosis of tuberculosis and failure to implement established infection control practices played a major

role in allowing the spread of multidrug-resistant tuberculosis in the outbreaks that have been described. Note also that many clinics and hospitals, as well as institutions in which individuals with tuberculosis may reside, lack facilities that are in compliance with recommendations for the isolation of individuals with infectious tuberculosis or those at high risk for tuberculosis.

The CDC published updated guidelines in 1990 for the prevention of tuberculosis transmission, with emphasis on the health care setting (74). These guidelines are summarized in Table 16A.7. Most of these guidelines reiterate long-standing recommendations for preventing tuberculosis transmission, with increased emphasis on outpatient and home care settings and specific attention to cough-inducing procedures including administration of aerosolized pentamidine, sputum induction, and bronchoscopy.

Among the most important aspects of these recommendations are early diagnosis and treatment of both active tuberculosis and asymptomatic infection. Tuberculin

Table 16A.7.   Summary of Recommendations for Preventing Transmission of Tuberculosis in Health Care Settings[a]

Early identification and treatment of persons with active TB
  Maintain a high index of suspicion for TB to identify cases rapidly
  Promptly initiate effective multidrug anti-TB therapy on the basis of clinical and drug resistance surveillance data

Prevention of spread of infectious droplet nuclei by source control methods and by reduction of microbial contamination of indoor air
  Initiate AFB isolation precautions immediately for all patients who have suspected or confirmed active TB and who may be infectious (AFB isolation precautions include use of a private room with negative pressure in relation to surrounding areas and at least six air exchanges per hour; room air should be exhausted directly to outside; use of ultraviolet lamps and high-efficiency particulate air filters to supplement ventilation may be considered)
  Persons entering the AFB isolation room should use disposable particulate respirators that fit snugly around the face
  Continue AFB isolation precautions until there is clinical evidence of reduced infectiousness (cough has substantially decreased and the number of organisims on sequential sputum smears is decreasing); if drug resistance is suspected or confirmed, continue AFB precautions until sputum smear is negative for AFB
  Use special precautions during cough-inducing procedures

Surveillance for TB transmission
  Maintain surveillance for TB infection among health care workers by routine, periodic tuberculin skin testing; recommend appropriate preventive therapy for health care workers when indicated
  Maintain surveillance for TB cases among patients and health care workers
  Promptly initiate contact investigation procedures among health care workers, patients, and visitors exposed to an untreated or ineffectively treated infectious TB patient for whom appropriate AFB procedures are not in place; recommend appropriate therapy or preventive therapy for contacts with disease or TB infection without current disease; therapeutic regimens should be chosen on the basis of the clinical history and local drug resistance surveillance data

[a]TB, tuberculosis; AFB, acid-fast bacilli. From Centers for Disease Control. Nosocomial transmission of multidrug-resistant tuberculosis among HIV-infected persons—Florida and New York, 1988–1991. MMWR 1991;40:586.

screening of all HIV-infected persons and consideration of pulmonary tuberculosis in all patients presenting with pulmonary disease are essential to this approach. Further, tuberculin testing of household and other close contacts when an HIV-infected adult or child is identified is essential to limiting the spread of tuberculosis in the community.

In addition to isolation with appropriate ventilation (negative pressure, more than six air exchanges per hour with external exhausting) for patients with, or suspected of having, active tuberculosis, establishment of adequate ventilation or use of supplemental measures such as high efficiency filtration in areas such as waiting rooms or emergency rooms should be instituted in areas where there is a high prevalence of tuberculosis. Although the incidence and infectivity of tuberculosis is lower in children than adults, this recommendation is also relevant in the pediatric setting, because many HIV-infected children will be accompanied by an adult in a high-risk group for tuberculosis. Recommendations for cough-inducing procedures focus on ventilation and the use of disposable particulate respirators, similar to surgical masks but more efficient at filtering small particles including droplet nuclei. The National Institute of Occupational Safety and Health has recommended the use of power respirators for those working with patients with infectious tuberculosis. This recommendation is considered to be excessive by many experts, although the use of such devices may be warranted in unusual circumstances where the risk of aerosolization of tubercle bacilli is exceptionally high, such as during bronchoscopy of a patient with newly diagnosed or suspected tuberculosis.

In addition to diagnosis and treatment and environmental measures, the third major component of tuberculosis infection control is surveillance of transmission among hospital workers. Surveillance is essential to document adequacy of infection control practice, to identify areas of high risk for transmission, and to identify workers who become infected so that appropriate medical management may be instituted.

The appropriateness of the application of isolation guidelines to HIV-infected children with documented or suspected pulmonary tuberculosis is unclear. In general pediatric

pulmonary tuberculosis has not been considered to be infectious, and isolation has not been recommended (75). The frequency of sputum acid-fast stain positivity, a finding that correlates strongly with infectivity in adults, is not explicit in the two small pediatric series of tuberculosis and HIV infection but is probably low. Nevertheless, a case of cavitary pulmonary disease in a 5-year boy with AIDS, with documented nosocomial transmission, indicates that pediatric tuberculosis may be infectious in children with AIDS (39). In addition, the high infectivity of tuberculosis in HIV-infected adults without cavitary disease suggests that HIV-infected children with tuberculosis who present with cough and pulmonary infiltrates may indeed be infectious. Thus it seems prudent to take an approach to HIV-infected children with pulmonary tuberculosis that is similar to the approach taken to adults with pulmonary tuberculosis. HIV-infected children with newly diagnosed pulmonary tuberculosis who have a cough or undergo cough-inducing procedures should be considered infectious. Patients who have begun appropriate antituberculous therapy and have had a definite clinical response (diminished cough and fever) are probably no longer infectious. If sputum samples can be obtained, diminished numbers of bacilli on acid-fast stain support this conclusion, and the absence of bacilli for 3 consecutive days confirms it. In adults this response may require 2–3 weeks or longer. In the HIV-infected child with drug-susceptible tuberculosis, response should occur in a matter of days. The more stringent criterion of three negative sputum smears has been recommended for determining that adults with multidrug-resistant tuberculosis are not infectious (53).

The emergence of multidrug-resistant tuberculosis and the high risk of nosocomial spread of this pathogen together with the lack of adequate isolation facilities in many institutions have led to the consideration of establishment of specialized facilities for the treatment of patients with multidrug-resistant tuberculosis. Such facilities would be designed to minimize the risk of transmission to other patients and health care workers. Clear evidence of nosocomial infection of health care workers and the risk of severe disease from multidrug-resistant tuberculosis in those who are immunocompromised have led to consideration of new policies for such employees, including those with HIV infection, who work in settings with a high risk of exposure to multidrug-resistant tuberculosis (66).

Interruption of tuberculosis transmission in the community relies on effective case management including assurance of completion of treatment, with directly observed therapy if necessary. In addition to treatment, the other central component of case management is contact tracing. This is especially true when a case of pediatric tuberculosis is diagnosed. Rather than finding contacts to determine exposure to and potential infection from the index case, the pediatric index case may be the result of a recent infection from an infectious case in the home or community environment of the infected child. This infectious case should be found so that treatment can be initiated for the benefit of that individual, other contacts can be evaluated for infection and active disease, and further transmission from this infectious individual does not occur.

PREVENTION

In the United States the approach to the prevention of tuberculosis has been one of active case finding, treatment, and contact tracing. Although there is no rationale to change this approach in the setting of the HIV epidemic, the need for greatly increased resources and commitment to successfully implement this approach has become apparent (10, 66). The limitations of vaccination with BCG, including tuberculin test conversion and uncertain efficacy, have resulted in this vaccine not being used routinely in the United States (76). The emergence of multidrug-resistant tuberculosis, however, has led to reconsideration of the use of this vaccine in health care workers at high risk for exposure to multidrug-resistant tuberculosis (66). Although revised recommendations will not be formulated by the CDC until a new analysis of existing data on the efficacy of BCG has been completed in mid-1993, the use of this vaccine in immunocompetent health care workers in settings with a high risk of exposure to multidrug-resistant tuberculosis must be considered.

In less-developed countries of the world where tuberculosis is prevalent, BCG vaccination to prevent tuberculosis has been standard practice, as recommended in the Expanded Program on Immunization of the World Health Organization. This recommendation has not changed in areas of high prevalence of HIV infection except that the World Health Organization recommends against vaccination with BCG in children with symptomatic HIV infection (77, 78). Although several reports have documented the occurrence of disseminated BCG infection in vaccinated adults and children with HIV infection (79–83), this complication has not been reported as a frequent occurrence in HIV-endemic areas where BCG vaccination of children is practiced. Preliminary reports from areas of Africa with high incidences of both tuberculosis and HIV infection indicate that complications of BCG vaccination in HIV-infected infants are uncommon (84, 85). One report also notes the significantly decreased response (measured by reaction to follow-up tuberculin testing) of HIV-infected infants relative to those who are uninfected. In this context it is important to note that the efficacy of BCG vaccination in preventing tuberculosis in HIV-uninfected populations is controversial, and its efficacy in people who are HIV-infected is unknown. A more extensive discussion of BCG vaccination in the setting of HIV infection is provided in Ref. 86.

FUTURE RESEARCH

There are abundant needs for basic and applied research relevant to mycobacterial disease in HIV-infected and uninfected patients. The emergence of multidrug-resistant tuberculosis has accentuated this need, and the National Action Plan to Combat Multidrug-Resistant Tuberculosis details research priorities in the areas of epidemiology, laboratory diagnosis, therapy, infection control, drug development, vaccine development, and the basic biology and immunology of *M. tuberculosis* and tuberculous disease (66).

Perhaps the most urgent needs, in addition to better basic understanding of the organism and disease mechanisms, are in the areas of diagnosis, treatment, and prevention. Tuberculin testing has served a central function for several decades but is insensitive in immunocompromised patients with HIV infection and is not specific for active disease. Similarly, the sensitivity and specificity of acid-fast stain and culture are inadequate, and culture is extremely slow. Improved culture methods and the development of sensitive, specific, and rapid diagnostic techniques such as the polymerase chain reaction, which could be applied directly to clinical samples, will be an important step in improving the care of patients with mycobacterial disease.

In the realm of therapy, the development and clinical testing of new antimycobacterial agents has become a pressing need with the emergence of multidrug-resistant tuberculosis. Better understanding of the biology of mycobacteria and mechanisms of resistance to existing drugs will be essential to the timely development of new agents (87). The inadequacies of BCG vaccination are apparent, and the need for a safe and effective vaccine to prevent infection or disease is even more urgent because of multidrug-resistant tuberculosis. Central to the development of candidate vaccines is a much clearer understanding of the nature of immunity to tuberculosis and the interaction of the bacillus and the immune system that alternatively results in clearance of infection, latency, or development of active disease.

SUMMARY

Tuberculosis, on its way to becoming eliminated as a major cause of disease in the developed world in the early 1980s, has re-emerged with a vengeance. The confluence of the AIDS epidemic, diminished tuberculosis control resources, and deteriorating social and economic conditions has resulted in a progressive increase in new cases of tuberculosis and tuberculosis transmission in adults and children in the United States. Worldwide, these same forces have not only resulted in increased transmission but increased morbidity and mortality among those with concomitant HIV and tuberculous infection. The marked increase in the incidence of multidrug resistance has added greatly to the difficulties in combating this disease.

Indeed the ancient plague of tuberculosis, in concert with the modern scourge of HIV infection, appears eager to reclaim its role as "captain of all these men of death" (cited in Ref. 12). Greatly increased resources and the dedicated efforts of researchers, clinicians, and public health workers must be mobilized if this is to be prevented from occurring.

References

1. Bloom B, Godal T. Selective primary health care: Strategies for control of disease in the developing world. Rev Infect Dis 1983;5:765–779.
2. Daniel T, Robert Koch, tuberculosis and the subsequent history of medicine [Editorial]. Am Rev Respir Dis 1982;125(suppl 2):1–3.
3. Dubos R, Dubos J. The white plague: Tuberculosis, man and society. Boston: Little Brown, 1952.
4. Centers for Disease Control. Tuberculosis, final data—United States, 1986. MMWR 1988;36:817–820.
5. Centers for Disease Control. Tuberculosis morbidity in the United States: Final data, 1990. MMWR CDC Surveill Summ 1991;40:23–27.
6. Centers for Disease Control. Tuberculosis morbidity—United States, 1991. MMWR 1992;41:240.
7. Centers for Disease Control. Tuberculosis—United States, 1985—and the possible impact of human T-lymphotropic virus type III/lymphadenopathy-associated virus infection. MMWR 1986;35:74–76.
8. Centers for Disease Control. Tuberculosis and acquired immunodeficiency syndrome—New York City. MMWR 1987;36:785–794.
9. Snider DJ, Hopewell P, Mills J, Reichman L. Mycobacterioses and the acquired immunodeficiency syndrome. Am Rev Respir Dis 1987;136:492–496.
10. Snider D, Roper W. The new tuberculosis. N Engl J Med 1992;326:703–705.
11. Brudney K, Dobkin J. Resurgent tuberculosis in New York City: Human immunodeficiency virus, homelessness and the decline of tuberculosis control programs. Am Rev Respir Dis 1991;144:745–749.
12. Bloom B, Murray C. Tuberculosis: Commentary on a reemergent killer. Science 1992;257:1055–1064.
13. Centers for Disease Control. Nosocomial transmission of multidrug-resistant tuberculosis among HIV-infected persons—Florida and New York, 1988–1991. MMWR 1991;40:585–591.
14. Centers for Disease Control. Transmission of multidrug-resistant tuberculosis among immunocompromised persons in a correctional system—New York, 1991. MMWR 1992;41:507–509.
15. Edlin B, Tokars J, Grieco M, et al. An outbreak of multidrug-resistant tuberculosis among hospitalized patients with the acquired immunodeficiency syndrome. N Engl J Med 1992;326:1514–1521.
16. Pearson M, Jereb J, Frieden T, et al. Nosocomial transmission of multidrug-resistant Mycobacterium tuberculosis. Ann Intern Med 1992;117:191–196.

17. Mann J, Snider D, Francis H, et al. Association between HTLV-III/LAV infection and tuberculosis in Zaire [Letter]. JAMA 1986;256:346.
18. Meeran K. Prevalence of HIV infection among patients with leprosy and tuberculosis in rural Zambia. Br Med J 1989;298:364–365.
19. Harries A. Tuberculosis and human immunodeficiency virus infection in developing countries. Lancet 1990;335:387–390.
20. Batungwanayo J, Taelman H, Dhote R, et al. Pulmonary tuberculosis in Kigali, Rwanda. Am Rev Respir Dis 1992;146:53–56.
21. Long R, Scalcini M, Mafreda J, et al. Impact of human immunodeficiency virus type 1 on tuberculosis in rural Haiti. Am Rev Respir Dis 1991;143:69–73.
22. Pean C, Pape J, Deschamps M-Mea. Natural history of M. leprae and HIV co-infection [Abstract ThBP 70]. Fifth International Conference on AIDS, Montreal, Jun 1989.
23. Turk J, Rees R. AIDS and leprosy [Editorial]. Lepr Rev 1988;59:193–194.
24. American Thoracic Society. Diagnostic standards and classification of tuberculosis. Am Rev Respir Dis 1990;142:725–735.
25. Centers for Disease Control. Tuberculosis and acquired immunodeficiency syndrome—Florida. MMWR 1986;35:587–590.
26. Pitchenik A, Cole C, Russell B, et al. Tuberculosis, atypical mycobacteriosis, and the acquired immunodeficiency syndrome among Haitian and non-Haitian patients in South Florida. Ann Intern Med 1984;101:641–645.
27. Handwerger S, Mildvan D, Senie R, McKinley F. Tuberculosis and the acquired immunodeficiency syndrome at a New York City hospital: 1978–1985. Chest 1987;91:176–180.
28. Selwyn P, Hartel D, Lewis V, et al. A prospective study of the risk of tuberculosis among intravenous drug users with human immunodeficiency virus infection. N Engl J Med 1989;320:545–550.
29. Starke J, Jacobs R, Jereb J. Resurgence of tuberculosis in children. J Pediatr 1992;120:839–855.
30. Moss W, Dedyo T, Suarez M, Nicholas S, Abrams E. Tuberculosis in children infected with human immunodeficiency virus: A report of five cases. Pediatr Infect Dis J 1992;11:114–120.
31. Khouri Y, Mastrucci M, Hutto C, Mitchell C, Scott G. Mycobacterium tuberculosis in children with human immunodeficiency virus type 1 infection. Pediatr Infect Dis J 1992;11:950–955.
32. Centers for Disease Control. Tuberculosis and human immunodeficiency virus infection: Recommendations of the advisory committee for the elimination of tuberculosis (ACET). MMWR 1989;38:236–238, 243–250.
33. Centers for Disease Control. Revision of the CDC surveillance case definition for acquired immunodeficiency syndrome. MMWR 1987;36:1s–5s.
34. Centers for Disease Control. Screening for tuberculosis and tuberculous infection in high-risk populations and the use of preventive therapy for tuberculous infection in the United States. MMWR 1990;39:1–12.
35. Lincoln E, Sewell E. Tuberculosis in Children. New York: McGraw-Hill, 1963.
36. Comstock G, Livesay V, Woolpert S. The prognosis of a positive tuberculin reaction in childhood and adolescence. Am J Epidemiol 1974;99:131–138.
37. Centers for Disease Control. Tuberculosis outbreak among persons in a residential facility for HIV-infected persons—San Francisco. MMWR 1991;40:649–652.
38. Daley C, Small P, Schecter G, et al. An outbreak of tuberculosis with accelerated progression among persons infected with the human immunodeficiency virus. N Engl J Med 1992;326:231–235.
39. Varteresian-Karanfil L, Josephson A, Fikrig S, Kauffman S, Steiner P. Pulmonary infection and cavity formation caused by Mycobacterium tuberculosis in a child with AIDS. N Engl J Med 1988;319:1018–1019.
40. Pitchenik A, Rubinson H. The radiographic appearance of tuberculosis in patients with the acquired immune deficiency syndrome (AIDS) and pre-AIDS. Am Rev Respir Dis 1985;131:393–396.
41. Louie E, Rice L, Holzman R. Tuberculosis in non-Haitian patients with acquired immunodeficiency syndrome. Chest 1986;90:542–545.
42. Chaisson R, Schecter G, Theuer C, et al. Tuberculosis in patients with the acquired immunodeficiency syndrome. Am Rev Respir Dis 1987;136:570–574.
43. Long R, Maycher B, Scalcini M, Manfreda J. The chest roentgenogram in pulmonary tuberculosis patients seropositive for human immunodeficiency virus type 1. Chest 1991;99:123–127.
44. Sunderam G, McDonald R, Maniatis T, et al. Tuberculosis as a manifestation of the acquired immunodeficiency syndrome (AIDS). JAMA 1986;256:362–366.
45. Small P, Schecter G, Goodman P, et al. Treatment of tuberculosis in patients with advanced human immunodeficiency virus infection. N Engl J Med 1991;324:289–294.
46. Berenguer J, Moreno S, Laguna F, et al. Tuberculosis meningitis in patients infected with the human immunodeficiency virus. N Engl J Med 1992;326:668–672.
47. Saltzman B, Motyl M, Friedland G, McKitrick J, Klein R. Mycobacterium tuberculosis bacteremia in the acquired immunodeficiency syndrome [Case report]. JAMA 1986;256:390–391.
48. Barnes P, Arevalo C. Six cases of Mycobacterium tuberculosis bacteremia. J Infect Dis 1987;156:377–379.
49. Bishburg E, Sunderam G, Reichman L, Kapila R. Central nervous system tuberculosis with the acquired immunodeficiency syndrome and its related complex. Ann Intern Med 1986;105:210–213.
50. Pitchenik A, Burr J, Suarez M, et al. Human T-cell lymphotropic virus-III (HTLV-III) seropositivity and related disease among 71 consecutive patients in whom tuberculosis was diagnosed. Am Rev Respir Dis 1987;135:875–879.
51. Centers for Disease Control. Purified protein derivative (PPD)-tuberculin anergy and HIV infection: Guidelines for anergy testing and management of anergic persons at risk of tuberculosis. MMWR 1991;40:27–32.

52. Pitchenik A, Burr J, Cole C. Tuberculin testing for persons with positive serologic studies for HTLV-III [Letter]. N Engl J Med 1986;314:447.
53. Centers for Disease Control. Prevention and control of tuberculosis in facilities providing long-term care to the elderly. MMWR 1990;39:7–13.
54. Hoyt L, Oleske J, Holland B, Connor E. Nontuberculous mycobacteria in children with acquired immunodeficiency syndrome. Pediatr Infect Dis J 1992;11:354–360.
55. Lewis L, Butler K, Husson R, et al. Defining the population of human immunodeficiency virus-infected children at risk for Mycobacterium avium-intracellulare. J Pediatr 1992;121:677–683.
56. Salzman S, Schindel M, Aranda C, Smith R, Lewis M. The role of bronchoscopy in the diagnosis of pulmonary tuberculosis in patients at risk for HIV infection. Chest 1992;102:143–146.
57. Starke J, Taylor-Watts K. Tuberculosis in the pediatric population of Houston, Texas. Pediatrics 1989;84:28–35.
58. Miro A, Gibilara E, Powell S, Kamholz S. The role of fiberoptic bronchoscopy for diagnosis of pulmonary tuberculosis in patients at risk for AIDS. Chest 1992;10:1211–1214.
59. de Blic J, Azeuedo J, Burren C, et al. The value of flexible bronchoscopy in childhood pulmonary tuberculosis. Chest 1991;100:688–692.
60. Toppet M, Malfroot A, Derde M, et al. Corticosteroids in primary tuberculosis with bronchial obstruction. Arch Dis Child 1990;65:1222–1226.
61. Brisson-Noel A, Gicquel B, Lecossier D, et al. Rapid diagnosis of tuberculosis by amplification of mycobacterial DNA in clinical samples. Lancet 1989;2:1069–1071.
62. Eisenach K, Cave M, Bates J, Crawford J. Polymerase chain reaction amplification of a repetitive DNA sequence specific for Mycobacterium tuberculosis. J Infect Dis 1990;161:977–981.
63. Committee on Infectious Diseases, American Academy of Pediatrics. Chemotherapy for tuberculosis in infants and children. Pediatrics 1992;89:161–165.
64. American Thoracic Society. Treatment of tuberculosis and tuberculosis infection in adults and children. Am Rev Respir Dis 1986;134:355–363.
65. American Thoracic Society. Mycobacterioses and the acquired immunodeficiency syndrome. Am Rev Respir Dis 1987;136:492–496.
66. Centers for Disease Control. National action plan to combat multidrug-resistant tuberculosis. MMWR 1992;41(RR-11):1–48.
67. Smith M, Marquis J. Tuberculosis and other mycobacterial infection. In: Feigin RD, Cherry JD, eds. Textbook of pediatric infectious diseases. 2nd ed. Philadelphia: WB Saunders, 1987:1370–1373.
68. Centers for Disease Control. Management of persons exposed to multidrug-resistant tuberculosis. MMWR 1992;41(RR-11):59–71.
69. Centers for Disease Control. Meeting the challenge of multidrug-resistant tuberculosis. MMWR 1992;41:49–57.
70. Centers for Disease Control. Nosocomial transmission of multidrug-resistant tuberculosis to health-care workers and HIV-infected patients in an urban hospital—Florida. MMWR 1990;39:718–722.

71. Fischl M, Daikos G, Uttamchandani R, et al. Clinical presentation and outcome of patients with HIV infection and tuberculosis caused by multiple-drug-resistant bacilli. Ann Intern Med 1992;117:184–190.
72. Fenlon C, Cynamon M. Comparative in vitro activities of ciprofloxacin and other 4-quinolones against Mycobacterium tuberculosis and Mycobacterium intracellulare. Antimicrob Agents Chemother 1986;29:386–388.
73. Gorzynski E, Gutman S, Allen W. Comparative antimycobacterial activities of difloxacin, temaloxacin, enoxacin, pefloxacin, reference fluoroquinolones, and a new macrolide, clarithromycin. Antimicrob Agents Chemother 1989;33:591–592.
74. Centers for Disease Control. Guidelines for preventing the transmission of tuberculosis in health-care settings, with special focus on HIV-related issues. MMWR 1990;39:1–29.
75. Report of Committee on Infectious Diseases. 22nd ed. Elk Grove Village, IL: American Academy of Pediatrics, 1991:505.
76. Centers for Disease Control. Use of BCG vaccines in the control of tuberculosis: A joint statement by the ACIP and the advisory committee for elimination of tuberculosis. MMWR 1988;37:663–675.
77. Von Reyn C, Clements C, Mann J. Human immunodeficiency virus infection and routine childhood immunization. Lancet 1987;2:669–672.
78. World Health Organization. Expanded programme on immunization: Global advisory group. Wkly Epidemiol Rec 1987;62:5–9.
79. Centers for Disease Control. Disseminated Mycobacterium bovis infection from BCG vaccination of a patient with acquired immunodeficiency syndrome. MMWR 1985;34:227–228.
80. Ninane J, Grymonprez A, Burtonboy G, Francois A, Cornu G. Disseminated BCG in HIV infection. Arch Dis Child 1988;63:1268–1269.
81. Houde C, Dery P. Mycobacterium bovis sepsis in an infant with human immunodeficiency virus infection. Pediatr Infect Dis J 1988;7:810–812.
82. Boudes P, Sobel A, Deforges L, Leblic E. Disseminated Mycobacterium bovis infection from BCG vaccination and HIV infection [Letter]. JAMA 1989;262:2386.
83. Armbruster C, Junker W, Vetter J, Jaksch G. Disseminated Bacille Calmette-Guerin in an AIDS patient 30 years after BCG vaccination [Letter]. J Infect Dis 1990;162:1216.
84. Colebunders R, Izaley L, Musampu M, et al. BCG vaccine abscesses are unrelated to HIV infection [Letter]. JAMA 1988;259:352.
85. Centers for Disease Control. BCG vaccination and pediatric HIV infection—Rwanda, 1988–1990. MMWR 1991;40:833–836.
86. Braun M, Cauthen G. Relationship of the human immunodeficiency virus epidemic to pediatric tuberculosis and bacillus calmette-guerin immunization. Pediatr Infect Dis J 1992;11:220–227.
87. Zhang Y, Heym B, Allen B, Young D, Cole S. The catalase-peroxidase gene and isoniazid resistance of Mycobacterium tuberculosis. Nature 1992;358:591–593.
88. Committee on Infections Diseases. Chemotherapy for tuberculosis in infants and children. Pediatrics 1992;89:161–165.

PART B / NONTUBERCULOUS MYCOBACTERIAL INFECTIONS

Linda L. Lewis

The nontuberculous or atypical mycobacteria were identified microbiologically not long after Koch described *M. tuberculosis* but were rarely considered responsible for serious, life-threatening infections in children in the pre-AIDS era. Before the 1980s, most nontuberculous mycobacterial infection reported in children appeared as localized, usually cervical, lymphadenitis or as bone or soft tissue infections complicating puncture wounds in otherwise normal hosts (1–3). Even these cases were relatively uncommon. With increasing numbers of HIV-infected patients, the most striking change has been the high frequency of disseminated infection with organisms in the *M. avium* (MAC) complex. Other nontuberculous mycobacteria also cause sporadic infection in individuals both with and without HIV infection but have not, to date, posed the clinical problems associated with tuberculosis or disseminated MAC infection.

Information regarding mycobacterial infection in HIV-infected children is often extrapolated from the larger population of adults with HIV infection. Recent investigations have attempted to address the similarities and differences of these infections in the pediatric group and help to identify specific pediatric needs for surveillance, prophylaxis, and therapy.

MYCOBACTERIUM AVIUM COMPLEX
Microbiology

M. avium, *M. intracellulare*, and unspeciated mycobacteria of the X cluster (4) are the species comprising MAC. Like *M. tuberculosis*, these organisms are slow-growing obligate aerobes, requiring 2–6 weeks for colony formation on solid media. Colonies are usually smooth but may be rough and can be transparent or opaque. MAC isolates are sometimes identified by the older Runyon classification system on the basis of growth and pigment characteristics. These organisms belong to group III or the non-photochromagens, organisms that grow slowly and do not produce pigment when cultured in either the presence or absence of light. Although these organisms will grow on various routine bacterial media, growth is enhanced with cultivation on selective mycobacterial media such as Lowenstein-Jensen medium or Middlebrook 7H10 and 7H11 agar. Like other mycobacteria, MAC organisms exhibit acid-fast staining caused by the cell wall mycolic acids that occur as esters bound to polysaccharides and as components of glycolipids.

Because of their morphologic and biochemical similarity, MAC isolates are often reported as *M. avium-intracellulare* without specific identification. Nucleic acid hybridization probes based on target sequences of ribosomal RNA are commercially available for rapid identification of clinical isolates (5, 6). However, currently available probes require growth of the organisms on solid medium or concentration from broth medium. MAC infection is most commonly diagnosed by culture of blood, bone marrow or other material in special liquid medium. By using the BACTEC system that detects growth of organisms by radiometrically measuring release of $^{14}CO_2$, positive cultures can be obtained in the range of 10 days to ≥3 weeks.

Antimicrobial susceptibility testing is not standardized for the nontuberculous mycobacteria and is usually performed only in research and reference laboratories. Until relatively recently the most commonly used method for testing susceptibility patterns for MAC isolates was the modified proportion method using solid agar medium and was based on methods, drug concentrations, and inoculum size described for *M. tuberculosis*. This method gives a qualitative result of sensitive or resistant according to the proportion of resistant bacteria in a given strain; resistance is usually defined as growth in the presence of the antimycobacterial agent greater than 1% of the growth of the control (7, 8). More recently, methods have been developed to determine the minimal inhibitory concentration, the concentration of drug required to inhibit 99% of the growth of a MAC isolate in broth medium. These methods may be based on a radiometric determination of a MAC isolate's growth index in a BACTEC system in the presence and absence of antimycobacterial drug or on a culturing organism in vials containing different concentrations of drug and then plating aliquots of medium for colony counts (9, 10). Unfortunately, interpreting results of any of these methods for MAC isolates has been hampered by a lack of clinical correlation of response to therapy and by wide variations in sensitivity patterns of MAC strains compared with *M. tuberculosis* strains. Data from non-HIV-infected adults with pulmonary MAC infection suggest that those individuals whose isolates were susceptible to several antimycobacterial agents responded more favorably to therapy than did patients whose isolates were resistant to many drugs (11).

Although there are some geographic differences, microbiologists noted that most MAC strains isolated from adult AIDS patients could be identified as either serotype 4 or serotype 8, whereas no predominant serotype has been identified in non-AIDS patients (12, 13). Using genetic probes, researchers have found that 97–98% of MAC isolates from AIDS patients were *M. avium*, in contrast to the 32–40% of MAC organisms isolated from non-AIDS patients that were *M. intracellulare* (13, 14). Investigators in England, using restriction fragment length polymorphism analysis, found that 79% of AIDS patients with disseminated MAC infection from Europe and the United States harbored a single strain of MAC organism (15). Virulence in MAC may be related to the presence of plasmids (16, 17). Although these data suggest the possibility of species or strain-specific virulence of these organisms among AIDS patients, there is at least some evidence that isolates from this patient population are not uniformly more virulent in a beige mouse model (18) (Table 16B.1). Further investigation is required to confirm and extend these observations.

Epidemiology

M. avium and *M. intracellulare* were recognized before the AIDS epidemic as uncommon causes of human illness in immunologically normal hosts and disseminated infection in some immunocompromised patients (19, 20). In nonimmunodeficient adult patients, lung disease has been the major manifestation of MAC infection and most of these patients have had underlying chronic lung disease. A recent report highlights the facts that not all patients with MAC infection have either deficient immunity or underlying lung disease and that the incidence of this infection in apparently

Table 16B.1. Microbiologic and Epidemiologic Features of MAC Infection

Characteristic	*M. avium* Complex
Gram smear	Weakly Gram-positive beaded rods or invisible
Acid-fast staining	Positive
Growth rate	Slow (>7 days to form colonies)
Colony characteristics	Usually smooth and transparent
Isolation from respiratory specimens	Variable, may represent colonization
Isolation from blood	Common; ~3–5% as AIDS-defining illness, 12–24% of patients with advanced HIV
Isolation from other sites	Common; lymph nodes, liver, spleen, bone marrow, gastrointestinal tract
High-risk groups	HIV-infected persons with low CD4 counts
Environmental sources	Soil, water, possibly aerosols above water
Transmission	Ingestion, inhalation probably less important, no documented person to person

normal adult hosts may be increasing (21, 22). The increase in numbers of pediatric AIDS cases has resulted in a dramatic increase in reports of disseminated MAC in this age group and heightened awareness of this pathogen in other immunocompromised children (23, 24).

Among patients with HIV infection, disseminated infection with MAC organisms was noted early in the AIDS epidemic (25, 26), and it remains among the most common opportunistic infections in United States patients with AIDS after *P. carinii* pneumonia. Approximately 6% of adult and 4% of pediatric AIDS patients reported to the Centers for Disease Control as of December 1992 had disseminated MAC infection as their AIDS-indicator disease (27). Autopsy series suggest that this infection is present in 20–50% of HIV-infected patients at the time of death (28–30); studies of clinic populations from across the country indicate that the infection probably occurs in 12–24% of adults with advanced HIV infection or AIDS (31–33). Investigators following a large cohort of HIV-infected adults in Dallas determined the incidence of disseminated MAC infection by prospectively monitoring blood cultures when patients developed CD4 counts of ≤200 cells/mm^3. Of 1006 patients in their cohort who had an AIDS-defining illness during the study period 191 developed MAC bacteremia, and for these individuals median survival after diagnosis of MAC was 134 days. After 12 months monitoring, 21% of the adults in this series had developed MAC bacteremia, and the incidence increased to 41% by 24 months (34). The geographic distribution of AIDS patients with disseminated MAC infection indicates that this infection occurs in all regions in the United States, so these data are probably widely applicable.

In contrast to tuberculosis, there do not appear to be particular high-risk subgroups for MAC infection among HIV-infected patients (32, 33) in terms of route of HIV acquisition or sex, a finding that is not surprising for these widely distributed environmental microorganisms. The incidence of MAC infection among HIV infected patients in less-developed countries, where tuberculosis is more of a problem, is unknown, but at least one reported series

failed to identify MAC bacteremia in a cohort of Ugandan AIDS patients (35). The incidence rate among AIDS patients in most European countries appears to be comparable with the United States rate, although one recent series from Italy documents nontuberculous mycobacterial disease in only 12.4% of 250 consecutive autopsies (36). It has been speculated that the apparently lower rate of MAC infection among Swedish AIDS patients may be a result of BCG vaccination early in life among most of these individuals (37).

Reviews of MAC infection in adult patients have identified low CD4 counts as the major risk factor for both pulmonary (38) and disseminated disease (39–41). In two prospective studies in adults CD4 counts of <100 cells/mm^3 and anemia were significantly associated with the development of MAC infection (33), and one of these studies also identified interruption of zidovudine as an independent risk factor (32). Although there are no similar prospective data available for children, the proportion of pediatric AIDS cases with disseminated MAC infection at the time of AIDS diagnosis appears to be comparable with or slightly greater than that found in adults (27, 42). Two retrospective reviews of MAC infection in large pediatric HIV clinic populations have also identified CD4 counts of <100 cells/mm^3 as the primary risk factor for this opportunistic infection (43, 44) In these studies 11–14% of HIV-infected children in clinic were found to have MAC infection; this proportion increased to 24% in the subset of children followed at the National Cancer Institute with <100 CD4 cells/mm^3 (44). As in the adult series, no difference in frequency of MAC infection was detected related to sex, race, or route of HIV transmission. In infants and young children, the possibility that MAC infections will occur at higher CD4 levels (because of age-specific differences in CD4 counts) must also be anticipated.

Pathogenesis, Clinical Presentation, and Natural History

Although a great deal remains to be learned about MAC infection in HIV-infected patients, many facts are known. As noted above, in the HIV-negative host, the most common manifestation of MAC infection is pulmonary disease; localized lymphadenitis is less common, and disseminated disease rarely occurs (3, 45). Many of these patients have other underlying disease processes: prior tuberculosis or other chronic lung disease has been associated with pulmonary MAC, and other causes of immune deficiency, especially corticosteroid use, have been identified in patients with disseminated infection. In HIV-infected patients, localized disease is relatively unusual and may represent the stage of infection before dissemination occurs in patients with higher CD4 counts. True pulmonary disease with MAC presenting as diffuse interstitial infiltrates or nodular, endobronchial, or even cavitary lesions has been reported but is uncommon in HIV-infected patients and, when present, is generally associated with nonpulmonary disease. MAC infections localized to the lungs, gastrointestinal tract, skin, and lymph nodes have all been described in AIDS patients, but long-term follow-up of these patients frequently reveals subsequent evidence of disseminated infection.

MAC organisms are common environmental organisms present in soil and water (and aerosols above water); MAC has been isolated from hospital water supplies and domesticated animal and patient household environments. Respiratory and gastrointestinal portals of entry have been proposed based on the environmental locations of these organisms and the histopathologic findings of infected patients. Humans are thought to be frequently colonized, although extensive data are lacking, and it is generally assumed that colonization precedes dissemination in AIDS patients. In one cohort of HIV-infected adults followed prospectively with mycobacterial cultures of blood, stool, and induced sputum, it was observed that patients who had MAC isolated from stool or sputum were much more likely to become bacteremic than those who did not have mycobacteria isolated from other body sites. However, of the patients who developed MAC bacteremia during the study period only 38% had a prior positive culture from one site (46). To date there is no evidence to support person to person

transmission of MAC. Factors leading to progression from colonization to disseminated infection are not defined, but in AIDS patients this progression is probably related to the degree of immunodeficiency, particularly diminished cell-mediated immunity.

Once an individual with AIDS is infected with MAC, persistent infection with continuous bacteremia and multiple organ involvement is the rule (47, 48). There have been reports of false-positive cultures related to laboratory contamination of specimens (49), although these events probably represent rarely encountered problems. Transient bacteremia was identified in 12% of adult patients enrolled in a MAC treatment protocol (50) and has been documented in two of 22 children who enrolled in antiretroviral protocols (44). Follow-up cultures documented subsequent bacteremia in all but one adult after 4–42 weeks of sterile cultures, but both children remain culture negative after more than 2 years.

In both adults and children disseminated MAC infection is characterized by fever, night sweats, malaise, and weight loss, often with anemia and neutropenia. The extent to which these nonspecific findings are directly attributable to MAC infection is difficult to ascertain. In patients with low CD4 counts and persistent fever without another apparent source, MAC infection can often be documented if looked for aggressively. Severe anemia, independent of leukopenia or thrombocytopenia, has been associated with presence of MAC bacteremia in large studies investigating the incidence and natural history of disseminated MAC (32, 33), and at least one series suggested that hematocrit of <25% was a poor prognostic indicator (51). Bone marrow involvement is common and may contribute to the anemia, leukopenia, and thrombocytopenia that are commonly observed in HIV-infected patients who have disseminated MAC infection.

In some individuals, disseminated MAC infection is characterized by gastrointestinal symptoms. Patients may have chronic diarrhea, abdominal pain, colitis, and malabsorption, often along with systemic symptoms (52–54); rarely, a patient may present with symptoms suggestive of an acute surgical abdominal process (55) or gastrointestinal bleeding (56). In the setting of chronic diarrhea and malabsorption, endoscopy and biopsy findings can be similar to those seen in Whipple's disease (57). Another reported gastrointestinal syndrome is that of extrahepatic biliary obstruction secondary to periportal lymphadenopathy. There is usually significant lymphadenopathy present elsewhere as well, and there is often associated hepatosplenomegaly. Although hepatosplenomegaly is common in patients with HIV and MAC infection, hepatic transaminases are infrequently increased, but elevations of alkaline phosphatase have been associated with disseminated MAC infection.

The symptoms associated with MAC infection in children appear to be similar to those found in adults. Most commonly these children exhibit fever, weight loss or failure to thrive, and gastrointestinal complaints ranging from anorexia to persistent, massive diarrhea (Table 16B.2) (43, 44). Unfortunately, many of these symptoms are also seen in HIV-infected children in whom MAC cannot be documented, and no single symptom or symptom complex can distinguish children with MAC bacteremia from those who have negative cultures for mycobacteria. In a small number of reported autopsy cases of children with MAC infection, prominent involvement of the abdominal lymph nodes was noted as well as involvement of the liver, spleen and intestinal tract (43, 58).

Organ tissue, particularly of the reticuloendothelial system, may provide a reservoir for mycobacteria and may contain 10^5–10^6 more organisms/g than blood samples (48). The organs most commonly infected include lymph nodes, spleen, and liver, with bone marrow, gastrointestinal tract, lungs, adrenals, kidneys, and other tissues less often affected. Histopathologic findings in AIDS patients may differ from those of immunocompetent individuals with MAC infection; there is often little inflammatory response to histiocytes filled with large numbers of organisms, and granulomata, when present, are poorly formed (28, 59, 60). Biopsy or autopsy specimens of patients who exhibit severe gastrointestinal symptoms may reveal aggregates of foamy macrophages containing clusters of acid-fast bacilli within the lamina propria of the intestine (52).

The contribution of MAC infection to mortality in AIDS patients was not clear in early studies, and some experts felt that this infection represented primarily a marker of profound immunodeficiency rather than a major contributor to morbidity or mortality in these patients (61, 62). There is now little disagreement that MAC is an important cause of morbidity in AIDS patients of all ages, and recent data confirm its contribution to shortened survival in patients with advanced HIV disease (32, 40–42). As noted previously, two series have identified severe anemia as an additional contributory event to poor survival in patients with MAC infection.

Table 16B.2.   Symptoms and Signs Present in Children with Documented MAC Infection

Symptoms and Signs Present	Hoyt et al. (43)		Lewis et al. (44)	
	N	%	N	%
Fever	16	80	19	86
Night sweats	5	25	7	32
Weight loss/failure to thrive	20	100	14	64
Abdominal pain	18	90	6	27
Diarrhea	12	60	2	9
Anemia	14	70	3	14
Anorexia	18	90	2	9
Neutropenia			12	55
Hepatosplenomegaly			10	45
Abnormal LFT[a] or jaundice			4	18
Joint pain	3	15		

[a]LFT, liver function tests.

Differential Diagnosis

The differential diagnosis of MAC infection depends on the clinical syndrome being investigated. The fever and other systemic symptoms associated with MAC can also be caused by various bacterial, viral, fungal, and parasitic organisms. In patients with diarrhea and/or malabsorption, bacterial stool pathogens (e.g., *Salmonella, Shigella*); *Cryptosporidium, Isospora* and other parasites; cytomegalovirus, rotavirus, and other gastrointestinal viruses; and nonspecific diarrhea must all be considered. Diffuse adenopathy may be caused by HIV infection itself, cytomegalovirus, Epstein-Barr virus, and tumor. Hematologic abnormalities that may be caused by MAC involvement of the bone marrow may also be the result of bone marrow involvement by other infectious and noninfectious processes (e.g., HIV, cytomegalovirus), as well as by increased consumption by autoimmune or other mechanisms. Pulmonary disease is much more likely to be caused by other processes, most commonly *P. carinii*, or other bacterial or viral etiologies. Because of the difficulty in treating MAC infections, other more treatable etiologies of any of these clinical syndromes should be sought. Symptoms suggestive of disseminated MAC may reflect relentless progression of HIV disease, and changes in antiretroviral therapy may be warranted if investigation fails to identify MAC or other secondary infections.

Diagnosis

Acid-fast staining and mycobacterial culture are the available means for diagnosing MAC infection. Culture is more sensitive than an acid-fast stain and is essential for identifying the mycobacterial species. Culture in mycobacterial isolation media is ideal; however, MAC organisms will grow in other fungal and bacterial media as well. Persistent bacteremia is common in disseminated MAC infection, and cell lysis blood culture techniques appear to increase the sensitivity blood cultures for MAC organisms (48). Although the optimal number and sites of cultures for recovery of MAC are still being evaluated there is some evi-

dence that obtaining two blood cultures for mycobacteria at different times is sufficient to detect almost all MAC bacteremic episodes (63). Isolation of MAC from nonsterile sites such as stool and respiratory secretions must be assessed together with symptoms since colonization may precede invasive infection by months. The finding of acid-fast bacilli in smears of unconcentrated stool may be more useful; this finding accurately predicted disseminated infection in one group of patients (52). Since symptoms attributed to MAC infection may involve many organs, histopathologic examinations of biopsy material should be directed toward those systems that seem to be affected in patients without detectable bacteremia. MAC, *M. tuberculosis*, and other mycobacteria are indistinquishable by smear or stained tissue specimens and the identity of any acid-fast bacillus must be confirmed by growth of the organism in culture and its speciation.

Treatment

Initial reports of treatment trials of MAC infection in patients with AIDS were extremely disappointing (52, 64). In vitro susceptibility testing, although not standardized, suggests that most MAC isolates are resistant to many antimycobacterial agents currently available. Correlation between in vitro susceptibility and clinical response has not been effectively documented, possibly because of large differences in drug levels required for killing as opposed to inhibition of these organisms (65). The agents to which in vitro sensitivity has been demonstrated for a significant proportion of isolates, and which have been used in vivo, include rifampin, rifabutin (ansamycin), amikacin, ethambutol, ethionamide, cycloserine, clofazamine, imipenem, several quinolone antibiotics (particularly ciprofloxacin and sparfloxacin), and two macrolide antibiotics (clarithromycin and azithromycin). Other antituberculosis agents including isoniazid and pyrazinamide are generally inactive in vitro.

Recently many combination regimens have been used to treat MAC infections, and results have been more encouraging. The first optimistic report described clearing of MAC bacteremia and improvement in symptoms in six of seven patients treated with a combination of rifabutin, clofazimine, ethambutol, and isoniazid (66). A larger Australian study evaluating this same drug combination documented microbiologic clearing of infection for at least 4 weeks in 22 of 25 patients and resolution of symptoms in 18 of these responders. Interestingly, microbiologic and clinical improvement did not correspond to susceptibility testing since most isolates initially recovered from patients on study were resistant to one or more of the drugs used (39). An initial trial by the California Collaborative Treatment Group employed the combination of amikacin, ethambutol, rifampin, and ciprofloxacin, and although five of the 17 patients enrolled in the trial were withdrawn from study before completing 12 weeks of therapy because of intolerance or hepatic toxicity a reduction in bacteremia and clinical improvement was observed, although this was not associated with improved survival (67). A second California Collaborative Treatment Group trial substituted clofazimine for amikacin and documented similar microbiologic and clinical effects. Although a significant number of patients were intolerant of the drug regimen, this study and another suggested a survival benefit from the treatment (40, 68).

Clarithromycin and azithromycin, two of the new generation of macrolide antibiotics with in vitro bactericidal activity against MAC, have been evaluated in clinical trials. Although minimal inhibitory concentrations of both these antibiotics against MAC are at or slightly above clinically achievable serum levels, these agents are concentrated in tissues and within macrophages. Clarithromycin has been evaluated as single agent therapy for adult AIDS patients with disseminated MAC in a small, randomized trial conducted in France; significant decreases in quantitative blood culture were achieved with a dose of 1000 mg twice daily, and improvements in fever and performance were documented (69). A larger, multicenter United States study evaluating three dose levels of clarithromycin confirmed reduction or clearing of bacteremia and improved quality of life at all doses, but an increased number of adverse events oc-

curred at the highest dose level. All MAC isolates were initially susceptible to clarithromycin, but over the 12-week study in vitro resistance developed in 22% (70). Side effects of clarithromycin reported in these trials were predominately gastrointestinal, and there was at least one case of mild hearing loss. An uncontrolled pilot study of arithromycin as single agent therapy for MAC bacteremia also showed reduction in bacteremia and clinical improvements in almost 75% of those patients treated for at least 20 days. Side effects in this study were relatively minor but again included gastrointestinal complaints. Although MAC strains isolated during this relatively short study remained susceptible to azithromycin, the investigators speculate that the longer duration of treatment necessary for successful treatment of disseminated MAC may lead to emergence of resistance to this agent (71).

Many agents evaluated for use in adults with MAC bacteremia have never been evaluated in children and are unavailable in formulations appropriate for young children. For some antimycobacterial agents such as amikacin and rifampin, pediatric experience with the drugs comes from other infectious processes; other agents such as ciprofloxacin and ethambutol have previously been considered contraindicated in children. Recently a pediatric trial of clarithromycin in HIV-infected children with MAC bacteremia was completed by the Pediatric Branch of the National Cancer Institute. Children on a stable antiretroviral regimen received clarithromycin at one of three doses over a 12-week study. Decreased fever, night sweats, and increased activity were observed at all dose levels; quantitative cultures showed consistent reductions after 6 and 12 weeks only at the highest dose of 30 mg/kg/day. The drug was well tolerated with only mild adverse reactions including one patient who experienced high-frequency hearing loss while on study. However, symptoms recrudesced in most patients during the study period, and increasing MICs were documented in MAC isolates from patients on study (72). Table 16B.3 includes suggested drug dosages for many antimicrobial agents used in the treatment of nontuberculous mycobacterial infections.

Table 16B.3.   Drugs Useful in Treatment of Nontuberculous Mycobacterial Infections

Drug	Formulations	Dosage	Maximum Dose
		mg/kg/day	*per day*
Amikacin	100, 500 mg; 1-g vials	15–30 divided q8–12 hr, IM or IV	1.5 g
Azithromycin	250-mg capsules	No pediatric dose established	500 mg
Cefoxitin	1- and 2-g vials	80–160 divided q 4–6 hr, IM or IV	12 g
Ciprofloxacin[a]	250-, 500-, 750-mg tablets 200- and 400-mg vials	20–30 divided q 12 hr, PO or IV	1.5 g
Clarithromycin	250- and 500-mg tablets 125 mg/5 ml suspension	30 divided q 12 hr, PO	2 g
Clofazamine	50- and 100-mg capsules	1–2 daily, PO	100 mg
Doxycycline	50- and 100-mg capsules 50 mg/5 ml syrup	2–4 divided q 12 hr, PO	200 mg
Erythromycin	Multiple tablet, capsule, and suspension formulations	40 divided q 6 hr, PO	2–4 g
Ethambutol	100- and 400-mg tablets	15–25 daily, PO	2.5 g
Ethionamide	250-mg tablets	10–20 divided q 8–12 hr, PO	1 g
Rifabutin[b]	150-mg tablets	300 mg total daily dose (not per kg), PO	
Rifampin	150- 300-mg capsules; syrup can be formulated from capsules, 600-mg vials	10–20 daily, PO or IV	600 mg
Streptomycin	1- and 5-g vials	20–40 daily, IM	1 g

[a]Not recommended for growing children.
[b]Currently recommended for prophylaxis in adults.

Concern about rapid emergence of resistance to the macrolides and other agents has led to the suggestion that this infection not be treated with a single agent. Most experts now recommend that treatment should be offered to all patients with MAC bacteremia should include at least two antimycobacterial agents, one of which should be a macrolide. Multiple drug regimens, however, may increase intolerance and toxicity. Specific criteria in terms of response and toxicity should be set, so patients in whom treatment is undertaken, but who do not respond, do not receive therapy from which they are not benefiting for prolonged periods. The need for new, more active agents is apparent. Earlier diagnosis, allowing earlier therapy at a time when the HIV-related immunodeficiency is not so profound, might result in more favorable response in some patients.

Prophylaxis

Two large, blinded, placebo-controlled trials of oral rifabutin at 300 mg/day have documented delay and prevention of MAC bacteremia in adults with CD4 counts of <200 cells/mm^3. These trials, conducted over 3 years, showed almost twice as many cases of MAC bacteremia developing in patients given placebo compared with those given rifabutin. Except for urine discoloration, there was no difference in the total proportion of patients in each group reporting adverse events; however, there was increased incidence of granulocytopenia and rashes in patients receiving rifabutin (73, 74).

In December 1992, a Task Force organized by the United States Public Health Service met to formulate recommendations for prophylaxis and treatment of MAC infection in AIDS patients. Although there was considerable debate among participants regarding treatment for documented MAC infection, the Task Force recommended that patients with CD4 counts of <100 cells/mm^3 receive rifabutin as prophylaxis for disseminated infection (75). Trials of other potentially useful prophylactic agents are in progress and may provide more options in the future. Studies evaluating the optimal dose and toxicity profile of rifabutin in children are underway.

Future Research

Among the highest priorities is the development of rapid diagnostic tests that are both sensitive and specific for the pathogenic mycobacterial species. Polymerase chain reaction techniques have been applied to both detection of MAC and other mycobacteria in clinical specimens and to more rapid, nonradiometric speciation of isolate (76–78). High-performance liquid chromatography has also been evaluated as a method of rapid identification of mycobacterial species and in experienced hands may be less expensive than identification using gene probes (79–81).

In vitro susceptibility testing also must be improved and standardized so that clinical correlation can be made. There is an urgent need for the development of new antimycobacterial agents active against MAC organisms and/or new methods of drug delivery that may enhance in vivo potency. Novel drug delivery systems such as liposome-encapsulated antimycobacterial agents have been applied to aminoglycosides and rifampin (82–84) in a beige mouse model and have been shown to decrease bacterial counts in blood, liver, and spleen at doses ineffective for free drug (85). Some guidelines for the evaluation of new antimycobacterial agents have been suggested by members of the Infectious Diseases Society of America and supported by the Food and Drug Administration (86). Promising new agents should be evaluated in children, particularly for pharmacokinetic profiles and optimal dosing, as soon as preliminary safety data are available from adult trials.

New approaches to treatment must also be undertaken. Biological response modifiers may have a significant role in the treatment of MAC infection, for example by stimulating mycobactericidal activity of phagocytic cells. The potential for this sort of approach has been demonstrated by the response of lepromatous leprosy, another mycobacterial disease with a high organism burden and depressed host immunity, to interferon-γ (87). Although it would seem logical that cytokines that activate macrophages might enhance killing of intracellular mycobacteria, in vitro studies using these agents in experimental MAC infection have been contradictory and inconclusive. Available clinical data consist only of case reports of a small number of adult

AIDS patients with MAC bacteremia who have been given interferon-γ as adjunctive therapy with variable results (88, 89). Various cytokines may have activity in decreasing or enhancing killing of MAC within phagocytic cells but may also affect production of other cytokines through the immune network.

OTHER NONTUBERCULOUS MYCOBACTERIA

Although the overwhelming proportion of nontuberculous mycobacterial infections occurring in HIV-infected patients are from MAC, many other species have caused infection in AIDS patients, most commonly, *M. kansasii* but also *M. xenopi*, *M. gordonae*, *M. chelonei*, *M. fortuitum*, and *M. bovis* (42, 90–93). These mycobacteria have generally caused infectious syndromes similar to those seen with MAC organisms, with widespread dissemination and systemic symptoms, although more limited local infections may also occur. Diagnostic considerations are generally the same as for MAC infection, but *M. kansasii* may be identifiable on smear by virtue of its rather distinctive size and staining properties. *M. kansasii* is not usually an environmental organism and should not be considered a colonizing organism when found in respiratory secretions, particularly in the setting of cavitary lung lesions; it remains an important cause of treatable pulmonary disease in AIDS patients (3, 94).

In some instances mycobacteria that could not be clearly speciated using routine laboratory methods have been identified in adult patients with AIDS and a syndrome of fever, diarrhea, and weight loss (95, 96). This organism has subsequently been identified as a new species of mycobacterium by a process of amplifying and sequencing species-specific ribosomal RNA genes and is tentatively named "*Mycobacterium genavense*" (97). This organism has also been identified in a small series of children (98) and may account for a significant number of cases of previously unidentifiable but clinically suspected mycobacterial infections.

Local infection by rapidly growing mycobacteria, *M. chelonei* and *M. fortuitim*, at central venous catheter exist sites, as has been described in pediatric cancer patients (99), has not yet been reported in AIDS patients. Bacteremia with these organisms associated with central venous catheters has also been reported in cancer patients (100) and HIV-infected patients (101). Given the prevalence of mycobacterial disease in these patients and the large number of HIV-infected children with central venous catheters, it seems likely that these complications may increase. Acid-fast staining and mycobacterial culture of specimens obtained from infected catheter exit sites should be considered when other pathogens have not been identified, and there is a poor response to conventional antibacterial therapy.

Some of these non-MAC, nontuberculous mycobacteria, including *M. kansasii, M. gordonnae, M. xenopi,* are sensitive to standard antituberculous agents, whereas others, *M. chelonei* and *M. fortuitum,* are not. The rapidly growing mycobacteria may, however, be susceptible to other available antimicrobial agents such as amikacin, cefoxitin, doxycycline, trimethoprim-sulfamethoxazole, imipenem, or the macrolides. Susceptibility testing and attempts at treatment are warranted in the case of infection by one of these organisms. As with MAC infection treatment should be with multiple drug regimens except in the case of superficial *M. marinum* infection, which can usually be successfully treated with a single agent.

SUMMARY

Nontuberculous mycobacterial infections have emerged as an important cause of morbidity in children with HIV infection. Recent advances in the understanding of the epidemiology, pathogenesis, and manifestations of disseminated MAC infection have led to increased awareness of this complication of late HIV-associated immunosuppression. Strategies for prophylaxis of the population at risk for MAC and improved options for therapy continue to evolve. Other mycobacteria are also emerging as important opportunistic pathogens in patients with HIV infection, and the clinician must remain alert to their potential impact in these severely immunocompromised children. New developments in diagnosis, rapid identification, susceptibility testing, and treatment are likely to provide significant benefit for children with mycobacterial infections in the future.

References

1. Margileth A. Management of nontuberculous (atypical) mycobacterial infections in children and adolescents. Pediatr Infect Dis J 1985;4:119–121.
2. Starke JR. Nontuberculous mycobacterial infections in children. In: Aronoff SC, Hughes WT, Kohl S, Speck WT, Wald ER, eds. Advances in pediatric infectious diseases. St. Louis: Mosby, 1992;7:123–159.
3. Wolinsky E. Mycobacterial diseases other than tuberculosis. Clin Infect Dis 1992;15:1–12.
4. Wayne LG, Good RC, Krichevsky MI, et al. Fourth report of the cooperative, open-ended study of slowly growing mycobacteria by the International Working Group on Mycobacterial Taxonomy. Int J System Bacteriol 1991:41:463–472.
5. Musial CE, Tice LS, Stockman L, Roberts GD. Identification of mycobacteria from culture by using the Gen-Probe rapid diagnostic system for *Mycobacterium avium* complex and *Mycobacterium tuberculosis* complex. J Clin Microbiol 1988;26:2120–2123.
6. Lim SD, Lopez J, Ford E, Janda JM. Genotypic identification of pathogenic *Mycobacterium* species by using a nonradioactive oligonucleotide probe. J Clin Microbiol 1991;29:1276–1278.
7. Heifets L. Qualitative and quantitative drug-susceptibility tests in mycobacteriology. Am Rev Respir Dis 1988;137:1217–1222.
8. Inderlied CB, Young LS, Yamada JK. Determination of *in vitro* susceptibility of *Mycobacterium avium* complex isolates to antimycobacterial agents by various methods. Antimicrob Agents Chemother 1987;31:1697–1702.
9. Heifets LB, Iseman MD, Lindholm-Levy PJ. Determination of MICs of conventional and experimental drugs in liquid medium by the radiometric method against *Mycobacterium avium* complex. Drugs Exp Clin Res 1987;13:529–538.
10. Heifets L. MIC as a quantitative measurement of the susceptibility of *Mycobacterium avium* strains to seven antituberculosis drugs. Antimicrob Agents Chemother 1988;32:1131–1136.
11. Horsburgh CR, Mason UG, Heifets LB, Southwick K, Labrecque J, Iseman MD. Response to therapy of pulmonary *Mycobacterium avium-intracellulare* infection correlates with results of *in vitro* susceptibility testing. Am Rev Respir Dis 1987;135:418–421.
12. Kiehn TE, Edwards FF, Brannon P, et al. Infections caused by *Mycobacterium avium* complex in immunocompromised patients: Diagnosis by blood culture and fecal examination, antimicrobial susceptibility tests, and morphological and seroagglutination characteristics. J Clin Microbiol 1985;21:168–173.

13. Yakrus MA, Good RC. Geographic distribution, frequency and specimen source of *Mycobacterium avium* complex serotypes isolated from patients with acquired immunodeficiency syndrome. J Clin Microbiol 1990;28:926–929.

14. Guthertz LS, Damsker B, Bottone EJ, et al. *Mycobacterium avium* and *Mycobacterium intracellulare* infections in patients with and without AIDS. J Infect Dis 1989;160:1037–1041.

15. Hampson SJ, Portaels F, Thompson J, et al. DNA probes demonstrate a single highly conserved strain of *Mycobacterium avium* infecting AIDS patients. Lancet 1989;1:65–68.

16. Crawford JT, Bates JH. Analysis of plasmids in *Mycobacterium avium-intracellulare* from persons with acquired immunodeficiency syndrome. Am Rev Respir Dis 1986;134:659–661.

17. Gangadharam PRJ, Perumal VK, Crawford JT, Bates JH. Association of plasmids and virulence of *Mycobacterium avium* complex. Am Rev Respir Dis 1988;137:212–214.

18. Gangadharam PRJ, Perumal VK, Jairam BT, Podapati NR, Taylor RB, LaBrecque JF. Virulence of *Mycobacterium avium* complex strains from acquired immune deficiency syndrome patients: Relationship with characteristics of the parasite and host. Microb Pathog 1989;7:263–278.

19. Wolinsky E. Nontuberculous mycobacteria and associated diseases. Am Rev Respir Dis 1979;119:107–159.

20. O'Brien RJ, Geiter LJ, Snider DE Jr. The epidemiology of nontuberculous mycobacterial diseases in the United States (results from a national survey). Am Rev Respir Dis 1987;135:1007–1014.

21. Prince DS, Peterson DD, Steiner RM, et al. Infection with *Mycobacterium avium* complex in patients without predisposing conditions. N Engl J Med 1989;321:863–868.

22. Iseman MD. *Mycobacterium avium* complex and the normal host. The other side of the coin. N Engl J Med 1989;321:896–897.

23. Ozkaynak MF, Lenarsky C, Kohn D, Weinberg K, Parkman R. *Mycobacterium avium-intracellulare* infections after allogeneic bone marrow transplantation in children. Am J Pediatr Hematol Oncol 1990;12:220–224.

24. Stone AB, Schelonka RL, Drehner DM, McMahon DP, Ascher DP. Disseminated *Mycobacterium avium* complex in non-human immunodeficiency virus-infected pediatric patients. Pediatr Infect Dis J 1992;11:960–964.

25. Greene JB, Sidhu GS, Lewin S. *Mycobacterium avium-intracellulare*: A cause of disseminated life-threatening infection in homosexuals and drug abusers. Ann Intern Med 1982;97:539–546.

26. Zakowski P, Fligiel S, Berlin GW, Johnson BL. Disseminated *Mycobacterium avium-intracellulare* infection in homosexual men dying of acquired immunodeficiency. JAMA 1982;248:2980–2982.

27. Centers for Disease Control and Prevention. HIV/AIDS Surveillance Rep 1993; Feb:1–23.

28. Reichert CM, O'Leary TJ, Levens DL, Simrell CR, Macher AM. Autopsy pathology in the acquired immune deficiency syndrome. Am J Pathol 1983;112:357–382.

29. Welch K, Finkbeiner W, Alpers CE, et al. Autopsy findings in the acquired immune deficiency syndrome. JAMA 1984;252:1152–1159.

30. Wilkes MS, Fortin AH, Felix JC, Godwin TA. Value of necropsy in acquired immunodeficiency syndrome. Lancet 1988;2:85–88.

31. Horsburgh CR Jr. *Mycobacterium avium* complex infection in the acquired immunodeficiency syndrome. N Engl J Med 1991;324:1332–1338.

32. Chaisson RE, Moore RD, Richman DD, Keruly J, Creagh T, Zidovudine Epidemiology Study Group. Incidence and natural history of *Mycobacterium avium*-complex infections in patients with advanced human immunodeficiency virus disease treated with zidovudine. Am Rev Respir Dis 1992;146:285–289.

33. Havlik JA Jr., Horsburgh CR, Metchock B, Williams PP, Fann SA, Thompson SE III. Disseminated *Mycobacterium avium* complex infection: Clinical identification of epidemiologic trends. J Infect Dis 1992;165:577–580.

34. Nightingale SD, Byrd LT, Southern PM, Jockusch JD, Cal SX, Wynne BA. Incidence of *Mycobacterium avium-intracellulare* complex bacteremia in human immunodeficiency virus-positive patients. J Infect Dis 1992;165:1082–1085.

35. Okello DO, Sewankambo N, Goodgame R, et al. Absence of bacteremia with *Mycobacterium avium-intracellulare* in Ugandan patients with AIDS. J Infect Dis 1990;162:208–210.

36. d'Arminio Monforte A, Vago L, Lazzarin A, et al. AIDS-defining diseases in 250 HIV-infected patients: A comparative study of clinical and autopsy diagnoses. AIDS 1992;6:1159–1164.

37. Kallenius G, Hoffner SE, Svenson SB. Does vaccination with Bacille Calmette-Guerin protect against AIDS? Rev Infect Dis 1989;11:349–350.

38. Masur H, Ognibene FP, Yarchoan R, et al. CD 4 counts as predictors of opportunistic pneumonias in human immunodeficiency virus (HIV) infection. Ann Intern Med 1989;111:223–231.

39. Hoy J, Mijch A, Sandland M, Grayson L, Lucas R, Dwyer B. Quadruple-drug therapy for *Mycobacterium avium-intracellulare* bacteremia in AIDS patients. J Infect Dis 1990;161:801–805.

40. Horsburgh CR, Havlik JA, Ellis DA, et al. Survival of patients with acquired immune deficiency syndrome and disseminated *Mycobacterium avium* complex infection with and without antimycobacterial chemotherapy. Am Rev Respir Dis 1991;144:557–559.

41. Jacobson MA, Hopewell PC, Yajko DM, et al. Natural history of disseminated *Mycobacterium avium* complex infection in AIDS. J Infect Dis 1991;164:994–998.

42. Horsburgh CR, Selik RM. The epidemiology of disseminated nontuberculous mycobacterial infection in the acquired immunodeficiency syndrome (AIDS). Am Rev Respir Dis 1989;139:4–7.

43. Hoyt L, Oleske J, Holland B, Connor E. Nontuberculous mycobacteria in children with acquired immunodeficiency syndrome. Pediatr Infect Dis J 1992;11:354–360.

44. Lewis LL, Butler KM, Husson RN, et al. Defining the population of human immunodeficiency

virus-infected children at risk for *Mycobacterium avium-intracellulare* infection. J Pediatr 1992; 121:677–683.

45. Horsburgh C, Mason UI, Farhi D, Iseman M. Disseminated infection with *Mycobacterium avium-intracellulare:* A report of 13 cases and a review of the literature. Medicine 1985; 64:36–48.

46. Chin DP, Hopewell PC, Yajko DM, Hadley WK, Horsburgh CR, Reingold AL. *Mycobacterium avium* complex (MAC) in the respiratory or gastrointestinal tract precedes MAC bacteremia [Abstract 6]. Eighth International Conference on AIDS, Amsterdam, Jul 1992.

47. Macher AM, Kovacs JA, Gill V, et al. Bacteremia due to *Mycobacterium avium-intracellulare* in the acquired immunodeficiency syndrome. Ann Intern Med 1983;99:782–785.

48. Wong B, Edwards FF, Kiehn TE, et al. Continuous high-grade *Mycobacterium avium-intracellulare* bacteremia in patients with the acquired immune deficiency syndrome. Am J Med 1985;78:35–40.

49. Graham L Jr, Warren NG, Tsang AY, Dalton HP. *Mycobacterium avium* complex pseudobacteriuria from a hospital water supply. J Clin Microbiol 1988;26:1034–1036.

50. Kemper CA, Havlir D, Bartok AE, et al. Transient *Mycobacterium avium* bacteremia in patients with AIDS [Abstract 14]. Frontiers in mycobacteriology: *M. avium,* the modern epidemic, Vail, CO, Oct 1992.

51. Sathe SS, Gascone P, Lo W, Pinto R, Reichman LB. Severe anemia is an important negative predictor for survival with disseminated *Mycobacterium avium-intacellulare* in acquired immunodeficiency syndrome. Am Rev Respir Dis 1990;142:1306–1312.

52. Hawkins CC, Gold JWM, Whimbey E, et al. *Mycobacterium avium* complex infections in patients with the acquired immunodeficiency syndrome. Ann Intern Med 1986;105:184–188.

53. Jacobson MA, Mycobacterial diseases. Tuberculosis and *Mycobacterium avium* complex. Infect Dis Clin North Am 1988;2:465–474.

54. Wolke A, Meyers S, Adelsberg BR, et al. *Mycobacterium avium-intracellulare*-associated colitis in a patient with the acquired immunodeficiency syndrome. J Clin Gastroenterol 1984; 6:225–229.

55. Patrick C, Hawkins E, Guerra I, Taber L. A patient with leukemia in remission and acute abdominal pain. J Pediatr 1987;111:624–629.

56. Cappell MS, Gupta A. Gastrointestinal hemorrhage due to gastrointestinal *Mycobacterium avium-intracellulare* or esophageal candidiasis in patients with the acquired immunodeficiency syndrome. Am J Gastroenterol 1992;87:224–229.

57. Gillin JS, Urmacher C, West R, Shike M. Disseminated *Mycobacterium avium-intracellulare* infection in acquired immunodeficiency syndrome mimicking Whipple's disease. Gastroenterology 1983;85:1187–1191.

58. Joshi V, Oleske J, Saad S, Connor E, Rapkin R, Minnefor A. Pathology of opportunistic infections in children with acquired immune deficiency syndrome. Pediatr Pathol 1986;6:145–150.

59. Amberson JB, DiCarlo EF, Metroka CE, Koizumi JH, Mouradian JA. Diagnostic pathology in the acquired immunodeficiency syndrome. Arch Pathol Lab Med 1985;109:345–351.

60. Klatt EC, Jensen DF, Meyer PR. Pathology of *Mycobacterium avium-intracellulare* infection in acquired immunodeficiency syndrome. Hum Pathol 1987;18:709–714.

61. Young LS. *Mycobacterium avium* complex infection. J Infect Dis 1988;157:863–867.

62. Chaisson RE, Hopewell PC. Mycobacteria and AIDS mortality. Am Rev Respir Dis 1989;139: 1–3.

63. Yagupsky P, Menegus MA. Cumulative positivity rates of multiple blood cultures for *Mycobacterium avium-intracellulare* and *Cryptococcus neoformans* in patients with the acquired immunodeficiency syndrome. Arch Pathol Lab Med 1990;114:923–925.

64. Masur H, Tuazon C, Gill V, et al. Effect of combined clofazimine and ansamycin therapy on *Mycobacterium avium-intracellulare* bacteremia in patients with AIDS. J Infect Dis 1987; 155:127–129.

65. Yajko D, Nassos PS, Hadley WK. Therapeutic implications of inhibition versus killing of *Mycobacterium avium* complex by antimicrobial agents. Antimicrob Agents Chemother 1987;31: 117–120.

66. Agins BD, Berman DS, Spicehandler D, El-Sadr W, Simberkoff MS, Rahal JJ. Effect of combined therapy with ansamycinn, clofazimine, ethambutol and isoniazid for *Mycobacterium avium* infection in patients with AIDS. J Infect Dis 1989; 159:784–786.

67. Chiu J, Nussbaum J, Bozzette S, et al. Treatment of disseminated *Mycobacterium avium* complex infection in AIDS with amikacin, ethambutol, rifampin and ciprofloxacin. Ann Intern Med 1990;113:358–361.

68. Kemper C, Meng T, Nussbaum J, et al. Treatment of *Mycobacterium avium* complex bacteremia in AIDS with a four-drug oral regimen: Rifampin, ethambutol, clofazimine and ciprofloxacin. Ann Intern Med 1992;116:466–472.

69. Dautzenberg B, Truffot C, Legris S, et al. Activity of clarithromycin against *Mycobacterium avium* infection in patients with the acquired immune deficiency syndrome: A controlled clinical trial. Am Rev Respir Dis 1991;144:564–569.

70. Chaisson RE, Benson C, Dube M, et al. Clarithromycin therapy for disseminated *Mycobacterium avium*-complex (MAC) in AIDS [Abstract 891]. 32nd Interscience Conference on Antimicrobial Agents and Chemotherapy, Anaheim, 1992.

71. Young LS, Wiviott L, Wu M, Kolonoski P, Bolan R, Inderlied CB. Azithromycin for treatment of *Mycobacterium avium-intracellulare* complex infection in patients with AIDS. Lancet 1991;338: 1107–1109.

72. Husson R, Ross L, Sandelli S, et al. A phase I study of clarithromycin for the treatment of systemic *Mycobacterium avium* complex (MAC) infection in children with AIDS. Eighth International Conference on AIDS, Amsterdam, Jul 1992.

73. Cameron W, Sparti P, Pietroski N, et al. Rifabutin prevents *M. avium* complex (MAC) bacteremia in patients with AIDS and CD4 ≤200 [Abstract 888]. 32nd Interscience Conference on Antimicrobial Agents and Chemotherapy, Anaheim, 1992.

74. Gordin F, Nightingale S, Wynne B, et al. Rifabutin monotherapy prevents or delays *Mycobacterium avium* complex (MAC) bacteremia in patients with AIDS [Abstract 889]. 32nd Interscience Conference on Antimicrobial Agents and Chemotherapy, Anaheim, 1992.

75. US Public Health Service Task Force on Prophylaxis and Therapy for *Mycobacterium avium* Complex. Recommendations for prophylaxis and therapy for *Mycobacterium avium* complex for adults and adolescents infected with human immunodeficiency virus. MMWR, in press.

76. Young KKY, Robinson E, Dare A, Fiss EH. Detection of Mycobacteria by PCR and species identification by reverse dot blot hybridization [Abstract U-60]. General Meeting of American Society for Microbiology, New Orleans, 1992.

77. Fiss E, York MK, Brooks GF. Detection of *Mycobacterium kansasii* from a brain lesion and *Mycobacterium avium* from blood of an AIDS patient using PCR and reverse dot blot hybridization [Abstract U-62]. General Meeting of American Society for Microbiology, New Orleans, 1992.

78. Telenti A, Gerber C, Marchesi M, Bodmer T. Rapid typing of mycobacteria by the polymerase chain reaction [Abstract U-58]. General Meeting of American Society for Microbiology, New Orleans, 1992.

79. Thibert L, Lapierre S. Field evaluation of reverse phase high performance liquid chromatography (HPLC) for mycobacteria identification [Abstract U-8]. General Meeting of American Society for Microbiology, New Orleans, 1992.

80. Jost KC, Dunbar D. Automated identification of mycobacteria by high performance liquid chromatography using computer-aided pattern recognition algorithms [Abstract U-69]. General Meeting of American Society for Microbiology, New Orleans, 1992.

81. Guthertz LS, Lim SD, Jang Y, Duffey PS. The utility of high performance liquid chromatography for the identification of mycobacteria in extent 4 laboratories [Abstract U-70]. General Meeting of American Society for Microbiology, New Orleans, 1992.

82. Bermudez LEM, Wu M, Young LS. Intracellular killing of *Mycobacterium avium* complex by rifapentine and liposome-encapsulated amikacin. J Infect Dis 1987;156:510–513.

83. Klemens SP, Cynamon MH, Swenson CE, Ginsberg RS. Liposome-encapsulated-gentamicin therapy of *Mycobacterium avium* complex infection in beige mice. Antimicrob Agents Chemother 1990;34:967–970.

84. Saito H, Tomioka H. Therapeutic efficacy of liposome-entrapped rifampin against *Mycobacterium avium* complex infection induced in mice. Antimicrob Agents Chemother 1989;33:429–433.

85. Bermudez LE, Yau-Young AO, Lin J-P, Cogger J, Young LS. Treatment of disseminated *Mycobacterium avium* complex infection of beige mice with liposome-encapsulated aminoglycosides. J Infect Dis 1990;161:1262–1268.

86. Hopewell P, Cynamon M, Starke J, Iseman M, O'Brien R. Evaluation of new anti-infective drugs for the treatment and prevention of infections caused by the *Mycobacterium avium* complex. Clin Infect Dis 1992;15(suppl 1):S296–S306.

87. Nathan CF, Kaplan G, Levis WR, et al. Local and systemic effects of intradermal recombinant interferon-gamma in patients with lepromatous leprosy. N Engl J Med 1986;315:6–15.

88. Squires KE, Murphy WF, Madoff LC, Murray HW. Interferon-γ and *Mycobacterium avium-intracellulare* infection. J Infect Dis 1989;159:599–600.

89. Squires K, Rowland V, Fassyuk E, et al. Interferon-γ (IFN-γ) for *Mycobacterium avium-intracellulare* (MAI) bacillemia in AIDS [Abstract]. Clin Res 1990;38:561A.

90. Sherer R, Sable R, Sonnenberg M, et al. Disseminated infection with *Mycobacterium kansasii* in the acquired immunodeficiency syndrome. Ann Intern Med 1986;105:710–712.

91. Chan J, McKitrick JC, Klein RS. *Mycobacterium gordonae* in the acquired immunodeficiency syndrome. Ann Intern Med 1984;101:400.

92. Eng RH, Forrester C, Smith SM, Sobel H. *Mycobacterium xenopi* infection in a patient with acquired immunodeficiency syndrome. Chest 1984;86:145–147.

93. Houde C, Dery P. *Mycobacterium bovis* sepsis in an infant with human immunodeficiency virus infection. Pediatr Infect Dis J 1988;7:810–812.

94. Levine B, Chaisson RE. *Mycobacterium kansasii*: A cause of treatable pulmonary disease associated with advanced human immunodeficiency virus (HIV) infection. Ann Intern Med 1991;114:861–868.

95. Hirschel B, Chang HR, Mach N, et al. Fatal infection with a novel, unidentified mycobacterium in a man with the acquired immunodeficiency syndrome. N Engl J Med 1990;323:109–113.

96. Wald A, Coyle MB, Carlson LC, Thompson RL, Hooton TM. Infection with a fastidious mycobacterium resembling *Mycobacterium simiae* in seven patients with AIDS. Ann Intern Med 1992;117:586–589.

97. Bottger EC, Teske A, Kirschner P, et al. Disseminated "*Mycobacterium genavense*" infection in patients with AIDS. Lancet 1992;340:76–80.

98. Nadal D, Caduff R, Kraft R, et al. Invasive infection with *Mycobacterium genavense* in three children with the acquired immunodeficiency syndrome. Eur J Clin Microbiol Infect Dis 1993;12:37–43.

99. Flynn PM, Van Hooser B, Gigliotti F. Atypical mycobacterial infections of Hickman catheter exit sites. Pediatr Infect Dis J 1988;7:510–513.

100. Hoy JF, Rolston KVI, Hopfer RL, Bodey GP. *Mycobacterium fortuitum* bacteremia in patients with cancer and long-term venous catheters. Am J Med 1987;83:213–217.

101. Brady MT, Marcon MJ, Maddux H. Broviac catheter-related infection due to *Mycobacterium fortiutum* in a patient with acquired immunodeficiency syndrome. Pediatr Infect Dis J 1987;6:492–494.

17
Fungal Infections Complicating Pediatric HIV Infection

Thomas J. Walsh

Fungal infections have become important causes of morbidity and mortality in immunocompromised children, including those with AIDS. Although significant therapeutic advances are being made in the field of antiretroviral therapy (1–4), parallel advances must be attained in the secondary infectious complications, including those caused by fungi. Medical knowledge must advance in understanding the fungal infections in children in order that potential therapeutic interventions might be optimized and associated morbidity curtailed. The purpose of this chapter is to review the current understanding of fungal infections in human immunodeficiency virus (HIV)-infected children, to compare the patterns of mycoses encountered with those of adults with AIDS, and to address the potential problems of these infections in this rapidly expanding population.

GENERAL CONCEPTS OF EPIDEMIOLOGY OF MYCOSES IN HIV-INFECTED CHILDREN

Several similarities and differences in fungal complications between children and adults with AIDS were described by Selik et al. (5) in a review of the first 30,632 AIDS patients from the United States reported to the Centers for Disease Control. Esophageal candidiasis occurred in 15.4% of 350 children (age <13 years) with AIDS and 10.6% of all adult AIDS patients. By comparison, extrapulmonary cryptococcosis oc-

curred in only 0.6% of children in comparison with 6.8% of the total population and in 5.2–11.5% of subpopulations of adult AIDS patients. The basis for these differences in susceptibility has not been well studied but is most likely related to the lack of exposure of most HIV-infected children to these fungal pathogens.

Disseminated histoplasmosis has become increasingly recognized in the adult population with AIDS, especially in those patients from endemic regions of the United States (6–8). Studies of histoplasmosis in HIV-infected adults from Indiana suggest that progression from primary acquisition, rather than reactivation, is the principal mechanism of infection in this population. Histoplasmosis has rarely been reported in HIV-infected children. Those who reside in endemic areas are also at risk. *Coccidioides immitis* is another endemic fungal pathogen of emerging importance in patients with AIDS in the southwestern United States (9–11). Virtually all cases of coccidioidomycosis reported thus far in AIDS have been observed in adults; most cases were disseminated infection or progressive pneumonia. Because coccidioidomycosis is well described in non-HIV-infected children (12, 13), there is a high probability that it will develop in children with AIDS who reside in regions endemic for *C. immitis*. The frequency of coccidioidomycosis in AIDS patients in Arizona approximates the rate of seropositivity in the general population, suggesting that HIV-infected patients with latent coccidioidomycosis have a high frequency of reactivation. Primary infection has also been observed in HIV-positive patients developing coccidioidomycosis after moving to Arizona from a nonendemic location. Given that HIV-infected children will likely not have encountered *C. immitis* previously, progressive primary infection may be more likely to develop than reactivation.

ESSENTIAL CLINICAL MICROBIOLOGICAL CHARACTERISTICS

Understanding the essential clinical microbiological features of the diverse group of fungi encountered in HIV-infected patients facilitates understanding the pathogenesis, diagnosis, and treatment of these mycoses (14, 15). These features are summarized in Table 17.1.

PATHOGENESIS OF MYCOSES IN HIV-INFECTED PATIENTS

Candida

Profound depletion of cell-mediated immunity is the central immunological deficit leading to increased risk of mucosal candidiasis, cryptococcosis, histoplasmosis, and coccidioidomycosis. The possible immunopathogenesis of several key mycoses is outlined in Figure 17.1. A recent study (16) found that impairment of helper T cell functions in HIV-infected children correlated with an increased risk of opportunistic infections, including persistent oropharyngeal and esophageal candidiasis. Although mucocutaneous candidiasis with marked oropharyngeal and esophageal involvement is common in HIV-infected children, disseminated candidiasis is unusual in the natural history of HIV infection, unless the there is a concomitant risk for nosocomial disseminated candidiasis (17).

Little is known about the mechanisms of defective systemic cell-mediated immunity that lead to defective mucosal immunity. Studies of experimental mucosal candidiasis reveal that parenterally administered corticosteroid therapy, which markedly impairs cellular immunity and T lymphocyte immunoregulation, leads to a marked increase in esophageal and gastrointestinal candidiasis in comparison with saline-treated controls (18). In further examining the mechanisms of impaired systemic cell-mediated immunity on mucosal immunity, a recent study (19) found that rabbits treated with parenteral corticosteroid had profound depletion of gut-associated lymphoid tissue. Lymphoid domes and follicles were considerably reduced in size, and the dome epithelial layer was markedly depleted of M cells and lymphocytes. There were numerous open lesions at the luminal surface of dome epithelium, consistent with necrosis of M cells, as well as depletion of follicular B cell and T cell regions. The involution of gut-associated lymphoid tissue in the these corticosteroid-treated animals was similar to that observed in patients with advanced HIV infection. Mucosal candidiasis, particularly oral and esophageal candidiasis, often develops in children receiving systemic or inhalational corticosteroids.

The immunopathogenesis of mucosal candidiasis is not understood, especially regarding the mechanism by which a defect in systemic cellular immunity may lead to a defective mucosal immunity. Nevertheless, some insight may be gained by considering chronic mucocutaneous candidiasis (CMC) of children, since this syndrome bears similarities to HIV-associated mucosal candidiasis. Oropharyngeal and esophageal candidiasis in patients with CMC are recurrent and severe (20). This heterogeneous condition is characterized by exuberant proliferation of *Candida* spp along the mucocutaneous surfaces of the mouth, perineum, hands, and nails. A key immunological deficit in CMC is the inability of T lymphocytes to recognize, process, or respond to *Candida* antigens. Whether similar impairments of cellular immunity are present in HIV-infected children remains to be determined.

The syndrome of severe combined immunodeficiency (SCID) is a particularly applicable relevant model of HIV infection. As a group of immune disorders, SCID consists of a global T and B cell deficiency and a complete absence of all adaptive response, leading to life-threatening infections (21). Unless immunological reconstitution is achieved, death from infection is inevitable. Similar to children with HIV infection, those with SCID suffer persistent infections

Table 17.1.   Essential Microbiological Characteristics of Fungi Infecting HIV-infected Patients

Organism	Morphological Features	Biochemical, Immunological, or Molecular Diagnostic Characteristics	Comments
Candida sp	Budding yeasts (blastoconidia) with pseudohyphae and hyphae; *C. albicans* identified by germ-tube production; morphology on cornmeal agar with Tween-80 identifies different *Candida* spp	Assimilation and fermentation patterns are utilized to distinguish *Candida* spp that not are *albicans*	Different species of *Candida* have different virulence potentials and susceptibility to antifungal agents
T. glabrata	Small budding yeast that does not produce germ tubes, pseudohyphae, or hyphae	Assimilation and fermentation patterns	Must be distinguished from other yeast-like fungi
C. neoformans	Encapsulated yeast	Urease activity and phenol oxidase activity distinguish *C. neoformans;* assimilation pattern identifies nonneoformans spp of *Cryptococcus*	Presumptive diagnosis can be made on direct examination of India ink preparation of CSF
H. capsulatum	Dimorphic fungus: yeast-form at 37°C (including tissue) and filamentous form at 20–30°C[a]	RNA hybridization studies or exoantigen identification of isolated organism by immunodiffusion	*H. capsulatum* grows slowly (4–6 weeks) in conventional media but may be recovered within 1–3 weeks from lysis centrifugation or mycobacterial radiometric blood culture systems
C. immitis	Dimorphic fungus: spherule in tissue (37°C) and filamentous form (arthroconidia and hyphae) at 20–30°C in culture[a]	RNA hybridization studies or exoantigen identification of isolated organism by immunodiffusion	Caution for clinical laboratory workers in handling organisms
S. schenckii	Dimorphic fungus growing within 3–5 days at 25°C as a hyaline mould and can be converted to a cigar-shaped yeast at 37°C[a]	Not routinely used	Biopsy of infected tissue is often negative; culture is preferred means of microbiological diagnosis
Aspergillus spp	Angular branching hyphae in tissue and characteristic vesicle, phialides, and conidia	Not routinely used	Conidia, vesicles, and phialides are not produced in tissue
M. furfur	Identified by skin scrapings as a characteristic cluster of blastoconidia and hyphae; flask-shaped blastoconidia are found in culture	Supplementation of the agar plate with olive oil or other C_{12}–C_{24} oil is necessary to promote growth of this lipophilic yeast	Distinguish from other yeast-like fungi if recovered from blood

[a]Living filamentous forms of these dimorphic fungi (*H. capsulatum, C. immitis,* and *S. schenckii*) are highly infectious and are examined only within a biosafety cabinet

from *C. albicans, Pneumocystis carinii,* varicella, cytomegalovirus, and other opportunistic pathogens. Profound lymphpenia, absent lymphocyte-proliferative responses, and delayed cutaneous anergy all indicate severe impairment of infants with SCID.

The pathogenesis of esophageal candidiasis in HIV infection is not well understood but likely includes one or more factors of depressed mucosal immunity, decreased gastric acidity, gastroesophageal reflux, concomitant virus esophagitis, foreign bodies (e.g., nasogastric tubes), and possibly altered epithelial attachment sites. Unlike granulocytopenic cancer patients with esophageal candidiasis, patients with HIV infection usually do not develop disseminated candidiasis arising from the gastroin-

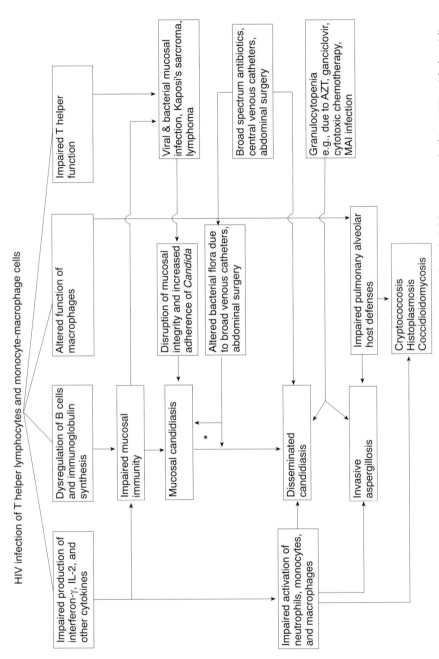

Figure 17.1. Model of possible immunopathogenesis of mycoses in HIV-infected children. *IL*, interleukin; *AZT*, azidothymidine.

testinal tract unless there is a concurrent problem of granulocytopenia, broad spectrum antibiotics, or severe mucosal disruption.

The mediators of surface mucosal immunity against *Candida* potentially may include IgA, interleukin-2, interferon-γ, other cytokines, and salivary and cell-surface glycoproteins, all of which may be depleted or altered in patients with HIV infection (21–24). The specific role of these and other putative factors in mucosal host defense require further study in experimental and clinical investigations.

Once colonization and superficial infection by *Candida* is established, deeper penetration into submucosal tissue may be facilitated by concomitant mucosal infections caused by herpes simplex virus (HSV) and other mucosal pathogens (25–27). The polymorphonuclear leukocyte (PMNL) is critical in host defense against tissue invasion by *Candida* blastoconidia, pseudohyphae, and hyphae (28). Although the absolute neutropenia would clearly increase the risk of deep mucosal and disseminated candidiasis in HIV-infected patients, subtle functional deficits in PMNLs from HIV-infected patients may also lead to significant deep mucosal infection.

Disseminated candidiasis is uncommon in the natural history of HIV-infected children, unless there are major quantitative or qualitative defects in circulating neutrophils or factors that are known to predispose to disseminated candidiasis, such as chronic indwelling venous catheters, broad spectrum antibiotics, or abdominal surgery. By contrast, granulocytopenic children with cancer have a comparatively higher risk of disseminated candidiasis. Although other factors, such as mucositis, vascular catheters, and broad spectrum antibiotics, may also predispose to disseminated candidiasis in these patients, the quantitative deficit of neutrophils is clearly an important risk factor in cancer patients.

Cryptococcus neoformans and Dimorphic Fungi

Human systemic mycoses caused by *C. neoformans* or the dimorphic fungi, *Histoplasma capsulatum* and *C. immitis*, are initiated in most cases when aerosolized conidia are inhaled to reach the lower respiratory tract, including the alveolar air spaces. Upon entry into the lower respiratory tract conidia are initially contained by alveolar macrophages, which are modulated by T lymphocytes.

More than 95% of cases of histoplasmosis and coccidioidomycosis are estimated to be self-limiting and produce minimal symptoms. In most cases, the only evidence of infection is the development of an immune response, which is manifested by conversion to a positive delayed-tape skin reaction and the production of specific precipitins and complement-fixing antibodies. Similarly exposure to *C. neoformans* is common, although, development of clinically overt infection is unusual. The small percentage of episodes that advance to progressive pulmonary infection or clinically overt disseminated infection is often associated with substantial deficits in cell-mediated immunity.

Numerous studies have demonstrated the critical role of cell-mediated immunity lymphocytes in host defense against disseminated cryptococcosis, histoplasmosis, and coccidioidomycosis, all of which are significantly increased in patients with HIV infection (28–30). Central to host defense against these infections are T lymphocytes, particularly T helper cells. Monocytes, activated macrophages, and natural killer cells also have been identified as being involved in conferring protection against these mycoses. That patients with HIV infection and T helper cell depletion suffer a predilection to cryptococcosis, histoplasmosis, and coccidioidomycosis is predictable.

Aspergillus

The increased of development of opportunistic mycoses caused by filamentous fungi, particularly *Aspergillus* spp, has been less predictable. Host defense against aspergillosis normally depends upon pulmonary alveolar macrophages that prevent germination of *Aspergillus* conidia and PMNLs that directly damage hyphal elements. Invasive pulmonary aspergillosis complicating HIV infection has been reported from various centers (31–34). Yet approximately half of these HIV-infected patients with invasive aspergillosis did not have the conventionally recognized risk factors of neutropenia or corticosteroid therapy, which are observed in patients receiving antineoplastic therapy (35). Indeed, considerable controversy has been generated by the possible pathogenesis of aspergillosis (36) in HIV infection, leading one investigator to propose that a new paradigm for understanding the pathogenesis of aspergillosis was necessary (37). A more recent study (38) demonstrated that PMNLs from HIV-infected children were less able to damage nonopsonized hyphae of *A. fumigatus* when the patients' age-adjusted CD4 count was <25% of normal median for age. Patients with CD4 counts ≥25% of normal for age had normal antifungal activity compared with healthy seronegative controls. This PMNL functional defect was dependent on serum from HIV-infected patients and was partially corrected by pretreatment with granulocyte-colony stimulating factor. The serum dependent effects of impaired PMNL activity were not replicated by preincubation of PMNLs with gp120, gp41, and p24 anti-

gens in normal serum. This deficit may reflect the lack of activation of PMNLs by HIV serum and/or the presence of a circulating inhibitory factor. Circulating peripheral blood mononuclear cells from HIV-infected patients do not appear to possess this functional deficit (39). Conversely, peripheral blood mononuclear cell-derived macrophages appear to possess a functional deficit in inhibition of germination of *Aspergillus* conidia. Thus functional deficits in PMNLs and possibly macrophages against *Aspergillus* may explain in part the emergence of invasive aspergillosis in HIV-infected patients without granulocytopenia or corticosteroid therapy. Patterns of fungal infections in children with selected immunological deficits are summarized in Table 17.2.

CLINICAL MANIFESTATIONS

Candidiasis

Oral Candidiasis

Oropharyngeal candidiasis occurs with such frequency among immunocompetent

Table 17.2.   Patterns of Fungal Infections in Children with Selected Immunological Deficits

Immunological Disorder	Fungal Infections	Proposed Mechanism(s)
Phagocytic cells[a]		
Chronic granulomatous disease	Invasive aspergillosis[b]	Defective intracellular killing; decreased peroxide and superoxide
Myeloperoxidase deficiency	Candidiasis	Defective intracellular killing
Granulocytopenia (chemotherapy-induced)	Invasive aspergillosis, candidiasis, and other opportunist fungi, e.g., zygomycosis, trichosporonosis, fusariosis, and pseudallescheriasis	Quantitative deficit in phagocytic cells
B lymphocyte defects	Usually none, unless associated with a concomitant disorder of T lymphocytes[c] or phagocytic cells	Role of Ig in host defense against fungi possibly important but not well understood
T lymphocyte defects		
SCID	Candidiasis	Severe impairment of T cell and B cell response to *Candida*
DiGeorge's syndrome	Cryptococcosis; histoplasmosis; candidiasis	Thymic hypoplasia
Chronic mucocutaneous candidiasis	Mucosal candidiasis	Impaired recognition or T cell response to *Candida* antigens
AIDS	Mucosal candidiasis; less commonly cryptococcosis, aspergillosis, histoplasmosis, and coccidioidomycosis	Defective cell-mediated immunity against intracellular fungi; impaired neutrophil function (secondary to defective systemic cytokine production?)

[a]Polymorphonuclear leukocytes and/or monocytes and macrophages.
[b]Nocardiosis, although not a fungus, may complicate the course of patients with chronic granulomatous disease and mimic clinical features of invasive aspergillosis.
[c]Severe combined immunodeficiency syndrome or Wiskott-Aldrich syndrome.

infants that it might be considered a normal event. *Candida* is initially acquired by many infants during passage through the birth canal. It may also be acquired from mothers during breast feeding. *Candida* can be recovered from the oropharynx as early as the first day of life. The incidence of *Candida* colonization increases gradually over the following few weeks such that over 80% of infants can be expected to be colonized by age 4 weeks (40, 41). However, symptomatic thrush may readily develop within days of colonization. In the immunocompetent child, however, this is an entity that is often mild and is readily amenable to treatment. Although *Candida* diaper dermatitis can remain a problem throughout infancy, oral candidiasis in the absence of specific predisposing factors such as antibiotic therapy is rarely encountered beyond the first 6 months of life.

Oral candidiasis occurs in at least 15–40% of children with HIV infection. Studies in adults found that the presence of oropharyngeal candidiasis in the absence of previous antibiotic usage was predictive of HIV infection (42). Similarly one could reasonably anticipate that children who are born to parents at risk for HIV infection and who present with oropharyngeal candidiasis beyond infancy may be immunocompromised and potentially HIV infected.

The clinical manifestations of oral candidiasis in HIV infected children are variable, including a punctate mucosal erythema, a diffuse mucosal erythema, angular chelitis, and the more classical white-beige pseudomembranous plaques on the buccal mucosa, hard palate, oropharyngeal mucosa, and gingivae (27, 43, 44). These lesions may become confluent plaques, involving extensive regions of the mucosa of the oral cavity. Such plaques can be removed with difficulty to reveal a granular base that bleeds easily. A more chronic form of oropharyngeal candidiasis may develop on the dorsum of the tongue, appearing as an erythematous lesion associated with the loss of papillae. The lesions may become sufficiently severe as to impair alimentation. Oral candidiasis in both neutropenic and HIV-infected children may be complicated by extension to laryngeal candidiasis or *Candida* epiglottitis, which may

cause hoarseness or threaten patency of the airway (45–47).

Leggott et al. (48) compared the oral manifestations of children with HIV infection with a combination of similar features found in children afflicted either with primary T cell defects (e.g., CMC) or with phagocytic defects (e.g., chronic granulomatous disease). Children with T cell disorders were found to have oral mucosal candidiasis, HSV infections, and recurrent aphthous ulcerations. By comparison, children with primary disorders of phagocytosis had problems with gingivostomatitis, periodontitis, and parotitis but not oral mucosal candidiasis. Children with HIV infection had a combination of these oral manifestations, indicating deficits in both T cells and phagocytic cells. Whether HIV-infected children have an increased risk of periodontitis and gingivostomatitis, however, is controversial.

The differential diagnosis of oropharyngeal candidiasis includes oral hairy leukoplakia (49–51). This lesion, which develops in the early phase of HIV infection, appears as a white, finely filamentous to papillary lesion along the lateral margins of the tongue. Oral hairy leukoplakia is thought to be due to intraepithelial proliferation of Epstein-Barr virus (51). Although oral hairy leukoplakia has been most frequently described in adults, a recent report of a child with this lesion (52) underscores the need to establish a firm microbiological diagnosis of oral candidiasis in a high-risk child. The lesions may regress during antiretroviral therapy and concurrent improvement of cellular immunity. The syndrome of chronic mucocutaneous candidiasis should be considered in any case of extensive oropharyngeal candidiasis in a child. Highlighting the need for recognition of CMC as a distinct entity are conditions associated with CMC, such as thymoma and endocrinopathies (hypoparathyroidism and adrenal insufficiency), which carry different therapeutic implications than does HIV-associated mucocutaneous candidiasis.

Esophageal Candidiasis

Esophageal candidiasis is a diagnostic indicator disease for AIDS. As such, one should have a high index of suspicion of this infection in high-risk patients. Esophageal candidiasis may coexist or occur without oropharyngeal candidiasis. The absence of oropharyngeal candidiasis does not exclude presence of esophageal candidiasis. Conversely, the presence of symptoms of esophagitis in a patient with AIDS and oropharyngeal candidiasis carries a high predictive value for the presence of esophageal candidiasis.

The frequency of esophageal candidiasis in HIV-infected children is not well-defined. Because of the variation in inter-institutional expertise in performing endoscopy in a pediatric population, a diagnosis may not always be definitive. However, given the importance of establishing the first index condition leading to a diagnosis of AIDS, children presenting symptoms of esophageal candidiasis should have a definitive diagnosis proven by endoscopy.

Symptoms of esophageal candidiasis may consist of substernal pain, dysphagia, or odynophagia. The patient may be able to localize symptoms to a given location in the epigastrium or substernal region. However, some patients with esophageal candidiasis may be entirely asymptomatic. The natural history of esophageal candidiasis in HIV infection is generally not one of dissemination.

Disseminated Candidiasis

Disseminated candidiasis is unusual in HIV-infected children. There have been several cases of catheter-associated fungemia in more than 150 symptomatic HIV-infected children followed in the Pediatric Branch of the National Cancer Institute during the past 4 years. However, deeply invasive tissue-proven candidiasis did not develop, and there were no fatalities from fungemia in these patients. By comparison, a retrospective study of 156 HIV-infected children during a 7.5-year period revealed that 11 (7%) of these patients had disseminated candidiasis (53). All but one of these cases was nosocomially acquired candidiasis. Eight (73%) of these 11 patients had central venous catheters as possible portals of entry. Two of the 11 patients had neutropenia. The predominant organism was *C. albicans*. Four (36%) of these patients with disseminated

candidiasis were not diagnosed until postmortem examination and received no antifungal therapy. The frequency of dissemination in this series is relatively high and likely reflects the susceptibility of this population in a hospital setting, where the risk for nosocomial candidiasis is relatively high. A review of the literature indicates a paucity of individual reported cases and emphasizes the relative infrequency with which deeply invasive candidiasis develops in HIV-infected patients (54–57).

Nevertheless, patients with HIV infection may develop disseminated candidiasis in cases where well-known predisposing factors may be present. Those factors predisposing to disseminated candidiasis in immunocompromised children have been detailed elsewhere (58–60) and include very low birth weight, central venous catheters, total parenteral nutrition, broad spectrum antibiotic therapy, aggressive surgical interventions, and granulocytopenia. HIV-infected children with none of these risk factors may rarely present with candidemia. Certainly very low birth weight infants and seriously ill full-term neonates carry a high risk for mucosal and disseminated candidiasis (59). If such neonates are also HIV infected, they would have at least the same risk of developing disseminated candidiasis as would their HIV-negative counterparts. Whether in fact that risk might be increased remains to be determined.

The complications of disseminated candidiasis have been detailed elsewhere (59–62). Common complications of invasive candidiasis in nonneutropenic patients include *Candida* endophthalmitis, renal candidiasis, arthritis, osteomyelitis, and vascular catheter-associated fungemia. Neonates and infants not infrequently develop *Candida* meningitis as a complication of disseminated candidiasis. Granulocytopenic patients may develop other patterns of infection, such as hepatosplenic candidiasis or *Candida* myositis with disseminated cutaneous lesions.

Cutaneous Candidiasis

Cutaneous candidiasis may develop as a diaper dermatitis or as a more generalized cutaneous eruption. These cutaneous forms of candidiasis in HIV-infected children are often recurrent and require protracted therapy.

Candida *Onychomycosis*

Occasionally, children with HIV infection and oral candidiasis may have a concomitant *Candida* onychomycosis. These lesions are often refractory to topical therapy. Depending upon the degree of nail involvement warranting systemic therapy, ketoconazole may be effective in ameliorating *Candida* onychomycosis in this patient population, although, the condition rarely clears completely. Onychomycosis caused by dermatophytes, particularly *Trichophyton* spp, also may develop as a recurrent process.

Cryptococcosis

Meningoencephalitis caused by *C. neoformans* occurs in ~6–13% of HIV-infected adults, whereas it is less common in children with HIV infection (63–70). Leggiadro and colleagues (68) surveyed investigators from 38 institutions concerning their experience with extrapulmonary cryptococcosis. Investigators from 33 (87%) of the institutions responded, resulting in data on 13 patients from 11 centers. Meningitis was the most common manifestation of extrapulmonary cryptococcosis, occurring in 8 (62%) of the 13 patients. Extrapulmonary cryptococcosis was the AIDS indicator disease in 9 (69%) of the 13 patients. The median age was 8 years with a range of 2–17 years. The spectrum of infection of cryptococcosis in these patients included a rapidly fatal fungemia to chronic meningitis to an indolent fever of unknown origin.

Fever, headache, and altered mental status in cryptococcal meningoencephalitis are usually indolent, often evolving over the course of weeks to months. Unlike some central nervous system (CNS) mycoses, such as aspergillosis, cryptococcal meningoencephalitis seldom presents with focal neurological deficits (71). Cryptococcal meningoencephalitis in HIV-infected patients often has few clinically overt signs early in infection but may present in some patients with meningismus, photophobia, and seizures. For example, one report described

fever and seizures as the initial manifestations of disseminated cryptococcosis in a 9-year HIV-infected boy (72). Cutaneous lesions may develop as a manifestation of disseminated cryptococcosis, as described in a 16-year HIV-infected male whose lesions caused by *C. neoformans* mimicked molluscum contagiosum (73). It should be anticipated that as children with HIV infection survive longer, cryptococcal infection may develop further in their course.

Histoplasmosis

Although *H. capsulatum* is well described as an infectious agent in children, particularly in infants (74), only limited data exist regarding its role in HIV-infected children (75, 76). One infant, who presented with a 2-week history of fever, was found to have disseminated histoplasmosis as the AIDS-defining illness (76). *H. capsulatum* is recoverable from bone marrow and blood cultures in HIV-infected patients with disseminated histoplasmosis (14). A distinctive syndrome of severe disseminated histoplasmosis can consist of cutaneous lesions, pulmonary infiltrates, and thrombocytopenia, which may progress to septic shock in HIV-infected patients (6, 77).

Coccidioidomycosis

Infection caused by *C. immitis* is usually self-limiting in >95% of infected cases in endemic areas. Patients with HIV infection in endemic areas appear to be at particularly high risk for development of disseminated coccidioidomycosis. Symptoms of disseminated coccidioidomycosis in adults have included fever, chills, weight loss, cough, chest pain, headache, altered sensorium, and skin rashes, corresponding to involvement of lungs, brain, skin, and other tissue sites. Although immunocompetent children have been reported with isolated organ disease, the presentation of coccidioidomycosis in an HIV-infected child is more likely to become manifest as progressive pneumonia or disseminated infection.

Aspergillosis

Among HIV-infected patients with granulocytopenia and thrombocytopenia, the clinical manifestations are similar to those patients with neoplastic diseases and can include hemorrhagic infarcts, pleuritic pain, and hemoptysis (31–34). Patients without marrow aplasia tend to have a more chronic bronchopneumonia, and some have been described as producing large intrabronchial mucus plugs containing hyphae (32). Among the conditions of invasive aspergillosis that may be encountered in HIV-infected patients are pulmonary aspergilloma, necrotizing tracheobronchitis, paranasal sinusitis, disseminated infection, and soft tissue aspergillosis (78–81). The functional deficits of PMNLs and the propensity for chronic respiratory aspergillosis in nonneutropenic HIV-infected patients are reminiscent of chronic granulomatous disease (82). Chest radiograph may initially fail to detect or may underestimate infiltrates caused by invasive pulmonary aspergillosis. A computerized tomography scan may facilitate initial detection of these infiltrates in high risk patients and more accurately characterize the extent of pulmonary infiltrates. A definitive microbiological diagnosis is established by bronchoalveolar lavage or open lung biopsy.

Other Mycoses

Malassezia furfur, a lipophilic yeast, causes tinea versicolor, an infectious folliculitis, and catheter-associated fungemia (83). The folliculitis caused by *M. furfur* is a pruritic, papular to papulosquamous eruption distributed most prominently on the facial and neck areas and may respond to topical imidazole therapy. Of note, fungemia caused by *M. furfur* has occurred in children receiving lipid supplemented total parenteral nutrition via central venous catheters (84).

Dermatophyte infections are common in patients with HIV infection (85) and include onychomycosis, periungual dermatophytosis, tinea pedis, and tinea manum. These infections tend to be extensive and severe; e.g., patterns of proximal white subungual onychomycosis and hypertrophic onychomycosis are unusual in normal hosts but are commonly encountered in HIV-infected patients.

Sporothrix schenckii most commonly causes a subcutaneous mycosis. Among immunocompromised hosts, however, *S. schenckii* may cause pulmonary or disseminated sporotrichosis. Given that cases of disseminated sporotrichosis have already been described in HIV-infected adults (86, 87), a reasonable probability exists that as the population of pediatric HIV infection expands and survives longer, pulmonary or disseminated sporotrichosis likely will appear in this younger population.

Trichosporon beigelii, which is an uncommon but serious cause of disseminated infection in neutropenic patients, has been reported as a cause of catheter-associated fungemia in HIV-infected patients (88, 89). The presence of deeply invasive *Trichosporon* infection may result in false-positive cryptococcal antigen reaction caused by cross-reacting antigen.

DIAGNOSIS

Table 17.3 summarizes salient features of the diagnostic approach toward selected mucocutaneous and systemic mycoses encountered in HIV-infected children.

Candidiasis

Although oral candidiasis is usually a clinical diagnosis, examination of wet mounts of swabs or scrapings of the lesions with identification of blastoconidia (budding yeast forms), pseudohyphae, and hyphae provides definitive confirmation. *C. albicans* is most common but other *Candida* spp and *Torulopsis glabrata* may also be identified. Isolation of *T. glabrata* may occur especially when the patient has been previously treated with an imidazole compound, such as ketoconazole, to which the fungus may be resistant. Unlike, *Candida* spp, *T. glabrata* does not produce pseudohyphae or hyphae, and thus appears on wet mount only as blastoconidia.

Culture and histopathology of an esophageal mucosal biopsy is the most definitive means by which to establish a diagnosis of esophageal candidiasis. A barium swallow is neither sensitive nor specific in establishing a diagnosis of esophageal candidiasis. Connolly et al. (90) reviewed 45 episodes of upper gastrointestinal symptoms in 43 HIV-infected patients. A diagnosis was established in 43 episodes (95%) by endoscopy

Table 17.3.   Diagnosis of Selected Fungal Infections Complicating Pediatric AIDS[a]

Infection	Physical Findings	Laboratory Studies
Candidiasis		
Oral candidiasis	Mucosal erythema, beige plaques	KOH prep, Gram stain; culture
Esophageal candidiasis	Mucosal erythema, beige plaques	Endoscopy: mucosal brushings and biopsy; direct exam, cultures, and histopathology
Disseminated candidiasis	Fever, cutaneous lessions, endophthalmitis, candiduria	Blood cultures, biopsy of normally sterile tissue site; antigen and metabolite detection are investigational
Pulmonary, meningeal, or disseminated cryptococcosis	Fever, cutaneous lesions, headache, confusion, lethargy	Chest radiograph; CT scan of head, cultures of sputum, blood, CSF, and urine; LCAT on blood and CSF
Histoplasmosis	Fever, pulmonary infiltrates, cutaneous lesions, septic shock	Chest radiograph; CT scan; sputum induction, BAL; biopsy of lung, bone marrow, or skin; blood cultures; antigen in serum and urine
Coccidioidomycosis	Fever, pulmonary infiltrates, cutaneous lesions	Chest radiograph; CT scan; sputum induction, BAL; biopsy of lung, or skin
Pulmonary aspergillosis	Fever, pulmonary infiltrates, pleuritic pain, cough, hemoptysis	Chest radiograph; CT scan; sputum induction, BAL; biopsy; serology; investigational antigen levels
Malassezia dermatitis	Papular, papulosquamous, follicular eruptions	Wet mount of skin scraping revealing hyphae and clusters of yeasts

[a]CT, computerized tomography; LCAT, latex cryptococcal antigen test; BAL, bronchoalveolar lavage.

but in only 14 (31%) by barium swallow. Bonacini and colleagues (91) conducted a prospective clinical case study of the causes of esophageal symptoms in 110 HIV-infected adults: 72 (65%) of the 110 patients had a total of 100 esophageal infections; 33 (30%) of the 110 patients had *Candida* alone, 22 (20%) had *Candida* and cytomegalovirus (CMV), 2 (1.8%) had *Candida*, CMV, and HSV, 7 (6%) had HSV alone, and 2 (1.8%) had both HSV and CMV. The sensitivity of brushings (95%) was superior to that of mucosal biopsy (70%) in detection of *Candida*. Oral candidiasis had a sensitivity of 53% and a positive predictive value of 77% for *Candida* esophagitis. That 24 (42%) of the 57 patients with esophageal candidiasis had concomitant viral infections underscores the need for considering endoscopy and culture in adults receiving antifungal therapy for presumptive candidiasis of the esophagus. Considerably less is known about the causes of esophageal symptoms in HIV-infected children. If endoscopy is performed, visual inspection brushings and cultures are warranted, especially because

other infectious agents, including HSV, CMV, and bacteria, may mimic or coexist with esophageal candidiasis (91–93).

Diagnosis of disseminated candidiasis in critically ill children can be elusive and may not be discovered until autopsy (94). Use of lysis centrifugation blood cultures has been found to detect more patients with fungemia and to detect them earlier in comparison with conventional broth techniques (95–97). Systems for detection of *Candida* antigen (e.g., enolase and mannans), metabolites (e.g., D-arabinitol), and genomic DNA, (using polymerase chain reaction) remain investigational for diagnosis of disseminated candidiasis (98, 99). Diagnostic imaging methods, including computerized tomographic scans, magnetic resonance imaging scans, and ultrasonography, may reveal abscesses in deep visceral organs. Lesions in non-neutropenic patients tend to localize to kidneys in comparison with those with neutropenia, where lesions may also be found in liver and spleen (100). Lesions of disseminated candidiasis that are ≤0.5 cm in diameter, however, may be below the threshold of detection of such imaging techniques.

Cryptococcosis

Diagnosis of cryptococcal meningitis in HIV infection can usually be established by a combination of direct examination of CSF on a wet mount, including India ink preparations, CSF culture, and cryptococcal capsular polysaccharide antigen detection in CSF, serum, and other normally sterile body fluids. The organism usually appears as an encapsulated budding yeast. However, capsules of some capsule-deficient strains have been reported in patients with HIV infection (101). These strains may be misdiagnosed upon direct exam as other yeasts or as contaminating particles. The CSF cell count, glucose, and protein in patients with HIV infection may be virtually normal, apparently because of the paucity of an effective inflammatory response. Staining with periodic acid-Schiff biopsy specimens of suspicious skin lesions may reveal the encapsulated budding yeast cells. Mucicarmine or Alcian blue stains can be used to specifically stain the mucopolysaccharide capsule. Although a computerized tomography scan is usually nonspecific in most cases of CNS cryptococcosis, it may reveal hydrocephalus or cryptococcomas. Other concomitant CSN processes such as toxoplasmosis or lymphoma, which may resemble cryptococcomas, may also be detected.

Several features are more distinctive in cryptococcal meningitis in HIV infection in comparison with other immunocompromised populations, such as those with cancer or organ transplants. The CSF antigen from HIV-infected patients with meningeal involvement tends to be substantially higher, often exceeding 1:1024 in seriously ill patients. Consistent with these serological findings, the concentration of organisms in CSF of patients with HIV infection tends to be substantially higher than that of patients with cryptococcal meningitis who do not have HIV infection; India ink preparation is usually positive in patients with HIV infection and cryptococcal meningitis. Culture and cryptococcal antigen titers by latex agglutination should confirm the diagnosis. Cultures and latex cryptococcal anti-

gen test should be performed on peripheral blood and CSF. During therapy, these titers and CSF culture results should be monitored.

Histoplasmosis

Culture and examination of bone marrow aspirate and biopsy is among the most reliable methods to establish the diagnosis of disseminated histoplasmosis in HIV-infected patients. Direct examination by Giemsa or Wright stains of touch preps, smears, paraffin-embedded clot sections, or decalcified biopsy reveals small 2–4-μm diameter yeast-like cells within the cytoplasm of macrophages. Blood cultures, using the lysis centrifugation blood culture system, also may recover the organism. Biopsy of lesions of the skin, lung, liver, and lymph nodes may demonstrate noncaseating and caseating granulomas with intracytoplasmically located blastoconidia within macrophages.

The chest radiograph in histoplasmosis in HIV-infected hosts may demonstrate various patterns, including reticulonodular, miliary, and lobar infiltrates. Organisms may be identified on bronchoalveolar lavage, or lung biopsy. Differentiating nonbudding yeast cells of *H. capsulatum* from the cysts of *P. carinii* may be difficult. Use of calcofluor white and monoclonal antibodies may facilitate this differential diagnosis. Circulating antibodies by complement fixation or by immunodiffusion may be undetectable in disseminated histoplasmosis complicating HIV-infection, most probably because of impaired antibody production. However, recent studies identified *H. capsulatum* antigen in urine and serum as a valuable marker in diagnosis and therapeutic monitoring of disseminated histoplasmosis (102).

Coccidioidomycosis

The diagnosis of coccidioidomycosis in HIV-infected patients can usually be established by direct examination and culture of respiratory secretions or by biopsy of suspicious pulmonary or cutaneous lesions to reveal characteristic spherules. Culture of specimens will reveal a fine hyaline mould that later demonstrates characteristic barrel-shaped arthroconidia. Serological tests, including complement fixation, tube precipitation, and immunodiffusion assays, are important in the diagnosis and monitoring of patients with disseminated coccidioidomycosis. These tests reveal a variable antibody response in HIV-infected patients, suggesting impaired antibody response.

Aspergillosis

Diagnosis of invasive aspergillosis is best established by biopsy and culture of suspicious pulmonary or cutaneous lesions. Recovery of *A. fumigatus* and *A. flavus* in respiratory secretions of HIV-infected patients with pulmonary infiltrates should be seriously considered as representing invasive aspergillosis, particularly in patients who are neutropenic.

TREATMENT WITH SYSTEMIC ANTIFUNGAL AGENTS

This decade is witnessing advances in application of novel antifungal compounds for mucosal and systemic mycoses complicating HIV infection and other immunocompromised conditions. Several reviews of antifungal agents provide a detailed account of these new compounds (103–106). Tables 17.4 and 17.5 summarize dosages, routes of administration, availability, and utilization of antifungal agents in managing fungal infections complicating HIV-infected children.

Amphotericin B Desoxycholate (Fungizone)

Amphotericin B desoxycholate (Fungizone) is the gold standard of efficacy for most disseminated mycoses, particularly in immunocompromised hosts. This parenterally administered compound has a long plasma half-life permitting once daily to once every other day dosing. Rigor, chills, fever, and phlebitis are among the acute complications of amphotericin B infusion. Azotemia, hypokalemia, hyperchloremic metabolic acidosis, hypomagnesemia, anemia, and weight loss can complicate chronic administration of amphotericin B.

There are several lipid formulations of amphotericin B being evaluated in the United States and Europe: amphotericin B lipid complex (ABLC), amphotericin B colloidal dispersion (ABCD, Amphocil), small unilameller vesicle amphotericin B (SUV, AmBisome) (106). These compounds enable amphotericin B to be administered in higher doses (2–5 mg/kg/day) with less

Table 17.4. Antifungal Agents Used in Treatment of Mucosal and Systemic Fungal Infections Complicating Pediatric AIDS

Class of Compound	Total Daily Dosage	Frequency
Orally administered		
Nystatin[a]	Four 2- to 6-ml doses (100,000 units/ml)	q 6 hr
Clotrimazole[b]	Five 10-mg troches	≤5/day
Ketoconazole[c]	5–10 mg/kg	q 24–q 12 hr
5-Fluorocytosine[g]	50–150 mg/kg[g]	q 12–q 6 hr[g]
Fluconazole[d, e, g]	2–8 mg/kg[g]	q 24 hr[g, i]
Itraconazole[c, f]	2–5 mg/kg	q 24 hr–q 12 hr
Parenterally administered		
Amphotericin B	0.5–1.5 mg/kg	q 24 hr–q 72 hr[h]
5-fluorocytosine[f–h]	50–150 mg/kg[g]	q 12–q 6 hr[g]
Fluconazole[e, g]	2–8 mg/kg[g]	q 24 hr[g]
Miconazole[a]	7–13 mg/kg	q 8 hr

[a]Nonabsorbable.
[b]Minimally absorbable.
[c]Absorption impaired by reduced gastric acidity.
[d]Well absorbed.
[e]Investigational in children ≤12 years at the time of this writing.
[f]Parenteral formulation not available in the United States.
[g]Dosage adjustment required for decreased creatinine clearance; plasma levels of 5-fluorocytosine should be monitored.
[h]Intervals of ≥72 hr have been used for maintenance of remission of cryptococcosis and other mycoses in HIV-infected patients.
[i]Fluconazole for life-threatening infections in children may require twice daily dosage.

**Table 17.5.   Summary of Initial Therapy and Maintenance Therapy
of Fungal Infections Complicating Pediatric AIDS[a]**

Fungal Infection	Initial Therapy	Maintenance Therapy
Oral candidiasis	Nystatin Clotrimazole Ketoconazole Fluconazole	Nystatin Clotrimazole
Esophageal candidiasis	Ketoconazole Fluconazole Amphotericin B	Nystatin Clotrimazole Ketoconazole Fluconazole
Disseminated candidiasis	Amphotericin B ±5-Fluorocytosine	Unknown at this time
Cutaneous candidiasis	Nystatin cream or powder; miconazole cream	Nystatin cream or powder; miconazole cream
Cryptococcal pneumonia and meningitis	Amphotericin B with or without flucytosine	Fluconazole
Disseminated histoplasmosis	Itraconazole Amphotericin B[1]	Itraconazole Amphotericin B
Disseminated coccidioidomycosis	Amphotericin B Itraconazole	Amphotericin B Itraconazole Fluconazole
Disseminated sporotrichosis	Amphotericin B	Amphotericin B (?) Itraconazole (?)
Pulmonary and/or disseminated aspergillosis	Amphotericin B	Amphotericin B Itraconazole
Malassezia dermatitis	Ketoconazole	Miconazole cream Ketoconazole

[a]Refer to text for details of selection of appropriate antifungal agents for individual mycoses.

nephrotoxicity and bone marrow suppression in comparison to that of conventional amphotericin B. Each lipid formulation of amphotericin B is being evaluated separately because of its distinct pharmacokinetic and pharmacodynamic properties. The role of these liposomal formulations of amphotericin B and other novel compounds in managing the fungal infections of HIV-infected children will require thoughtfully designed clinical trials based upon a firm pharmacokinetic and pharmacodynamic foundation.

Antifungal Imidazoles

The antifungal azoles are fungistatic compounds that include the imidazoles (e.g., clotrimazole, miconazole, and ketoconazole) and triazoles (e.g., fluconazole, itraconazole). Saperconazole is an investigational triazole undergoing preclinical investigation. In comparison with the systemically administered imidazoles (miconazole and ketoconazole), the more recently developed antifungal triazoles as a group have longer half-lifes, improved CNS penetration with better activity against CNS mycoses, and broader spectrum of activity. Fluconazole also had the flexibility of oral and parenteral administration.

Ketoconazole is an orally administered imidazole active against various yeast-like fungi, including *Candida* spp, *H. capsulatum,* and *C. neoformans.* However, because of the lack of CNS penetration, ketoconazole should not be used for treatment for cryptococcal infections. This agent has been an important advance in the effective treatment of chronic mucocutaneous candidiasis in children, oral and esophageal candidiasis, refractory dermatophytoses, infections from *M. furfur,* and selected conditions of endemic mycoses, including histoplasmosis, blastomycosis, coccidioidomycosis, and paracoccidioidomycosis. Ketoconazole is administered orally twice daily, but its absorption may be impaired by elevated gastric pH from oral antacids, H_2 receptor blocking agents, or intrinsic gastric achlorhydria. Patients taking concomitant rifampin or isoniazid may have reduced serum levels caused by acceleration of hepatic metabolism of ketoconazole. Ketoconazole is generally well tolerated by children at dosages of ≤5 mg/kg/day; dosages exceeding this level may be more commonly associated with anorexia, nausea, and vomiting as dose-limiting symptoms, although, some children may tolerate ketoconazole at 10 mg/kg/day without intolerance. Ketoconazole is approved by the Food and Drug Administration for children over 2 years old. Hepatotoxicity is a feature common to all antifungal azoles. Approximately 5% of patients receiving ketoconazole will have reversible elevation of hepatic transaminases as the drug is continued. Some patients will have continued elevation of serum transaminases requiring discontinuation of the compound. Caution should be exerted in using any antifungal triazole in patients with extant liver disease. Because ketoconazole can inhibit mammalian cytochrome P-450-dependent enzymes, steroidogenesis may be inhibited, resulting in transient, dose-dependent suppression of serum testosterone and cortisol. The latter effect has rarely caused adrenal insufficiency.

Fluconazole was recently approved for use against cryptococcosis and candidiasis in the United States. Fluconazole achieves high concentrations in the CSF and in multiple tissue sites relative to plasma concentrations. Its long plasma half-life (~30 hr) in adult patients permits once daily dosing. Fluconazole has not been approved by the Food and Drug Administration for use in children. An initial study of 6 mg/kg/day fluconazole for treatment of candidiasis in immunocompromised children, including those with HIV infection, suggested good activity against mucosal infection, particularly oral candidiasis and urinary tract infection (106). However, an increase to 12 mg/kg was required in two patients in this study with fungemia from *C. parapsilosis*. A recent phase I–II pharmacokinetic study of fluconazole in febrile neutropenic children revealed that the plasma half-life of fluconazole was only approximately half that of a comparable adult population (107). These findings led to an ongoing study of fluconazole with a dosing regimen of 12 mg/kg in two divided doses for treatment of deeply established mycoses in children to compensate for this greater clearance rate.

Itraconazole is a new orally administered antifungal triazole with activity against *Candida* spp, *C. neoformans*, *Aspergillus* spp, *H. capsulatum*, *S. schenckii*, *Blastomyces dermatitidis*, and *C. immitis*. Itraconazole also appears to be effective in the suppression of cryptococcal meningitis in patients with HIV infection. Itraconazole has a long plasma half-life in humans that permits once or twice daily oral dosing. Since bioavailability of itraconazole is markedly reduced in patients with gastric achlorhydria, caution should be used in treatment of invasive mycoses in patients who are dependent on antacids or who may have intrinsic achlorhydria. An aldosterone-like effect of hypokalemia has been observed in some recipients of itraconazole. There is a paucity of data on the safety, tolerance, pharmacokinetics, or efficacy of itraconazole in children.

5-Fluorocytosine

5-Fluorocytosine is a fluorinated pyrimidine with antifungal activity against *Candida* spp, *C. neoformans*, and other systemic fungal pathogens. The pharmacologic and therapeutic properties of 5-fluorocytosine are discussed in a recent review (108). Because resistance may emerge rapidly when this agent is used alone, flucytosine is combined with amphotericin B to augment antifungal activity, provide better CNS and renal concentrations of an antifungal agent, and, depending on dose of amphotericin B, have an amphotericin B sparing effect. 5-Fluorocytosine is administered orally (parenteral formulation has been withdrawn from United States) and has a short plasma half-life, requiring three to four times per day administration with normal renal function. The compound is completely cleared by the kidneys, and the dosage must be adjusted for impaired renal clearance. Toxicity includes bone marrow suppression, diarrhea, and hepatitis. Myelosuppression is the most common side effect and is dose dependent. Because plasma concentrations of flucytosine in plasma of >100 µg/ml are associated with increased toxicity, plasma concentrations should be monitored to maintain levels between 40 and 60 μg/ml. These levels exceed by at least 10-fold the minimal inhibitory concentrations of most susceptible fungi.

TREATMENT OF SPECIFIC MYCOSES IN HIV-INFECTED CHILDREN

Candidiasis

Oral Candidiasis

Treatment of oropharyngeal candidiasis may be initially accomplished by administration of nystatin suspension or clotrimazole troches (109–111). Compliance in younger children with nystatin suspension or clotrimazole troches is often difficult. More severe or refractory cases can be managed by use of ketoconazole or fluconazole. However, data regarding the use of fluconazole in children are minimal. Parenterally administered amphotericin B occasionally may be needed for treatment of refractory oropharyngeal candidiasis, particularly if esophageal extension is suspected. Some children with refractory oropharyngeal or mucosal candidiasis may require chronic intermittent amphotericin B.

Oral and esophageal candidiasis, as well as many other mycoses in HIV infection, have a high propensity for relapse unless suppressive maintenance antifungal therapy is continued. Maintenance therapy of mucosal candidiasis can usually be achieved by administration of nystatin, clotrimazole, ketoconazole, or fluconazole.

Esophageal Candidiasis

Treatment of esophageal candidiasis has been attempted with nystatin suspension, clotrimazole troches, ketoconazole, fluconazole, and amphotericin B. Our experience indicates that neither nystatin nor clotrimazole is reliably effective in treatment of esophageal candidiasis. Occasional responses of presumptive esophageal candidiasis to nystatin or clotrimazole are observed. However, esophageal candidiasis also may develop in patients already receiving nystatin or clotrimazole for oral candidiasis. Endoscopy may be performed in an HIV-infected child with esophageal symptoms for 1) proving the presence of esophageal candidiasis as the first opportunistic infection that substantiates a diagnosis of HIV infection and, 2) esophageal symptoms refractory to oral therapy. Treatment of esophageal candidiasis in HIV infection is based on several factors: 1) severity of symptoms, especially restricting the ability to maintain adequate fluid intake, 2) history of previous or current antifungal therapy, 3) compliance with oral medications, 4) additional immunocompromised conditions (e.g., neutropenia), and 5) concomitant infections. For example, for patients with few symptoms who are not receiving antifungal therapy, and who have no problems of compliance, neutropenia, or concomitant infections, a systemic azole (ketoconazole or fluconazole) would be appropriate. By comparison, for patients who have severe symptoms impairing adequate hydration and who may already be receiving an oral agent, intravenous amphotericin B is the most appropriate choice. Those patients who may have been receiving an antifungal azole (e.g., clotrimazole, ketoconazole or fluconazole) may develop esophageal infection from *T. glabrata*, many strains of which are resistant to these compounds. Amphotericin B is the most appropriate agent for *T. glabrata* esophagitis, especially in patients previously treated with antifungal azoles. Obviously, noncompliance with oral medications would require a parenteral antifungal compound. Concomitant granulocytopenia in a febrile patient also warrants administration of amphotericin B because of the potential risk of deep visceral or disseminated candidiasis.

If there is progression of symptoms, 5 mg/kg/day ketoconazole, or 3–6 mg/kg fluconazole should be administered until resolution of symptoms. We then continue a maintenance regimen of clotrimazole or nystatin indefinitely. Amphotericin B should be considered in lieu of oral therapy of esophageal candidiasis in HIV-infected patients in the following conditions: 1) lack of response to oral therapy, 2) inability to tolerate oral medications (e.g., odynophagia), 3) risk of disseminated candidiasis (e.g., granulocytopenia), 4) development of esophageal candidiasis during oral antifungal therapy for mucosal candidiasis, 5) *T. glabrata* esophagitis, 6) fungemia, and 7) microbiological resistance to azoles. If there is progression of symptoms refractory to ketoconazole, endoscopy is performed, if possible, and intravenous amphotericin B is initiated at 0.5 mg/kg/day and continued until resolution of symptoms.

Resolution of symptoms does not reliably indicate eradication of infection; biopsy of patients treated for esophageal candidiasis and whose symptoms have resolved may reveal residual fungi. Routinely performing endoscopy on children to confirm resolution of esophageal candidiasis is not warranted, but a reasonable strategy is to maintain suppressive therapy indefinitely.

Fluconazole has been increasingly used in adults for chronic suppression of oropharyngeal and esophageal candidiasis (112–115). This chronic usage has been more recently associated with the emergence of resistance of *C. albicans* to fluconazole (116–119).

Cutaneous (Diaper) Dermatitis

Diaper dermatitis in HIV-infected children merits special comments. Fundamental to the treatment of diaper dermatitis is the frequent changing of diapers to prevent cutaneous maceration. Antifungal therapy with miconazole or Lotrimin cream or nystatin cream or powder with each diaper change may effect improvement. Chronic use of topical corticosteroids can lead to cutaneous atrophy and generally is to be discouraged. However, if used sparingly during the first few days of therapy, they can provide an anti-inflammatory effect. The simultaneous administration of oral antifungal agents, such as nystatin, may contribute to further reducing *Candida* colonization. Treatment of generalized cutaneous candidiasis entails maintaining good hygiene and application of topical antifungal creams, as previously mentioned. Ketoconazole (Nizoral) cream may also be useful for generalized cutaneous candidiasis.

Disseminated Candidiasis

Treatment of choice for disseminated candidiasis is amphotericin B. The dosage, duration, and use of combinations of antifungal compounds depends on the host factors and pattern of invasive infection. For example, 0.5–1.0 mg/kg/day for 2 weeks is usually an effective range for uncomplicated catheter-associated fungemia caused by *C. albicans* in a non-neutropenic child, provided that the infected catheter is removed. By comparison, disseminated *C. tropicalis* fungemia complicated by cutaneous lesions, and renal impairment in a neutropenic child usually requires a more aggressive approach with 1.0–1.5 mg/kg/day amphotericin B for 4–8 weeks. Development of hepatosplenic candidiasis may require a protracted duration of amphotericin B therapy of 4–6 months (60–100 mg/kg/day). 5-Fluorocytosine may be useful in combination with amphotericin B when there is involvement of the CNS (e.g., *Candida* meningitis or endophthalmitis), hepatosplenic candidiasis, or renal candidiasis. 5-Fluorocytosine levels should be followed carefully, and dosages should be adjusted to maintain peak serum concentrations at approximately 40–60 µg/ml. Serum levels of >100 µg/ml are associated with bone marrow suppression. Given the diminished bone marrow reserve of many patients with HIV infection, especially those receiving azidothymidine, close monitoring of flucytosine serum levels is even more imperative. Reduction of peak serum concentrations to 30–40 µg/ml and addition of granulocyte-colony stimulating factor may be required in some HIV-infected children.

Cryptococcosis

The current treatment of choice for initial treatment of cryptococcal meningitis is amphotericin B with or without 5-fluorocytosine, recognizing that fluconazole and itraconazole have been reported for use as first-line therapy (63–67, 73, 120–130). The role of flucytosine in combination with amphotericin B in HIV infection is controversial because of suppression of hematopoiesis. This combination has been used in non-HIV-infected patients but has been supplanted in HIV-infected patients in many centers by amphotericin B alone. Titers of cryptococcal antigen should decline in the CSF during therapy. Patients who respond well to therapy usually have a decline in CSF titers to ≤1:8. Persistence of an elevated titer may presage refractory or recurrent infection.

Amphotericin B, 0.5–1.0 mg/kg/day with or without 5-fluorocytosine for 4–8 weeks, is the preferred agent for initial treatment of cryptococcal meningitis. A recent controlled trial of fluconazole (200 mg/day) vs. amphotericin B (mean daily dose 0.4–0.5 mg/kg/day) for primary treatment of CNS cryptococcosis observed that high-risk patients had a trend toward higher mortality because of neurological deterioration in the fluconazole arm (131). These findings and those of Larsen et al. (124) underscore the importance of amphotericin B with or without 5-fluorocytosine in the initial management of high-risk HIV-infected patients with cryptococcal meningitis. Patients with altered mental status, evidence of increased intracranial pressure (e.g., papilledema), seizures, and focal deficits are considered to be at particularly high risk for sudden death from CNS cryptococcosis.

Maintenance therapy for prevention of recurrence of CNS cryptococcosis is necessary (65). A recently completed controlled trial found that fluconazole (200 mg/day PO) was clearly superior to amphotericin B (1 mg/kg/week IV) in preventing relapse of cryptococcal meningitis in HIV-infected adults. Children who initially receive an "induction" of remission of CNS cryptococcosis with amphotericin B may be placed on a maintenance regimen of fluconazole of 3–6 mg/kg/day (132). Fluconazole and itraconazole are being compared in adults for maintenance of remission of CNS cryptococcosis.

Histoplasmosis

The treatment of choice for severe disseminated histoplasmosis is amphotericin B. Itraconazole has been recently approved by the Food and Drug Administration in adults for treatment of stable disseminated histoplasmosis and is a reasonable alternative to amphotericin B in patients with fever and fungemia but no clinically overt CNS infection or hemodynamic deterioration (133). Although short courses of amphotericin B have been advocated for disseminated histoplasmosis of infancy, an indefinite course of antifungal therapy will likely be necessary for treatment of disseminated histoplasmosis complicating HIV infection

(134). Such a course may follow the pattern of an induction regimen with amphotericin B, as in treatment of cryptococcal meningitis, followed by a maintenance course of amphotericin B or an antifungal imidazole or triazole. Recent advances in antigen detection systems for *H. capsulatum* offer the potential for noninvasive monitoring of antifungal therapy.

Aspergillosis

Amphotericin B is the drug of choice for invasive aspergillosis. Doses of 1.0–1.5 mg/kg/day may be required in granulocytopenic patients (135). Because of a paucity of clinical data, the use of rifampin and/or flucytosine in combination with high dosages of amphotericin B is unclear at this time. Encouraging reports by Denning and Stevens (136) of itraconazole in treatment of invasive pulmonary aspergillosis indicate that this agent may be useful in management of selected patients with this infection (136).

Other Mycoses

Topical azoles (clotrimazole and miconazole) are the cornerstone of management of cutaneous infections from dermatophytes and cutaneous infections from *M. furfur.* More refractory cutaneous mycoses and onychomycosis may be managed by griseofulvin, ketoconazole, or fluconazole. *M. furfur* fungemia is treated by discontinuing parenteral lipids and removing the catheter. Immunocompromised children with *M. furfur* fungemia also may be benefited by a course of ketoconazole.

FUTURE DIRECTIONS

As patients with HIV infection survive longer, newer approaches to mucosal candidiasis become increasingly important as emergence of resistance to systemic azoles becomes more prevalent. Treatment of mucosal candidiasis is amenable to novel strategies of mucosal blockade as adjuncts to antifungal therapy. Advances in antifungal chemotherapy with novel mechanisms of action will afford new approaches to management of both refractory and early mycoses.

Augmentation of host defenses can continue to be develop through improvements in antiretroviral therapy and in selective uses of recombinant cytokines. For example, granulocyte-colony stimulating factor is used to manage azidothymidine-induced or ganciclovir-induced granulocytopenia, thus preventing infections as the result of quantitative defects in circulating neutrophils. However, increasing in vitro and experimental animal data suggest that granulocyte-colony stimulating factor may augment the functional activity of circulating neutrophils against fungi such as *Aspergillus* spp. Caution is mandated, however, in employing recombinant cytokines that may activate monocytes or macrophages. Because these cells of the monocyte-macrophage lineage contain HIV, cytokines may lead to proliferation of virus in activated cells. Vaccines against selected pathogenic fungi (e.g., *C. neoformans*, *H. capsulatum*, and *C. immitis*) are yet another potential strategy for prevention of invasive mycoses that has witnessed substantial preclinical development and early phase I trials. New diagnostic strategies including improved culture techniques, new methods for detection of fungal antigens and metabolites, and development of molecular diagnostic techniques, such as polymerase chain reaction, will improve the early recognition and therapeutic monitoring of opportunistic mycoses in HIV-infected children.

References

1. Pizzo PJ, Eddy J, Falloon F, et al. Effect of continuous intravenous infusion of zidovudine (AZT) in children with symptomatic HIV infection. N Engl J Med 1988;319:889–896.
2. Pizzo PA. Considerations for the evaluation of antiretroviral agents in infants and children with human immunodeficiency virus: A perspective from the National Cancer Institute. Rev Infect Dis 1990;12(suppl 5):S561–S569.
3. Katz SL, Wilfert CM. Human immunodeficiency virus infection of newborns [Editorial]. N Engl J Med 1989;320:1687–1689.
4. Pizzo PA. Pediatric AIDS: Problems within problems. J Infect Dis 1990;161:316–325.
5. Selik R, Starcher E, Curran J. Opportunistic diseases reported in AIDS patients: Frequencies, associations, and trends. AIDS 1987;1:175–182.
6. Wheat LJ, Connolly-Springfield PA, Baker RL, et al. Disseminated histoplasmosis in the acquired immune deficiency syndrome: Clinical findings, diagnosis, and treatment, and review of the literature. Medicine 1990;69:361–364.
7. Graybill JR: Histoplasmosis and AIDS. J Infect Dis 1988;158:623–626.
8. Johnson PC, Khardori N, Najjar AF, Butt F, Mansell PWA, Sarosi GA. Progressive disseminated histoplasmosis in patients with acquired immunodeficiency syndrome. Am J Med 1988; 85:152–158.
9. Roberts C. Coccidioidomycosis in acquired immune deficiency syndrome. Depressed humoral as well as cellular immunity. Am J Med 1984;76:734–736.
10. Abrams DI, Robia M, Blumenfeld W, Simonson J, Cohen M, Hadley K. Disseminated coccidioidomycosis in AIDS. N Engl J Med 1984;310:986–987.
11. Bronniman D, Adam R, Galgiani J, et al. Coccidioidomycosis in the acquired immunodeficiency syndrome Ann Intern Med 1987;106:372–379.
12. Harrison H, Galgiani J, Reynolds A, et al. Amphotericin B and imidazole therapy of coccidioidal meningitis in children. Pediatr Infect Dis J 1983;2:216–221.
13. Shehab Z, Britton H, Dunn J. Imidazole therapy of coccidioidal meningitis in children. Pediatr Infect Dis J 1989;7:40–44.
14. Walsh TJ, Mitchell T. Dimorphic fungi causing systemic mycoses. In: Manual of clinical microbiology. 5th ed. Washington DC: American Society for Microbiology, 1991:630–658.
15. Kaufman L, Standard PG. Specific and rapid identification of medically important fungi by exoantigen detection. Annu Rev Microbiol 1987;41:209–225.
16. Roilides E, Clerici M, DePalma L, Rubin M, Pizzo PA, Shearer GM. Helper T-cell responses in children infected with human immunodeficiency virus type 1. J Pediatr 1991;118:724–730.
17. Walsh T, Pizzo P. Nosocomial fungal infections: A classification for hospital-acquired fungal infections and mycoses arising from endogenous flora or reactivation. Annu Rev Microbiol 1988;42:517–545.
18. Walsh TJ, Pizzo PA. Experimental gastrointestinal and disseminated candidiasis in immunocompromised animals. Eur J Epidemiol 1992;8:477–483.
19. Roy MJ, Walsh TJ. Histopathological and immunohistochemical changes in gut-associated lymphoid tissues following treatment of rabbits with dexamethasone. Lab Invest 1992;64:437–443.
20. Kobayashi RH, Rosenblatt HM, Carney JM, et al. *Candida* esophagitis and laryngitis in chronic mucocutaneous candidiasis. Pediatrics 1980;66:380–384.
21. Buckley RH. Immunodeficiency diseases. JAMA 1992;268:2797–2806.
22. Lane HC, Masur H, Edgar LC, Whalen G, Rook AH, Fauci AS. Abnormalities of B-cell activation and immunoregulation in patients with the acquired immunodeficiency syndrome. N Engl J Med 1983;309:453–458.
23. Lane HC, Depper JM, Greene WC, Whalen G, Rook AH, Fauci AS. Quantitative analysis of immune function in patients with the acquired immunodeficiency syndrome: Evidence for a selec-

tive defect in soluble antigen recognition. N Engl J Med 1985;313:79–84.

24. McCarthy GM. Host factors associated with HIV-related oral candidiasis. Oral Surg Oral Med Oral Pathol 1992;73:181–186.

25. Scully C. Oral manifestations of HIV infection and their management. I. More common lesions. Oral Surg Oral Med Oral Pathol 1991;71:158–166.

26. Scully C. Oral manifestations of HIV infection and their management. I. More common lesions. Oral Surg Oral Med Oral Pathol 1991;71:167–171.

27. Leggott PJ. Oral manifestations of HIV infection in children. Oral Surg Oral Med Oral Pathol 1992;73:187–192.

28. Walsh TJ, van Cutsem J, Polak A, Graybill JR. Pathogenesis, immunomodulation, and antifungal therapy of experimental invasive candiadiasis, histoplasmosis, and aspergillosis: Recent advances and concepts. J Med Vet Mycol 1992;30(suppl 1):225–240.

29. Kappe R, Levitz SM, Cassone A, and Washburn RG: Mechanisms of host defense against fungal infection. J Med Vet Mycol 1992;30(suppl 1):167–177.

30. Modlin RL, Segal GP, Hofman FM, et al. In situ localization of T lymphocytes in disseminated coccidioidomycosis. J Infect Dis 1985;151:314.

31. Woods GL, Goldsmith JC. Aspergillus infection of the central nervous system in patients with acquired immunodeficiency syndrome. Arch Neurol 1990;47:181–184.

32. Denning DW, Follansbee SE, Scolaro M, Norris S, Edelstein H, Stevens DA. Pulmonary aspergillosis in the acquired immunodeficiency syndrome. N Engl J Med 1991;324:654–662.

33. Minamoto GY, Barlam TF, Van der Els NJ. Invasive aspergillosis in patients with AIDS. Clin Infect Dis 1992;14:66–74.

34. Purcell KJ, Telzak EE, Armstrong D. Aspergillus species colonization and invasive disease in patients with AIDS. Clin Infect Dis 1992;14:141–148.

35. Walsh TJ. Invasive aspergillosis in patients with neoplastic diseases. Sem Respir Infect 1990;5:111–122.

36. Schaffner A. Pulmonary aspergillosis in AIDS [Letter]. N Engl J Med 1991;325:355.

37. Stevens DA, Denning DW. Pulmonary aspergillosis in AIDS [Letter]. N Engl J Med 1991;325:356–357.

38. Roilides E, Holmes A, Blake C, Pizzo PA, Walsh TJ. Impairment of neutrophil fungicidal activity in HIV-infected children against Aspergillus fumigatus hyphae. J Infect Dis 1993;167:905–911.

39. Washburn RG, Tuazon CU, Bennett JE. Phagocytic and fungicidal activity of monocytes from patients with acquired immunodeficiency syndrome. J Infect Dis 1985;151:565–566.

40. Russell C, Lay K. Natural history of Candida species and yeasts in the oral cavities of infants. Arch Oral Biol 1973;18:957–962.

41. Baley J, Kliegman R, Boxerbaum B, et al. Fungal colonization in the very low birth weight infant. Pediatrics 1986;78:225–232.

42. Klein RS, Harris CA, Small CB, Moll B, Lesser M, Friedland GH. Oral candidiasis in high-risk patients as the initial manifestation of the acquired immunodeficiency syndrome. N Engl J Med 1984;311:354–311.

43. Ketchem L, Berkowitz RJ, McIlveen L, Forrester D, Rakusan T. Oral findings in HIV-seropositive children. Pediatr Dent 1990;12:143–146.

44. Samaranayake LP. Oral mycoses in HIV infection. Oral Sur Oral Med Oral Pathol 1992;73:171–180.

45. Hass A, Hyatt AC, Kattan M, Weiner M, Hodes DS. Hoarseness in immunocompromised children: Association with invasive fungal infection. J Pediatr 1987;111:731–733.

46. Walsh T, Gray W. Candida epiglottitis in immunocompromised patients. Chest 1987;91:482–485.

47. Balsam D, Sorrano D, Barax C. Candida epiglottitis presenting as stridor in a child with HIV infection. Pediatr Radiol 1992;22:235–236.

48. Leggott P, Robertson P, Greenspan D, Wara D, Greenspan J. Oral manifestations of primary and acquired immunodeficiency diseases in children. Pediatr Dent 1987;9:98–104.

49. Roberts M, Brhim J, Rinne N. Oral manifestations of AIDS: a study of 84 patients. J Am Dent Assoc 1988;116:863–867.

50. Greenspan D, Hollander H, Friedman-Kien A, Freese U, Greenspan J. Oral hairy leucoplakia in two women, a hemophiliac, and a transfusion recipient. Lancet 1986;2:987–989.

51. De Souza Y, Greenspan D, Felton J, Hartzog G, Hammer M, Greenspan J. Localization of Epstein-Barr virus DNA in the epithelial cells of oral hairy leukoplakia by in situ hybridization on tissue sections. N Engl J Med 1989;320:1559–1560.

52. Greenspan JS, Mastrucci MT, Leggott PJ, et al. Oral hairy leukoplakia in a child [Letter]. AIDS 1988;2:143.

53. Leibovitz E, Rigaud M, Chandwani S, et al. Disseminated fungal infection in children with human immunodeficiency virus. Pediatr Infect Dis J 1991;10:888–894.

54. Alsina A, Mason M, Uphoff R, Riggsby S, Becker J, Murphy D. Catheter-associated Candida utilis fungemia in a patient with acquired immunodeficiency syndrome: Species verification with a molecular probe. J Clin Microbiol 1988;26:621–624.

55. Stellbrink HJ, Albrecht H, Fenske S, Koperski K. Candida krusei sepsis in HIV infection. AIDS 1992;6:746–748.

56. Meyer RD, Gaut PL. Candidal pyarthrosis in an AIDS patient. Scand J Infect Dis 1990;22:607–610.

57. Bruinsma-Adams IK. AIDS presenting as Candida albicans meningitis: A case report. AIDS 1991;5:1268–1269.

58. Stiehm ER. New and old immunodeficiencies. Pediatr Res 1993;33(suppl):S2–S8.

59. Butler K, Baker C. Candida: An increasingly important pathogen in the nursery. Pediatr Clin North Am 1988;35:543–563.

60. Lecciones JA, Lee JW, Navarro E, et al. Vascular catheter-associated fungemia in cancer patients: Analysis of 155 episodes. Rev Infect Dis 1992;14:875–883.

61. Odds F. *Candida* and candidosis. 2nd ed. Philadelphia: Bailliere Tindall, 1988.
62. Bodey GP, Fainstein V, eds. Candidiasis, New York: Raven, 1985.
63. Dismukes W. Cryptococcal meningitis in patients with AIDS. J Infect Dis 1988;157:624–628.
64. Kovacs J, Kovacs A, Polis M, Wright W, et al. Cryptococcosis in the acquired immunodeficiency syndrome. Ann Intern Med 1985;103:533–538.
65. Zuger A, Louie E, Holzman R, Simberkoff M, Rahal J. Cryptococcal disease in patients with the acquired immunodeficiency syndrome. Diagnostic features and outcome of treatment. Ann Intern Med 1986;104:234–240.
66. Eng R, Bishburg E, Smith S, Kapila R. Cryptococcal infections in patients with acquired immune deficiency syndrome. Am J Med 1986;81:19–23.
67. Leggiadro R, Kline M, Hughes W. Extrapulmonary cryptococcosis in children with AIDS. Pediatr Infect Dis J 1991;10:658–662.
68. Leggiadro R, Barrett F, Hughes W. Extrapulmonary cryptococcosis in immunocompromised infants and children. Pediatr Infect Dis J 1992;11:43–47.
69. Allende M, Horowitz M, Pass HI, Pizzo PA, Walsh TJ. Pulmonary cryptococcosis presenting as metastases in children with sarcoma. Pediatr Infect Dis J 1993;12:240–243.
70. Baldwin S, Stagno S, Odrezin G, Kelly D, Whitley R. Isolated *Cryptococcus neoformans* osteomyelitis in an immunocompetent child. Pediatr Infect Dis J 1988;7:289–292.
71. Walsh TJ, Hier DB, Caplan LR. Fungal infections of the central nervous system: Analysis of risk factors and clinical manifestations. Neurology 1985;35:1654–1657.
72. Pippard M, Dalgleish A, Gibson P, Malkovsky M, Webster A. Acquired immunodeficiency with disseminated cryptococcosis. Arch Dis Child 1986;61:289–302.
73. Jimenez-Acosta F, Casado M, Borbujo J, Soto-Melo J, Viguer J, Sanjurjo M. Cutaneous cryptococcosis mimicking molluscum contagiosum in a haemophiliac with AIDS. Clin Exp Dermatol 1987;12:446–450.
74. Leggiadro R, Barrett F, Hughes W. Disseminated histoplasmosis of infancy. Pediatr Infect Dis J 1988;7:799–805.
75. Schutze GE, Tucker NC, Jacobs RF. Histoplasmosis and perinatal human immunodeficiency virus [Letter]. Pediatr Infect Dis J 1992;11:501–502.
76. Byers M, Feldman S, Edwards J. Disseminated histoplasmosis as the acquired immunodeficiency syndrome-defining illness in an infant. Pediatr Infect Dis J 1992;11:127–128.
77. Hazelhurst J, Vismer H. Histoplasmosis presenting with unusual skin lesions in acquired immunodeficiency syndrome. West J Med 1985;113:345–348.
78. Henochowicz S, Mustafa M, Lawrinson W, et al. Cardiac aspergillosis in acquired immune deficiency syndrome. Am J Cardiol 1985;55:1239.
79. Jones P, Cohen R, Batts D, et al. Disseminated histoplasmosis, invasive pulmonary aspergillosis, and other opportunistic infections in a homosexual patient with the acquired immune deficiency syndrome. Sex Transm Dis 1983;10:202–204.
80. Lombardo G, Anadarao N, Lin C, et al. Fatal hemoptysis in a patient with AIDS-related complex and pulmonary aspergilloma. NY State J Med 1987;87:306–308.
81. Pervez N, Kleinerman J, Kattan M, et al. Pseudomembranous necrotizing bronchial aspergillosis. A variant of invasive aspergillosis in patient with hemophilia and acquired immune deficiency syndrome. Am J Med 1985;131:961–963.
82. Cohen MS, Isturiz RE, Malech HL, et al. Fungal infection in chronic granulomatous disease. The importance of the phagocyte in defense against fungi. Am J Med 1981;71:59–66.
83. Klotz S. *Malassezia furfur*. Infect Dis Clin North Am 1989;3:53–64.
84. Redline R, Redline S, Boxerbaum B, et al. Systemic *Malassezia furfur* infections in patients receiving intralipid therapy. Hum Pathol 1985;16:815–822.
85. Daniel CR, Norton LA, Scher RK. The spectrum of nail disease in patients with human immunodeficiency virus infection. J Am Acad Dermatol 1992;27:93–97.
86. Bibler M, Luber H, Glueck H, et al. Disseminated sporotrichosis in a patient with HIV infection after treatment for acquired factor VIII inhibitor. JAMA 1986:3125–3126.
87. Lipstein-Kresch E, Isenberg H, Singer C, et al. Disseminated *Sporothrix schenckii* infection with arthritis in a patient with acquired immunodeficiency syndrome. J Rheumatol 1985;12:805–808.
88. Leaf H, Simberkoff M. Invasive trichosporonosis in a patient with the acquired immunodeficiency syndrome. J Infect Dis 1989;160:356–357.
89. Walsh TJ, Melcher GP, Lee JW, Pizzo PA: Infections due to *Trichosporon* species: New concepts in mycology, pathogenesis, diagnosis, and treatment. Curr Top Med Mycol 1993, in press.
90. Connolly G, Forbes A, Gleeson J, Gazzard B. Investigation of upper gastrointestinal symptoms in patients with AIDS. AIDS 1989;3:453–456.
91. Bonacini M, Young T, Laine L. The causes of esophageal symptoms in human immunodeficiency virus infection: A prospective study of 110 patients. Arch Intern Med 1991;151:1567–1572.
92. Walsh T, Belitsos N, Hamilton S. Bacterial esophagitis in immunocompromised patients. Arch Intern Med 1986;146:1345–1348.
93. Walsh T, Hamilton S, Belitsos N. Esophageal candidiasis. Diagnosis and treatment of an increasingly recognized fungal infection. Postgrad Med J 1988;84:193–205.
94. Walsh T, Hutchins G. Postoperative fungal infections of the heart in children. J Pediatr Surg 1980;15:325–331.
95. Bille J, Stockman L, Roberts G, et al. Evaluation of a lysis centrifugation system for recovery of yeasts and filamentous fungi from blood. J Clin Microbiol 1983;18:469–471.
96. Bille J, Edson R, Roberts G, et al. Clinical evaluation of the lysis centrifugation blood culture system for the detection of fungemia and compari-

son with a conventional biphasic broth blood culture system. J Clin Microbiol 1984;19: 126–128.

97. Brannon P, Kiehn T. Clinical comparison of lysis centrifugation and radiometric resin systems for blood culture. J Clin Microbiol 1986;24:886–887.

98. Walsh TJ, Pizzo PA. Laboratory diagnosis of candidiasis. In: Bodey GP, ed. Candidiasis. 2nd ed. New York: Raven, 1993:109–136.

99. de Repentigny L. Serodiagnosis of candidiasis, aspergillosis, and cryptococcosis. Clin Infect Dis 1992;14:S11–S22.

100. Thaler M, Pastakia B, Shawker T. Hepatic candidiasis in cancer patients: The evolving picture of the syndrome. Ann Intern Med 1988;108: 88–100.

101. Bottone E, Wormser G. Capsule-deficient cryptococci in AIDS. Lancet 1985;2:553.

102. Wheat L, Kohler R, Tewari R. Diagnosis of disseminated histoplasmosis by detection of Histoplasma capsulatum antigen in serum and urine specimens. N Engl J Med 1986;314:83–88.

103. Walsh T, Pizzo P. Treatment of systemic fungal infections: Recent advances and current problems. Eur J Clin Microbiol Infect Dis 1988;7:460–475.

104. Graybill J. Systemic fungal infections diagnosis and treatment I: Therapeutic agents. Infect Dis Clin North Am 1988;2:805–825.

105. Saag M, Dismukes WE. Azole antifungal agents: Emphasis on new triazoles. Antimicrob Agents Chemother 1988;32:1–8.

106. Lyman C and Walsh TJ: Systemically administered antifungal agents: a review of clinical pharmacology and therapeutic applications. Drugs 1992;44:9–35.

106. Viscoli C, Castagnola E, Fioredda F, Ciravegna B, Barigione G, Terragna A: Fluconazole in the treatment of candidiasis in immunocompromised children. Antimicrob Agents Chemother 1991;35: 365–367.

107. Lee JW, Amantea MA, Seibel NI, Whitcomb P, Pizzo PA, Walsh TJ. Safety, tolerance, and pharmacokinetics of fluconazole in children with neoplastic diseases J Pediatr 1992;120:987–993.

108. Francis P, Walsh TJ. The evolving role of flucytosine in immunocompromised patients: New insights into safety, pharmacokinetics, and antifungal therapy. Rev Infect Dis 1992;15:1003–1018.

109. Lalor E, Rabeneck L. Esophageal candidiasis in AIDS. Dig Dis Sci 1991;36:279–281.

110. Larsen RA. Azoles and AIDS. J Infect Dis 1990; 162:727–730.

111. Odds FC: Candida infections in AIDS. Int J STD AIDS 1992;3:157–160.

112. Just-Nubling G, Gentschew G, Dohle M, Bottinger C, Helm EB, Stille W. Fluconazole in the treatment of oropharyngeal candidosis in HIV-positive patients. Mycoses 1990;33: 435–440.

113. Nathwani D, Green ST, McGuire W, Goldberg DJ, Kennedy DH. New triazole antifungal agents (fluconazole and itraconazole) in the treatment of HIV-related gastrointestinal candidiasis. Scand J Infect Dis 1989;21:355–356.

114. Cirelli A, Rossi F, Ciardi M. Treatment of oropharyngeal and esophageal candidiasis with a new antifungal agent, fluconazole, in HIV-infected patients. Curr Ther Res Clin Exp 1990;47:81–87.

115. Esposito R, Castagna A, Foppa CU. Maintenance therapy of oropharyngeal candidiasis in HIV-infected patients with fluconazole. AIDS 1990;4: 1033–1034.

116. Fox R, Neal KR, Leen CLS, Ellis ME, Mandal BK. Fluconazole-resistant Candida in AIDS. J Infect 22:201–204.

117. Kitchen VS, Savage M, Harris JRW. Candida albicans resistance in AIDS. J Infect 1991;22:204–205.

118. Troilet N, Drussel C, Bille J, Glauser MP, Chave Chuv JP. Fluconazole-resistant oral candidiasis in HIV-infected patients: In vitro–in vivo correlation [Abstract 1202]. 32nd Interscience Conference on Antimicrobial Agents and Chemotherapy, Anaheim, 1992.

119. Dupont B, Improvisi L, Eliaszewicz M, Pialoux G, et al. Resistance of Candida albicans to fluconazole in AIDS patients [Abstract 1203]. 32nd Interscience Conference on Antimicrobial Agents and Chemotherapy, Anaheim, 1992.

120. Holmberg K, Meyer RD. Fungal infections in patients with AIDS and AIDS-related complex. Scand J Infect Dis 1986;18:179–192.

121. Diamond RD. The growing problem of mycoses in patients infected with the human immunodeficiency virus. Rev Infect Dis 1991;13:480–486.

122. Viviani MA. Opportunistic fungal infections in patients with acquired immune deficiency syndrome. Chemotherapy 1992;38(suppl):35–42.

123. Viviani MA, Tortorano AM, Carbonera GP, et al. Itraconazole for cryptococcal infection in the acquired immunodeficiency syndrome. Ann Intern Med 1987;106:166.

124. Larsen RA, Leal MAE, Chan LS. Fluconazole compared with amphotericin B plus flucytosine for cryptococcal meningitis in AIDS. A randomized trial. Ann Intern Med 1990;113:183–187.

125. Denning DW, Tucker RM, Hanson LH, Hamilton JR, Stevens DA. Itraconazole therapy for cryptococcal meningitis and cryptococcosis. Arch Intern Med 1989;149:2301–2308.

126. Chuck SL, Sande MA. Infections with Cryptococcus neoformans in the acquired immunodeficiency syndrome. N Engl J Med 1989; 321:794–799.

127. Pippard MJ, Dalgleish A, Gibson P, Malkovsky M, Webster ADB. Acquired immunodeficiency with disseminated cryptococcosis. Arch Dis Child 1986;61:289–302.

128. Ting SF, Glader BE, Prober CG. Cryptococcus infection in a nine year old child with hemophilia and acquired immunodeficiency syndrome. Pediatr Infect Dis J 1991;10:76–77.

129. Dozic S, Suvakovic V, Cvetkovic D, Jevtovic DJ, Skender M. Neoplastic angioendotheliomatosis (NAE) of the CNS in a patient with AIDS subacute encephalitis, diffuse leukoencephalopathy, and meningocerebral cryptococcosis. Clin Neuropathol 1990;9:284–289.

130. Rubin LG, Gleit-Caduri D, Krilov LR. Multiple opportunistic infections in an adolescent with AIDS, with recovery. Child Hosp Q 1989;1:299–303.

131. Saag MS, Powderly WG, Cloud GA, et al. Comparison of amphotericin B with fluconazole

in the treatment of acute AIDS associated crypto-coccal meningitis. N Engl J Med 1992;326:83–89.

132. Powderly WG, Saag MS, Cloud GA, et al. A controlled trial of fluconazole or amphotericin B to prevent relapse of cryptococcal meningitis in patients with the acquired immunodeficiency syndrome. N Engl J Med 1992;326:793–798.

133. Wheat LJ, Hafner RE, Ritchie M, Schneider D. Itraconazole is effective treatment for histoplasmosis in AIDS: Prospective multi-center non-comparative trial [Abstract 1206]. 32nd Interscience Conference on Antimicrobial Agents and Chemotherapy, Anaheim, 1992.

134. Fosson A, Wheeler W. Short-term amphotericin B treatment of severe childhood histoplasmosis. J Pediatr 1975;86:32–36.

135. Burch PA, Karp JE, Merz WG, Kuhlman J, Fishman E. Favorable outcome of invasive aspergillosis in patients with acute leukemia. J Clin Oncol 1987;5:1985–1993.

136. Denning DW, Tucker RM, Hanson LH, Stevens DA. Treatment of invasive aspergillosis with itraconazole. Am J Med 1989;86:791–800.

18

Herpesvirus Infections in Children with Human Immunodeficiency Virus

Sue Jue and Richard J. Whitley

Herpesviruses are a common cause of infections in humans and pose unique challenges to the clinician because they result in a spectrum of illness ranging from that which is totally asymptomatic to life-threatening disease. These organisms establish latency and can recur periodically throughout life. Most infections from these viruses occur early in childhood and are asymptomatic, but clinical illness throughout childhood and adulthood occurs. Transmission requires inoculation of infected secretions from one person into a susceptible individual. The seven human herpesviruses are cytomegalovirus (CMV), varicella-zoster virus (VZV), herpes simplex virus types 1 and 2 (HSV-1 and HSV-2), Epstein-Barr virus (EBV), and human herpesvirus types 6 and 7 (HHV-6 and HHV-7).

These viruses cause significant morbidity and mortality in adults and children who are immunosuppressed, including those with human immunodeficiency virus (HIV) infection (Table 18.1). The disease burden caused by herpesviruses in children with HIV infection can be the consequence of congenital, perinatal, or primary infection in addition to reactivation of latent infection. For example, infants born with HIV infection may have concomitant CMV infection acquired either congenitally or postnatally (breast feeding, transfusion, day care acquisition, etc.) (1). Mothers who are HIV infected are also immune deficient and may be more likely to transmit a herpesvirus such as CMV or HSV to their infants, although this is not proven. The potential role of all the herpesviruses as a cofactor in the development of AIDS has been postulated but warrants further evaluation (2, 3). This chapter will focus on the unique manifestations of herpesvirus infections, particularly CMV, VZV, and HSV, in children with HIV infection. Attention will be devoted to

Table 18.1. Target Organs and Disease Syndromes of Herpes Group Viruses

Virus	Target Organs	Disease Syndromes
HSV-1 and -2	Mucous membranes (oralabial and genital), skin, cornea, brain, perianal	Oral and genital mucocutaneous lesions, retinitis, esophagitis keratitis, encephalitis chorioretinitis, hepatitis, pneumonitis
CMV	Lung, liver, retina, gastrointestinal tract, brain	Chorioretinitis, esophagitis, pneumonitis, hepatitis, colitis encephalitis
VZV	Mucous membranes, skin, lung, brain, liver	Chickenpox, shingles, recurrent or chronic varicella, pneumonitis hepatitis esophagitis, meningoencephalitis
EBV	Lymph nodes, liver, spleen, lung, B cells	Mononucleosis, lymphocytic interstitial pneumonia, hairy leukoplakia, lymphomas

the natural history, diagnosis, and treatment of CMV, VZV, and HSV infections in particular. Diagnostic tests for the herpes group viruses are shown in Table 18.2. Very little is known about HHV-6 and HHV-7 in the HIV-infected child and, therefore, will only be very briefly mentioned. A more detailed discussion of EBV appears in Chapter 25.

The human herpesviruses are enveloped double-stranded DNA viruses. They are classified into three subfamilies according to host range and other biologic properties. The first subfamily consists of HSV-1 and -2 and VZV that grow rapidly in cell culture in a wide range of tissues, efficiently destroying host cells. CMV is a member of the second subfamily and is characterized by slow growth in very restricted types of cells. Finally, EBV grows slowly in and immortalizes lymphoid cells of the natural host.

The prototype of the human herpesviruses is HSV, and it is composed of an inner core containing linear double-stranded DNA surrounded concentrically by an icosahedral capsid of ~100 nm, an amorphous material (tegument), and an outer envelope composed of lipids and glycoproteins. CMV, EBV, and VZV resemble HSV morphologically but vary in size and genomic structure.

Virus replication in eukaryotic cells is associated with coordinately regulated expression of designated classes of virus genes (α, β, γ) resulting in the synthesis of immediate, early, and late proteins, including proteins involved in DNA replication, glycoproteins, and structural proteins of the viral capsid. Assembly of the virus core and capsid occurs within the nucleus; envelopment occurs at the nuclear membrane, and egress from the nucleus is through the endoplasmic reticulum and Golgi. Mature virions are transported to the outer membrane of the host cell within vesicles. The release of progeny virus is accompanied by lysis of the host cell and cell death.

CYTOMEGALOVIRUS INFECTION
Background

As with the other herpesviruses, CMV is a ubiquitous organism commonly spread

Table 18.2. Diagnostic Tests for Herpes Group Virus Infection[a]

Virus	Virus Culture		Histology		DNA Probes
	Routine	Rapid (shell vial)[b]	Indirect (FA/ immunonoperoxidase[b])	Direct[c]	
HSV-1 and -2	24–72 hr from lesions, throat, eye, tissue, CSF (rarely)	24-hr tissue culture stain by FA or immunoperoxidase	Cells from base of lesions stained with monoclonal Ab	Tzanck smear (giant cells)	HSV-DNA probes; tissue in situ hybridization or immuno-peroxidase; detection of DNA by PCR[d]
CMV	24 hr–6 wk from urine, tissue PBL (buffy coat), BAL	24-hr stain tissue culture by FA or immunoperoxidase	CMV immunoper-oxidase staining BAL/tissue	CMV inclusions H&E	DNA probe, in situ hybridi-zation, tissue and buffy coat; detection of DNA by PCR[d]
VZV	7–10 days from lesions, base vesicular fluid CSF, buffy coat		FA on base of lesions poly or monoclonal Ab to VZV	Tzanck smear (giant cells)	In situ hybridi-zation, cDNA on tissue, immuno-peroxidase staining (PCR[d] in development)

[a]FA, fluorescent antibody; PBL, peripheral blood leukocyte; BAL, bronchoalveolar lavage; H&E, hematoxylin and eosin; Ab, antibody; PCR, polymerase chain reaction.
[b]Preferred.
[c]Not specific.
[d]Experimental.

among humans. Disease associated with CMV can occur in newborns and immuno-compromised patients, such as transplant recipients and individuals with AIDS, resulting in significant morbidity and mortality. Humans are the only known reservoir for CMV infection. Transmission can either be vertical (mother to baby) or horizontal (person to person). Sources of CMV for infection of the susceptible individual include blood, urine, saliva, tears, stool, and genital secretions. Factors that influence the incidence of infection include age, socioeconomic status, and housing conditions with the highest seroprevalence rates in the lower socioeconomic groups of more developed countries. Horizontal transmission of CMV most commonly occurs as a result of salivary contamination, but contact with infected urine can also result in infection. An example of horizontal transmission of CMV is that which occurs between children attending day care centers from the sharing and mouthing of toys. Under the latter circumstances, CMV excretion rates approach 70% for children 1 3 years old. Young children can, then, transmit CMV to their parents and other care takers. In adolescents and adults, sexual transmission occurs, and CMV can be isolated from semen and cervical secretions.

Vertical transmission is best exemplified by maternal to fetal infection, resulting in congenital CMV infection. Congenital CMV infection is the most common intrauterine infection affecting ~1% of all live-born infants (4). Symptomatic CMV infection occurs in 5 10% of these cases and is associated with a high incidence of mental retardation, sensorineural hearing loss, chorioretinitis, and neurologic defects. Ninety percent of these infants have no clinical manifestations at birth, but 5 15% may develop hearing loss as a late appearing abnormality usually within the first 2 years of life (4). An additional 5% of the infants in this group develop microcephaly with degrees of mental retardation and neuromuscular defects (4).

Infection of the fetus in utero can occur whether the mother experiences a primary (first exposure) or recurrent (reactivated) infection. Preexisting maternal immunity does not prevent the transmission of CMV to the fetus but provides substantial protection against symptomatic congenital infection (5). Congenital infections resulting from recurrence of CMV during pregnancy are less likely to be clinically apparent than maternal primary infection. Most congenitally infected infants who are symptomatic at birth and/or develop sequelae are thought to result from primary maternal CMV infection.

Vertical transmission also can lead to perinatal infection, namely an infection acquired at delivery by exposure to CMV-infected maternal genital secretions or ingestion of infected breast milk. Overall, perinatal CMV infection occurs in ~40 60% of infants of seropositive mothers who are breast fed for more than 1 month (6) and 25 50% of those exposed to CMV in the birth canal (7). Although the quantity of virus excreted by infants with perinatal infection is less than that found with congenital infection, the infection is chronic because virus is shed for years. Other routes of CMV transmission include blood transfusion or receipt of an organ transplant from an infected donor. By adulthood 60 100% of individuals have been infected with CMV.

Pathogenesis

Many host and virus factors are associated with pathology after CMV infection. Although infection with CMV is common, especially early in life as described above, associated disease is a relatively exceptional event, occurring rarely in immunocompetent infants, children, and adults. Disease can result as a major complication in the premature, immunodeficient, or immunosuppressed host and usually reflects the site(s) of virus replication. Thus, CMV can be found to replicate in multiple body sites including salivary glands, prostate, cervix, testes, and possibly peripheral blood lymphocytes. The site of latency is unknown but may occur in peripheral blood lymphocytes.

Under conditions of immune compromise, especially impairment of cell-mediated immunity, virus may reactivate to produce various clinical syndromes including chorioretinitis, esophagitis, colitis, pneumonia, encephalitis, and adrenalitis (8). In the context of HIV infection, disease pathogenesis likely varies between adults and children. For adults, primary CMV infection occurred before HIV infection, and these individuals can be infected by multiple CMV strains (9). In contrast, infants and children may be more likely to be infected with HIV before experiencing primary CMV infection.

Host defense mechanisms against CMV include humoral and cellular immune responses. Humoral immunity provides the best evidence of prior infection and, hence, the ability to transmit infection. There is some evidence that passive administration of antibodies modifies or possibly prevents disease in both mice and humans.

Clinical Manifestations

The clinical impact of CMV infection differs according to the time of acquisition. If clinical illness occurs in an immunocompetent host, a heterophile negative mononucleosis syndrome may ensue with fever, myalgia, and asthenia. However, in the HIV-infected individual CMV infection is more commonly associated with disease than in the normal host. Numerous studies have documented an extremely high prevalence of CMV infection in most adult HIV-infected patient populations: ≥90% of adult patients with AIDS had culture-proven or histologic evidence of CMV infection at autopsy; ≥25% may experience life- or sight-threatening infection (10). For children, nearly 60% with AIDS have either systemic CMV disease or asymptomatic shedding (11 15). Clinical manifestations of CMV disease in children with HIV infection include interstitial pneumonia, encephalitis, hepatitis, gastritis, colitis, and chorioretinitis.

CMV Pneumonitis

Pneumonia attributed to CMV is considered to result in a diffuse interstitial process. Isolation of CMV from bronchoalveolar lavage or lung biopsy specimens from both adults and children with AIDS is relatively common, but the true pathogenic role of the virus is unclear. Many HIV patients with pulmonary disease and CMV isolated from their lungs have concomitant infection with other pathogens such as *Pneumocystis carinii* and may respond to *P.*

carinii therapy alone. Hypoxemia is usually present, with patient complaints of gradual worsening shortness of breath and a dry nonproductive cough. Differential diagnosis of children presenting with interstitial pneumonia includes *P. carinii* pneumonia, CMV, lymphoid interstitial pneumonia, tuberculosis, chlamydia, and other respiratory viruses as well as mycobacterial, fungal, and bacterial infections.

Chorioretinitis

Clinical evidence of CMV retinitis in adults with AIDS occurs in at least 5 10% with autopsy studies indicating retinitis in up to 30% of patients (16). In adult patients, retinitis is occasionally the presenting manifestation of AIDS, but it more commonly presents months to years after the diagnosis of HIV. Although well recognized in adults, CMV retinitis in the pediatric HIV population is becoming more common as the diagnosis is pursued (see Chapter 24). Ophthalmologic examination reveals large white perivascular exudates and hemorrhages with a cottage cheese and catsup appearance. Lesions initially involve the periphery of the retina but may progress to involve the macula and optic disc. Diagnosis of CMV retinitis must be made clinically because patients may or may not have positive CMV cultures from blood or urine. Other causes of chorioretinitis to be considered include infection with toxoplasmosis, syphilis, toxocara, and HSV.

Gastrointestinal Disease

CMV colitis occurs in at least 5 10% of adult patients with AIDS with complaints of diarrhea, pain, weight loss, anorexia, and fever. The true frequency of CMV colitis in HIV-infected children is not well established. Differential diagnosis of colitis includes infection from *Cryptosporidium*, giardiasis, *Mycobacterium avium* complex, *Salmonella*, *Entamoeba histolytica*, *Isospora*, *Shigella*, *Campylobacter*, or *Clostridium difficile*. Infection may compromise mucosal barriers and predispose to infection with other pathogens as well. Children with HIV with or without CMV may exhibit failure to thrive caused by malabsorption and/or intractable diarrhea requiring supplemental nutritional support.

Esophagitis in AIDS patients is primarily due to *Candida albicans* or HSV but can also be caused by CMV. Frequently, large shallow ulcerations are present in the esophagus, but single ulcers have also been reported. Diagnosis is usually made by endoscopy with biopsy showing histologic evidence of intranuclear inclusions, positive viral culture, or detection of CMV antigen in tissue.

Histologic evidence of CMV hepatitis is found in nearly half of HIV-infected children who have evidence of hepatic infection. Although most HIV-infected children will develop hepatosplenomegaly and elevated liver enzymes, clinical symptoms are uncommon. Differential diagnosis of hepatitis includes HIV and drug reactions as well as hepatitis A, B, and C. Liver biopsy with specific histopathological change (multinucleated giant cells) from CMV may be helpful in diagnosis. Other hepatic manifestations include cholangitis, papillary stenosis, and acalculous cholecystitis.

Central Nervous System Disease

Children with AIDS develop a progressive encephalopathy, pyramidal tract abnormalities, and microcephaly (17). Subacute encephalitis may occur in HIV-infected children with CMV, but it is difficult to determine whether brain involvement is due to CMV, HIV, or both. Fever, altered mental status, personality changes, headaches, confusion, and somnolence are frequent symptoms regardless of the etiology. Cultures of cerebrospinal fluid (CSF) in adults have yielded HIV in two-thirds of seropositive patients and CMV in rare cases with neurologic symptoms (18). Diagnosis can be suspected from CSF cultures but is confirmed only by brain biopsy with evidence of CMV inclusions, isolation of virus, or identification of viral antigen or nucleic acid in tissue.

Diagnosis

Diagnosis of CMV infection in children and adults, whether healthy or immunosuppressed, requires laboratory confirmation and cannot be made on clinical grounds.

Laboratory diagnosis of CMV depends on either isolation of the virus (optimal), antigen detection, or demonstration of a serologic rise in antibodies (seroconversion). Because CMV is common in normal children, infection must be distinguished from disease. Diagnosis is therefore based on histopathologic or other evidence of disease at the organ sites involved along with isolation of the virus. Since children may acquire HIV perinatally, it might be prudent to obtain a CMV urine culture within the first 3 weeks of life for babies born to HIV-infected women to exclude concomitant CMV infection. In general, culture of the urine is the most consistent site for virus isolation with culture of saliva yielding nearly the same order of sensitivity.

Diagnosis of CMV infections is not always straightforward. For example, the diagnosis of pneumonia is made by a combination of factors: positive CMV culture from lung tissue or bronchoalveolar lavage; presence in tissue of pathognomonic cells with intranuclear inclusion bodies or CMV antigen by immunoperoxidase, cDNA probes, etc.; absence of other pathogens. Buffy coat cultures may document viremia.

Virus Isolation

Virus may be recovered from body fluids or from tissues obtained from either biopsy or at autopsy. In addition to urine, CMV can be isolated from blood, throat washings, saliva, tears, milk, semen, stool, and vaginal/cervical secretions. Specimens are inoculated into susceptible cell lines of human origin, such as human fibroblasts, and observed for cytopathogenic effect that occurs in 1 4 weeks. Unfortunately, isolation of virus in these fluids in immunocompromised patients may offer little information about the severity of infection. Cultures from bronchoalveolar lavage, biopsy material, and blood are more indicative of disease. Viremia is considered a marker of active infection and has been shown to correlate with significant CMV disease (19, 20).

Antigen Detection

Because of the prolonged time for the results of virus culture, more rapid methods of virus detection have been developed. A modification of conventional technique (centrifuging sample onto cells and utilizing monoclonal antibody to directly detect CMV antigens in cell culture by immunofluorescence) can document the presence of CMV within 12 24 hr of inoculation. The shell vial technique has a sensitivity that approaches 100% but falls to 70% in populations in which clinical specimens contain low quantities of virus.

DNA hybridization techniques, including hybridization of nucleic acids and direct in situ hybridization, remain in use only in research laboratories. The introduction of polymerase chain reaction has provided a means for the rapid and early detection of CMV, but it is not widely available.

Serologic Evaluation

Serologic diagnosis in infants may be difficult to interpret because maternal transplacental antibody may persist for 6 9 months. Various serologic assays, including complement fixation, latex agglutination, indirect hemagglutination, immunofluorescence, enzyme-linked immunosorbent assay (ELISA), and immunoassays, have been used to detect IgG antibodies reactive with CMV and IgM antibody detection is particularly important in infants.

Therapy

Although various antiviral agents have been used to treat symptomatic CMV infection, only ganciclovir (cytovene), an analogue of acyclovir and foscarnet, have been shown to have potent activity against CMV in vitro and in vivo. The triphosphate derivative of ganciclovir inhibits CMV DNA polymerase.

Although there is limited experience with the use of ganciclovir in children, favorable clinical responses to ganciclovir therapy have been reported in adult patients with AIDS suffering from CMV retinitis and gastrointestinal disease and other immunocompromised patients with life-threatening CMV manifestations. The usual dosage of ganciclovir is 7.5 15 mg/kg/day divided into two or three doses for 10 21 days. For patients with chorioretinitis, this regimen results in an initial clinical response consisting of improvement in visual acuity and/or appearance of the retina in 80% of adult AIDS patients with CMV retinitis (21, 22). Once therapy is discontinued, however, relapse is common. Ganciclovir reduces or eliminates virus excretion and viremia during administration, but both return at variable intervals after cessation of therapy. Therefore maintenance therapy (5 10 mg/kg/day) is required. For patients who continue to progress on maintenance therapy, reinduction or an increase in maintenance dose appears warranted. The most significant toxicity is bone marrow suppression, which prevents maintenance therapy in upward of 38% of patients (23 26), with dose reduction or interruption of therapy necessary in up to 50% of patients because of anemia, neutropenia, or thrombocytopenia. Other adverse side effects include central nervous system or gastrointestinal dysfunction, thrombophlebitis, and azoospermia in animals (27). Parenthetically, an oral formulation of ganciclovir is under evaluation in adults and children with HIV infection to determine if the reactivation of CMV and associated disease (e.g., chorioretinitis) can be prevented.

The pharmacokinetics of ganciclovir in newborns with symptomatic congenital CMV disease was evaluated in 27 babies using either 4 or 6 mg/kg/day every 12 hr for 6 weeks (28). The plasma half-life was similar to that found in adult studies, namely 2.5 hr, with peak and trough levels predictable from earlier investigations. The volume of distribution was 669 – 70 ml/kg for the 4-mg/kg group and 749 – 59 ml/kg for the 6-mg/kg group. The drug clearances for the 4- and 6-mg/kg groups were 189 – 28 and 213 – 21 ml/hr/kg, respectively. Pharmacodynamically, therapy resulted in improved hearing (38%) and growth (60%) and an increased platelet count (45%). All babies experienced a decrease in the quantity of virus excreted in the urine; however, all had return of viral excretion at near original levels in the urine within 2 weeks of cessation of therapy. In addition, retinal hemorrhage occurred in four babies, but it was unclear if this was due to drug administration, reactivation of CMV, or both. In one case, a 6-month infant with AIDS and CMV retinitis was treated with ganciclovir at 5 mg/kg every 12 hr for 21 days with ocular improvement and was discharged on maintenance therapy. This patient later succumbed to *P. carinii* pneumonia, and on the day of his death both urine and blood cultures were negative for CMV (29). This child had no adverse reactions to therapy.

One major problem in treating CMV disease in HIV-infected patients is that hematologic toxicity appears to be exacerbated by the concomitant administration of zidovudine and ganciclovir. One approach to this problem is administration of hematologic growth factors such as granulocyte macrophage-colony stimulating factor or granulocyte-colony stimulating factor in combination with ganciclovir (30). Preliminary studies using this regimen in adult AIDS patients have suggested that leukopenic patients who are intolerant of ganciclovir were able to continue therapy with continual daily doses of granulocyte macrophage-colony stimulating factor. Ganciclovir neutropenia is usually reversible once therapy is discontinued or the dosage reduced. Ganciclovir resistant strains of CMV have been isolated from immunosuppressed patients receiving long-term therapy (31). Therefore alternative therapies for CMV must be developed.

Foscarnet is an alternative therapeutic to ganciclovir. All tested herpesvirus DNA polymerases are inhibited by foscarnet, which reversibly and noncompetitively inhibits the activity of CMV DNA polymerase. Controlled trials in HIV-infected patients have shown it to be efficacious in treating CMV retinitis (32, 33). The major toxicity is renal, and it is not associated with myelosuppression. Foscarnet has also been found to sequester in bone and cartilage where it can reside for months. Foscarnet has been administered by intermittent infusion to adult AIDS patients with CMV retinitis (34). The dose of foscarnet used was 60 mg/kg/body weight three times a day (induction regimen) followed by a maintenance regimen of 90 mg/kg once a day. The dose in children has not been established.

Although ganciclovir and foscarnet are effective for the treatment of CMV retinitis in patients, the benefits are limited. A child

with HIV infection and CMV retinitis that progressed despite therapy with either agent alone received the combination of the two drugs, resulting in a sustained clinical response (35). The approach of combination therapy in the future will, most assuredly, be evaluated.

High doses of polyclonal immunoglobulin when administered intravenously and prophylactically to CMV-seronegative bone marrow transplant recipients may have an effect in modifying the severity of CMV infection. The role for this prophylactic in the treatment of CMV infection in AIDS patients has not been determined. CMV immunoglobulin, a hyperimmune CMV globulin, also has clinical utility in the prevention of CMV infection in seronegative renal transplant recipients who receive a graft from a seropositive donor. The effectiveness of CMV IgG in other settings, such as in HIV-infected patients, is unproven.

Prevention

In general, CMV is not very contagious, and its transmission requires close direct contact with infected secretions. Prevention is dependent on knowledge of the sources of infection in the environment. Asymptomatic infection is extremely common in newborns and during infancy and early childhood. Infants younger than 2 years in day care are at high risk for acquisition of CMV. This fact should be remembered in the placement of HIV-infected infants in a day care setting, but it is not a contraindication to their placement. Principle sources of CMV infection among women of childbearing age are sexual contacts and exposure to children excreting CMV. Commonsense measures such as thorough hand washing and avoiding contact with secretions should help prevent acquisition of infection. Transmission of CMV via blood transfusion to premature neonates can be virtually eliminated by the use of CMV-seronegative blood products, filtered blood, or deglycerolized, frozen red blood cells (36, 37). In addition, breast feeding is also a means of transmission for CMV and HIV. Currently breast feeding is not recommended in the United States for HIV-infected mothers a recommendation that should also reduce the risk of CMV acquisition. The classic strategy of prevention is immunization. There are two live CMV vaccines under study. The Towne live attenuated vaccine has been found to partially protect seronegative renal transplant patients from severe CMV disease, but it does not protect from infection (38). The most important use of a successful CMV vaccine would be for the immunization of women before pregnancy to prevent serious consequences of congenital CMV infection. In 22 women immunized with the AD169 vaccine and followed for 8 years, antibody and lymphocyte responses disappeared in 50% of the women (39). The use of a live CMV vaccine is controversial because of concern regarding reactivation. It is not approved for any use in the United States.

Future Considerations

Diagnostic techniques that distinguish infection from disease more precisely and allow rapid quantitation of viral load are essential for early diagnosis of CMV infection and assessment of therapeutic efficacy. Development of antiviral agents with less toxicity and more manageable treatment regimens (oral bioavailability) would be of great benefit.

VARICELLA-ZOSTER VIRUS
Background

Varicella (chickenpox) is usually a benign exanthematous illness characterized by a diffuse vesicular rash caused by primary infection with VZV. Overall, chickenpox is a disease of childhood since 90% of cases occur in children younger than 15 years. Approximately 10% of individuals over age 15 remain susceptible to VZV infection. Varicella is usually acquired by contact with other infected children either via the respiratory route or by direct contact with cutaneous lesions. The incubation is 2 weeks for both the normal and immunocompromised child with a range of 10 21 days. Secondary infection rates among susceptible household contacts approach 90% (40, 41). Children may also contract varicella from an adult with herpes zoster (shingles), which is the reactivated form of VZV infection.

VZV infections are usually self-limited in normal children, but complications can include secondary bacterial infections, pneumonitis, cerebellar ataxia, transverse myelitis, and encephalitis (42, 43). The frequency of complications and severity of disease increases in immunocompromised children and adults, as will be described below. Children infected with HIV represent the largest reservoir of VZV-susceptible immunodeficient children in the world. Because most HIV-infected children acquire HIV perinatally, primary infection with VZV usually occurs in the context of preexisting HIV infection. In contrast, VZV disease in immunocompetent adults is usually due to reactivation of latent virus causing herpes zoster that, obviously, preceded infection with HIV.

Herpes zoster caused by reactivation of latent VZV typically affects the elderly but is seen with increased frequency among immunodeficient patients, particularly those with deficiencies in cell-mediated immunity. Among children with AIDS, the interval between chickenpox and shingles may be reduced to weeks or months, instead of decades (44, 45). The appearance of shingles in children and young adults serves as a clinical marker for HIV infection in high-risk groups and may be an indicator of both disease progression and further suppression of cell-mediated immunity in those individuals already infected with HIV (46, 47).

Pathogenesis and Natural History
Chickenpox

Acquisition of VZV occurs by airborne transmission or contact with infected skin lesions (shingles) by the susceptible host. After a 2-week incubation, chickenpox in the immunocompetent host is associated with a prodrome lasting 1 2 days, followed by the appearance of a generalized pruritic vesicular rash and relatively few systemic manifestations. The characteristic vesicular lesions appear on the face and trunk and spread centripetally to involve the extremities. The lesions progress to pustules and form crusts. Duration of illness is generally 3 7 days with a period of vesicle formation lasting 2 5 days. Severity of skin lesions is variable, but most children have <400 lesions/m^2. New lesions rarely appear after the 7th day in the immunocompetent child (48).

Infection with VZV can cause significant morbidity and mortality in certain high-risk groups such as neonates exposed shortly after birth, adults, and the immunocompromised host. In immunocompromised children with impaired cellular immunity such as those with leukemia, lymphoma, or HIV, progressive varicella characterized by continuing eruption of lesions and high fever persisting into the second week of illness can occur. Duration of lesion formation averages more than 2 weeks in untreated patients, pneumonia develops in over 25% of patients, encephalitis occurs in 6% of patients, and hepatitis in nearly 20% of patients in the absence of therapy. Overall, half of immunocompromised children with chickenpox will have a visceral complication. In the absence of therapy, mortality has been reported to be 15 20% (43). For HIV-infected children, persistent lesion formation can continue intermittently for months despite antiviral therapy.

Varicella in children with HIV may resemble progressive varicella in children with malignancy and is associated with pneumonitis, hepatitis, thrombocytopenia, disseminated intravascular coagulation, and encephalitis (42). HIV patients with low CD4 counts and varicella infection typically have >400 lesions/m^2 and exhibit extensive cutaneous and mucous membrane disease with persistent new vesicle formation synonymous with prolonged virus excretion (44). The course of disease in these children tends to be chronic, progressive, and recurrent. HIV-infected children can suffer from chronic and persistent VZV infection. Visual impairment and blindness can rarely occur as a consequence of VZV infection because of acute cortical necrosis.

Herpes Zoster

Herpes zoster is unusual in normal children, with an estimated annual rate of 1 case per 1000 children between the ages of 1 and 19 years (43). The incidence is 20-fold higher in the immunocompromised host. The younger the immunocompetent

child at the time of chickenpox (especially younger than 2 years), the more likely that the child will develop herpes zoster later in childhood. Rather than the lower thoracic and upper lumbar dermatomes of involvement, sites common in adults, zoster in younger children often occurs in dermatomes supplied by the cervical and sacral dermatomes. In children with HIV infection, the appearance of herpes zoster may occur within months of varicella (45). These children are at high risk for cutaneous dissemination and visceral involvement. Although second episodes of herpes zoster are uncommon in other immunocompromised patients, recurrent or persistent herpes zoster is common in HIV-infected patients adults and children alike. Herpes zoster can produce disseminated lesions involving multiple dermatomes or a varicella-like eruption in the HIV population (see also Chapter 28).

Complications

Virus pneumonitis and life-threatening bacterial infections such as sepsis, skin infections, or osteomyelitis may be more common among HIV-infected children. In a study by Jura et al. (44), four of eight children with perinatally acquired HIV infection and varicella had evidence of bacteremia with staphylococci or streptococci as well as Gram-negative organisms such as *Pseudomonas* and *Salmonella*. One patient died from enterococcal sepsis. Two patients had symptomatic and radiographic evidence of osteomyelitis. All eight patients had virus pneumonitis. Broad spectrum antibiotic coverage is indicated when bacterial sepsis is suspected in HIV infected children. Scrupulous attention to closely cropped nails, administration of antipyretics, and clinical examination for skin infection is warranted.

Pneumonitis

Varicella pneumonia is more common during chickenpox but may occur in an immunocompromised patient with zoster because of virus dissemination. Patients may exhibit mild respiratory symptoms to severe hypoxemia and respiratory failure.

Diagnosis may be complicated because of secondary bacterial or viral pathogens.

Central Nervous System Disease

Neurologic complications of VZV infections are well recognized. Clinical manifestations may vary from acute cerebellar ataxia or aseptic meningitis to fulminating encephalitis. Other neurologic complications such as transverse myelitis and Guillain-Barre syndrome have also been described. These complications may occur in otherwise healthy children, albeit at a low incidence. Children with AIDS may be at greater risk for central nervous system disease and may develop acute encephalitis from active VZV replication in the brain. Although cerebral vasculitis with ischemic infarcts, a complication of zoster in the elderly, has not been previously described in children, there has been a case reported in a child with HIV and varicella (49). The actual spectrum of VZV manifestations of brain disease in HIV-infected children with chickenpox or shingles remains to be defined.

Diagnosis

Diagnosis of chickenpox is usually made clinically by recognition of the characteristic vesicular lesions seen in a child with a history of exposure to an infected sibling or playmate. In children with HIV, diagnosis may be more difficult because of the atypical appearance of VZV lesions, which have been described as necrotic, ulcerated, hyperkeratotic, or hemorrhagic. New lesions may appear over a prolonged interval. Other pathogens such as HSV can also cause widely distributed cutaneous lesions and could be confused with VZV. Differential diagnosis of varicella includes impetigo, HSV, atypical measles, insect bites, scabies, rickettsialpox, and enterovirus infections (Coxsackievirus A).

Virus Isolation

VZV may be isolated from vesicular fluid obtained within the first 3 4 days of rash with inoculation into human embryonic fibroblast tissue cultures. In patients with progressive varicella and in normal children before onset of the rash, virus has also been isolated from peripheral white blood cells (50, 51). Virus has not been isolated from the respiratory tract before appearance of vesicular lesions, although infection is communicable before visible rash.

Antigen Detection

Rapid diagnosis of VZV can also be accomplished by direct detection of antigen in lesion scrapings by immunofluorescence with a monoclonal antibody to VZV or immunoprecipitation. Direct immunofluorescence should be confirmed by virus culture if possible. It is more difficult to isolate VZV than HSV in tissue culture, and the time for the appearance of cytopathic effect is longer.

Other Antigen Detection-Histopathologic Assays

Tzanck smears (multinucleated giant cells containing intranuclear inclusions) indicate a herpesvirus infection but are not specific for VZV infection. Visualization of herpesvirus virions by electron microscopy does not distinguish VZV from other herpesviruses such as HSV, CMV, or EBV.

Serologic Evaluation

Various serologic techniques are available for demonstrating antibody to VZV. For confirmation of herpes zoster or varicella, the complement fixation test has been available for decades; however, it is not suitable for determining immune status because of poor sensitivity. More sensitive tests such as demonstration of antibody membrane antigen by fluorescence micropsy, immune adherence hemagglutination, or ELISA should be used to determine susceptibility to VZV infection. The ELISA is generally available and used most frequently for demonstration of antibody. Some children with HIV may not develop VZV IgG antibodies after varicella, and their antibody titers may decline to undetectable levels over time (44). The VZV immune status of children with HIV should be documented if possible.

Therapy

Medical management of chickenpox and shingles in the normal host is directed toward avoiding known complications, and specific antiviral therapy is usually not indicated despite availability. However, because of the high risk of dissemination after chickenpox in children with HIV-1 infection, antiviral chemotherapy is warranted.

Both acyclovir and intravenous vidarabine are effective in treating varicella or herpes zoster in immunocompromised patients. However, a randomized trial between acyclovir and vidarabine in the treatment of bone marrow transplant recipients who presented within 72 hours of onset of infection showed acyclovir to be superior to vidarabine (52). In addition to efficacy, acyclovir is considered the drug of choice owing to less toxicity and ease of administration. The dose of acyclovir administered to children for the treatment of VZV infection is 500 mg/m^2/dose every 8 hr IV (total daily dose 1500 mg/m^2/day) usually for 7 days (Table 18.3). The duration of therapy may be prolonged according to clinical response. The utility of orally administered acyclovir to treat VZV in HIV-infected children is not established. Although dosages of 20 mg/kg/8 hr have been employed in the normal child with disease lasting <24 hr, the value of this approach in the HIV-infected child is unproven. Regardless, after initial intravenous therapy of varicella, many clinicians have resorted to long-term suppressive acyclovir administration because of continued lesion recurrences. Oral therapy is contradicted in immunocompromised patients with severe and progressive disease because of the poor oral bioavailability of acyclovir.

Intravenous acyclovir therapy has been used in the treatment of adult AIDS patients with herpes zoster. In many of these patients, lesions remain confined to a dermatomal distribution. Chronic herpes zoster may also occur with individuals sustaining new lesion formation in the absence of healing of existing lesions. Herpes zoster has been associated with isolation of VZV resistant to acyclovir (53). Acyclovir therapy of 30 mg/kg/day IV or 800 mg PO five times daily in HIV-infected adults has been successfully used for minimally immunocompromised adults. The treatment of shingles in the child with HIV infection remains unstudied. It would be prudent to administer acyclovir at dosages equivalent to those studies for chickenpox in the management of this disease.

Many AIDS patients children and adults alike with localized herpes zoster will not be ill enough to require hospitalization. The decision to hospitalize an individual patient must be based on several factors, including severity of infection, immune status of host, and whether visceral or cutaneous dissemination has occurred. All AIDS patients, including children, with disseminated VZV infection, either cutaneous or visceral, probably should be hospitalized initially and treated with acyclovir 500 mg/m^2 IV every 8 hr for at least 7 days or until all external lesions are crusted, although no clinical trials yet support this approach. Benefit should include a reduction in the duration of virus shedding, new lesion formation, frequency of dissemination, and mortality (52, 54). With persistent and/or recurrent cutaneous lesion formation, oral acyclovir therapy (at the above dosages) may be valuable.

Steroids are not of proven value in adults or children with AIDS with herpes zoster. Some HIV-infected children with herpes zoster require chronic therapy with acyclovir to suppress symptomatic recurrences or prevent dissemination. Management of these patients may be difficult because of the poor oral bioavailability of acyclovir and the emergence of VZV strains resistant to acyclovir.

Table 18.3. Management of VZV Infections in AIDS

Clinical Presentation	Treatment
Chickenpox	Acyclovir 500 mg/m^2/dose q 8 hr for 7–10 days or 20 mg/kg PO four times daily not to exceed 800 mg four times daily for 5–7 days
Shingles	20 mg/kg PO four times daily not to exceed 800 mg four times daily for 5–7 days
Disseminated infection	Acyclovir 500 mg/m^2/dose IV q 8 hr × 7 days

Prevention

Recognize that patients with VZV infection, regardless of immune status, who require hospitalization should be placed in strict isolation to prevent nosocomial spread of infection. Patients with herpes zoster are also contagious and must be isolated as well. The risk of contracting infection by susceptible nurses and other medical personnel providing care to infected individuals is high. Fortunately 90% of adults are not susceptible. Susceptible and at risk HIV-infected children should be given varicella-zoster immune globulin if significant personal contact with a person infected with VZV occurs, preferably within 96 hr of exposure. The dose of varicella-zoster immuneglobulin is one vial (1.25 ml) for each 10 kg body weight. Varicella-zoster immune globulin may not prevent infection, but it can help to modify or decrease severity of infection in immunocompromised hosts (55). Patients receiving monthly treatments of high dose intravenous immunoglobulin (100 400 mg/kg) should be protected and do not require varicella-zoster immune globulin if the last dose of immunoglobulin was given within 3 weeks of exposure. Some children with HIV infection may develop severe varicella despite timely administration of varicella-zoster immune globulin.

A live attenuated varicella vaccine has been found to be immunogenic both in immunocompromised children with leukemia and in normal healthy children. Once a VZV vaccine is licensed in the United States, it may be prudent to vaccinate susceptible healthy contacts in an HIV family to minimize household exposures to varicella. The value of vaccination of HIV-infected children may vary depending on the degree of immune compromise and is being considered for investigation.

Future Considerations

Newer antiviral medications with improved bioavailability, such as bromovinyl arabinosyl uracil, are being investigated. Preliminary experience with bromovinyl arabinosyl is encouraging. A prodrug of acyclovir may prove valuable in the treatment of VZV infection as will a similar compound famciclovir. The best protection for immunosuppressed children, such as those with HIV infection, may be vaccination, especially immunocompetent siblings and schoolmates. Duration of immunity and effect of vaccination on the epidemiology of varicella are unanswered questions.

HERPES SIMPLEX VIRUS
Background

Infections caused by HSV-1 and -2 are recognized worldwide. These infections usually occur asymptomatically and generally are limited to the skin and mucous membranes. However, in immunocompromised hosts, such as HIV-infected adults and children, infection can be severe and prolonged and involve other organs. Transmission of HSV most often occurs in association with intimate personal contact with infected secretions. HSV-1 is transmitted primarily by oral secretions and HSV-2 by genital secretions.

Primary HSV-1 infection in the child is limited to the oropharynx and may manifest as gingivostomatitis. Primary infection in young adults has been associated with pharyngitis and often a mononucleosis-like syndrome (56). Seroprevalence studies indicate that acquisition of HSV is inversely related to age and socioeconomic status. Antibodies to HSV, indicative of past infection, are present in as many as 75 90% of individuals from lower socioeconomic groups by the end of the first decade of life. In contrast, only 30 40% of individuals from middle to upper socioeconomic groups are seropositive by the middle of the second decade of life (57 60). Currently most HIV-infected children who are of lower socioeconomic status acquire HSV infection before the age of 10 15 years.

Because infections with HSV-2 are usually acquired through sexual contact, antibodies to this virus are rarely found until the age of onset of sexual activity. Acquisition of HSV-2 is also related to socioeconomic status, with 50 60% of the lower socioeconomic population having antibodies to HSV-2. In contrast, only 10 30% of individuals in higher socioeconomic groups are seropositive (61, 62). The number of sexual contacts is an important risk factor for acquisition of HSV-2 as well as for HIV infection. Since the seroprevalence of HSV is as high as 30 60% in pregnant women, women with HIV are also at risk of perinatal transmission of HSV to their infants.

Infection with HSV-1 or HSV-2 may be asymptomatic or present as gingivostomatis or genitalis, after which the virus becomes latent and may later reactivate. Reactivation of HSV is enhanced by immunosuppression and is clinically more severe in immunocompromised patients. Both adults and children with HIV may have clinically severe, chronic, and frequent recurrences of either oral or genital herpes. Recurrent HSV infections in AIDS patients result in extensive tissue destruction and prolonged virus shedding.

Pathogenesis and Natural History

In normal immunocompetent children, primary gingivostomatitis is associated with high fever and extensive mucosal ulcerations and in severe cases may require hospitalization because of dehydration. Onset of symptoms may be abrupt or insidious and is accompanied by fever, mucosal ulcers, drooling, and anorexia. With inoculation into the skin or mucous membranes, HSV replicates in epithelial cells; incubation is 4 6 days. As replication occurs, cell lysis and local inflammation ensue, resulting in the characteristic vesicles on an erythematous base. Viremia and visceral dissemination may develop depending on the immunologic competence of the host. Histologic examination of scrapings of viral lesions demonstrate multinucleated giant cells and intranuclear inclusion bodies (Cowdry s type A bodies), which are suggestive but not diagnostic of HSV infection. In the immunocompetent host, the illness usually lasts 10 14 days.

Oropharyngeal Herpes

The most common manifestation of recurrent HSV infection in the normal host is herpes labialis (cold sores or fever blisters). Herpes labialis is estimated to occur in 25 50% of infected individuals and often occurs as a consequence of febrile illness, local trauma, sun exposure, or menstruation. The natural history of recurrent herpes labialis has been described in adults (63, 64), but no similar data are available for children, least of all those with HIV infection. Most individuals experience a prodrome (pain, burning, tingling, or itching) at the site lasting 6 hr to several days. Vesicles typically appear at the vermilion border of the lips and are associated with considerable pain. Vesicles progress to ulcers and then finally to crusts over 2 4 days. Most lesions are healed within 5 10 days. Orolabial recurrences in AIDS patients may increase in frequency and severity as immunosuppression increases. Although oral lesions in the normal host usually heal over 7 10 days, AIDS patients, if untreated, may have chronic ulcerative lesions with persistent virus shedding for weeks (65). From 5 to 10% of children with AIDS and primary gingivostomatitis (66, 67) have frequent HSV recurrences associated with severe ulcerative herpetic lesions and several recurrent bouts of oral gingivostomatitis normally encountered only with primary infection (68 70). In immunocompromised patients such as transplant recipients, those with malignancies and those infected with HIV-1, HSV can spread from the oropharynx to the esophagus or become disseminated either cutaneously or to other visceral organs. For adults, HSV lesions lasting more than 1 month in individuals with no other reason for immunodeficiency are considered a criterion for diagnosis of AIDS by the Centers for Disease Control (71).

Esophagitis

Esophagitis from HSV infection has rarely been reported in normal children (72, 73) but is a relatively common occurrence in immunocompromised patients. Pathologic studies have suggested that ~25% of cases of autopsy-proven esophagitis in adults are secondary to HSV infection (74), with 20 58% of these patients having involvement elsewhere (lungs, trachea, skin). The incidence of esophagitis in HIV-infected children is undetermined. Symptoms of esophagitis include retrosternal pain and odynophagia. Herpetic lesions in the oropharynx may not be present, and the clinical picture is often confused with *C. esophagitis.* Esophagoscopy with biopsy and virus culture will be diagnostic and help exclude other common causes of esophagitis including CMV, other fungal/bacterial infections, and chemotherapy-induced complications (74, 75). This diagnostic approach should be applied to HIV-infected children since the results will guide therapy.

Genital Infection

Primary herpetic vulvovaginitis rarely occurs in young immunocompetent infants and children unless HSV is introduced inadvertently when handling the genital area with contaminated hands. There is a paucity of data concerning the incidence of genital herpes in children, especially those with HIV infection. In adolescents, symptoms of genital herpes include fever, pain from ulcers on the genital-perirectal area, itching, dysuria, vaginal, or urethral discharge and tender inguinal adenopathy. Lesions tend to last 2–3 weeks before complete healing (mean 19 days). Virus shedding occurs for a mean 11.5 days (68, 76). Other venereal diseases should be excluded including chancroid, syphilis, erythema multiforme, and local moniliasis. Although primary infections are usually in perioral, ocular, or genital areas, any skin site may be involved. Primary HSV infection may be extensive and mimic herpes zoster, although usually not in a dermatomal distribution and the pain is less severe.

Recurrent genital HSV infection in the normal host is probably the second-most common manifestation of disease and is much more common after primary HSV-2 (90%) than HSV-1 (55%) infection (77). From 5 to 12% of individuals with recurrent genital HSV have constitutional symptoms. Local symptoms include pain, itching, dysuria, and adenopathy. Symptoms are generally milder and of shorter duration than in primary genital disease. As with orolabial herpes, the frequency and severity of genital recurrences in adult AIDS patients may increase with increasing immunosuppression. No data exist from prospective studies on the natural history of recurrent genital HSV infection in children and adolescents

with HIV infection. Prolonged virus shedding, progressive tissue destruction, and persistent local pain occur for several weeks in HIV-infected adults (78, 79).

Central Nervous System Disease

Although it occurs infrequently, HSV encephalitis is a life-threatening complication of HSV infection in patients with AIDS. Although HSV-1 is the principal causal agent beyond the neonatal period, both HSV-1 and HSV-2 have been identified in brain tissue of AIDS patients (80, 81). The temporal lobe is the principle target of the virus, and a necrotizing hemorrhagic encephalitis results. Headache, fever, behavioral disorders, and focal seizures are prominent features along with abnormal CSF. Additionally, both generalized and chronic manifestations of central nervous system disease have been reported in adults with HIV infection. Infectious virus is rarely present in CSF during disease, and brain biopsy with appropriate histologic and culture techniques is the most reliable way to make the diagnosis (82–85). The clinical diagnosis of HSV encephalitis is extremely difficult because other central nervous system infections including HIV encephalopathy and infections with *Cryptococcus neoformans* and *Toxoplasma gondii* may present in an identical fashion (these latter infections are rare in children with HIV). In addition, tuberculous and fungal meningitis, brain abscess, cerebral vascular accident, and brain tumors should be included in the differential diagnosis (86).

Disseminated Disease

The most severe form of HSV in the immunocompromised host is that of widely disseminated disease involving the liver, adrenals, lungs, spleen, kidney, and brain. Cutaneous dissemination of HSV may involve a widespread vesicular eruption looking much like varicella or may involve more localized, large hemorrhagic vesicles and bullae. Patients may exhibit hepatitis, pneumonia, shock, hemorrhage, disseminated intravascular coagulation, seizures, renal failure, and death in days to weeks. Even with antiviral therapy, death can occur (87).

Patients compromised by immunodeficiency or immunosuppression, by malnutrition, or by disorders of skin integrity (burns, eczema) are at greater risk of developing severe HSV infection.

Other Manifestations

Herpetic Whitlow can also occur in infants with gingivostomatitis by autoinoculation of fingers. HSV may also infect the eyes, causing keratitis, blepharitis, or keratoconjunctivitis. Prophylactic antivirals may be warranted, but steroid use is contraindicated.

Diagnosis

Diagnosis of HSV infection is usually suspected clinically by the appearance of vesicles, ulcers, or maculopapular lesions on mucous membranes or skin. In immunocompromised patients, these lesions may be atypical in nature and can present as deep necrotic ulcers or can be hemorrhagic or hyperkeratotic. Differential diagnosis of a newborn with a vesicular rash includes neonatal melanosis, acrodermatitis enteropathica, varicella, enteroviral infection, cutaneous candidiasis, congenital syphilis, and staphylococcal skin infection.

Virus Isolation

Isolation of the virus remains the definitive diagnostic method. In addition to scrapings of skin vesicles, other sites from which virus may be isolated include the CSF, stool, urine, throat, and conjunctivae. It may also be useful in infants with hepatitis or other gastrointestinal abnormalities to obtain and culture duodenal aspirates for HSV. Typing of an isolate can be performed by techniques available primarily in research laboratories. Outcome with treatment does not appear to be related to the type of HSV.

Histopathologic Evaluation

In the absence of facilities for diagnostic virology, cytologic examination of cells from sites involved may be used. The presence of intranuclear inclusions and multi-nucleated giant cells indicates herpes virus infection.

Antigen Detection

Immunoflourescence or immunoprecipitation can be performed for the detection of HSV antigens. In addition the detection of HSV DNA by polymerase chain reaction in CSF may prove useful but is still experimental.

Serologic Evaluation

The use of serologic diagnosis for HSV infection is less than optimal. Inability of commonly available assays to distinguish between antibodies to HSV-1 and HSV-2 or to detect the presence of transplacentally acquired virus-specific maternal IgG makes assessment of neonatal antibody status difficult. The most commonly used tests for measurement of antibody to HSV include complement fixation, passive hemagglutination, neutralization, immunofluorescence, and ELISA.

Treatment

The prompt institution of antiviral therapy for pediatric and adult AIDS patients with acute HSV infection reduces morbidity and the risk of serious complications. Symptomatic HIV-infected children with primary gingivostomatitis may have the potential for local or visceral dissemination. It would therefore seem reasonable to treat with acyclovir at 250 mg/m^2/dose IV every 8 hr or 250 mg/m^2/dose PO every 6 hr. Children presenting with evidence of disseminated infection should be treated with a higher intravenous dose, 500/mg/m^2 every 8 hr for at least 10 days or until healing occurs. In addition, children with ocular involvement from HSV should receive a topical ophthalmic drug such as 1 2% trifluridine, 1% iododeoxyuridine, or 3% vidarabine. Infants with neonatal herpes should be treated with acyclovir 30 mg/kg/day IV divided into three doses for 10 21 days (Table 18.4).

Recurrences of oral or genital HSV are common in adult AIDS patients, and many patients require chronic suppressive therapy with oral acyclovir. For children with se-

Table 18.4.   Management of HSV Infection in AIDS

Clinical Presentation	Treatment
Gingivostomatitis	Acyclovir 250 mg/m^2/dose IV q 8 hr or 250 mg/m^2/dose PO q 6 hr for 5–7 days
Disseminated infection (visceral)	Acyclovir 500 mg/m^2/dose IV q 8 hr for 10 days
Keratoconjunctivitis	1% trifluridine (viroptic) topically one drop in affected eye q 2 hr while awake
Severe recurrent mucocutaneous infection	Acyclovir 300 mg/m^2/dose POQ 6 hr for 5–7 days
Neonatal herpes (SEM, central nervous system, disseminated)	Acyclovir 30 mg/kg/d IV q 8 hr for 10–21 days

vere mucocutaneous recurrences, oral therapy with acyclovir at 300 mg/m2/dose every 6 hr for at least 5 7 days may be considered. Daily suppression with acyclovir may be considered for children with frequent recurrences (six or more per year). These regimens are based on studies of adults with genital herpes (88).

If healing does not occur or lesions progress while on therapy, virus cultures should be repeated, and acyclovir-resistant strains should be eliminated. Patients with acyclovir-resistant strains of HSV may respond to vidarabine at 15 mg/kg in a 12-hr infusion for 10 days. In addition, foscarnet is another alternative that is successful in adults with acyclovir-resistant strains (89).

Prevention

Although much progress has been made since the advent of antiviral therapy for the treatment of life-threatening HSV infections, the best approach is that of prevention. Infants with perinatal HIV infection are also at risk for acquisition of HSV at the time of birth if their mothers are excreting HSV. In women with active genital herpetic lesions at the time of delivery, it is recommended that cesarean section be performed within 4 hr of rupture of membranes to decrease the risks of transmission to their infants (90). However, cases of neonatal HSV infection can still occur; cesarean section has not proven efficacious when membranes have been ruptured for a longer period. There is no licensed vaccine for prevention of HSV infection and no studies to determine if prophylaxis with either acyclovir or intravenous globulin would prevent infection if exposed. Caretakers should be aware of the potential risks of exposure of an HIV-infected child to HSV and perform thorough hand washing whenever fever blisters or cutaneous HSV lesions are present.

Future Considerations

A phase III clinical trial using oral acyclovir to suppress local recurrencers of HSV in infants is underway. The emergence of acyclovir-resistant strains is a potential problem in pediatrics because it has already been observed in adult AIDS patients with chronic genital and perianal herpes. Development of newer drugs that can be administered orally and are effective against acyclovir-resistant strains are needed. Evaluation of a vaccine against HSV might also be beneficial.

OTHER HERPESVIRUSES

HHV-6 was first isolated from human lymphocyte cultures in 1986 (91). It has now been found to be the etiologic agent of exanthem subitum (roseola), a common infection in childhood. Essentially all adults have antibody to HHV-6, so newborns are all antibody positive. Efficient transmission of the virus occurs with the median age of acquisition being ~9 months. By the age of 2 years, over 90% of children have antibody to HHV-6. Although HHV-6 commonly infects children in early life, its role in HIV-1-infected children is unclear. HHV-6 and HIV can replicate in the same cell. If HHV-6 influences the course of HIV infection this will be determined in studies of infants who are acquiring this virus. Studies relating HHV-6 acquisition and its effect on HIV infection are in progress. Little is known about the clinical manifestations of the most recently discovered herpesvirus, HHV-7.

Primary infection with EBV usually occurs in early childhood as well and is usually asymptomatic but may be associated with signs and symptoms common to other viral agents. Some EBV infections in children may present as classic infectious mononucleosis as seen typically in young adults (93). However, the disease in young children may be atypical with an increased frequency of rash, significant neutropenia, and hepatosplenomegaly. Findings of failure to thrive, otitis media, and episodes of recurrent tonsillopharyngitis are more closely associated with childhood disease. Infection with EBV has been linked to lymphoproliferative disorders of children with AIDS (see Chapter 33). The DNA and nuclear antigens of EBV have been detected in tissue specimens on non-Hodgkin s lymphoma and lymphocytic interstitial pneumonitis from patients with AIDS and may be involved in the development of these disorders (94).

SUMMARY

Herpesvirus infections cause substantial morbidity and mortality among immunocompromised patients, including adults and children with HIV-1 infection. Early diagnosis and treatment with available antiviral drugs is essential. The development of new antiviral drugs that are less toxic and can be given orally would greatly simplify long-term maintenance regimens. The value of adjunctive therapies such as hyperimmunoglobulin for CMV disease is still under investigation. Future interventions for prevention of herpesvirus infections such as antibody prophylaxis and development of vaccines must be addressed.

References

1. Adler SP. Cytomegalovirus and child day care. Evidence for an increased infection rate among day-care workers. N Engl J Med 1989;321:1290–1296.
2. Skolnik PR, Kosloff BR, Hirsch MS. Bidirectional interactions between human immunodeficiency virus Type 1 and cytomegalovirus. J Infect Dis 1988;157:508–513.
3. Elfassi E, Michelson S, Backerlerie F, Arenzana-Seusdedos F, Virelizier JL. Transactivation of human immunodeficiency virus long terminal repeat during the early phases of human cytomegalovirus infection. Ann Virol (Inst Pasteur) 1987;138:461–470.
4. Stagno S, Pass RF, Dworsky ME, Britt WJ, Alford CA. Congenital and perinatal cytomegalovirus infections: Clinical characteristics and pathogenic factors. Birth Defects 1984;20:65–85.
5. Fowler KB, Stagno S, Pass RF, Britt WJ, Boll TJ, Alford CA. The outcome of congenital cytomegalovirus infection in relation to maternal antibody status. N Engl J Med 1992;326:663–667.
6. Stagno S, Pass RF, Dworsky ME, Alford CA. Congenital and perinatal cytomegalovirus infections. Semin Perinatol 1983;7:31–42.
7. Reynolds DW, Stagno S, Hosty TS, Tiller M, Alford CA. Maternal cytomegalovirus excretion and perinatal infection. N Engl J Med 1973;289:1–5.
8. Armstrong D, Gold JWM, Dryjanski J. Treatment of infections in patients with the acquired immunodeficiency syndrome. Ann Intern Med 1985;103:738–743.
9. Drew WL, Sweet ES, Miner RC, Morarski ES. Multiple infection by cytomegalovirus in patients with AIDS. J Infect Dis 1984;150:952–953.
10. Reichert CM, O'Leary TJ, Levens DL, Simrell CR, Macher AM. Autopsy pathology in the acquired immune deficiency syndrome. Am J Pathol 1983;112:357–382.
11. Scott GB, Buck BE, Leterman JG, et al. Acquired immunodeficiency syndrome in infants. N Engl J Med 1984;310:76–81.
12. Shannon KM, Ammann AJ. Acquired immune deficiency syndrome in childhood. J Pediatr 1985;106:332–342.
13. Oleske J, Minnefor A, Cooper R, et al. Immune deficiency syndrome in children. JAMA 1983;249:2345–2349.
14. Pawha S, Kaplan M, Fikrig S, et al. Spectrum of human T-cell lymphotropic virus type III infection in children. JAMA 1986;255:2299–2305.
15. Daus W, Zimmer KP, Moller P. Beidseitige Zytomegalie-Retinitis bei einem Saugling mit letal verlaufenem konnatalen AIDS. Klin Monatsbl Augenheilkd 1986;188:604–609.
16. Drew WL. Cytomegalovirus infection in patients with AIDS. J Infect Dis 1988;158:449–455.
17. Wiley CA, Nelson JA. Role of human immunodeficiency virus and cytomegalovirus in AIDS encephalitis. Am J Pathol 1988;133:73–81.
18. Levy JA, Shimabukuro J, Hollander H, Mills J, Kaminsky L. Isolation of AIDS-associated retrovirus from cerebrospinal fluid and brain of patients with neurologic symptoms. Lancet 1985;2:586–588.
19. Gadler H, Tillegard A, Groth CG. Studies of cytomegalovirus infection in renal allograft recipients virus isolation. Scand J Infect Dis 1982;14:81–87.
20. Rubin RH, Colvin RB. Cytomegalovirus infection in renal transplantation; clinical importance and control. In: Williams GM, Burdick JF, Solez K eds. Kidney transplant rejection. New York: Marcel Dekker, 1986;283–304.
21. Collaborative DHPG Treatment Study Group. Treatment of serious cytomegalovirus infections with 9-(1,3 dihydroxy-2-propoxy methyl) guanine in patients with AIDS and other immunodeficiencies. N Engl J Med 1986;314:801–805.

22. Mills J, Jacobson MA, O'Donnell JJ, Cederberg D, Holland GM. Treatment of cytomegalovirus retinitis in patients with AIDS. Rev Infect Dis 1988;10:S522–S531.

23. Henderly DE, Freeman WR, Causey DM, Rao NA. Cytomegalovirus retinitis and response to therapy with ganciclovir. Ophthalmology 1987;94:425–434.

24. Holland GN, Sidikaro Y, Kreiger AE, Et al. Treatment of cytomegalovirus retinopathy with ganciclovir. Ophthalmology 1987;94:815–823.

25. Jabs DA, Newman C, DeBustros S, Polk BF. Treatment of cytomegalovirus retinitis with ganciclovir. Ophthalmology 1987;94:824–830.

26. Orellana J, Teich SA, Friedman AH, et al. Combined short and long term therapy for the treatment of cytomegalovirus retinitis using ganciclovir (BW B759U). Ophthalmology 1987;94:831–838.

27. Mills J. 9-(1,3-dihydroxy-2-propoxymethyl) guanine (DHPG) for treatment of cytomegalovirus infections. In: Mills J, Corey L, eds. Antiviral chemotherapy: New directions for clinical application and research. New York: Elsevier, 1986:199–208.

28. Trang JM, Kidd L, Gruber W, et al. Linear single-dose pharmacokinetics of ganciclovir in newborns with congenital cytomegalovirus infections. NIAID Collaborative Antiviral Study Group. Clin Pharmacol Ther 1933;53:15–21.

29. Levin AV, Zeichner S, Duker JS, Starr SE, Augsburger JJ, Kronwith S. Cytomegalovirus retinitis in an infant with acquired immunodeficiency syndrome. Pediatrics 1989;84:683–687.

30. Grossberg HS, Bonnem EM, Buhles WC Jr. GM-CSF with ganciclovir for the treatment of CMV retinitis in AIDS [Letter]. N Engl J Med 1989;320:1560.

31. Drew WL, Miner RC, Busch DF, et al. Prevalence of resistance in patients receiving ganciclovir for serious cytomegalovirus infection. J Infect Dis 1991;163:716–719.

32. Walmsley SL, Chew E, Read SE, et al. Treatment of cytomegalovirus retinitis with trisodium phosphonoformate hexahydrate (Foscarnet). J Infect Dis 1988;157:569–572.

33. Studies of Ocular Complications of AIDS Research Group, in Collaboration with AIDS Clinical Trials Group. Mortality in patients with the acquired immunodeficiency syndrome treated with either foscarnet or ganciclovir for cytomegalovirus retinitis. N Engl J Med 1992;326:213–220.

34. Palestine AG, Polis MA, DeSmet MD, et al. A randomized controlled trial of foscarnet in the treatment of cytomegalovirus retinitis in patients with AIDS. Ann Intern Med 1991;115:665–673.

35. Butler KM, DeSmet MD, Husson RN, et al. Treatment of aggressive cytomegalovirus retinitis with ganciclovir in combination with foscarnet in a child infected with human immunodeficiency virus. J Pediatr 1992;120:483–486.

36. Yeager AS, Grumet C, Hafleigh EB, et al. Prevention of transfusion-acquired cytomegalovirus infection in newborn infants. J Pediatr 1981;98:281–287.

37. Brady MT, Milam JD, Anderson DC, et al. Use of deglycerolized red blood cells to prevent post-transfusion infection with cytomegalovirus in neonates. J Infect Dis 1984;150:334–339.

38. Plotkin SA, Friedman HM, Fleisher GR, et al. Towne-vaccine-induced prevention of cytomegalovirus disease after renal transplants. Lancet 1984;1:528–530.

39. Stern H. Live cytomegalovirus vaccination of healthy volunteers: Eight year follow-up studies. Birth Defects 1984;20:263–269.

40. Ross AH. Modification of chickenpox in family contacts by administration of gamma globulin. N Engl J Med 1962;267:369–376.

41. Weller TH. Varicella: Herpes zoster virus. In: Evans AS, ed. Viral infections of humans. New York: Plenum, 1982:569–595.

42. Preblud SR. Varicella: Complications and cost. Pediatrics 1986;72:728–735.

43. Whitley RJ. Varicella-zoster virus infections. In: Galasso G, Merigan T, Whitley RJ ed. Antiviral agents and viral diseases of man. New York: Raven, 1990:235–263.

44. Jura E, Chadwick EG, Josephs SH, et al. Varicella-zoster virus infections in children infected with human immunodeficiency virus. Pediatr Infect Dis J 1989;8:586–590.

45. Patterson LE, Butler KM, Edwards MS. Clinical herpes zoster shortly following primary varicella in two HIV-infected children. Clin Pediatr 1989;28:354.

46. Colebunders R, et al. Herpes zoster in African patients: A clinical predictor of HIV. J Infect Dis 1988;157:314–318.

47. Friedman-Kien AE, Lafleur FL, Gendler E, et al. Herpes zoster: A possible early clinical sign for development of acquired immunodeficiency syndrome in high-risk individuals. J Am Acad Dermatol 1986;14:1023–1028.

48. Dunkle LM, Arvin AM, Whitley RJ, et al. A controlled trial of acyclovir for chickenpox in normal children. N Engl J Med 1991;325:1539–1544.

49. Frank Y, Lim W, Kahn E, et al. Multiple ischemic infarcts in a child with acquired immunodeficiency syndrome, varicella zoster infection, and cerebral vasculitis. Pediatr Neurol 1989;5:64–67.

50. Feldman S, Chaudary S, Ossi M, et al. A viremic phase for herpes zoster in children with cancer. J Pediatr 1977;91:597–600.

51. Feldman S, Epp E. Isolation of varicella-zoster virus from blood. J Pediatr 1976;88:265–267.

52. Shepp D, Dandliker PS, Meyers JD. Treatment of varicella-zoster virus in severely immunocompromised patients: A randomized comparison of acyclovir and vidarabine. N Engl J Med 1986;314:208–212.

53. Drew WL, Buhles W, Erlich KS. Herpesvirus infections (cytomegalovirus, herpes simplex virus, varicella-zoster virus). How to use ganciclovir (DHPG) and acyclovir. Infect Dis Clin North Am 1988;2:495–509.

54. Balfour HH, Bean B, Laskin OL, et al. Acyclovir halts progression of herpes zoster in immunocompromised patients. N Engl J Med 1983;308:1448–1453.

55. Zaia JA, Levis MJ, Preblud SR, et al. Evaluation of varicella-zoster immune globulin: Protection of immunosuppressed children after household ex-

posure to varicella. J Infect Dis 1983;147: 737–743.

56. Glezen WP, Fernald GW, Lohr JA. Acute respiratory disease of university students with special references to the etiologic role of Herpesvirus hominis. Am J Epidemiol 1975;101:111–121.

57. McClung H, Seth P, Rawls WE. Relative concentrations in human sera of antibodies to cross-reacting and specific antigens of herpes simplex virus types 1 and 2. Am J Epidemiol 1976;104:192–201.

58. Smith IW, Peutherer JF, MacCallum FO. The incidence of Herpesvirus hominis antibody in the population. J Hyg (Lond) 1967;65:395–408.

59. Wentworth BB, Alexander ER. Seroepidemiology of infections due to members of the herpesvirus group. Am J Epidemiol 1971;94:496–507.

60. Nahmias AJ, Josey WE, Naib ZM, Luce CF, Duffey C. Antibodies to Herpesvirus hominis types 1 and 2 in humans. I. Patients with genital herpetic infections. Am J Epidemiol 1970;91:539–546.

61. Stavraky KM, Rawls WE, Chiavetta J, Donner AP, Wanklin JM. Sexual and socioeconomic factors affecting the risk of past infections with herpes simplex virus type 2. Am J Epidemiol 1983;118: 109–121.

62. Bryson Y, Arvin A. Herpes group virus infection in HIV-1 infected infants, children and adolescents. In: Pizzo PA, Wilfert CM, eds. Pediatric AIDS: The challenge of HIV infection in infants, children, and adolescents. Baltimore: Williams & Wilkins, 1991;245–265.

63. Bader C, Crumpacker CS, Schnipper LE, et al. The natural history of recurrent facial-oral infection with herpes simplex virus. J Infect Dis 1978;138:897–905.

64. Spruance SL, Overall JC, Kern ER, et al. The natural history of recurrent herpes simplex labialis: Implication for antiviral therapy. N Engl J Med 1977;297:69–75.

65. Straus SE, Smith HA, Brickman C, et al. Acyclovir for chronic mucocutaneous herpes simplex virus infection in immunosuppressed patients. Ann Intern Med 1982;96:270–277.

66. Erice A, Chou S, Biron KK, et al. Progressive disease due to ganciclovir-resistant cytomegalovirus in immunocompromised patients. N Engl J Med 1989;320:289–293.

67. Scott GB, Buck BE, Leterman JG, et al. Acquired immunodeficiency syndrome in infants. N Engl J Med 1984;310:76–81.

68. Corey L, Adams HG, Brown AZ, et al. Genital herpes simplex virus infections, clinical manifestations, course, and complication. Ann Intern Med 1983;98:958–972.

69. Rubinstein A. Pediatric aids. In: Current problems in pediatrics. Chicago: Year Book, 1986;362–409.

70. Pahwa S, Kaplan M, Fikrig S, et al. Spectrum of human T-cell lymphotropic virus type III infection in children: Recognition of symptomatic, asymptomatic, and seronegative patients. JAMA 1986;255:2299–2305.

71. Centers for Disease Control. Revision of the CDC surveillance case definition for acquired immunodeficiency syndrome. MMWR 1987;36:1S–15S.

72. Bastain JF, Kaufman IA. Herpes simplex esophagitis in a healthy 19 year old boy. J Pediatr 1982; 100:426–427.

73. Owensby LC, Stammer JL. Esophagitis associated with herpes simplex infection in an immunocompetent host. Gastroenterology 1978;74:1305–1306.

74. Nash G, Ross JS. Herpetic esophagitis, a common cause of esophageal ulceration. Hum Pathol 1974;5:339–345.

75. Buss DH, Scharyj M. Herpesvirus infection of the esophagus and other visceral organs in adults: Incidence and clinical significance. Am J Med 1979;66:457–462.

76. Corey L, Holmes KK. Genital herpes simplex infections: Current concepts in diagnosis, therapy and prevention. Ann Intern Med 1983;98: 973–983.

77. Reeves WC, Corey L, Adams HG, et al. Risk of recurrence after first episodes of genital herpes. Relation to HSV type antibody response. N Engl J Med 1981;305:315–319.

78. Armstrong D, Gold JWM, Dryjanski J, et al. Treatment of infections in patients with the acquired immunodeficiency syndrome. Ann Intern Med 1985;103:738–743.

79. Whitley RJ, Levin M, Barton N, et al. Infections caused by herpes simplex virus in the immunocompromised host: Natural history and topical acyclovir therapy. J Infect Dis 1984;150:323–329.

80. Dix RD, Bredesen DE, Erlick KS, Mills J. Recovery of herpesvirus from cerebrospinal fluid of immunodeficient homosexual men. Ann Neurol 1985; 18:611–614.

81. Dix RD, Waitzman DM, Follansbee S, et al. Herpes simplex virus type 2 encephalitis in two homosexual men with persistent adenopathy. Ann Neurol 1985;17:203–206.

82. Hinthorn RD, Baker LH, Romig DA. Recurrent conjugal neuralgia caused by Herpesvirus hominis type 2. JAMA 1976;236:587–588.

83. Whitley RJ, Soong S-J, Dolin R, et al. Adenine arabinoside therapy of biopsy proven herpes simplex encephalitis. N Engl J Med 1977;297:289–294.

84. Whitley RH, Soong SJ, Hirsch MS, et al. Herpes simplex encephalitis. Vidarabine therapy and diagnostic problems. N Engl J Med 1981;304: 313–318.

85. Whitley RJ, Tilles J, Linneman CR Jr, et al. Herpes simplex encephalitis. Clinical assessment. JAMA 1982;246:317–320.

86. Hirsch MS. Herpes simplex virus. In: Mandell GL, ed. Principles and practice of infectious diseases. 3rd ed. New York: Churchhill-Livingstone, 1991: 1144–1153.

87. Whitley RJ, Gnann JW. The epidemiology and clinical manifestations of herpes simplex virus infections. In: Roizman B, Whitley RJ, eds. Herpesviruses: Biology, pathogenesis and treatment. New York: Raven in press.

88. Douglas JM, Critchlow C, Bernedetti J, et al. A double-blind study of oral acyclovir for suppression of recurrences of genital herpes simplex virus infection. N Engl J Med 1984;310:1551–1556.

89. Erlich KS, Mills J, Chatis P, et al. Acyclovir-resistant herpes simplex virus infections in patients with the acquired immunodeficiency syndrome. Med Intelligence 1989;320:293–296.

90. Nahmias AJ, Visintine AM. Perinatal herpes simplex virus infection. In: Remington J, Klein J, eds.

Congenital and perinatal infection. Philadelphia: Saunders, 1974:156–196.

91. Salahuddin SZ, Ablashi DV, Markham PD, et al. Isolation of a new virus, HBLV, in patients with lymphoproliferative disorders. Science 1986;234: 596–601.

92. Pietroboni GR, Harnett GB, Farr TJ, Bucens MR. Human herpes virus type 6 (HHV-6) and its in vitro effect on human immuno-deficiency virus (HIV). J Clin Pathol 1988;41: 1310–1312.

93. Baehner RL, Shuler SE. Infectious mononucleosis in childhood. Clin Pediatr 1967;6:393–399.

94. Katz BZ, Berkman AB, Shapiro ED. Serologic evidence of active Epstein-Barr virus infection in Epstein-Barr virus associated lymphoproliferative disorders of children with AIDS. J Pediatr 1992;120:228–232.

19
Respiratory Virus Infections

Kenneth McIntosh

Acute lower respiratory tract infections (LRTI) are among the most common clinically significant illnesses among children with human immunodeficiency (HIV) infections. Although certain opportunistic organisms such as *P. carinii*, cytomegalovirus and other herpes viruses, and atypical mycobacteria have received considerable attention as causes of LRTI in children and adults with AIDS, common respiratory viruses have been almost totally neglected. This is despite the fact that infections are frequent, their features differ in certain important ways from infections in normal hosts, and their clinical consequences are often quite significant.

In normal children respiratory viruses are the most commonly identified cause of LRTI (1 3). There are certain important underlying illnesses that predispose to severe and complicated viral respiratory infections (4), and several of these are common in AIDS, including cellular immunodeficiency, chronic pulmonary disease, and congestive heart failure.

Measles virus is also included in this review since it has many features in common with the respiratory viruses and is itself a major respiratory pathogen.

MICROBIOLOGY AND EPIDEMIOLOGY OF RESPIRATORY VIRUSES

The principal viruses causing acute LRTI in children are shown in Table 19.1. Respiratory syncytial virus (RSV) is the most frequent lower respiratory tract pathogen in childhood, causing principally bronchiolitis

Table 19.1. Respiratory Viruses

Virus	Family	Genus	No. of Types	Nucleic Acid	Respiratory Illnesses Caused in Infants and Children
RSV	Paramyxoviridae	*Pneumovirus*	2 subtypes	RNA	URI[a], bronchiolitis, pneumonia
Parainfluenza virus	Paramyxoviridae	*Paramyxovirus*	4 (only 3 cause LRTI)	RNA	URI, croup, pneumonia bronchiolitis
Influenza virus	Orthoyxoviridae	*Myxovirus*	2, many subtypes	RNA (segmented)	URI, pneumonia, croup
Adenovirus	Adenoviridae	*Adenovirus*	45+ (2 enteral)	DNA	URI, pharyngitis, pneumonia, conjunctivitis
Rhinovirus	Picornaviridae	*Rhinovirus*	100+	RNA	URI
Coronaviruses	Coronaviridae	*Coronavirus*	3–4 (1–2 enteral)	RNA	URI
Measles virus	Paramyxoviridae	*Morbillivirus*	1	RNA	Measles, pneumonia, croup

[a]URI, upper respiratory infection.

365

and pneumonia in infants younger than 1 year. In temperate climates it is epidemic in the colder seasons of the year. Immunity following natural infection in the normal host is both temporary and incomplete, and reinfection, with significant disease, is common even in normal children.

There are four types of parainfluenza viruses, but only the first three are of clinical importance in LRTI. Types 1 and 2 principally cause croup, but they can also produce pneumonia and do so frequently in children with underlying immunologic defects. Type 3 is the second most frequent cause (after RSV) of pneumonia in children. These viruses have a complex epidemiology, with types 1 and 2 being epidemic in the fall and early winter and type 3 being epidemic in the winter and spring in some years and endemic in others.

Two major influenza virus types, A and B, cause significant LRTI. Whereas these viruses are clearly the most important respiratory viruses in adults, they are much less so in children. They tend to produce febrile respiratory disease, but pneumonia is uncommon. They also predispose to bacterial superinfection in normal children. They are epidemic in cold weather, and their incidence varies markedly from year to year, depending on the pattern of prevalent serotypes and the level of immunity in the population.

Adenoviruses are common causes of upper respiratory tract illness in children and rare causes of severe LRTI. They replicate readily in the gut, and some serotypes cause primarily diarrhea. They also sometimes cause viremia, even in the immunologically normal host, with consequent symptoms such as meningitis, encephalitis, rash, and fever.

Both rhinoviruses and coronaviruses require mention for the sake of completeness, but both are primarily causes of upper respiratory tract illness. Although infection is common, and although both virus groups have occasionally been found in association with lower respiratory tract illness in normal children (5, 6), evidence of their involvement in HIV-infected patients has not thus far been presented.

Measles virus, although it may be classed as a respiratory virus, belongs in a separate category for two major reasons. The first is that, unlike infections by the viruses discussed above, measles is universally accompanied by viremia. This is reflected clinically in the longer incubation and the presence of systemic symptoms and signs such as rash, fever, and a septic appearance. The second reason is that cell-mediated immunity is more critical in recovery from measles than from other respiratory viral diseases (7 9). In this respect measles is more akin to herpesvirus infections than to the other respiratory viruses. Nevertheless, measles virus replicates readily in the epithelial cells of the respiratory tract, including the conjunctivae, and produces widespread destruction very similar to that produced by influenza virus. The consequence of this is an illness characterized by conjunctivitis, cough, coryza, and, in a proportion of cases, croup or pneumonia. Perhaps because of the destructive nature of the infection, measles, like influenza virus, probably predisposes to bacterial superinfection more readily than the other respiratory viruses.

The epidemiology of several respiratory viruses can be considered to change in certain microenvironments as a consequence of chronic shedding by immunodeficient patients, including children with AIDS and HIV infection. For example, because of chronic shedding, several viruses, including particularly RSV, parainfluenza viruses, and influenza A virus, are recognized outside their usual seasonal epidemics. This unusual epidemic behavior applies not only to children with HIV infection, in whom these viruses may be found as presumed causes of lower respiratory tract disease at unusual times of year, but also to other children in their environments (hospital, school, day care) in whom institutional cross-infection may occur.

IMMUNOLOGIC CONSIDERATIONS

In Table 19.2 is a summary of certain aspects of immunity to the respiratory viruses that are pertinent to their pathogenicity in children with HIV infection. As with other infectious diseases, the mechanisms of protection against respiratory virus infection are frequently not the same as the mecha-

Table 19.2.   Immunologic Mechanisms and Consequences of HIV Infection

Virus	Likely Protective Immune Mechanism	Likely Curative Immune Mechanism	In HIV Infection	
			Disease of Increased Severity	Prolonged Excretion
RSV	Serum antibody	Cellular immunity ? Serum antibody ? Secretory antibody	Yes	Yes
Parainfluenza virus	Serum and secretory antibody	Cellular immunity	?Yes	Yes
Influenza virus	Serum and secretory antibody	Cellular immunity	?Yes	Yes
Adenovirus	Serum antibody	Cellular immunity ? Serum antibody	?Yes	No
Rhinovirus	Serum and secretory antibody	? Serum antibody	No	No
Coronaviruses	?	?	No	No
Measles virus	Serum antibody ? Cellular immunity	Cellular immunity	Yes	No

nisms of recovery from infection. Note also that animal model investigations, as well as analysis of infections in patients with immunodeficiencies, have shown quite convincingly that clinical manifestations of respiratory viral infections are a combination of virus cytopathic (i.e., cell destructive) effects and the consequences of the immune response. For this reason, we can expect that infections in immunodeficient hosts may differ from those in normal hosts in their clinical expression in certain more or less obvious ways. And infections in patients with immunologic *dys*regulation, which is the condition of many individuals with AIDS, may manifest themselves in complex ways that are difficult to predict.

Respiratory Syncytial Virus

Infections by RSV have been studied more thoroughly than those by most other respiratory viruses. The evidence favors a protective role for high titers (but not low titers) of neutralizing serum IgG antibody (10). There is also some evidence that secretory antibody is protective (11). Recovery is probably mediated largely through cell-mediated mechanisms, as demonstrated by the prolongation and, in some instances, intensification of infection in a few patients specifically lacking T cells (12). Instances of severe infection in deficient hosts have been observed primarily in children with defects in

both B and T cell function and rarely in children with primary antibody deficiencies. In addition, both animal (13) and human (14) studies have shown that large doses of immunoglobulin administered systemically can shorten the course of infection. Thus it is difficult to eliminate entirely a role for circulating antibody in natural recovery. Finally, disappearance of virus in infants coincides with the appearance of secretory IgA antibody in the nasopharynx (15), and in animal models intratracheally administered IgG functions quite efficiently to eliminate virus from the respiratory tract (16). Thus recovery may be multifactorial, but the best evidence indicates that cellular mechanisms are paramount. Immunopathology during infections with RSV is widely assumed (17), and may also be due to multiple mechanisms; IgE production (18), type IV cellular mechanisms (19), and immune complex disease (15) have all been postulated.

Children and adults with cancer or who have been pharmacologically immunosuppressed also illustrate the increased pathogenicity of RSV in the presence of defects in B or T cell function (20 22). Virus excretion is prolonged, and illness more severe in this group. In addition, immunosuppressed adults, at an age when lower tract pathology with RSV infections is uncommon, may develop extensive or even fatal pneumonia.

Parainfluenza Viruses

Although parainfluenza viruses have not been as well studied, it seems likely that, because of their structural similarity to RSV, the mechanisms of protection, recovery and immunopathology are quite similar (12). Instances of prolonged excretion and progressive pathology in children lacking cell-mediated immunity, either through congenital defects (23) or immunosuppression (24), are common.

Animal model experiments (25), a very large experience with protection through parenteral inoculation of inactivated virus vaccines, and some experience in immunodeficient hosts (12) suggest that influenza also shares similar mechanisms of protection and recovery.

Adenoviruses

The immunology of adenovirus infections is complex and has not been thoroughly studied. In immunized individuals, antibody correlates with protection. Case reports would indicate that severe pulmonary infections occur on rare occasions in agammaglobulinemic patients (26) and somewhat more commonly in those with defects in both antibody production and cell-mediated immunity (27). Immunocompromised patients with cancer (28) and with organ transplants (29 31) have been described with both severe pneumonia and fatal hepatitis. Thus, it appears likely that both antibody and cellular immunity are important in recovery from adenoviral infections.

Rhinoviruses and Coronaviruses

Little is known about the important immunologic mechanisms in either rhinovirus or coronavirus infection. There is evidence that secretory (and probably systemic) antibody is protective against rhinovirus infection (32). Rhinoviruses, being structurally similar to enteroviruses, may share their susceptibility to the curative effects of antibody, either circulating or secretory (33).

Measles

Measles can be protected against by circulating antibody, as demonstrated clearly by the capacity of maternally transmitted IgG to protect against natural infection and immunization. Untreated children with congenital agammaglobulinemia recover from measles in an ordinary fashion, and there are no records of recurrent disease on repeat exposure even before the prophylactic use of replacement immunoglobulin (34). Thus cell-mediated immunity can probably prevent disease even in the absence of antibody, as well as promoting recovery. Measles infection in patients lacking T cells, either through congenital defects (8), through the presence of malignancy (7), or through iatrogenic immunosuppression (9), is severe and also different, in that there is often no associated rash and giant-cell pneumonia is frequent and often fatal.

CLINICAL PRESENTATION

There is one prospective survey of respiratory viral infections in HIV-infected infants and children (35). Respiratory virus cultures were obtained at 3-month intervals from 50 children born to HIV-infected mothers, of whom five were themselves infected. Cultures from the five infected children more frequently grew a virus than those from the 45 uninfected, and the infected children had more frequent symptomatic episodes. Because of the small numbers of children and illnesses studied, however, little could be concluded from this survey.

Because of the lack of published literature on the presentation of respiratory virus infections in children with HIV infection, an informal survey of the experience of clinicians in the major pediatric centers who have cared for large numbers of HIV-infected infants and children in the United States was performed in preparation for the first edition of this book. Much information in the following section is based on this informal survey, as well as personal experience. Attribution is made wherever appropriate to those individuals who kindly shared their experience with us.

Respiratory Syncytial Virus

Published information on clinical presentation of RSV LRTI in subjects with HIV infection consists of a case series (36) and several case reports (37 39). The series describes 10 children, six of whom were younger than 1 year and the remainder between 2 and 4 years. Seven were treated with ribavirin, and two died, both infants younger than 9 months and both with advanced immunodeficiency. The most unusual aspect of the ten infections was the distinct rarity of wheezing (one of ten) despite the severity of illness in a few. This clinical feature was associated with a lack of both acute and convalescent secretory IgE. Excretion of RSV in three children with serial antigen measurements was prolonged: more than 80 days in one case; total CD4 cell count in this child was 1415/mm^3.

The other notable feature of these published cases was the presence, in the two cases with advanced immunodeficiency and a fatal outcome, of important coinfecting pathogens: in one, *P. carinii* and *Pseudomonas aeruginosa* (the latter in postmortem lung cultures) and in the other *P. aeruginosa* in blood cultures and lung at autopsy and *P. carinii* at autopsy.

There is one published account of interstitial pneumonia caused by RSV infection in an adult with HIV infection (39).

Several additional cases of RSV upper or lower respiratory infection were described by those answering the survey. None were remarkable.

We have observed 16 cases of RSV infection at Children's Hospital in Boston, all but one in vertically infected infants. Most have been unremarkable in their clinical presentation. Excretion of virus has been prolonged in some children (up to 56 days), and the cases were generally unresponsive to ribavirin treatment. We have also seen two fatal cases, one complicated by cytomegalovirus and *P. aeruginosa* pneumonia. One other fatal case in a 16-month child was apparently not superinfected (autopsy was not performed). This child presented with bronchiolitis and was found as part of his general work-up to have HIV infection. He was profoundly immunodeficient, with CD4 cells of 16/mm^3, and died of progressive respiratory failure.

One near-fatal infection occurred in a child with severe cardiomyopathy and chronic pulmonary disease probably secondary to lymphocytic interstitial pneumonia (40). Parainfluenza virus type 3 (PIV3) was also present in the respiratory secretions, although this had been present on a previous occasion 7 months earlier. Illness was characterized by severe bronchospasm and required prolonged intubation and ventilation. This child was 16 months old at the time, with a total CD4 cell count of 1664/mm3.

Parainfluenza Viruses

As might be expected, parainfluenza virus infection is common in children with HIV infection. One published report (41) describes two children with prolonged PIV3 excretion (for 1 and 3 months, respectively). In both children, as in the children with RSV infection described above, other respiratory pathogens were isolated along with PIV3 from upper respiratory or bronchial cultures (*P. carinii*, *Candida*, influenza A, RSV, other viruses). In both cases, the pathogenic role of PIV3 was unclear. Another report describes a child with interstitial pneumonia from whom *P. carinii*, *Legionella*, and PIV3 were recovered by bronchoalveolar wash (38). Finally, a case of fatal measles giant cell pneumonia was described in which both cytomegalovirus and PIV3 were present, but of unknown pathogenicity, during the illness and were found again at autopsy (42).

Our informal survey recovered many important and illustrative cases. The most remarkable was a child (E. R. Stiehm, personal communication, 1989) who had been vertically infected by HIV and who presented with progressive immunologic deficiency and a long history of asthma. At the age of 6 years, while on treatment with monthly intravenous immunoglobulin and oral and aerosolized asthma medications, he was hospitalized in status asthmaticus and required intubation. PIV2 was isolated from the respiratory tract at that time and remained present throughout hospitalization. His CD4 lymphocyte count was 4/mm^3. He was rehospitalized for acute asthma 5 months later, and PIV2 was again recovered. Moreover, about 1 year after his first hospitalization, PIV2 was still consistently recoverable. The only symptoms referable to the viral infection were wheezing and rales throughout his chest.

We have also cared for a child with AIDS who has intermittently excreted PIV3 (along with cytomegalovirus) for 9 months, apparently without symptoms, as well as a child with essentially absent T4 lymphocytes who had intermittent symptoms of wheezing and a persistent lower lobe pulmonary infiltrate accompanying PIV3 excretion for at least 2 months.

Two other illustrative cases (J. F. Modlin, personal communication, 1989) are those of a 4-month child with PIV3 pulmonary infection accompanying fatal *P. carinii* pneumonia, as well as an 18-month child with histologically proven lymphoid interstitial pneumonitis accompanied by PIV3. The virus was isolated from a lung biopsy obtained during an exacerbation of symptoms.

Influenza Virus

There is one case report of an adult with HIV infection and influenza virus pneumonia (43). The illness was self-limited and not severe, although it was accompanied by hypoxia. Influenza virus A was found in the lung of one child who died of pneumonia caused by *P. carinii* and histologically proven cytomegalovirus (44). Aside from a single report of asymptomatic carriage of influenza virus A (41), there are no other published descriptions of influenza virus infection in HIV-infected children.

We have seen one HIV-infected child from whom influenza virus B was isolated at the time of a febrile seizure. This child's CD4 lymphocyte percentage was low (9%), but recovery from this illness was uneventful, and although it was accompanied by otitis, pneumonia did not occur.

Another child with advanced HIV infection and biopsy-proven cytomegalovirus myocarditis under treatment with ganciclovir presented during a prolonged hospitalization with worsening respiratory symptoms, wheezing, and persistent pulmonary interstitial infiltrates. Even though the season was midsummer, influenza A virus (H3N2, Washington/15/91-like) was grown from the respiratory tract for at least 3.5 weeks. The child developed progressive respiratory failure despite treatment first with oral amantadine and then with aerosolized ribavirin. She died 1 day after bronchoalveolar lavage yielded fluid from which the same influenza virus was grown as the sole pathogen. *P. carinii* was not found. Two buffy coat cultures failed to grow cytomegalovirus during her final illness, and her cytomegalovirus retinitis was stable during this time, probably because of continuing ganciclovir suppressive treatment. Although an autopsy was not performed, it appears likely that influenza virus was the primary respiratory pathogen and was responsible for her death.

Adenovirus

Adenoviruses from hemagglutinin group B and most closely resembling types 34 and 35 have been isolated from urine in a surprisingly large proportion of adults with AIDS (45), and group D strains have been isolated frequently from stools. In most circumstances, these viruses have not been considered to have any pathogenic role in this setting, and in particular they have not been associated with respiratory illness. However, one adult has been described in whom adenovirus type 29 was recovered from alveolar washings during a fatal illness that was, on histologic grounds, probably a combination of *P. carinii* and adenovirus pneumonia (46).

A recent review of disseminated adenovirus infections with hepatic necrosis includes three with underlying HIV infection, two of whom were children, aged 6 months and 7 years (47). Types 1, 2, and 3 were involved, and all cases were fatal. In all instances pneumonia was present, but fulminant hepatic failure was the determining factor in the clinical evolution. In one, a 7-year boy, *P. carinii* pneumonia and *Candida* blood stream infection were present at death.

The informal mail survey turned up one interesting case (M. Horwitz, personal communication, 1989). A 6-month baby with presumed HIV infection (mother HIV antibody positive, clinical course in child consistent with HIV infection) died of progressive pneumonia. A lung biopsy a few days before death grew both RSV and adenovirus type

5, and postmortem examination of the lungs demonstrated interstitial pneumonia, interstitial fibrosis, and widespread "smudge" cells consistent with adenovirus infection. Bacteria, mycobacteria, fungi, and *P. pneumoniae* were not found.

Measles Virus

It should not come as a surprise that measles is a severe illness in children with HIV infection, particularly those with advanced immunodeficiency. It is generally accepted that the clinical expression of measles is more susceptible to the level of cellular immunity than that of the respiratory viruses discussed above, and the case reports of measles in HIV-infected children confirm this impression.

There are eleven cases of measles in HIV-infected individuals described in literature from the United States (42, 48 52), eight of which were in children younger than 13 years. Five childhood cases were hospital acquired. Pneumonia, with typical giant cell histology in instances where tissue was examined, occurred in six. Five had absent, delayed, or atypical rashes. Ribavirin was administered by aerosol to most children with pneumonia. Despite this, two of these children died of pneumonia. A recent case in a 26-year hemophiliac complicated by both respiratory failure and measles encephalitis was treated wtih intravenous ribavirin and high-dose intravenous immunoglobulin and survived without sequelae (51).

Several of the cases described had received vaccine previously, but there was no firm evidence that antibody was still present at the time of exposure. Two had received immunoglobulin to prevent the infection, but in neither instance was the timing of this prophylaxis ideal: one was receiving regular doses of intravenous immunoglobulin, but the most recently administered dose was 3 weeks before the onset of illness; the other was given varicella-zoster immunoglobulin a few days before onset of measles.

There are two case series from central Africa (53, 54). In both series many children were younger than 1 year, and there was uncertainty about the diagnosis of HIV infection. Moreover, the background fatal-

ity rate of hospitalized measles in that setting was high enough so that increased morbidity was difficult to demonstrate. Nevertheless, there was a trend toward higher mortality, largely from pneumonia, in somewhat older children with proven HIV infection and measles (53). The important observation was also made that the attack rate of measles before routine vaccination at 9 months in offspring of HIV-infected mothers was higher than that in control infants, with an odds ratio of 3.8 (95% confidence interval, 1.2 13.2) (54). The impression that such infants are at increased risk because of lower antibody titers was confirmed by another study in Rwanda showing a significantly lower prevalence of detectable measles antibody in such children at age 6 months than in control children (55). It is reassuring that in that study the infected offspring of HIV-infected mothers responded to vaccine as briskly as uninfected children.

Other Respiratory Viruses

There are no reports of infections with either rhinoviruses or coronaviruses. We have seen one child with a rhinovirus infection who did not have an unusual illness.

LABORATORY DIAGNOSIS

Laboratory diagnosis of respiratory virus infection in infants and children with HIV infection is similar to that in normal children (56). The mainstay of such diagnosis is detection of the virus in a sample of respiratory secretion, rather than measurement of antibody in serum. In normal children IgM antibody is not dependably made during the acute phase of respiratory viral infection, and the usefulness of acute and convalescent serum specimens is limited to retrospective diagnosis. Nevertheless, finding a rise of antibody in a convalescent sample can be useful in certain instances. For adenovirus infection it can help to distinguish prolonged carriage from acute infection. In influenza virus infection, it is probably more sensitive than virus isolation in normal children.

In immunodeficient children there is more reason to use virus detection for laboratory diagnosis, because antibody rises become even less reliable. The case descriptions above, however, emphasize that finding virus in the upper respiratory tract does not necessarily indicate that the recovered virus is the cause of the disease in question. Thus, viruses should be sought, whenever possible, from lung tissue directly or, failing this, from bronchial washes.

Methods of virus detection are well described (57). Culture is slow but sensitive and reliable. Immunofluorescence has the advantage of wide applicability (it is as sensitive as culture for RSV, more sensitive for measles, and acceptably sensitive for the parainfluenza viruses). Enzyme-linked immunosorbent assays (ELISAs) are commercially available only for RSV but are quite acceptable both in sensitivity and specificity.

MANAGEMENT
Chemotherapy

There are two licensed chemotherapeutic agents for the treatment of respiratory viral infection: ribavirin aerosol for RSV (57) and amantadine for influenza A (58). Ribavirin aerosol has also demonstrated efficacy in the treatment of influenza A and B in adults (59), and it shows activity against parainfluenza viruses and measles *in vitro* that is comparable with that seen for RSV (60, 61). Although there has been some experience in treatment of measles infections with oral ribavirin in normal hosts (61), it has not been sufficient to judge efficacy.

There have been several reports of the use of aerosolized ribavirin in the treatment of respiratory viral infection in immunodeficient hosts, including children with AIDS (36, 49, 62, 63). Although no controlled studies exist, several patients with severe combined immunodeficiency syndrome have been described where PIV3 or RSV have been eliminated from the respiratory tract during ribavirin treatment. Most clinicians would agree that treatment is probably indicated in instances where infection is symptomatic and persistent or progressive (64).

It is useful to differentiate between measles and other respiratory viruses since measles in children with advanced HIV infections, because of its poor prognosis and rapid course, should probably be treated as early as possible. In contrast, judging from the accumulated experience of multiple centers, in other respiratory virus infections there is usually time to evaluate the patient, assure (if possible) that the offending virus is a major cause of the illness, and then initiate therapy. Therapy with ribavirin should be given in the usual dose (20 mg/ml in reservoir) for 16 20 of each 24 hr for at least 5 days and longer if virus and symptoms persist. Because of concerns about the expense of administration and possible hazards to people in the environment, ribavirin has recently been administered at a higher dose (60 mg/ml in reservoir) over shorter periods (aerosol administered over 2 hr at 8-hr intervals) for 5 days (65). Although evidence from rodent models indicates that this treatment is effective (66), there have not been controlled trials in infected children. The more traditional administration is therefore recommended.

Immunotherapy

Immunotherapy in the form of very high doses of intravenous immunoglobulin has been successfully administered to normal infants with RSV infections, with an apparent therapeutic effect quite equivalent to that of aerosolized ribavirin (14). It seems logical to suppose that such therapy would offer some benefit if used in severe respiratory viral infections of children with AIDS, particularly those with far advanced immunodeficiency. It may be assumed that commercial lots of intravenous immunoglobulin will have high titers of antibody to all major respiratory viruses since such antibody is essentially universal in the general population. This has been verified for RSV.

General Management

Probably the most important lesson from the various cases presented above is that when respiratory viral infections in HIV-infected children are accompanied by severe symptoms there is frequently some coinfecting microorganism present. Thus, the search for etiology should not necessarily stop when a respiratory virus has been found. Nevertheless, in many instances it seems likely that the respiratory viral infection, even when not the sole cause of symptoms, was an important contributor, and management and therapy directed at these organisms should be logical and aggressive.

It is also clear from the experience thus far that the clinical response of an HIV-infected child to respiratory viral infection is exceedingly variable and that it is difficult to predict what that response will be on the basis of measurements of immunity, such as absolute CD4 lymphocyte count, or the presence of underlying conditions, such as chronic pulmonary disease or myocardiopathy.

PREVENTION

The important modes of prevention of respiratory viruses are epidemiologic barrier methods (of prime importance in the hospital), passive immunization, and chemoprophylaxis.

Epidemiologic Methods

Respiratory viruses spread by three major routes of transmission: fomite transfer, large-particle aerosols, and small-particle aerosols. The present evidence is that the most important routes for respiratory viruses (excluding measles) are the first two (67). Measles, which is one of the most contagious viruses known, spreads through small-particle aerosols (68), and there is some evidence that, at least under certain circumstances, influenza does too (69).

The importance of the distinction between small-particle aerosol and the other two modes of spread involves the barriers used in the hospital setting. RSV has been successfully contained by the use of contact precautions alone, particularly gloves and gowns (70). Some additional protection can probably be afforded by the use of goggles to prevent inoculation of caretakers' conjunctivae (71). Single rooms are not necessary for infected children.

In contrast, measles virus frequently (68), and influenza virus at times (69), will spread widely and rapidly in indoor settings, even in the absence of close face-to-face contact. Thus, single rooms with control of airflow are recommended for hospitalized patients with measles and influenza. All caretakers should have definite evidence of immunity to measles and be immunized against influenza on a yearly basis.

There is little information about the route of spread of parainfluenza viruses and adenovirus. Thus, a logical approach is not possible, and single room isolation is probably warranted when infections are recognized.

Passive Immunization

Measles can be prevented or modified by administration of sufficient antibody in the form of intramuscular or intravenous immunoglobulin within several days of exposure. In infants and children with HIV infection, intramuscular antibody should be given (0.5 ml/kg, maximum 15 ml) as soon as possible after bona fide exposure to measles regardless of *whether the child has received vaccine before* (49). Because such antibody would appear to have at least some chance of modifying the course of the illness, it should be administered even if 6 days have elapsed since exposure.

The use of prophylactic immunoglobulin is not normally considered upon exposure to other respiratory viruses (see Chapter 45). It is, however, evident that circulating antibody in sufficient quantity can ameliorate or prevent infection (10). Thus, it seems likely, and limited experience would confirm, that respiratory virus infections under the umbrella of regularly administered intravenous immunoglobulin might be less severe. Conversely, this is rarely of sufficient consequence to stand on its own as a compelling rationale for administration of intravenous immunoglobulin. In the recent controlled study of intravenous immunoglobulin in pediatric HIV infection, respiratory virus infections as a group and RSV infections in particular were not found to be prevented by intravenous immunoglobulin (72).

Chemoprophylaxis

There is good evidence that amantadine and its presently unlicensed congener, rimantidine, are highly efficient in the prevention of influenza A infections when taken at the time of exposure (73, 74). The usefulness of these drugs has been limited because of their narrow spectrum of activity. The circumstances under which their use would appear to be clinically indicated would be a known outbreak of influenza A, a high-risk setting (such as a hospital or day care center), and a child with both HIV infection and either severe immunodeficiency or underlying pulmonary disease. In that circumstance, amantadine (4 mg/kg/day PO divided every 12 hr) should be administered during the time significant exposure is expected to occur.

References

1. Paisley JR, Lauer BA, McIntosh K et al. Pathogens associated with acute lower respiratory tract infection in young children. Pediatr Infect Dis J 1984; 3:14–19.
2. Ramsey BW, Marcuse EK, Foy HM et al. Use of bacterial antigen detection in the diagnosis of pediatric lower respiratory tract infections. Pediatrics 1986;78:1–9.
3. Turner RB, Lande AE, Chase P, et al. Pneumonia in pediatric outpatients: Cause and clinical manifestations. J Pediatr 1987;111:194–200.
4. Dennehy PH, McIntosh K. Viral pneumonia in childhood. In: Weinstein L, Fields BN, eds. Seminars in infectious diseases, New York: Academic, 1983.
5. Krilov L, Pierik L, Keller E, et al. The association of rhinoviruses with lower respiratory tract disease in hospitalized patients. J Med Virol 1986;19: 345–352.
6. McIntosh K, Chao RK, Krause HE, Wasil R, Mocega HE, Mufson MA. Coronavirus infection in acute lower respiratory tract disease of infants. J Infect Dis 1974;130:502–507.
7. Enders JF, McCarthy R, Mitus A, Cheatham WJ. Isolation of measles virus at autopsy in cases of giant cell pneumonia without rash. N Engl J Med 1959;261:875–879.
8. Nahmias AJ, Griffith D, Salsbury C, Yoshida K. Thymic aplasia with lymphopenia, plasma cells, and normal immunoglobulins: relation to measles virus infection. JAMA 1967;201:729–734.
9. Lewis MJ, Cameron AH, Shah KJ, Purdham DR, Mann JR. Giant cell pneumonia caused by measles and methotrexate in childhood leukemia in remission. Br Med J 1978:1:330–331.
10. Glezen WP, Paredes A, Allison JE, et al. Risk of respiratory syncytial virus infection for infants from low-income families in relationship to age, sex, ethnic group and maternal antibody level. J Pediatr 1981;98:708–715.
11. Mills J, Van Kirk JE, Wright PF, Chanock RM. Experimental respiratory syncytial virus infection of adults. J Immunol 1971;107:123–130.
12. Fishaut M, Tubergen D, McIntosh K. Cellular response to respiratory viruses with particular reference to children with disorders of cell-mediated immunity. J Pediatr 1980:96:179–186.
13. Prince GA, Hemming VH, Horswood RL, Chanock RM. Immunoprophylaxis and immunotherapy of respiratory syncytial virus infection in the cotton rat. Virus Res 1985;3:193–206.
14. Hemming VG, Rodriguez W, Kim HW, et al. Intravenous immunoglobulin treatment of respiratory syncytial virus infections in infants and young children. Antimicrob Agents Chemother 1987; 31:1882–1886.
15. McIntosh K, Masters HB, Orr I, Chao RK, Barkin RM. The immunologic response to infection with respiratory syncytial virus in infants. J Infect Dis 1978;138:24–32.
16. Prince GA, Hemming VH, Horswood RL, Baron PA, Chanock RM. Effectiveness of topically administered neutralizing antibodies in experimental immunotherapy of respiratory syncytial virus infection in cotton rats. J Virol 1987;61: 1851–1854.
17. McIntosh K, Fishaut JM. Immunopathologic mechanisms in lower respiratory tract disease of infants due to respiratory syncytial virus. Prog Med Virol 1980;26:94–118.
18. Welliver RC, Wong DT, Sun M, Middleton E, Vaughn RS, Ogra PL. The development of respiratory syncytial virus-specific IgE and the release of histamine in nasopharyngeal secretions after infection. N Engl J Med 1981;305:841–846.
19. Welliver RC, Kaul LA, Ogra PL. Cell-mediated immune response to respiratory syncytial virus infection: relationship to the development of reactive airway disease. J Pediatr 1979;94:370–375.
20. Hall CB, Powell KR, Macdonald NE, et al. Respiratory syncytial viral infection in children with compromised immune function. N Engl J Med 1986;315:77–81.
21. Englund JA, Sullivan CJ, Jordan MC, Dehner LP, Vecellotti GM, Balfour HH Jr. Respiratory syncytial virus infection in immunocompromised adults. Ann Intern Med 1988;109:203–208.
22. Sinnott JT, Cullison JP, Sweeney MS, Hammond M, Holt DA. Respiratoryt syncytial virus pneumonia in a cardiac transplant recipient. J Infect Dis 1988;158:650–651.
23. Delage G, Brochu P, Pelletier M, Gasmin G, Lapointe N. Giant-cell pneumonia caused by parainfluenza virus. J Pediatr 1979;94:426–429.
24. Weintrub PS, Sullender WM, Lombard C, Link MP, Arvin A. Giant Cell pneumonia caused by parainfluenza type 3 in a patient with acute myelomonocytic leukemia. Arch Pathol Lab Med 1987;111:569–570.
25. Ada GL, Jones PD. The cell-mediated and humoral responses to influenza virus infection in the mouse lung. Adv Exp Med Biol 1987;216:1033–1042.
26. Siegel FP, Dikman SH, Arayata RB, Bottone EJ. Fatal disseminated adenovirus 11 pneumonia in an agammaglobulinemic patient. Am J Med 1981; 71:1062–1067.
27. Wigger HJ, Blanc WA. Fatal hepatic and bronchial necrosis in adenovirus infection with thymic alymphoplasia. N Engl J Med 1966;275:870–874.
28. Zahradnik JM, Spencer MJ, Porter DD. Adenovirus infection in the immunocompromised patient. Am J Med 1980;68:725–732.

29. Koneru B, Jaffe R, Esquivel CO, et al. Adenoviral infections in pediatric liver transplant recipients. JAMA 1987;258:489–492.

30. Myerowitz Rl, Stalder H, Oxman MN, et al. Fatal disseminated adenovirus infection in a renal transplant recipient. Am J Med 1975;59:591–598.

31. Shields AF, Hackman RC, Fife KH, Corey L, Meyers JD. Adenovirus infections in patients undergoing bone-marrow transplantation. N Engl J Med 1985;312:529–533.

32. Perkins JC, Tucker DN, Knopf HLS, Wenzel RP, Kapikian AZ, Chanock RM. Comparison of protective efficacy of neutralizing antibody in serum and nasal secretions in experimental rhinovirus type 13 illness. Am J Epidemiol 1969;90:519–526.

33. Wlfert CM, Buckley RH, Mohanakumar T, et al. Persistent and fatal central-nervous-system echovirus infections in patients with agammaglobulinemia. N Engl J Med 1977;296:1485–1489.

34. Rosen FS, Janeway CA. The gamma globulins. III. The antibody deficiency syndromes. N Engl J Med 1966;275:709–715.

35. Hague RA, Burns SE, Hargreaves FD, Mok JYQ, Yap PL. Virus infections of the respiratory tract in HIV-infected children. J Infect 1992;24:31–36.

36. Chandwani S, Borkowsky W, Krasinski K, Lawrence R, Welliver R. Respiratory syncytial virus infection in human immunodeficiency virus-infected children. J Pediatr 1990;117:251–254.

37. Bye MR, Bernstein L, Shah K, Ellaurie M, Rubinstein A. Diagnostic bronchoalveolar lavage in children with AIDS. Pediatr Pulmonol 1987;3:425–428.

38. de Blic J, Blanche S, Danel C, Le Bougeois M, Caniglia M, Scheinmann P. Bronchoalveolar lavage in HIV infected patients with interstitial pneumonia. Arch Dis Child 1989;64:1246–1250.

39. Murphy D, Rose RC. Respiratory syncytial virus pneumonia in a human immunodeficiency virus-infected man [Letter]. JAMA 1989;261:1147.

40. Centers for Disease Control. Classification system for human immunodeficiency virus (HIV) infections in children under 13 years of age. MMWR 1987;36:225–236.

41. Josephs S, Kim HW, Brandt CD, Parrott RH. Parainfluenza 3 virus and other common respiratory pathogens in children with human immunodeficiency virus infection. Pediatr Infect Dis J 1988;7:207–209.

42. Nadel S, McGann K, Hodinka RL, Rutstein R, Chatten J. Measles giant cell pneumonia in a child with human immunodeficiency virus infection. Pediatr Infect Dis J 1991;10:542–544.

43. Thurn JR, Henry K. Influenza A pneumonitis in a patient infected with the human immunodeficiency virus (HIV). Chest 1989; 95:807–810.

44. Cohen-Abbo A, Wright PF. Complex etiology of pneumonia in infants perinatally infected with human immunodeficiency virus 1. Pediatr Infect Dis J 1991;10:545–547.

45. Flomenberg PR, Chen M, Munk G, Horwitz MS. Molecular epidemiology of adenovirus type 35 infections in immunocompromised hosts. J Infect Dis 1987;155:1127–1134.

46. Valainis GT, Carlisle JT, Daroca PJ, Goh RS, Enelow TJ. Respiratory failure complicated by adenovirus serotype 29 in a patient with AIDS. J Infect Dis 1989;160:349–351.

47. Krilov LR, Rubin LG, Frogel M, et al. Disseminated adenovirus infection with hepatic necrosis in patients with human immunodeficiency virus infection and other immunodeficiency states. Rev Infect Dis 1990;12:303–307.

48. Centers for Disease Control. Measles in HIV-infected children, United States. MMWR 1988;37:183–186.

49. Krasinski K, Borkowsky W. Measles and measles immunity in children infected with human immunodeficiency virus. JAMA 1989;261:2512–2516.

50. Markowitz LE, Chandler FW, Rolden EO, et al. Fatal measles pneumonia without rash in a child with AIDS. J Infect Dis 1988;158:480483.

51. Ross LA, Kim KS, Mason WH Jr, Gomperts E. Successful treatment of disseminated measles in a patient with acquired immunodeficiency syndrome: Consideration of antiviral and passive immunotherapy. Am J Med 1990;88:313–314.

52. Kaplan LJ, Daum RS, Smaron M, McCarthy CA. Severe measles in immunocompromised patients. JAMA 1992;267:1237–1241.

53. Sension MG, Quinn TC, Markowitz LE, et al. Measles in hospitalized African children with human immunodeficiency virus. Am J Dis Child 1988;142:1271–1272.

54. Embree JE, Datta P, Stackiw W, et al. Increased risk of early measles in infants of human immunodeficiency virus type 1-seropositive mothers. J Infect Dis 1992;165:262–267.

55. Lepage P, Dabis F, Msellati P, et al. Safety and immunogenicity of high-dose Edmonston-Zagreb measles vaccine in children with HIV-1 infection. A cohort study in Kigali, Rwanda. Am J Dis Child 1992;146:550–555.

56. McIntosh K. Diagnostic virology In: Fields BN, ed. Virology. 2nd ed. New York: Raven, 1989:411–440.

57. Hall CB, McBride JT, Walsh EE, et al. Aerosolized ribavirin treatment of infants with respiratory syncytial virus infection. N Engl J Med 1983;308:1443–1447.

58. Wingfield WL, Pollack D, Grunert RR. Therapeutic efficacy of amantadine HCl and rimantadine HCl in naturally occurring influenza A2 respiratory illness in man. N Engl J Med 1969;281:579–584.

59. Gilbert BE, Wilson SZ, Knight V, et al. Ribavirin small-particle aerosol treatment of infections caused by influenza virus strains A/Victoria/7/83 (H1N1) and B/Texas/1/84. Antimicrob Agents Chemother 1985;27:309–313.

60. Sidwell RW, Huffman JH, Khare GP. Broad-spectrum antiviral activity of virazole: 1-beta-D-ribofuranosyl-1,2,4-triazole-3-carboxamide. Science 1972;177:705–706.

61. Banks SG, Fernandez H. Clinical use of ribavirin in measles. A summarized review. In: Smith RA, Knight V, Smith JAD, eds. Clinical applications of ribavirin. Orlando: Academic, 1984:203–209.

62. McIntosh K, Kurachek S, Cairns LM, Burns JC, Goodspeed B. Teatment of respiratory viral infection in an immunodeficient infant with ribavirin aerosol. Am J Dis Child 1984;138:305–308.

63. Gelfand EW, McCurdy D, Rao CP, Middleton PJ. Ribavirin treatment of viral pneumonitis in severe combined immunodeficiency disease. Lancet 1983;2:732–733.

64. Committee on Infectious Disease. Ribavirin therapy of respiratory syncytial virus. Pediatrics 1987; 79:475–478.

65. Englund JA, Piedra PA, Jefferson LS, Wilson SZ, Taber LH, Gilbert BE. High-dose, short-duration ribavirin aerosol therapy in chldren with suspected respiratory syncytial virus infection. J Pediatr 1990;117:313–320.

66. Wyde PR, Wilson SZ, Petrella R, Gilbert BE. Efficacy of high dose-short duration ribavirin aerosol in the treatment of respiratory syncytial virus infected cotton rats and influenza B virus infected mice. Antiviral Res 1987;7:211–220.

67. Hall CB, Douglas RG. Modes of transmission of respiratory syncytial virus. J Pediatr 1981;99:100–103.

68. Remington PL, Hall WN, Davis IH, Herald A, Gunn RA. Airborne transmission of measles in a physicians office. JAMA 1985;253:1574–1577.

69. Moser MR, Bender TR, Margolis HS, et al. An outbreak of influenza aboard a commercial airliner. Am J Epidemiol 1979;110:1–6.

70. LeClair MM, Freeman J, Sullivan BF, Crowley CM, Goldmann DA. Prevention of nosocomial respiratory syncytial virus infections through compliance with glove and gown isolation precautions. N Engl J Med 1987:317:329–334.

71. Gala CL, Hall CB, Schnabel MA, et al. The use of eye-nose goggles to control nosocomial respiratory syncytial virus infection. JAMA 1986;256: 2706–2708.

72. Mofenson LM, Moye J Jr, Bethel J, et al. Prophylactic intravenous immunoglobulin in HIV-infected children with CD4+ counts of 0.20×10^9/L or more: Effect on viral, opportunistic, and bacterial infections. JAMA 1992;268:483–488.

73. Centers for Disease Control. Measles prevention: Recommendations of the Immunization Practices Advisory Committee (ACIP). MMWR 1989;38(suppl 9):1–18.

74. Dolin R, Reichman RC, Madore HP, Maynard R, Linton PN, Webber-Jones J. A controlled trial of amantadine and rimantadine in the prophylaxis of influenza A infection. N Engl J Med 1982;307: 580–584.

20

Infections of the Gastrointestinal Tract

Larry K. Pickering

Gastrointestinal tract manifestations that occur in persons with AIDS include diarrhea, anorexia, abdominal pain, malabsorption, weight loss, and in certain instances vomiting, dysphagia, odynophagia, jaundice, proctitis, and death (1–17). Pathologic changes in the gastrointestinal tract of a patient with human immunodeficiency virus (HIV) infection can be produced by various infectious agents including bacteria, viruses, parasites, and fungi. In addition, malignancies, HIV infection of intestinal tract tissue, or a combination of these conditions occur (11). Many investigators report that diarrhea is a complication of HIV infection in 30–60% of adult patients with AIDS in industrialized countries (2, 16, 17) and in 60–90% of adult patients with AIDS from Haiti (18) or Africa (19–21). Depending on the specific cause and the immunologic status of a patient, clinical manifestations may be acute or chronic with significant weight loss and debilitation. Diagnosis and therapy are often frustrating and difficult because of the diversity of agents that can produce infection, the frequent finding of more than one potential cause, and the devastation of the immune system that often makes resolution difficult. Despite these problems associated with establishing a diagnosis, prospective studies of diarrhea in patients with AIDS have identified enteric pathogens in 75–85% of cases (22–26). Enteropathogens that infect individuals infected with HIV will be similar worldwide, but the frequency will generally depend on the age of the patient, the underlying immune status, and the geographic location

and exposure of individuals. This chapter will deal with infections of the gastrointestinal tract in patients with HIV infection.

ETIOLOGY

Infectious and noninfectious causes of gastrointestinal tract disease in children with AIDS can be divided into several major categories based on the microbiologic classification of infectious causes (bacteria, viruses, parasites, fungi), region of the digestive tract involved (esophagus, stomach, intestine, liver, or gallbladder), pathophysiology of disease produced, and host response to individual agents. Division among these various classifications is often blurred because many enteropathogens produce disease in several areas of the gastrointestinal tract, several agents often simultaneously infect an individual, and host responses to many infectious and noninfectious agents appear clinically similar.

Limited data are available to describe the range of enteric pathogens that infect children with HIV infection. Most published literature dealing with gastrointestinal tract disease in patients with AIDS describes patients in whom various enteropathogens, including unusual opportunistic gastrointestinal tract pathogens (8), have been found (Table 20.1). Although many enteropathogens have been associated with diarrhea in immunocompetent children (10), there are relatively few articles describing the cause of diarrhea in pediatric patients with AIDS (6, 27–29). The eight organisms that infect the gastrointestinal tract and fulfill the Centers for Disease Control and

Table 20.1.   Infections of Gastrointestinal Tract in Patients with AIDS

Sites of Infection	Signs and Symptoms	Common Organisms	Uncommon Organisms
Esophagus	Dysphagia, odynophagia, retrosternal pain	C. albicans, CMV herpes simplex	H. capsulatum L. donovani N. asteroides Toxoplasma gondii
Stomach	Abdominal pain	CMV MAC	L. donovani
Liver and gallbladder	Abdominal pain, jaundice, biliary colic	CMV, Cryptosporidium, Hepatrotropic viruses, MAC	T. gondii Rochalimaea quintana-like organism Pneumocystis carinii E. cuniculi Adenovirus P. marneffei L. donovani
Small intestine	Diarrhea, abdominal pain, weight loss, nausea, vomiting	Campylobacter sp, Cryptosporidium, CMV, E. bieneusi, G. lamblia, I. belli, MAC, Salmonella, S. stercoralis	A. hydrophila B. hominis Campylobacter species Chlorella-like organisms (blue green algae) Enteric adenovirus H. capsulatum
Large intestine	Diarrhea, abdominal pain, tenesmus	C. jejuni, C. difficile, CMV, E. histolytica, herpes simplex, MAC, Salmonella sp, Shigella sp	

Prevention revised classification system for HIV infection and expanded AIDS surveillance case definition for adolescents and adults include *Candida, Cryptosporidium,* cytomegalovirus (CMV), herpes simplex virus, *Histoplasma capsulatum, Isospora, Mycobacterium avium* complex (MAC), and *Salmonella* (30, 31). Although only those organisms that involve the gastrointestinal tract are listed in the Centers for Disease Control and Prevention case definition, many other organisms can produce disease in children with HIV infection. With a wider application of sophisticated laboratory techniques, future studies in various populations of children and adults with AIDS will increase our knowledge about the causes of gastrointestinal tract disease in this population and will provide data that may result in an expanison of organisms in the classification system. Pathogens that involve the gastrointestinal tract in the major classes of bacteria, viruses, and parasites will be considered below.

Bacteria

The major bacterial enteric pathogens associated with acute infectious diarrhea include *Aeromonas hydrophila, Campylobacter* species, *Clostridium difficile, Escherichia coli, Salmonella* species, *Shigella* species, *Vibrio cholerae, V. parahaemolyticus, Yersinia enterocolitica,* and MAC. Although any bacterial pathogen can infect an individual with AIDS, *Campylobacter* species (32–38), *Salmonella* (39–42), *Shigella* (43–45), and MAC (46, 47) have been the most frequently reported, with MAC and *Salmonella* being listed on the Centers for Disease Control and Prevention AIDS surveillance case definition (30, 31). It is estimated that ~40% of patients with AIDS have disseminated infections caused by MAC. Diseases from other bacterial enteropathogens including *Aeromonas* (48, 49), *E. coli* (43, 50), and blue-green algae (cyanobacteria) (51) have been reported in HIV-infected persons.

Viruses

Acute infectious diarrhea of virus origin is generally a self-limited disease associated with one of the following agents: rotavirus, enteric adenovirus, astrovirus, and calicivirus (10). All these viruses generally infect infants and young children, but any can involve the gastrointestinal tracts of older children and adults. These viruses have not been reported to cause diarrhea in children with AIDS at a rate disproportionate to that in the general population. Adenovirus was detected by electron microscopy and/or culture in five of 51 adults with AIDS and chronic diarrhea (52). In Australia, adenovirus was detected in 17 of 50 patients with advanced AIDS, and rotavirus was detected in 26 of these patients (53). In another study from Australia, rotavirus was detected in 18% of homosexual males infected with HIV who had diarrhea (54). Viruses were detected in 35% of 109 HIV-infected adults with diarrhea and included astrovirus, picobirnavirus, caliciviruses, small round structured viruses and, adenovirus (55). CMV frequently coinfects HIV-seropositive adults and can be found in the gastrointestinal tract of 15–45% of adults with AIDS (56–58), but its role in pediatric gastrointestinal tract disease has not been delineated. Approximately 5–10% of these adults exhibit pathologic evidence of disease that most commonly manifests as esophagitis or colitis (58–61). Herpes simplex virus has been associated with esophagitis and proctitis, with the latter generally occurring in homosexual males.

Adults with HIV infection often have been or become infected with one of the hepatotrophic viruses, which include hepatitis viruses A, B, C, D, and E (62). HIV can influence the course of prior, simultaneous, or subsequent infection by several of these hepatotropic viruses. Similarly, the effects of HIV infection can be modified by coinfection with several hepatotropic viruses.

Parasites

With the advent of HIV, there has been a renewed interest in protozoan organisms that involve the gastrointestinal tract. Organisms in this category associated with diarrhea in patients with HIV infection include *Cryptosporidium* (6, 7, 24, 27, 63–67), *I. belli* (7, 63, 68–72), *Giardia lamblia* (22, 23, 73–75), Microsporidia (18, 24, 76–86), and *Strongyloides stercoralis*. *Entamoeba histolytica* has been identified in homosexual men (22, 73, 74, 87). Parasitic diseases of the gastrointestinal tract included in the CDC surveillance definition for AIDS are *Cryptosporidium* and *Isospora* (30, 31). The Centers for Disease Control and Prevention reports that 3–4% of patients with AIDS in the United States have had cryptosporidial enteritis, but rates of 10–20% have been reported from some centers in the United States (16). *Isospora* is more common in tropical and subtropical climates and has been encountered in 15% of Haitian patients with AIDS but <0.2% of patients in the United States (68). *Giardia* has been found in 4–70% of patients with AIDS in the United States (22, 23, 73, 75) and in patients with AIDS from Europe (74). Microsporidia refers to a complex group of unicellular parasites that have been recognized as human pathogens. *Enterocytozoon bieneusi* is the species of microsporidia associated with diarrhea in patients with HIV infection. Prevalences of microsporidiosis among AIDS patients were found to be 10–16% in European studies (88). The importance of other parasites that infect the gastrointestinal tract such as *Blastocystis hominis*, *Dientamoeba fragilis*, *Balantidium coli*, nonpathogenic *Entamoeba* strains, and "cyanobacterium-like bodies" (organisms of the genus cyclospora) in patients with AIDS is unknown (2, 89–94). Other organisms including *Leishmania* (95, 96) have been reported to involve the gastrointestinal tract of patients infected with HIV. Fungal infections of the small and large intestine are unusual, but disseminated histoplasmosis may involve this organ (97).

EPIDEMIOLOGY

The incidence of gastrointestinal tract disease by specific enteropathogens varies by geographic location, mode of transmission, age and sex of infected individuals, degree of immune suppression, complexity of the laboratory evaluation of patients studied, and presence of continuing risk factors. The occurrence of chronic diarrhea and perhaps malabsorption will depend on the immune status of the host as well as the virulence properties of the enteropathogen. There are several general concepts that can be applied to the epidemiology of organisms that infect the gastrointestinal tract: 1) most infections of intestine occur via the fecal-oral route; 2) the dose of organisms necessary to produce an infection varies but is lower in patients with immunodeficiency; 3) there is often overlap in the clinical manifestations of infection by various enteropathogens; 4) enteropathogens may be acquired from non-human animals and contaminated food or water, and some are transmitted easily from person to person; and 5) the hepatotropic viruses may be immunopathic (hepatitis B virus (HBV)) or cytopathic (hepatitis C (HCV)) and (hepatitis E (HEV) viruses) in patients with HIV infection. Specifics of the epidemiology of each group of enteropathogens are given below.

Bacteria

The principal reservoirs for bacterial enteropathogens are animals including poultry, livestock and pets; other sources include contaminated animal and meat products, contaminated water, and infected humans. For *Shigella* species and *S. typhi*, infected humans are the only reservoir because no animal reservoir is known. Modes of transmission include ingestion of contaminated food or water, contact with infected animals, person to person transmission via the fecal-oral route, and contact with a contaminated environment or contaminated inanimate objects. Predisposing factors include crowded living conditions, low hygienic standards, closed population groups with substandard environmental sanitation, improper food preparation or storage, and travel to or living in countries with low standards of food hygiene. Water supply is thought to be the usual source of MAC, and the intestine is believed to be the usual portal of entry.

Viruses

Most human infections with rotavirus and enteric adenovirus result from contact with infected humans via the fecal-oral route. Person to person transmission of Calicivirus and astrovirus occurs, but transmission via contaminated food and water also has been reported. Herpes simplex and CMV can be transmitted both horizontally (by direct person to person contact with virus-containing secretions) and vertically.

Several viruses can infect the liver. With regard to hepatitis A virus (HAV), there is no convincing evidence that a person infected with HIV has more severe infection or subsequent loss of immunity during or after infection by HAV. There is a high prevalence of HBV infection in individuals infected with HIV. There is evidence at the molecular level that interactions between HIV and HBV alter the pathogenesis and clinical manifestations of the diseases they cause. The major modes of HBV transmission are through contact with blood and through sexual activity. Over 70% of adult intravenous drug users with AIDS were reported to have past or current HBV infection (98, 99). In a report from the multicenter AIDS Cohort Study (100) of homosexual men, 20% of the HBV-seronegative group became infected with HBV and 8% of the initially HIV-negative group became HIV positive during a 30-month follow-up; suggesting that HBV was transmitted 8.6 fold more efficiently than HIV among homosexual men. Perinatal transmission of HBV can occur when mothers are hepatitis B surface antigen (HbsAg) positive with transmission usually occurring at the time of delivery. When women also are hepatitis B e antigen (HBeAg) positive, 70–90% of their offspring not receiving appropriate immunoprophylaxis will acquire HBV at birth and become chronic carriers.

HCV infection is recognized in persons with HIV, particularly in intravenous drug users and recipients of blood products (98). Transmission of HCV can occur by parenteral administration of or exposure to blood or blood products with up to 90% of intravenous drug users having anti-HCV antibodies (98, 99). In nondrug users the prevalence of anti-HCV was <10% (101), and in multiply transfused thalassemia patients it was 33% (102), indicating the population-based differences. Perinatal transmission is uncommon and appears more likely if the mother is coinfected with HIV (103), but the risks are not fully defined. Although sexual transmission is reported for HCV, it is much less frequent than with HBV or HIV (101, 104). Hepatitis delta virus (HDV) is a unique defective or incomplete virus that requires the "helper" function of HBV. It circulates in the bloodstream in a subpopulation of HbsAg particles in persons who are HbsAg positive. HDV can cause an infection at the same time as the initial HBV infection (coinfection), or it can infect an individual already chronically infected with HBV (superinfection). Transmission is similar to that of HBV, except that transmission from mother to newborn is uncommon. HEV infection appears to explain many epidemics of enterically transmitted non-A, non-B hepatitis that occur worldwide. Little is known about the effects of chronic HIV infection on disease outcome of infection from HEV, although immunosuppression could or has been reported in pregnant women (105). Herpes simplex virus and CMV mainly are associated with hepatitis in the presence of significant immunosuppression, as occurs in postorgan transplantation. Although CMV-associated biliary tract disease is common in HIV infection, CMV hepatitis is less common in this setting. CMV and herpes simplex virus persist in latent forms after a primary infection; reactivation can occur years later, particularly under conditions of immunosuppression.

Parasites

Cryptosporidium has been identified in various hosts including birds, reptiles, and mammals throughout the world. Infection occurs after ingestion and possibly inhalation of oocysts (66, 67). Person to person and animal to human transmission have been documented and can result in outbreaks of disease as has been reported in child day care centers where person to person transmission occurs. In addition, spread can occur via water and food that is fecally contaminated. The parasite is resistant to chlorine, and therefore water filtration systems are important for public water supplies. Humans are the only known host of *I. belli*. The organism is acquired through ingestion of sporulated oocysts, but the infective dose for humans is unknown. *G. lamblia* is a common cause of enteritis and is found with increased frequency in children in day care centers, travelers to endemic areas, and male homosexuals. Transmission occurs via the fecal-oral route by passage of infectious cysts from person to person or by ingestion of fecally contaminated food or water (106). Microsporidia are obligate intracellular spore-forming protozoan parasites that have been recognized in various animals, particularly invertebrates (63). Immunosuppression probably is important for human infection. Information about the epidemiology and frequency of disease is limited. *S. stercoralis* transmission occurs via contaminated soil. The worm burden depends on the size of larval inoculation and on the degree of autoinfection. People with compromised immune systems may have enhanced autoinoculation and develop overwhelming infection that may lead to death (107).

PATHOPHYSIOLOGY

Enteropathogens produce disease in the gastrointestinal tract by several mechanisms, including enterotoxin production, cytotoxin production, epithelial cell invasion, adherence, and translocation (10). Various host factors such as gastric hypoacidity have been associated with quantitative bacterial overgrowth and opportunistic enteric infections and may be important in pathophysiology of the chronic diarrhea seen in some patients with AIDS (108). Enterotoxin producing *E. coli* and some other enteric organisms are examples of enteropathogens that can produce one or more enterotoxins that induce sodium and water secretion by small intestinal enterocytes by activation of adenylate cyclase in a manner similar to that of heat labile cholera enterotoxin or by activation of guanylate cyclase by a heat stable toxin. Cytotoxins do not cause active fluid secretion but bind to globotriaosylceramide and act by inhibiting protein synthesis. Several organisms including *S. dysenteriae* type 1, *C. difficile* and *E. coli* 0157:H7 produce cytotoxins. The enteric viruses, *G. lamblia*, *Cryptosporidium*, *Isospora*, and *E. bieneusi* produce a noninflammatory insult to absorptive surfaces of the small intestine resulting in watery diarrhea and carbohydrate malabsorption. With most enteric pathogens the ability to colonize a relevant region of the intestine is as important in causing disease as production of a toxin. An inflammatory response of the distal small and large intestine can be produced by organisms that invade the epithelial cells of the intestine and include *Salmonella, Shigella, C. jejuni, Y. enterocolitica,* and invasive *E. coli.*

For clinical consideration these pathophysiologic mechanisms can be grouped into one of three categories. The first consists of episodes of diarrhea that are noninflammatory, usually occurring in the upper small intestine and resulting from the action of an enterotoxin or other process that specifically alters the absorptive function of the villous tip, such as occurs with enteropathogenic *E. coli* and most enteric viruses and parasites. The second type of disease is termed inflammatory and usually occurs in the large intestine from an invasive process and/or cytotoxin production, such as ocurs with *Shigella, Salmonella, C. jejuni, E. coli* 0157:H7, and *E. histolytica.* A third type of infection occurs when organisms enter Peyer's patches and regional lymph nodes and results in a systemic infection such as occurs with *S. typhi* and other *Salmonella* species, *C. fetus,* and *Y. enterocolitica.* Although most enteropathogens generally are restricted to the intestine, many will involve other areas, especially in patients with AIDS who have a severe immunodeficiency.

Evidence of liver cell damage, spotty necrosis, and inflammatory cell infiltrates are the characteristic findings of acute virus hepatitis. The extent of necrosis and inflammatory cell infiltration varies from lobule to lobule. Although differences in the histologic features of hepatitis A, B, and non-A, non-B have been described, these differences are generally not sufficiently distinctive to be diagnostic in an individual and are not a substitute for serologic studies. The liver is not considered a target organ in HIV infection. The presence of CD4 has not been described on the surface of hepatocytes, although CD4 receptors have been described on the cytoplasmic membranes of Kupffer cells and endothelial cells (109). Although these cells may serve as reservoirs of HIV, the role of the liver in the natural history of HIV infection needs clarification.

Herpes simplex virus, CMV, and *C. albicans* produce gastrointestinal tract disease in patients with AIDS, but rarely involve the intestinal tract of persons who are not immunocompromised. These organisms usually produce ulceration and extensive acute inflammatory changes (Figs. 20.1–20.3). Intestinal biopsy of patients with CMV colitis reveals vasculitis, neutrophilic infiltration, and nonspecific inflammation. The presence of CMV inclusions is important in helping establish the diagnosis. The histologic changes caused by most enteropathogens often are similar in patients with AIDS and in other immunocompromised patients. One notable exception is MAC infections in which the usual granulomatous reaction is conspicuously absent with only mild crypt atrophy and increased chronic inflammatory cells, particularly histiocytes, seen in the lamina propria in routine paraffin sections (Fig. 20.4A). Special histochemical strains reveal numerous microorganisms (Fig. 20.4B). Infection of the same organ by more than one opportunistic agent seems to occur more frequently in patients wiht AIDS than other types of immunocompromised patients (Fig. 20.2).

In most patients with AIDS and diarrhea, an opportunistic pathogen will be detected if an appropriate evaluation has been performed (22, 26). However, villous atrophy and malabsorption occur in the absence of identifiable pathogens (16, 17, 22, 110). Although one explanation for this finding is that enteropathogens are missed or have not yet been identified as pathogens, HIV may be directly responsible for signs and symptoms of disease. In one study (110) either reduced or normal levels of vitamin B_{12} with abnormal Schilling test results were found in a group of patients with AIDS who did not have gastrointestinal tract symptoms, weight loss, or detectable intestinal pathogens. The patients had mild chronic inflammation of the duodenal mucosa that often was associated with partial villous atrophy (110), suggesting that patients with AIDS can occasionally manifest villous atrophy and malabsorption in the absence of identifiable pathogens (16, 110, 111). Ullrich and associates (112) found that patients with enteric infection had villous atrophy and crypt hyperplasia, whereas those without such infection had normal crypt depth, slightly reduced villous surface area, reduced numbers of mitotic figures per crypt, and lactase deficiency, providing additional evidence that patients with AIDS

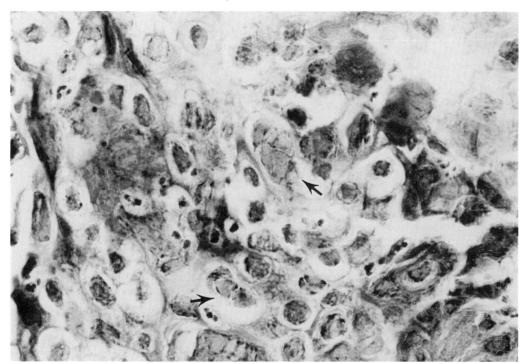

Figure 20.1. Herpes simplex virus in esophageal mucosa forming multinucleated cells with characteristic intranuclear inclusions (*arrow*). Hematoxylin and eosin. ×480.

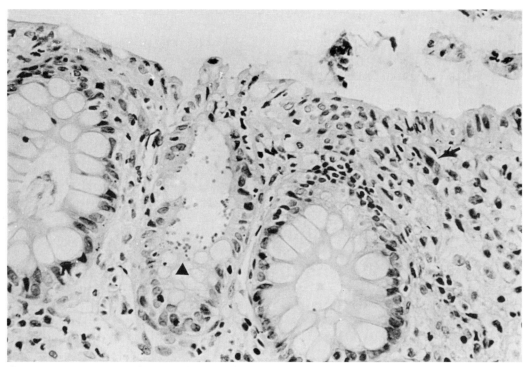

Figure 20.2. *Cryptosporidia* along the brush border and CMV with characteristic intranuclear and intracytoplasmic inclusions (*arrowhead*) in lamina propria of colon. Hematoxylin and eosin. ×480.

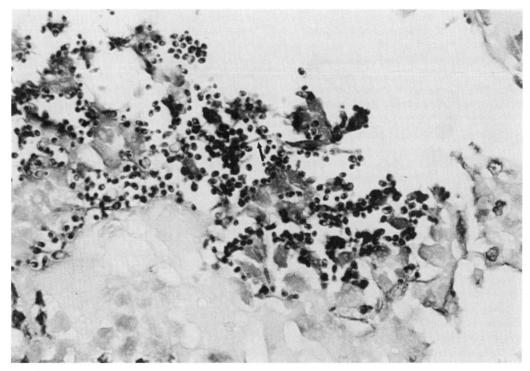

Figure 20.3. *C. albicans* with yeast forms and pseudohyphae (*arrow*) in duodenal mucosa. Hematoxylin and eosin. ×125.

may develop an "enteropathy" in the absence of detectable enteric infection. These subtle morphologic changes were more evident in patients whose lamina propria contained HIV p24 antigen, suggesting that the enteropathy was caused by HIV (112). The role of the HIV receptor, galactosyl ceramide, which is found on colonic mucosal cells, in gastrointestinal tract disease caused by HIV is unknown (113).

Another explanation of gastrointestinal tract disease in the absence of an identifiable cause is that low-grade bacterial overgrowth may contribute to the enteropathy (22, 114). Because excessive numbers of bacteria in the small intestine, particularly anaerobes, are associated with malabsorption, low-grade bacterial overgrowth could contribute to the malabsorption that characterizes patients with AIDS, particularly those with enteropathy. Altered IgA production, together with the impaired gastric-acid secretion reported to occur in HIV infection (108), leads to small intestine colonization with increased numbers of bacteria, which may contribute to mucosal inflamma-

tion. The chronic mucosal inflammation promotes villous atrophy, which together with low-grade bacterial overgrowth leads to malabsorption. In addition, changes in the mucosal immune system occur in HIV infection. These changes are similar to those present in patients with common variable immunodeficiency that also manifest as mild bacterial overgrowth, villous atrophy, and malabsorption.

CLINICAL PRESENTATION

The most common clinical presentations of the gastrointestinal tract that occur in children with AIDS are esophagitis, acute diarrhea, chronic diarrhea, failure to thrive, and hepatobiliary tract disease. Many diseases that involve various parts of the digestive tract can be rapidly evaluated, diagnosed, and treated; other conditions such as weight loss, failure to thrive, chronic diarrhea, and malabsorption are difficult conditions in which to establish a diagnosis and to specifically treat. It has been observed that patients with AIDS who develop diar-

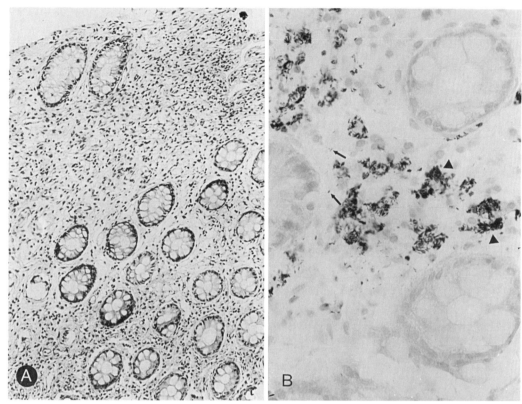

Figure 20.4. **A,** colonic mucosa with crypt atrophy and increased histiocytes in lamina propria. Hematoxylin and eosin. ×480. **B,** same as *panel A.* Numerous acid-fast bacteria are present as single forms (*arrows*) and in clumps (*arrowheads*). Ziehl-Neelson. ×480.

rhea have a greater weight loss and a higher incidence of extraintestinal opportunistic infections than those without diarrhea (22, 115). Each clinical presentation will be discussed below.

Esophageal Symptoms

Patients with involvement of the pharynx and esophagus present with odynophagia, dysphagia, and/or retrosternal esophageal pain. The most common esophageal complaint is dysphagia, and the most frequently identified organism associated with dysphagia is *C. albicans.* Odynophagia and retrosternal pain with dysphagia occur more frequently in patients with herpes simplex and CMV esophagitis than with *C. albicans.* In addition to erosive esophagogastritis, colitis is another common manifestation of CMV involvement of the gastrointestinal tract (56, 57, 59, 116). Other less frequent organisms or conditions that involve the

esophagus include histoplasmosis, *Nocardia, L. donovani,* primary lymphoma, Kaposi's sarcoma, squamous cell carcinoma, peptic acid reflux, idiopathic ulcerations, and ulcers from medication (95–97, 117, 118).

Diarrhea

Most episodes of diarrhea that occur during infancy and childhood are acute, self-limited episodes. However, in children with AIDS, infection with any enteropathogen can result in prolonged diarrhea and malabsorption with subsequent malnutrition, recurrence of infection after a course of appropriate antimicrobial therapy (32), and bacteremia associated with diarrhea (34, 43, 50). Children with small bowel disease generally have abdominal pain, weight loss, and watery diarrhea of large volume. Large bowel disease is manifest by small volume stools, lower quadrant pain, tenesmus, bloody diarrhea containing mucus, and fever. Severity of gastrointestinal tract disease in adults with AIDS was illustrated in one study in which 96% of individuals with AIDS and gastrointestinal tract manifestations had weight loss (17). In another study adults with AIDS suffered a mean weight loss from preillness to death of 11.8 ± 8 kg (119). Differential diagnosis of prolonged diarrhea is similar to that for chronic diarrhea of childhood (120) and generally occurs because of persistence of an enteropathogen or secondary to damage to the gastrointestinal tract that persists after the organism is no longer present.

Several cases of recurrent, persistent, and multiply resistant infection with *C. jejuni,* *Campylobacter*-like organisms such as *Helicobacter cinaedi* and *H. fennelliae* (32–35), and *Shigella* (45) have been reported. In one study *Campylobacter*-specific antibody titers were found to be low or absent and may have been important in the persistence of this pathogen (32). Chronic diarrhea in HIV-infected persons can be caused by *Campylobacter* species, and recurrent antibiotic therapy may result in development of antibiotic resistance. Infection of the gastrointestinal tract with MAC usually is associated with chronic diarrhea, abdominal pain, malabsorption, and marked wasting (46, 47).

In patients with normal immune systems, infections with parasitic organisms generally are short and respond to therapy when available, but in patients with AIDS, the clinical course may be protracted. *Cryptosporidium* causes self-limited, watery diarrhea, abdominal pain, weight loss, and anorexia in persons who are immune competent, but *Cryptosporidium* has been associated with voluminous, profuse watery diarrhea, anorexia, profound weight loss, and even death in patients with AIDS (6). Stool contains mucus but no blood or leukocytes. The severity and duration of illness depends on the degree of immune incompetence (121). A similar clinical presentation occurs in other individuals with defects in cell-mediated or humoral immunity. The CD4 count has been shown to be useful in predicting the course of *Cryptosporidium* infection in patients with AIDS, as it is with other opportunistic infections (Fig. 20.5).

Infection with *Isospora* is characterized by profuse watery diarrhea without blood or polymorphonuclear leukocytes, crampy abdominal pain, weight loss, malaise, and flatulence. Fever and leukocytosis are uncommon. Diarrhea usually is self-limited but chronic; relapsing infection has been reported in patients with AIDS (71, 72). Clinical symptoms in individuals infected with *Giardia* are similar to those in immunocompetent individuals and consist of an acute diarrheal illness characterized by nausea, bloating, and abdominal cramps or chronic illness manifested by a protracted, intermittent, frequently debilitating disease (106). Malabsorption and anorexia that occur can result in significant failure to thrive and weight loss (22, 23, 74). However, if diagnosed, prolonged infections with the parasite are uncommon because effective therapy is available.

It was initially thought that infections with microsporidia in patients with AIDS consisted of either small intestinal infection associated with diarrhea (*E. bieneusi*) or keratitis (*E. cuniculi*); however, hepatitis, myositis, and disseminated infection have been reported (83, 84, 86). Clinical manifestations associated with gastrointestinal tract involvement include chronic diarrhea and weight loss. This organism may be involved

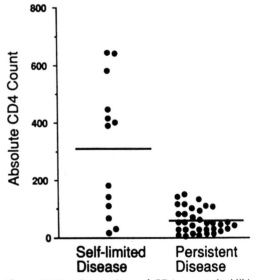

Figure 20.5. Comparison of CD4 counts in HIV-positive persons with self-limited (*n* = 13) compared with persistent (*n* = 34) cryptosporidiosis. From Flanigan T, Whalen C, Turner J, et al. *Cryptosporidium* infection and CD4 counts. Ann Intern Med 1992;116:841.

in patients with HIV wasting syndrome. Microsporidia are now recognized more frequently as a cause of diarrhea in this population (24, 76, 78, 86).

Clinical symptoms in patients infected with *S. stercoralis* can range from asymptomatic infection in one-third of patients to death. The type of symptomatology will depend on the stage of infection. Skin and pulmonary disease consists of pruritus, papula erythematous rash, and a Löffler-like syndrome of eosinophilia. Signs and symptoms associated with the intestinal phase of disease include abdominal pain, diarrhea containing mucus, and occasionally nausea, vomiting, weight loss, and malabsorption. When infection occurs, particularly in immunocompromised individuals, signs and symptoms include generalized abdominal pain, diffuse pulmonary infiltrates, ileus, and meningitis or sepsis from Gram-negative bacilli.

Complications of intestinal infection including intestinal perforation or hemorrhage, peritonitis, and bacteremia have been associated with amebiasis, shigellosis, salmonellosis, *C. difficile*, *E. coli* 0157:H7, and CMV infection of the ileocecal region. Appendicitis (122), pancreatitis (123), and discrete mass lesions are infrequent gastrointestinal manifestations of CMV infection in patients with AIDS (59, 60, 122–129). Pneumocystis has been shown to involve the small intestine (130). Complications must be recognized and appropriately diagnosed so correct therapy can be administered.

Neutropenic enterocolitis (typhlitis) is a clinical entity that occurs most commonly among patients with hematologic malignancies and chemotherapy-induced neutropenia. This entity has been described in patients with AIDS (131). Manifestations include fever, abdominal pain, and diarrhea that occur in a granulocytopenic host.

Hepatobiliary Tract

Abnormalities of the hepatobiliary tract in patients with HIV infection are common and result in clinical manifestations ranging from mild abdominal pain with minimal elevations of liver function tests to hepatic failure and death. Involvement of the liver includes nonspecific abnormalities that occur in chronic illness (132) as well as involvement by malignancies and infection with HAV, HBV, HCV, HDV, MAC, *M. tuberculosis*, *H. capsulatum*, *C. neoformans*, CMV, and *T. gondii* (62, 132). Several less common pathogens have been associated with hepatitis or hepatomegaly, including the organism responsible for bacillary peliosis hepatis (133, 134), *P. carinii* (135–137), *E. cuniculi* (65), *Penicillium marneffei* (138), *Leishmania* (139, 140), and adenovirus (141), which caused disseminated hepatic necrosis in three children. The organism associated with bacillary peliosis hepatis may be the same one that is associated with bacillary angiomatosis (134) and cat-scratch disease. These reports illustrate the fact that an unusual, diverse group of organisms can infect patients with AIDS (8). Clinical manifestations include hepatomegaly, right upper quadrant pain, and/or tenderness and jaundice. The extent and causes of liver disease in children with AIDS is unknown.

Because the liver is not considered a primary target organ in HIV infection, most hepatic symptoms observed in patients with AIDS are related to opportunistic infections, drug toxicity, or neoplasms. Clinical and laboratory manifestations of infection with the hepatotropic viruses including HBV, HCV, and HDV have been reviewed in many textbooks and review articles. The effects of these viruses on HIV infection and the effect of HIV infection on the clinical manifestations of these viruses will be considered here. The effects of HBV on HIV replication have been studied in vitro (62). Proteins encoded by the HBV genome have been shown to have a direct effect on HIV replication, but the role this has on enhancing HIV replication in vivo in cells containing both HIV and HBV is unknown. Although studies indicate that activation of HIV by HBV could occur in vivo, clinical studies do not support this (142, 143). In a study of a cohort of homosexual men, HBV infection did not lead to a more rapid decline of T helper cells and was not associated with an increased incidence of AIDS at 2.5 years follow-up (142). The effect of immunosuppression from HIV on HBV carriers also has been studied. Data indicate that when immunosuppression from HIV occurs in HBV carriers, HBV replication increases, but liver inflammation lessens and transaminase values decrease (144, 145).

Studies have shown that the risk of chronic HBV infection is greater in HIV-positive compared with HIV-negative homosexual men (146–148). The HIV-positive subjects who cleared HBV tended to have higher CD4 counts than those who became carriers. However, histologically and biochemically, the liver disease in patients with HBV and HIV coinfection was less severe than, or the same as, patients with HBV infection who were HIV negative (146, 149–151). It appears that HIV-infected individuals will develop a high carrier state but manifest less severe histopathologic changes and lower transaminase concentrations when infected with HBV. However, because of greater viral replication these individuals may be more contagious (151). Several cases of HBV reactivation have been recorded in patients with HIV infection (152, 153, 154). In HIV and HBV coinfected patients, severe liver damage can be present in the setting of reactivation in patients with low CD4 counts (152). Four cases were described in an earlier study in which HBsAg reappeared despite circulating anti-HBc antibodies (153), indicating that the presence of circulating anti-HBc antibodies in an immunodeficient host does not protect against either reinfection or reactivation of latent infection.

HCV in contrast to HBV is cytopathic rather than immunopathic. Coinfection with HIV does not appear to reduce hepatic inflammation. In one study three patients with probable HCV and HIV infection developed symptomatic cirrhosis within 3 years of the onset of hepatitis (155), suggesting a more rapid progression of disease than what occurs in HIV-negative patients with chronic HCV.

HDV is, like HCV, thought to be cytopathic. HIV coinfection leads to a worsening of liver disease (156). In HIV-seronegative individuals, HDV is thought to have an inhibitory effect on the replication of HBV in both coinfection (157) and superinfection (158). HIV appears to alter the inhibitory effect of HDV on HBV replication (159, 160). One report (160) described superinfection of an HBV carrier with both

HIV and HDV. Increasing levels of HDV antigen suggested reactivation of HDV infection. HDV infection was studied in intravenous drug users (161). δ-Antigen was detected in 6% of the AIDS group and 0.8% of the non-AIDS group, whereas anti-HDV was detected in none of the AIDS group and 21% of the non-AIDS group. Despite a 90% prevalence of anti-HBc antibodies in both groups, more in the AIDS groups had HBsAg (15%) compared with the non-AIDS group (5%). This study suggests that persistence or reactivation of HBV and HDV is common in this group of patients.

Biliary tract abnormalities are complications that occur in patients with AIDS. Reports have described biliary tract abnormalities including cholecystitis, papillary stenosis, and sclerosing cholangitis (61, 124–129), with the latter two complications of certain opportunistic infections referred to as AIDS cholangiopathy. Clinical manifestations include epigastric and/or right upper quadrant pain, fever, nausea, emesis, and right upper quadrant tenderness that are often associated with markedly elevated levels of alkaline phosphatase and minimal elevations of aminotransferase. The most common etiology has been CMV infection; however, cryptosporidiosis, MAC, malignancy, and direct involvement by HIV with a local atypical immune response have been reported (128). Acalculous cholecystitis has been associated with chronic illness, with both CMV and *Cryptosporidium* implicated as causative agents (61, 124, 126, 127).

DIAGNOSTIC CONSIDERATIONS

Individuals with AIDS who have either acute or chronic diarrhea should be thoroughly evaluated to determine the cause, since a specific pathogen can be identified in most patients and because specific therapy can often reduce the volume and/or frequency of diarrhea (22, 23). In addition, nutrition assessment should be performed on a routine basis to identify and treat new problems that may arise. In many patients with AIDS and gastrointestinal tract disease, the causative event is no longer present when the child is evaluated, but residual damage to the intestine persists. In children with AIDS a subset of the causes of chronic diarrhea will often need to be considered in the differential diagnosis (120). History and physical examination should provide information to help direct laboratory evaluation. Diagnosis should be approached in a stepwise manner with the initial evaluation to include culture and microscopy and further evaluation to include endoscopy for biopsy and culture (Table 20.2).

Strategies for evaluation and management of diarrhea in adults with AIDS have been proposed (9, 162). In children, a logical approach consists of obtaining at least two stool cultures for *Salmonella, Shigella,* and *C. jejuni* as well as for organisms that require special laboratory techniques. Commercially available enzyme-linked immunosorbent assays (ELISA) can detect rotavirus, enteric adenovirus, and the toxins of *C. difficile* and *G. lamblia.* Microscopy should be performed to detect fecal leukocytes and parasites. Stools should be prepared using saline, iodine, trichrome, and acid-fast stains. If the patient is febrile, then blood cultures for bacteria, mycobacteria, and CMV should be ordered. If a diagnosis is not established and a response to symptomatic treatment is not achieved, then esophagogastroduodenoscopy and/or colonoscopy could be performed to visualize the mucosa and to obtain biopsy specimens and luminal fluid.

Acute Diarrhea

The causes of acute diarrhea are numerous and include infectious and noninfectious etiologies. Identifying the cause of diarrhea in patients with AIDS is dependent on many factors including availability of laboratory technology. In several studies, microscopic examination and culture of stool and duodenal fluid followed by duodenal and/or colonic biopsy lead to a diagnosis in 85% of patients studied (22–26). The initial evaluation of children with AIDS and gastrointestinal tract involvement is outlined above and in Table 20.2. Blood cultures should be obtained from febrile patients for bacteria, mycobacteria, and CMV. Other tests that should be reserved for patients with more persistent episodes in which a diagnosis is not established include sigmoidoscopy, barium enema, intestinal biopsy, and tests for malabsorption. Children with persistent diarrhea will need periodic reevaluation of stool specimens. Details of the specific evaluation of children for bacterial, parasitic, viral, and fungal causes of infectious diarrhea are discussed below.

Chronic Diarrhea

Children with AIDS often develop chronic diarrhea or are recognized as failing to thrive. In the diagnostic approach to these children, a hierarchy of tests and pro-

Table 20.2.   Diagnostic Evaluation of Patients with Diarrhea and HIV Infection

Test	Organisms Detected
Level 1: Microscopy and culture	
Stool culture	
Routine	*Shigella, Salmonella C. jejuni*
Specialized	*Aeromonas,* Diarrhea-associated *E. coli,* MAC, other *Campylobacter* species, *Vibrio* species, *Y. enterocolitica*
ELISA	Rotavirus, enteric adenovirus *C. difficile* toxins, *G. lamblia*
Microscopy	
Fecal leukocytes	Invasive bacteria
Ova and parasite	*Giardia, E. histolytica*
Trichrome stain	Microsporidia
Acid-fast stain	*Cryptosporidium, I. belli,* MAC, blue-green algae
Blood culture (if febrile)	Bacteria, mycobacteria, CMV
Level 2: Endoscopy for biopsy, histology and culture	
Esophagogastroduodenoscopy	See Table 20.1
Colonoscopy	See Table 20.1
Electron microscopy	*E. bieneusi*

cedures must be established. The impact of the illness on the health and development of the child should be continually reassessed. Important aspects of care of children with AIDS and chronic diarrhea, malabsorption, and failure to thrive are observation of weight gain, status of the height and weight curves, and stool pattern. Infectious causes of diarrhea should be evaluated. These initial tests should include evaluation of stool specimens and blood. Stool cultures, ova and parasite examination, and fecal leukocyte testing may yield an infectious cause of the episode (10). Diagnosis of each category of diarrhea is listed below. In several studies of chronic diarrhea in adults with AIDS, *Cryptosporidium,* microsporidia, CMV, and MAC were the most frequently isolated organisms (22, 24–26).

Esophageal Involvement

In adults with HIV infection and odynophagia or dysphagia, the sensitivity of endoscopic brushings (95%) was better than that of histologic examination (70%) in the diagnosis of *Candida* esophagitis. Histopathology has been used to demonstrate tissue-invasive pseudomycelia. Barium contrast radiography may support but not document the diagnosis of *Candida* esophagitis. If a patient with AIDS has thrush and dysphagia, endoscopy may not be needed to document esophageal involvement, unless treatment fails to produce improvement. For CMV and herpes simplex, virus cultures of brushings or biopsy specimens were more sensitive (67%) than histologic examination (35%) for virus esophagitis (15). Diagnosis of herpes simplex by histopathology is made by visualizing giant cells and less commonly Cowdry's type A intranuclear inclusions in infected cells, although similar findings can be seen with CMV and varicella-zoster virus. Virus culture is confirmatory. Demonstration of CMV-infected endothelial cells is the hallmark of CMV disease in patients with AIDS. Tissue cultures positive for CMV alone do not prove CMV is causing disease. Although CMV and herpes simplex ulcerations are sometimes indistinguishable when visualized, herpes simplex ulcers are generally

fewer, smaller, and deeper than those of CMV. Cloned subgenomic probes are available for diagnosis of CMV.

Liver

Most individuals with AIDS have abnormalities of liver function tests during their illness. Because the liver is not considered a target organ in HIV, most of these abnormalities are related to opportunistic infections, hepatotropic viruses, neoplasms, or medications. Serologic tests are available commercially for diagnosis of hepatitis A, B, C, and D. Research-based serologic tests are available to test for antibody to HEV (anti-HEV). Serologic assays detect anti-HAV and IgM-specific anti-HAV antibodies. Tests for HBV antigens include HBsAg and HBeAg and for HBV antibody assays for antibody to HBsAg (anti-HBs), antibody to HBsAg (anti-HBc), and antibody to HBeAg (anti-HBe) are available. The presence of HBsAg indicates acute or chronic infection. The presence of IgM antibody to the HBV core antigen (IgM anti-HBc) is specific for diagnosis of acute or recent HBV infection. In some cases of acute infection serum HBsAg will have disappeared and antibody to surface antigen has not yet appeared; in these cases IgM anti-HBc may be present. Anti-HBc is detectable in many persons with prior hepatitis B infection and indicates past infection.

A serologic test for anti-HCV is available. Antibodies may be absent during the acute illness and may only become detectable 6 months after onset of illness. A positive anti-HCV serologic test does not necessarily indicate continuing infection. A test for anti-HDV antibody is commercially available. Tests for IgM-specific anti-HDV antibody and δ-antigen are research procedures. If markers of HDV infection exist, coinfection with HBV can usually be differentiated from superinfection of an established HBsAg carrier by testing for hepatitis B core antibody of the IgM class (IgM anti-HBc). Absence of markers of acute hepatitis B infection in a patient with HDV infection suggests that the person is an HBsAg carrier. A problem of loss of immunity and reactivation has occurred, especially in individuals with low CD4 counts. A rapid decline in antibodies to HBsAg levels with time has been reported in HIV-seropositive individuals with a history of HBV (163, 164) and HCV (98). A similar phenomenon is reported in HIV-infected individuals who initially responded to HBV vaccination (165, 166). In a study of HIV-infected hemophilia patients, 20% demonstrated antibody loss to HBV and/or did not respond to hepatitis vaccine (167).

In most instances parenchymal liver disease in patients with AIDS represents a manifestation of a previously diagnosed, widely disseminated disease process or infection with one hepatotropic virus, and liver biopsy usually does not document a new diagnosis, making liver biopsy unnecessary in most patients with abnormal liver function tests (168). Studies have demonstrated the most common histologic abnormalities to be steatosis, portal inflammation, and noncaseating poorly formed granuloma. Diagnostic yield of liver biopsy has been reported to be as low as 25% among HIV-infected patients, although diagnostic yields of 50% (18 of 36 patients) have been reported (168). A biopsy was more likely to be diagnostic when a patient had a preexisting diagnosis of AIDS, a longer duration of AIDS, a greater number of previous opportunistic infections, and more markedly elevated alkaline phosphatase levels (168).

Whereas liver biopsy generally is not indicated in patients with AIDS and liver function abnormalities, obstructive biliary tract disease should be thoroughly and rapidly evaluated by ultrasound, computerized tomography scan, and/or endoscopic cholangiography. Most patients with AIDS and biliary tract disease will be noted by ultrasound or computerized tomography to have prominent or dilated intrahepatic or extrahepatic bile ducts. However, in one study, 75% of patients with cholangiopathy who had abnormal cholangiograms had grossly normal noninvasive studies including abdominal ultrasonography and computerized tomography. Twenty (77%) of these 26 patients had abnormal findings on endoscopic retrograde cholangiopancreatography (125). The several patterns of abnormal cholangiograms noted included papillary stenosis, sclerosing cholangitis, and long extrahepatic bile duct strictures.

Bacteria

Most bacterial enteropathogens can be identified by standard diagnostic or modified diagnostic stool cultures, although other detection methods including serotyping, tissue culture assays, ELISA, and gene probes are available (10). Standard microbiologic cultures will detect *Shigella* species, *Salmonella* species, and *C. jejuni*. If other bacterial agents are suspected, laboratory personnel must be notified so that modified laboratory procedures can be used for identification. Bacterial enteropathogens in this category include pathogenic *E. coli*, *Vibrio* species, *Campylobacter* species (excluding *C. jejuni*), *Y. enterocolitica*, *C. difficile*, and *Aeromonas*. Diagnosis of MAC is by use of acid-fast stain and by cultures of stool and blood. The preferred method of diagnosis is small bowel biopsy to demonstrate the pathologic changes and the presence of organisms on acid-fast stain. Biopsy specimens of the small intestine usually show changes similar to those seen in Whipple's disease (169).

Viruses

Commercially available assays can be used to detect rotavirus and enteric adenovirus. Diagnostic methods that are used to detect other enteric viruses are less suitable for routine use and include gel electrophoresis, polymerase chain reaction, electron microscopy, ELISA, radioimmunoassay, and virus culture (10). In patients with CMV colitis, sigmoidoscopy will reveal areas that range from diffuse or focal mucosal erythema to extensive, deep, friable ulcerations with clearly defined borders and nonpurulent bases (119, 170, 171), although 10% of patients with histologic evidence of CMV colitis may have a grossly normal appearing mucosa. Barium radiographs may demonstrate diffuse abnormalities ranging from edema, mucosal fold thickening, and superficial erosions to deep ulcerations (170). When the disease occurs in the atrium of the stomach, lack of distensibility of the stomach may occur (172), and terminal ileal involvement may appear indistinguishable from Crohn's disease (173). Focal mass lesions are rare and must be distinguished from malignancies (126). Computerized tomography may reveal diffuse bowel wall thickening, luminal narrowing, and inflammatory changes in the surrounding mesenteric and pericolonic fat (174). The presence of giant cells CMV and inclusions in the biopsy is the most important evidence to support diagnosis of CMV colitis. The presence of CMV antigen, a positive culture of biopsy tissue, or both can help substantiate the diagnosis.

Parasites

Diagnosis of parasitic causes of diarrhea generally depends on microscopy, although rapid diagnostic tests are available for several parasitic enteropathogens. Diagnosis of infection with *Cryptosporidium* is made by identification of the oocyst form of the parasite by microscopic examination of stool or by histologic examination of tissue sections. Stool specimens are concentrated using either the sucrose Sheather flotation technique or formalinethyl acetate concentration methods followed by staining with a modified Kinyoun acid-fast stain, which permits differentiation of acid-fast cryptosporidial oocysts from yeasts (Table 20.3). The auramine O fluorescent stain is a rapid, sensitive screening procedure used to detect oocysts. Patients with AIDS and diarrhea caused by *Cryptosporidium* often excrete high numbers of oocysts, frequently making concentration of stool unnecessary to establish a diagnosis. Organisms also may be identified in jejunal or rectal biopsy specimens and in aspirated duodenal contents. Cryptosporidial oocysts also can be detected using an indirect immunofluorescent detection procedure in which monoclonal antibody binds to the cell wall of the oocysts

Table 20.3.   Diagnosis of Parasitic Causes of Diarrhea[a]

Organism	Size	Specimen	Recommended Diagnostic Procedure	Comment
	μm			
Cryptosporidum	Oocysts 4–6	Stool	Wet preparation, acid-fast stains, mAb-based assays (IF-α, ELISA)	Concentration methods may be needed (see text); auramine-rhodamine stains may be used, but positive results should be confirmed by one recommended procedure
		Intestinal or tissue biopsy	Histology, EM	
I. belli	Oocysts 20–30 by 10–19	Stool	Wet preparation, acid-fast stains	Same comments as for *Cryptosporidium*; biopsy may be positive, whereas stool exam is negative
		Intestinal biopsy	Histology, EM	
E. bieneusi	Spores 1–5 by 2–7	Intestinal or or tissue biopsy and touch preps	Histology, EM	Identification by histology may be difficult; EM is required to classify species
		Stool	Giemsa stain, modified trichrome stain, EM	
G. lamblia	8–12 by 7–10 cyst 9–21 by 5–15 (trophozoite)	Stool or duodenal aspirate	Wet prepartion, Giemsa stain, ELISA	Concentration technique may be necessary; ELISA more sensitive
S. stercoralis	200–300	Stool duodenal material	Wet preparation	Rhabditiform larvae

[a]mAb, monoclonal antibody; If, immunofluorescence; EM, electron microscopy.

(Merifluor-*Cryptosporidium*, Meridian Diagnostics, Cincinnati, OH). Although not helpful in rapid diagnosis, an ELISA technique that detects IgG and IgM antibodies in serum has been used (175). Radiographic studies show barium flocculation, mucosal thickening, and small bowel dilatation.

Diagnosis of *Isospora* is made by finding oocysts in stool specimens. Oocysts of *I. belli* are acid-fast and can be distinguished easily from *Cryptosporidia* by their ellipsoidal shape and larger size (20–30 μm by 10–20 μm compared with 2–5 μm diameter cryptosporidial oocysts) (176). The oocysts may be in the stool for as long as 120 days after infection, but they are few and shed intermittently. Because of the low number of organisms shed, use of concentration methods may improve the yield. Oocysts of *Isospora* do not stain well with methods frequently used for diagnosis of other intestinal protozoa. Oocysts often can be seen in duodenal aspirate and small bowel biopsy material.

Conformation of infection by *Giardia* depends on demonstration of cysts or trophozoites by microscopic examination of stool, duodenal aspirate, or biopsy material. Merthiolate-iodine Formalin concentration technique improves the sensitivity of stool examination when compared with use of Lugol's iodine and methylene blue wet mounts. Rapid diagnostic tests that detect *Giardia* antigens in stool specimens also are available (177). Patients with AIDS generally do not suffer prolonged diarrhea if treated, because available therapy is effective and there is some indication that prior exposure to the organism confers a protective immunity (75).

Diagnosis of microsporidia infection is difficult since the parasites are easily overlooked in routine tissue examinations because they are small, stain poorly with the commonly used stains, and evoke little or no tissue response. Proper identification requires careful attention to the preparative technique. Orenstein and colleagues (76) used both light microscopy and transmission electron microscopy to review intestinal biopsy specimens from 67 persons with HIV disease and chronic diarrhea. This study documented *E. bieneusi*, the most common species causing diarrhea in patients with AIDS, in 20 (30%) of the 67 patients; microspora were more likely to be identified in jejunal samples than in samples from other intestinal sites. Although electron microscopy appears to be the most sensitive method for identification of microsporidia, *E. bieneusi* and its spores were identified by light microscopy in 19 of 20 cases of microsporidiosis documented by electron microscopy (76). The identification of intracellular and luminal spores can facilitate diagnosis and can be best accomplished with the use of Brown-Brenn and acid-fast stains (76). A method whereby microsporidial spores can be visualized using modified trichrome staining of stool specimens has been developed (178). This method simplifies diagnosis of intestinal microsporidiosis and reduces or eliminates the need for small intestinal biopsies. Electron microscopy can be used to detail the presence of the organism, which permits appropriate classification (18).

Diagnosis of *Strongyloides* depends on demonstration of rhabditiform larvae in feces or duodenal fluid. Rhabditiform larvae are products of ova produced by parasitic females in the small intestine of infected persons. The eggs hatch deep in the mucosa of the duodenum and are almost never identified in stool. Stool should be examined after being subjected to a concentration technique such as zinc sulfate. Repeat examinations of concentrated stool specimens are often necessary. Serodiagnosis can be useful but is limited in availability, and cross-reaction with antigens of filarial worms occurs, limiting the sensitivity. Figure 20.6 shows oocysts of *Cryptosporidium* and *Isospora*, trophozoite and cyst forms of *G. lamblia*, and rhabditiform larvae of *Strongyloides* as they appear in stool specimens.

TREATMENT

Treatment of patients with acute diarrhea includes replacement and maintenance of fluid and electrolytes (179) and early reintroduction of normal nutrients. In addition, nonspecific therapy of patients with refractory watery diarrhea, especially those without identifiable pathogens, may

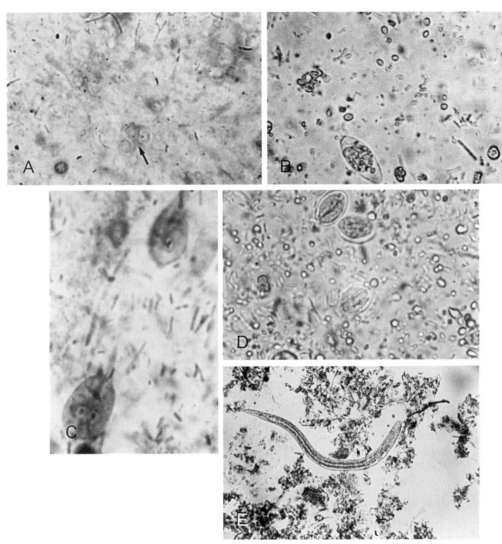

Figure 20.6.   *Cryptosporidium* oocysts (**A**, ×1000), *I. belli* oocysts (**B**, ×1000), *G. lamblia* trophozoites (**C**, ×1000) and cysts (**D**), and rhabditiform larvae of *S. stercoralis* (**E**, ×400). All organisms were identified in stool specimens from patients with AIDS.

respond favorably to octreotide (somatastatin) (180). Specific causes of fever, diarrhea, decreased intake, and feeding problems should be sought and treated. Infectious and noninfectious agents or diseases that involve the gastrointestinal tract or other organ systems, such as pneumonia, may contribute to decreased intake and malnutrition. Studies have demonstrated severe, progressive malnutrition in adult patients with AIDS, with the lowest measures of lean body mass occurring in those patients close to death. Although studies of nutritional status of pediatric patients with AIDS are limited, weight loss, decreased intake, feeding problems, and malnutrition are all well recognized to occur (181). In patients in whom no specific etiology can be identified, symptomatic treatment is the mainstay of therapy. In general, nutritional support is an essential component of the long-term management of all children with AIDS. Chapter 27 provides information about supportive care including nutritional support. Specific therapy is available for treatment of persons infected with certain enteropathogens.

Bacteria

Antimicrobial therapy is administered to selected patients with bacterial gastroenteritis to abbreviate the gastrointestinal tract illness and/or decrease fecal shedding of the causative organism (10). Stool cultures should be obtained to identify the enteropathogen and provide an organism on which antimicrobial susceptibility testing can be performed. Table 20.4 outlines recommended antimicrobial therapy for commonly encountered enteropathogens. Considerations of therapy should include whether dissemination has occurred and whether another enteropathogen is coinfecting the patient. Therapy may need to be administered for a period longer than what is recommended. Treatment of MAC has been problematic because of the relative resistance of this organism to most drugs, although clarithromycin or azithromycin in combination with either ethambutol, clofazimine, or other antimycobacterial agents may have potential benefit (182).

Viruses

Specific therapy is unavailable for treatment of patients infected with virus enteropathogens except CMV and herpes simplex virus. Nutrition must be considered in all persons with liver disease and avoidance of hepatotoxic compounds and drugs is critical. Interferon-α has been used in patients with HBV and HCV infection. It was apparent from early interferon-α trials for chronic HBV infection that underlying immunosuppression was associated with a poor response to therapy. It has subsequently been confirmed that patients with HIV and HBV coinfection are unlikely to clear HBV infection when interferon is prescribed (183–185). Zidovudine has been shown to have an inhibitory effect on the replication of duct hepatitis B virus (186). The results against human HBV have been somewhat disappointing (187). In one study HBV DNA levels and HBV DNA polymerase activity were measured in 14 male homosexual patients with chronic HBV infection and symptomatic HIV infection who were prescribed zidovudine. In the 13 patients with detectable baseline HBV DNA or HBV DNA polymerase, no significant change was noted in either viral marker during the first 16 weeks of therapy. In a study of six patients (188) the combination of interferon and zidovudine also appeared to be of no benefit for HIV and HBV coinfection. Other reverse transcriptase inhibitors, including 2´,3´-dideoxycytidine,

Table 20.4. Antimicrobial Therapy for Children with Bacterial Enteropathogens

Organism	Indication for Antimicrobial thearpy	Antimicrobial Agent
Aeromonas	Dysentery-like illness, prolonged diarrhea	TMP-SMX[a]
Campylobacter	Early in course of illness	Erythromycin
C. difficile	Moderate to severe antimicrobial associated colitis	Vancomycin or metronidazole
E. coli		
Enterotoxigenic	Severe or prolonged illness	TMP-SMX
Enteropathogenic	Nursery epidemics, life-threatening illness	TMP-SMX
Enteroinvasive	All cases	TMP-SMX
Salmonella	Gastroenteritis in infants <3 mo and in immunodeficient patients, typhoid fever, bacteremia, dissemination with localized suppuration	Ampicillin, chloramphenicol, TMP-SMX, cefotaxime, or ceftriaxone
Shigella	All cases	TMP-SMX
	Resistant strains	Nalidixic acid
	Resistant strains in persons older than 17 yr	Ciprofloxacin or ofloxacin
V. cholerae	All symptomatic cases	Tetracycline or TMP-SMX

[a]TMP-SMX, trimethoprim-sulfamethoxazole.

remain under investigation. Many trials of interferon-α for chronic HCV infection have excluded patients with HIV coinfection, and therefore there are few data examining this issue. It has been shown that patients with HCV and HIV coinfection have a reduction in aminotransferase levels when treated with zidovudine (189). It is impossible from these clinical studies to determine whether this is a direct antiviral effect of zidovudine against HCV or whether the anti-HIV effect leads to an improvement in immune function and a secondary effect on HCV.

Esophagitis or colitis from CMV may improve with ganciclovir therapy (190, 191). Neutropenia is a dose-limiting adverse effect of ganciclovir. Relapses or recurrences are common, and maintenance therapy is often necessary. There has not been a placebo-controlled study of foscarnet in the treatment of CMV gastrointestinal tract disease. Patients with herpes esophagitis usually respond to acyclovir, but maintenance therapy is often needed to prevent relapses.

Parasites

Enteric infections from protozoal organisms are not always self-limiting in children with AIDS, do not always respond to specific therapy if available, and frequently relapse after an appropriate therapeutic course. Nonspecific therapy and careful attention to dietary intake and nutrition can provide relief for some patients and help prevent the malnutrition and wasting that so frequently occur.

Specific antimicrobial therapy for *Cryptosporidium* is unavailable. Spiramycin has been used with varied response (192) but generally is thought to be ineffective (Table 20.5). Orally administered bovine transfer factor, hyperimmune bovine colostrum and cow's milk immunoglobulin are all being evaluated (14, 193, 194). Immune bovine colostral whey has been shown to neutralize *C. parvum* sporozoites and to partially protect mice against oral challenge with *C. parvum* oocysts (195). Management includes fluid therapy, nutritional support, and use of antidiarrheal agents. In patients with AIDS or scleroderma and large volume intractable diarrhea, octreotide (somatostatin) has controlled diarrhea but not infection (129, 196, 197). Octreotide is thought to work through a nonspecific inhibitory effect on gastrointestinal tract fluid and electrolyte secretion. Paromomycin may be helpful in some patients.

Unlike *Cryptosporidium, Isospora* responds to treatment with oral trimethoprim-sulfamethoxazole; however, recurrent symptomatic disease occurs in 50% of patients (68). Recurrent disease may be prevented by use of prophylaxis with trimethoprim-sulfamethoxazole, which in immunocompromised patients may need to be continued indefinitely (198). In sulfonamide-sensitive patients, pyrimethamine daily has been effective in adults (199). Both these compounds are considered investigational for isosporiasis by the Food and Drug Administration. Patients receiving either compound should be carefully monitored for bone marrow suppression, skin reactions, and allergic manifestations (200). Metronidazole (Flagyl) and pyrimethamine (50–75 mg daily for adults) (Daraprim) also have been reported to be effective in a limited number of patients (199) and may be considered an alternate therapy in sulfa-allergic individuals.

Quinacrine (Atabrine), metronidazole (Flagyl), and furazolidone (Fruoxone) are

Table 20.5. Treatment of Protozoa That Cause Diarrhea in Patients with AIDS

Organism	Treatment
Cryptosporidium	None proven; octreotide may decrease diarrhea
I. belli	Trimethoprim-sulfamethoxazole (Bactrim, Septra)
G. lamblia	Quinacrine HC1 (Atabrine)
	Furazolidone (Furoxone)
	Metronidazole (Flagyl)
E. bieneusi	None proven, octreotide may decrease diarrhea
S. stercoralis	Thiabendazole

specific therapies for patients with *G. lamblia.* Furazolidone is the only drug available in liquid suspension for use in young children (106). Metronidazole is not approved for treatment of patients with giardiasis in the United States, but it is widely used. Tinidazole and ornidazole are as effective as and better tolerated than metronidazole but are unavailable for use in the United States. Quinacrine has frequent toxic side effects including yellow discoloration of skin and sclerae, nausea and vomiting, toxic psychosis, and exfoliative dermatitis. Both metronidazole and quinacrine have an unpleasant taste that precludes ingestion by children. Relapse is common in immunocompromised patients, and therapy in these individuals may need to be prolonged. There is no known effective therapy for microsporidia, although in small uncontrolled studies metronidazole and albendazole alleviated symptoms in some cases (77, 78). Octreotide has provided symptomatic relief in adults with AIDS (180).

Individuals infected with *S. stercoralis* should be treated with thiabendazole (Mintezol) (200); ivermectin and albendazole also have been used. Patients with the hyperinfection syndrome should receive therapy for at least 5 days, but mortality is high despite treatment (107). Patients with a past history of infection with *S. stercoralis* should receive a thorough examination and treatment before receiving immunosuppressive therapy.

Fungi

Patients with thrush and/or esophagitis from *C. albicans* usually respond to a 7- to 14-day course of ketoconazole or fluconazole. If this therapy fails, other causes should be sought before considering therapy with amphotericin B. Esophageal lesions may not completely resolve in patients who have a favorable clinical response despite months of therapy.

PREVENTION

The public health measures of improved water supply and sanitation facilities are important for control of most enteric infections. Use of appropriate hygiene measures, especially hand washing, and careful preparation of food will further decrease the occurrence of enteric infection. Attention to nutritional status will help offset the debilitation that frequently occurs in children with AIDS. Vaccines against rotavirus, *Salmonella, Shigella,* and diarrhea-producing *E. coli* strains are being tested but are not available. There are no effective vaccines against parasitic enteric infections. Pharmacologic antagonists to microbial adherence or toxin action are being evaluated.

Prevention of spread of enteropathogens to contacts of infected persons can occur by use of enteric precautions in the hospital and home environments. To ensure protection of health care professionals as well as patients, universal precautions must be practiced as well as appropriate disinfection or sterilization of equipment used on all patients. Guidelines for prevention of transmission of HIV and HBV to and from health care workers have been published (201, 202).

Although HBV vaccine is recommended for individuals at high risk, poor response rates to HBV vaccination occurred in HIV-infected individuals (164, 166, 203). In one study of homosexual men (166), only one of 18 HIV-negative men failed to respond compared with 8 of 17 seropositive subjects. Hadler et al. (148) also found that HBV vaccination was much less likely to provide protection in those who were HIV positive. They also reported a high HBV carriage rate in those HIV-positive individuals who were infected with HBV around the time of an HBV vaccine dose. Simultaneous HBV infection and vaccination was associated with a carriage rate in 8 of 10 (80%) of those infected at the time of the first vaccine dose and in 5 of 9 (56%) at the time of the second dose. However, in the Hadler et al. study (148) the HIV group who failed to respond to HBV vaccination had no higher subsequent HBV carriage rates than the unvaccinated group. In children with hemophilia immunized with HBV, the antibody titers to HBsAg were lower in children with HIV-1 antibodies than in those without antibodies, and postimmunization anti-HBs levels fell more quickly in seropositive HIV-infected children (204).

References

1. Cello JP. Gastrointestinal manifestations of HIV infections. Infect Dis Clin North Am 1988;2:387–396.
2. Lane GP, Lucas CR, Smallwood RA. The gastrointestinal and hepatic manifestations of the acquired immunodeficiency syndrome. Med J Aust 1989;150:139–143.
3. Janoff EN, Smith PD. Perspectives on gastrointestinal infections in AIDS. Gastroenterol Clin North Am 1988;17:451–463.
4. Smith PD, Janoff EN. Infectious diarrhea in human immunodeficiency virus infection. Gastroenterol Clin North Am 1988;17:587–598.
5. Doyle MG, Pickering LK. Gastrointestinal tract infections in children with AIDS. Semin Pediatr Infect Dis 1990;1:64–72.
6. McLoughlin LC, Nord KS, Joshi VV, Oleske JM, Connor EM. Severe gastrointestinal involvement in children with the acquired immunodeficiency syndrome. J Pediatr Gastroenterol Nutr 1987;6:517–524.
7. Soave R. Cryptosporidiosis and isosporiasis in patients with AIDS. Infect Dis North Am 1988;2:485–493.
8. Gradon JD, Timpone JG, Schnittman SM. Emergence of unusual opportunistic pathogens in AIDS: A review. Clin Infect Dis 1992;15:134–157.
9. Smith PD, Quinn TC, Strober W, Janoff EN, Masur H. Gastrointestinal infection with AIDS. Ann Intern Med 1992;116:63–77.
10. Pickering LK, Cleary TG. Approach to patients with gastrointestinal tract infections and food poisoning. In: Feign RD, Cherry JD, eds. Textbook of pediatric infectious diseases. 3rd ed. Philadelphia: WB Saunders, 1992:565–596.
11. Bartlett JG, Belitsos PC, Sears CL. AIDS enteropathy. Clin Infect Dis 1992;15:726–735.
12. Peña JM, Martinez-López MA, Arnalich F, Barbado FJ, Vázquez JJ. Esophageal candidiasis associated with acute infection due to human immunodeficiency virus: Case report and review. Rev Infect Dis 1991;13:872–875.
13. Law CLH, Qassim M, Cunningham AL, Malhall B, Grierson JM. Nonspecific proctitis: Association with human immunodeficiency virus infection in homosexual men. J Infect Dis 1992;165:150–154.
14. Melamed I, Griffiths AM, Rolfman CM. Benefit of oral immune globulin therapy in patients with immunodeficiency and chronic diarrhea. J Pediatr 1991;119:486–489.
15. Bonacini M, Young T, Laine L. The causes of esophageal symptoms in human immunodeficiency virus infection: A prospective study of 110 patients. Arch Intern Med 1991;151:1567–1572.
16. Kotler DP, Gaetz HP, Lange M, Klein EB, Holt PR. Enteropathy associated with the acquired immunodeficiency syndrome. Ann Intern Med 1984;101:421–428.
17. Dworkin B, Wormser GP, Rosenthal WS, et al. Gastrointestinal manifestations of the acquired immunodeficiency syndrome: A review of 22 cases. Am J Gastroenterol 1985;80:774–778.
18. Malebranche R, Arnoux E, Guerin JM, et al. Acquired immunodeficiency syndrome with severe gastrointestinal manifestations in Haiti. Lancet 1983;2:873–878.
19. Piot P, Quinn TC, Taelman H, et al. Acquired immunodeficiency syndrome in a heterosexual population in Zaire. Lancet 1984;2:65–69.
20. Conlon CP, Pinching AJ, Perera CU, Moody A, Luo NP, Lucas SB. HIV-related enteropathy in Zambia: A clinical, microbiological and histological study. Am J Trop Med Hyg 1990;42:83–88.
21. Quinn TC, Mann JM, Curran JW, Piot P. AIDS in Africa: An epidemiologic paradigm. Science 1986;234:955–963.
22. Smith PD, Lane HC, Gill VJ, et al. Intestinal infections in patients with the acquired immunodeficiency syndrome (AIDS): Etiology and response to therapy. Ann Intern Med 1988;108:328–333.
23. Laughon BE, Druckman DA, Vernon A, et al. Prevalence of enteric pathogens in homosexual men with and without acquired immunodeficiency syndrome. Gastroenterology 1988;94:984–993.
24. Kotler DP, Francisco A, Clayton F, Scholes J, Orenstein J. Small intestinal injury and parasitic diseases in AIDS. Ann Intern Med 1990;113:444–449.
25. Greenson JK, Belitsos PC, Yardley JH, Bartlett JG. AIDS enteropathy: Occult enteric infections and duodenal mucosal alterations in chronic diarrhea. Ann Intern Med 1991;114:366–372.
26. Madi K, Trajman A, daSilva CF, et al. Jejunal biopsy in HIV infected patients. J Acquir Immune Defic Syndr 1991;4:930–937.
27. Berkowitz CD, Seidel JS. Spontaneous resolution of cryptosporidiosis in a child with acquired immunodeficiency syndrome [Letter]. Am J Dis Child 1985;139:967.
28. Lim W, Kahn E, Gupta A, et al. Treatment of cytomegalovirus enterocolitis with ganciclovir in an infant with acquired immunodeficiency syndrome. Pediatr Infect Dis J 1988;7:354–357.
29. Schettini F, DeMattia D, Fumarola D, et al. Lymphadenopathy syndrome and HIV infection in multi-transfused beta-thalassemia child. Boll Ist Sieroter Milan 1987;66:235–238.
30. Centers for Disease Control. Revision of the CDC surveillance case definition for acquired immunodeficiency syndrome. MMWR 1987;36:1S–15S.
31. Centers for Disease Control. 1993 Revised classification system for HIV infection and expanded surveillance case definition for AIDS among adolescents and adults. MMWR 1992;41(RR-17):1–19.
32. Perlman DM, Ampel NM, Schifman RB, et al. Persistent *Campylobacter jejuni* infections in patients infected with human immunodeficiency virus (HIV). Ann Intern Med 1988;108:540–546.
33. Dworkin B, Wormser GP, Abdoo RA, Cabello F, Aguero ME, Sivak SL. Persistence of multiply antibiotic-resistant *Campylobacter jejuni* in a patient with the acquired immune deficiency syndrome. Am J Med 1986;80:965–970.
34. Sacks LV, Labriola AM, Gill VJ, Gordin FM. Use of ciprofloxacin for successful eradication of bacteremia due to *Campylobacter cinaedi* in a human immunodeficiency virus-infected person. Rev Infect Dis 1991;13:1066–1068.

35. Aboulafia D, Mathisen G, Mitsuyasu R. Case report: Aggressive Kaposi's sarcoma and *Campylobacter* bacteremia in a female with transfusion associated AIDS. Am J Med Sci 1991;301: 256–258.

36. Sorvillo FJ, Lieb LE, Waterman SH. Incidence of campylobacterosis among patients with AIDS in Los Angeles County. J Acquir Immune Defic Syndr 1991;4:598–602.

37. Totten PA, Fennell CL, Tenover FC, et al. *Campylobacter cinaedi* (sp. nov.) and *Campylobacter fennelliae* (sp. nov.): Two new *Campylobacter* species associated with enteric disease in homosexual men. J Infect Dis 1985;151:131–139.

38. Laughon BE, Vernon AA, Druckman DA, et al. Recovery of *Campylobacter* species from homosexual men. J Infect Dis 1988;158:464–467.

39. Levine WC, Buehler JW, Bean NH, Tauxe RV. Epidemiology of non-typhoidal *Salmonella* bacteremia during the human immunodeficiency virus epidemic. J Infect Dis 1991;164:81–87.

40. Salmon D, Detruchis P, Leport C, et al. Efficacy of zidovudine in preventing relapses of *Salmonella* bacteremia in AIDS. J Infect Dis 1991;163:415–416.

41. Celum CL, Chaisson RE, Rutherford GW, Barnhart JL, Echenberg DF. Incidence of salmonellosis in patients with AIDS. J Infect Dis 1987;156:998–1002.

42. Sperber SJ, Schleupner CJ. Salmonellosis during infection with human immunodeficiency virus. Rev Infect Dis 1987;9:925–934.

43. Gilks CF, Brindle RJ, Leaber LS, et al. Life threatening bacteremia in HIV-1 seropositive adults admitted to hospital in Nairobi, Kenya. Lancet 1990;336:545–549.

44. Blaser MJ, Hale TL, Formal SB. Recurrent shigellosis complicating human immunodeficiency virus infection: Failure of pre-existing antibodies to confer protection. Am J Med 1989;86:105–107.

45. Baskin DH, Lax JD, Barenberg D. Shigella bacteremia in patients with acquired immunodeficiency syndrome. Am J Gastroenterol 1987;82: 338–341.

46. Hawkins CC, Gold JW, Whimbey E, et al. *Mycobacterium avium* complex infections in patients with the acquired immunodeficiency syndrome. Ann Intern Med 1986;105:184–188.

47. Horsburgh CR Jr. *Mycobacterium avium* complex in the acquired immunodeficiency syndrome. N Engl J Med 1991;324:1332–1338.

48. Liao WC, Cappell MS. Treatment with ciprofloxacin of *Aeromonas hydrophilia* associated colitis in a male with antibodies to the human immunodeficiency virus. J Clin Gastroenterol 1989;11:552–554.

49. Roberts IM, Parenti DM, Albert MB. *Aeromonas hydrophilia*-associated colitis in a male homosexual. Arch Intern Med 1987;147:1502–1503.

50. Bessesen MT, Wang E, Echeverria P, Blaser MJ. Enteroinvasive *Escherichia coli:* A cause of bacteremia in patients with AIDS. J Clin Microbiol 1991;29:2675–2677.

51. Long EG, Ebrahimzadeh A, White EH, Swisher B, Callaway CS. Alga associated with diarrhea in patients with acquired immunodeficiency syndrome and in travelers. J Clin Microbiol 1990;28: 1101–1104.

52. Janoff EN, Orenstein JM, Manischewitz JF, Smith PD. Adenovirus colitis in the acquired immunodeficiency syndrome. Gastroenterology 1991; 100:976–979.

53. Hierholzer JC, Wigand R, Anderson LJ, Adrian T, Gold JWM. Adenoviruses from patients with AIDS: A plethora of serotypes and a description of five new serotypes of subgenes D (types 43-47). J Infect Dis 1988;158:804–813.

54. Cunningham AL, Grohman GS, Harkness J, et al. Gastrointestinal viral infections in homosexual men who were symptomatic and seropositive for human immunodeficiency virus. J Infect Dis 1988;158:386–391.

55. Grohmann GS, Glass RI, Pereira HG, et al. Enteric viruses and diarrhea in HIV-infected patients. N Engl J Med, in press.

56. Klatt EC, Shibata D. Cytomegalovirus infection in the acquired immunodeficiency syndrome. Arch Pathol Lab Med 1988;112:540–544.

57. Dannenberg AJ, Margulis SJ. Cytomegalovirus infection of the gastrointestinal tract in AIDS [Abstract]. Gastroenterology 1987;92:1362.

58. Freedman PG, Weiner BC, Balthazar EJ. Cytomegalovirus esophagogastritis in a patient with acquired immunodeficiency syndrome. Am J Gastroenterol 1985;80:434–437.

59. Ferrell LD. Gastrointestinal pathology of AIDS. Semin Gastrointest Dis 1991;2:37–48.

60. Kotler DP. Intestinal and hepatic manifestations of AIDS. Adv Intern Med 1989;34:43–71.

61. Kavin H, Jonas RB, Chowdhury L, Kabins S. Acalculous cholecystitis and cytomegalovirus infection in the acquired immunodeficiency syndrome. Ann Intern Med 1986;104:53–54.

62. McNair ANB, Main J. Thomas HC. Interactions of the human immunodeficiency virus and the hepatotropic viruses. Semin Liver Dis 1992;12: 188–196.

63. O'Ryan M, Owen RL, Pickering LK. *Cryptosporidium, Isospora* and Microsporidium. In: Feigin RD, Cherry JC, eds. Textbook of pediatric infectious diseases. Philadelphia: WB Saunders, 1992:1939–1952.

64. Connolly GM, Dryden MS, Shanson DC, Gazzard BG. Cryptosporidial diarrhea in AIDS and its treatment. Gut 1988;29:593–597.

65. Andreani T, Modigliani R, Charpentier YL, et al. Acquired immunodeficiency with intestinal cryptosporidiosis: Possible transmission by Haitian whole blood. Lancet 1983;1:1187–1191.

66. Pitlik SD, Fainstein V, Garza D, et al. Human cryptosporidiosis: Spectrum of disease. Report of six cases and review of the literature. Arch Intern Med 1983;143:2269–2275.

67. Janoff EN, Reller LD. *Cryptosporidium* species, a protean protozoan. J Clin Microbiol 1987;25: 967–975.

68. DeHovitz JA, Pape JW, Boney M, Johnson WD Jr. Clinical manifestations and therapy of *Isospora belli* infection in patients with the acquired immunodeficiency syndrome. N Engl J Med 1986; 35:87–90.

69. Whiteside ME, Barkin JS, May RG, Weiss SD, Fischl MA, MacLeod CL. Enteric coccidiosis among patients with the acquired immunodeficiency syndrome. Am J Trop Med Hyg 1984;33: 1065–1072.

70. Trier JS, Moxey PC, Schimmel EM, Robles E. Chronic intestinal coccidiosis in man: Intestinal morphology and response to treatment. Gastroenterology 1974;66:923–935.

71. Forthal DN, Guest SS. *Isospora belli* enteritis in three homosexual men. Am J Trop Med Hyg 1984;33: 1060–1064.

72. Restrepo C, Macher AM, Radany EH. Disseminated extraintestinal isosporiasis in a patient with acquired immunodeficiency syndrome. Am J Clin Pathol 1987;87:536–542.

73. Quinn TC, Stamm WE, Goodnell SE, et al. The polymicrobial origin of intestinal infections in homosexual men. N Engl J Med 1983;309:576–582.

74. Connolly GM, Shanson D, Hawkins DA, Webster JNH, Gazzard BG. Noncryptosporidial diarrhoea in human immunodeficiency virus (HIV) infected patients. Gut 1989;30:195–200.

75. Janoff EN, Smith PD, Blaser MJ. Acute antibody responses to *Giardia lamblia* are depressed in patients with AIDS. J Infect Dis 1988;157:798–804.

76. Orenstein JM, Chiang J, Steinberg W, Smith PD, Rotterdam H, Kotler DP. Intestinal microsporidiosis as a cause of diarrhea in human immunodeficiency virus-infected patients: A report of 20 cases. Hum Pathol 1990;21:475–481.

77. Blanshard C, Peacock C, Ellis D, Gazzard B. Treatment of intestinal microsporidiosis with albendazole [Abstract WB 2265]. Seventh International Conference on AIDS, Florence, Jun 1991.

78. Eeftinck-Schattenkerk JKM, van Gool T, van Ketel RJ, et al. Clinical significance of small intestinal microsporidiosis in HIV-1-infected individuals. Lancet 1991;337:895–898.

79. Ripstra AC, Canning EU, Van-Ketel RJ, Eeftinck-Schattenkerk JKM, Laarman JJ. Use of light microscopy to diagnose small intestinal microsporidiosis in patients with AIDS. J Infect Dis 1988;157:827–831.

80. Curry A, McWilliam LJ, Haboubi NY, Mandal BK. Microsporidiosis in a British patient with AIDS. J Clin Pathol 1988;41:477–478.

81. Modigliani R, Bories C, LeCharpentier Y, et al. Diarrhea and malabsorption in acquired immunodeficiency syndrome: A study of four cases with special emphasis on opportunistic protozoan infestations. Gut 1985;26:179–187.

82. Dobbins WO, Weinstein WM. Electron microscopy of the intestine and rectum in acquired immunodeficiency syndrome. Gastroenterology 1985;88:738–749.

83. Terada S, Reddy KR, Jeffers LJ, Cali A, Shiff ER. Microsporidian hepatitis in the acquired immunodeficiency syndrome. Ann Intern Med 1987; 107:61–62.

84. Ledford DK, Overman MD, Gonzalvo A, Cali A, Mester SW, Lockey RF. Microsporidiosis myositis in a patient with the acquired immunodeficiency syndrome. Ann Intern Med 1985;102:628–630.

85. Shadduck JA. Human microsporidiosis and AIDS. Rev Infect Dis 1989;2:203–207.

86. Orenstein JM, Tenner M, Cali A, Kotler DP. A microsporidian previously described in humans, infecting enterocytes and macrophages associated with diarrhea in an AIDS patient. Hum Pathol 1992;23:722–728.

87. Henry MC, DeClerg D, Lokombe B, et al. Parasitologic observations of chronic diarrheoa in suspected AIDS adult patients in Kinshasa (Zaire). Trans R Soc Trop Med Hyg 1986;80:309–310.

88. Bernard E, Michiels JP, Durant J, et al. Prevalence in AIDS patients of intestinal microsporidiosis due to *Enterocytozoon bieneusi* in the south of France [Abstract MB 2216]. Seventh International Conference on AIDS, Florence, Jun 1991.

89. Rolston KV, Hoy J, Mansell PWA. Diarrhea caused by "nonpathogenic amoebae" in patients with AIDS [Letter]. N Engl J Med 1986;315:192.

90. Garavelli PL, Orsi P, Scaglione L. *Blastocystis hominis* infection during AIDS [Letter]. Lancet 1988;2:1364.

91. Rolston KVI, Winans R, Rodriguez S. *Blastocystis hominis*: Pathogen or not? Rev Infect Dis 1989; 11:661–662.

92. Caravelli PL, Libanore M. Blastocystis in immunodeficiency diseases [Letter]. Rev Infect Dis 1990;12:158.

93. Llibre JM, Tor J, Manterola JM, Carbonell C, Foz M. *Blastocystis hominis* chronic diarrhoea in AIDS patients [Letter]. Lancet 1989;1:221.

94. Ortega YR, Sterling CR, Gilman RH, Cama VA, Díaz F. Cyclospora species—a new protozoan pathogen of humans. N Engl J Med 1993;328: 1308–1312.

95. Berenguer J, Moreno S, Cercenado E, et al. Visceral leishmaniasis in patients infected with human immunodeficiency virus (HIV). Ann Intern Med 1989;111:129–132.

96. Delsedime L, Coppola F, Mazzucco G. Gastric localization of systemic leishmaniasis in a patient with AIDS. Histopathology 1991;19:93–95.

97. Wheat LJ, Connolly-Stringfield PA, Baker RL, et al. Disseminated histoplasmosis in the acquired immunodeficiency syndrome. Medicine (Baltimore) 1990;69:361–374.

98. Sonnerborg A, Abebe A, Strannegard O. Hepatitis C virus infection in individuals with or without human immunodeficiency virus type 1 infection. Infection 1990;18:347–351.

99. Zeldis JB, Jain S, Kuramoto IK, et al. Seroepidemiology of viral infections among intravenous drug users in northern California. West J Med 1992;156:30–35.

100. Kingsley LA, Rinaldo CR Jr, Lyter DW, et al. Sexual transmission efficiency of hepatitis B virus and human immunodeficiency virus among homosexual men. JAMA 1990;264:230–234.

101. Corona R, Prignano G, Mele A, et al. Heterosexual and homosexual transmission of hepatitis C virus: Relation with hepatitis B virus and human immunodeficiency virus type 1. Epidemiol Infect 1991;107:667–672.

102. de Montalembert M, Costagliola DG, Lefrere JJ, et al. Prevalence of markers for human immunodeficiency virus types 1 and 2, human T-lymphotropic virus type I, cytomegalovirus, and hepatitis B and C virus in multiply transfused

thalassemia patients. Transfusion 1992;32: 509–512.

103. Giovanninni M, Tagger A, Ribero ML, et al. Maternal-infant transmission of hepatitis C virus and HIV infections; a possible interaction [Letter]. Lancet 1990;335:1166.

104. Tamura I, Koda T, Kobayashi Y, et al. Prevalence of four bloodborne viruses (HBV, HCV, HTLV-1, HIV-1) among haemodialysis patients in Japan. J Med Virol 1992;36:271–273.

105. Myint H, Soe MM, Khin T, et al. A clinical and epidemiological study of an epidemic of non-A, non-B hepatitis in Rangoon. Am J Trop Med Hyg 1985;34:1183–1189.

106. Pickering LK, Engelkirk PG. *Giardia lamblia.* Pediatr Clin North Am 1988;35:565–567.

107. Neva FA. Biology and immunology of human stronglyloidiasis. J Infect Dis 1986;153:397–406.

108. Belitsos PC, Greenson JK, Yardley JH, Sisler JR, Bartlett JG. Association of gastric hypoacidity with opportunistic enteric infections in patients with AIDS. J Infect Dis 1992;166:277–284.

109. Lafon ME, Kirn A. Human immunodeficiency virus infection of the liver. Semin Liv Dis 1992; 12:197–204.

110. Harriman GR, Smith PD, Horne MK, et al. Vitamin B12 malabsorption in patients with acquired immunodeficiency syndrome. Arch Intern Med 1989;149:2039–2041.

111. Gillin JS, Shike M, Alcock N, et al. Malabsorption and mucosal abnormalities of the small intestine in the acquired immunodeficiency syndrome. Ann Intern Med 1985;102:612–622.

112. Ullrich R, Zeitz M, Heise W, L'age M, Hoffken G, Riecken EO. Small intestinal structure and function in patients infected with human immunodeficiency virus (HIV): Evidence for HIV-induced enteropathy. Ann Intern Med 1989;111:15–21.

113. Yahi N, Baghdiguian S, Moreau H. Galactosyl ceramide is the receptor for human immunodeficiency virus type 1 on human colon epithelial HT29 cells. J Virol 1992;66:4848–4854.

114. Budhraja M, Levendoglu H, Kocka F, Mangkornkanok M, Sherer R. Duodenal mucosal T cell subpopulation and bacterial cultures in acquired immune deficiency syndrome. Am J Gastroenterol 1987;82:427–431.

115. Grunfield C, Feingold KR. Metabolic disturbances and wasting in the acquired immunodeficiency syndrome. N Engl J Med 1992;327:329–337.

116. Wilcox CM, Diehl DL, Cello JP, Margaretten W, Jacobson MA. Cytomegalovirus esophagitis in patients with AIDS: A clinical, endoscopic and pathologic correlation. Ann Intern Med 1990; 113:589–593.

117. Kim J, Minamoto GY, Grieco MH. Nocardia infection as a complication of AIDS: Report of six cases and review. Rev Infect Dis 1991;13: 624–629.

118. Indorf AS, Pegram S. Esophageal ulceration related to zalcitabine (ddC). Ann Intern Med 1992;117:133–134.

119. Garcia ME, Collins CL, Mansell PA. The acquired immune deficiency syndrome: Nutritional complications and assessment of body weight status. Nutr Clin Pract 1987;2:108–111.

120. Lo CW, Walker WA. Chronic protracted diarrhea of infancy: A nutritional disease. Pediatrics 1983;72:786–800.

121. Flanigan T, Whalen C, Turner J, et al. *Cryptosporidium* infection and CD4 counts. Ann Intern Med 1992;116:840–842.

122. Dieterich DT, Kim MH, McMeeding A, Rotterdam H. Cytomegalovirus appendicitis in a patient with acquired immune deficiency syndrome. Am J Gastroenterol 1991;86:904–906.

123. Wilcox CM, Forsmark CE, Grendell JH, Dorragh TM, Cello JP. Cytomegalovirus-associated acute pancreatic disease in patients with acquired immunodeficiency syndrome: Report of two patients. Gastroenterology 1991;99:263–267.

124. Saraux JL, Lenoble L, Toublanc M, Smiejan JM, Dombret MC. Acalculous cholecystitis and cytomegalovirus infection in a patient with AIDS [Letter]. J Infect Dis 1987;155:829.

125. Schneiderman DJ, Cello JP, Liang FC. Papillary stenosis and sclerosing cholangitis in the acquired immunodeficiency syndrome. Ann Intern Med 1987;106:546–549.

126. Rich JD, Crawford JM, Kazanjian SN, Kazanjian PH. Discrete gastrointestinal mass lesions caused by cytomegalovirus in patients with AIDS: Report of three cases and review. Clin Infect Dis 1992; 15:609–614.

127. Blumberg RS, Kelsey P, Perrone T, Dickersin R, Laquaglia M, Ferruci J. Cytomegalovirus- and cryptosporidium-associated acalculous gangrenous cholecystitis. Am J Med 1984;76: 11187–1123.

128. Cello JP. Acquired immunodeficiency syndrome cholangiopathy: Spectrum of disease. Am J Med 1989;86:539–546.

129. Jacobson MA, Cello JP, Sande MA. Cholestasis and disseminated cytomegalovirus disease in patients with the acquired immunodeficiency syndrome. Am J Med 1988;84:218–224.

130. Carter TR, Cooper PH, Petri WA Jr, Kim CK, Walzer PD, Guerrant RL. *Pneumocystis carinii* infection of the small intestine in a patient with acquired immune deficiency syndrome. Am J Clin Pathol 1988;89:679–683.

131. Cutrona AF, Blinkhorn RJ, Crass J, Spagnuolo PJ. Probable neutropenic enterocolitis in patients with AIDS. Rev Infect Dis 1991;13:828–831.

132. Lebovics E, Dworkin BM, Heier SK, Rosenthal WS. The hepatobiliary manifestations of human immunodeficiency virus infection. Am J Gastroenterol 1988;83:1–7.

133. Perkocha LA, Geaghan SM, Yen TSB, et al. Clinical and pathological features of bacillary peliosis hepatitis in association with human immunodeficiency virus infection. N Engl J Med 1990; 323:1581–1586.

134. Relman DA, Loutit JS, Schmidt TM, Falkow S, Tompkins LS. The agent of bacillary angiomatosis: An approach to the identification of uncultured pathogens. N Engl J Med 1990;323: 1573–1580.

135. Poblete RB, Rodriguez K, Foust RT, Reddy KR, Saldana MJ. *Pneumocystis carinii* hepatitis in the acquired immunodeficiency syndrome (AIDS). Ann Intern Med 1989;110:737–738.

136. Raviglione MC. Extrapulmonary pneumocystosis: The first 50 cases. Rev Infect Dis 1990;12: 1127–1138.

137. Hagopian WA, Huseby JS. Pneumocystis hepatitis and choroiditis despite successful aerosolized pentamidine pulmonary prophylaxis. Chest 1989;96:949–951.

138. Tsang DNC, Li PCK, Tsui MS, Lau YT, Ma KF, Yeoh EK. *Penicillium marneffei*: Another pathogen to consider in patients infected with human immunodeficiency virus. Rev Infect Dis 1991;13:766–767.

139. Wilkins MJ, Lindley R, Dourakis SP, Goldin RD. Surgical pathology of the liver in HIV infection. Histopathology 1991;18:459–464.

140. Datry A, Similowski T, Jais P, et al. AIDS-associated leishmaniasis: An unusual gastro-duodenal presentation. Trans R Soc Trop Med Hyg 1990; 84:239–240.

141. Krilov LR, Rubin LG, Frogel M, et al. Disseminated adenovirus infection with hepatic necrosis in patients with human immunodeficiency virus and other immunodeficiency states. Rev Infect Dis 1990;12:303–307.

142. Solomon RE, VanRaden M, Kaslow RA, et al. Association of hepatitis B surface and core antibody with acquisition and manifestations of human immunodeficiency virus type 1 infection. Am J Public Health 1990;80:1475–1478.

143. Koblin BA, Taylor PE, Rubinstein P, Stevens CE. Effect of duration of hepatitis B virus infection on the association between human immunodeficiency virus type-1 and hepatitis B viral replication. Hepatology 1992;15:590–592.

144. Perrillo RP, Regenstein FG, Roodman ST. Chronic hepatitis B in asymptomatic homosexual men with antibody to human immunodeficiency virus. Ann Intern Med 1986;105:382–383.

145. Krogsgaard K, Lindhardt BO, Nielson JO, et al. The influence of HTLV III infection on the natural history of hepatitis B virus infection in male homosexual HBsAg carriers. Hepatology 1987;7: 37–41.

146. Bodsworth NJ, Cooper DA, Donovan B. The influence of human immunodeficiency virus type 1 infection on the development of the hepatitis B virus carrier state. J Infect Dis 1991;163: 1138–1140.

147. Scharschmidt BF, Held MJ, Hollander HH, et al. Hepatitis B in patients with HIV infection: Relationship to AIDS and patient survival. Ann Intern Med 1992;117:837–838.

148. Hadler SC, Judson FN, O'Malley PM, et al. Outcome of hepatitis B virus infection in homosexual men and its relation to prior human immunodeficiency virus infection. J Infect Dis 1991;163:454–459.

149. Goldin RD, Fish DE, Hay A, et al. Histological and immunohistochemical study of hepatitis B virus in human immunodeficiency virus infection. J Clin Pathol 1990;43:203–205.

150. Housset C, Pol S, Carnot F, et al. Interactions between human immunodeficiency virus-1, hepatitis delta virus and hepatitis B virus infections in 260 chronic carriers of hepatitis B virus. Hepatology 1992;15:578–583.

151. Bodsworth N, Donovan B, Nightingale BN. The effect of concurrent human immunodeficiency virus infection on chronic hepatitis B: A study of 150 homosexual men. J Infect Dis 1989;160: 577–582.

152. Levy P, Marcellin P, Martinot-Peignoux M, et al. Clinical course of spontaneous reactivation of hepatitis B virus infection in patients with chronic hepatitis B. Hepatology 1990;12:570–574.

153. Waite J, Gilson RJC, Weller IVD, et al. Hepatitis B virus reactivation or reinfection associated with HIV-1 infection. AIDS 1988;2:443–448.

154. Lazizi Y, Grangeot-Keros L, Delfraissay JF. Reappearance of hepatitis B virus in immune patients infected with the human immunodeficiency virus type 1. J Infect Dis 1988;158:666–667.

155. Martin P. DiBiseglie AM, Kassianides C, et al. Rapidly progressive non-A, non-B hepatitis in patients with human immunodeficiency virus infection. Gastroenterology 1989;97:1559–1561.

156. Govindarajan S, Cassidy WM, Valinluck B, Redeker AG. Interactions of HDV, HBV and HIV in chronic B and D infections and in reactivation of chronic D infection. Prog Clin Biol Res 1991; 364:207–210.

157. Morante AL, De La Cruz F, De Lope CR, et al. Hepatitis B virus replication in hepatitis B and D co-infection. Liver 1989;9:65–70.

158. Govindarajan S, Valinluck B, Peters RL. Relapse of acute B viral hepatitis: Role of delta agent. Gut 1986;27:19–22.

159. Govindarajan S, Valinluck B. Serum hepatitis B virus DNA in chronic hepatitis B and delta infection. Arch Pathol Lab Med 1985;109:398–399.

160. Shattock AG, Finlay H, Hillary IB. Possible reactivation of hepatitis D with chronic delta antigenaemia by human immunodeficiency virus. Br Med J 1987;294:1656–1657.

161. Kreek MJ, Des Jarias DC, Trepo CL, Novick DM, Abdul-Quader A, Raghunath J. Contrasting prevalence of delta hepatitis markers in parenteral drug abusers with and without AIDS. J Infect Dis 1990;162:538–541.

162. Johanson JF, Sonnenberg A. Efficient management of diarrhea in the acquired immunodeficiency syndrome (AIDS). A medical decision analysis. Ann Intern Med 1990;112:942–948.

163. Laukamm-Josten U, Muller O, Bienzie U, et al. Decline of naturally acquired antibodies to hepatitis B surface antigen in HIV-1 infected homosexual men with AIDS. AIDS 1988;2:400–401.

164. Biggar RJ, Goedert JJ, Hoofnagle J. Accelerated loss of antibody to hepatitis B surface antigen among immunodeficient homosexual men infected with HIV. N Engl J Med 1987;316:630–631.

165. Loke RH, Murray-Lyon IM, Coleman JC, et al. Diminished response to recombinant hepatitis B vaccine in homosexual men with HIV antibody; an indicator of poor prognosis. J Med Virol 1990; 31:109–111.

166. Carne CA, Weller IVD, Waite J, et al. Impaired responsiveness of homosexual men with HIV antibodies to plasma derived hepatitis B vaccine. Br Med J 1987;294:866–868.

167. Drake JH, Parmley RT, Britton HA. Loss of hepatitis B antibody in human immunodeficiency virus-

positive hemophilia patients. Pediatr Infect Dis J 1987;6:1051–1054.

168. Cappell MS, Schwartz MS, Biempica L. Clinical utility of liver biopsy in patients with serum antibodies to the human immunodeficiency virus. Am J Med 1990;88:123–130.

169. Relman DA, Schmidt TM, MacDermott RP, Falkow S. Identification of the uncultured bacillus of Whipple's disease. N Engl J Med 1992;327:293–301.

170. Edwards P, Thompson IL, Wodak A, Penny R, Cooper DA. The gastrointestinal manifestations of AIDS. Aust N Z J Med 1990;20:141–148.

171. Frager DH, Frager JD, Wolf EL, et al. Cytomegalovirus colitis in acquired immune deficiency syndrome: Radiologic spectrum. Gastrointest Radiol 1986;11:241–246.

172. Balthazar EJ, Megibow AJ, Hulnick DH. Cytomegalovirus esophagitis and gastritis in AIDS. Am J Roentgenol 1985;144:1201–1204.

173. Wajsman R, Cappell MS, Biempica L, Cho KC. Terminal ileitis associated with cytomegalovirus and the acquired immune deficiency syndrome. Am J Gastroenterol 1989;84:790–793.

174. Teixidor HS, Honig CL, Norsoph E, Albert S, Mouradian JA, Whalen JP. Cytomegalovirus infection of the alimentary canal: Radiologic findings with pathologic correlation. Radiology 1987;163:317–323.

175. Ungar BL, Soave R, Fayer R, Nash TE. Enzyme immunoassay detection of immunoglobulin M and G antibodies to *Cryptosporidium* in immunocompetent and immunocompromised patients. J Infect Dis 1986;153:570–578.

176. Ng E, Markell EK, Fleming RL, Fried M. Demonstration of *Isospora belli* by acid-fast stain in a patient with acquired immune deficiency syndrome. J Clin Microbiol 1984;20:384–386.

177. Knisley CV, Englekirk PG, Pickering LK, West MS, Janoff EN. Rapid detection of *Giardia* antigen in stool using enzyme immunoassays. Am J Clin Pathol 1989;91:704–708.

178. Weber R, Bryan RT, Owen RL, et al. Improved light-microscopical detection of microsporidia spores in stool and duodenal aspirates. N Engl J Med 1992;326:161–166.

179. Duggan C, Santosham M, Glass RI. The management of acute diarrhea in children: Oral rehydration, maintenance, and nutritional therapy. MMWR 1992;41:1–20.

180. Cello JP, Grendell JH, Basuk P, et al. Effect of octreotide on refractory AIDS-associated diarrhea. Ann Intern Med 1991;115:705–710.

181. Bentler M, Standish M. Nutritional support of the pediatric patient with AIDS. J Am Diet Assoc 1987;87:488–491.

182. Anonymous. The choice of antibacterial drugs. Med Lett Drugs Ther 1992;34:49–56.

183. McDonald JA, Caruso L, Karayiannis P, et al. Diminished responsiveness of male homosexual chronic hepatitis B virus carriers with HTLV III antibodies to recombinant interferon. Hepatology 1987;7:719–723.

184. Brook MG, Chan G, Yap I, et al. Randomised controlled trial of lymphoblastoid interferon alfa in European men with chronic hepatitis B virus infection. Br Med J 1989;299:652–656.

185. Perillo RP, Regenstein FG, Peters MG, et al. Prednisone withdrawal followed by recombinant alpha interferon in the treatment of chronic type B hepatitis. Ann Intern Med 1988;109:95–100.

186. Haritami H, Uchida T, Okuda Y, Shikata T. Effect of 3' azido-3' deoxythymidine on replication of duck hepatitis B virus in vivo and in vitro. J Med Virol 1989;29:244–248.

187. Gilson RJ, Hawkins AE, Kelly GK, et al. No effect of zidovudine on hepatitis B virus replication in homosexual men with symptomatic HIV-1 infection. AIDS 1991;5:217–220.

188. Hess G, Rossol S, Voth R, et al. Treatment of patients with chronic type B hepatitis and concurrent human immunodeficiency virus with a combination of interferon alpha and azidothymidine. Digestion 1989;43:56–59.

189. Garofano T, Vento S, Di Perri G, et al. Zidovudine induces remission of chronic active hepatitis C in HIV carriers [Abstract WB 89]. Seventh International Conference on AIDS, Florence, Jun 1991.

190. Chachoua A, Dieterich D, Krasinski K, et al. 9-(1,3-dihydroxy-2-propoxymethyl)guanine (ganciclovir) in the treatment of cytomegalovirus gastrointestinal disease with the acquired immunodeficiency syndrome. Ann Intern Med 1987;107:133–137.

191. Kotler DP. Cytomegalovirus colitis and wasting. J Acquir Immune Defic Syndr 1991;4(suppl):S36–S41.

192. Pilla AM, Rybak MJ, Chandrasekar PH. Spiramycin in the treatment of cryptosporidiosis. Pharmacotherapy 1987;7:188–190.

193. Louie E, Borkowsky W, Klesius PH, et al. Treatment of cryptosporidiosis with oral bovine transfer factor. Clin Immun Immunopathol 1987;44:329–334.

194. Tzipori S, Roberton D, Chapman D. Remission of diarrhoea due to cryptosporidiosis in an immunodeficient child treated with hyperimmune bovine colostrum. Br Med J 1986;293:1276–1277.

195. Perryman LE, Riggs MW, Mason PH, Foyer R. Kinetics of *Cryptosporidium parvum* sporozoite neutralization by monoclonal antibodies, immune bovine serum and immune bovine colostrum. Infect Immun 1990;58:257–259.

196. Cook DJ, Kelton JG, Stanisz AM, Collins SM. Somatostain treatment of cryptosporidial diarrhea in a patient with the acquired immunodeficiency syndrome (AIDS). Ann Intern Med 1988;108:708–709.

197. Katz MD, Erstad BL, Rose C. Treatment of severe *Cryptosporidium*-related diarrhea with octreotide in a patient with AIDS. Drug Intelligence Clin Pharm 1988;22:134–136.

198. Pape JW, Verdier RI, Johnson WD. Treatment and prophylaxis of *Isospora belli* infection in patients with the acquired immunodeficiency syndrome. N Engl J Med 1989;320:1044–1047.

199. Weiss LM, Perlman DC, Sherman J, Tanowitz H, Wittner M. *Isospora belli* infection: Treatment with pyrimethamine. Ann Intern Med 1988;109:474–475.

200. Anonymous. Drugs for parasitic infections. Med Lett Drugs Ther 1992;34:17–26.

201. Polder JA, Bell DM, Curran J, et al. Recommendations for preventing transmission of human immunodeficiency virus and hepatitis B virus to patients during exposure-prone invasive procedures. MMWR 1991;40:1–9.

202. Mullan RJ, Baker EL, Hughes JM, et al. Guidelines for prevention of transmission of human immunodeficiency virus and hepatitis B virus to health care and public safety workers. MMWR 1989;38:1–37.

203. Collier AC, Corey L, Murphy VL, Handsfield HH. Antibody to human immunodeficiency virus (HIV) and suboptimal response to hepatitis B vaccination. Ann Intern Med 1988;109:101–105.

204. Chan W, Petric M, Wang E, Koren G, Read S, Blanchette V. Response to hepatitis B immunization in children with hemophilia: Relationship to infection with human immunodeficiency virus type 1. J Pediatr 1990;117:427–430.

21
Pneumocystis carinii Pneumonia

Walter T. Hughes

AIDS was discovered in 1980 because of *Pneumocystis carinii* pneumonia. Over several decades *P. carinii* had become recognized and established as a cause of an acute, diffuse, and life-threatening pneumonitis. Uniquely, the pneumonitis had occurred only in severely immunocompromised individuals. Thus, when previously healthy young men began to appear in New York and California with *P. carinii* pneumonitis, attention was immediately directed to the search for an underlying immunodeficiency. Before a dozen cases had occurred, AIDS had been recognized as a new entity. Without *P. carinii*, when would AIDS have been discovered?

More than 40 yr before the epidemic of AIDS began, an epidemic of *P. carinii* pneumonitis was ongoing in Europe. The disease occurred exclusively in infants. Although the provocative factor was often attributed to malnutrition, no proof was ever established. After World War II those epidemics, having affected several thousand infants, subsided. In light of current understanding of the pathogenesis of human immunodeficiency virus (HIV) infection, one might hypothesize that the infantile epidemics could also have been associated with a retrovirus infection. However, there is no evidence for or against this speculation.

Beginning in the mid-20th century, *P. carinii* pneumonitis began to be recognized in adults and children who were immunocompromised because of cancer chemotherapy, organ transplantation, and congenital immunodeficiency disorders. Clinical features and histopathology of the

epidemic infantile type of *P. carinii* pneumonitis differs somewhat from those in the sporadic adult-childhood cases. In the former the onset is subtle without fever but with cough, tachypnea, dyspnea, and cyanosis and is characterized by an interstitial plasma cell pneumonitis. The latter type usually begins abruptly with fever, cough, and tachypnea and progresses to dyspnea, cyanosis, and death. Histologically the disease is a severe diffuse alveolitis.

P. carinii pneumonitis in AIDS differs in some minor aspects from that in non-AIDS patients, and the pneumonitis in adult AIDS patients differs slightly from that in infants with AIDS. These features are discussed in this chapter.

MICROBIOLOGY

The taxonomy of *P. carinii* has not been firmly established as either a fungus (1, 2) or a protozoan (3). Recent studies of DNA homology suggests *P. carinii* is a fungus. Analysis of sequences of a single ribosomal gene (1) and seven contiguous mitochondrial genes (4) indicates a fungal nature of the organism. A recent study shows it closely related to the ustomycetous red yeast (5). Unlike the dihydrofolate reductase of protoza, that of *P. carinii* is not a bifunctional polypeptide with thymidylate synthetase. The cell wall contains chitin and β-1,3 glucan, which are found more often in fungi than protozoa.

Unlike fungi, however, *P. carinii* cell membranes do not contain ergosterol and the characteristic protein elongation factor

(6). Drugs known to be effective against fungi (amphotericin B, ketoconazole, nystatin, 5-flucytosine, and miconazole) have no effect against *P. carinii* infection. However, drugs with known effects against protozoa (pentamidine, fansidar, trimethoprim-sulfamethoxazole, clindamycin-primaquine, atovaquone) are effective anti-*P. carinii* agents. Morphologically it more closely resembles a protozoan than a fungus, thus accounting for the terms used in protozoology to designate development stages of the organism (7). The "cyst" form is a thick-walled structure measuring 5–8 μm in diameter. Its form may be round, cup-shaped, or crescent-shaped. The cell wall stains with toluidine blue O (Fig. 21.1), methenamine silver nitrate (Grocott-Gomori), or Gram-Weigert methods but stains poorly or not at all with polychrome stains, such as that of Giemsa. Within the cyst are up to eight small pleomorphic cells termed "sporozoites." These measure 1–2 μm and are often crescent-shaped to round, conforming to their positions within the cyst. These appear with Giemsa stain (Fig. 21.2) as delicate cells with pale cytoplasm and an eccentric chromatid body, presumably the nucleus.

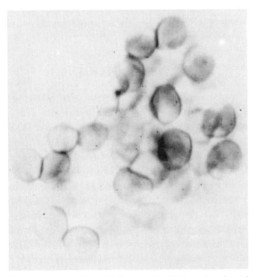

Figure 21.1. *P. carinii* cysts in BAL stained with toluidine blue O. Stain impregnates cyst wall, demonstrating round, oval, and cup-shaped cells and turns them blue-lavender. No budding occurs. Trophozoites and sporozoites cannot be seen with this stain.

The "trophozoite" is an extracystic form of the organism, measuring 2–5 μm in diameter. This cell is pleomorphic with a delicate cell wall and pale purple cytoplasm accented with a dark reddish-purple nucleus when stained with Giemsa, Wright, or other polychrome stains. The trophozoite does not stain with toluidine blue O or Grocott-Gomori stains. Trophozoites are much more numerous than cysts in infected lungs.

P. carinii can be propagated with brief periods in culture with cell lines such as chick embryonic epithelial, Vero, and WI-38 cells. However, in vitro cultivation for prolonged periods is not possible.

EPIDEMIOLOGY AND RISK FACTORS

It is generally believed that most individuals in most parts of the world are infected with *P. carinii* early in life and that these infections are asymptomatic. Residual organisms persist in a latent state unless the host experiences impairment of the immune system. Especially with a serious compromise in cell-mediated immunity, pneumonitis from *P. carinii* occurs. The latency concept is supported by studies showing that over 75% of normal children in the United States (8) and Europe (9) have acquired antibody to *P. carinii* by the age of 4 years. Cases of *P. carinii* pneumonitis have been reported from most countries of the world. Furthermore, a high proportion of lower mammals are latently infected with *P. carinii* (7).

Even at the beginning of the AIDS epidemic it was obvious that *P. carinii* was a highly prevalent companion infection (10). In a sense, the epidemiology of *P. carinii* pneumonitis has become the epidemiology of AIDS.

Many studies have consistently shown that about 75% of adults with AIDS will have *P. carinii* pneumonitis. Information on the incidence of *P. carinii* pneumonia in children with AIDS is fairly sparse. However, data culled from several studies of children with AIDS give some indication of the risk for *P. carinii* pneumonitis in children (Table 21.1). Overall, one may expect ~50% of children with AIDS to have *P. carinii* pneumoni-

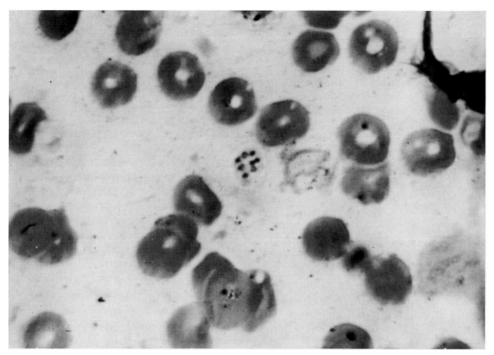

Figure 21.2. *P. carinii* stained with Giemsa method. Cyst wall does not stain, leaving a clear zone around cluster of intracellular sporozoites, which are round to crescent-shaped and measure 1–2 μm in diameter. Trophozoite is extracystic and has a delicate cell wall with a punctate nucleus.

Table 21.1.   Proportion of Pediatric AIDS Patients with *P. carinii* Pneumonia

Reference	Age	No. of Cases Studied	% with PCP[a]
Scott et al., 1984 (13)	<3 yr	14	29
Shannon and Amman, 1985 (50)	mean 5 mo (1–21 mo)	36	33
Silverman and Rubinstein, 1985 (23)	mean 36 mo (9–72 mo)	17	18
Joshi et al., 1986 (19)	73% <2 yr (3 mo–10 yr)	15	47
Rubinstein et al., 1986 (22)	mean 26 mo (4–68 mo)	15	53
Bye et al., 1987 (26)	mean 22 mo (2–54 mo)	29	50
Rogers et al., 1987 (51)	80% <3 yr	307	53
Vernon et al., 1988 (52)	mean 10.4 mo 97% <3 yr	31	42
Kovacs et al., 1991 (15)	<1 yr	68	29
Total		532	39

[a]PCP, *P. carinii* pneumonia.

tis. In the 307 children reported to the Centers for Disease Control (CDC) by 1985, those younger than 1 year were more likely to have *P. carinii* pneumonitis (72%) compared with older children (38%) (*P* < 0.001) (10). By September 1992, 3838 pediatric pa-tients (<13 years old) have been reported to the CDC. A recent report from the CDC shows a decrease in *P. carinii* pneumonitis as an AIDS-defining illness from 66% in 1988 to 49% of the cases with AIDS in homosexual and bisexual men in 1990 (11). Similar data for children are not yet available. Federal guidelines for adults in 1989, and infants and children in 1991, likely will impact further on the incidence of this pneumonitis in HIV-infected individuals. However, unless infants are screened for HIV at birth or early in life and, if infected, placed on appropriate prophlaxis, it is still likely that *P. carinii* pneumonia will be an AIDS-identifying illness during infancy.

The risk for a first episode of *P. carinii* pneumonitis in adults with AIDS has been well defined by the Multicenter AIDS Cohort Study (12). There was a close correlation ($P < 0.001$) between T helper lymphocytes (CD4+ cells) and the incidence of *P. carinii* pneumonia. For example, of those with CD4+ cell counts of $<200/mm^3$, 13, 24, and 39% had developed pneumonitis by 6, 12, and 36 months, respectively. In other studies of adults with AIDS who had one episode of *P. carinii* pneumonitis, 50% had a second episode within 8 months (12). Such studies are unavailable for infants and children. However, the studies by Scott et al. (13) and Kovacs et al. (15) show that a CD4+ cell count of $<500/mm^3$ is not a sensitive indicator for *P. carinii* pneumonitis in infants with AIDS. Four infants with *P. carinii* pneumonitis in the first report and 11 infants in the second report had CD4 counts greater than 500 mm^3 (13, 15). The age-appropriate norms for CD4 cells in infants younger than 1 year appear to be considerably higher than adult values. Until 1992, little information was available regarding the quantity and distribution of T lymphocyte subsets for healthy infants and children of various ages. Denny et al. (14) studied 208 children aged 1–59 months and found the CD4 lymphocyte count or percentage to be highly age dependent. Median CD4 counts (5th and 95th percentiles) for children aged 2–3, 4–8, 12–23, and 24–59 months were 2.83 (1.46–5.22), 2.95 (1.69–4.61), 2.07 (1.02–3.60), and 1.80 (0.90 to 2.86) $\times 10^9$/liter, respectively. The CD4 T lymphocyte count, or percentage, has provided a basis for administration of chemoprophylaxis for *P. carinii* pneumonitis described later in this chapter.

P. carinii pneumonitis has been reported in immunocompromised hosts in most countries of the world. However, there is some evidence to suggest that the pneumonitis is infrequently encountered in AIDS patients in central Africa (16) (see also Chapter 3).

The mode of transmission of *P. carinii* in humans has not been established. However, in animal studies transmission of the organism by the airborne route from animal to animal occurs (7). The only habitat of *P. carinii* identified to date is animal reservoirs.

PATHOGENESIS

It has been presumed that *P. carinii* is acquired by the airborne route. The stage of the life cycle of the organism at which transmission and infection occurs is unknown. Once in the alveolus the organism adheres to the epithelial cell surface. Replication occurs in the alveolus. It is generally believed that normal competent hosts undergo an asymptomatic infection with few if any signs and symptoms of illness and that the organism persists indefinitely. If the individual's immune system becomes compromised, the organism replicates, and pneumonitis ensues. In the infantile epidemic type seen in European cases the disease is an interstitial plasma cell pneumonitis. In the sporadic form occurring in immunocompromised children and adults with cancer, organ transplantation, congenital immune deficiency syndromes, and so forth, a diffuse alveolopathy occurs.

In AIDS patients with symptomatic pneumonitis diffuse alveolar damage is found, characterized by an exudative phase with interstitial edema and hyaline membranes and a proliferative phase with regeneration of alveolar epithelium, interstitial inflammation, and fibrosis (17). Pathologic studies of infants and children with AIDS and *P. carinii* pneumonitis are limited, but Joshi and coworkers (18, 19) found the expected foamy alveolar exudate with abundant organisms in histopathologic studies of seven patients. There are no studies to indicate whether the pneumonitis in infants with AIDS is a primary de novo infection or reactivation of an earlier infection with *P. carinii*. It seems reasonable to expect that the pneumonitis in infants younger than 6 months is primary infection.

Recent studies by Wakefield et al. (20) using a polymerase chain reaction with oligonucleotide primers that specifically amplify *P. carinii* DNA suggest that the pneumonitis in immunocompromised patients may be due to a de novo infection acquired from the environment, rather than recrudescence of a latent infection.

CLINICAL FEATURES

P. carinii pneumonitis is characterized by a tetrad of signs: tachypnea, dyspnea, fever, and cough. These clinical manifestations occur with *P. carinii* pneumonitis in infants, children, and adults with AIDS and with non-AIDS immunocompromising diseases. However, the magnitude of these signs varies among patients. Some patients may not be febrile, but almost all patients will have tachypnea once the pneumonitis is evident by radiograph.

Blood gas values are especially useful in evaluating the extent of *P. carinii* pneumonitis. In a study of children with AIDS the arterial oxygen tension (Pao_2) ranged from 34 to 73 mm Hg (in room air) at the time of presentation (21), and all children had alveolar-arterial oxygen gradients of >30 mm Hg.

The lactate dehydrogenase activity is usually increased, with levels ranging from 320 to 2000 units/liter (mean 922), in children with AIDS and *P. carinii* pneumonitis (21–23). However, this abnormality is not specific for *P. carinii* and may be associated with other causes of pneumonitis.

The chest radiograph reveals bilateral diffuse alveolar disease. The earliest infiltrates are usually perihilar, progressing peripherally but sparing until the last the apical portions of the lungs. Various atypical lesions caused by *P. carinii* have been described but are rare. These have included lobar, miliary, coin, cavitary, and nodular lesions. Pleural effusion may be seen but is usually small. In the study of 27 children with *P. carinii* pneumonitis and AIDS, Conner et al. (24) found the HIV-associated conditions that frequently antedated the diagnosis of the pneumonitis included failure to thrive (70%), persistent oral or esophageal candidiasis (67%), neurodevelopmental disorders (52%), hypergammaglobulineamia

(59%), diarrhea (7%), and cytomegalovirus pneumonia (4%).

Extrapulmonary disease caused by *P. carinii* has been described more frequently in AIDS patients than in non-AIDS patients. Furthermore, most of such cases have been in adults, with only seven cases having been reported in children and none in children with AIDS. Extrapulmonary sites that have been reported include the liver, heart, adrenal glands, kidneys, brain, spleen, lymph nodes, bone marrow, pancreas, thymus, retina, appendix, middle ear, mastoid choroid, thyroid, and external otic canal. The use of aerosolized pentamidine for prophylaxis may be associated with such extrapulmonary replication.

The clinical course of *P. carinii* pneumonitis is progressive, if untreated the patient becomes markedly tachypneic, dyspneic, and cyanotic because of severe hypoxemia; death occurs in ~100% of cases.

DIAGNOSTIC CONSIDERATIONS

When an infant or child with AIDS presents with tachypnea, cough, dyspnea, and fever and the chest radiograph reveals a diffuse bilateral alveolar disease, several organisms must be considered as causative agents. In addition to *P. carinii*, cytomegalovirus, *Mycobacterium avium-intracellulare*, Epstein-Barr virus, and lymphoid interstitial pneumonitis have been implicated as causes of diffuse pneumonia in pediatric AIDS (see Chapters 16, 18, and 25). Clearly the two most frequent causes are *P. carinii* pneumonitis and lymphoid interstitial pneumonitis (pulmonary lymphoid hyperplasia). Careful clinical evaluation is very helpful in differentiating these two entities, even though histologic examination is necessary for a firm diagnosis.

The CD4+ lymphocyte count or percentage suggests the relative susceptibility to *P. carinii* pneumonia, so the age-related values mentioned in the section on prophylaxis may be of help in suspecting the diagnosis of *P. carinii* pneumonitis.

Lymphoid interstitial pneumonitis occurs in older infants and children and is subtle in onset with a slowly progressive pneumonic disease and mild to moderate hypoxemia (see Chapter 25). Fever is usually absent or low grade; the salivary glands are often enlarged; hilar nodes may be enlarged; and ditial clubbing may be evident. The chest radiograph is characterized by reticulonodular infiltrates and hilar node enlargement, findings not seen with *P. carinii* pneumonia (22). Hilar adenopathy and nodular infiltrates may occur as a result of coinfection with *P. carinii* caused by infections such as histoplasmosis, cryptococosis, or tuberculosis.

Gallium scintigraphy of the chest offers little useful information in determination of the cause of diffuse pneumonitis because both *P. carinii* pneumonia and lymphoid interstitial pneumonitis exhibit increased radionuclide concentration throughout the lungs (25). This procedure may be useful for the unusual case of early *P. carinii* pneumonitis with a normal chest radiograph. The gallium scan may reveal the pneumonitis in such cases.

A definitive diagnosis of *P. carinii* pneumonitis requires demonstration of the organism in pulmonary parenchyma or in secretions from the lower respiratory tract, along with clinical manifestations of pneumonitis (Fig. 21.3). Lung specimens obtained by open lung and transbronchial biopsy provide the most sensitive and specific findings. However, specimens obtained by bronchoscopy and bronchoalveolar lavage (BAL) or by procedures to induce sputum are often diagnostic for *P. carinii* pneumonitis. Although these latter two procedures will not serve to diagnose lymphoid interstitial pneumonitis, they may be used for patients whose clinical features strongly suggest *P. carinii* pneumonia. Failure to establish a diagnosis by these relatively simple and safe procedures may lead to use of open lung biopsy. Since BAL and induced sputum methods have been used predominantly in adults with AIDS, a brief description is given here for these diagnostic procedures in children with AIDS.

Bronchoalveolar Lavage

Bye and colleagues (26) studied 29 infants and children aged 2–54 months with AIDS or AIDS-related complex and pneumonitis. *P. carinii* was identified in 14 of these patients. The method is as follows.

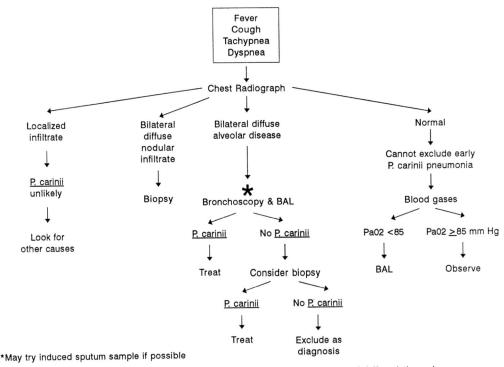

*May try induced sputum sample if possible

Figure 21.3.   Suggested scheme for establishing diagnosis of diffuse bilateral pneumonitis in immunosuppressed children.

1) Premedicate with atropine 0.01 mg/kg IM before the procedure, and at time procedure starts give meperidine 3.0 mg/kg IV. Administer supplemental oxygen, and apply topical anesthesia with 1% lidocaine to nose, pharynx, vocal cords, and tracheobronchial tree.
2) Insert flexible bronchoscope transnasally or, if intubated, through the endotracheal tube.
3) Examine airway, and wedge bronchoscope into a subsegment of the right middle or right lower lobe.
4) Begin BAL by instilling 2.0 ml/kg sterile normal saline (without preservative) not to exceed a total of 10 ml.
5) After a few seconds aspirate saline with a syringe attached to suction port. This procedure may be repeated five to seven times, depending on the amount of fluid aspirated and patient tolerance.
6) Process specimen for cytology and cultures.

A nonbronchoscopic BAL procedure has been described for children requiring mechanical ventilation (27). A No. 8 French polyethylene feeding catheter is used through the endotracheal tube to lavage 5-ml aliquots of saline.

Transbronchial Lung Biopsy

Transbronchial lung biopsy is often performed along with BAL. The biopsy expands the information obtained and is highly dependable when properly done. The biopsy specimen should contain at least 20 alveoli to be adequate for diagnosis (28).

Induced Sputum

This procedure is less sensitive than BAL. Nine episodes of *P. carinii* pneumonitis were documented in 20 episodes of pneumonia in pediatric patients aged 2–13 years using the procedure described by Ognibene and coworkers (29).

1) Food is withheld for 4 hr before procedure.
2) Rinse mouth with 3.0% saline (up to 50 ml) to remove oral contaminants.

3) Have patient inhale a nebulized mist of 3% saline delivered from an ultrasonic nebulizer (Ultra-Neb 100, De Vilbiss Health Care, Somerset, PA).
4) Some patients require 20–30 min for saline inhalation.
5) Expectorated sputum is collected in specimen cups and diluted 1:1 with sterile water.
6) Specimens are then digested with dithiothreitol and processed for culture and cytology.

Open Lung Biopsy

An open lung biopsy provides the most sensitive method for diagnosis of *P. carinii* pneumonitis. However, the procedure requires a general anesthetic, an operating room, and a surgical team. Some impairment of pulmonary function may follow the surgery. The major complications are pneumothorax, pneumomediastinum, and bleeding, but these occur infrequently. Generally less-invasive procedures such as induced sputum and BAL are performed first, and if the diagnosis is not forthcoming a biopsy is indicated (Fig. 21.3). A biopsy is necessary for the diagnosis of lymphoid interstitial pneumonitis, and it is essential for appropriate therapy to differentiate this pneumonitis from that caused by *P. carinii* because treatments are strikingly different.

Stains

At least three stains should be used.

1) Grocott-Comori methenamine silver nitrate: stains *P. carinii* cyst brownish black with a green background. Trophozoite does not stain.
2) Toluidine blue O: stains cyst blue to lavender; does not stain trophozoite (Fig. 21.1).
3) Giemsa: stains trophozoite and sporozoite but not cyst. Organisms have pale blue cytoplasm with punctate reddish nucleus (Fig. 21.2).

Other stains may also be used if available. These include the use of a monoclonal antibody in an indirect fluorescent antibody technique or stains with acridine orange,

Gram-Weigert, Papanicolaou, and periodic acid-Schiff (7).

The indirect immunofluorescent monoclonal antibody method is highly sensitive and is now available commercially (Merifluor, Meridian Diagnostics, Cincinnati, OH). Use of oligonucleotide primers to amplify DNA sequences by the polymerase chain reaction offers great promise for the identification of *P. carinii* in clinical specimens but is not yet appropriate for general use (5, 20, 30).

TREATMENT

Once *P. carinii* has become evident from chest radiograph and clinical signs, the outcome is fatal in ~100% of cases, if untreated. Two drugs are in general use for therapy. They are equally effective, but trimethoprim-sulfamethoxazole is preferred over pentamidine because of differences in adverse effects. However, in AIDS patients

tolerance to either drug is less than in non-AIDS patients. The adverse effects of both drugs are less frequent in infants and children in AIDS than adults with AIDS (31); ~15% of children with AIDS have significant adverse reactions from trimethoprim-sulfamethoxazole.

Trimethoprim-sulfamethoxazole is recommended for the initial treatment of *P. carinii* pneumonitis (see Fig. 21.4). The intravenous dose is trimethoprim 15–20 mg and sulfamethoxazole 75–100 mg/kg day divided in three to four equal doses. Each dose is infused over 1 hr. The intravenous solution requires that 80 mg trimethoprim and 400 mg sulfamethoxazole (one 5.0-ml vial) be added to at least 125 ml of 5% dextrose in water. In all but the mildest cases the initial doses of the drugs should be given intravenously. Once the pneumonitis is resolving, trimethoprim-sulfamethoxazole may be administered orally. Either tablets or suspension may be used in the dose of 20

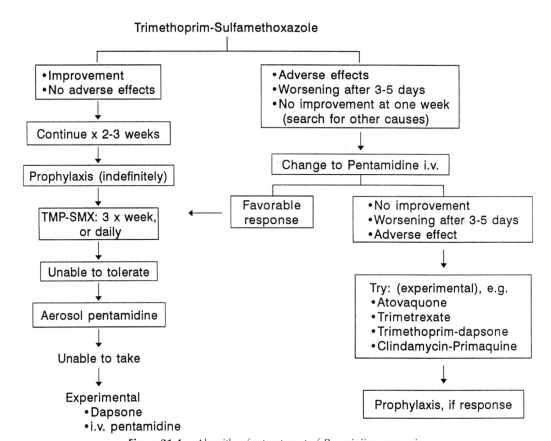

Figure 21.4. Algorithm for treatment of *P. carinii* pneumonia.

mg trimethoprim and 100 mg sulfamethoxazole per kilogram per day in three or four equally divided doses. The course of treatment is 2–3 weeks. At the completion of therapy the drugs are reduced to prophylactic doses, which are continued indefinitely.

Adverse effects from trimethoprim-sulfamethoxazole occur when the drugs are given by either the oral or the intravenous route. A transient erythematous maculopapular rash is the most frequent side effect. Usually withdrawal of the drug until the rash resolves, then readministration of the drug, permits continuation without recurrence of the rash. If an urticarial rash or the rash of Stevens-Johnson syndrome occurs, the drugs should be discontinued and not administered again. Less frequent adverse effects are nausea, vomiting, neutropenia, diarrhea, megaloblastic anemia, aplastic anemia, methemoglobinemia, and toxic nephrosis. As a general rule if no improvement is evident after 5–7 days trimethoprim-sulfamethoxazole therapy, the drugs should be changed to pentamidine.

Patients who cannot tolerate trimethoprim-sulfamethoxazole or who fail to respond to this therapy must be treated with pentamidine isothionate. The dose is 4.0 mg/kg/day IV. The drug can be given intramuscularly, but the intravenous route is preferred to minimize adverse effects. Usually 2–3 weeks of treatment are needed. Adverse effects are frequent and include hepatic and renal toxicity, hypotension, hypo- or hyperglycemia, rash, thrombocytopenia, anemia, and injection site reactions. These adverse reactions in children with AIDS are described elsewhere (31).

In a recent double-blind study of 322 adults with *P. carinii* pneumonia and AIDS, atovaquone, a new hydroxynaphthoquinone, compared favorably with trimethoprim-sulfamethoxazole (32). The drug was found to be remarkably safe, although somewhat less effective than the combination. Phase I studies in infants and children have demonstrated safety similar to adults. Atovaquone was approved by the Food and Drug Administration in 1992 for the treatment of mild to moderate *P. carinii* pneumonitis in adults who are intolerant of trimethoprim-sulfamethoxazole. Preliminary pharmacokinetic studies in infants and children suggest

the dose of 40 mg/kg/day PO would be appropriate, but efficacy studies in children have not been performed.

Other drugs with some promise for efficacy are under clinical investigation for treatment of *P. carinii* pneumonitis in AIDS. These include trimethoprim-dapsone, trimetrexate the leucovorin, pyrimethamine-sulfadiazine, aerosolized pentamidine and clindamycin plus primaquine. However, these investigations have been limited to adults.

Most patients require oxygen therapy, and some may require assisted ventilation. Pao$_2$ should be maintained above 70 mm Hg. Avoid oxygen toxicity. The fraction of inspired oxygen should be kept below 50 vol% if possible. Assisted ventilation is usually indicated when the Pao$_2$ cannot be maintained at 60 mm Hg or greater with inspired oxygen fraction of 50% or greater. Patients with alveolar-arterial gradients of <30 mm Hg at the time therapy is started generally have a better prognosis than those with values of ≥30 mm Hg.

Paradoxically, corticosteriods, known to promote *P. carinii* pneumonitis, have been recently advocated by some investigators for use in the therapy of acute pneumonitis. Studies in adults show sufficient efficacy to recommend the use of prednisone with the onset of antimicrobial therapy of *P. carinii* pneumonitis in those patients with disease advanced to the stage where Pao$_2$ is <70 mm Hg or the alveolar-arterial gradient is >35 mm Hg (33). Although no similar studies have been completed for infants and children, it seems reasonable to consider corticosteriods for the more severe pediatric cases. The initial dose recommended for adults for oral prednisone is 40 mg twice daily for 5 days, once daily for 6 through 10 days, and 20 mg daily for 11 through 21. One must be very cautious to exclude concomitant infections, such as tuberculosis, that might become worse because of corticosteroid administration.

In the study of Bernstein and coworkers (21) of 18 children with AIDS and *P. carinii* pneumonitis, 60% required intubation; 39% died during the initial hospitalization; and of the 11 surviving the episode of pneumonitis, five were dead within 1 year after recovery. Most deaths were in very young infants. Six (55%) children who recovered from the first episode of *P. carinii* pneu-monitis had a recurrence of the pneumoni-tis within 15 months of the initial illness. This remarkably high rate of recurrence emphasizes the need for chemoprophylaxis.

During the early days of treatment clinical response is best judged by blood gas studies (Pao_2, alveolar-arterial gradients, arterial CO_2 tension, and pH). The chest radiograph is less precise in revealing improvement or worsening of the pneumonitis.

PREVENTION

Effective chemoprophylaxis is now avail-able for *P. carinii* pneumonitis. Treatment with zidovudine does not prevent the infec-tion. Studies of adults with AIDS reveal a strong correlation between the T4 lympho-cyte (CD4+) count and the risk for *P. carinii* pneumonitis (12). For example, when the CD4+ count is ≤200 cells/mm³ *P. carinii* pneumonitis will occur in 18–24% of cases within 12 months. Similar data are not available for infants and children. However, by reviewing age-related CD4 lymphocyte counts and percentages in nor-mal infants and children, the counts and percentages in infants and children with AIDS and *P. carinii* pneumonitis and the age of occurrence of the pneumonia, rea-sonable estimates can be made for risk fac-tors in the younger age group. Guidelines have been established by an expert committee under the auspices of the National Pediatric HIV Resource Center at Children's Hospital of New Jersey and CDC (34) and will be described here. It must be emphasized that these recommendations are based on a consensus of opinion based on review of CD4 counts available when the HIV-infected child had developed *P. carinii* pneumonitis. Studies on the chemoprophy-laxis of non-AIDS immunocompromised children provide useful information on ef-ficacy of trimethoprim-sulfamethoxazole (35, 36).

Indications for Prophylaxis in HIV-infected Infants and Children

1) Any child who has had an episode of *P. carinii* pneumonitis, regardless of age or CD4 lymphocyte count.

2) Low age-adjusted CD4 lymphocyte count:
   - <1500 cells/mm³ for infants 1–11 months
   - <750 cells/mm³ for children 12–23 months
   - <500 cells/mm³ for children 24 months through 5 years
   - <200 cells/mm³ for children 6 years and older

   (a CD4 lymphocyte percentage of <20% is an indication for prophylaxis regard-less of absolute count).

3) Infants of HIV-infected mothers:
   - Indeterminate infection: start prophy-laxis as if HIV infected until state of infectivity is established.
   - Prophylaxis is usually not necessary during the first month of life because *P. carinii* pneumonitis rarely occurs at this age
   - If CD4 lymphocyte counts are not below threshold risk levels mentioned above, repeat the count at least every 3 or 4 months until prophylaxis is begun.

4) May consider in certain unusual circum-stances such as a constellation of HIV-related symptoms, even if CD4 lympho-cyte counts are normal or if reliable counts are unavailable.

Chemoprophylaxis Regimens from CDC Guidelines (34)

1) Recommended regimen (≥1 month old): trimethoprim-sulfamethoxazole 150 mg trimethoprim/M²/day with 750 mg sul-famethoxazole/M²/day PO in divided doses BID, three times per week on con-secutive days, e.g., Mon–Tue–Wed. Acceptable alternative trimethoprim-sulfamethoxazole dosage schedules:
   - 150 mg trimethoprim/M²/day with 750 mg sulfamethoxazole/M²/day PO as a single daily dose, three times per week on consecutive days (e.g., Mon–Tue–Wed)
   - 150 mg trimethoprim/M²/day with 750 mg sulfamethoxazole/M²/day PO divided BID and given 7 days/week
   - 150 mg trimethoprim/M²/day with 750 mg sulfamethoxazole/M²/day PO divided BID and given three times per

week on alternate days (e.g., Mon–Wed–Fri).

2) Alternative regimens, if trimethoprim-sulfamethoxazole not tolerated:
Aerosolized pentamidine (≥5 years old) 300 mg given via Respirgard II inhaler once monthly. Katz and Rosen (37) have administered aerosol pentamidine to infants as young as 8 months. Infants are held in the caretaker's lap, and the medication is administered via a cushioned face mask with at least 30 airflow changes/hour. No efficacy studies have been performed in infants. Dapsone (≥1 month old) 1 mg/kg (not to exceed 100 mg) PO once daily. If neither aerosolized pentamidine nor dapsone is tolerated, some clinicians use intravenous pentamidine (4 mg/kg) given every 2 or 4 weeks. Mueller et al. (38) found breakthrough episodes of *P. carinii* pneumonitis in 3 of 100 (3%) HIV-infected children receiving trimethoprim-sulfamethoxazole, 4 of 26 cases (15%) given dapsone, 5 of 34 cases (15%) given aerosol pentamidine, and 6 of 24 children (25%) given intravenous pentamidine prophylaxis. Recent observations suggest that breakthrough infections with dapsone may be higher than previously suggested.

Trimethoprim-sulfamethoxazole is highly effective in the prevention of *P. carinii* pneumonitis when given daily (35) or only 3 days a week (36). In a controlled study Fischl and coworkers (39) randomized 60 AIDS patients to receive either trimethoprim-sulfamethoxazole daily or no drug for prophylaxis over 2 years. Whereas 53% of the no-drug group developed *P. carinii* pneumonitis, none of the 30 patients who received the drug combination developed the pneumonitis. Five patients required discontinuation of the drug because of adverse effects. Although infants and children with AIDS have not been studied in prospective trials for *P. carinii* prophylaxis, there is no reason to believe that efficacy differs from other immunocompromised children at risk for the pneumonitis. A major disadvantage of trimethoprim-sulfamethoxazole prophylaxis is the high rate of adverse reactions in AIDS patients. The reason HIV-infected patients have exaggerated adverse reactions is unknown, but children with AIDS have fewer reactions than adults (31).

Aerosolized pentamidine is in general use for the prevention of *P. carinii* pneumonitis in adults. However, no studies have been reported on the use of this regimen for infants and children. Two large studies in adults with AIDS demonstrate efficacy for *P. carinii* prophylaxis with aerosolized pentamidine. One study used the Respirgard II nebulizer (Marquest Medical Products, Englewood, CO) with doses of 30 or 150 mg pentamidine every 2 weeks or 300 mg once a month (40). The 300-mg dose was more effective than the others. No comparison was made with no prophylaxis. This latter dose is now approved by the Food and Drug Administration for prophylaxis. The second-largest study determined the efficacy of aerosolized pentamidine for secondary prophylaxis in a double-blinded, placebo-controlled, randomized study using the Fisoneb ultrasonic nebulizer (Fisons, Bedford, MA) to deliver a dose of 60 mg every 2 weeks after initial loading doses. Thirty-five percent of the 78 placebo-managed patients developed recurrent *P. carinii* pneumonia compared with 6% of the 84 patients receiving pentamidine (41). The major adverse reactions are due to irritation of the airway, resulting in cough and bronchospasm. No systemic toxicity has been described. The AIDS Clinical Trials Group 021 study showed trimethoprim-sulfamethoxazole to be about three times more effective in the prevention of *P. carinii* pneumonia (12). Few data are available for the use of aerosolized pentamidine in infants and children by age-appropriate delivery devices; it seems reasonable to use this method for older children and adolescents who cannot take trimethoprim-sulfamethoxazole and who can cooperate with the procedure. Doses of 300 mg pentamidine with the Respirgard II monthly may be used as tolerated. Orcutt et al. (42) treated 22 patients aged 3–15 years with this dose and found it well tolerated, and no patients developed *P. carinii* pneumonitis. Prophylaxis does not assure complete protection from *P. carinii* pneumonitis (43), and protection is afforded only as long as the drug is administered.

For children who have adverse reactions to trimethoprim-sulfamethoxazole and are in an age group for which aerosolized pentamidine is not feasible, the alternatives are limited, and none has been adequately tested for prophylaxis in children. If the adverse reaction is the usual maculopapular rash, fever, neutropenia, or other reactions other than urticaria, Stevens-Johnson syndrome, and hypotensive episodes, trimethoprim-sulfamethoxazole can be stopped until the reaction has resolved and the drug can be tried again. Frequently the reaction will not recur. Desensitization has been effective in some cases. Gluckstein and coworkers (44) could desensitize all of seven AIDS patients who had experienced rash, fever, and anaphylactoid reactions. They administered trimethoprim-sulfamethoxazole in increasing amounts of total hourly doses of 0.004, 0.04, 0.4, 4, 40, and 160 mg trimethoprim (plus five times this amount for sulfamethoxazole).

Parenteral pentamidine has been used in uncontrolled studies to prevent *P. carinii* pneumonitis. Biweekly or monthly intramuscular or intravenous doses have prevented some but not all cases of *P. carinii* pneumonitis (45–47). The adverse effects were similar to but less intense than daily therapeutic regimens. All studies have been with adult patients. A monthly dose of 200 mg was effective. A dose of 4.0 mg/kg monthly or biweekly would be a comparable dose for infants and children.

Other drugs have been effective in the prevention of *P. carinii* pneumonitis. These include Fansidar (pyrimethamine and sulfadoxine) (48) and dapsone with or without trimethoprim (49). None of these have been studied in infants and children with AIDS, but investigations in adult patients with AIDS suggest efficacy as prophylactic agents.

No vaccine is available for *P. carinii* infection.

AREAS FOR FUTURE RESEARCH

A precise and sensitive noninvasive test for *P. carinii* pneumonitis is one of the greatest pragmatic needs for the management of infants and children with AIDS. Research into the structure and biology of *P. carinii* will provide knowledge with which to approach the development of diagnostic tests. Basic to such studies is the capability to cultivate *P. carinii* in culture, preferably in cell-free culture media, to obtain purified isolates of *P. carinii*. Once this is accomplished, currently available technology such as the polymerase chain reaction to amplify DNA sequences should permit rapid development of new techniques for diagnostic application.

New drugs are needed for both treatment and prophylaxis in patients who cannot tolerate or who do not respond to trimethoprim-sulfamethoxazole and pentamidine.

References

1. Edman JC, Kovacs JA, Masur H, Santi DV, Elwood HJ, Sogin ML. Ribosomal RNA sequence shows *Pneumocystis carinii* to be a member of the fungi. Nature 1988;334:519.
2. Sogin ML, Edman JC. A self-splicing intron in the small subunit rRNA gene of *Pneumocystis carinii*. Nucleic Acids Res 1989;17:5349.
3. Hughes WT. *Pneumocystis carinii*: Taxing the taxonomy. Eur J Epidemiol 1989;5:265.
4. Pixley FJ, Wakefield AE, Banerji S, Hopkins JM. Mitochondrial gene sequences show fungal homology for *Pneumocystis carinii*. Mol Microbiol 1991;5:2347–1351.
5. Wakefield AE, Peters SE, Banerji S, et al. *Pneumocystis carinii* shows DNA homology with ustomycetous red yeast fungi. Mol Microbial 1992;6:1903–1911.
6. Jackson HC, Colthrust D, Hancock V, Marriott MS, Tuite MF. No detection of characteristic fungal protein elongation factor EF-3 in *Pneumocystis carinii*. J Infect Dis 1991;163:675–677.
7. Hughes WT. *Pneumocystis carinii* pneumonitis. Boca Raton, FL: CRC Press, 1987.
8. Pifer LL, Hughes WT, Stagno S, Woods D. *Pneumocystis carinii* infection: Evidence of high prevalence in normal and immunosuppressed children. Pediatrics 1978;61:35–40.
9. Meuwissen JHE Th, Tauber, Leeuwenberg ADEM, Beckers PJA, Sieben M. Parasitology and serologic observation of infection with *Pneumocystis carinii* in humans. J Infect Dis 1977;136:43–48.
10. Rogers MA. AIDS in children: A review of the clinical, epidemiologic and public health aspects. Pediatr Infect Dis J 1985;4:230–236.
11. Ciesielski CA, Fleming PA, Berkklamn RL. Changing trends in AIDS-indicator diseases in the U.S.—role of therapy and prophylaxis [Abstract 254]. 31st Interscience Conference on Antimibrobial Agents and Chemotherapy, Chicago, Oct 1991.
12. Centers for Disease Control. Recommendation for prophylaxis against *Pneumocystis carinii* pneumonitis for adults and adolescents infected with human immunodificiency virus. MMWR 1992; 41:1–11.

13. Scott GB, Buck BE, Leterman JG, Bloom FL, Parks WP. Acquired immunodeficiency syndrome in infants. N Engl J Med 1984;310:76–81.

14. Denny T, Yogev R, Gelman R, Skuza C, Oleske J, et al. Lymphocyte subsets in healthy children during the first 5 years of life. JAMA 1992;267:2484–2488.

15. Kovacs A, Frederick T, Church J, Eller A, Oxtoby M, Mascola L. CD4 T-lymphocyte counts and *Pneumocystis carinii* pneumonia in pediatric HIV infection. JAMA 1991;265:2698–2703.

16. Elvin KM, Lumbwe CM, Luo NP, Bjorkman A, Kallnius G, Linder E. *Pneumocystis carinii* is not a major cause of pneumonia in HIV infected patients in Lusaka, Zambia. Trans R Soc Trop Med Hyg 1989;83:553–555.

17. Wallace JM, Hannah JB. Pulmonary disease at autopsy in patients with the aquired immunodeficiency syndrome. West J Med 1988;149:167–171.

18. Joshi VV, Oleske JM, Minnefor AB. Pathologic pulmonary findings in children with the acquired immunodeficiency syndrome: A study of ten cases. Hum Pathol 1985;16:241–246.

19. Joshi W, Oleske JM. Pathology of opportunistic Pulmonary lesions in children with acquired immunodeficiency syndrome. Hum Pathol 1986;17:641–642.

20. Wakefield AE, Peters SE, Hopkin JM, Moxon ER. Epidemiology of *Pneumocystis carinii* infection; a molecular approach [Abstract P38]. British Pediatric Association, Coventry, England, Apr 7–10, 1992.

21. Bernstien LJ, Bye MR, Rubinstein A. Prognostic factors and life expectancy in children with acquired immunodeficiency syndrome and *Pneumocystis carinii pneumonia*. Am J Dis Child 1989;143:775–778.

22. Rubinstein A, Moreckis R, Silverman B, et al. Pulmonary disease in children with acquired immunodeficiency syndrome and AIDS-related complex. J Pediatr 1986;108:498–503.

23. Silverman BA, Rubinstein A. Serum lactate dehydrogenase levels in adults and children with acquired immunodeficiency syndrome (AIDS) and AIDS-related complex: Possible indicator of B cell lymphoproliferation and disease activity. Am J Med 1985;78:726–736.

24. Conner E, Bagarazzi M, McSherry G, Oleske J. Clinical and laboratory correlates of *Pneumocystis carinii* pneumonia in children infected with HIV. JAMA 1991;265:1693–1697.

25. Schiff RG, Kabat L, Kamani N. Gallium scanning of lymphoid interstitial pneumonitis of children with AIDS. J Nucl Med 1987;28:1915–1919.

26. Bye MR, Bernstein L, Shah K, Ellawie M, Rubinstein A. Diagnostic bronchoalveolar lavage in children with AIDS. Pediatr Pulmonol 1987;3:425–428.

27. Amaro-Galvez R, Rao M, Abadco D, Kravath RE, Steiner P. Nonbronchoscopic bronchoalveolar lavage in ventilated children with acquired immunodeficiency syndrome: A simple and effective diagnostic method for *Pneumocystis carinii* infection. Pediatr Infect Dis J 1991;10:473–475.

28. Fraire AE, Cooper SP, Greenberg SD, Rowland LP, Langston C. Transbronchial lung biopsy. Chest 1992;102:748–752.

29. Ognibene FP, Gill VJ, Pizzo PA, et al. Induced sputum to diagnose *Pneumocystis carinii* pneumonia in immunosuppressed pediatric patients. J Pediatr 1989;115:430–433.

30. Kitada K, Oka S, Kimwa S, Shimada K, Serikawa T. Detection of *Pneumocystis carinii* sequences by polymerase chain reaction: Animal models and clinical application to noninvasive specimens. J Clin Microbial 1992;29:1985–1990.

31. McSherry G, Wright M, Oleske J, Connor E. Frequency of serious adverse reactions to trimethoprim-sulfamethoxazole and pentamidine among children with human immunodeficiency virus [Abstract 1357]. 28th Interscience Conference on Antimicrobial Agents and Chemotherapy, Los Angeles, Oct 1988.

32. Hughes WT, Leoung G, Kramer F. Bozzette S. Framer P. Comparison of Atovaquon 566C80 and trimethoprim-sulfamethoxazole to treat *P. carinii* pneumonitis in patients with AIDS. N Engl J Med 1993;328:1521–1527.

33. National Institutes of Health—University of California Expert Panel for Corticosteroids as Adjunctive Therapy for *Pneumocystis carinii*. Consensus statement on the use of corticosteroids as adjunctive therapy for pneumocystis pneumonia in the acquired immunodeficiency syndrome. N Engl J Med 1990; 323:1500–1504.

34. Centers for Disease Control. Guidelines for prophylaxis against *Pneumocystis carinii* pneumonia in children infected with human immunodeficiency virus. MMWR 1991;40:1–13.

35. Hughes WT, Kuhn S, Chaudhary S, et al. Successful chemoprophylaxis for *Pneumocystis carinii* pneumonitis. N Engl J Med 1977;297:1419–1426.

36. Hughes WT, Rivera GK, Schell MJ, Thornton D, Lott L. Successful intermittent chemoprophylaxis for *Pneumocystis carinii* pneumonia. N Engl J Med 1987;316:1627–1632.

37. Katz BZ, Rosen C. Aerosolized pentamidine in young children. Pediatr Infect Dis J 1991;12:958.

38. Mueller BU, Steinberg S, Pizzo P. Failure of intravenous pentamidine prophylaxis for *Pneumocystis carinii* pneumonia. [Letter]. J Pediatr 1993;122:163–164.

39. Fischl MA, Dickinson GM, La Voie L. Safety and efficacy of sulfamethoxazole and trimethoprim chemoprophylaxis for *Pneumocystis carinii* pneumonia in AIDS. JAMA 1988;259:1185–1189.

40. Leoung GS, Montgomery AB, McGinty E, Feigal DW. Double-blinded randomized trial of aerosol pentamidine for secondary prophylaxis of *Pneumocystis carinii* pneumonia [Abstract TBP 78]. Fifth International Conference on AIDS, Montreal, Jun 1989.

41. Montaner JSG, Lawson L, Falutz J, et al. Aerosolized pentamidine for the second prophylaxis of *Pneumocystis carinii* pneumonia in the acquired immune deficiency syndrome: A report from the Canadian cooperative trial [Abstract TBP 54]. Fifth International Conference on AIDS, Montreal, Jun 1989.

42. Orcutt TA, Godwin CR, Pizzo P, Ognibene FP. Aerosolized pentamidine: A well-tolerated mode of prophylaxis against *Pneumocystis carinii* pneu-

monia in older children with human immunodeficiency virus infection. Pediatr Infect Dis J 1991; 11:290–294.

43. Mueller BU, Butler KM, Husson RN, Pizzo P. *Pneumocystis carinii* pneumonia despite prophylaxis in children with human immunodeficiency virus infection. J Pediatr 1991;119:992–994.

44. Gluckstein D, Ruskin J, Neilsen D. Oral desensitization to trimethoprim-sulfamethoxazole in hypersensitive AIDS patients: Utility in T/S prophylaxis of *Pneumocystis carinii* pneumonia [Abstract 7176]. Fourth International Conference on AIDS, Stockholm, Jun 1988.

45. Winslow D, Bincsik A, Lincoln P, Smolka H, Holloway W. Secondary prophylaxis of *Pneumocystis carinii* pneumonia with systemic pentamidine [Abstract TBP 45]. Fifth International Conference on AIDS, Montreal, Jun 1989.

46. Karaffa C, Rehm S, Calabrese L. Efficacy of monthly pentamidien infusion in preventing recurrent *Pneumocystis carinii* pneumonia in AIDS patients [Abstract 690]. 26th Interscience Conference on Antimicrobial Agents and Chemotherapy, New Orleans, Sep 1986.

47. Miller S, Lifris D. Efficacy of intramuscular pentamidine in the prophylaxis of recurrent *Pneumocystis carinii* pneumonia [Abstract TBP 60]. Fifth International Conference on AIDS, Montreal, Jun 1989.

48. Madoff LC, Scavuzzo D, Roberts RB. Fansidar secondary prophylaxis of *Pneumocystis carinii* pneumonia in acquired immunodeficiency syndrome patients [Abstract]. Clin Res 1986;34: 524A.

49. Metroka CE, Jacobus D, Lewis N. Successful chemoprophylaxis for pneumocystis with dapsone or bactrim [Abstract TBO 4]. Fifth International Conference on AIDS, Montreal, Jun 1989.

50. Shannon Km, Ammann AJ. Acquired immune deficiency syndrome in childhood. J Pediatr 1985;106:332–342.

51. Rogers MF, Thomas PA, Starcher ET, Noa MC, Bush TJ, Jaffee HW. Acquired immunodeficiency syndrome in children: Report of the Centers for Disease Control National Surveillance, 1982 to 1985. Pediatrics 1987;79:1008–1014.

52. Vernon DD, Holzman BH, Lewis P, Scott GB, Birriel JA, Scott MB. Respiratory failure in children with acquired immunodeficiency syndrome and acquired immunodeficiency syndrome complex. Pediatrics 1988;82:223–228.

22
Toxoplasmosis

Charles D. Mitchell

Although *Toxoplasma gondii* has received considerable attention in the literature as a common opportunistic infection among adult AIDS patients (1–7), there is a paucity of published information in the pediatric literature because of the apparent rarity of its occurrence in children. *Toxoplasma* encephalitis and systemic toxoplasmosis have not been commonly reported in children with symptomatic human immunodeficiency virus (HIV)-1, which has fostered the impression that these infections do not occur. Clinical toxoplasmosis occurs among these children, and although the number of recognized cases reported thus far is few, the actual number of cases may be considerably higher. As opposed to the adult experience where most cases occur secondary to reactivation of previously acquired infection (1–5), a major mode of acquisition in children is congenital.

MICROBIOLOGY

T. gondii is an obligate, intracellular protozoan parasite that has a diverse range of hosts including most species of mammals, birds, and some reptiles. Phylogenetically, the organism is classified within the same subclass Coccidia as two other protozoa that are commonly associated with opportunistic infections in AIDS patients: *Cryptosporidium* species and *Isospora belli* (8). As a group, the coccidia are characterized by an apical complex of organelles that are generally present at some stage of their life cycle (hence the phylum name Apicomplexa), locomotion of the mature organism by body flexion or un-

dulation of longitudinal ridges, and an alteration in generations that includes both a sexual and asexual phase (8).

The sexual phase of the life cycle of *T. gondii* occurs within the gut epithelium of members of the cat family, which are the only known definitive hosts (Fig. 22.1). After the invasion of the lining epithelium by the proliferative form (the trophozoite or tachyzoite), gametogony ensues with the formation of the micro (male)- and macro (female)-gametocyte. The union of the gametocytes results in the formation of a fertilized zygote that is shed in the fecal stream as an unsporulated oocyst after the formation of a protective, thin cyst wall (9). Sporulation and the development of an infective oocyst occurs after 1–5 days in the environment. The fully sporulated oocyst may remain viable in warm, moist soil >1 year (10).

Although the asexual phase (schizogony) may also occur in the definitive host, it is the only phase to occur in the intermediate host (humans, other mammals, birds, and reptiles). Only two morphological stages of the life cycle are found in the intermediate host: the proliferating, motile tachyzoite that is evident during the early acute phase of infection and the tissue cyst that is found during the chronic phase of infection. Formed within the host cell, the tissue cyst may vary widely in size relative to the number of bradyzoites or slowly replicating organisms contained within the cyst.

Acquired human infection occurs after ingestion of undercooked meat containing viable tissue cysts or any food contaminated

419

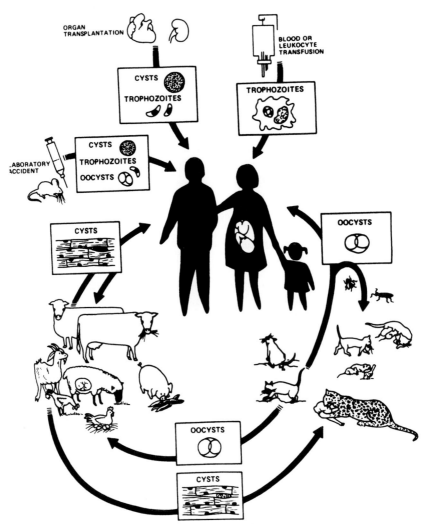

Figure 22.1.   Life cycle of *T. gondii*. From Remington JS, McLeod R. Toxoplasmosis. In: Braude AI, ed. International textbook of medicine: Medical microbiology and infectious disease. Philadelphia: WB Suanders, 1981;II:1818.

with the sporulated oocysts (10). Although the relative importance of the oocyst to human transmission has yet to be determined, it is probable that it is vital. The seroprevalence of *Toxoplasma* in human populations has been found to be higher when cats are present and epidemics of toxoplasmosis have been associated with exposure to domestic cats. Horizontal infection may also occur via blood or leukocyte transfusion and via transplantation of a solid organ that contains tissue cysts into a previously uninfected recipient. Laboratory workers can acquire infection by accidental self-inoculation with the organism (2).

The overwhelming majority of cases of congenital toxoplasmosis result from the occurrence of primary maternal *Toxoplasma* infection during pregnancy (10, 11). The few cases of congenital infection documented to have occurred with chronic or latent maternal infection have usually been associated with maternal immunosuppression.

EPIDEMIOLOGY

T. gondii has a ubiquitous global distribution with serological evidence of human infection being found on at least five different continents (10). In general, the seroprevalence of *Toxoplasma* among various human populations increases with increasing age as a result of horizontal acquisition. Congenital infection and parenteral inoculation from either transfusion or from the transplantation of an infected organ account for a comparatively small number of cases. The estimated incidence of congenital toxoplasmosis in the United States has been reported to vary between 0.1 and 1.3 cases/1000 live births (12). A similar frequency has been observed in studies from Europe. The rate of infection among various adult populations has been noted to vary considerably among geographical areas (10). Data obtained from different patient populations in the United States, Europe, and Africa illustrate this latter point (Table 22.1). This variance is most likely secondary to differences among human populations in their relative exposure to either soil contaminated with infectious oocysts or meat containing viable tissue cysts.

Until recently, there was a paucity of data regarding the seroprevalence of *Toxoplasma* among populations who are either at risk for or infected with HIV-1. Because the importance of cerebral toxoplasmosis as an opportunistic infection in AIDS patients has been recognized, there have been a growing number of reports describing the epidemiology of *Toxoplasma* in these patients. Among HIV-1-infected patients in New York, London, and San Francisco, the seroprevalence has recently been reported to be 32 (13), 27 (14), and 16% (15), respectively. The annual rate of seroconversion of *Toxoplasma*-specific IgG among the population in London was calculated to be 75/1000 patients. Comparable data from Central Africa have demonstrated a similar variability in the seroprevalence for *Toxoplasma*. Among HIV-1-infected patients in Nairobi (16), the seroprevalence was 54%. In Uganda (17) and Zaire (18), the

Table 22.1. Seroprevalence of *T. gondii* among Various Patient Populations[a]

Region	Patient Population	No. Tested	%Seropositive
North America			
Denver	OB	120	3
Palo Alto	OB	500	10
Chicago	OB	2,000	12
Boston	Cord[b]	92,000	14
Birmingham	OB	8,140	30
Miami	M-II	124	35
Caribbean basin			
San Juan	HIV	100	43.2
Jamaica	OB	1,604	57
Europe			
London	OB	196	21
Stuttgart	OB	200	36
Vienna	OB	52,000	48
Brussels	OB	2,986	53
Padua	OB	200	56
Paris	OB	200	72
Africa			
Zambia	OB	497	23
Nairobi, Kenya	HIV	180	54
Gabon	OB	268	60
Central African Republic	OB	32	81
Other			
Melbourne, Australia	OB	3,463	4
Santiago, Chile	OB	833	59
Panama City	OB	124	63
Belo Horizonte, Brazil	OB	187	65

[a]OB, pregnant and/or nonpregnant women of childbearing age; M-II, 124 women of Haitian birth known to be infected with HIV-1. Adapted with modifications from Ref. 12.
[b]Data derived from cord blood obtained at delivery.

seroprevalence was 34 and 24%, respectively. The seroprevalence of *Toxoplasma* among Zambian patients infected with HIV-1 was considerably lower (4%) (17), although additional data reported in edition 1 of this book cited 23% as the seroprevalence of *Toxoplasma* among pregnant women in Zambia (12).

Based upon survival analysis, Grant el al. (13) have previously estimated that the probability of an adult AIDS patient who is seropositive for *T. gondii* ever developing *Toxoplasma* cerebritis is 28%. Given this observation and the appreciable seroprevalence of *Toxoplasma* among certain adult populations in the United States, the projection made by Israelski and Remington (19) that by 1991 there would be at least 20,000 cases of reactivated *Toxoplasma* encephalitis in patients with AIDS is not surprising. Corresponding data regarding the frequency of *Toxoplasma* encephalitis in Africa are unavailable. Although the frequency of this opportunistic infection among African AIDS patients may be lower, toxoplasmosis is probably underdiagnosed because of the absence of adequate laboratory facilities and the possible masking of this diagnosis by other intercurrent infections such as tuberculosis (20).

There is little published information regarding the seroprevalence of *T. gondii* among infants and children (21–25) and what little there is has originated from Africa, Europe, or South America. Azara et al. (24) screened some 1500 children, aged 3–18 years, in Italy and discovered an overall seroprevalence of 17.9%. Only 4.7% of the children 4–6 years old were seropositive. Huldt et al. (23) found that antibodies to *Toxoplasma* are uncommon in small children in Sweden, with only 8% of the children younger than 10 years being infected. Corresponding data from Somalia suggest that although an appreciable percentage of children acquire *Toxoplasma* by the end of the first decade of life (55 of 185 or 29.7% by age 10 were seropositve) the rate of horizontal acquisition under age 5 was much less (5/57 or 8.7%). The rate of congenital infection in this same population was not specified. Despite the apparent differences in the rate of acquisition between age 5 and 10 years in Sweden vs. Somalia (which the

authors of the latter study attribute to climate and more frequent contact with soil contaminated with oocysts), the frequency of horizontal infection in children under age 5 in both areas was low. This observation is supported by studies in Miami on 68 infants born to mothers who lack antibodies to *Toxoplasma*. None of these infants acquired *Toxoplasma* infection during the first 12–24 months of life (C. Mitchell, unpublished observations). There are no other comparable data from the United States, and there are yet no published data regarding the seropositivity rate among children infected with HIV-1. Consequently there is no information by which to assess the risk of reactivated toxoplasmosis in this latter group of children. The sporadic occurrence of reactivated toxoplasmosis among HIV-1-infected young children is very likely secondary to the lower seroprevalence of *Toxoplasma* in those age groups most affected by perinatally acquired HIV-1.

Although toxoplasmosis is not as frequent an opportunistic infection among HIV-1 infected children as it is among adult AIDS patients, there appears to be a growing number of cases (see "Clinical Manifestations"). Perhaps more significantly is the recognition that it can assume two forms. Like adults, toxoplasmosis may present as an encephalitis presumably secondary to reactivation of latent tissue cysts within the central nervous system. Toxoplasmosis may also present in perinatally HIV-1 infected children during the first months of life with severe systemic manifestations as a result of congenital infection (26).

To assess the risk of congenital toxoplasmosis among infants born to mothers who are dually infected with both HIV-1 and *T. gondii*, the seroprevalence of *Toxoplasma* among pregnant women in areas with a high endemic rate of HIV-1 must first be determined. The overall incidence of HIV-1 infection in an obstetrical population in Miami during 1989 was reported to be 2.3% (27). If the seroprevalence of *Toxoplasma* among pregnant women in Miami is 33% (Table 22.2), then the percentage of mothers who are dually infected with both HIV-1 and *T. gondii* is 0.33 × 0.023 or 0.7%. That the seroprevalence of *Toxoplasma* among

Table 22.2. Seroprevalence of HIV-1 and *Toxoplasma* in Three Different Obstetrical Populations

Region	Rate of Seropositivity for		Estimated Rate of Dual Infection/1000 Patients
	HIV-1	*T. gondii*	
	%		
Miami	2.3[a]	33.2	7
San Juan	0.17	41.6	0.7
Cite Soleil, Port-au-Prince	10.0[b]	51.0	51

[a]Ref. 27.
[b]Ref. 29.

pregnant women known to be HIV-1 infected in Miami is 35% suggests that there is no significant difference in the seroprevalence between HIV-1-infected and uninfected women (Tables 22.1 and 22.2). Although the seroprevalence of HIV-1 in an obstetrical population in San Juan was previously found to be relatively low (0.17%, C. Diaz, personal communication, 1993) Puerto Rico has one of the fastest growing rates of pediatric AIDS cases in the United States (28), implying a corresponding increase in the rate of HIV-1 infection among Puerto Rican women. Because the reported seroprevalence of HIV- 1 in San Juan is low, there are as yet very few women who are infected with both agents (Table 22.2). In contrast, corresponding data (29) from Cite Soleil (an economically depressed section of Port-au-Prince, Haiti) suggest that the frequency of women infected with both HIV-1 and *Toxoplasma* may be as high as 5% (Table 22.2). If the risk of congenital toxoplasmosis in infants born to mothers dually infected with both agents is considerably higher than the background rate and congenital toxoplasmosis is not clinically recognized, then congenital *Toxoplasma* infection in perinatally HIV-1-exposed infants may be more common than presently thought and may be associated with significant early morbidity and mortality. The proof of this hypothesis will require a prospective cohort study comparing the incidence of congenital toxoplasmosis in mothers infected with both HIV-1 and *Toxoplasma* v. mothers infected with *Toxoplasma* alone. It is probable that the risk of maternal to fetal transmission of *Toxoplasma* will be highest in obstetrical populations where a significant percentage of mothers who are dually infected with both agents exists and there are a sizable proportion of HIV-1-infected mothers with advanced HIV-1 disease who are more immunosuppressed.

PATHOGENESIS AND NATURAL HISTORY

Most cases of acquired toxoplasmosis occur as a result of the ingestion of either viable oocysts or the consumption of inadequately cooked meat containing intact tissue cysts. Occasionally *Toxoplasma* is transmitted by the inadvertent transfusion of blood or blood products containing viable tachyzoites or after transplantation of an organ from a seropositive donor to a seronegative recepient (10). After oral ingestion and disruption of the protective cyst wall, sporozoites are released into the small bowel lumen from the oocysts while bradyzoites are released from the degraded tissue cysts. Infection of the epithelial lining cells of the gut ensues. Intracellularly both the sporozoites and bradyzoites become proliferating tachyzoites. After disruption of the initially parasitized cells and local invasion, hematogenous dissemination ensues, resulting in the spread of the parasite to several different organs. The acute phase of the primary infection is superseded by the chronic phase as the host's immune response attempts to halt the continued replication of the protozoa. Tachyzoites are eventually replaced by the slowly replicating bradyzoites. Tissue cysts develop as a result of the continued intracellular division of the bradyzoite and the formation of a protective cell wall that does not elicit a protective inflammatory response. These arise in multiple organs (most notably brain, heart, and skeletal muscle) during the first weeks after acute infection. The continued latency of the organism within the tissue cysts characterizes the chronic phase of this infection in the immunocompetent host (9).

developed cerebritis gave birth to five children. The first, second, third, and fifth baby of this mother were perinatally infected with HIV-1 and have died of AIDS. The third and fifth infants were simultaneously infected with congenital toxoplasmosis. The fourth infant had neither HIV-1 nor toxoplasmosis (26).

DIAGNOSIS

Toxoplasmosis may induce various nonspecific laboratory abnormalities including eosinophilia, monocytosis, leukocytosis, or leukopenia. In congenital infection, thrombocytopenia is common in neonates and infants both with or without objective evidence of infection. Cerebrospinal fluid xanthochromia and mononuclear pleocytosis are also frequently found in infants with congenital toxoplasmosis.

Multiple assays have been developed to detect *Toxoplasma*-specific antibodies. Among the assays for the detection of *Toxoplasma*-specific IgG are the Sabin-Feldman dye test, indirect immunofluorescence, direct agglutination, and an antibody-capture enzyme-linked immunosorbent assay (ELISA) (10). The Sabin-Feldman dye test has been considered the reference standard against which most assays have been compared to determine their sensitivity and specificity. Because of the technical difficulty in adopting this test to the clinical laboratory (viable tachyzoites harvested from the peritoneal cavity of infected mice are necessary for the performance of this assay), other IgG assays have been adopted by many clinical laboratories. Previous data have indicated a 95% overall agreement in results between the Sabin-Feldman dye test and the indirect immunofluorescence antibody assay (36). Because of the ease of use and capability to perform multiple specimens simultaneously, ELISA has become increasingly popular. Preliminary data using one commercial ELISA assay for *Toxoplasma* IgG in Miami have suggested a 95% overall agreement between this assay and indirect immunoflourescence antibody assay.

Similarly there are many different assays that have been developed to detect *Toxoplasma*-specific IgM. Among these are the following: an indirect immunofluorescent IgM antibody test, a conventional IgM capture ELISA, a double sandwich IgM ELISA, and an immunosorbent agglutination assay (10). Although all of these assays are useful for detecting an IgM response associated with acquired infection, only the double sandwich IgM ELISA and the immunosorbent agglutination assay possess sufficient sensitivity(75–80%) to diagnose most cases of congenital toxoplasmosis. The sensitivity of both the immunofluorescent assay and the conventional ELISA for detecting the IgM response associated with congenital infection are only 25 and 50%, respectively. For a comprehensive discussion of the various serological means that have been used to diagnose toxoplasmosis, refer to Ref. 10.

Recent data (37) have suggested that the detection of *Toxoplasma*-specific IgA (by a double sandwich ELISA) may facilitate diagnosis of congenital toxoplasmosis. However, there is no published experience with this assay in HIV-1-infected patients.

Diagnosis of *Toxoplasma* encephalitis in an HIV-1-infected patient in many instances is based on the detection of *Toxoplasma* IgG in a patient who presents with either clinical and/or radiologic evidence of intracerebral mass lesions. Unfortunately serological tests cannot be used in most AIDS patients to reliably distinguish those patients with active toxoplasmosis from those patients who are chronically infected (3). This is probably because of the associated immunosuppression and the fact that most cases are secondary to reactivated infection. Some AIDS patients with *Toxoplasma* encephalitis may be seronegative for *T. gondii* (33). Congenital toxoplasmosis in infants born to mothers dually infected with both *Toxoplasma* and HIV-1 can be diagnosed serologically. Two of the seven cases identified to date in Miami and followed prospectively developed a positive IgM response (at birth to 2–3 months) and an elevated IgG titer. Alternatively, some of these infants lose *Toxoplasma* IgG antibodies despite developing clinically active disease (26).

Because diagnosis of active toxoplasmosis cannot always be made serologically in HIV-1-infected patients, additional means of detecting this infection (i.e., histological diagnosis, isolation, antigen detection) may need to be employed. When indicated, clinical specimens should be referred to a reference laboratory experienced with these assays to facilitate diagnosis of active infection. Although the demonstration in pathological specimen (12) of tachyzoites suggests active *Toxoplasma* infection, the presence of tissue cysts alone does not, unless there is associated inflammation and necrosis. The importance of histological diagnosis is underscored by the fact that three of seven cases of congenital toxoplasmosis in HIV-1-infected infants in Miami were diagnosed at autopsy after microscopic examination of the central nervous system. Many additional cases may be missed because these infants may die at an early age with nonspecific signs and symptoms and do not receive a complete postmortem examination.

Although there have been reports of successful isolation of *T. gondii* from AIDS patients with encephalitis using tissue culture (38), mouse inoculation remains the most sensitive assay available for isolating the parasite from clinical specimens (10). Although parasitemia has been demonstrated in these patients, there are no published data about its frequency or duration. There are also no corresponding data from infants who have both perinatal HIV-1 infection and congenital toxoplasmosis.

Toxoplasma-specific lymphocyte transformation has previously been shown to help document congenital infection (39), but there are no data to assess its usefulness in HIV-1-infected infants at risk for congenital toxoplasmosis. However, these infants may be able to mount an antigen-specific lymphocyte blastogenic response early in their course before significant immune impairment secondary to HIV-1 develops.

Although various methods of detecting *Toxoplasma* antigens in bodily fluids have been described (10, 40, 41), these assays are available in only a few research laboratories. Their sensitivity may be limited by the binding of circulating antigens by their respective antibodies, thus masking their presence in clinical specimens.

There is a growing body of literature regarding the diagnostic utility of the polymerase chain reaction when employed with primers specific for a genomic segment of *T. gondii* (42–46). Recently Grover et al. (43) demonstrated that the *Toxoplasma*-specific polymerase chain reaction could be used to diagnose congenital toxoplasmosis prenatally. Holliman et al. (46) using a polymerase chain reaction assay to detect *Toxoplasma* nucleic acid in brain tissue could confirm the clinical diagnosis of cerebral toxoplasmosis in two AIDS patients. Preliminary data from Minnesota (G. Felice, J. Hitt, personal communication, 1993) have suggested that the polymerase chain reaction assay can detect parasitemia in seropositive AIDS patients with and without clinical encephalitis. Further studies obviously are needed to determine sensitivity and specificity of the *Toxoplasma*-specific polymerase chain reaction assay relative to mouse inoculation as a means of documenting active infection.

TREATMENT

The combination of pyrimethamine and a sulfonamide (usually sulfadiazine) administered orally remains the standard regimen for treatment of active toxoplasmosis in patients with AIDS. Supplemental folinic acid is usually prescribed to prevent potential bone marrow toxicity. Presently the recommended oral doses of these agents for children are as follows: pyrimethamine 15 mg/m^2/day or 1 mg/kg/day (maximum daily dose 25 mg) with double dose being given during the first 2 days of therapy; sulfadiazine 85 mg/kg/day two to four times a day, and folinic acid 5 mg every three days (this may be increased to 10 mg every 3 days in the event of bone marrow toxicity). In very young infants, folinic acid should be given intramuscularly (10). The recommended duration of primary therapy for adult AIDS patients with *Toxoplasma* cerebritis is 6 weeks (3). Because of the high frequency of relapse, these patients should continue to be treated with the combination of pyrimethamine and sulfadiazine given daily in the same dosagaes described above as chronic suppressive therapy. Alternative suppressive regimens that have been proposed include the combination of pyrimethamine and clindamycin, pyrimethamine in higher doses alone, and the combination of pyrimethamine and sulfadoxine three times a week. Although the incidence of relapse may be higher with these latter regimens, there are few data available to determine which is the optimal choice for suppressive therapy. Because of the continuing immunocompromise, this maintenance (i.e., suppressive) regimen should be continued indefinitely. Of concern is a recent report (47) which suggests that concomitant zidovudine therapy may antagonize the therapeutic efficacy of the above regimen against *Toxoplasma*. The same therapeutic strategem consisting of both a primary phase for the acute illness followed by a chronic suppressive phase should be employed for older children and adolescents with reactivated central nervous system disease. Both adults and older children with *Toxoplasma* cerebritis should also be treated with short courses of corticosteroids if there is associated cerebral edema. Although the standard regimen of pyrimethamine and sulfadiazine (in conjunction with folinic acid) should be used to treat HIV-1-exposed infants who have congenital toxoplasmosis, the duration is controversial. Twelve months have been suggested as the appropriate length of therapy for non-HIV-1-infected infants with congenital infection (12). Two infants in our population whose congenital toxoplasmosis was diagnosed serologically and were begun on therapy early have not had a clinical reoccurrence despite receiving <12 months of treatment. Because of the paucity of data regarding this question, however, no firm recommendations can be made. The minimum length of therapy, however, should probably be at least 6 months. If the infant is severely immunosuppressed, chronic suppressive therapy should probably be continued indefinitely.

Because of the significant hematologic and dermatologic adverse effects associated with the standard regimen, additional agents are being evaluated for their effectiveness against *T. gondii*. Clindamycin has been found to be an effective agent in a murine model of *Toxoplasma* encephalitis, and there are several anecdotal and at least one retrospective report suggesting that clindamycin may be effective for both acute and chronic maintenance treatment phases (3, 48, 49). Apparent side effects include di-

arrhea, reversible granulocytopenia, and skin rashes. The role of clindamycin should be more clearly defined after completion of the currently ongoing large scale clinical trials sponsored by the AIDS Clinical Trials Group.

Additional classes of drugs that are also being evaluated as possible anti-*Toxoplasma* agents include, macrolide antibiotics (roxithromycin, azithromycin), folic acid antagonists (piritrexim, trimetrexate), purine analogues (arprinocid), and immunomodulators (interferon-γ) (3, 50). Using an animal model, Araujo et al. (50) found that azithromycin was superior to roxithromycin and spiramycin in protecting mice against death from acute toxoplasmosis. The hydroxynaphthoquinone, 566C80 or atovaquone, was recently shown to possess significant in vitro and in vivo (in preliminary animal work) activity against both the tachyzoite and tissue cysts of various strains of *T. gondii* (51). Clinical trials of this agent in adult AIDS patients for the treatment of both *T. gondii* (and *P. carinii*) are underway. Although data is limited in adults and there are none in children, this agent may prove to be especially useful for the treatment of toxoplasmosis if it can eliminate both the tachyzoite and cyst form of the organism and thus eliminate the need for suppressive therapy.

PREVENTION

The standard measures proscribed to prevent horizontal acquisition of *T. gondii* have been previously well described by Remington and Desmonts (10). These can be summarized as follows: wash hands thoroughly and avoid mucous membrane contact during and after handling raw meat, and also wash all working surfaces that have been in contact with raw meat; meat should always be cooked until well-done, or meat can be smoked or cured in brine; prevent access of copraphagic insects to all foods and wash fruits and vegetables thoroughly before eating; and avoid direct contact with cat feces or soil that may be contaminated with cat feces. Although there are no means by which to predict which patient will develop *Toxoplasma* encephalitis, all known HIV-1-infected infants and children should have an antibody determination for *Toxoplasma* performed. Those HIV-1-infected patients found to be seropositive should have their absolute CD4 count monitored closely to identify those children who are severely immunosuppressed (CD4 count <200 cells/mm³) and who probably have a higher risk of developing clinical toxoplasmosis. These patients should be carefully followed for clinical evidence of *Toxoplasma* encephalitis and/or chorioretinitis. Although administration of trimethoprim-sulfamethoxazole to prevent *P. carinii* pneumonitis may also reduce the possibility of toxoplasmosis, this question must be studied on a prospective basis before this strategem is accepted.

The macrolide antibiotic spiramycin, although ineffective as either a therapeutic or prophylactic agent against reactivated toxoplasmosis in AIDS patients, has been shown

to effective in reducing the incidence of congenital infection after primary maternal infection (3, 10). However, before any recommendations can be made about which mothers infected with both *Toxoplasma* and HIV-1 should be treated with this agent, additional information should be obtained to define which mothers are most at risk for delivering an infant who has congenital toxoplasmosis. Table 22.3 contains a proposed schema for the management of mothers (and their infants) known to be infected with both HIV-1 and *Toxoplasma*.

FUTURE AREAS OF RESEARCH

The actual risk of congenital toxoplasmosis among infants born to mothers who are dually infected with *T. gondii* and HIV-1 must be assessed in a prospective format both in the United States and in geographi-

Table 22.3. Management of Obstetrical Patients Dually Infected with HIV-1 and *T. gondii* and Their Infants

1. All HIV-1-infected pregnant women should be tested for *Toxoplasma*-specific IgG. They should also have an absolute CD4 cell count, %T4, and T4:T8 ratio determined to assess their immunological status. A baseline obstetrical ultrasound should be performed to eliminate hydrocephalus, myocardial dilatation, and intraabdominal calcifications in the fetus.
2. All *Toxoplasma* IgG positive patients should have a *Toxoplasma* IgM performed to determine if the mother has been recently infected.
3. All HIV-1-positive pregnant women with chronic *Toxoplasma* infection should be followed for clinical evidence of reactivated toxoplasmosis, particularly encephalitis.
4. If there is any clinical evidence of reactivated maternal toxoplasmosis, or mother appears to have primary maternal infection, the fetus should be followed with sequential ultrasounds to detect congenital infection. Whether amniocentesis with or without fetal blood sampling increases risk of perinatal HIV-1 infection is unknown, and the decision to perform these procedures to diagnose congenital toxoplasmosis must be made in light of this potential risk. Risks of these procedures must be reviewed with the mother before they are performed.
5. If it is decided that an amniocentesis and/or fetal blood sampling is clincially indicated, then arrangments should be made with a referal laboratory that is competent in performing mouse inoculation for isolation of *Toxoplasma*. Assays for *Toxoplasma* specific IgM and IgG should be performed if fetal blood is obtained. IgM assay on fetal blood should be performed perferably by double sandwich IgM ELISA or immunoabsorbent agglutination and not by Immunofluorescence.
6. Infant should be examined carefully at birth for signs of congenital toxoplasmosis. For infants who have objective signs of infection at birth or if mother has *Toxoplasma* cerebritis at delivery, a complete workup for congenital toxoplasmosis should be performed: 1) computerized axial tomography with contrast, 2) opthalmologic examination, 3) *Toxoplasma* specific IgG, IgA, IgE, and IgM, and 4) mouse inoculation for *Toxoplasma* isolation.
7. If infant has objective evidence of toxoplasmosis at delivery or if above work-up suggests active infection, therapy should be started with pyrimethamine and sulfadiazine (with folinic acid supplementation) (see "Treatment").
8. All infants should have follow-up *Toxoplasma*-specific IgG and IgM titers performed to determine if they retain or lose *Toxoplasma* IgG antibody. They should also be followed for the possibility of concomitant perinatally acquired HIV-1 infection.

cal regions of the developing world where the seroprevalence of HIV-1 and *Toxoplasma* is high. If the frequency of congenital toxoplasmosis is increased several-fold in this population, than an examination of maternal determinants as well as the potential interaction between congenital *Toxoplasma* infection and perinatal HIV-1 infection should be attempted. What measures are necessary to block transplacental passage of the parasite should then be examined. Additional, more readily available methods for detecting parasitemia must also be developed to facilitate diagnosis of congenital infection and reactivated clinical disease.

References

1. Kovacs JA. Toxoplasmosis in patients with the acquired immunodeficiency syndrome. In: Leoung G, Mills J, eds. Opportunistic infections in patients with the acquired immunodeficiency syndrome. New York: Marcel Dekker, 1989;341–354.

2. McCabe RE, Remington JS. Toxoplasma gondii. In: Mandell GL, Douglas RG, Bennett JE, eds. Principles and practice of infectious diseases. New York: Churchill Livingstone, 1990:2090–2103.

3. Isrealski DM, Remington JS. Toxoplasmic encephalitis in patients with AIDS. Infect Dis Clin North Am 1988;2:429–445.

4. Luft BJ, Brooks RG, Conley FK, McCabe RE and Remington JS. Toxoplasmic encephalitis in patients with acquired immune deficiency syndrome. JAMA 1984;252:913–917.

5. Wong B, Gold JWM, Brown AE, et al. Central nervous system toxoplasmosis in homosexual men and parenteral drug abusers. Ann Intern Med 1984;100:36–42.

6. Gold JWM, Armstrong D. Opportunistic infections in homosexual men. In: Ma P, Armstrong D, eds AIDS and infections of homosexual men. Boston: Butterworths, 1987:325–335.

7. Isrealski DM, Remington JS. Toxoplasmosis encephalitis in patients with AIDS. In: Sande MA, Volberding PA, eds. The medical management of AIDS. Philadelphia: WB Saunders, 1990:319–345.

8. Beaver PC, Jung RC, Cupp EW. Clinical parasitology. Philadelphia: Lea and Febiger, 1984:149–173.

9. Frenkel JK. Toxoplasmosis: Parasite life cycle, pathology, and immunology. In: Hammond DM, ed. The Coccidia. Baltimore: University Park, 1973:343–410.

10. Remington JS, Desmonts G. Toxoplasmosis. In: Remington JS, Klein J, eds. Infectious diseases of the fetus and newborn. Philadelphia: WB Saunders, 1990:89–195.

11. Couvreur J, Desmonts G. Toxoplasmosis. In: MacLeod C, ed. Parasitic infections in pregnancy and the newborn. Oxford: Oxford University, 1988:112–142.

12. Miller MJ, Remington JS. Toxoplasmosis in infants and children with HIV infection or AIDS. In: Pizzo PA, Wilfert CM, eds. Pediatric AIDS: The Challenge of HIV Infection in Infants, Children, and Adolescents. Baltimore: Williams & Wilkins, 1991:299–307.

13. Grant IH, Gold JW, Rosenblum M, Niedzwiecki D, Armstrong D. Toxoplasma gondii serology in HIV-infected patients: The development of central nervous system toxoplasmosis in AIDS. AIDS 1990; 4:519–521.

14. Hullman R. Serological study of the prevalence of toxoplasmosis in asymptomatic patients infected with human immunodeficiency virus. Epidemiol Infect 1990;105:415–418.

15. Darmemann B, Isrealski D, Leoung GS, McGraw T, Mills J, Remington J. Toxoplasma serology, parasitemia, and antigenemia in patients at risk for Toxoplasmic encephalitis. AIDS 1991;5:1363–1365.

16. Bundle R, Holliman R, Gilks C, Kinyanjuni M. Toxoplasma antibodies in HIV-positive patients from Nairobi. Trans R Soc Trop Med Hyg 1991; 85:750–751.

17. Zumla A, Savva D, Wheeler RB, et al. Toxoplasma serology in Zambian and Ugandan patients infected with the human immunodeficiency virus. Trans R Soc Trop Med Hyg 1991;85:227–229.

18. De Clercq D, Henry MC, Lokombe B. Serological observations on toxoplasmosis in zairian AIDS patients. Trans R Soc Trop Med Hyg 1986;80: 613–614.

19. Isrealski DM, Remington JS. Toxoplasmic encephalitis in patients with AIDS. Infect Dis Clin North Am 1988;2:429–445.

20. Lucas SB. AIDS in Africa—clinopathological aspects. Trans R Soc Trop Med Hyg 1988;82:801–802.

21. Ahmen HJ, Mohammed HH, Yusuf MW, Ahmed SF, Huldt, G. Human toxoplasmosis in Somalia. Prevalence of Toxoplasma antibodies in a village in the lower Scebelli region and in Mogadishu. Trans R Soc Trop Med Hug 1988;82:330–332.

22. Dumas N, Cazaux M, Carme B, Seguela JP, Charlet JP. Toxoplasmosis in the Congo Republic. Seroepidemiological study. Bull Soc Pathol Exot Filiales 1990;83:349–359.

23. Haldt J, Lagercrantz R, Sheehe, PR. On the epidemiology of human toxoplasmosis in Scandinavia especially in children. Acta Paediatr Scan 1979;68:745–749.

24. Azara A, DeMattia D, Chiaramonte M, Rigo G, Scarpa B. Prevalence of Toxoplasma gondii antibodies among children and teenagers in Italy. Microbiologica 1991;14:229–234.

25. Jamra L, Guimaraes, E. Conversao sorologica para Toxoplasmose em criancas de um centro de saude de Sao Paulo. Rev Inst Med Trop Sao Paulo 1981; 23:133–137.

26. Mitchell CD, Erlich S, Mastrucci M, Hutto SC, Parks WP, Scott G. Congenital toxoplasmosis occuring in infants perinatally infected with human immunodeficiency virus 1. Pediatr Infect Dis J 1990;9:512–518.

27. O'Sullivan MJ, Fajardo A, Ferron P, Efantis J, Senk C, Duthely M. Seroprevalence in a pregnant, multi-ethnic population [Abstract MBP 23]. Fifth International Conference on AIDS, Montreal, Jun 1989.

28. Centers for Disease Control. HIV/AIDS Surveillance, Oct 1992.

29. Halsey N, Boulos R, Holt E, et al. Transmission of HIV-1 infections from mother to infants in Haiti. JAMA 1990;264:2088–2092.

30. Sothi KK, Pickarski G. Immunological aspects of toxoplasmosis. In: Soulsby EJB, ed. Immune response in parasitic infections. Baton Raton, FL: CRC Press, 1987:314–336.

31. Wilson CB, Remington JS, Stagno S, Reynolds DW. Development of adverse sequelae in children born with subclinical congenital *Toxoplasma* infection. Pediatrics 1980;66:767–774.

32. Luft JB, Remington JS. Toxoplasmic encephalitis. J Infect Dis 1988;157:1–6.

33. Porter SB, Sande MA. Toxoplasmosis of the central nervous system in the acquired immunodeficiency syndrome. N Engl J Med 1992;327:1643–1648.

34. Oksenhendler E, Cadranel J, Sarfate C, et al. *Toxoplasma gondii* pneumonia in patients with the acquired immunodeficiency syndrome. Am J Med 1990;88(suppl):18–21.

35. Obhen-Addad NE, Joshi VV, Sharer LR, Epstein LG, Gubitosi TA, Oleske JM. Congenital acquired immunodeficiency syndrome and congenital toxoplasmosis: Pathologic support for a chronology of events. J Perinatol 1988;8:328–331.

36. Walton BC, Benchoff BM, Brooks WH. Comparison of the indirect fluorescent antibody test and methylene blue dye test for detection of antibodies to *Toxoplasma gondii*. Am J Trop Med Hygiene 1966;15:149–152.

37. Stipick-Biek P, Thulliez P, Araujo FG, Remington JS. IgA antibodies for diagnosis of acute congenital and acquired toxoplasmosis. J Infect Dis 1990;162:270–273.

38. Hofflin JM, Remington JS. Tissue culture isolation of toxoplasma from blood of a patient with AIDS. Arch Intern Med 1985;145:925–926.

39. Wilson CB, Desmonts G, Couvreur J, Remington JS. Lymphocyte transformation in the diagnosis of congenital *Toxoplasma* infection. N Engl J Med 1980;302:785–788.

40. Brooks RG, Sharma SD, Remington JS. Detection of *Toxoplasma gondii* antigens by a dot-immunobinding technique. J Clin Microbiol 1985;21:113–116.

41. Hassl A, Aspock H, Flamm H. Circulating antigen of *Toxoplasma gondii* in patients with AIDS: Significance of detection and structural properties. Zentralbl Bakt Hyg 1988;A270:302–309.

42. van de Ven E, Melchers W, Galama J, Camps W, Meuwissen J. Identification of *Toxoplasma gondii* infections by B1 gene amplification. J Clin Microbiol 1991;29:2120–2124.

43. Grover C, Thulliez P, Remington JS, Boothroyd JC. Rapid prenatal diagnosis of congenital *Toxoplasma* infection by using polymerase chain reaction and amniotic fluid. J Clin Microbiol 1990;28:2207–2301.

44. Weiis LM, Udem SA, Salgo M, Tanowitz HB, Wittner M. Sensitive and specific detection of *Toxoplasma* DNA in an experimental murine model: Use of *Toxoplasma gondii*-specific cDNA and the polymerase chain reaction. J Infect Dis 1991;163:180–186.

45. Burg JL, Grover CM, Pouletty P, Boothroyd JC. Direct and sensitive detection of a pathogenic protozoan. *Toxoplasma gondii* by polymerase chain reaction. J Clin Microbiol 1989;27:1787–1792.

46. Holliman RE, Johnson JD, Savva D. Diagnosis of cerebral toxoplasmosis in association with AIDS using the polymerase chain reaction. Scan J Infect Dis 1990;22:243–244.

47. Israelski DM, Tom C, Remington JS. AZT antagonizes pyrimethamine (PYR) in experimental infection with *Toxoplasm gondii* (TG) [Abstract 349]. 28th Conference on Antimicrobial Agents and Chemotherapy, Los Angeles, Oct 1988.

48. Hofflin JM, Remington JS. Clindamycin in a murine model of Toxoplasma encephalitis. Antimicrob Agents Chemother 1986;31:492–496.

49. Dannemann BR, Israelski DM, Remington J.S. Treatment of toxoplasmic encephalitis with intravenous clindamycin. Arch Intern Med 1988;148:2477–2482.

50. Amujo FG, Shepard RM, Remington JS. In vivo activity of the macrolide antibiotics azithromycin, roxithromycin, and spiramycin against *Toxoplasma gondii*. Eur J Clin Microbiol Infect Dis 1991;10:519–524.

51. Amujo FG, Huskinson J, Remington JS. Remarkable in vivo and in vitro activities of the hydrogynaphthoquinone 566C80 against tachyzoites and tissue cysts of *Toxoplasma gondii*. Antimicrob Agents Chemother 1991;35:293–299.

23

Central Nervous System Involvement: Manifestations, Evaluation, and Pathogenesis

Pim Brouwers, Anita L. Belman, and Leon Epstein

Soon after the initial descriptions of pediatric AIDS, central nervous system (CNS) involvement was recognized as a frequent manifestation. A progressive encephalopathy with cognitive, behavioral, and motor deficits was described (1, 2), as was more static neurologic impairment (2, 3). It subsequently became clear that in most children neurologic dysfunction could not be explained by CNS infection with opportunistic or common pathogens, CNS neoplasm, or stroke (4–6). It also became clear that by the time human immunodeficiency virus type 1 (HIV-1) infection advanced to severe symptomatic stages, cognitive and motor impairment of varying severity, duration, and progression were common findings (5, 7). Compelling evidence had also been accumulated indicating that the CNS is directly infected by HIV-1 (5, 8, 9–12) and that neuropathologic changes associated with HIV-1 can be identified (2, 4, 6, 13–15). When and how HIV-1 infects the CNS of infants and children and the relation among virus invasion, latency, and subsequent course of CNS manifestations, however, remain unclear and will undoubtedly vary with subsets of patients.

This chapter summarizes the current knowledge of clinical (neurologic and neuropsychologic), neuroimaging, and pathologic studies of HIV-related CNS disease in infants and children. Based on our current understanding of pathogenetic mechanisms and the natural history of HIV-1 infections in children, areas for future research and speculation are indicated.

NATURAL HISTORY AND CLINICAL PRESENTATION

Neuroepidemiology

Compelling evidence that CNS dysfunction may occur in a large percentage of HIV-infected infants and children has been provided by numerous studies (2, 3, 5, 7, 16–18). The true incidence of HIV-1-related CNS disease in infants and children, however, is unknown. In the early years of the epidemic a 50–62% prevalence of progressive encephalopathy was estimated from clinical series of patients with advanced symptomatic HIV-1 disease (AIDS as defined by the 1985 criteria of Centers for Disease Control) (5, 7, 19). More recently a 30–40% prevalence rate was estimated at the National Cancer Institute in the cohort of symptomatic children referred for antiretroviral therapy (20). In series that included asymptomatic, mildly symptomatic children, and children with advanced disease, a 19.6% prevalence rate is reported (21–24).

The earlier studies may have overestimated prevalence rates of CNS disease because they were drawn from samples in which children had more severely progressed disease, whereas preliminary data from prospective studies, based on both relatively small cohort size and young age of patients, may be an underestimate (24–26).

Two factors seem to influence the incidence of encephalopathy in pediatric AIDS disease stage and age of the child. There appears to be a trend for HIV-1-related CNS disease to parallel progression and severity of systemic disease and immunodeficiency in all age groups. However, it is also appears that some patients will develop HIV-1-related CNS disease as a first or only sign and in the absence of other major AIDS-defining illnesses or severe immunodeficiency (27, 28). Some degree of neurologic and neuropsychologic impairment, however, is probably found in most symptomatic HIV-1-infected children (1–3, 5, 18).

The incidence of progressive encephalopathy is greater for infants and young children. Encephalopathy was reported as a first manifestation for 12% of perinatally infected children with symptomatic HIV-1 infection (22). A recent study however, suggested that the outlook for children with vertically acquired HIV infection is better than previously thought (29).

Less epidemiologic data regarding HIV-1 CNS disease are available for later childhood. In some children with vertically acquired HIV infection signs of CNS impairment may not be manifest until middle childhood or later (30–32). In fact the precise number of children with asymptomatic or mildly symptomatic infection remains unknown because many of these children may not yet have been identified (33). It has not yet been conclusively documented whether older, asymptomatic pediatric patients may have subtle deficits in CNS function (34) similar to those reported for asymptomatic adult patients (35, 36).

Static encephalopathy as evidenced by nonprogressive cognitive and/or motor deficits has been observed in ~25% of symptomatic children (3, 18).

Also it is important to remember that the natural history and incidence of pediatric HIV-1-related CNS disease may be changing with the introduction of antiviral therapy. This has been suggested for AIDS dementia complex in adults (37).

Terminology

HIV-1-related CNS disease is a clinical syndrome complex, manifested by varying and sometimes discrepant degrees of cognitive, motor, and behavioral impairment. The rate of neurologic deterioration and the severity of dysfunction varies among patient subsets (5, 7, 38, 39). Additionally, some patients may have severe and progressive motor dysfunction, compared with more stable (although impaired) cognitive, behavioral, or socially adaptive skills (2, 7, 39). Conversely, some children show greater cognitive impairment than motor deficits.

Differences in the onset and subsequent rate of CNS disease progression may be associated with the exact timing and the route of HIV infection and further influenced by genetic, environmental, and other cofactors.

Initially two forms of encephalopathy were described: progressive and static (2, 7). Progressive encephalopathy was further divided based on rapidity of progression and severity of neurologic deficits using the clinically descriptive terms subacute progressive course and plateau course (7) (Fig. 23.1).

In a recent consensus report on nomenclature (40), it was proposed that the term "HIV-associated progressive encephalopathy of childhood" replace the various other terms found in the literature. Clinical and research observations of children followed longitudinally, however, suggest that there is a spectrum of CNS disease related (either directly or indirectly) to HIV-1 CNS infection and that a more differentiated and clinically descriptive terminology remains useful in characterizing levels of impairment and disease patterns.

CLINICAL FEATURES AND FINDINGS

HIV-1-associated Progressive Encephalopathy of Childhood

This is considered the most severe manifestation of HIV-1 CNS disease. In contrast to the less severe minor cognitive/motor disorder, the impact has to be sufficient to interfere with activities of daily living, which for children include social, developmental, and educational domains. The most severe but not most common form has a subacute progressive course mostly seen in infants or young children (1, 2, 5, 7). It is characterized by progressive deterioration in cognitive, motor, language, and adaptive func-

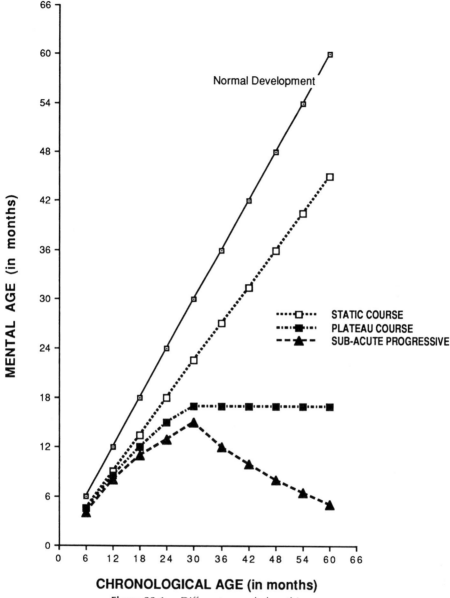

Figure 23.1.   Different encephalopathic courses.

tion with the loss of previously acquired milestones or skills and decreased gestures and vocalizations (7), often accompanied at end stage by apathy and loss of interest in the environment or increased hyperactivity and emotional lability. In the severe infantile form of the illness, spastic quadriparesis, with or without pseudobulbar signs, is common. Additional neurologic changes include impaired cranial growth resulting in acquired microcephaly, cerebral atrophy, enlargement of the ventricles, and bilateral calcifications in the basal ganglia. Clinically, extrapyramidal and delays or regression in motor development have been described particularly in children younger than age 5 and cerebellar signs usually in older children (1–3, 5, 7, 18, 41). Severely affected infants and young children may develop a characteristic "mask-like" facial appearance with an alert, wide-eyed expression and a paucity of spontaneous facial movements

(7). Level of psychological functioning is in general pervasively and globally impaired (42). The rate of neurologic deterioration is variable and may be rapid over 1–2 months or episodic, with periods of deterioration interrupted by variable periods of relative neurologic stability.

A more frequent and possibly less severe form of encephalopathy has a more indolent plateau course. Children gain little or no further developmental skills over time, resulting in a decline in IQ scores, but loss of milestones or previously acquired abilities is not observed. New milestones are either not acquired or the rate of acquisition is markedly slow, deviating not only from the norm but also from the child's previous rate of progress, resulting in a decline in IQ scores (7, 18, 39, 43). Motor deficits are common during this phase, but progression and severity may vary from concurrent cognitive development (2, 44). As HIV disease advances, patients with the plateau course may have further neurologic deterioration (5, 7, 17, 45). During plateau phase longitudinal measurement of head circumference also shows poor brain growth with loss of percentile rank (5, 7).

Children with static encephalopathy continue to acquire skills and abilities at rates consistent with their impaired initial level of functioning, alhough still below the normal expected rate (2). That is, their functioning appears lowered possibly because of the results of concurrent or previous effects of HIV infection on the CNS. There is, however, no progressive decline or halting of development. Initial levels of functioning may vary from the low average range to moderate to mild degrees of mental retardation, and these levels remain relatively stable over time (3, 5, 7). Many of these patients also have varying degrees of motor involvement.

Neuropsychological Impairments

In children with symptomatic HIV disease but without a diagnosis of progressive encephalopathy who function within the normal range (i.e., IQ > 80) various profiles of impaired and preserved cognitive abilities have been reported. Selective weaknesses or deficits in perceptual motor functioning (5), gait and motor coordination (43), attentional functioning (46, 47) and expressive language (2, 48) have been described.

Two domains of cognitive function appear the most susceptible to the effects of HIV infection on the CNS in children: attentional processes and expressive behavior.

Attention

Attention deficits have been widely recognized in patients with pediatric HIV disease. Behavioral ratings and assessments have indicated increased distractibility, excitability, and impulsiveness (30, 47). In an analysis of the subscales of the IQ tests a relative weakness on the following subtest has been documented: digit span (repeat string of numbers either in same order or reversed), coding (insert geometric codes that are on a one-to-one basis associated with numbers or shapes), and arithmetic (simple auditory mental computation and manipulation of numbers) (46). It is unclear, however, whether attentional problems are directly attributable to HIV. In addition, on an individual basis, the base rate for the development of attention deficit disorders (ADD) is not negligible for a group of young children aged 4 to 8 years. Moreover, further research has suggested that a subgroup of roughly one-fourth of the HIV-1 patients seem to display a characteristic ADD pattern with significantly decreased scores on the freedom from distractability factor. When this group is included in the sample, it may be responsible for the appearance of an overall attentional deficit profile (42).

Expressive Behavior

Expressive behavior appears to be affected more than other domains of functioning in pediatric HIV patients (3, 5, 7, 18, 30, 47–49).

Language.   In children with symptomatic HIV-1 disease (AIDS) speech and language abilities frequently become impaired. Children may regress from speaking in full sentences to using single words. The children's receptive language (the ability to understand language) during this decline in expressive skills is often retained or less impaired. Delayed development of expressive language (the ability to produce language) may be seen in infants, despite apparently age-appropriate or mildly delayed development of receptive language abilities (3, 7, 18). Overall it can be stated that deficits in expressive language are more common and of greater severity than delays in receptive language (5, 48, 50).

Motor. Deficits in motor functioning are frequently observed in infants and children with symptomatic HIV infection. Infants may exhibit delayed overall motor development and abnormalities in muscle tone. Older preschool and school-age children are more likely to develop disturbances in balance and gait, and in some cases they may lose the ability to walk (3, 18, 47–49). The presence and severity of these motor abnormalities may be independent from possible cognitive deficits.

Social Adaptive Skills and Affect. Some HIV-infected children with less severe forms of CNS compromise may also exhibit behaviors that resemble symptoms of depression. They are observed to become more socially withdrawn, with loss of initiative and interest in participating in activities, show symptoms of fatigue, lethargy, and inattentiveness, and also may exhibit decreased expression of feelings and emotions both verbally and nonverbally. Some children may become irritable, while others display unmodulated activity levels, short attention spans, and uncooperative and resistant behaviors (7, 18, 30, 48).

Apparently Normal Functioning

HIV-positive children may be unimpaired on neuropsychologic evaluation and have no neurologic abnormalities even if they previously had opportunistic infections or chronic bacterial infections. Two subgroups may be identified. In the first, subjective changes in psychomotor speed, fatigue, and mood have been observed by parents and caretakers in many such children (44). Furthermore, significant improvements with zidovudine therapy were seen in the patients whose baseline functioning was in the average range (85 < full scale intelligence quotient < 115) (51). Thus these children appear normal only because their previous unrecorded level of functioning was in the high average or superior range.

Another subgroup, whom we assume are not CNS compromised, are patients who score more than one standard deviation above their age norm (full scale intelligence quotient >115) and who do not have any documented evidence of decline in their functioning. In a study evaluating the benefits of didanosine (20) these patients were analyzed separately. Their level of performance over 6- and 12-month follow-up has basically remained unchanged (52), which may suggest that these patients did not experience measurable effects of HIV infection on the CNS.

Behavior

HIV infection in children and adolescents may influence their behavior; effects may be primary or direct, caused by HIV-associated CNS manifestations as described above, or secondary or indirect as reactions to social and illness-related experiences. The child's developmental stage may determine some secondary effects of having HIV. The cognitive framework for organizing the consequences of having a chronic life-threatening illness, understanding the necessity of invasive medical procedures, and coping with the variation in feelings of well-being will change with further mental development. Younger children are more sensitive to issues regarding separation and physical injury. Peer relations and social acceptance are more likely to be of concern between ages 6 and 11 years. The adolescent is more preoccupied with the consequence of the disease on the development and expression of independence, on sexual behavior, and on their future. Deficits in physical growth are also common among HIV-infected children (53) and may lead to poor self-image, particularly among school-age children and adolescents. Despite the many stressors, during periods when older HIV-infected children are relatively symptom free they show few signs of adjustment difficulties related to their illness, even though privately they may be trying to cope with their illness and feel under great tension. They seem able to effectively focus on typical everyday activities and engage in appropriate social interactions with peers and adults.

Hyperactivity and attentional difficulties may be due to HIV-1 infection or other causes. Many children that exhibit these problems in the hospital or testing setting also are reported to exhibit learning and behavior problems in school. It is not yet clear whether hyperactivity and attention deficits noted in these children are a direct manifestation of HIV-1-compromised CNS.

NEUROIMAGING FINDINGS

Computed tomographic (CT) examinations of the head show variable degrees of cerebral atrophy and decreased attenuation in the white matter (1, 2, 5–7, 54). In some patients, bilateral symmetrical calcification of the basal ganglia and, less frequently, calcification of the frontal white matter may be noted (1, 2, 5, 7, 16). Serial studies in children with HIV-1-associated progressive encephalopathy often show progressive atrophy, progressive white matter abnormalities, and in some cases progressive calcification of the basal ganglia (2, 6, 7) (Fig. 23.2). Improvements on serial CT scan evaluations, however, have been reported after antiretroviral therapy (55). Bilateral symmetrical calcification of the basal ganglia may be considered a marker of HIV-1-related CNS disease in an infant or child with HIV-1 infection (when other causes of calcification have been excluded) (7).

Note that in a subset of children serial neuroimaging studies may show no change, even though poor brain growth is demonstrated by serial head circumference measurements and serial clinical examinations show a plateau in developmental progress or severe developmental delays in mental function (with or without progressive motor deficits) (56, 57).

Magnetic resonance imaging may reveal atrophy and may show abnormal signal intensity in the white matter and/or basal ganglia. In one study (58), magnetic resonance imaging abnormalities (increased signal intensity in the white matter) were detected in 40% of children with HIV-1 disease. Because these abnormalities were present in both neurologically asymptomatic and symptomatic children the investigators suggested this may reflect HIV-1 CNS infection. However, patients with clinical evidence of HIV-1 related CNS disease were found to also have leukomalacia and cerebral atrophy.

Magnetic resonance imaging is more sensitive for imaging abnormalities of the white matter and for showing patterns of myelination. CT is more sensitive for demonstrating calcification. Cerebral atrophy is well detected by both techniques (54, 59, 60).

CEREBROSPINAL FLUID FINDINGS

Abnormal CSF profiles (mild pleocytosis and elevated protein content) are uncommon, although these abnormalities may be seen during the later stages of progressive encephalopathy and seem to correlate with very severe white matter abnormalities as imaged on CT (27, 39).

Intrathecal (or intra-blood-brain barrier) synthesis of anti-HIV-1 antibody, detectable levels of cytokines, and isolation of HIV-1 from the CSF have been reported in children with progressive encephalopathy (subacute progressive and plateau course), in children with static encephalopathy, and in some neurologically normal children (5, 7, 16, 23, 61) and provide additional evidence for primary HIV-1 infection of the CNS.

HIV-1-specific p24 core antigen is found in the CSF of some children with progressive encephalopathy (7, 16, 62). Tardieu and colleagues (62), however, found HIV-1 p24 positivity in the CSF in only 6.5% of their patients but in 52% of the matched serum samples. Thus HIV-1-specific p24 in the CSF may not be a helpful early prognostic marker of progressive encephalopathy in children.

NEUROPATHOLOGICAL FINDINGS

Gross inspection of brains at postmortem in children with AIDS has shown variable degrees of cerebral atrophy, ventricular enlargement, widening of sulci, and attenuation of deep cerebral white matter (4, 7, 63–65).

Recently an attempt has been made to arrive at consensus for the terminology used to describe neuropathologic changes associated with AIDS (66). This classification of the microscopic findings applies well to both adult and pediatric brains, with some caveats described below. The distinction is

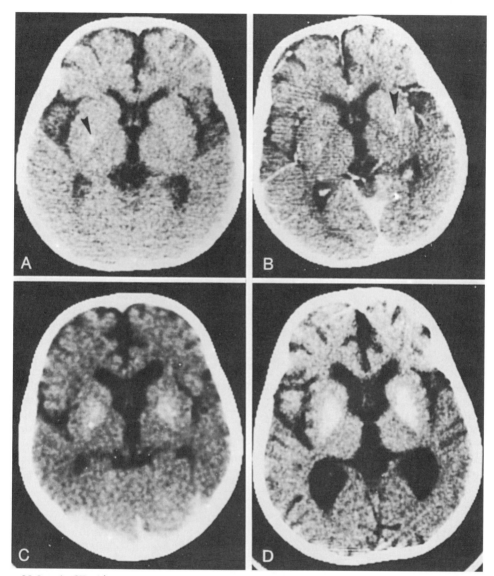

Figure 23.2. **A,** CT without contrast in a patient at age 15 months shows a punctate area of increased density in the posterolateral lenticular region (*arrow*) as well as sulcal and ventricular enlargement. **B,** after intravenous injection of contrast material, there is clear evidence of contrast enhancement in left basal ganglia region (*arrow*), medial to enhancing middle cerebral arterial branches in left sylvian fissure. **C,** 7 months later, punctate and diffuse zones of calcification are present bilaterally in basal ganglia. There is evidence of progressive cerebral atrophy. **D,** after an additional 8 months CT without contrast shows that both basal ganglia calcification and cerebral atrophy have increased. From Belman AL, Lantos G, Horoupian D, et al. AIDS: Calcification of the basal ganglia in infants and children. Neurology 1986;36:1194.

made between HIV-1 encephalitis, HIV-1 leukoencephalopathy, and diffuse poliodystrophy (66). HIV-1 encephalitis is characterized by multiple disseminated foci of inflammatory cells composed of microglia, macrophages, and multinucleated giant cells (MGC) found primarily in white matter, deep gray matter, and cortex (67). In the absence of MGC the presence of HIV-1 antigen or nucleic acids must be demonstrated by immunocytochemistry or in situ hybridization (67). HIV leukoencephalopathy is described as diffuse damage to white matter including myelin loss, reactive astrogliosis, macrophages, and MGC but no distinct inflammatory infiltrates (66). In young children (younger than 3 years), myelin pallor may be difficult to appreciate because of incomplete myelination (4, 63–65). Diffuse poliodystrophy is characterized by reactive astrogliosis and microglial activation in cerebral gray matter including cortex, basal ganglia, and brainstem nuclei (66). There may be associated neuronal loss (68–70) or damage to dendritic processes (70) and, in severe cases, spongioform changes (67). Although this classification may be extremely useful in correlating clinical syndromes, neuropathological findings, and pathogenetic mechanisms, it remains possible that considerable overlap will be found between the entities described above.

Unique to pediatric AIDS is a calcific vasculopathy of the basal ganglia, and in some cases centrum semiovale, perhaps the most frequent neuropathological finding in children (4, 6, 7, 65). Mineralization is most often found in the walls of small blood vessels, but calcific deposits may be seen in walls of vessels of all sizes including large arteries (4, 6, 7, 13, 65). Calcific vasopathy may coexist with HIV-1 encephalitis, but in many cases basal ganglia calcification is present without appreciable inflammatory CNS disease.

The neuropathological findings in the spinal cord of children with HIV-1 infection differ in some respects from those reported in adult AIDS patients. Vacuolar myelopathy, a common finding in adults (71), has been observed infrequently in children (63, 72, 73), whereas inflammatory changes (myelitis) similar to those described as HIV-1 encephalitis, have been observed more frequently (67, 72, 73). In addition bilateral and symmetrical pallor localized to the corticospinal tracts has been reported (74). Two forms of corticospinal tract degeneration have been described: an axonopathy type, with both axonal and myelin loss, and a myelinopathy type, with disproportionate pallor of myelin with respect to axons (73, 74). Children with the axonopathy type often had marked cerebral pathology (HIV encephalitis) (72, 74). This suggests that the corticospinal tract degneration in these cases may be secondary to axonal injury in the brain (72, 74). The myelinopathy type

of degneration may be due to a delay in normal myelination or the effects of a myelinotoxic factor or cytokine in the tracts that are the last to myelinate (73, 74)

SECONDARY COMPLICATIONS

Infants and children with HIV-1 infection may develop neurological complications secondary to immunodeficiency. Cerebrovascular complications may also occur and in general are related to infection or other AIDS-associated illnesses including cardiomyopathy. Clinically these secondary complications can usually be distinguished from the more insidious and stereotypic cognitive and motor manifestations characteristic of HIV-1-related CNS disease. It is not uncommon for children to develop more than one CNS secondary complication. More recently, secondary CNS complications have been noted in older children with asymptomatic, mildly symptomatic, as well as more advanced systemic systemic HIV-1 disease (7, 75, 76).

Secondary CNS complications must be considered in the differential diagnosis of the child with HIV-1 infection who presents with a new onset of focal neurologic deficits, seizures, headache, or abrupt changes in mental status.

CNS Neoplasm

Primary CNS lymphoma and systemic lymphoma metastatic to the CNS are now well recognized secondary complications in children with HIV-1 infection (7, 77). Primary lymphoma, a heretofore exceedingly rare neoplasm of childhood, is the most common cause of CNS mass lesions in children in the United States with AIDS, although it is still much less common than in adults with AIDS. Age at presentation has ranged from 6 months to 10 years, with most patients older than 1 year. Neurologic deterioration is often rapidly progressive. Children usually present with the new onset of focal neurologic deficits, seizures, or changes in behavior and mental status.

CT characteristics of lymphoma are variable and include hyperdense mass lesions with or without surrounding edema that may be enhanced after administration of contrast material. Other presentations include isodense to slightly dense lesions that may exhibit contrast enhancement, ring and periventricular enhancement, or diffusely infiltrating contrast-enhancing lesions. Multiple lesions with a predilection for the basal ganglia and periventricular areas have also been observed.

CSF profiles suggested CNS lymphoma include mild to moderate pleocytosis, elevated protein content, and a hypoglycorrhachia. An initial partial response to cranial radiation with reduction in tumor mass has been reported, but long-term survival has not yet been noted.

Cerebrovascular Complications

Cerebrovascular complications may also complicate the course of HIV-1 infection in children. Both hemorrhagic and nonhemorrhagic strokes have been reported (7, 78, 79). The new onset of focal neurological deficit (most commonly hemiparesis), at times associated with seizures, is the most common presentation.

Intracerebral hemorrhage usually occurs in a setting of immune-mediated thrombocytopenia. Clinical presentation is variable, reflecting the severity and location of the hemorrhage. Strokes may be catastrophic and fatal or clinically silent. Hemorrhage into tumor may also occur.

Ischemic infarctions have been associated with intrinsic disease of cerebral blood vessels, arteriopathies of the leptomeningeal arteries, or vasculitis associated with bacterial meningitis. Ischemic infarctions have also been associated with a cardiomyopathy (78–80). Clinical presentation is variable, again reflecting severity and location of the stroke.

Neuroradiologic findings are those typical of cerebrovascular accident (bland infarction, hemorrhagic infarction, or intracranial hemorrhage).

CNS Infections

Infants and children with HIV-1 infection are at risk for developing CNS infections caused by various pathogens. Serious bacterial infections, including sepsis and meningitis, have been reported in HIV-1-infected children (see Chapter 13). Although infrequent, congenital CNS infections (toxoplasmosis, cytomegalovirus and syphilis) have also been reported in infants with vertically transmitted HIV-1 infection (81, 82).

Unlike adult patients with HIV-1-infection, CNS opportunistic infections are uncommon in HIV-1-infected infants and young children. Cytomegalovirus encephalitis and Candida albicans meningitis and microabscesses are the most frequent CNS opportunistic infections reported (2, 4, 7, 17). Remember that most CNS opportunistic infections in adults are caused by reactivation of previously acquired infection such as toxoplasmosis, cytomegalovirus, and JC virus infection. Reactivation of latent agents would not be expected in infants and young children. However, because of more aggressive medical management as well as antiretroviral and immunomodulating therapy, children with HIV-1 infection and AIDS are living longer. Thus CNS infections common to HIV-1-infected adults can now be anticipated to occur in children and adolescents and must be considered in the differential diagnosis. Note that progressive multifocal leukoencephalopathy, a devastating demyelinating disease of the brain caused by JC virus, has recently been reported in three children with HIV-1 infection (75, 83). Furthermore, in one of these children, progressive multifocal leukoencephalopathy was the first major AIDS-defining illness.

Secondary Effects and Predisposing Conditions

Children with AIDS form a heterogeneous group with very different social and environmental backgrounds as well as predisposing medical conditions. In addition, most children older than 10 will tend to have transfusion-acquired HIV disease and be male, whereas children younger than 8 will have vertically acquired HIV, although these divisions will alter over time with the changing face of the epidemic. The negative effects of HIV on the behavioral, neuropsychological, and neurological development of the child may thus be confounded with environmental and medical factors as well as the age of the child.

In patients with vertical infection, the adverse effect of in utero exposure to drugs must be considered for infants whose mothers have a history of drug abuse. The negative effects of maternal drug abuse on the newborn have been reported among others for heroin (84), cocaine (85, 86), and alcohol (87, 88). In the first years of life, neurobehavioral abnormalities observed in children born to HIV-positive mothers (89) are rather similar to symptoms associated with substance abuse during pregnancy. Differentiating between the contributions of HIV and of prenatal drug exposure to neurobehavioral dysfunctioning would be very complex (90).

The home environment in which some patients with vertically acquired HIV-1 are growing up may also negatively influence development of the child. The negative influences of impoverished home environments and other adverse conditions on psychosocial adjustment, mental growth, and development have been well documented (91).

Children who acquired HIV through blood product or coagulation factor transfusion may be affected by potential adverse CNS sequelae of the medical condition that initially required transfusion. For example, late adverse effects of premature birth (92), CNS bleeds in hemophiliacs, cardiac surgery (93), and some forms of childhood cancer (94) have been reported. It may be difficult to distinguish between these late effects and the more acute CNS manifestations of HIV. Regarding their home environment, children infected through transfusion tend to more often come from intact stable families with better economic and social support systems than vertically infected children. In addition, these families often have had to cope with chronic potentially life-threatening medical illness before (hemophilia, cancer, major surgery, etc.) and may have grown somewhat accustomed to the stress and uncertainties associated with such conditions.

ASSESSMENT

Comprehensive psychological assessment of children with HIV-1 infection remains critical because of the likelihood of HIV-1-associated neurodevelopmental abnormalities. Standard test instruments, similar to those used with other pediatric populations, should be employed to evaluate possible interval change in these patients. In addition, more experimental measures to better define the neurocognitive profiles of these patients at different developmental stages and various phases of the disease process may be developed and added (95). Testing chronically ill children is complicated by concerns about reliability and validity. There is an added difficulty in assessing very young infants who may be functioning significantly below their chronological age. Three logistic issues of assessment should continue to be addressed: 1) what to measure and how to measure it, 2) when to test and how frequently, and 3) how to handle unstandardized administration.

What to Measure and How to Measure It

The primary focus in the assessment of children with HIV-1 disease should be on psychological functions (e.g., intelligence, memory, attention, psychomotor function) and secondarily on the instruments with which to measure them. Stability of psychological functions over time and at different age ranges also must be considered since changes with further mental development may occur. For example, age-related changes in memory may not simply reflect increased capacity but also the development of different strategies to remember (96).

It is important to distinguish between two levels of measurement in the evaluation of therapy-related neurobehavioral change, particularly when associated with nonpsychological interventions: the global and the specific level (97). On the global level, interval change that is clinically and/or ecologically significant (i.e., within the total pattern of relations between the person and environment) must be demonstrated. The measurement of this global change does not necessarily have to indicate the underlying mechanisms (in functional neuropsychological terms) of this change. That is the object of the specific level of measurement where a more microscopic investigation of the observed changes are conducted. The reason that both levels of measurement are needed is that, for example, significant change on a specific micromeasure (i.e., improved response times in a reaction time task) may not be sufficient to provide strong evidence for the activity of a treatment. In combination with a global change (i.e., a significant rise in IQ), however, it will strengthen the evidence for the efficacy. In addition it will indicate a possible mechanism of the effect (i.e., improved attention) that otherwise would have been unknown.

For children, the use of the IQ from a standardized common intelligence test as a measure of general level of cognitive functioning seems valid. In addition, tests in the areas of social and everyday behavior (e.g., Vineland Adaptive Behavior Scales (98)), despite their shortcomings, and of academic achievement (e.g., Wide Range Achievement Test Revised (99)) are also valid indicators of relevant ecological behavior in children. Domains of human psychological functioning on a more specific level that could or should be evaluated are illustrated in an example of a comprehensive psychological test battery (Table 23.1) that has been used in clinical trials with HIV-1-infected children (20, 44, 51, 53). A standard or core evaluation battery should thus at least include an age-appropriate intelligence test as a measure of general level of cognitive functioning for measurement at the global level. These tests will provide summary scores that are rather stable over most follow-ups encountered in current protocols and have acceptable predictive reliabilities and relatively constant construct validity (100). There is a wide range of standardized and broadly used instruments assessing general level of cognitive functioning including the Bayley Scales of Infant Development, the McCarthy

Table 23.1. Comprehensive Test Battery for Pediatric AIDS Patients

Function Measured	Test[a]	Age Range[c]
		yr
General intelligence	Bayley mental scales	0–2.5
	McCarthy scales	2.5–8
	WISC-R	6–16
	Stanford-Binet IV[b]	2–23
	Merrill-Palmer	18–63
Language	Peabody PVT-R	2.5–40
	Gardner naming	2–16
	Verbal fluency	>2.5
Visuospatial perception	Beery VMI	4–17
	Rey-Osterrieth	>8
Memory and learning (verbal and nonverbal)	Rey Auditory verbal	>6
	McCarthy memory	2.5–8
	Rey Osterrieth	>8
	Wechsler designs[b]	
	S-B IV memory[b]	2–23
Attention	Target detection[b]	
	Trail making[b]	
	Reaction time[b]	
Motor function	Bayley motor scale	0–2.5
	Peabody motor scale	0.5–6
	Bruininks-Oseretsky	>5.5
	Grip strength	>5
	Grooved pegboard[b]	>5
Concept formation	Ravens matrices	>5.5
Behavior and personality	Vineland	0–19
	Behavior ratings[b]	
	Video recordings[b]	

[a]WISC-R, Wechsler intelligence scale for children, revised.
[b]Optional or alternative test.
[c]Age range for which test is standardized.

Scales of Children's Abilities, the Wechsler Intelligence Scale for Children (either Revised or III), and the Wechsler Adult Intelligence Scale-Revised.

In addition, subtest scores on the intelligence test may highlight strengths and weaknesses in the psychometric profile indicative of more focal deficits. They also may indicate, on the more specific level, the possible underlying mechanisms of impairment or change and provide a basis for selecting further neuropsychological tests. Furthermore, to obtain a comprehensive picture, neuropsychological functions that are ambiguously measured with standard intelligence tests should be evaluated. It is very helpful if these tests also can generate IQ equivalent (i.e., standard) scores to facilitate comparisons across domains of functions and analysis of the results.

The fact that children are constantly developing, either attaining new abilities or further mastering already existing skills, complicates evaluation of young patients with HIV-1. If serial assessments are administered, interval change has must be measured against a background of normally occurring developmental growth, possible deterioration associated with the natural history of the disease, and variable rates of development associated with socioeducational environmental factors. Appropriate measurement of psychological functioning is very dependent on having reliable age norms, preferably with small age range increments. The choice of standardized tests over experimental or novel instruments is thus essential to reliably document cognitive functioning unless large control groups can be concurrently serially evaluated (see also Ref. 101 for possible other approaches).

When to Test and How Frequently

The goal of assessment should be to reliably estimate the child's optimal level of functioning. Therefore scheduling testing after upsetting or painful medical procedures as well as after the use of sedatives or after pupil dilation should be avoided.

Furthermore, patients should not be tested when they are sick and/or are febrile. Confounding medical factors must be controlled because otherwise changes

over time may just reflect the resolution of these factors.

Longitudinal designs require repeated testing; unfortunately few psychological tests have multiple or even alternate forms. The possibility of considerable practice effects with repeated administration of similar tests are a significant limitation. We reviewed, in the first edition, the factors affecting the magnitude of practice effects (e.g., rate of development of the child, its comparative level of functioning (102), health status (103, 104), and potential for latent learning (105)) in more detail.

Testing frequency should be limited as much as possible. Since there have been significant changes in the prognosis for pediatric patients with HIV-1 disease a more individualistic approach to neurobehavioral monitoring of patients is needed. A critical determinant of testing frequency and schedule, which may differ according to the therapy is the expectancy of when reliable and possibly optimal effects can be observed. Treatment can have two different modes of action, interventive and preventive. When the CNS of the patient is compromised by HIV-1 leading to (progressive) neuropsychological deficits an interventive mode of therapy is required. Treatment may result in the change in this condition, possibly leading to improvement in function, and frequent assessments to capture this interval change or to detect further decline in function and respond appropriately is required. If the patient is functioning in or above the normal range and it is assumed that the CNS is not yet compromised, treatment in a preventive mode may protect against the development of neurocognitive abnormalities. A less frequent monitoring may be sufficient to appropriately follow these patients. Many different pediatric subgroups with varying likelihood for the development of HIV-1-associated CNS manifestations can be distinguished. Separation is conditional on the age and extent of HIV-1 disease of the patient, and these subgroups will require different types of assessment schedules and possibly different forms of treatment. In decreasing order of severity and/or likelihood of developing CNS manifestations these subgroups follow: group 1, patients with evidence of HIV-1-

associated CNS abnormalities or symptomatic (here not meaning CNS per se) children younger than 2.5 years; group 2, symptomatic patients between 2.5 and 6 years, no evidence of CNS abnormalities; group 3, asymptomatic patients younger than 3 years; group 4, symptomatic patients 6 years and older, no evidence of CNS abnormalities; group 5, asymptomatic patients, 3 years and older. A proposed testing schedule for these groups is illustrated in Table 23.2. This evaluation design requires a comprehensive assessment at baseline and at the (study) end point (and other critical timepoints) with interim monitoring using a smaller test battery at the in-between time points. Use of a monitoring battery, which is less sensitive to practice effects, also reduces the more likely practice effects on the comprehensive assessment by reducing the number of times it is administered. This monitoring exam that can be based on an evaluation of clinical events (milestones) or a formal assessment can also be used as a screening, which may trigger administration of a comprehensive exam. The considera-

tions discussed above are incorporated in the battery shown in Table 23.3 and is suggested as a good minimum or core design to investigate changes in neuropsychological status associated with treatment or natural history (see also Chapter 35).

How to Handle Unstandardized Administration

Besides cognitive deficits of varying degrees of severity, children with AIDS may also exhibit behavioral problems, physical impairments, and medical complications that may require novel approaches or modification of common psychological testing procedures. Floor effects (situations in which the subject is scoring so low on the test that no variability can be measured) are common in very young chronically ill children who function below their expected chronological age level. These effects occur especially when the child just enters the lower age limit of a new test. The child may even be unable to obtain any score on some age appropriate tests because the skill has not

Table 23.2. Neuropsychychology Test Schedule[a]

Group	Baseline	3 mo	6 mo	9 mo	12 mo	15 mo	18 mo	24 mo	30 mo	36 mo	48 mo
Group 1	Co	Mo	Co	Mo	Co	Mo	Co	Co	Mo	Co	Co
Group 2	Co		Mo		Co		Mo	Co		Mo	Co
Group 3	Co		Mo		Co		Mo	Co		Co	Co
Group 4	Co		Mo		Co			Co			Co
Group 5	Co				Co			Co			Co

[a]Co, comprehensive (macro) exam; Mo, monitoring battery (micro) exam.

Table 23.3. Monitoring and Core Battery[a]

Age Range at Baseline	Monitoring Tests	Core Battery Tests
Birth–28.5 mo	Bayley scales (MDI)	Bayley scales (MDI)
28.5 mo–6 yr	PPVT-R Gardner naming Beery VMI McCarthy: Numeric memory forward	McCarthy scales
6 yr and older	PPVT-R Gardner naming Beery VMI Ravens colored or standard WISC-R: Digit span WISC-R: Alternate form coding Grip strength and pegboard Verbal Fluency	WISC-R

[a]MDI, mental developmental index; PPVT-R, Peabody picture vocabulary test, revised; VMI, visual motor integration; WISC-R, Wechsler intelligence scale for children, revised.

yet been developed. An alternative to obtain a usable estimate to evaluate interval change for such children is to employ a test instrument more suited to their developmental rather than age level, and it is normally administered to younger children or infants. By estimating a mental age or age equivalent one can then obtain a ratio IQ (rather than a deviation IQ). Under such circumstances the next follow-up should also use the same test and ratio IQ for evaluation of interval change.

One may also encounter patients with verbal, motor, or sensory (visually or auditory) impairments owing to HIV-1, opportunistic infections, or other non-HIV-1-related causes. Alternative test instruments (indicated in Table 23.1) should be employed to obtain the best possible estimate of level of functioning, and these same instruments should again be used at follow-up even when significant gains have been made. Utilizing these "special" tests will help ensure that the child's physical problems are not interfering with the evaluation of his or her mental abilities.

Owing to fatigue and/or behavioral problems it is often necessary to use multiple test sessions with lenient administration. Testing limits and assessing the process by which the child proceeds is also valuable. If multiple sessions are used, the tester should take the time on follow-up to reestablish rapport and familiarize the patient with the testing situation and materials. Particularly younger children can be frightened by the hospital setting and may need initial "play" time with the examiner before testing begins. Moreover, as more younger vertically infected children are identified, the importance and need for highly qualified examiners with the necessary skills to evaluate such young children and infants becomes more apparent. These professionals not only should have a full knowledge of various tests to best measure areas of behavioral, social, affective, and cognitive functioning but also clinical skills in managing behaviorally difficult children.

For some test instruments, such as WISC, one has to decide whether to include all subtests, particularly the optional subtests (e.g., digit span and mazes subtests on Wechsler). We think that evaluation of at-

tentional functioning is critical in HIV-1 infection since it has been frequently reported as affected. Therefore the digit span subtests or its equivalent definitely should be included in any assessment.

PATHOLOGY AND PATHOGENESIS
Neuroinvasion: HIV-1 Entry into CNS and Cell Tropisms

The exact timing of HIV invasion into the CNS in infants and children is unknown and may vary in subsets of patients. Early invasion of the CNS has been suggested by studies in both adults and children, demonstrating synthesis of HIV-1 antibodies (5, 16, 106, 107) and isolation of HIV-1 from the CSF in neurologically symptomatic and asymptomatic adults at the time of, or subsequent to, seroconversion (108, 109). There is one report of an individual with a transient peak of HIV-1 antigen in the CSF before seroconversion (110). These findings are fortified by observations of infection of brain parenchyma as early as 2 weeks after experimental inoculation of Rhesus macaques with simian immunodeficiency virus (111).

HIV-1 is similar to other lentiviruses in requiring macrophage tropism for tissue invasion (112, 113). Only blood derived macrophages, resident microglia, and MGC formed by the fusion of these cell types have been found to harbor productive HIV-1 infection (4, 63, 64, 114, 115) (see below). Macrophage tropism is determined by the V3 domain of the HIV-1 envelope glycoprotein (116, 117). In both HIV-1 and simian immunodeficiency virus infection, subsequent selection occurs in the host for a subset of macrophage-tropic virus that invades the brain (118, 119). Evidence for direct invasion of the CNS by cell free virus remains minimal, although in vitro studies indicate that choroid plexus cells are susceptible to HIV-1 infection (120). Infection of endothelial cells in postmortem brain has been observed (15) but remains controversial (63, 115).

Viral Persistence in CNS

HIV-1 like other members of the lentivirus subfamily uses various mechanisms to evade immune clearance including rapid mutation of the immunodominant external envelope glycoprotein recognized by neutralizing antibodies and the ability to establish latent or restricted infection in selected cells (64, 121). The primate lentiviruses HIV and simian immunodeficiency virus also cause profound immunodeficiency (64, 121). The brain is a common site for persistent lentiviral infection (121). Studies using molecular techniques have consistently identified brain tissue as a reservoir of HIV-1 provirus and unintegrated viral DNA (9, 122) even in brains with minimal neuropathological findings (4, 9). In situ hybridization with RNA probes found only infrequent cells with macrophage-microglia-MGC morphology expressing HIV-1 mRNAs (15, 72). These observations are consistent with previous studies that localized HIV-1 p24/25 to the same population of monocyte derived cells (64, 72, 123). Although several investigators have demonstrated infection of neuronal or glial cell lines (12, 124, 125) reviewed in Ref. 64), evidence of in vivo infection of neuroectoderm derived cells has been lacking. Recent observations, however, suggest that restricted infection in astrocytes occurs in vitro (126) and in postmortem brain tissue (B. Blumberg and E. Major personal communications 1992 and B. Blumberg unpublished data, 1992). These in situ hybridization studies employed probes containing HIV-1 nef, which appears to be present as overexpressed early spliced mRNAs (127). The nef is one of many regulatory genes of HIV whose mRNA appears before the mRNA for the HIV-1 structural proteins. Hence detection methods that search for structural proteins will not identify the products of these early regulatory proteins. The nef reading frame was found to be open in pathological brain tissue, predicting that the nef gene product would be expressed (128). Expression of nef may serve as a marker for restricted infection. These data suggest that altered astrocyte function may be involved in HIV-1 neuropathogensis.

MECHANISM OF TISSUE DAMAGE IN HIV-1 INFECTION OF CNS

Virus-mediated Factors

Other lentiviruses, including visna and SIV, show differences in neurovirulence between characterized isolates (64, 121, 129). Studies of serial HIV-1 isolates from individuals suggest that HIV-1 variants with increased virulence emerge over time and that in vitro cytopathicity (syncytium formation) and efficient replication correlate with in vivo virulence and disease progression (129, 130). Most HIV-1 isolated from brain tissues or characterized after PCR amplification appears to be macrophage-tropic. However, distinctly neurovirulent strains of HIV-1 have not yet been identified.

No studies have convincingly demonstrated HIV-1 infection of neurons or oligodendrocytes to explain the neuronal loss or myelin pallor observed neuropathologically (reviewed in Refs. 63 and 64). Studies above (12) suggest that restricted HIV-1 infection of astrocytes occurs. This could disrupt astrocyte functions that might then secondarily result in neuronal dysfunction. Other recent reports indicate that HIV-1 may interact with neuronal or oligodendroglial membranes via the β-galactosidase (131) or other receptors (132), which could disturb cellular pocesses even if infection is not established.

In vitro studies have suggested that the HIV-1 envelope glycoprotein gp120 or a smaller peptide fragment (133) of this protein is toxic to neurons and associated with an influx of calcium in primary cultures of rodent brain. Subsequent reports by Lipton (134) indicate that the toxicity associated with gp120 is only observed in the cultures containing monocytes and glial components, suggesting an intermediate step and possibly the participation of cell-derived factors (reviewed in Ref. 134 and see below).

Host-mediated Factors

Indirect Effects Mediated by Cellular Products

Studies of other lentivirus encephalitides suggest that immune mediated mechanisms of tissue damage may be operative in HIV-1 infection (64, 121, 135). Further, a discrepancy has been noted between the number of cells in the CNS harboring productive HIV-1 infection and the magnitude of pathological damage (myelin pallor, astrogliosis, and neuronal loss) (67–70, 136) focusing attention on indirect mechanisms mediated by cytokines or other cellular products involved in the inflammatory response (54, 137). Early studies suggested that cytokines such as tumor necrosis factor-α might be important (138) (reviewed in Ref. 137). Recently Tyor et al. (139) have demonstrated diffuse immune activation, with the up-regulation of major histocompatibility complex class ll antigen, in the CNS of AIDS patients, despite the paucity of productively infected (p24 and p25 bearing) cells.

Complementary to the above observations, several investigators have implicated cytokines or other cell derived factors in supernatants from HIV-1-infected monocytes as neurotoxic factors in human brain aggregates (140) and primary chick (141) and rodent brain cultures (137). Other studies, however, indicate that HIV-1-infected human monocytes do not produce excess cytokines or neurotoxins (142). Recent studies suggest that a cell to cell interaction between the HIV-1-infected monocyte and astroglia are required for production of neuronotoxins (143, 144). These studies indicate an autocrine loop established between HIV-1-infected monocytes and astrocytes that involves induction of high levels of tumor necrosis factor-α and interleukin-1β proteins, as well as metabolites of the arachidonic acid cascade (143, 144). Further, supernatants from HIV-1-infected monocyte and astrocyte cocultures result in glial proliferation as well as neuronal loss (143). This may be important both because diffuse astrogliosis is a prominent neuropathological finding in HIV-1 infection and because astrocytes may participate in the pathogenetic process. Overall the effects of this macrophage and astrocyte interaction might be to amplify the induction of cytokines, recruit additional inflammatory cells into the brain, and activate HIV-1 replication in macrophage or microglia and/or in astrocytes (145, 146).

These findings are consistent with the work of Tardieu et al. (147) who could not replicate that supernatants from the HIV-infected monocyte cell line U937 were toxic to neurons, previously reported by Giulian et al. (141) (1990) but found that direct cell to cell contact was necessary for the neu-

ronotoxic effects (147). Furthermore, they observed some morphological alterations in the astrocytes that they interpreted as suggesting that the cytopathic changes depend on the release of viral antigens associated with adherence to the astrocyte membrane (147). Overall these findings tend to support a role for cell to cell interactions with the HIV-infected monocyte as the initiator and other cells, in particular the astrocyte, implicated as possible contributors to the pathologic process.

NMDA Receptor as Final Common Pathway

Lipton et al. (134, 148, 149) have proposed that HIV-1-associated neuronal damage is mediated via activation of the N-methyl-D-aspartate (NMDA) receptor. These NMDA receptors, which are receptors for excitatory amino acids in the brain, have been previously implicated in the final common pathway of many neuropathological processes leading to neuronal demise (134). Data to support this theory come from the observation that the neuronal death caused by HIV-1 gp120 can be ameliorated by calcium channel blockers such as nimodipine and nifedipine (148), and by antagonists of the NMDA receptor channel complex such as D-2-amino-5-phosphono-valerate and dizocilpine (149). However, further experiments demonstrated that HIV-1 gp120 alone does not appear to be a glutamate-like agonist of the NMDA receptor, whereas depletion of endogenous glutamate from the cultures protects neurons from gp120-induced toxicity (134, 149). These observations suggest that gp120, perhaps in concert with other factors secreted from HIV-1-infected cells, may sensitize the neuronal membrane to the then damaging effects of excitatory amino acids such as glutamate.

Additional support for the biological relevance of this theory is provided by the studies of Heyes et al. (150, 151) on quinolinic acid, an excitotoxic metabolite of L-tryptophan, and an agonist of the NMDA receptors. Quinolinate was markedly elevated in CSF of AIDS patients, correlated with the severity of the dementia, and diminished coincident with antitviral therapy and clinical improvement in neurological signs.

Conclusions

Virus factors probably determine neuroinvasiveness and possibly contribute to neurovirulence. Tissue damage in the CNS including white matter pallor and neuronal loss is probably initiated by the HIV-1-infected macrophage and microglia and amplified by cell to cell interactions with astrocytes that may harbor restricted HIV-1 infection, resulting in the production of high levels of cytokines and metabolites of the arachidonic acid cascade (143, 144). Myelin damage may be associated with the local action of high levels of cytokines (152), whereas neuronal damage and loss is likely mediated by activation of the NMDA receptor by excitatory amino acids (134, 148–151).

Implicating the NMDA receptor as the final common pathway for neuronal dysfunction, and ultimate loss, offers a plausible explanation for the apparent selection of a subpopulation of neurons responsible for the "subcortical" dementia, as well as the reversibility of neurologic signs earlier in the disease in both adult and pediatric patients. The description of macrophage and astrocyte interactions suggests multiple sites for potential therapeutic intervention by blocking specific cytokines, arachidonic acid metabolites, or the NMDA receptor.

PREVENTION OF HIV-ASSOCIATED CNS PATHOLOGY

It must be assumed that, when left untreated, HIV-1 infection of the CNS will eventually result in irreversible lesions in many children. Two approaches seem appropriate to prevent HIV-associated CNS pathology: 1) interventions aimed at reducing viral load within the CNS and 2) interventions targeted at blocking viral or cellular products that mediate neuronal damage.

Antiretroviral therapy has been associated with significant improvements in CNS function and even with some reversals in the progression of the encephalopathy (44). Concurrent decreases in the size of enlarged ventricles and subarachnoid space dilation on CT scan with zidovudine (55) have been reported. These changes have been of a larger magnitude for agents with good CNS permeability zidovudine (44, 51, 153) and less for agents with poor CNS permeability (dideoxycytidine) (53) (see also Chapters 34 and 35).

As mentioned in "Host-mediated Factors," there is a new understanding of the pathogenic mechanisms that may lead to neuronal damage. In particular, neurotoxins, including cytokines and metabolites at the arachidonic acid pathway, have been suggested to be involved in the pathogenesis (143, 144). In addition, there is an increasing understanding of the role of excitatory amino acids, and particularly the NMDA receptor, as a possible final common pathway for neuronal damage (134, 149). There are agents available that can modify these pathways or that can block the NMDA receptor or interfere with the calcium influx (134). These agents may mediate the negative effects of the neurotoxins. In fact, a phase I–II study of one such agent (nimodipine), a calcium-channel blocker, is underway in adult patients with the AIDS dementia complex (134).

Detailed clinical neurological and neuropsychological assessments, which have been shown to be sensitive indicators of HIV-associated CNS pathology particularly if longitudinal serial assessments are administered, will be needed to evaluate change in response to these types of therapies.

Recent clinical studies suggest that the incidence of encephalopathy could be significantly reduced with early antiviral therapy, but long-term neurologic outcomes are still uncertain (37) (see also Chapter 35).

FUTURE RESEARCH

Although there is now ample evidence indicating that CNS impairment is related to HIV-1 brain infection, questions concerning routes of CNS invasion, pathogenesis, and natural history remain unanswered.

Prospective Natural History Studies

Prospective studies to identify correlations between distinct clinical neurologic syndromes, HIV-1 activity in the CSF, and host immune responses still must be completed. In addition, neuropathologic investigations, including in situ studies of HIV-1 infection, must be conducted with special attention to the distribution of virus antigens and host derived cytokines. In addition, prospective studies must identify the earliest clinical, neuroimaging, and neurophysiologic manifestations of HIV-1-related CNS disease. Staging of CNS disease with identification of prognostic correlates clearly deserves attention (29). Surrogate markers of HIV-related CNS disease should be identified. Uniform measures of mental and motor assessment should be established and large multicenter and even international collaborative studies undertaken so that we can better understand the effects of HIV on the developing nervous system and better define stages of HIV-1-related CNS disease (39).

Anti-HIV Therapy Studies

Longitudinal studies are critical for the design of therapeutic protocols, in determining prognostic factors, and as possible historical controls against which interval changes associated with treatment can be compared. Objective measures of CNS functioning, which also reliably document interval changes, can be obtained as described previously. The use of CNS-related variables as markers to measure efficacy of therapeutic regimens for children with HIV disease is of great value because the CNS is a major target for HIV-1. In fact, clinical trials of pharmacologic agents that block factors leading to CNS damage may provide some confirmation of proposed mechanisms of neuropathogenesis, based on animal models or in vitro studies. Second, the CNS may form a sanctuary for HIV-1 against systemic treatment. Finally, CNS involvement significantly reduces the quality of life of children with HIV-1 infection .

References

1. Epstein LG, Sharer LR, Joshi VV, Fojas M, Koenigsberger MR, Oleske JM. Progressive encephalopathy in children with acquired immune deficiency syndrome. Ann Neurol 1985;17:488–496.
2. Belman AL, Ultmann MH, Horoupian D, et al. Neurologic complications in infants and children with acquired immune deficiency syndrome. Ann Neurol 1985;18:560–566.
3. Ultmann MH, Belman AL, Ruff HA, et al. Developmental abnormalities in infants and children with acquired immune deficiency syndrome (AIDS) and AIDS-related complex. Dev Med Child Neurol 1985;27:563–571.
4. Sharer LR, Epstein LG, Cho ES, et al. Pathologic features of AIDS encephalopathy in children: Evidence for LAV/HTLV-III infection of the brain. Hum Pathol 1986;17:271–284.
5. Epstein LG, Sharer LR, Oleske JM, et al. Neurologic manifestations of human immunodeficiency virus infection in children. Pediatrics 1986;78:678–687.
6. Belman AL, Lantos G, Horoupian D, et al. AIDS: Calcification of the basal ganglia in infants and children. Neurology 1986;36:1192–1199.
7. Belman AL, Diamond G, Dickson D, et al. Pediatric acquired immune deficiency syndrome: Neurologic syndromes. Am J Dis Child 1988; 142:29–35.
8. Gajdusek DC, Amyx HL, Gibbs CJ, et al. Infection of chimpanzees by human T-lymphotropic retroviruses in brain and other tissues from AIDS patients. Lancet 1985;1 :55–56.
9. Shaw GM, Harper ME, Hahn BH, et al. HTLV-III infection in brains of children and adults with AIDS encephalopathy. Science 1985;227:177–181.
10. Epstein LG, Sharer LR, Cho S-E, Meyenhofer MF, Navia BA, Price RW. HTLV-111/LAV-like retrovirus particles in the brains of patients with AIDS encephalopathy. AIDS Res 1985;1:447–454.
11. Resnick L, DiMarzo-Veronese RF, Schuphach J, et al. Intra-blood-brain barrier synthesis of HTLV-III specific IgG in patients with neurologic symptoms associated with AIDS or AIDS-related complex. N Engl J Med 1985;313:1498–1504.
12. Dewhurst S, Sakai K, Bresser J, Stevenson M, Evinger-Hodges MJ, Volsky DJ. Persistent productive infection of human glial cells by human immunodeficiency virus (HIV) and by infectious molecular clones of HIV. J Virol 1987;61:3774–3782.
13. Sharer LR, Cho ES, Epstein LG. Multinucleated giant cells and HTLV-III in AIDS encephalopathy. Hum Pathol 1985;16:760.
14. Navia BA, Jordon BD, Price RW. The AIDS dementia complex. I. Clinical features. Ann Neurol 1986;19:517–524.
15. Wiley CA, Schrier RD, Nelson JA, Lampert PW, Oldstone MB. Cellular localization of human immunodeficiency virus infection within the brains of acquired immune deficiency syndrome patients. Proc Natl Acad Sci USA 1986;83: 7089–7093.
16. Epstein LG, Goudsmit J, Paul DA, et al. Expression of human immunodeficiency virus in cerebrospinal fluid of children with progressive encephalopathy. Ann Neurol 1987;21:397–401.
17. Epstein LG, Sharer LR, Goudsmit J. Neurological and neuropathological features of HIV in children. Ann Neurol 1988;23(suppl):S19–S23.
18. Ultmann MH, Diamond G, Ruff HA, Belman AL, et al. Developmental abnormalities in infants and children with acquired immune deficiency syndrome (AIDS): A follow up study. Int J Neurosci 1987;32:661–667.

19. Centers for Disease Control Revision of the case definition of acquired immunodeficiency syndrome for national reporting—United States. MMWR 1985;34:373–377.

20. Butler KM, Husson RN, Balis FM, et al. Dideoxyinosine (ddI) in symptomatic HIV-infected children: A phase I-II study. N Engl J Med 1991;324:137–144.

21. Centers for Disease Control. Classification system for human immunodeficiency virus (HIV) infection in children under 13 years of age. MMWR 1987;103:665–670.

22. Scott G, Hutto C, Makuch RW, et al. Survival in children with perinatally acquired human immunodeficiency virus type infection. N Engl J Med 1989;321:1791–1796.

23. Blanche S, Tardieu M, Duliege AM et al. Longitudinal study of 94 symptomatic infants with perinatally acquired human immunodeficiency virus infection: Evidence for a bimodal expression of clinical and biological symptoms. Am J Dis Child 1990;144:1210–1215.

24. Cogo P, Laverda AM, Ades AE. European Collaborative Study: Neurologic signs in young children with human immunodeficiency virus infection. Pediatr Infect Dis J 1990;9:402–406.

25. Blanche S, Rouzioux C, Guihard ML, et al. A prospective study of infants born to women seropositive for human immunodeficiency virus type 1. N Engl J Med 1989;320:1643–1648.

26. Mok JQ, Gianquinto C, DeRossi A, Ades AE, Grosch-Worner I, Peckman CS. Infants born to mothers seropositive for human immunodeficiency virus. Lancet 1987;1:1164–1168.

27. Belman AL, Calvelli T, Nozyce M. Neurologic and immunologic correlates in infants with vertically transmitted HIV infection [Abstract]. Neurology 1990;40(suppl 1):409.

28. Calvelli TA, Belman AL, Bueti C. Divergence of onset of neurologic and immunologic impairment in infants born to HIV seropositive mothers. [Abstract TBP 184]. Fifth International Conference on AIDS, Montreal, Jun 1989.

29. Tovo PA, deMartino M, Gabiano C, et al. Prognostic factors and survival in children with perinatal HIV-I infection. Lancet 1992;339:1249–1253.

30. Moss H, Wolters P, Eddy J. The effects of encephalopathy and AZT treatment on the social and emotional behavior of pediatric AIDS patients [Abstract TBP 248]. Fifth International Conference on AIDS, Montreal, Jun 1989.

31. Moss H, Brouwers P, Wolters P, El-Amin D, Butler K, Pizzo P. Gender differences in neuropsychological vulnerability of children with vertically-acquired HIV infection [Abstract MB 2012]. Seventh International Conference on AIDS, Florence, Jun 1991.

32. Persaud D, Sulachni C, Rigaud M, et al. Delayed recognition of human immunodeficiency virus infection in preadolescent children. Pediatrics 1992;90:688–691.

33. Krasinski K, Borkowsky W, Holzman R. Prognosis of human immunodeficiency virus in children and adolescents. Pediatr Infect Dis J 1989;8:216–220.

34. Cohen SL, Mundy T, Karassik B, et al. Neuropsychological functioning in human immunodeficiency virus type 1 seropositive children infected through neonatal blood transfusion. Pediatrics 1991;88:58–68.

35. Grant I, Atkinson JH, Hesselink JR, et. al. Evidence for early central nervous system involvement in the acquired immunodeficiency syndrome (AIDS) and other human immunodeficiency virus infections. Ann Intern Med 1987; 107: 828–836.

36. Wilkie F, Eisdorfer C, Morgan R, Lowenstein D, Szapocznik J. Cognition in early human immunodeficiency virus infection. Arch Neurol 1990; 47:433–440.

37. Portegies P, DeGans J, Lange J, et al. Declining incidence of AIDS dementia complex after introduction of zidovidine treatment. Br Med J 1989; 299 :819–821.

38. Rogers M, Thomas P, Starcher E, Noa M, Bush T, Jaffe H. Acquired immunodeficiency syndrome in children: Report of the Centers for Disease Control National Surveillance, 1982 to 1985. Pediatrics 1987;79:1008–1014.

39. Belman AL. AIDS and pediatric neurology. Neurol Clin 1990;8:571– 603.

40. American Academy of Neurology AIDS Task Force. Nomenclature and research case definitions for neurologic manifestations of human immunodeficiency virus-type 1 infection. Ann Neurol 1991;41:778–785.

41. Falloon J, Eddy J, Wiener L, Pizzo PA. Human immunodeficiency virus infection in children. J Pediatr 1989;114:1–30.

42. Brouwers P, Moss H, Wolters P, El-Amin D, Tassone E, Pizzo P. Neurobehavioral typology of school-age children with symptomatic HIV disease [Abstract]. J Clin Exp Neuropsychol 1992;14:113.

43. Diamond GW, Kaufman J, Belman AL, et al. Characterization of cognitive functioning in a subgroup of children with congenital HIV infection. Arch Clin Neuropsychol 1987;2:1–16.

44. Pizzo PA, Eddy J, Falloon J, et al. Effect of continuous intravenous infusion of zidovudine (AZT) in children with symptomatic HIV infection. N Engl J Med 1988;319:889–896.

45. Belman AL, Diamond G, Park Y, et al. Perinatal HIV infection: A prospective longitudinal study of the initial CNS signs. Neurology 1989;39(suppl): 278–279.

46. Brouwers P, Moss H, Wolters P, Eddy J, Pizzo P. Neuropsychological profile of children with symptomatic HIV infection prior to antiretroviral therapy [Abstract TBP 179]. Fifth International Conference on AIDS, Montreal, Jun 1989.

47. Hittelman J, Willoughby A, Mendez H, et al. Neurodevelopmental outcome of perinatally-acquired HIV infection on the first 24 months of life [Abstract TUB 37]. Seventh International Conference on AIDS, Florence, Jun 1991.

48. Wolters P, Moss H, Eddy J, Pizzo P, Brouwers P. The adaptive behavior of children with symptomatic HIV infection and the effects of AZT therapy [Abstract MBO 43]. Fifth International Conference on AIDS, Montreal, Jun 1989.

49. Hittelman J. Neurodevelopmental aspects of HIV infection. In: Kozlowski PB, Snider DA, Vietze

PM, Wisneiwski HM, eds. Brain in pediatric AIDS. Basel: Karger, 1990:64–71.

50. McCardle P, Nannis E, Smith R, Fischer G. Patterns of perinatal HIV-related language deficit [Abstract WB 2021]. Seventh International Conference on AIDS, Florence, Jun 1991.

51. Brouwers E, Moss H, Wolters P, et al. Effect of continuous-infusion zidozudine therapy on neuropsychologic functioning in children with symptomatic human immunodeficiency virus infection. J Pediatr 1990;117:980–985.

52. Wolters P, Brouwers P, Moss H, et al. The effect of dideoxyinosine on the cognitive functioning of children with HIV infection after 6 and 12 months of treatment [Abstract WB 2051]. Seventh International Conference on AIDS, Florence, Jun 1991.

53. Pizzo PA, Butler K, Balis F. Dideoxycytidine alone and in an alternating schedule with zidovudine in children with symptomatic human immunodeficiency virus infection. J Pediatr 1990;117:7991808.

54. Price RW, Brew B, Sidtis J, Rosenblum M, Scheck AC, Cleary P. The brain in AIDS: Central nervous system infection and AIDS dementia complex. Science 1988;239:586–592.

55. DeCarli C, Fugate L, Falloon J, et al. Brain growth and cognitive improvement in children with human immunodeficiency virus-induced encephalopathy after 6 months of continuous infusion zidovudine therapy. J Acquir Immune Defic Syndr 1991;4:585–592.

56. Belman AL. Acquired immunodeficiency syndrome and the child's central nervous system. Pediatr Clin North Am 1992;39:691–714.

57. Wiley CA, Belman AL, Rubinstein DD, Nelson JA. Human immunodeficiency virus within the brains of children with AIDS. Clin Neuropathol 1990;9:1–6.

58. Tardieu M, Blanche W, Brunelle F. Cerebral magnetic resonance imaging studies in HIV-1 infected children born to seropositive mothers [Abstract]. Neuroscience of HIV-1 infection. Satellite Conference of Seventh International Conference on AIDS, Padova, 1991:60.

59. Chamberlain MC, Nichols SL, Chase CH. Pediatric AIDS: Comparative cranial MRI and CT scans. Pediatr Neurol 1991;7:357–362.

60. Kauffman WM, Sivit CJ, Fitz CR, Rakusan TA, Herzog K, Chandra RS. CT and MR evaluation of intracranial involvement in pediatric HIV infection: A clinical-imaging correlation. Am J Neuroradiol 1992;13:949–957.

61. Gallo P, Laverda AM, DeRossi A. Immunological markers in the cerebrospinal fluid of HIV-1 infected children. Acta Pediatr Scand 1991;80: 659–666 .

62. Tardieu M, Blanche S, Deliege A, Rouzioux, Griscelli G. Neurological involvement and prognostic factors after materno-fetal infection [Abstract MB 039]. Fifth International Conference on AIDS, Montreal, Jun 1989.

63. Sharer LR. Pathology of HIV-1 infection of the central nervous system. J Neuropathol Exp Neurol 1992;51:3–11.

64. Michaels J, Sharer LR, Epstein LG. Human immunodeficiency virus type 1 (HIV-1) infection of

the nervous system: A review. Immunodeficiency Rev 1988;1:71–104.

65. Dickson DW, Belman AL, Park YD, et al. Central nervous system pathology in pediatric AIDS: An autopsy study. Acta Pathol Microbiol Immunol Scand 1989;8 (suppl):40–57.

66. Budka H, Wiley CA, Kleihues P. A HIV-associated disease of the nervous system: Review of nomenclature and proposal for neuropathology-based terminology. Brain Pathol 1991;1:143–152.

67. Budka H. Neuropathology of human immunodeficiency virus infection. Brain Pathol 1991; 1:163–175.

68. Ketzler S, Weis S, Haug H, Budka H. Loss of neurons in the frontal cortex in AIDS brains. Acta Neuropathol 1990;80:92–94.

69. Everall IP, Luthert PJ, Lantos PL. Neuronal loss in the frontal cortex in HIV infection. Lancet 1991; 337:1119–1121.

70. Wiley CA, Masliah E, Morey M, et al. Neocortical damage during HIV infection. Ann Neurol 1991; 29:651–657.

71. Petito CK, Navia BA, Cho ES, et al. Vacuolar myelopathy pathologically resembling subacute combined degeneration in patients with the acquired immunodeficiency syndrome. N Engl J Med 1985;312:874–879.

72. Sharer LR, Dowling PC, Michaels J, Cook SD, Blumberg BM, Epstein LG. Spinal cord disease in children with HIV-1 infection: A combined molecular and neuropathological study. Neuropathol Appl Neurobiol 1990;16:317–331 .

73. Dickson DW, Belman AL, Kim TS, Horoupian D, Rubinstein A. Spinal cord pathology in pediatric acquired immunodeficiency syndrome. Neurology 1989;39:227–235.

74. Weidenheim KM, Kure K, Belman AL, Dickson DW. Pathogenesis of corticospinal tract degeneration in pediatric AIDS [Abstract 251]. J Neuropathol Exp Neurol 1989;48:384.

75. Berger JR, Scott G, Albrecht J, Belman AL, Tornatore C, Major EO. Progressive multifocal leukoencephalopathy in HIV-1-infected children. AIDS 1992;6:837–841.

76. Burger H, Belman AL, Grimson R. Long HIV-1 incubation periods and dynamics of transmission within a family. Lancet 1990;336:134–136.

77. Epstein LG, Dicarlo F, Joshi V, et al. Primary lymphoma of the central nervous system in children with acquired immunodeficiency syndrome. Pediatrics 1988;82:355–363.

78. Park Y, Belman AL, Dickson DW, et al. Stroke in pediatric acquired immunodeficiency syndrome. Ann Neurol 1990;28:303–311.

79. Frank Y, Lim W, Kahn E, et al. Multiple ischemic infarcts in a child with AIDS, varicella zoster infection and cerebral vasculitis. Pediatr Neurol 1989;5:64–67.

80. Dickson DW, Llena JF, Weidenheim KM. Central nervous system pathology in children with AIDS and focal neurologic signs—stroke and lymphoma. In: Kozlowski P, eds. Brain behavior and pediatric AIDS. Basel: Karger, 1990:147–157.

81. Shanks GD, Redfield RR, Fischer GW. Toxoplasma encephalitis in an infant with ac-

quired immunodeficiency syndrome. Pediatr Infect Dis J 1987;6:70–71.

82. Biggemann B, Voit T, Neuen E. Neurological manifestations in three German children with AIDS. Neuropediatrics 1987;18:99–106.

83. Vandersteenhoven JJ, Dbaibo G, Boyko OB, Huletta CM, Anthony DC, Wilfert C. Progressive multifocal leukoencephalopathy in pediatric acquired immunodeficiency syndrome. Pediatr Infect Dis J 1992;11:232–237.

84. Naeye R, Blanc W, Leblanc W, Khatamee M. Fetal complications of maternal heroin addiction: Abnormal growth, infections, and episodes of stress. J Pediatr 1973;83:1055–1061.

85. Chasnoff I, Griffith D, MacGregor S, Dirkes K, Burns K. Temporal patterns of cocaine use during pregnancy. JAMA 1989;261:1741–1744.

86. MacGregor S, Keith L, Chasnoff I, et al. Cocaine use during pregnancy: Adverse perinatal outcome. Am J Obstet Gynecol 1987;157:686–690.

87. Iosub S, Fuchs M, Bingol N, Gromisch DS. Fetal alcohol syndrome revisited. Pediatrics 1981;68: 475–479.

88. Day N, Jasperse D, Richardson G, et al. Prenatal exposure to alcohol: Effect on infant growth and morphologic characteristics. Pediatrics 1989;84: 536–541.

89. Marion RW, Wiznia AA, Hutcheon RG, Rubinstein A. Human T-cell lymphotropic virus type III (HTLV-III) embryopathy. Am J Dis Child 1986;140:638–640.

90. Fulroth R, Phillips B, Durand D. Perinatal outcome of infants exposed to cocaine and/or heroin in utero. Am J Dis Child 1989;143:905–910.

91. Capron C, Duyme M. Assessment of effects of socio-economic status on IQ in a full cross-fostering study. Nature 1989;340:552–554.

92. Spreen O, Tupper D, Risser A, Tuokko H, Edgell D. Human Developmental Neuropsychology. New York: Oxford University Press, 1984.

93. Terplan J. Patterns of brain damage in infants and children with congenital heart disease: Association with catherization and surgical procedures. Am J Dis Child 1973;125:175–185.

94. Poplack DG, Brouwers P. Adverse sequalae of central nervous system therapy. Clin Oncol 1985; 4:263–285.

95. Albert MS. Criteria for the choice of neuropsychological tests in clinical trials. In: Mohr E, Brouwers P, eds. Handbook of clinical trials: The neurobehavioral approach. Amsterdam: Swets & Zeitlinger, 1991:131–139.

96. Kail R. The development of memory in children. San Francisco: WH Freeman, 1984.

97. Brouwers P, Mohr E. Design of clinical trials. In: Mohr E, Brouwers P, eds. Handbook of clinical trials: The neurobehavioral approach. Amsterdam: Swets & Zeitlinger, 1991:45–66.

98. Sparrow S, Balla D, Cicchetti D. Vineland Adaptive behavior scales. Circle Pines, MN: American Guidance Service, 1984.

99. Jastak S, Wilkinson G. Wide range achievement test—revised. Wilmington: Jastak Associates, 1984.

100. Appelbaum AS, Tuma JM. Social class and test performance: Comparative validity of the Peabody with the WISC and WISC-R for two socioeconomic groups. Psychol Rep 1977;40: 139–145.

101. Fletcher J, Francis D, Pequegnat W, et al. Neurobehavioral outcomes in diseases of childhood: Individual change models for pediatric human immunodeficiency viruses. Am Psychol 1991;46:1267–1277.

102. Tuma JM, Appelbaum AS. Reliability and practice effects of WISC-R, IQ estimates in a normal population. Educ Psychol Meas 1980;40:671–678.

103. Moss HA, Nannis ED, Poplack DG. The effects of prophylactic treatment of the central nervous system on the intellectual functioning of children with acute lymphocytic leukemia. Am J Med 1981;71:47–52.

104. Farwell JR, Lee YJ, Hirtz DG Sulzbacher SI, Ellenberg JH, Nelson KB. Phenobarbital for febrile seizures—effects on intelligence and on seizure recurrence. N Engl J Med 1990;322:364–369.

105. Tuma JM, Appelbaum AS, Bee DS. Comparability of the WISC and the WISC-R in normal children of divergent socioeconomic backgrounds. Psychol Schools 1978;15:339–346.

106. Goudsmit J, Wolters EC, Bakker M, et al. Intrathecal synthesis of antibodies to HTLV-III in patients without AIDS or AIDS related complex. Br Med J 1986;292: 1231– 1234.

107. Resnick L, Berger JR, Shapshak P, Tourtellotte WW. Early penetration of blood-brain-barrier by HIV. Neurology 1988;38:9–14.

108. Ho DD, Rota TR, Schooley RT, et al. Isolation of HTLV-III from CSF and neural tissues of patients with AIDS related neurologic syndromes. N Engl J Med 1985;313:1493–1497.

109. Hollander H, Levy JA. Neurologic abnormalities and recovery of human immunodeficiency virus from the cerebrospinal fluid. Ann Intern Med 1987;106:692–695.

110. Goudsmit J, de Wolf F, Paul DA, et al. Expression of human immunodeficiency virus antigen (HIV-ag) in serum and cerebrospinal fluid during acute and chronic infection. Lancet 1986;2:177–180.

111. Sharer LR, Michaels J, Murphey-Corb M, et al. Serial pathogenesis study of SIV brain infection. J Med Primatol 1991;20:211–217.

112. Peluso R, Haase A, Stowring L, Edwards M, Ventura P. A Trojan horse mechanism for the spread of visna virus in monocytes. Virology 1985;147:231–236.

113. Desrosiers RC, Hansen-Moosa A, Mori K, et al. Macrophage-tropic variants of SIV are associated with specific AIDS-related lesions but are not essential for the development of AIDS. Am J Pathol 1991;139:29–35.

114. Koenig S, Gendelman HE, Orenstein JM, et al. Detection of AIDS virus in macrophage in brain tissue from AIDS patients with encephalopathy. Science 1986;233:1089–1093.

115. Michaels J, Price RW, Rosenblum MK. Microglia in the giant cell encephalitis of AIDS: Proliferation, infection and fusion. Acta Neuropathol 1988;76:373–379.

116. Westervelt P, Gendelman HE, Ratner L. Identification of a determinant within the human immunodeficiency virus 1 surface envelope glyo-

protein critical for productive infection of primary monocytes. Proc Natl Acad Sci USA 1991;88:3097–3101.

117. Westervelt P, Trowbridge DB, Epstein LG, et al. Macrophage tropism determinants of human immunodeficiency virus type 1 in vivo. J Virol 1992;66:2577–2582.

118. Epstein LG, Kuiken K, Blumberg BM, et al. HIV-1 V3 domain variation in brain and spleen of children with AIDS: Tissue specific evolution within host-determined quasi species. Virology 1991;180:583–I590.

119. Sharma DP, Zink MC, Anderson M, et al. Derivation of neurotropic simian immunodeficiency virus from exclusively lymphocytetropic parental virus: Pathogenesis of infection in macaques. J Virol 1992;66:3550–3556.

120. Harouse JM, Wroblewska Z, Laughlin MA, Hickey WF, Schonwetter BS, Gonzalez-Scarano F. Human charoid plexus cells can be latently infected with human immunodeficiency virus. Ann Neurol 1989;25:406–411.

121. Narayan O, Clements JE. Biology and pathogenesis of lentiviruses. J Gen Virol 1989;70:1617–1639.

122. Pang S, Koyanagi Y, Miles S, Wiley C, Vinters HV, Chen I. High levels of unintegrated HIV-1 DNA in brain tissue of AIDS dementia patients. Nature 1990;343:85–89.

123. Pumarola-Sune T, Navia BA, Cordon-Cardo D, et al. HIV antigen in the brains of patients with the AIDS dementia complex. Ann Neurol 1987;21:490–496.

124. Harouse JM, Kunsch C, Hartle HT, et al. CD4-independent infection of human neural cells by human immunodeficiency virus type 1. J Virol 1989;63:2527–2533.

125. Shapshak P, Sun HCS, Resnick L, et al. HIV-1 propogates in human neuroblastoma cells. J Aquir Immune Defic Syndr 1991;4:228–237.

126. Brack-Werner R, Kleinschmidt A, Ludvigsen A, et al. Infection of human brain cells by HIV-1: Restricted virus production in chronically infected human glial cell lines. AIDS 1992;6:273–285.

127. Schwartz S, Felber BK, Benko DM, Fenyo E-M, Pavlakis GN. Cloning and functional anaylsis of multiply spliced mRNA species of human immunodeficiency virus type 1. J Virol 1990;64:2519–2529.

128. Blumberg BM, Epstein LG, Saito Y, Chen D, Sharer LR, Anand R. Human immunodeficiency virus type 1 nef quasispecies in pathological tissue. J Virol 1992;66:5256–5264.

129. Cheng-Mayer C, Weiss C, Seto D, Levy JA. Isolates of human immunodeficiency virus type 1 from the brain may constitute a special groups of the AIDS virus. Proc Natl Acad Sci USA 1989;86:8575–8579.

130. Tersmette M, Gruters RA, deWolf F, et al. Evidence for a role of virulent human immunodeficiency virus (HIV) variants in the pathogenesis of acquired immunodeficiency syndrome: Study on sequential HIV isolates. J Virol 1989;63:2118–2125.

131. Harouse JM, Bhat S, Spitalnik SL, et al. Inhibition of entry of HIV-1 in neural cell lines by antibodies against galactosyl ceramide. Science 1991;253:320–323.

132. Mizrachi Y, Zeira M, Shahabuddin M, Li G, Sinangil F, Volsky DJ. Efficient binding, fusion and entry of HIV1 into CD4-negative neural cells: A mechanism for neuropathogenesis in AIDS. Bull Inst Pasteur 1991;89:81–96.

133. Brenneman DE, Westbrook GL, Fitzgerald SP, et al. Neuronal cell killing by the envelope protein of HIV and its prevention by vasoactive intestinal peptide. Nature 1988;335:639–642.

134. Lipton SA. Models of neuronal injury in AIDS: Another role for the NMDA receptor? Trends Neurosci 1992;15:75–79.

135. Sharer LR, Baskin GB, Cho ES, Murphey-Corb M, Blumberg BM, Epstein LG. Comparison of SIV and HIV encephalitides in the immature host. Ann Neurol, 1 988;23(suppl) S108–S112.

136. Vazeus R, Croxchiudo CL, Blanche S. Low levels of human immunodeficiency virus replication in brain tissue of children with severe AIDS encephalopathy. Am J Pathol 1992;140:137–144.

137. Merrill JE, Chen ISY. HIV-1, macrophages, glial cells, and cytokines in AIDS nervous system disease. FASEB J 1991;5:2391–2397.

138. Mintz M, Rapaport R, Oleske JM, et al. Elevated serum levels of tumor necrosis factor are associated with progressive encephalopathy in children with acquired immunodeficiency syndrome. Am J Dis Child 1989;143:771–774.

139. Tyor WR, Glass JD, Griffin JW. Cytokine expression in the brain during the acquired immunodeficiency syndrome. Ann Neurol 1992;31:349–360.

140. Pulliam L, Herndier BG, Tang NM, McGrath MS. Human immunodeficiency virus-infected macrophages produce soluble factors that cause histological and neurochemical alterations in cultured human brains. J Clin Invest 1991;87:503–512.

141. Giulian D, Vaca K, Noonan CA. Secretion of neurotoxins by mononuclear phagocytes infected with HIV-1. Science 1990;250:1593–1596.

142. Bernton E, Bryant H, Decoster M, et al. No direct neuronotoicity by HIV-1 virions or culture fluids from HIV-1 infected T-cells or monocytes. AIDS Res Hum Retroviruses 1992;8:495–503.

143. Gendelman HE, Genis P, Jett M, et al. Experimental model systems for studies of HIV-associated CNS disease. In: Montagnier L, Gougeon ML, eds. New concepts in AIDS pathogenesis. New York: Marcel Dekker, in press.

144. Genis P, Jett M, Bernton EW, et al. Cytokines and arachidonic metabolites produced during human immunodeficiency virus (HIV)-infected macrophage-astroglial interactions: Implications for the neuropathogenesis of HIV disease. J Exp Med 1992;176:1703–1718.

145. Tornatore C, Nath A, Amemiya K, Major EO. Persistent HIV-1 infection in human fetal glial cells reactivated by T-cell factor(s) or by the cytokines tumor necrosis factor alpha and interleukin 1 beta. J Virol 1991;65:6094–6100 .

146. Griffin DE, McArthur JC, Cornblath DR. Neopterin and interferon-gamma in serum and cerebrospinal fluid of patients with HIV associ-

ated neurologic disease. Neurology 1991;41: 69–74.

147. Tardieu M, Hery C, Peudenier S, Boespflug O, Montagnier L. Human immunodeficiency virus type 1-infected monocytic cells can destroy human neural cells after cell-to-cell adhesion. Ann Neurol 1992;32:11–17.

148. Dreyer EB, Kaiser PK, Offerman JT, Lipton SA. HIV-1 coat protein neurotoxicity prevented by calcium channel antagonists. Science 1990;248: 364–367.

149. Lipton SA, Sucher NJ, Kaiser PK, Dreyer EB. Synergistic effects of the HIV coat protein and NMDA receptor-mediated neurotoxicity. Neurology 1991;7:111–118.

150. Heyes MP, Rubinow D, Lane C. Cerebrospinal fluid quinolinic acid concentrations are increased in acquired immune deficiency syndrome. Ann Neurol 1989;26:275–277.

151. Heyes MP, Brew BJ, Martin A. Quinolinic acid in cerebrospinal fluid and serum in HIV-1 infection: Relationship to clinical and neurological status. Ann Neurol 1991;29:202–209.

152. Selmaj KW, Raine CS. TNF mediates myelin and oligodendrocyte damage in vitro. Ann Neurol 1988;23:339–346.

153. McKinney RE Jr, Maha MA, Connor EM, et al. A multicenter trial of oral zidovudine in children with advanced human immunodeficiency virus disease. N Engl J Med 1991;324:1018–1025.

scheme is proposed after a discussion of most common sight threatening entities.

HIV induced immunosuppression leads to a depression of cellular immunity that predisposes patients to opportunistic infections. Bacterial (syphilis, tuberculosis), viral (CMV, herpes zoster, herpes simplex), and protozoal (toxoplasmosis, *Pneumocystis carinii*) infections are the most common sight threatening ocular pathogens seen in adults with AIDS. Most opportunistic ocular infections occur as a result of a systemic infection, although in many patients the systemic infection may be dormant or asymptomatic, whereas the ocular disease is active and problematic. In immunocompetent individuals, it is often possible to make a diagnosis of an ocular opportunistic infection by noting the presence of a systemic infection (e.g., tuberculosis) and then inferring that the ocular lesions are a localized manifestation of the same systemic problem. This same approach can also be used in AIDS; 40% of patients, with ocular toxoplasmosis, for example, also have brain lesions. However, it must be emphasized that AIDS patients frequently have multiple infections. Hence, knowledge of both the serology and systemic infection is often insufficient to specify the nature of the ocular disease. Diagnosis must then be based on clinical correlations made from available pathologic material, and on the extent of the patient's immunosuppression (4). In adults, toxoplasmosis appears with CD4 counts below 200, but CMV is generally not found until the CD4 count drops well below 100. In children with HIV infection, congenital toxoplasmosis may result in ocular lesions. Both active ocular toxoplasmosis and CMV retinitis are devastating when they occur, but they appear to be less common in children compared with adults. Note that the risk for these infections, as reflected by the patient's CD4 count, may also differ in children because of age-related differences in the CD4 count.

On occasion it is necessary to make a tissue diagnosis to institute appropriate therapy. In most cases, this is only when there is sight threatening bilateral disease. If one eye is already blind, one can propose enucleation of the blind eye. This is the preferred approach because it guarantees that the lesion will not be missed and that there will be enough tissue available for all laboratory tests. If there is still residual vision, a retinal or chorioretinal biopsy can be performed that when well planned can yield the appropriate diagnosis (5). One must secure a piece of tissue that contains both healthy and diseased retina and ensure that the pathologist can make a diagnosis on limited tissue. In general, only a pathologist with extensive training in cytopathology will be competent enough to make a diagnosis (6). Newer techniques of molecular biology, including in situ hybridization, and polymerase chain reaction, will certainly change our diagnostic approach in years to come (7).

CLINICAL MANIFESTATIONS OF HIV

Noninfectious Manifestations

Ocular manifestations of HIV can be divided into those caused by opportunistic pathogens and those that are a consequence of the HIV virus itself. Opportunistic infections often have characteristic clinical appearances irrespective of the patient's age. The more common infections, particularly CMV and toxoplasmosis, will be discussed in the next sections. The most common manifestation of the HIV virus in adults is the cotton wool spot. This microvascular occlusion is present in 60–70% of patients and first appears in patients with AIDS-related complex (8). It is rarely seen in the pediatric population, and is only seen in children older than 8–10 years of age. Cotton wool spots are the result of a microvascular infarct of the nerve fiber layer leading to retinal edema. It usually resolves in 4–6 weeks, in contradistinction to a CMV lesion that would increase in size during the same time (9). Other vascular phenomena include retinal hemorrhages, and retinal arterial or venous occlusions. The latter can lead to significant visual loss, but once again these rare manifestations appear to be restricted to the older children and adults.

In children younger than 8 years, we have observed few signs attributable to HIV infection. Vascular sheathing is only occasionally seen in North America and Europe but is a frequent finding among African children infected with HIV (10, 11). An increased incidence of optic nerve pallor and atrophy has been reported in up 18% of children (2), but this has not been our experience. An asymptomatic dry eye syndrome has also been reported (10). It is of concern if an HIV-infected child develops a corneal ulcer. The antibiotic drops that are used can cause a corneal epithelial breakdown that can result in corneal perforation if not carefully monitored (12). In children with congenitally acquired HIV, an increase in the incidence of strabismus has also been noted. It appears to be 6% in congenitally infected children compared with 2–4% in the general population. Untreated, strabismus can lead to amblyopia and a permanent loss of vision to the 20/200 level. This loss is preventable and reversible in the early stages of amblyopia, if it is dealt with as soon as possible after it develops and before the visual system has reached maturity. All children younger than 8 years should be periodically checked for the presence of strabismus and referred to a pediatric ophthalmologist if an eye deviation is observed.

CMV Retinitis

CMV retinitis is the most common pediatric ocular infection in AIDS. The overall incidence in the pediatric population appears to be much lower than in adults. In 220 patients with HIV infection with a Centers for Disease Control classification P-2 or worse followed over the last 4 years by the National Cancer Institute and the National Eye Institute, we have noted an overall incidence of CMV retinitis of 1.6% compared with 20% in the adult population (1, 13). The incidence increases ten-fold when the CD4 count falls below 100 and then affects about 16% of patients. This incidence is lower than the 50% incidence found in the adult population with a similar CD4 count.

Adult patients with CMV retinitis often have no complaints unless the central vision of one eye is affected. Patients only rarely notice the presence of increased floaters or a diminution of peripheral vision. CMV retinitis is never associated with ocular pain or external signs of involvement. Because the symptoms are so rare and nonspecific, we can rarely make an early diagnosis of CMV

retinitis in children. Indeed, children typically present with bilateral involvement, often with central disease in one eye. Early detection depends on adequate screening by physicians and parents alike (see below).

Diagnostic features of CMV retinopathy are well described (9, 14–18) and will only be summarized here. The most characteristic presentation is that of a white granular lesion with irregular borders, often associated with satellite lesions beyond the leading edge and hemorrhage if the lesion is close to the vascular arcades or the optic nerve (Fig 24.1 and 24.2). The involved areas become necrotic, leaving behind an atrophic gliotic membrane that has no visual potential and is associated with an absolute scotoma. In the zones of atrophy, the underlying retinal pigment epithelium often has a granular appearance. This atrophic retina is prone to retinal detachment that occurs in up to 30% of adult CMV patients when extensive disease is present, particularly along the vitreous base. Inflammation in the anterior chamber or the vitreous is generally minimal or nonexistent, although a breakdown of the blood-ocular barrier

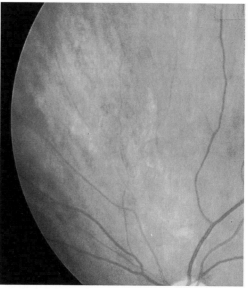

Figure 24.1. Typical early CMV retinitis lesion. Lesion is centered around a blood vessel. Note white granular nature of leading edge of lesion. Lesion progresses by extension into healthy retina, away from the presently affected retina. In its wake is left a thin atrophic retina. There is little or no vitreal inflammation present.

Figure 24.3. sion of a CMV rophic periphe right eye after ciclovir. **B,** pat active lesion ar tried on indu

Ocular to common oc Its overall America (25 ocular toxop it can occur (congenital) ular scar is Involvemer focus, or s ent. Bilatera of patients. an associate to different 24.4) (9). T diffuse mal pole very h above the t will have co

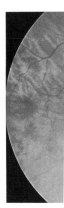

Figure 24.2.
ble affectin
CMV lesion
associated
spots are se

can be d
tometry (]
CMV r
lessly, adv
if left unt
tive to in
tinitis is d
ral agent
Neither
therapy r
the patie
ministere
bloodstre
The latte
practical
must be
Recently
oped usi
can be ir
cavity. It
gression
in a grou
designec
months
approac
other for

Ganci
minister
2–3 week
empirica
Unfortu
and car
cases. G
of 5 mg
mainten

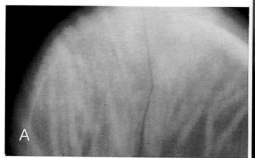

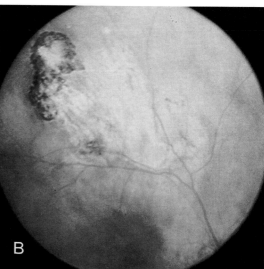

Figure 24.4.   **A,** active toxoplasmosis lesion. Notice presence of vitreal haze on this picture overlying the area of retinitis. This limited inflammatory response overlying an area of retinitis is typical of toxoplasmosis lesions in AIDS. **B,** acquired toxoplasmosis lesions in AIDS. This picture was taken after the toxoplasmosis retinitis was treated. Notice complete atrophy of retina and choroid, allowing underlying sclera to be seen as a very white layer. Along superior and temporal margins of lesion, there is increased pigmentation as a result of retinal pigment epithelial proliferation. Another very common manifestation of ocular toxoplasmosis.

P. carinii (31, 32), and herpes zoster or herpes simplex (33). All have characteristic clinical pictures. Syphilis is being increasingly recognized in the adult population. It is very frequently associated with optic neuritis or optic perineuritis and must be aggressively treated using the same treatment regimens as for neurosyphilis because it can otherwise lead to severe permanent visual loss. *P. carinii* is characterized by a yellowish choroidal infiltrate with indistinct borders that rarely will cause a significant decrease in vision (Fig. 24.5). *P. carinii* choroiditis is a sign of a disseminated systemic infection, and it usually responds well to standard systemic therapy with complete or near complete resolution of the choroidal lesions. Herpetic retinal infections from either herpes zoster or herpes simplex are of greater concern since they will lead to bilateral blindness in a few days unless they are recognized early and intravenous therapy is instituted immediately. Both viruses are thought to present the same clinical picture, although retinal infections with herpes zoster are more frequent. The lesions can present as a white confluent necrotic peripheral lesion (Fig. 24.6) or as punctate outer retinal

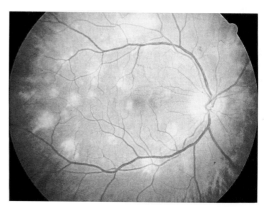

Figure 24.5.   *P. carinii* choroiditis in an adult patient. Lesions are yellow-white with indistinct borders. There is no vitreal inflammation, and the overlying retina is normal. Notice that retinal vessels are visible above lesions.

lesions (Fig. 24.7) (33). Both acyclovir and ganciclovir have been tried with moderate success. In AIDS patients, therapy must be continued for a prolonged period. Rapid visual loss has been observed when the therapy is switched from an intravenous formulation to oral. Thus the patients must be carefully monitored for any signs of progression or visual loss when they are switched to

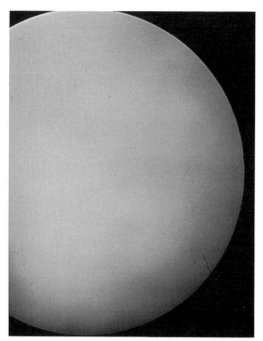

Figure 24.6.   Herpes zoster retinitis in a child with AIDS. Notice confluent nature of retinitis with a sharp demarcation border. This is typical of acute retinal necrosis syndrome of which this is an example.

oral therapy. Even when the switch is successful, it is probably wise to keep the patients on continuous anti-viral therapy.

Drug Toxicities

In addition to sight threatening retinal infections, patients may develop ocular complications as a result of the chemotherapeutic agents used to treat their infections. Patients being treated for tuberculosis with ethambutol, for example, can develop optic neuritis and should have their vision frequently monitored. In children that are old enough, vision should be checked on a monthly basis for the first 6 months of therapy and include a color vision test. In younger children, the optic nerve can be examined for signs of neuritis. Clofazimine used to treat atypical mycobacteria has been associated with macular pigmentary changes in a retinal bull's-eye configuration (34, 35). The exact incidence of this complication is unknown.

Recently we have become aware of the retinopathic effect of 2',3'-dideoxyinosine (ddI) (36). In a phase I-II study conducted

at the National Institute of Health, 43 children with symptomatic HIV infection (stage P-2) were entered in a dose escalation study. Three children developed a peripheral retinopathy when treated at 360 mg/m²/days or more, This dose is higher than the currently suggested daily dose of ddI. Lesions started to appear as early as 36 weeks after initiating therapy with ddI and did not cease until therapy was discontinued. Lesions were bilateral, located in the mid to far periphery of the eye, and characterized by small circumscribed areas of retinal and retinal pigment epithelium atrophy (Fig. 24.8). Sometimes they were sur-

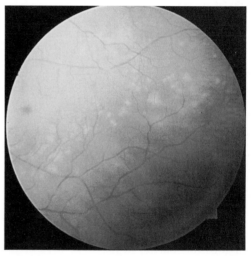

Figure 24.7.   Herpes zoster retinitis in a child with AIDS. Here there are multiple lesions located in deep retina. This particular form is often associated with severe compromise of retinal circulation and appearance of a cherry red spot in macula.

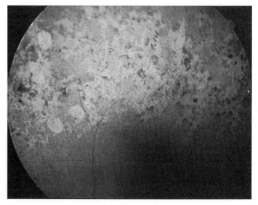

Figure 24.8.   Peripheral retinal and retinal pigment epithelial atrophy in a child being treated with ddI.

rounded by a ring of pigment hypertrophy, particularly in the case of older lesions. With time, the peripheral lesions tended to coalesce, whereas new lesions appeared more centrally. The electro-oculogram, a measure of retinal pigment epithelial function, was abnormal in one patient, indicating that the toxic effect of ddI was not restricted to the abnormal areas. We have not observed these changes at the lower ddI doses. We have also examined all adult patients treated at the National Institutes of Health with ddI and not found any retinal abnormalities. Nevertheless, all patients on ddI should be monitored periodically for signs of toxicity.

PREVENTION

Prevention of the ocular infections described above is not yet feasible. However, with proper screening and monitoring of the visual loss may be limited. Proper screening and monitoring require a close collaboration between all health professionals, the patient, and family. For each patient, the approach will need to be tailored to age and level of comprehension. Children must be monitored for signs of sight threatening infections, but also for evidence of aberrant visual development. Visual maturation is only achieved at age 8 years. Before then, any obstruction of the visual pathway or the appearance of an ocular deviation (strabismus) will lead to amblyopia. If noticed early enough, it can be corrected through a combination of means including glasses, patching, and eye muscle surgery.

Monitoring for signs of sight threatening disease is more difficult. Based on our experience at the National Institutes of Health, there is little likelihood of an older child developing CMV retinitis until his absolute T helper cell count falls below 100. Younger children may of course be at risk at higher absolute CD4 counts because of the age-specific differences in CD4 numbers. The probability of developing another type of retinal infection is so low that repeated screening of asymptomatic children is not cost effective and may give a false sense of security. However, once the CD4 count falls below 100, it is wise to be examined by an ophthalmologist to eliminate the presence of ocular

pathology. This is also a good time to instruct the parents on the early signs and manifestations of visual loss, and to teach them how to screen their child for the appearance of these signs. We suggest that these tests be performed on a weekly basis, but they can be performed more frequently since they do not require much time. Since the incidence of ocular complications is low, a dilated fundus exam is probably only required every 6 months, unless a patient develops visual complaints or shows signs of disease in other organs. We have seen patients, both adults and children with CMV pneumonitis, whose retinal infection went unrecognized for several weeks.

Infants cannot indicate that they have lost vision. An easy and useful exam of central visual function is to alternatively cover one eye then the other with the palm of a hand (or an opaque occluder). If the child has a significant visual impairment, he or she will either start to cry or try to push away the occluding hand when the unaffected eye is covered. The same test can be used in toddlers and young children who will not notice a unilateral visual impairment unless the normal eye is covered. Upon covering the eye, the child should be asked to describe what he or she is able to see. It is best for the examiner to cover the child's eye, because most children will otherwise try to cheat during the exam, and peak around their hand or through their fingers. Older children can perform the exam on their own, looking for the presence of an alteration in either the peripheral or central field of vision. This is best performed against a background with a grid-like quality. For distance, a newspaper held at arms' length may be useful, and an Amsler chart (Fig. 24.9) can be used to test the central visual field. Any distortion or fading of the lines indicates a potential problem. In all of these tests, remember that each eye must be tested independently since the visual fields of both eyes overlap in the central 90° of field.

FUTURE RESEARCH

Better antiviral agents are needed to treat patients with CMV retinitis. Agents that can be administered orally or subcutaneously would represent a major advance. Even

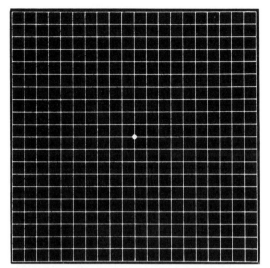

Figure 24.9. Amsler's chart. This grid can be used to test central visual field. Any distortion or disappearance of squares is an indication that there is retinal pathology.

more useful would be the development of a prophylactic because agent that could prevent the development of CMV retinitis because it is unlikely that a drug that will affect latent virus will be developed in the near future. Identification of risk factors may assist in deciding which patients would benefit from a periodic eye exam. Appropriate screening and monitoring schemes are also needed to follow and treat an increasingly diverse group of children infected with AIDS.

References

1. de Smet MD, Butler KM, Rubin Bl, et al. The ocular complications of HIV in the pediatric population. In: Dernouchamps JP, Verougstraete C, Caspers-Velu L, Tassignon MJ, eds. Recent advances in ureitus. Amsterdam: Kugler, 1993:315–320.
2. Chiama M, Blini M, Marchisio P, Plebani A, Bertoni G. Ophthalmic problems in pediatric patients with HIV infection [Abstract HB 2406]. Eighth International Conference on AIDS, Florence, Jun 1991:283.
3. Dennehy PJ, Warman R, Flynn JT, Scott GB, Mastrucci MT. Ocular manifestations in pediatric patients with acquired immunodeficiency syndrome. Arch Ophthalmol 1989;107:978–982.
4. Crowe SM, Carlin JB, Stewart Kl, Lucas CR, Hoy JF. Predictive value of CD4 lymphocyte numbers for the development of opportunistic infections and malignancies in HIV infected persons. J Acquir Immune Defic Syndr 1991;4:770–776.
5. Chan CC, Palestine AG, Davis JL, et al. Role of chorioretinal biospy in inflammatory eye disease. Ophthalmology 1991;98:1281–1286.
6. Davis JL, Nussenblatt RB, Bachman DM, Chan CC, Palestine AG. Endogenous bacterial retinitis in AIDS. Am J Ophthalmol 1989;107:613–623.
7. Brezin AP, Egwuagu CE, Burnier MJ, et al. Identification of toxoplasma gondii in paraffin embedded sections by polymerase chain reaction. Am J Ophthalmol 1990;110:599–604.
8. Brezin A, Girard B, Rosenheim M, Marcel P, Gentilini M, Le Hoang P. Cotton-wool spots and AIDS related complex. Int Ophthalmol 1990;14: 37–41.
9. de Smet MD, Nussenblatt RB. Ocular manifestations of AIDS. JAMA 1991;266:3019–3022.
10. Kestelyn P, Lepage P, Stevens AM, Van de Perre P. Ophthalmic manifestations of HIV infection in an African pediatric population. [Abstract TBP 203]. Fifth International Conference on AIDS, Montreal Jun 1989:321.
11. Kestelyn P, Lepage P, Van de Perre P. Perivasculitis of the retinal vessels as an important sign in children with AIDS-related complex. Am J of Ophthalmol 1985;100:614–615.
12. Belfort R Jr, de Smet M, Whitcup SM, et al. Ocular complications of Stevens Johnson syndrome and toxic epidermal necrolysis in patients with AIDS. Cornea 1991;10:536–538.
13. Jabs DA, Enger C, Bartlett JG. Cytomegalovirus retinitis and acquired immunodeficiency syndrome. Arch Ophthalmol 1989;107:75–80.
14. de Smet MD. Differential diagnosis of retinitis and choroiditis in patients with acquired immunodeficiency syndrome. Am J Med 1992;92:17–21.
15. Holland GN, Pepose JS, Pettit TH, Gottlieb MS, Yee RD, Foos RY. Acquired immune deficiency syndrome: Ocular manifestations. Ophthalmology 1983;90:859–873.
16. Palestine AG, Rodrigues MM, Macher AM, et al. Ophthalmic involvement in acquired immunodeficiency syndrome. Ophthalmology 1984;91: 1092–1099.
17. Pepose JS, Holland GN, Nestor MS, Cochran AJ, Foos RY. Acquired immune deficiency syndrome: Pathogenic mechanisms of ocular disease. Ophthalmology 1985;92:472–484.
18. Freeman WR, Lerner CW, Mines JA, et al. A prospective study of the ophthalmologic findings in the acquired immune deficiency syndrome. Am J Ophthalmol 1984;97:133–142.
19. Muccioli C, Belfort R Jr, Lottemburg C, et al. Quantitive assessment of aqueous flare in HIV infected patients with and without CMV retinitis. 3rd International Symposium on Uveitis, Brussels, 1992.
20. Palestine AG, Polis MA, de Smet MD, et al. A randomized, controlled trial of foscarnet in the treatment of cytomegalovirus retinitis in patients with AIDS. Ann Intern Med 1991;115:665–673.
21. Cochereau-Massin I, LeHoang P, Lautie-Frau M, et al. Efficacy and tolerance of intravitreal ganciclovir in cytomegalovirus retinitis in acquired immune deficiency syndrome. Ophthalmology 1991;98:1348–1353.
22. Smith TJ, Pearson PA, Blanford DL, et al. Intravitreal sustained-release ganciclovir. Arch Ophthalmol 1992;110:255–258.

23. Sanborn GE, Anand R, Torti RE, et al. Sustained-release ganciclovir therapy for treatment of cytomegalovirus retinitis. Use of an intravitreal device. Arch Ophthalmol 1992;110:188–195.

24. Butler KM, de Smet MD, Husson RN, et al. Treament of aggressive CMV retinitis with ganciclovir in combination with foscarnet in a child with human immunodeficiency virus infection. J Pediatr 1992;120:483–485.

25. Gagliuso DJ, Teich SA, Friedman AH, Orellana J. Ocular toxoplasmosis in AIDS patients. Trans Am Ophthalmal Soc 1990;80:63–86.

26. Holland GN. Ocular toxoplasmosis in the immunocompromised host. Int Ophthalmol 1989;13:399–402.

27. Cochereau-Massin I, LeHoang P, Lautier-Frau M, et al. Ocular toxoplasmosis in human immunodeficiency virus-infected patients. Am J Ophthalmol 1992;114:130–135

28. Lopez JS, de Smet MD, Masur H, Mueller BU, Pizzo PA, Nussenblatt RB. Orally administered 566C80 for treatment of ocular toxoplasmosis in a patient with the aquired immunodeficiency syndrome. Am J Ophthalmol 1992;113:331–333.

29. McLeish WM, Pulido JS, Holland S, Culbertson WW, Winward K. The ocular manifestations of syphilis in the human immunodeficiency virus type 1-infected host. Ophthalmology 1990;97:196–203.

30. Passo MS, Rosenbaum JT. Ocular syphilis in patients with human immunodeficiency virus infection. Am J Ophthalmol 1988;106:1–6.

31. Freeman WR, Gross JG, Labelle J, Oteken K, Katz B, Wiley CA. Pneumocystis carinii choroidopathy. A new clinical entity. Arch Ophthalmol 1989;107:863–867.

32. Rao NA, Zimmerman PL, Boyer D, et al. A clinical, histopathologic, and electron microscopic study of, *Pneumocystis carnii* choroiditis. Am J Ophthalmol 1989;107:218–228.

33. Margolis TP, Lowder CY, Holland GN, et al. Varicella-zoster virus retinitis in patients with the acquired immunodeficiency syndrome. Am J Ophthalmol 1991;112:119–131.

34. Craythorn JM, Swartz M, Creel DJ. Clofazimine-induced bull's-eye retinopathy. Retina 1986;6:50–52.

35. Cunningham CA, Friedberg DN, Carr RE. Clofazamine-induced generalized retinal degeneration. Retina 1990;10:131–134.

36. Whitcup SM, Butler KM, Caruso R, et al. Retinal toxicity in human immunodeficiency virus-infected children treated with 2',3'-dideoxyinosine. Am Ophthalmol 1992;113:1–7.

25
Lymphoid Interstitial Pneumonitis

Edward M. Connor and Warren A. Andiman

INTRODUCTION AND BACKGROUND

The initial clinical description of AIDS in infants and children included pulmonary diseases that were both severe and unique (1, 2). Among the first ten patients identified in Newark, three died of *Pneumocystis carinii* pneumonia (PCP) and/or cytomegalovirus pneumonitis, four had lymphoid interstitial pneumonitis (LIP), and three had desquamative interstitial pneumonia (DIP). As the number of human immunodeficiency virus-infected children increased, experience confirmed the initial observation that the respiratory tract is commonly affected in AIDS, second only to the immune system.

Pulmonary disease and progressive respiratory failure continue to contribute significantly to the morbidity and mortality of pediatric patients with HIV infection. Data collected prospectively document that over 80% of HIV-infected children develop lung disease at some time during their illness (3–5). These include acute, usually infectious, diseases (e.g., PCP, bacterial pneumonitis, etc.) and chronic pulmonary diseases (e.g., LIP, pulmonary lymphoid hyperplasia (PLH), etc.). In the discussion that follows we will focus on the latter of these groups, in particular LIP.

Overall, the chronic pulmonary diseases seen in children with HIV infection can be divided into two categories based on pathologic criteria: lymphoid lesions and nonlymphoid lesions.

Lymphoid Pulmonary Lesions

The group of diseases characterized principally by lymphoid infiltrates in the lung are common among HIV-infected children and represent a continuum from focal lymphocytic infiltration of lung paranchyma (PLH), to more diffuse infiltration of alveolar septae (LIP), and finally to neoplastic or paraneoplastic lymphoproliferative disease (e.g., polyclonal polymorphic B cell lymphoproliferative disorder).

Recently, it has been suggested that PLH/LIP may progress to neoplastic disease. Two patients from Newark have been described who initially had histologically proven PLH/LIP and at subsequent biopsy and autopsy were shown to have a polyclonal B cell lymphoproliferative disorder (6–8). A more recent report describes a 33-month child who developed disseminated Burkitt's lymphoma with lung involvement 11 months after he was first diagnosed with LIP (9.) It is unknown whether PLH/LIP complex will evolve to neoplastic lymphoproliferative disorders in greater numbers of children as they grow older, but the recognition of polyclonal B cell lymphoproliferative disorder suggests the possibility of this type of progression.

Before the recognition of pediatric AIDS, PLH/LIP was rare, having been described in only a few adults with autoimmune diseases, such as Sjögren's syndrome (10). Since the start of the AIDS epidemic in children, PLH/LIP has been frequently found in biopsy and autopsy specimens of lung tissue. As experience from multiple centers caring for children has increased, PLH/LIP has been recognized as a common and distinctive marker for HIV infection. As a result, PLH/LIP has now been included in the Centers for Disease Control (CDC) criteria for AIDS in children (11). PLH/LIP is now the most commonly described lesion seen in open lung biopsy and autopsy specimens from pediatric AIDS patients (12).

Nonspecific Nonlymphoid Pulmonary Lesions

DIP was one of the first lesions to have been reported in pediatric patients with AIDS (1). Although DIP was first thought to be part of the PLH/LIP complex, it is now considered a nonspecific pathologic process associated with lung injury. DIP has been described in cases of PCP and cytomegalovirus pneumonia as well as in cases of PLH/LIP. DIP is characterized by large intra-alveolar collections of mononuclear cells and cuboidal metaplasia of alveolar lung epithelium (12, 13). There are minimal to mild alveolar septal lymphoplasmacytic infiltrates and fibrosis but no necrosis, hyaline membranes, granulomas, lymphoid nodules, or virus inclusion bodies.

Diffuse alveolar damage is a destructive inflammatory lesion seen in HIV-infected patients as a secondary phenomenon, often as a consequence of advanced pulmonary infection or oxygen toxicity. The pathology of diffuse alveolar damage is nonspecific, showing both exudative and organizing stages of inflammation (14). Chronic passive congestion (CPC) is another commonly recognized pathologic process found in lung specimens from HIV-infected children. In particular, CPC has been identified in patients with congestive heart failure and AIDS-associated cardiomyopathy (15).

ETIOLOGY, PATHOLOGY, PATHOGENESIS, AND NATURAL HISTORY

The etiology and pathogenesis of PLH/LIP are not well understood. Histopathologic examination of PLH/LIP lesions have failed to demonstrate evidence of virus inclusions, fungi, parasites, pyogenic bacteria, or acid-fast bacilli (3, 8, 16). Suggested etiologies of PLH/LIP have included 1) an exaggerated immunologic response to inhaled or circulating antigens and/or 2) primary infection of the lung with HIV, Epstein-Barr virus (EBV), or both, or by another agent yet to be identified.

Pathologic Findings

PLH is characterized by peribronchiolar lymphoid nodules that have germinal centers. These nodules contain mature and immature lymphoid cells in the germinal centers, and plasma cells at the periphery. LIP is characterized by diffuse infiltration of the alveolar septae by both mature and immature lymphocytes, plasmacytoid lymphocytes, plasma cells, and immunoblasts (Fig. 25.1). Nodular aggregates of these cells are found occasionally, but there is no involvement of blood vessels nor destruction of lung architecture. Granuloma, consisting of pale mononuclear cells and multinucleated giant cells, are also sometimes seen. In some cases, the lesions are so severe focally that they obscure and distort the normal pulmonary architecture. PLH and LIP may overlap to a considerable extent (17, 18). Therefore the two terms will be used together throughout the remainder of the text.

The lymphoid infiltrates in PLH/LIP include both B cells and T cells, with CD8+ cells prodominating. In a study in which postmortem lung specimens from children with PLH/LIP were examined to determine lymphocyte phenotype using flow cytometry, 46% were B cells, 25% T helper (CD4+) cells, and 40% T cytotoxic/supressor (CD8+) cells (12). Immunoperoxidase stains for κ- and λ-light chains of immunoglobulins and phenotyping of cells extracted from the pulmonary lymphoid infiltrates of PLH/LIP demonstrated that their origin was polyclonal (19).

Pathogenesis

Lymphoid tissue is initially absent from the lungs of newborn infants and only develops after exposure to inhaled and/or circulating antigens. Progression of this normal developmental process into a pathologic state similar to PLH/LIP has been de-

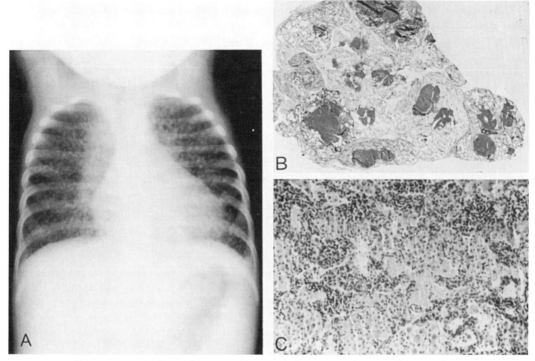

Figure 25.1. Radiographic (**A**) and histopathologic (**B, C**) features of PLH and LIP.

scribed in experimental animals exposed to aerosols of viruses and bacteria (20, 21). It has been postulated that PLH/LIP in patients with HIV infection may represent a delayed immunologic response to a circulating antigen or hypersensitivity to an inhaled antigen.

Immunologic Aspects

The HIV-infected child often displays significant immunologic abnormalities, including hypergammaglobulinemia, circulating immune complexes, and loss of immune regulation that occurs as a result of progressive depletion of CD4 lymphocyte function (1, 2, 16). In the immunocompromised child with repeated exposure to pulmonary infections, immune dysregulation may be involved in the development of the pathological lesions of PLH/LIP. The occurrence of PLH/LIP in some adults with autoimmune disorders (e.g., Sjögren's syndrome, systemic lupus, thyroiditis, myasthenia gravis, etc.) supports this immunologic theory.

Cytokines have been shown to play an important regulatory role in HIV replication and HIV pathogenesis. The role of cytokines in the pathogenesis of LIP is just beginning to be explored. Tumor necrosis factor (TNF) is known to up-regulate HIV replication, and overexpression of TNF has been described in adults with advanced disease and some children with encephalopathy (22–25). Recent studies, however, have shown TNF-α and interleukin-1 to be present in highest concentrations among pediatric patients with LIP (a relatively good prognostic indicator) when compared with other infected children (26, 27). It is unclear whether TNF-α is casually related to the pathogenesis of LIP or to the relatively good prognosis in these patients. TNF-α and interleukin-1 prime tissue macrophages for increased release of free oxygen radicals, and they may also be responsible for the enhanced production of immunoglobulins by B cells in children with LIP.

It has also been shown that children with LIP have much higher titers of a functional antibody that prevents HIV-1-induced syncytium formation when compared with children with opportunistic infections (28). Whether this is an epiphenomenon related to the hypergammaglobulinemia of pediatric AIDS or is an integral part of the pathogenesis of LIP is unknown.

Relationship among EBV, HIV-1, and LIP

There is evidence to suggest that the underlying cause of PLH/LIP may be primary infection of the lung with a specific infectious agent or combination of agents. In 1985, two reports appeared suggesting an association between EBV and the pathogenesis of LIP. Fackler et al. (29) described a 3-year girl who, at 11 months of age, developed tachypnea and diffuse pulmonary infiltrates (29). Examination of lung biopsy material revealed pathologic findings consistent with LIP, and EBV DNA was found in lung tissue by dot-blot hybridization using probes prepared from the Bam HI-W repeat fragment of the virus genome. Long-standing persistent infection with EBV was documented by identification of EBV DNA in her saliva at 7 months of age and repeated recovery of transforming virus from the patient's peripheral blood mononuclear cells over 2.5 years. Although the patient developed high titers of heterophile antibodies at 10 months of age, EBV-specific serologic responses were delayed until 14 months of age.

Andiman and coworkers (30) examined, by Southern blot hybridization, lung biopsy specimens from 17 patients with AIDS. In ten patients the histologic diagnosis was LIP, whereas in the remaining seven children, opportunistic pathogens were discovered. EBV DNA was discovered in eight of the ten biopsies showing LIP but in none of the seven biopsies from patients with opportunistic infections of the lung. Rubinstein et al. (3) have made similar observations. In some specimens the lymphoproliferations were shown to be polyclonal by the use of immunoblobulin gene probes. The group of patients with LIP also showed remarkable EBV antibody responses that were consistent with chronic active EBV infection, such as high levels of antibody to the replicative antigens of the virus (viz, viral capsid antigen and early antigen). In contrast, many children with LIP, was well as those with opportunistic infections of the lung, have defective serologic responses to the Epstein-Barr nuclear antigen, specifically that

component encoded by the Bam HI K fragment of the virus genome. This antigen is invariably recognized by normal EBV-seropositive individuals. That EBV is not merely a passenger virus associated with the florid lymphoproliferations so characteristic of LIP was shown more recently by Katz et al. (31). By using a case control method, it was shown that all ten children with lymphoproliferative disorders (LIP 7, nonHodgkin's lymphoma 3) had EB virus serologic profiles consistent with either a primary or reactivated EBV infection compared with only 15% of matched control patients. These data strongly suggest that active EBV infection occurs in children with AIDS whose tissue samples contain EBV genome material.

Viewed in toto these studies imply that EBV plays a significant pathogenetic role in LIP. LIP has long been considered to reflect the local response to a persistent antigenic stimulus; that stimulus might be EBV. EBV is a potent, polyclonal stimulus of B cells (32). Many of the cells found in hyperplastic areas of lung tissue from patients with LIP are B cells. The germinal follicles (the B cell cell areas) within lymph nodes from patients with LIP are almost always hyperplastic as well. The high antibody titers to the early and capsid antigens of EBV found so often in patients with LIP suggest that extensive viral replication is occurring, perhaps within epithelial or lymphoid cells in the lower respiratory tract. It is known that HIV replication is enhanced in EBV-transformed lymphoblasts and that HIV RNA has been found in lungs of patients with AIDS (33, 34). There is experimental evidence that EBV resides in the lung and that it may be associated with some episodes of pneumonitis of ill-defined etiology or with other unusual pulmonary conditions (35–37). HIV-1 has been found in pulmonary macrophages of patients with AIDS and infectious HIV, and HIV-specific immunoglobulin has been detected in bronchoalveolar lavage fluid from adult Haitian women with LIP (38). Coinfection of pulmonary macrophages by both EBV and HIV or of EBV-stimulated B cells by HIV may provide sufficient antigenic stimulation of surrounding cells to precipitate the progressive pathologic changes observed in patients with LIP (33, 34).

Finally, HIV is genetically related to maedi/visna, a pathogenic lentivirus that produces a chronic lymphocytic interstitial pneumonia of sheep. Maedi infection of the lung produces a proliferative lymphocytic and plasma cell infiltration of the lung parenchyma. Similarly, infected sheep have enlarged lymph nodes. Recently, alveolar macrophages have been implicated as important targets in the pathogenesis of ovine lentivirus-induced LIP (39). The number of infected alveolar macrophages and the virus load has been shown to reflect the severity and pathologic manifestations of LIP in sheep.

Whether PLH/LIP is an immunologic process or a primary pulmonary infection, studies to date suggest that its occurrence is over-represented among children with perinatal HIV rather than HIV that is acquired by other routes. PLH/LIP has been reported to occur in 25–40% of symptomatic children who acquire HIV perinatally. Conversely, autopsy studies of adults with HIV show that only 3% develop PLH/LIP (this may be an underestimate of the true incidence in this population) (40). It also appears that patients with transfusion-acquired HIV are less likely to develop PLH/LIP; among 25 cases of transfusion-acquired HIV in children followed in Newark, only three (12%) developed histologically confirmed PLH/LIP.

A discrepancy between the incidence of PLH/LIP in perinatal HIV infection vs. HIV infection acquired by other routes might, theoretically, be explained by direct intrauterine or intrapartum exposure of lung tissue to HIV or other agents. This concept is supported by data from the newborn lamb model in which, after direct intratracheal inoculation of ovine lentivirus, animals develop PLH/LIP. These newborn lambs subsequently have a clinical course typical of children with PLH/LIP (41). Animal models have also shown that the neonatal lung macrophage is immature, may be more permissive of HIV infection, and may serve as a reservoir for HIV (42).

Based on analysis of these collective data, one can speculate that PLH/LIP represents a primary infection of lung tissue, acquired either in utero or at the time of delivery, as a result of aspiration of HIV contained in amniotic fluid or in blood and genital secretions. Subsequent clinical and histopathological expression may be driven by postnatally acquired EBV infection, especially if such infections occur in the first several years of life.

Many pediatric patients in the United States at risk for PLH/LIP are of African-American decent, and many live in crowded urban settings. There may be genetic and socioeconomic factors in these at-risk populations that influence the development of PLH/LIP complex. Before the advent of the HIV epidemic, adult patients whose PLH/LIP occurred in association with autoimmune diseases were noted to be predominantly African-American (43). After assuming that EBV is involved in PLH/LIP pathogenesis, it is noteworthy that EBV infects many inner city children at a young age, corresponding to the time when PLH/LIP becomes clinically recognized for the first time. Data regarding the geographic variation of the incidence of PLH/LIP are limited. Experience has shown that PLH/LIP occurs among HIV-infected children in Europe and Africa, but details regarding the frequency and distribution of cases are not available. In one series of 107 HIV-infected pediatric patients from Rwanda, 24 (22.4%) were found to have radiographic evidence of LIP (44).

Natural History

The natural history of PLH/LIP is incompletely understood. Available data would suggest that early in the clinical course patients have histopathologic and radiographic evidence of pulmonary disease but may be asymptomatic. The rate at which patients progress from this initial stage to symptomatic disease is variable. Some remain clinically stable for long periods.

Many patients who develop symptoms have a course marked by slowly progressive chronic pulmonary disease, punctuated by the occurrence of intercurrent pulmonary infections that result in episodes of respiratory decompensation. Despite this, children with PLH/LIP have a relatively good prognosis compared with other children who meet the CDC surveillance definition of AIDS; several studies have demonstrated that children with PLH/LIP have a significant survival advantage over those with PCP. By using data from cohort studies in Miami, survival after the diagnosis of PLH/LIP has been estimated to be ~72 months (45). Figure 25.2 illustrates this survival advantage for children with LIP in a cohort followed at AIDS Clinical Trials Group centers before antiretroviral agents were available for treatment of children.

Although PLH/LIP causes substantial morbidity, the contribution that it makes to mortality among children with AIDS is uncertain. The cause of death among children with PLH/LIP is more often intercurrent infection, or other known complications of HIV, rather than PLH/LIP itself. Although some children who survive PCP may subsequently develop PLH/LIP, the reverse appears to be less common. This may reflect the more "normal" immunologic state of patients who present with PLH/LIP as their first manifestation of HIV infection rather than any intrinsic protection afforded by PLH/LIP against PCP. The long-term morbidity associated with PLH/LIP is now well

recognized. Some older survivors of PLH/LIP have been noted to develop pulmonary neoplasms (see "Introduction and Background"), and some have developed bronchiectasis (6, 46–50).

Although most children with PLH/LIP have a slowly progressive clinical course, it has recently been suggested that PLH/LIP may, on occasion, remit naturally. Longitudinal follow-up of children in Newark with radiographic evidence of PLH/LIP has identified several patients in whom the typical nodular pattern has resolved over time without treatment (51).

CLINICAL PRESENTATION

Table 25.1 lists the pulmonary lesions found in 40 children from the Children's Hospital AIDS Program in Newark who had lung biopsy and/or autopsy specimens obtained. In this program, before the introduction of antiretroviral therapy, PLH/LIP occurred in over 40% of symptomatic HIV-infected children at some time during their clinical course. Some children with acute

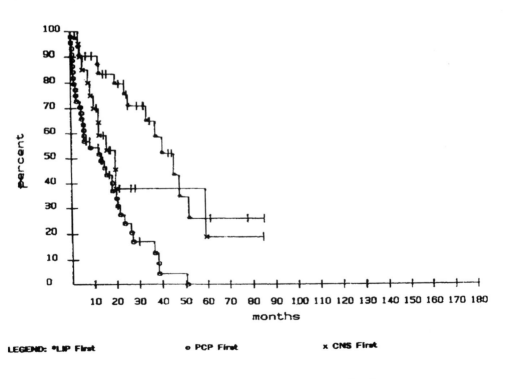

Figure 25.2.   Survival from diagnosis of HIV.

Table 25.1.   Types of Pulmonary Lesions in 40 HIV-infected Children with AIDS Based on Biopsy or Autopsy Specimens

Type of Lesions	Number of Cases[a]
PLH/LIP complex	22
Polyclonal polymorphic B cell lymphoproliferative disorders	2
DIP	5
Diffuse alveolar damage	7
Chronic passive congestion and/or edema	4
Nonspecific minimal abnormalities	2
B cell lymphoma	1
Bacterial pneumonia	1
Opportunistic infection	19
P. carinii	12
Cytomegalovirus	5
Aspergillus	2
Total	65

[a]Several cases had more than one diagnosis.

progressive pneumonia were selected for lung biopsy to confirm the presence of *P. carinii* or another infectious agent; other patients with chronic progressive pulmonary disease were evaluated because PLH/LIP was suspected on clinical grounds. The frequency of pulmonary diagnoses listed in Table 25.1 is similar to that reported from other large pediatric HIV centers (3, 45).

PLH/LIP may be the first clinical manifestation of HIV infection in children. Although described in infants as young as 2 months, PLH/LIP is usually diagnosed in children with perinatally acquired HIV who are older than 1 year. In contrast, PCP is diagnosed typically in the first year of life (47, 48).

Data obtained from prospective case series suggest that PLH/LIP initially presents as chronic infiltration of the lungs, unaccompanied by clinical symptoms. It often occurs in association with lymphoid proliferation and hypertrophy at other sites; typically patients with PLH/LIP have generalized lymphadenopathy and may also have hepatosplenomegaly and parotid enlargement (3, 50, 51). Pulmonary compromise occurs as a result of superimposed recurrent infections and progressive infiltration of the lung; these may be accompanied by right-sided heart failure. Tachypnea, cough, wheezing, and hypoxemia are usual signs of the fully expressed disease. In the absence

of superimposed acute bacterial pneumonia, rales are infrequent. Clubbing is a characteristic feature as PLH/LIP advances. Pulmonary function tests usually reveal impaired gas flow, a reduction in V_{max} as measured by partial forced exhalation and diminished lung compliance (52). Patients with PLH/LIP can progress to chronic respiratory failure.

Children who have had PLH/LIP for several years demonstrate progressive changes on chest X-ray that accompany their clinical deterioration. The radiographic characteristics of PLH/LIP are described below. Longstanding PLH/LIP may ultimately be associated with chronic bronchiectasis and may mimic end-stage cystic fibrosis. Chronic respiratory decompensation and hypoxemia are often associated with poor weight gain.

The evolution of PLH/LIP is typically more indolent and chronic than that of most opportunistic (e.g., PCP) and bacterial infections of the respiratory tract. At times, however, this clinical distinction may be difficult. CMV pneumonitis or pulmonary tuberculosis, for example, may present in a subacute or chronic manner, similar to that of PLH/LIP. Pulmonary infection with *Mycobacterium tuberculosis* shares many clinical and radiographic features of PLH/LIP, has commonly been found in adults with AIDS, and is being recognized with increasing frequency in HIV-infected children (53–56).

PLH/LIP may be complicated by superinfection with bacterial, viral, or other pathogens. Among the most common bacterial pathogens isolated have been *Hemophilus influenzae*, *Staphylococcus aureus*, and *Streptococcus pneumoniae*, and various enteric Gram-negative bacilli. These secondary bacterial infectious are usually associated with acute excacerbations in pulmonary symptoms. *Pseudomonas aeruginosa* has been isolated from fatal, necrotizing pneumonia at autopsy (57, 58).

Compared with the child with PCP, the child with PLH/LIP usually has a greater elevation in serum immunloglobulin levels and lower (but elevated over normal) levels of lactate dehydrogenase (46). Blood gas analysis and serial cutaneous oxygen saturation determinations reflect the clinical progression of this disease and the development of hypoxemia and respiratory alkalosis.

DIAGNOSTIC CONSIDERATIONS

Pulmonary diseases that occur in association with HIV infection encompass a wide spectrum from acute, often infectious processes to more indolent diseases such as PLH/LIP. The acute infectious pulmonary diseases seen in the HIV-infected child often have distinctive clinical presentations which help the clinician in diagnosis. In contrast, the chronic pulmonary diseases associated with HIV present a much greater diagnostic dilemma. As mentioned earlier, the chronic and acute patterns may overlap when the child with PLH/LIP develops acute symptoms from superimposed infection, cardiac decompensation, or fluid and electrolyte imbalances. The discussion below focuses on the specific diagnosis of PLH/LIP and the differentiation of PLH/LIP from other causes of subacute and chronic respiratory disease.

Clinical features alone are usually insufficient to differentiate PLH/LIP from other causes of pulmonary disease. Findings such as dyspnea, cough, abnormal chest X-ray, and a restrictive pulmonary pattern with hypoxia may be common to many processes (44, 59). In contrast, digital clubbing is found more specifically in the HIV-infected child with longstanding hypoxia caused by PLH/LIP.

Imaging Techniques

The chest X-ray is often the initial diagnostic procedure used to evaluate the child with suspected PLH/LIP. The CDC has set criteria for the radiographic diagnosis of PLH/LIP to be used for surveillance purposes. Here, the presence of a reticulonodular pattern, with or without hilar adenopathy, that persists on chest X-ray for 2 months or greater and that is unresponsive to antimicrobial therapy is considered presumptive evidence of PLH/LIP. Figure 25.1 illustrates the typical radiographic appearance of PLH/LIP. In clinical practice, interpretation of the chest X-ray vis-à-vis diagnosis of LIP may be difficult. Care must be taken to exclude other possible etiologies, and radiologic expertise with pediatric HIV cases is important.

Although the presence of a consistent and reproducible reticulonodular pattern has been shown to correlate with the pathologic diagnosis of PLH/LIP, the differentiation of PLH/LIP from other causes of pulmonary infiltrates cannot reliably be made using chest radiography alone (60). Consequently, additional studies are often required to eliminate alternative etiologies. Other imaging modalities have added little to the sensitivity and specificity of chest X-ray for the diagnosis of LIP. In most cases of PLH/LIP, gallium lung scans show increased uptake in affected areas and have been used to guide selection of a site for open lung biopsy. However, gallium scans may also be positive in patients with PCP and other infectious processes and are therefore nonspecific (61). The definitive diagnosis of PLH/LIP can only be made by histopathology (6, 12, 60, 62, 63). In some cases of histopathologically proven PLH/LIP, the chest X-ray may be normal despite the presence of significant symptomatology.

Examination of Respiratory Secretions

Examination of tracheal secretions, induced sputum, and bronchoalveolar lavage (BAL) fluid has been used successfully to establish the etiology of many pulmonary infections. Respiratory secretions should be obtained for histologic examination and culture in HIV-infected children with acute, subacute, or chronic abnormalities on chest X-ray in whom a diagnosis has not been established by other means. Material should be evaluated for a wide range of potential pathogens including *P. carinii*, bacteria, viruses, fungi, and acid-fast bacilli.

With the recent resurgence of tuberculosis, it is important that this diagnosis be carefully considered in all patients with pulmonary findings. Diagnostic workup should include the placement of purified protein derivative skin test with controls for anergy epidemiologic evaluation, and examination of gastric aspirates or respiratory secretions (depending on the age of the child) for acid-fast bacilli. Children should also be considered candidates for a diagnostic BAL.

Although respiratory secretions have sometimes contained HIV and/or HIV-specific antibodies, neither has proven to be useful in establishing the diagnosis of PLH/LIP (62–66). Studies from Paris have suggested that examination of BAL fluid from patients with PLH/LIP reveal significantly higher numbers of lymphocytes and significantly lower numbers of polymorphs than are found in association with PCP; in some PLH/LIP patients, BAL fluids also contain increased numbers of CD8+ cells (67, 68). Because these studies are preliminary, no criteria have been established to define PLH/LIP by this procedure. Thus, if infectious agents cannot be found in BAL fluid, one would normally need to plan a more invasive procedure for diagnosis.

Biopsy

Because currently available radiographic procedures and BAL fluids are not specific for PLH/LIP, definitive diagnosis requires a biopsy. If, in the HIV-infected child with pulmonary symptoms and an abnormal chest X-ray, an infectious etiology cannot be established by examination of respiratory secretions (tracheal aspiration, induced sputum, BAL) and the patient continues to have respiratory deterioration, an open lung biopsy should be performed. Histologic examination of lung biopsy specimens is also the only definitive means to evaluate the patient for pulmonary neoplasm, an uncommon but reported pulmonary complication of HIV infection.

Evaluation of HIV-infected children with pulmonary abnormalities requires a systematic and thorough approach. Figure 25.3 illustrates one possible approach to the HIV-infected child who presents with an abnormal chest X-ray.

MANAGEMENT AND TREATMENT

Once the diagnosis of PLH/LIP complex is established, management becomes a life-long challenge for the patient, medical personnel, and family. PLH/LIP can usually be treated in the outpatient setting. Currently, treatment consists of antiretroviral agents to control the underlying HIV infection, symptomatic pulmonary therapy, and the use of corticosteriods to suppress the pulmonary lymphocytic infiltration and, possibly, to modify cytokine production (69, 70).

Early in the course of PLH/LIP patients may fail to show respiratory symptoms and are managed expectantly. Throughout the course, general supportive care should be provided to optimize the health status of the patient and to minimize pulmonary damage from intercurrent infections and the complications of end-organ failure. Attention should be paid to the patient's overall nutritional status, and correctable causes of anemia (e.g., iron deficiency) should be addressed. In addition, measures directed at the prevention of respiratory infections, such as immunization against influenza, should be considered. Pneumococcal and *H. influenzae* type B conjugate vaccines should be given routinely. Intercurrent respiratory tract infections should be managed aggressively to minimize pulmonary injury and abnormalities of cardiac function. HIV-infected children should routinely be tested for tuberculosis, using purified protein derivative skin tests and appropriate anergy controls.

Anticipatory management also includes monitoring the patient for disease progression. This includes serial clinical evaluations, chest X-rays, pulse oximetry, and pulmonary function testing. As children with PLH/LIP progress, they may develop hypoxemia and require supplemental oxygen. This can usually be accomplished in the home setting.

Children with PLH/LIP are considered to have symptomatic HIV infection and, therefore, should receive antiretroviral treatment. The effects of antiretroviral therapy on the development of PLH/LIP and on the course of PLH/LIP are areas of current investigation. Such agents may have a direct beneficial effect, if PLH/LIP is driven by HIV, or may be indirectly effective if there is amelioration of the associated immunological abnormalities (71–73). In the years since primary therapy for HIV has become available for children, the frequency of LIP among children with AIDS (<13 years of age) reported to the CDC has declined from 27.7 to 20.6% (Fig. 25.4). It is unclear if this trend will be maintained and if it is a result of changes in reporting, alteration of disease manifestations, or a direct effect of antiretroviral treatment.

It had been proposed in the past that acyclovir might have a beneficial effect on the course of PLH/LIP by affecting the natural

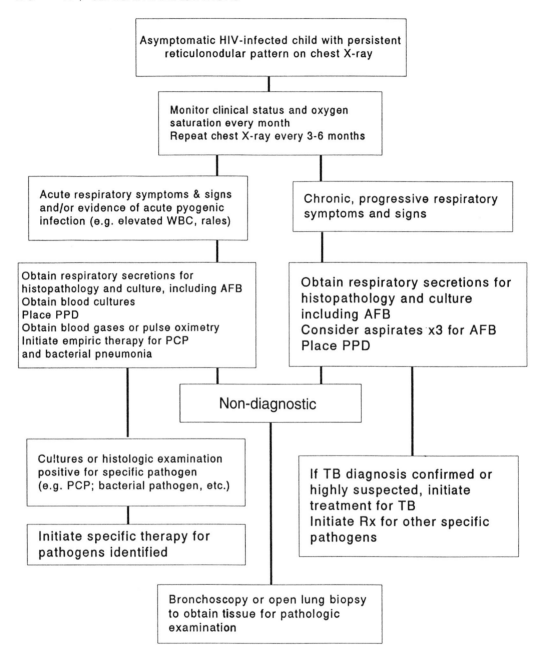

Figure 25.3.   General approach to evaluation of HIV-infected children with persistent reticulonodular pattern on chest X-ray. *WBC*, white blood cell; *AFB*, *TB*, tuberculosis; *PPD*, purified protein derivative.

course of the associated EBV virus infection. Acyclovir acts only during the lytic cycle of EBV infection, not on the latent phases. Thus, during EBV-associated infectious mononucleosis, acyclovir reduces oropharyngeal shedding of the virus but does not affect the number of immortalized B cells in the peripheral blood. There have been no formal studies on the state of the virus (i.e., EBV) in the lymphoid infiltrates of PLH/LIP. In addition, there have been no controlled, empiric trials of acyclovir in patients with PLH/LIP.

Although no controlled studies have been performed, there is a developing consensus that steroids are involved in the care

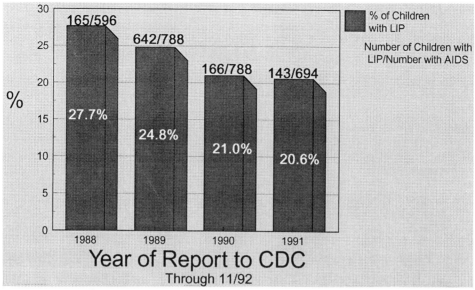

Figure 25.4.   LIP among pediatric AIDS cases reported to CDC.

of the child with progressive PLH/LIP. This therapy has been associated with improvement in respiratory symptoms and oxygenation (70, 72). At the Children's Hospital of New Jersey, in Newark, children with PLH/LIP are candidates for systemic corticosteroid therapy if they have signs and symptoms of chronic pulmonary disease (i.e., digital clubbing) and/or hypoxemia, as evidenced by arterial oxygen tension <85–90 mmHg. One such protocol includes an initial 4- to 12-week course of prednisone (2 mg kg/day) followed by a tapering dose, using O_2 saturation and clinical status as a guide to improvement (73). Many patients are then maintained on a chronic daily or every other day regimen of low dose prednisone (10–20 mg every day or every other day). It is important to use steroids with caution, especially in the setting of a changing respiratory picture where concurrent infections may be present. However, PLH/LIP patients who develop an acute exacerbation of their disease, especially as a result of superimposed viral pneumonia, often respond dramatically to a brief steroid burst (5–7 days), followed by a taper to their regular dose. One should only consider using steroids in patients with PLH/LIP that has been definitively diagnosed, and treatment should only be instituted by medical personnel experienced in the treatment of HIV-infected children. Children placed on systemic corticosteroid treatment for PLH/LIP should also be given PCP prophylaxis.

The role of anti-inflammatory agents other than glucocorticoids in the treatment of LIP is unknown. Theoretically, if elevated local cytokines (e.g., TNF) play a causal role in the development of PLH/LIP, agents that suppress their production could be of benefit. However, if increased cytokine production is related to longer survival of children with LIP, this approach may be counterproductive. Preliminary studies of the TNF inhibitor, pentoxifylline, as adjunctive therapy in adult patients with AIDS have shown promise. This agent and other anti-inflammatory agents have not been studied in children with AIDS.

Children with PLH/LIP who are receiving antiretroviral therapy and steroids and who continue to progress are candidates for re-evaluation of the etiology of their pulmonary disease, including consideration for repeat BAL or biopsy. If no new infectious etiologies are found, such patients may also be candidates for alternative antiretroviral therapy.

Although pulmonary function data from adults with PLH/LIP typically demonstrate a restrictive pattern, many children with PLH/LIP develop wheezing and evidence of an obstructive component to their pulmonary disease. Bronchodilator therapy using nebulized β_2 drugs, such as albuterol and metaproterenol, have proven beneficial in selected cases (52, 70).

Some long term survivors of PLH/LIP have progressed to a state of chronic respiratory insufficiency, similar to that seen in patients with cystic fibrosis. These children experience recurrent or chronic bacterial infections of the respiratory tract, and some have developed bronchiectasis and micro abscesses. Chronic antibiotic administration and chest physical therapy may be beneficial. The assistance of a pediatric pulmonologist is required by many children with advanced PLH/LIP.

In addition to infectious causes, acute respiratory deterioration of the child with PLH/LIP may occur because of episodes of pulmonary edema or congestive heart failure. Right-sided failure may occur as a result of ever increasing resistance in the pulmonary vascular bed. Cardiomyopathy has been documented to be a complication of HIV infection in children and may explain some of these episodes (15). Treatment consists of diuretics and, at times, inotropic drugs (e.g., digoxin).

Some children with PLH/LIP have exaggerated levels of γ-globulin that can result in hyperviscosity syndromes that may exacerbate the symptoms of PLH/LIP. There are no studies that have defined the frequency of hyperviscosity in HIV-infected children or its role in the pathogenesis of end-organ failure resulting from vaso-occlusive phenomena. In a small number of children, we have seen both clinical and X-ray evidence of pulmonary edema without underlying heart disease; this may be related to local pulmonary vascular hyperviscosity (74).

PREVENTION

Prevention of PLH/LIP is linked to the prevention of HIV infection itself; this subject is discussed elsewhere. Once HIV infection occurs, symptomatic PLH/LIP appears to be a late event in the clinical course of some children. Therefore, prevention of PLH/LIP could theoretically be accomplished by primary treatment of HIV infection with antiretroviral agents. If PLH/LIP

is the result of aspiration of the retrovirus in utero or at the time of delivery, as the lamb model might suggest, one could speculate about several additional potential preventive strategies. Expectant and vigorous antibiotic therapy and immunization against respiratory pathogens such as influenza, pneumococcus, and *H. influenzae* type B may prevent some infectious complications of PLH/LIP. Steroids may prevent or delay some late complications of the disease. Administration of intravenous γ-globulin may be used to prevent some respiratory infections in children with PLH/LIP (75, 76).

AREAS FOR FUTURE RESEARCH

Some questions regarding PLH/LIP that will require active research are practical, and some are theoretical. First, the etiology, pathogenesis, and natural history of PLH/LIP must be more fully investigated, and the role played by EBV requires further consideration. This is essential to devise targeted therapeutic approaches and to measure their efficacy. In addition, alternatives to the histopathologic diagnosis of PLH/LIP must be explored. Although the chest radiograph is used commonly as a diagnostic tool, there are no clearly established standards for radiographic interpretation. The application of molecular biologic techniques to the examination of lung tissue and of cells from bronchiolar lavage may be potentially useful in the diagnosis of PLH/LIP. Prognostic factors and/or staging of PLH/LIP would be helpful in selecting appropriate patients for therapeutic intervention (e.g., use of steroids, bronchodilators, prophylactic antibiotics, intravenous γ-globulin) and for predicting their course.

One could speculate about many novel approaches to the treatment of PLH/LIP. If PLH/LIP reflects, at least in part, a primary pulmonary infection by HIV, then the use of topically administered antivirals may be a less toxic alternative to systemic therapy. The role of inhaled steroids, as presently employed in asthma, may have a palliative role in the treatment of PLH/LIP while avoiding the potential side effects of systemic use.

The number of HIV-infected infants and children is expected to increase by

5000–8000 each year in the United States (77, 78). Current trends in treatment include institution of antiretroviral therapy early in HIV infection. The impact of early antiretroviral therapy on the development of PLH/LIP and its natural history is unknown and is an important area for clinical investigation.

References

1. Oleske J, Minnefor A, Cooper R, et al. Immune deficiency syndrome in children. JAMA 1983; 249:2345–2346.
2. Rubinstein A, Sislick M, Gupta A, et al. Acquired immunodeficiency with reversed T4/T8 ratios in infants born to promiscuous and drug-addicted mothers. JAMA 1983;249:2340–2346.
3. Rubinstein A, Morecki R, Silverman B, et al. Pulmonary disease in children with acquired immune deficiency syndrome and AIDS-related complex. J Pediatr 1986;108:498–503.
4. Centers for Disease Control. Update: Acquired immunodeficiency syndrome—United States. MMWR 1986;35:757–759.
5. Vernon DD, Holzman BH, Lewis P, et al. Respiratory failure in children with acquired immunodeficiency syndrome and acquired immunodeficiency syndrome related complex. Pediatrics 1988; 82:223–229.
6. Anderson VM, Lee H. Lymphocytic interstitial pneumonitis in pediatric AIDS. Pediatric Pathol 1988;8:417–421.
7. Joshi VV, Kauffman S, Oleske JM, el al. Polyclonal polymorphic B-cell lymphoproliferative disorder with prominent pulmonary involvement in children with AIDS. Cancer 1987;59:1455–1462.
8. Montes M, Tomasi TB, Noehren TH, Culver GJ. Lymphoid interstitial pneumonia with monoclonal gammopathy. Ann Rev Respir Dis 1968; 98:272–280.
9. Young SA, Crocker DW. Burkitt's lymphoma in a child with AIDS. Pediatr Pathol 1991;11:115–122.
10. Boccon-Gibod L, Sacre JP, Just J, et al. Lymphoid interstitial pneumonia in children with AIDS or AIDS-related complex. Pediat Pathol 1986;5:238–240.
11. Centers for Disease Control. Classification system for HIV infection in children under 13 years of age. MMWR 1987;36:225–236.
12. Joshi VV, Oleske JM, Minnefor AB, et al. Pathological pulmonary findings in children with the acquired immunodeficiency syndrome: A study of ten cases. Hum Pathol 1985;16:241–246.
13. Stillwell PC, Norris DG, O'Connell EJ, et al. Desquamative interstitial pneumonitis in children. Chest 1980;77:165–172.
14. Askin F, Katzenstein A. *Pneumocystis carinii* infection masquerading as diffuse alveolar damage. A potential source of diagnostic error. Chest 1981;79:420–423.
15. Joshi VV, Gadol C, Connor E, et al. Dilated cardiomyopathy in children with AIDS. Hum Pathol 1988;19:69–73.
16. Scott GB, Buck BE, Letterman JG, Bloom FL, Parks WP. Acquired immunodeficiency syndrome in infants. N Engl J Med 1984;310:76–81.
17. Kradin RL, Mark J. Benign lymphoid disorders of the lung, with a therapy regarding their development. Hum Pathol 1983;14:857–867.
18. Joshi VV, Morrison S, Connor EM, Marquis J, Oleske JM. Pulmonary pathology of acquired immune deficiency syndrome in children. In: Stocke JT, ed. Pediatric pulmonary disease. New York: Hemisphere Publishing, 1989:187–206.
19. Joshi VV, Oleske JM. Pulmonary lesions in children with the acquired immunodefciency syndrome: A reappraisal based on data in additional cases and follow-up study of previously reported cases. Hum Pathol 1986;17:641–642.
20. Milne RW, Bienerstock J, Perey DY. The influence of antigenic stimulation in the ontogeny of lymphoid aggregates and immunoglobulin-containing cells in mouse bronchial and intestinal mucosa. J Reticuloendothel Soc 1975;17:361–367.
21. Emery JL, Dinsdal F. Increased incidence of lymphoreticular aggregates in lungs of children found unsuspectedly dead. Arch Dis Child 1974;49:107–111.
22. Merrill, JE. Cytokines and retroviruses. Clin Immunol Immunopathol 1992;64:23–27.
23. Poli G, Fauci A. The effect of cytokines and pharmacologic agents on chronic HIV infection. AIDS Res Hum Retroviruses 1992;8:191–197.
24. Dezuke B, Pardee A, Beckett LA, et al. Cytokine dysregulation in AIDS: In vivo overexpression of mRNA of tumor necrosis factor-α and its correlation with that of the inflammatory cytokine GRO. J Acquir Immune Defic Syndr 1992;5:1099–1103.
25. Mintz M, Rapaport R, Olekse JM, et al. Elevated serum levels of tumor necrosis factor are associated with progressive encephalopathy in children with acquired immunodeficiency syndrome. Am J Dis Child 1989;143:771–774.
26. Ellaurie M, Rubinstein A. Tumor necrosis factor α in pediatric HIV-1 infection. AIDS 1992;6:1265–1268.
27. Arditi M, Kabat W, Yogev R. Serum tumor necrosis factor-alpha, interleukin 1-beta, p24 antigen concentrations and CD4+ cells at various stages of human immunodeficiency virus 1 infection in children. Pediatr Infect Dis J 1991;10:450–455.
28. Brenner TJ, Dahl KE, Olson B, et al. Relation between syncytium inhibition antibodies and clinical outcome in children. Lancet 1991;337:1001–1005.
29. Fackler JC, Nagel JE, Adler WH, et al. Epstein-Barr virus infection in a child with acquired immunodeficiency syndrome. Am J Dis Child 1985;139:1000–1004.
30. Andiman WA, Eastman R, Martin K, et al. Opportunistic lymphoproliferations associated with Epstein-Barr viral DNA in infants and children with AIDS. Lancet 1985;2:1390–1393.
31. Katz BZ, Berkman AB, Shapiro ED. Serologic evidence of active Epstein-Barr virus infection in Epstein-Barr virus-associated lymphoproliferative disorders of children with acquired immunodeficiency syndrome. J Pediatr 1992;120:228–232.

32. Chyat KJ, Harper ME, Marselle LM, et al. Detection of HTLV-III RNA in lungs of patients with AIDS and pulmonary involvement. JAMA 1986;256:2356–2359.

33. Lane HC, Mansur H, Edgar LC, et al. Abnormalities of B-cell activation and immunoregulation in patients with acquired immunodeficiency syndrome. N Engl J Med 1985;309:453–458.

34. Montagnier L, Gruest J, Chamaret S, et al. Adaption of lymphadenopathy associated virus (LAV) to replication in EBV-transformed B lymphoblastoid cell lines. Science 1984;225:63–66.

35. Lung ML, Lam WK, So SY, et al. Evidence that the respiratory tract is a major reservoir for Epstein-Barr Virus. Lancet 1985;1:889–892.

36. Vergnon JM, Vincent M, de The G, et al. Cryptogenic fibrosing alveolitis and Epstein-Barr virus: An association? Lancet 1984;2:768–770.

37. Andiman WA, McCarthy P, Markowitz R, et al. Clinical, virologic and serologic evidence of Epstein-Barr virus infection in association with childhood pneumonia. J Pediatr 1981;99:880–886.

38. Resnick L, Ptichenik AE, Fisher E, et al. Detection of HTLV-III/LAV-specific IgG and antigen in bronchoalveolar lavage fluid from two patients with lymphocytic interstitial pneumonitis associated with AIDS-related complex. Am J Med 1987;82:553–556.

39. Brodie SJ, Marcom LD, Pearson LD, et al. Effects of virus load in the pathogenesis of lymphoid interstitial pneumonitia. J Infect Dis 1992;166:531–541.

40. Marchesvsky A, Rosen MJ, Chrystal G, Kleinerman J. Pulmonary complications of the acquired immunodeficiency syndrome: A clinicopathologic study of 70 cases. Hum Pathol 1985;16:659–670.

41. Laimore MD, Rosadro RH, DeMortine JC. Ovine lentivirus lymphoid interstitial pneumonia—rapid indication in neonatal lambs. Am J Pathol 1986;125:177–181.

42. Beinestock J. Bronchus-associated lymphoid tissue. Int Arch Allergy Appl Immunol 1985;76 (suppl 1):62–69.

43. Lin RY, Gruber PJ, Saunder R, Perla EN. Lymphocytic interstitial pneumonitis in adult HIV infection. NY State J Med 1988;88:273–276.

44. Lepage P, Van de Perre P. Clinical manifestations in infants and children. Baillieres Clin Trop Med Commun Dis 1988;3:89–101.

45. Scott GB, Hutto C, Markuch RW, et al. Survival in children with perinatally acquired human immunodeficiency virus type 1 infection. N Engl J Med 1989;321:1971–1976.

46. Krasinski K, Borkowsky W, Bonk S, et al. Bacterial infections in human immunodeficiency virus-infected children. Pediatr Infect Dis J 1988;7:323–329.

47. Parks WP, Scott BG. An overview of pediatric AIDS: Approaches to diagnosis and outcome assessment. In: Broder S, ed. AIDS: Modern concepts and therapeutic hallogens. New York: Marcel Dekker, 1987:245–262.

48. Rogers MF, Thomas PA, Staricher ET, Nod MC, Bush TJ, Jaffe HW. Acquired immunodeficiency syndrome in children. Report of the CDC national surveillance, 1982 to 1985. Pediatrics 1987;79:1008–1014.

49. Thomas PA, O'Donnell RE, Lessner L. Survival analysis of children reported with AIDS in New York City, 1982-1986 [Abstract]. Third International Conference on AIDS, Washington, DC, Jun 1987.

50. Minnefor AB, Oleske JM. Pneumonitis in acquired immune deficiency syndrome (AIDS). In Hughes W, Laraya-Cuasay LR, eds. Interstitial lung diseases in children. vol 2. Boca Raton, FL: CRC Press, 1985:49–55.

51. Pahwa S, Kaplan M, Fikrig S, et al. Spectrum of human T-cell lymphotropic virus type III infection in children recognition of symptomatic, asymptomatic and seronegative patients. JAMA 1986;255:2299–2305.

52. Grieco MH, Chinoy-Acharya P. Lymphocytic interstitial pneumonia associated with the acquired immune deficiency syndrome. Am Rev Respir Dis 1985;131:952–955.

53. Sunderman G, McDonald RJ, Maniatis T, Oleske JM, Kapila R, Reichman LB. Tuberculosis as a manifestation of the acquired immunodeficiency syndrome. JAMA 1986;256:362–366.

54. McSherry G, Berman C, Aguila H, Oleske J, Santiago T, Connor E. Tuberculosis in HIV-infected children in Newark 1981–1992 [Abstract 905]. 32nd International Conference on Antimicrobial Agents and Chemotherapy, Anaheim, 1992.

55. Moss W, Dedyo T, Suarez M, Nicholas S, Abrams E. Tuberculosis in children infected with human immunodeficiency virus: A report of five cases. Pediatr Infect Dis J 1992;11:114–120.

56. Khouri Y, Mastrucci M, Hutto C, Mitchell C, Scott G. Mycobacterium tuberculosis in children with human immunodeficiency virus type 1 infection. Pediatr Infect Dis J 1992;11:950–955.

57. Vernon DD, Holzman BH, Lewis P, et al. Respiratory failure in children with acquired immunodeficiency syndrome and acquired immunodeficiency syndrome related complex. Pediatrics 1988;82:223–228.

58. Joshi VV, Oleske JM. Pathology of AIDS in children. In: Wormser GP, Stahl RE, Bottore EJ, eds. AIDS and their manifestations of HIV infection. Park Ridge, NJ: Noyes, 1987:915–934.

59. White DA, Matthaj RA. Noninfectious pulmonary complications of infection with the human immunodeficiency virus. Am Rev Respir Dis 1989;140:1763–1787.

60. Zimmerman BL, Haller JO, Price AP, Thelno WL, Fikrig S. Children with AIDS: Is pathologic diagnosis possible based on chest radiographs? Pediatr Radiol 1987;17:303–307.

61. Schiff RG, Kabal L, Kamani N. Gallium scanning in lymphoid interstitial pneumonitis of children with AIDS. J Nucl Med 1987;28:1915–1919.

62. Foglia RP, Shilyansky J, Fonkal EW. Emergency lung biopsy in immunocompromised pediatric patients. Ann Surg 1989;210:90–92.

63. Resnick L, Pitchenik AE, Fisher E, Croneg R. Detection of HIV-III/LAV specific IgG and antigen in bronchoalveolar lavage fluid from two patients

with LIP associated with AIDS-related complex. Am J Med 1987;82:553–556.

64. Teirstein AS, Rosen MJ. Lymphocytic interstitial pneumonia. Clin Chest Med 1988;9:467–471.

65. Bigby TD, Margolskee D, Curtis JL, et al. The usefulness of induced sputum in patients with the acquired immunodeficiency syndrome. Am Rev Respir Dis 1986;133:515–518.

66. Dean NC, Golden JA, Evans LA, et al. Human immunodeficiency virus recovery from bronchoalveolar lavage fluid in patients with AIDS. Chest 1988;93:1176–1179.

67. Solal-Celigny P, Couderc LK, Herman V, et al. Lymphoid interstitial pneumonitis in acquired immunodeficiency syndrome-related complex. Am Rev Respir Dis 1985;131:956–960.

68. deBlic J, Blanche S, Danel C, et al. Bronchoalveolar lavage in HIV infected patients with interstitial pneumonitis. Arch Dis Child 1989;64: 1246–1250.

69. Rubinstein A, Berstein LJ, Caytan M, Krieger BZ, Ziprkouski M. Corticosteroid treatment for pulmonary lymphoid hyperplasia in children with AIDS. Pediatr Pulmonol 1988;4:13–17.

70. Oleske JM, Connor EM, Minnefor AB, Graffino DB, Ugazio AG. AIDS: Treatment of HIV-infected infants and children. In: Stroder J, Meitens C, Eichenwald H, eds. Current therapy in pediatrics. 2nd ed. Philadelphia: BC Decker, 1989:476–480.

71. Bach MC. Zidovudine for lymphocytic interstitial pneumonia associated with AIDS. Lancet 1987; 2:655–661.

72. Kornstein MJ, Pietra GG, Hoxie JA, et al. The pathology and treatment of interstitial pneumonitis in two infants with AIDS. Am Rev Respir Dis 1986;133:1196–1198.

73. Oleske JM, Connor EM, Grabenau M, Minnefor AB. Treatment of HIV infected infants and children. Ann Pediatr 1988;17:332–339.

74. Lania-Howarth M, Graffino D, Oleske J, Connor E. Blood viscosity measurements in children with HIV infection. J Allergy Clin Immunol 1990;85: 148.

75. Siegal FP, Oleske JM. Management of the acquired immune deficiency syndrome: Is there a role for immune globulin? In: Morell A, Nydeggar AE, eds. Clinical use of intravenous immunoglobulins. London: Academic, 1986:373–384.

76. Calvelli T, Rubenstein A. Intravenous gamma-globulin in infant acquired immunodeficiency syndrome. Pediatr Infect Dis J 1986; 5:5207–5211.

77. Gwinn M, Robers M, Berkelman R, et al. Incidence of pediatric AIDS in the USA; predictions from seroprevalence data [Abstract]. Fifth International Conference on AIDS, Montreal, Jun 1989.

78. Oleske JM. The child with HIV infection: Dilemmas in management. AIDS Med Rep 1990; 3:19–22.

26
Cardiovascular Problems

Steven E. Lipshultz

Most clinical cardiovascular disease in human immunodeficiency virus (HIV)-infected children has been underreported and is often clinically occult, and signs and symptoms are erroneously attributed to other organ systems. Cardiac disease was initially noted in adults with HIV infection by echocardiography but was thought to be "clinically unobtrusive" and not related to mortality (1). Early adult autopsy series demonstrated unremarkable cardiovascular findings including uncommon patchy mononuclear infiltration of the heart or rare intracardiac infectious organisms (2). There remains a poor cardiac structure-function relation, although pathologic lesions of the heart in HIV infection encompass the entire range of cardiac involvement, from disease of the pericardium, epicardium, and myocardium to the endocardium. Cardiac involvement may occur at any stage of HIV infection, and although generally not clinically significant, it may result in life-threatening situations, and may be difficult to diagnose clinically. However, with increased length of survival of HIV-infected children there has been more cardiac morbidity and mortality detected. Quantitative testing of the cardiovascular system is helpful for patient management. Many protean cardiovascular manifestations that often become clinically significant are easily detected using proper technology (3). Over 90% of HIV-infected children have cardiovascular abnormalities on testing, although this figure may reflect patients referred for testing (4). The preclinical detection of cardiovascular abnor-

malities results in early therapeutic interventions and reduces cardiovascular morbidity and mortality. Cardiac disease may be important in the natural history and prognosis of HIV infection.

EPIDEMIOLOGIC CONSIDERATIONS
Congenital Structural Heart Defects

Noncardiac teratogenic effects of HIV resulting in a dysmorphic syndrome have been suggested but not proven (5, 6). One study, uncontrolled for other possible confounding factors (7), reported that the incidence of structural heart defects in infants born to HIV-seropositive mothers was significantly higher (2.8%) than in historical reports from populations studied before the HIV epidemic (0.8%) and included some children with defects requiring surgery (8, 9). Another pediatric center noted congenital heart disease in 4 of 133 HIV-infected patients (3%) (10). We have also detected congenital structural heart defects in children with perinatally acquired HIV infection. Several of our children have had congenital structural heart defects resulting in significantly increased blood flow to the lungs that contributed to increased difficulty improving from respiratory infections. It is unknown whether these congenital structural heart defects are more likely to cause problems in HIV-infected children compared with uninfected children whose mothers were infected or with non-HIV-infected children with similar defects. Whether the reported higher incidence of congenital structural heart defects is the re-

483

sult of fetal HIV infection during primary cardiac development (first trimester), the nonspecific response to a fetus developing within an HIV-infected mother, or the result of other maternal cofactors, such as cocaine use (7), malnutrition, sexually transmitted diseases, or smoking, is unknown.

Decisions regarding surgical management of HIV-infected children with significant congenital structural heart disease are difficult. Although palliative procedures and ligation of a patent ductus arteriosus should be performed as clinically warranted, it is less clear whether complete repair of complex heart disease should be performed in all HIV-infected children, especially when palliative options exist. Although an ethically correct position may be to simply treat all children the same without regard to HIV status, one must be careful to do no harm. HIV-infected patients appear at higher risk than uninfected patients for hemodynamically significant reactions with procedures and medications (4, 11–18). Further, questions have been raised whether the protracted severe immune dysregulation induced by cardiopulmonary bypass may render patients undergoing this procedure as part of a complete repair more susceptible to HIV infection or result in progression to more advanced HIV infection in those already infected (19–22). Clearly the risk-to-benefit ratio of performing complete definitive surgical repairs using cardiopulmonary bypass in children with complex heart disease is unknown at this time. Therefore, as Vogel (9) has stated, decisions regarding surgical options for such children should be made on an individual basis.

Left Ventricular Dysfunction

Figure 26.1 illustrates the changes in cardiac structure and function we have observed in HIV-infected children over time and compares them with changes in weight as a marker of HIV disease progression. These parameters are expressed as z scores, which allows standardization for children of different ages or body sizes to allow comparison of abnormalities with time. Figure 26.1 should be referred to throughout this chapter to more completely understand the in-

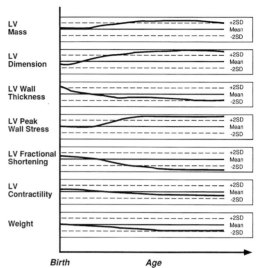

Figure 26.1. Changes in left ventricular (*LV*) structure and function in HIV-infected children as a function of age. Z scores are used for each parameter and indicate position of each measurement relative to normal population expressed as standard deviations from population mean. Reporting data as Z scores adjusts for effects of variation in age and body size. Body weight is listed as a noncardiac marker of stage of HIV disease. Data represent an assimilation of available information.

terrelatedness of these cardiovascular abnormalities and to appreciate that no incidence study thus far can adequately describe the degree of cardiovascular involvement in pediatric HIV because changes are progressive.

The Centers for Disease Control (CDC) did not feel in 1990 that the incidence of cardiovascular complications of HIV infection could be accurately assessed (23). Some investigators believe that the cardiac morbidity rate in adults with AIDS has remained constant at 6–7% since the epidemic began (24, 25). Another preliminary report suggested that over 4.5 years, 7.5% of 93 adults with AIDS developed congestive heart failure (26). A prospective study of 244 HIV-infected adults with initially normal echocardiograms indicated that during 640 patient-years of follow-up (21 months), 26% of patients developed new echocardiographic abnormalities each year that became clinically symptomatic with heart failure, pericardial effusion requiring drainage, obstructive intracardiac mass, symptomatic ventricular tachycardia, and aborted sudden death at a rate of 7% of all patients each year (27). Another prospective study confirmed that cardiac disease is more common in HIV-infected patients (28). The presence of any cardiac abnormality was detected in 40.6% of 101 HIV-infected adults vs. 12.5% in 24 healthy controls ($P = 0.003$), and echocardiographic abnormalities were noted in 28.7 vs. 12.5% ($P = 0.04$) (28).

Left ventricular dysfunction is emerging as the most important cardiac manifestation of HIV infection (29–35). At the Boston Children's Hospital, 29% of HIV-infected children (9/31) had a reduced left ventricular fractional shortening, and this was significantly more common with symptomatic HIV infection (4); 74% (17/23) of children with symptomatic HIV infection had left ventricular dysfunction, and 44% (10/23) had symptoms of cardiovascular compromise in another study (36). A follow-up study on 172 perinatally infected children noted "cardiomyopathy" (acute and subacute presentations characterized by heart failure, cardiomegaly, ventricular hypertrophy, and ST or T wave abnormalities) occurring at any time except initial presentation in 23 (14%) children with a median age at diagnosis of "cardiomyopathy" of 22 months (range 6–84 months) (37).

Left ventricular dilation with systolic dysfunction was noted in 45% of children with symptomatic HIV infection (38). In another series of HIV-infected children, left ventricular dilation was noted in 30%, left ventricular dysfunction in 18%, and congestive heart failure in 10% (6/61). This was associated with endomyocardial biopsy diagnoses of myocarditis in two, borderline myocarditis in one, and "dilated cardiomyopathy" in three children (39). Left ventricular dilation resolved in 33%, and the dysfunction improved in 25% of children. However, left ventricular abnormalities were more likely to persist and be associated with symptoms than right ventricular abnormalities or pericardial effusions (39). The 88 children with relatively advanced symptomatic HIV infection in the initial multicenter phase II evaluation of azidothymidine (AIDS Clinical Trials Group 043) underwent serial echocardiography, which demonstrated decreased ventricular function in 21% of children and ventricular dilation in 34%, and 14% of these children required medical therapy for cardiovascular abnormalities (40).

Hyperdynamic Left Ventricular Systolic Function

Forty-five percent (19/42) of HIV-infected children at Boston Childrens Hospital had hyperdynamic fractional shortening on initial evaluation (4, 41, 42). On follow-up 62% had a reduction in function. This pattern was noted in children at all stages of HIV infection and included all patients with high-grade ectopy, sudden unexplained death and four of five patients with evidence of cardiac or neural inflammation at autopsy. Unusual heart rate and blood pressure variability as well as exaggerated responses to medications were seen in these patients. Autonomic function testing in selected patients demonstrated enhanced sympathetic tone. This appears to be a common finding in early pediatric HIV infection, is often associated with autonomic instability, and may be a marker for arrhythmia or sudden death (4, 41). Hyperdynamic left ventricular function was also noted in 19% of children with early HIV infection by others (43).

Depressed Contractility

Autopsy studies note that up to 25% of HIV-infected adults had "dilated cardiomyopathy" (24) and up to 52% had myocarditis (44). Some studies have stated that 50% of HIV-infected adults with "dilated cardiomyopathy" will die within 6 months (45, 46). Left ventricular dysfunction in HIV-infected patients has frequently been referred to as "cardiomyopathy," which may be too general a term to use. We prefer to restrict the use of the term cardiomyopathy to conditions where primary heart muscle dysfunction (depressed left ventricular contractility) is present. Numerous other secondary causes of left ventricular dysfunction may not be due to depressed contractility but rather to the effects of other organ systems or noncardiac physiology on cardiac function, and therefore these causes do not represent cardiomyopathy or cardiac muscle dysfunction (47). Using measurements of ventricular function dependent on loading conditions, one group found that HIV-infected children were significantly more likely to have "cardiomyopathy" when HIV nephropathy or hemolytic anemia were present (10). Both these conditions are associated with markedly abnormal ventricular loading conditions, and it is therefore unclear if the term "cardiomyopathy" is justified in that case. For example, the natural history of changes in cardiac structure and function in HIV-infected children has been referred to as "dilated cardiomyopathy" because there was progressive left ventricular dilation that resulted in excess ventricular afterload, which reduced left ventricular function (48, 49). However, ventricular contractility remained normal, and therefore this was a secondary process and not a cardiomyopathy. The distinction is important because recommendations to obtain invasive endomyocardial biopsies or to withhold potentially lifesaving treatments can be based on the assumption that all ventricular dysfunction reflects primary myocardial disease and, most of the time, it does not (47). We reported that although 93% of HIV-infected children had abnormal ventricular function, only 26% actually had depressed contractility (4, 42).

Congestive Heart Failure

Stewart et al. (50) described two patterns of congestive heart failure in HIV-infected children. Children diagnosed with heart failure during severe, acute, systemic illness represented most patients followed. These patients were generally later in the course of HIV infection, had a more fulminant course at the time of diagnosis with congestive heart failure, and died 2 months after diagnosis of multisystem organ failure. Prompt treatment of congestive heart failure diagnosed during less severe illness resulted in a more indolent course with survival for >1 year after diagnosis with a significantly improved quality of life.

Acute extracardiac disease (e.g., renal failure with hypertension, adrenal insufficiency, adult respiratory distress syndrome, and bacterial sepsis) that could have af-

fected cardiac function has been noted at the time of diagnosis of congestive heart failure in some HIV-infected children (50). Ten percent of patients at Boston Children's Hospital exhibited transient congestive heart failure requiring treatment for <30 days and generally in the setting of other intercurrent illnesses (12, 13, 51).

Chronic congestive heart failure occurred in an additional 10% of patients at our institution (12, 13, 51). The fact that 20% of children at our center developed transient or chronic congestive heart failure is quite high. The cumulative incidence is so high that when some global projections for pediatric HIV incidence at the turn of the century are used (e.g., up to 10 million (52)), the incidence of congestive heart failure in this population might exceed the current rate of congestive heart failure in the entire adult population of the United States (53) by the year 2000. Risk factors for the development of congestive heart failure in HIV-infected adults have been reported (54).

Abnormalities of Cardiac Growth

At autopsy all 11 hearts from children with AIDS demonstrated hypertrophy and enlargement in weight and/or size (55–57). Hypertrophy was indicated by nuclear enlargement and increased diameter of myocardial fibers, and left ventricular endocardial thickening was detected (55–57). Mean heart weight from HIV-infected children at our institution was 184% of the predicted normal weight and was increased for all children despite all children being significantly malnourished (4, 42, 48, 58–61).

Arrhythmias and Electrocardiographic Abnormalities

Arrhythmias occurred in 35% of HIV-infected children followed at Boston Children's Hospital (12, 13, 51). The types of arrhythmias included atrial ectopy in 25%, premature junctional beats in 4%, premature ventricular beats in 15%, ventricular tachycardia in 2%, and ventricular fibrillation in 1%. Marked sinus arrhythmia was present in 17% of children. Ventricular tachycardia was documented in association with abnormal autonomic function in one patient (12, 13, 51). A wide range of other electrocardiographic findings were noted in children we have followed, including conduction disturbances, abnormalities of rate and chamber enlargement or hypertrophy, and ST and T wave abnormalities (4). At another center, significant arrhythmias were noted in three of 250 HIV-infected children and included second-degree atrioventricular block in a child with a nontoxic digoxin level; another child had frequent episodes of sinus arrest, and the third child had an automatic atrial tachycardia (9). Fifty-five percent of children with symptomatic HIV infection had electrocardiographic abnormalities that included ventricular hypertrophy in 36% of children and one child with complete right bundle branch block (38). Another study of electrocardiogram and Holter abnormalities in HIV-infected children suggested that routine electrical monitoring may be indicated to detect subclinical heart disease that might have been progressive (62). That study demonstrated that 6 of 15 patients had electrocardiographic abnormalities; for four of them there was no other evidence of cardiovascular involvement, and one of four children, who was otherwise asymptomatic from a cardiac perspective, subsequently developed congestive heart failure (62).

Electrocardiographic abnormalities were noted in 51% of children with symptomatic HIV-infection enrolled in a multicenter trial, ACTG 043, and included rhythm disturbances in 24%, atrial enlargement in 5%, conduction abnormalities in 48%, ventricular hypertrophy in 17%, and ST and T wave changes in 33% (40). Sixty-five percent (15/23) of HIV-infected children at one center had electrocardiographic abnormalities including left ventricular hypertrophy in six children, sinus tachycardia in six children, nonspecific ST and T wave changes in five children, right axis deviation in two children, right ventricular hypertrophy in six children, and right atrial enlargement in one child (63). Rhythm disturbances were noted in three patients and included frequent uniform ventricular premature beats (>250/hr), sick sinus syndrome, and second degree heart block (63). At another pediatric center 24 of 80 children (30%) had significant electrocardiographic abnormalities (20 ventricular hypertrophy, 1 right bundle branch block, 1 atrial flutter, 1 ventricular premature beats, 1 QTc prolongation) (43). Children with prenatal cocaine exposure and no known HIV infection have a 12-fold higher risk of cardiology consultation for arrhythmia compared with children without such exposure (64). Therefore, other factors must be considered before attributing arrhythmias in HIV-infected children to HIV. A prospective study of HIV-infected adults found no significant differences in abnormalities on the electrocardiogram when compared with healthy controls (28).

Hemodynamic Abnormalities

Abnormalities of heart rate also appeared in this population (4, 12, 13, 51). Resting sinus tachycardia was noted in 64% of 81 HIV-infected children followed serially and was felt to be an early finding in HIV disease. Sinus bradycardia was noted on serial evaluation in 11% of these patients. Nineteen percent of infected children at the Boston Children's Hospital had hypertensive episodes that were temporally associated with infection, medication, renal failure, central nervous system hemorrhage, or congestive heart failure. Twenty percent of patients we have followed had hypotension that was temporally related to infections, medications, respiratory arrest, and pericardial effusion with congestive heart failure, among other causes. Drug hypersensitivity reactions resulting in hemodynamic abnormalities have been noted in HIV-infected patients (65).

Unexpected Arrest

We have observed eight unexpected cardiorespiratory arrests in seven of the first 81 HIV-infected children (9%) at our center (12, 13, 51). One arrest was fatal and was associated with pericarditis, myocarditis, and inflammation of the cardiac conduction system (4). For other children, arrests were temporally related to flushing a central line, medications, respiratory infection, sepsis, or had no known association (12, 13, 51). Encephalopathy was the most significant correlate of cardiorespiratory arrest, perhaps reflecting autonomic nervous system dysfunction (12, 13, 51). Two HIV-infected children with cytomegalovirus (CMV) coinfection had an unanticipated cardiac arrest as a terminal event (21, 67). Seven other infected children were reported with sudden death (62, 66). Myocytes from some of these children were noted to have HIV, and there were histories of myo- and pericardial disease for all children (66). At autopsy that patient was noted to have CMV pancarditis including the intracardiac conduction system that was felt to relate to sudden death. Bharati et al. (56) have examined the hearts of six children who died of AIDS and noted abnormalities of the intracardiac conduction system consisting of vasculitis, myocarditis, or fragmentation of the bundle with lobulation and fibrosis. Sudden unexpected death has been noted in HIV-infected adults (44, 68). Sudden death was documented on Holter monitoring of an adult with HIV myocarditis and began as polymorphic ventricular tachycardia (69).

"Cardiac Death"

Although there are over 30 known causes of cardiac lesions in HIV-infected patients who have died, a pathogen is identified in less than one-third of documented cases (23). Thirty-seven percent of HIV-infected children we studied died during our study. For 33% of patients who died, death was associated with marked cardiac dysfunction; one child had a sudden death presumed secondary to dysrhythmia, and the remaining nine had significantly depressed ventricular function before death (13). Congestive heart failure in HIV-infected adults is fatal in 85% of cases (26). Adults with cardiac manifestations had greater mortality than those without cardiac involvement (70). The cardiac mortality rate associated with HIV infection in the United States is estimated to be 1–6% of infected patients (24). Cardiac abnormalities were seen in two-thirds of 700 HIV-infected patients at autopsy and could not be explained for the majority (71). Twenty-five percent of HIV-infected children who died at one center had an immediate cause of death of "cardiomyopathy" or sudden unexplained death. However, 83% of children that died at that same center had premorbid arrhythmias or "cardiomyopathy" (43).

Vascular Disease

Severe microvascular disturbances, characterized clinically by reduced microcirculatory perfusion, have been described in adults with HIV (72). We have had several HIV-infected children with peripheral vascular perfusion abnormalities clinically reminiscent of the vasospastic disorder, Raynaud's phenomenon. Vascular changes were found in all six hearts examined at autopsy from children with AIDS (56). Changes observed were detected in small arteries, arterioles, and venules. In the arteries, they involved the intima, media, and adventia and perivascular areas in a degenerative and inflammatory process. The elastic tissue was especially affected. Two types of arteriopathy were noted in HIV-infected children; inflammatory and fibrocalcific (73). The inflammatory arterial lesions were seen in the brain of children with HIV encephalopathy. The fibrocalcific lesions were noted in the heart and other organs and consisted of intimal fibrosis with elastic fragmentation and medial fibrosis and calcification resulting in luminal narrowing of small and medium-sized arteries and thought to be more common in children with longer survival times. Fusiform aneurysms of the coronary artery were seen with luminal thrombosis and fatal myocardial infarction (73). Striking coronary artery lesions, some proving fatal, were noted in eight young (23–31 years) HIV-infected adult patients (74). We have had two young HIV-infected children with myocardial infarction and have seen coronary artery dilation in other infected children that was accompanied by ventricular dysfunction. Endothelial cell dysfunction has been noted in HIV-infected patients (75), and we have noted what appears to be HIV-infected endothelial cells in an HIV-infected child with cardiovascular involvement (61). Recurrent Kawasaki disease, a syndrome of findings that includes vasculitis, was associated with coinfection with parvovirus B19 and HIV-1 in a child (76).

Pericardial Disease

Pericardial effusions resulting in tamponade and/or sudden death have been reported in several HIV-infected children and were associated with the presence of HIV (66). Most reports of pericardial disease are in children with relatively advanced HIV disease that may bias the data. Pericardial effusion was noted in 51% of HIV-infected children but was transient for over half of affected patients on serial echocardiography (39). The ACTG 043 study cohort had pericardial effusion noted in 16% of HIV-infected children (40). Five of 23 HIV-infected children (22%) in another study had moderate pericardial effusions associated with ventricular dysfunction (36). Pericardial effusion was noted in four of 22 children with symptomatic HIV infection (18%) (38). A recent large series noted pericardial effusion in 13–58% of HIV-infected children, and 69% of these children with effusion had associated cardiac abnormalities (ventricular dilatation and/or hypertrophy, myocarditis, or pericarditis) (77). Additionally, pericardial effusion was often seen in infected children with pleural effusion or ascites (77).

There is a high prevalence of pericardial disease in HIV-infected patients that may be associated with high morbidity or mortality but is frequently responsive to treatment or interventions when recognized early (1, 45, 54, 70, 77–85). Pericardial effusion has been described during all stages of HIV infection, both with and without opportunistic infections and with malignancy. Pericardial effusion with HIV is frequently seen, and its clinical spectrum is broad (86). Of 187 hospitalized adults with known pericardial effusion 7% were known to be HIV infected with small to large effusions or tamponade. Mortality for that group was 29%, and two patients had endocarditis, one had lymphoma, and one had a myocardial infarction. Twenty-eight percent of all adults undergoing pericardiocentesis recently at one urban hospital were HIV infected, and an etiology was established in 71% of infected patients, with mycobacterial disease occurring most frequently (78).

Cardiac Tumor

Primary cardiac lymphoma has been noted most commonly in the pericardium, but has also been seen in the myocardium or subendocardium, may result in conges-

tive heart failure or arrhythmias, and may be more common in patients with mononuclear infiltrative lung disease (87–94). Malignant lymphoma of the heart is rare but is being encountered with increased frequency and should be considered in HIV-infected patients with the sudden onset and rapid progression of cardiac symptoms (95). Metastatic cardiac involvement is seen in up to 20% of adults with lymphoma (96). Kaposi's sarcoma limited to the heart has been noted (97), but pericardial or cardiac involvement is more common in metastatic or disseminated Kaposi's sarcoma in adult HIV-infected patients (44, 70, 98–105). Cardiac localization of this malignancy has been reported in one child (106).

Endocarditis

For both adults and children the incidence of endocardial abnormalities is less than that of myocardial or pericardial findings with HIV. An HIV-infected child with congestive heart failure has been reported with endocarditis of the aortic valve at age 4 months (50), and another infected child had nonbacterial thrombotic endocarditis of the mitral valve (107). Similar findings of nonbacterial thrombotic endocarditis have been noted in HIV-infected adults (1, 98, 99). Fungal endocarditis (108, 109) and pyogenic bacterial endocarditis (2) have been noted in adults with HIV infection. Bacterial endocarditis in HIV-infected adults is often related to *Staphylococcus aureus* (over 75% of cases), *Streptococcus pneumoniae*, and *Haemophilus influenzae* (110). Fungal endocarditis is often spread from an extracardiac source and pathogens include *Aspergillus*, *Candida*, and *Cryptococcus neoformans* (71, 79). Patients with advanced HIV disease with endocarditis have a 40% mortality compared with a 10% in asymptomatic HIV-infected patients (110).

Pulmonary Hypertension

Pulmonary hypertension can occur secondary to left ventricular dysfunction, repeated respiratory infections, or thromboembolic disease. Two of 47 (4%) HIV-infected children had evidence of increased right ventricular pressure, but this was transient for both children and thought to be related to pulmonary complications (39). Pulmonary hypertension was noted in four children with symptomatic HIV infection and repeated pulmonary infections (17% of the cohort) (36). Another study found evidence of pulmonary hypertension in two of 22 (9%) infected children (38). Cor pulmonale and pulmonary hypertension were noted at the time of diagnosis in a 10-year child with perinatally acquired HIV infection (111). Severe pulmonary hypertension and cor pulmonale of unclear etiology, out of proportion to the mild restrictive lung disease, has been noted in some adults with AIDS (112).

RISK FACTORS

Stage of HIV Disease

The relationship of clinical cardiac symptoms and signs, congestive heart failure, and abnormalities on noninvasive testing to the stages of HIV infection remains incompletely elucidated. Prevalence and severity of cardiac abnormalities related to HIV infection may vary according to the stage of HIV infection (45). Adults with cardiac symptoms were more likely to have more advanced HIV infection (26, 113), female gender, and opportunistic infections (70). In adults the prevalence of echocardiographic abnormalities was similar in AIDS-related complex and AIDS patients except for pericardial effusion, which was more common with AIDS (70, 85). Dilated "cardiomyopathy" was more commonly noted in adults with advanced HIV disease in contrast to isolated dilatation of either ventricle, which generally occurred at an earlier stage of HIV infection and was transient (114). One study of infected adults showed no relation of left ventricular dysfunction with CD4 counts (115). For others, echocardiographic abnormalities were more common in adults with CD4 counts $\leq 100/mm^3$, in hospitalized patients, and in patients with *Pneumocystis* pneumonia (45, 84). However, there is conflict regarding the relationship between absolute CD4 counts and the incidence of cardiac abnormalities (45, 112). Another study of adults has found no correlation between HIV staging, CD4 cell count,

acute illness, or severity of illness and the presence of cardiac abnormalities (28).

We have found that the stage of pediatric HIV disease was associated with the occurrence of cardiovascular problems in infected children (12, 13, 51). Cardiac abnormalities were more frequent and severe in patients with advanced HIV disease. Asymptomatic status was not a significant correlate of any adverse cardiac event. AIDS-related complex, defined as symptomatic patients who did not fulfill CDC criteria for AIDS, had the greatest risk of marked sinus arrhythmia with marked heart rate variability and were likely to have tachycardia and bradycardia. The risk of cardiac arrest appeared to be increased in AIDS-related complex. AIDS-related complex did not correlate with blood pressure abnormalities, congestive heart failure, or death. Lymphocytic interstitial pneumonitis, CDC class P-2C, was associated with cardiac abnormalities seen early in HIV disease, including marked sinus arrhythmia, tachycardia, and cardiac arrest, but was not related to other outcomes. Nonneurologic, non-LIP AIDS, CDC class P-2D1 and P-2D2, was associated with many severe outcomes including death with cardiac dysfunction, hypotension, hypertension, and abnormalities of heart rate. The presence of HIV encephalopathy (CDC class P-2B) is associated with a poorer prognosis in children and was strongly associated with all adverse cardiac outcomes we examined. Encephalopathy was the strongest predictor of cardiac arrest and was the only AIDS-defining illness associated with chronic congestive heart failure. Encephalopathy may be an indicator of autonomic nervous system dysfunction. Thus children with AIDS and encephalopathy had a higher risk of adverse cardiac outcomes than AIDS patients without encephalopathy (13). At another center, progressive cardiac abnormalities were noted in HIV-infected children and were related to increasing severity of their HIV disease (43).

Length of Time Infected

In the early 1980s, children with AIDS frequently died of overwhelming infection before these cardiac manifestations became clinically obvious. With the advent of newer therapeutic modalities for treating infection it is likely that patients with HIV will survive longer and that cardiac involvement may become a more prominent part of the clinical picture (2). The increased success in reducing infections, improving nutrition, and slowing the progression of HIV may result in more patients with HIV-associated cardiac disease. Since there are more infected children surviving longer there may be a substantial increase in the incidence of HIV-associated heart disease. "Cardiomyopathy" was noted in none of the 12 HIV-infected children younger than 3 years and was more likely to be reversible in nonfatal "cardiomyopathy" in children younger than 3 years but was found in 31% of those dying after age 3 (10).

Coinfections

Infectious pathogens have been infrequently identified within myocardial cells, and their relation to heart disease in HIV-infected individuals has been mostly indirect. Myocarditis, characterized by mononuclear cellular infiltration and myocyte necrosis, is noted in some HIV-infected patients and may be associated with abnormalities of ventricular function or of an infectious etiology, but these associations have not been conclusively established.

Virus Infections

Possible infection with cardiotropic viruses and subsequent spontaneous improvement has been noted. We have found that Epstein-Barr virus coinfection in HIV-infected children increased the risk of abnormalities of heart rate and blood pressure, congestive heart failure, as well as cardiac, noncardiac, and total death (12, 13, 51). Coinfection with Epstein-Barr virus was the strongest predictor of chronic congestive heart failure and may identify HIV-infected children at especially high risk for adverse cardiac outcomes (12, 13, 51). Conversely, although CMV has been associated with myocarditis in HIV-infected patients, we found no evidence for an association between CMV infection and adverse cardiac events (12, 13, 51). Disseminated

CMV infection commonly occurs with HIV infection and may involve the heart (116). Five HIV-infected children with congestive heart failure were noted to have CMV myocarditis with necrosis of myocytes and CMV inclusions at autopsy (50, 57, 77, 107). We have also had an HIV-infected child with congestive heart failure and biopsy-proven CMV myocarditis at our center. Adult HIV-infected patients with congestive heart failure, arrhythmias, and electrocardiographic changes were noted to have CMV inclusions within myocytes (44, 102, 108, 117). The absence of CMV inclusions within myocytes does not exclude the presence of myocyte CMV infection. Wu et al. (117) demonstrated CMV immediate early gene transcripts with myocytes without intranuclear inclusions from HIV-infected adults with congestive heart failure by in situ hybridization, suggesting latent CMV infection. A recent study of HIV-infected adults found no serologic evidence of recent or past infection with CMV in patients with myocardial dysfunction (114). Pericarditis with tamponade caused by CMV has been reported in HIV-infected adults (118).

Another HIV-infected child at our center with disseminated adenovirus coinfection, which is thought to be a common cause of myocarditis in children (119), was symptomatic from frequent high-grade ventricular arrhythmias. Coxsackievirus is a common cardiotropic pathogen to the pericardium and myocardium and may be associated with dilated "cardiomyopathy," but this has not been widely reported in HIV-infected patients (120). There may be more Coxsackievirus cardiac involvement with HIV, but serologic assays used to establish this diagnosis may be less reliable and underestimate the prevalence in HIV-infected patients. Herpes viruses are uncommon cardiac pathogens but have been described in that role with HIV (121) in a patient with high-grade arrhythmias and pericardial involvement. We have had two children with rapidly fatal myocarditis associated with parvovirus B19, and this has been noted by others as a cause of myocarditis in children (122). Parvovirus B19 has been detected in an HIV-infected child with recurrent Kawasaki disease (76).

We have detected HIV RNA and DNA by in situ hybridization and polymerase chain reaction in the heart of a child with cardiovascular abnormalities (increased ventricular mass, hyperdynamic ventricular function, enhanced contractility, reduced afterload, and focal myocarditis and pericarditis) and perinatally infected AIDS (60, 61). Myocytes and endothelial cells appeared to be infected by an unknown mechanism since these cells are CD4 receptor negative. The number of infected cells was small and was not related to regions of myocarditis, suggesting that if HIV has a significant effect on cardiac structure or function it may be by an indirect mechanism such as the induction of cardiotoxic cytokines (123). Other indirect, immunologically mediated HIV mechanisms have been suggested to cause organ dysfunction (124). If HIV is a direct cardiac pathogen then there may be specific cardiotropic strains of HIV. Others have identified HIV within the heart as well and found dendritic cells to be another source of HIV-infected cells within the myocardium (125–130).

Fungal Infections

Candida endocarditis, myocarditis, or pericarditis may occur in the setting of this systemic coinfection in both children and adults (2, 77). Cardiac disease associated with aspergillosis in HIV-infected patients may result in endocarditis, intramyocardial abscesses, or purulent pericarditis, all of which may follow pulmonary aspergillosis (108, 109). Cryptococcal coinfection is common in adults with advanced HIV infection with central nervous system involvement or total systemic involvement. The central nervous system involvement may again predispose infected patients to arrythmias and hemodynamic instability. We have reported an HIV-infected patient with congestive heart failure, dilated "cardiomyopathy," and chronic cryptococcal disease (4). Myocardial, pericardial, and endocardial pathologic and clinical involvement have also been noted in adult HIV-infected patients with cryptococcal disease (105, 131–134).

Bacterial Infections

Ventricular dysfunction has been noted during *S. aureus* sepsis in HIV-infected patients (85), and pericarditis with the isolation of this organism from the pericardial fluid of HIV-infected patients has been reported (77, 135, 136). *S. epidermidis*, *Pseudomonas aeruginosa*, and *Enterococcus* have also been cultured from the pericardial fluid of HIV-infected children (77). Extrapulmonary manifestations of tuberculosis in HIV-infected patients may involve the pericardium or, less frequently, the myocardium (137–139). Tuberculous pericarditis may be less likely to respond to therapy than extracardiac tuberculosis (140). *Mycobacterium avium-intracellulare* (MAI) coinfection was associated with "cardiomyopathy" in seven of nine HIV-infected children (78%) (89). Most of our patients with known MAI coinfection developed progressive ventricular dysfunction and congestive heart failure. Although symptomatic heart failure improved with anti-infective and anticongestive treatment of MAI and heart failure, this was transient. Joshi et al. (57) described a 2-year child with AIDS, MAI coinfection and "dilated cardiomyopathy." Thirty-seven percent of adults with AIDS and MAI had positive MAI cultures from the heart (141). As children live longer with HIV infection the risk of MAI coinfection increases (142). Coinfection with MAI is difficult to establish (142). Children with advanced HIV infection presenting with unexplained symptomatic ventricular dysfunction should undergo assessment for the presence of MAI coinfection. It is unclear whether MAI directly and independently increases the incidence of ventricular dysfunction or whether MAI is a marker of advanced HIV disease that has already been associated with ventricular dysfunction. Pericardial disease has also been noted in HIV-infected patients with MAI, and MAI was seen in the pericardium of one child (77, 143). Pericardial and myocardial diseases have also been noted in HIV-infected patients with *Actinomycetales* and *Nocardia* infections (144).

Protozoan Infections

Although the heart is not usually directly involved during *P. carinii* pneumonia, the onset of this infection usually indicates advanced HIV disease, a state where abnormalities of the heart, pericardium, and pulmonary artery resistance are more likely (112). *P. carinii* has been demonstrated to be a cardiac pathogen with intramyocardial lesions diffusely consisting of myocyte necrosis and immunohistochemical and microscopic confirmation of the organism (25). *Toxoplasma gondii* is another important protozoan infection, although it appears to be far less common in children with HIV infection in the United States compared with adults. Nonetheless, an 11-week child with AIDS and unexplained hypertrophic "cardiomyopathy" was noted to have congenital cardiac toxoplasmosis at death (145). *Toxoplasma* myocarditis and intracardiac involvement have been described and related to ventricular dysfunction and are the most common documented infectious cause of myocarditis in adults with HIV (44, 98, 103, 146–149). However, a recent study of infected adults with ventricular dysfunction found no serologic evidence of recent or past infection with *T. gondii* (114).

Malnutrition

Possible etiologies for HIV-related cardiac disease include selenium deficiency (150, 151, 227) and malnutrition (152, 153). Abnormalities of growth and body composition are common and progressive in children with HIV infection (154). In the absence of HIV infection, malnutrition has been linked to decreases in left ventricular mass, left ventricular volume, ventricular function, and blood pressure (152, 153).

Cardiac infection with HIV or other viruses may indirectly affect the growth and dilatation of the heart in children by the activation of proto-oncogenes (48, 155) or changes in cytokines (48, 123, 156). Cytokines and growth factors are found in markedly abnormal concentrations in HIV-infected patients and may contribute to cardiovascular abnormalities (123, 155, 156).

Severe anemia may relate to HIV heart disease (157, 158) as might chronic lung disease, resulting in hypoxic myocardial damage, renal disease, or autonomic dysfunction.

Excess catecholamine stimulation may be a risk factor for HIV cardiac disease (159). Catecholamine-induced myocarditis and dilated "cardiomyopathy" have been reported to be caused by repeated transient focal or widespread ischemia resulting from episodes of microvascular spasm (160, 161).

Therapy

Life-threatening reactions requiring cardiopulmonary resuscitation after administration of trimethoprim-sulfamethoxazole have occurred in two HIV-infected children at our center and elsewhere (14, 65) (Table 26.1). Both children had evidence of cardiac abnormalities, suggesting a hyperadrenergic state before receiving the medication as well as having had a prior cutaneous reaction to this medication in the recent past. Hypersensitivity myocarditis (162) was suspected in these children. Intravenous pentamidine was associated with prolongation of the QTc interval and the reproducible development of symptomatic torsades de pointes (polymorphic ventricular tachycardia) in an HIV-infected patient we have followed with autonomic dysfunction (4). This has also been reported in HIV-infected adults receiving either intravenous or intramuscular pentamidine (16–18, 163–167). Ganciclovir has also been associated with

Table 26.1.   Therapy-related Cardiovascular Complications[a]

	Increased QT$_c$ Torsades de Pointes	Other Arrhythmias	Hemodynamic Abnormalities	Arrest	Cardiomyopathy LV dysfunction
TMP-SMZ	X		X	X	X
Pentamidine	X		X	X	
Ganciclovir		X	X		
Foscarnet				X	
Interferon-α					X
Amphotericin B		X	X	X	
Corticosteroids					X

[a]LV, left ventricular; TMP-SMZ, trimethoprim-sulfamethoxazole.

the development of ventricular tachycardia in adults with HIV infection (15). Foscarnet has been related to reversible ventricular dysfunction. Interferon-α therapy was associated with the development of reversible congestive "cardiomyopathy" in three adults with AIDS and Kaposi's sarcoma (168). Amphotericin B may cause arrhythmias, hypertension, and cardiac arrest if infused too rapidly (i.e., <1 hr) (140). Systemic corticosteroids are used to treat some infected children and may result in ventricular hypertrophy and ventricular dysfunction (169).

The potential cardiotoxic effects of zidovudine are controversial. Conflicting reports suggest a relationship between administration of zidovudine and an improvement (170), preservation (171), or deterioration (172, 173) of ventricular function in adults. Recent studies (25, 174–176) report cardiotoxic mitochondrial effects of zidovudine in rats. Zidovudine inhibits mitchondrial γ-DNA polymerase (177). Up to 78% of the mitochondrial DNA is reversibly depleted in zidovudine-associated skeletal myopathy (177). Despite experimental and human studies suggesting that zidovudine can cause myopathy, the patients we followed appeared to have normal ventricular contractility (48). The major cardiac abnormalities observed were progressive ventricular dilation and inadequate ventricular hypertrophy. However, these changes were no more marked with zidovudine than during the period before therapy in the same patients. This suggests that the cause is related to the primary disease process itself rather than to zidovudine therapy. Because of limitations of the comparison group, we could not evaluate the possibility that zidovudine slowed the rate of progression of cardiac abnormalities to that seen in an earlier phase of the disease. Interestingly, none of the zidovudine-treated children with advanced HIV disease we reported (48) had clinical congestive heart failure. That was surprising considering that 20% of HIV-infected children at our institution had either transient or chronic congestive heart failure (13). Recommendations (172) that antiretroviral therapy be interrupted in HIV-infected patients with evidence of "cardiomyopathy" or congestive heart failure may deny potentially beneficial, or even lifesaving, therapy.

Our patients would probably have had zidovudine therapy interrupted owing to this recommendation since measures of left ventricular dimension and load-dependent ventricular performance suggested a "dilated cardiomyopathy" associated with zidovudine. However, contractility remained normal, and the same progressive cardiac abnormalities were seen before initiation of zidovudine. Our data do not support the recommendation to withhold zidovudine in patients with reduced cardiac function. A recent study of infected adults also showed that treatment with zidovudine did not predispose toward the development of cardiac dysfunction (114). However, zidovudine overdose has been associated with hemodynamic abnormalities of heart rate and blood pressure (178).

PATHOGENESIS AND NATURAL HISTORY

Ventricular Dysfunction and Congestive Heart Failure

The pathogenesis "dilated cardiomyopathy" that has been observed may be multifactorial and related to myocardial inflammation resulting in injury to the myocyte, to HIV infection of cardiac tissues, or to the cardiotoxicities of therapeutic agents. Infection, postmyocarditis, immunologic factors, cytokines and other potential cardiac "toxins," anemia, deficiency of nutritional factor(s), and longer survival may be related to the pathogenesis. Although the relation of myocarditis to the development of "cardiomyopathy" has not been established, some reports suggest that there may be a continuum.

Three histopathologic patterns of myocardial involvement have been noted in HIV-infected patients: mononuclear infiltration with necrosis of myocytes (myocarditis), mononuclear infiltration without myocyte damage, and myocyte damage without infiltration (179–188). The significance of these different histologic patterns in terms of ventricular function or subsequent course is not clearly known. Lymphocytic infiltration of the heart was noted in 77% of HIV-infected adults, and 34% of the cohort had myocarditis, none of whom had cardiac symptoms (103). Myocarditis was seen in 52% of adult hearts in another series and included all patients (10%) with "dilated cardiomyopathy" and congestive heart failure (44). For 81% of these patients no etiology was established (44). Inflammatory infiltrate without necrosis was seen in an additional 14% of the hearts in this series, which was a comparable prevalence to that noted in non-HIV-infected patients dying of sudden traumatic death (44). In another series, 45% of adult hearts had myocarditis, and 58% of these hearts had clinical cardiac abnormalities vs. 19% of patients without myocarditis (102). Caution has been advised in attributing all pathologic cardiac abnormalities to HIV (188, 189). Major cardiac abnormalities were only observed in patients with myocarditis (102). The presence of myocarditis was similar in all intravenous drug users regardless of HIV status (57% infected vs. 44% not infected), as was the presence of ventricular dilation (190). Another study suggested an even higher incidence of myocarditis in HIV-negative intravenous drug users and suggested that intravenous drug use may contribute to the prevalence of myocarditis in AIDS (191). However, a recent report found that the frequency of left ventricular dysfunction in HIV-seronegative intravenous drug users was <4% compared with an incidence of 10–20% for "cardiomyopathy" among patients with AIDS, suggesting that intravenous drug use alone was insufficient to explain the frequency of "cardiomyopathy" among patients with AIDS (192). A dilated hypocontractile left ventricle in children and adults with HIV infection is generally progressive, although spontaneous regression may occur (193, 194).

Circulating antiheart antibodies may be involved in the development of myocarditis and "cardiomyopathy." Three HIV-infected children with myocardial or pericardial disease had elevated serum autoantibody titers against mitochondrial adenine nucleotide translocator and myosin, suggesting that cardiac involvement in pediatric HIV infection may be related to autoimmunity (195). At least one of three heart autoantibody titers were elevated in 80% of HIV-infected adults with heart disease, in contrast to 15% of HIV-infected adults without heart disease and 70% of younger, HIV-negative patients with idiopathic "cardiomyopathy," suggest-

ing an autoimmune-mediated phenomena (196). Monoclonal antibodies to HIV core proteins p17 and p24 reacted more strongly to antigenic molecules from cardiocytes of AIDS patients than non-AIDS patients (197). This suggested that some cardiac abnormalities in HIV-infected patients may relate to a direct effect of HIV proteins, but not necessarily the intact virus itself, on the metabolism and function within myocytes (23, 197). Alternatively, an autoimmune mechanism may be responsible whereby antibodies against HIV react with specific subcellular components of myocytes (23, 197). In addition, myocyte injury can be produced by sensitized cytotoxic T lymphocytes and result in contractile abnormalities (198).

Autonomic Dysfunction

HIV infection has been associated with a wide spectrum of central and peripheral nervous system disorders, including autonomic dysfunction, that may occur in patients at any stage of the infection and have a significant effect on cardiovascular reflexes (4, 11, 13, 199–203). Despite frequently detected abnormalities, no systematic, large scale or prospective study of autonomic function has been reported in HIV-infected patients.

Increased left ventricular performance, suggesting a hyperadrenergic state, was the most common echocardiographic finding that we noted in HIV-infected children (4, 41, 42, 47, 61). High-grade ectopy, sudden unexplained death and myocarditis, pericarditis, inflammation of the cardiac conduction tissue were more likely to occur in these patients. We have found clinically apparent autonomic dysfunction manifested by syncope, hypotension, abnormal hemodynamic responses to conventional therapeutic interventions, and even sudden death in children and adults at all stages of HIV infection. Autonomic dysfunction has been confirmed with formal autonomic function testing in selected patients. Because neural tissue is affected early in HIV infection, these cardiovascular effects may be manifestations of an autonomic neuropathy. We and others have noted inflammatory changes of the cardiac conduction tissue and peripheral nerves in HIV-infected children with autonomic dysfunction who have died (4, 56).

Chronic catecholamine excess, noted with an increased sympathetic state, is a potent stimulator of cardiac hyperplasia and hypertrophy. Inappropriate hypertrophy similar to that seen in hypertrophic "cardiomyopathy", with or without obstruction, is among the most common cardiac abnormalities we have found in HIV-infected children.

Our recent data indicate that the magnitude of clinical problems associated with autonomic dysfunction in children with symptomatic (CDC class P-2) HIV infection is significant. Hemodynamic abnormalities, dysrhythmias, unexplained arrest, and/or sudden death are common in the HIV-infected children we follow, especially when acute deterioration, interventions, or neurologic involvement is present (12, 13, 51). Limited data also suggest that abnormal cardiac autonomic regulation is a likely contributor to these problems and should be assessed prospectively.

Abnormal Cardiac Growth

We have found progressive abnormalities of left ventricular structure and function (4, 48, 58–61, 204). Figure 26.2 illustrates the probable sequence of events in zidovudine-treated HIV-infected children. Progressive left ventricular dilation resulted in wall thin-ning, a fall in the thickness-to-dimension ratio, and a rise in both peak systolic and end-systolic wall stress (afterload). The increased afterload was associated with decreased ventricular performance assessed by fractional shortening, although left ventricular contractility was not impaired. The rise in afterload correlated with left ventricular dilation and thinning of the left ventricular wall. Ventricular dilation progressed and, despite hypertrophy and normalization of the thickness-to-dimension ratio, elevation of peak systolic wall stress persisted. Left ventricular mass increased significantly during the study but failed to keep pace with ventricular dimension, consistent with inadequate left ventricular hypertrophy.

Figure 26.3 illustrates the normal hypertrophic cascade that is activated in response to an acute increase in hemodynamic load to the left ventricle. Initially, either a fall in the left ventricular thickness-to-dimension ratio or a rise in pressure results in a rise in peak systolic wall stress. Peak stress appears to be the principal transducer of mechanically induced hypertrophy, and when elevated, left ventricular hypertrophy results. Hypertrophy of the ventricle continues until peak systolic wall stress returns to normal at which point the hypertrophic response stops.

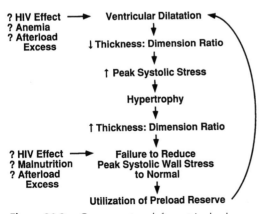

Figure 26.2. Compensatory left ventricular hypertrophy in response to changes in left ventricular load in children with symptomatic HIV infection.

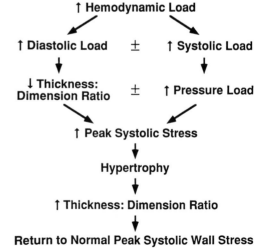

Figure 26.3. Compensatory left ventricular hypertrophy in response to changes in left ventricular load in normal children without HIV infection.

Figure 26.2 depicts what we have observed with HIV-infected children. Ventricular dilation of unclear and possibly multifactorial cause evokes the normal sequence of compensatory hypertrophy, resulting in a significant increase in left ventricular mass. However, unlike normal children, the magnitude of hypertrophy is inadequate to reduce peak systolic wall stress to normal. The continued afterload excess results in further utilization of preload reserve with progressive ventricular dilation. The continuing elevation of peak systolic wall stress indicates that the degree of left ventricular hypertrophy is inadequate for the progressively increasing left ventricular dimension. The ventricular dilation and compensatory rise in left ventricular mass in HIV-infected children appears unrelated to contractile state or congestive heart failure. The elevated left ventricular mass observed in these subjects (48) is corroborated by a separate study of HIV-infected children at our hospital who had a mean cardiac weight at autopsy 184% above normal (4, 48).

Figure 26.2 also suggests several possible mechanisms for the increased left ventricular dimension and mass in pediatric HIV infection. Anemia does not appear to be significant because hemoglobin levels, although less than normal, remained constant. Stable mild anemia would not be expected to cause the progressive ventricular dilation observed in this study.

HIV infection may directly affect cells of the pediatric heart. Elevation of peak systolic stress (afterload), observed in these HIV-infected children, results in proto-oncogene activation that appears to modulate the hypertrophic response. However, expression of some proto-oncogenes appears mediated by retroviruses (48, 155). This might alter the normal hypertrophic responses in children with HIV. Similarly, dramatic cellular shape changes can result from retroviral infection of cells in vitro. This also might be involved in the unexplained progressive dilation of the left ventricle in patients with HIV. We have demonstrated the presence of HIV RNA and DNA in cardiac cells in children with HIV infection (60, 61) so that such direct effects on ventricular dilation and hypertrophy are

possible. HIV infection also alters expression of cytokine growth factors. Cytokines are known to affect cardiac myocyte proliferation and DNA synthesis, as well as the expression of contractile proteins (48, 155). This effect might adversely influence the hypertrophic response to dilation.

Autonomic dysfunction is present even in early HIV infection. Increased sympathetic tone is associated with increased catecholamines, which are potent stimulators of myocardial hypertrophy. Increased ventricular mass for body surface area may relate to chronically increased sympathetic activity, which in part may be due to HIV infection of the nervous system, the effects of the elevated blood pressure observed in these children, malnutrition, or altered levels of cytokines. However, autonomic dysfunction does not explain the subnormal hypertrophy for left ventricular dimension.

Malnutrition was common in these patients at all ages. In the absence of HIV infection, malnutrition has been linked to decreases in left ventricular mass, decreased blood pressure and a fall in ventricular function. Yet, we found left ventricular mass increased or preserved in 71% of echocardiograms (204), blood pressure normal to elevated, and stable contractility indicating that some other agent overrode the usual effects of malnutrition (48). It remains possible that inadequate nutrition may have contributed to the subnormal hypertrophic responses relative to left ventricular dimension observed in these patients.

DIAGNOSTIC CONSIDERATIONS AND EVALUATION

We recommend that children with indeterminate HIV status (CDC class P-0) and seroreverters (CDC class P-3) undergo a cardiac evaluation as indicated by signs or symptoms of heart disease. We recommend that children with asymptomatic HIV infection receive a baseline cardiac evaluation, including electrocardiography and echocardiography, at diagnosis. Routine follow-up of these patients includes echocardiography every 6–12 months and electrocardiography with Holter monitoring at 1-year intervals. We recommend that follow-up echocardiography be considered with intercurrent illnesses, especially if accompanied by unexplained or unresponsive respiratory symptoms, persistent tachycardia and/or tachypnea, poor feeding, or poor perfusion or if the severity of these symptoms warrants hospitalization. Follow-up electrocardiography and Holter monitoring should be considered when there is an intercurrent illness, especially if there is a history of blue spells, seizures, syncope or if the severity of the illness warrants hospitalization. Children with symptomatic HIV infection (CDC class P-2) without cardiac abnormalities should also be monitored for the risk of developing cardiac disease with echocardiography every 3–6 months and electrocardiography and Holter monitoring every 6–12 months. Children with AIDS but no past history of cardiac involvement, especially with encephalopathy or other coinfections, should be tested at frequent intervals.

If any signs or symptoms listed below are noted in an HIV-infected child with a symptomatic intercurrent illness, a formal cardiac assessment is suggested.

If cardiac disease cannot be excluded, then further cardiac evaluation should be considered, as indicated by the algorithm in Figure 26.4. The algorithm is intended to maximize the possibility of making a diagnosis while minimizing invasive studies.

1) Unexpected or unresponsive respiratory symptoms lasting >7 days (e.g., oxygen desaturation, rales, cough).
2) Signs and/or symptoms suggestive of congestive heart failure (e.g., persistent tachycardia and/or tachypnea, poor feeding, poor perfusion).
3) Past history or presence of left ventricular dysfunction or dilation, structural abnormality, or pericardial effusion.
4) Past history or presence of frequent arrhythmias.
5) History or presence of cyanotic episodes, seizures, syncope, or autonomic dysfunction.
6) Severity of intercurrent illness warrants hospitalization.
7) Evidence of clinical coinfections (e.g., Epstein-Barr virus, CMV, MAI) present in symptomatic patient.
8) Evidence of HIV encephalopathy.
9) CDC-defined AIDS.
10) Therapy with intravenous pentamidine or ganciclovir.

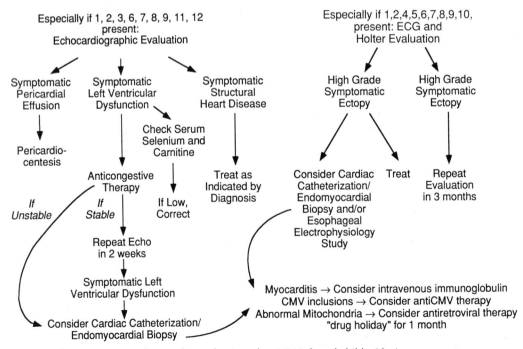

Figure 26.4. Cardiovascular evaluation of an HIV-infected child with signs or symptoms consistent with cardiovascular involvement.

11) Antiretroviral therapy for >1 year or interferon therapy.

12) Known selenium or carnitine deficiency.

Conditions 1–3, 6–9, 11, or 12 (Fig. 26.4) may be seen in HIV-infected patients with symptomatic pericardial effusion, left ventricular dysfunction, or structural heart disease. These disorders can be detected, if present, by an echocardiogram. Therefore, the presence of these conditions during an intercurrent illness should prompt this evaluation.

Similarly, conditions 1, 2, or 4–10 (Fig. 26.4) may be seen in HIV-infected patients with arrhythmias or conduction abnormalities. Arrhythmias and conduction abnormalities may be detected by electrocardiographic and Holter monitor evaluations. Therefore the presence of these conditions during an intercurrent illness should prompt this evaluation.

TESTS POTENTIALLY USEFUL FOR CARDIOVASCULAR ASSESSMENT

Cardiac Physical Exam

We have found that cardiovascular abnormalities can be difficult to recognize clinically. Because most patients also have hepatosplenomegaly, interstitial lung disease (205) and intermittent S_3 gallop at baseline and some may have renal disease, it can be difficult to establish the clinical diagnosis of congestive heart failure. In fact, some patients with the greatest myocardial impairment fail to show clinical evidence of cardiac involvement. Preexistent hepatosplenomegaly, fever, infection, and anemia can also result in physical findings that may mimic findings of heart failure, thereby masking the occurrence of cardiac dysfunction. It has been suggested that an S_3 gallop may indicate the presence of impaired heart function in this population when other clinical signs are masked (50). The presence of tachypnea, tachycardia, and a gallop rhythm may be helpful clinical indicators of congestive heart failure in HIV-infected children (9). Other signs and symptoms associated with congestive heart failure in young children include changes in feeding patterns, amount of formula consumed per feeding, feeding time, history of diaphoresis, growth failure, respiratory difficulties (symptoms and pattern), perfusion, edema, diastolic filling sounds, and hepatomegaly (206). Exercise dysfunction with a limitation of oxygen delivery to exercising muscles has been detected in HIV-infected adults and may represent an important and more accurate way to evaluate functional cardiovascular involvement in older children because that report showed a poor correlation between HIV-infected patients with cardiac symptoms and patients with exercise limitations (207).

Myocardial dysfunction related to HIV can be easily overlooked (208). Notably, in one series, children who were ultimately proved to have congestive heart failure had all their symptoms of respiratory distress attributed to other causes, often pneumonias (50). Accordingly, sensitive noninvasive echocardiographic indexes of myocardial function can assist in more accurate assessment of these patients.

Clinical signs and symptoms of significant pericardial disease (e.g., chest pain, sitting position, cough, dysphagia, dyspnea, poor perfusion, pulsus paradoxicus, jugular venous distension) may be difficult to detect in children with HIV because of the age of the child, chronicity of the process, low pressure tamponade, or concurrent signs and symptoms of other ongoing processes in the child.

Echocardiography

The echocardiogram remains the single most useful noninvasive diagnostic test to determine cardiac status in HIV-infected patients (209) and can help with the assessment of the following.

- *Ventricular Function.* HIV-infected children with congestive heart failure had depressed left ventricular fractional shortening in one study, although half of these patients had values that were within 2 percentage points of the lower limit of normal (50). After anticongestive therapy all patients demonstrated marked improvements in fractional shortening as well as clinical symptomatology, suggesting that, for at least half of these patients, multisystem noncardiac factors had a significant adverse effect on ventricular preload, heart rate, and afterload. Because half the children with HIV infection who have depressed shortening fraction have normal or enhanced contractility, we prefer the use of load-independent measurements of contractility for greater sensitivity and specificity (4, 41, 42, 47–49, 61). Echocardiography may be used to assess diastolic ventricular dysfunction that may also be found in HIV-infected patients.

- *Ventricular Structure.* Echocardiography can be used to assess ventricular thickness, dimension, and masses attached to catheter tips or the endocardium.
- *Cardiac Anatomy.* Structural defects, vegetations, thrombi, and abscesses can be detected by echocardiography. The sensitivity of transthoracic echocardiography in the detection of vegetations is ~75%, whereas transesophageal echocardiography has a sensitivity of up to 96% in high-risk populations (210). Transesophageal echocardiography has a higher rate of detection of ring abscesses (sensitivity 84% vs. 19%) (210). The importance of follow-up transesophageal echocardiographic examination when suspicion of endocarditis persists despite negative test results has been established (211).
- *Pericardial Disease.* Echocardiography is both sensitive and specific for detecting pericardial effusion and tamponade. Demonstration of right atrial compression or right ventricular diastolic collapse by echocardiography is seen with pericardial tamponade and suggests the need for a therapeutic intervention to relieve the tamponade. The presence of pericardial disease should result in skin testing for tuberculosis and consideration of other testing for infectious causes.
- *Coronary Arteries.* Echocardiography has been useful for assessing coronary dilation and aneurysms in HIV-infected children.

Electrocardiography

Electrocardiographic abnormalities of chamber enlargement or hypertrophy, as well as ST segment and T wave changes, have been frequently described in HIV-infected children with congestive heart failure (50). The electrocardiogram is useful in assessing heart rate, arrhythmias, atrial enlargement and ventricular hypertrophy, ischemic heart disease, the conduction system, and various ST and T wave changes, including ischemia and strain. In contrast, signal-averaged electrocardiograms were performed on HIV-infected adults to assess the relation between late potentials and ventricular dysfunction or arrhythmias without any significant relations noted (212).

Holter Monitor

Arrhythmias on physical exam or ectopy on the electrocardiogram should prompt Holter monitoring to determine heart rate, rhythm, and the presence and type of various arrhythmias, conduction defects, or ST and T wave changes (ischemia, strain).

Chest Radiography

Radiographic evidence suggestive of cardiac involvement can be difficult to discern (4, 50, 77) or can even be misleading (77). Pericardial effusion and cardiac disease should be suspected in HIV-infected children with radiographic signs of cardiomegaly, pleural effusions, or ascites, even if they have a normal cardiac silhouette, especially if the child has respiratory symptoms and is not showing clinical improvement (77).

Serum Selenium, Carnitine, and Other Micronutrients

Tissue micronutrient deficiencies are reportedly a reversible cause of ventricular dysfunction. However, it is unclear how tissue and serum micronutrient levels are related. Serum micronutrient level determination for the assessment of possible deficiency should be considered if ventricular dysfunction is noted.

Endomyocardial Biopsy

Because up to 52% of adults with HIV have myocarditis at autopsy, and for many of these patients treatable infections were detected, endomyocardial biopsy performed at a center experienced in their use in sick children may result in improved diagnosis and treatment of HIV-associated cardiac disease. The treatment of myocarditis in children is anecdotal, but promising new treatment options are available. Endomyocardial biopsy has identified potentially treatable infections with organisms such as *T. gondii* (146). The sensitivity of endomyocardial biopsy for detecting focal myocardial processes, or its relation to other less invasive diagnostic studies, is unknown. Repeat biopsy may still be warranted in patients with suspected myocarditis despite six to eight negative biopsy samples (213). There is poor correlation between the clinical and biopsy diagnoses of acute myocarditis in infants, children, and adolescents, emphasizing the importance of the biopsy in making this diagnosis (214). Caution should be exercised before subjecting HIV-infected pediatric patients to endomyocardial biopsy procedures or to experimental drug regimens that have not yet been shown to be efficacious. Therefore, we recommend endomyocardial biopsy for HIV-infected children with clinical congestive heart failure refractory to a trial of anticongestive therapy. The sensitivity of endomyocardial biopsy may be enhanced by techniques such as the polymerase chain reaction and in situ hybridization for HIV and other infectious pathogens. At this time, the endomyocardial biopsy may be helpful to diagnose the following conditions: inflammatory heart disease, a reversible mitochondrial myopathy of zidovudine, or infectious heart disease (e.g., CMV).

TREATMENT

General Supportive Care Issues

Francis (2) has emphasized several aspects of care to reduce cardiac problems in HIV-infected patients. For example, it is important to correct factors in HIV-infected children that might contribute to cardiac symptoms (e.g., anemia, dehydration, malnutrition, and electrolytes). Prompt identification and treatment of routine intercurrent pulmonary disease of childhood should reduce the likelihood of cardiac problems. Cardiac abnormalities may be reduced by the early initiation of empiric an-

timicrobial therapy, whereas awaiting culture results in potentially life-threatening situations. It is also essential to reassess the accuracy of diagnosis and efficacy of therapy frequently, because all symptoms in a HIV-infected patient being treated for an infection may not relate to that infection and because polymicrobial infections and relapses are common.

Specific Therapy

Anticongestive Treatment

HIV-infected adults and children demonstrate improved cardiac function with appropriate medical management (4, 50, 114, 115, 215). Transfusion of anemic patients, antipyrexic therapy, aggressive respiratory care, and oxygen therapy are beneficial for most children with clinical heart failure. Ionotropic support such as digoxin may be helpful for children with symptomatic depressed left ventricular contractility. Digoxin may improve the quality of life for a patient with congestive heart failure even if it does not prolong life. Minimally symptomatic children with depressed ventricular contractility should start digoxin at the maintenance dosage and should achieve steady-state levels in several days. Children with impaired renal function should receive a lower dosage. More symptomatic children may benefit from inpatient loading of digoxin with close monitoring of cardiac rhythm and electrolytes. Serum electrolytes should be measured regularly while on digoxin, and digoxin should not be given if serum potassium is lower than 3.0. Although there is no need to monitor digoxin levels in treated patients without toxicity, a level should be obtained if toxicity is suspected. Diuretic therapy is generally synergistic when given with digoxin to improve ventricular function in children with congestive heart failure, but combined therapy mandates regular assessment of serum electrolytes. Afterload reduction therapy with angiotensin converting enzyme inhibitors has been shown in adults with congestive heart failure to reduce progression to death, but this has not been studied in children with HIV infection. Although not approved by the Food and Drug Administration for children younger than

12 years, these agents are used widely in pediatrics and appear to have good safety records. In children with congestive heart failure or with excessively high afterload, these agents are initiated with careful monitoring of blood pressure. Dosages are adjusted based on reduction in clinical congestive heart failure, level of ventricular afterload, and blood pressure. Occasionally, patients with refractory severe symptomatic ventricular dysfunction despite maximal conventional anticongestive therapy will achieve improved ventricular performance and a better quality of life lasting occasionally for several weeks after several days of palliative inpatient intravenous dobutamine therapy. Other intensive care therapies for congestive heart failure are beyond the scope of this chapter.

Immunoglobulin Treatment

Children with Kawasaki syndrome treated with intravenous immunoglobulin during the acute phase have accelerated recovery of early abnormalities of left ventricular contractility and function (216). Preliminary retrospective data suggest that intravenous immunoglobulin treatment of children with acute congestive cardiomyopathy may result in improved recovery of left ventricular function and in improved survival (217). Some HIV-infected children with inflammatory heart disease detected by endomyocardial biopsy and congestive heart failure that is unresponsive to anticongestive therapy may improve with intravenous immunoglobulin therapy (218). Immunoglobulin therapy has also resulted in improvement for HIV-associated polymyositis, an inflammatory skeletal muscle disorder (219). Children with HIV infection and CD4 counts of $\geq 0.2 \times 10^9$/liter who were not consistently receiving zidovudine or trimethoprim-sulfamethoxazole had beneficial effects from intravenous immunoglobulin therapy that included reductions in serious bacterial and minor viral and bacterial infections (220, 221). The mechanism by which intravenous immunoglobulin results in cardiac improvements in children is unknown. However, it is postulated to alter the secretion or effects of excessively produced cytokines (222), which are known to significantly affect the cardiovascular system (123, 155).

Immunosuppression Treatment

One HIV-infected adult with endomyocardial biopsy-proven myocarditis and ventricular dysfunction showed resolution of myocarditis and was not on medication for this problem 15 months later after having been treated with prednisone plus azathioprine (69). Although a small uncontrolled trial of immunosuppressive therapy in the management of acute myocarditis in children found prednisone useful in improving the clinical course and cardiac function without adverse side effects (223), larger controlled trials in adults failed to find benefits from its use. It is unclear whether immunosuppressive therapy alters the course of myocarditis in this population.

Micronutrient Replacement Treatment

Selenium (150, 151, 227) and other micronutrient deficiencies (224) are frequently noted in malnourished HIV-infected patients. The major enzyme responsible for cellular peroxide elimination is selenium dependent. Therefore, it has been suggested that selenium deficiency may increase oxidative stress in HIV-infected patients, resulting in progression of HIV disease (225). Selenium deficiency in selected uninfected patients has also been associated with reversible ventricular dysfunction (226), perhaps by a similar mechanism. Several HIV-infected adults were noted to have reduced cardiac selenium content but did not have correlation with ventricular function (150). A selenium-deficient HIV-infected child with symptomatic ventricular dysfunction poorly responsive to conventional anticongestive therapy had improved cardiac function after selenium repletion (151), and this has been suggested for HIV-infected adults as well (228). We have prospectively assessed selenium levels, nutritional status, severity of HIV infection, and cardiac function in HIV-infected children (229). Although there were significant associations between selenium levels, nutritional status, and severity of HIV infection, there were non-significant positive associations between selenium and ventricular function and contractility (229). Similarly L-carnitine deficiency was noted in 72% of malnourished HIV-infected adults, some of whom had cardiac symptoms, in one study (224). Carnitine deficiency is another potentially reversible cause of symptomatic ventricular dysfunction in other populations (230). For HIV-infected children with worsening or symptomatic ventricular dysfunction it appears prudent to determine micronutrient status and, if reduced, initiate micronutrient replacement therapy. Although such a benign micronutrient replacement effort has not been demonstrated to be efficacious in HIV-infected patients, that is not the case in other micronutrient-deficient populations where replacement may reverse ventricular dysfunction.

Anti-infective Treatment

At least in the short term, it appears that some infectious causes of HIV-associated heart disease are amenable to anti-infective treatment. Significant improvements in cardiac status were reported in HIV-infected adults with cardiac symptoms who had tuberculous pericarditis, cryptococcal myopericarditis, or *Salmonella* endocarditis by conventional anti-infective therapy (140).

We have noted significant improvement in ventricular function and clinical heart failure in HIV-infected children with CMV coinfection after treatment of CMV with combinations of ganciclovir and CMV hyperimmunoglobulin. Preliminary results in adults with active myocarditis or dilated "cardiomyopathy" and identification of CMV by endomyocardial biopsy treated with CMV hyperimmunoglobulin had significant elimination of CMV from the myocardium (231).

Antiarrhythmia Treatment

Antiarrhythmic therapy in children with symptomatic arrhythmias is appropriate. Patients receiving intravenous or intramuscular pentamidine should have electrocardiographic measurement of QTc intervals at regular intervals. Prolongation of the QTc interval beyond 0.48 sec could cause the health care provider to consider holding further pentamidine until this is no longer prolonged to hopefully reduce the chance of the patient developing high-grade ventricular ectopy. Pentamidine-related torsades de pointes should be treated by drug termination and repletion of electrolyte deficiencies. Consideration should be given to the use of type 1B antiarrhythmics, overdrive atrial or ventricular pacing, or isoproterenol administration. Type 1A antiarrhythmics, quinidine and procainamide, should be avoided when the QTc interval is prolonged.

Antihypertension Treatment

Infected children at our center requiring intensive care support were significantly more likely to have hypertension, usually of unclear etiology, than children outside that setting (12, 13, 51). For several children at our center hypertension was quite refractory to manage and resulted in clinically significant hypertensive sequelae, including death. Antihypertensive therapy and search for treatable causes of hypertension are indicated in HIV-infected children because their cardiovascular substrate may be compromised and less able to utilize cardiovascular reserves necessary to maintain cardiac function in the setting of severe hypertension.

Pericardiocentesis

Pericardiocentesis is indicated for pericardial tamponade and may be used for diagnostic evaluation as well. In the absence of tamponade treatment is largely supportive and nonspecific for pericardial disease and may include aspirin or indomethacin for chest pain. The use of steroids or anticoagulants may be contraindicated for HIV-infected patients with pericardial involvement (2).

PREVENTION

Although little can be done to prevent cardiovascular abnormalities from developing in HIV-infected children other than, we hope, avoiding HIV disease progression and development of coinfections and maintaining a good nutritional balance, the monitoring program listed above should have a significant impact on avoiding development of symptomatic cardiac dysfunction in this population. The early identification of progressive cardiovascular disease in HIV-infected children permits early interventions to occur and can alter the subsequent course for many patients. Treating patients with less severe cardiac involvement results in greater improvements in ventricular function than trying to treat patients with severe ventricular dysfunction.

The pediatric HIV population should therefore undergo routine monitoring of left ventricular function for the following reasons. First, the prevalence of congestive heart failure is high in HIV-infected children and may increase dramatically (13, 114, 232). Second, symptomatic left ventricular dysfunction is underreported, unless ventricular function is monitored by echocardiography, because clinical signs of congestive heart failure are often incorrectly attributed to pulmonary or infectious causes (4). Third, most HIV-infected children respond well to anticongestive therapy especially if treatment is initiated early (4, 50). Fourth, because HIV-infected children are at risk for hemodynamic abnormalities with therapeutic interventions, we should try to avoid inappropriate treatment (4, 11–18, 51).

AREAS FOR FUTURE RESEARCH

Ventricular dysfunction in HIV-infected patients probably represents the synergistic and concomitant effects of many factors. There is a need to perform prospective studies to establish the true incidence, pathogenesis, and natural history of HIV-associated heart disease and relate this to external risk factors, individual susceptibility, and immunologic events. Randomized treatment trials of therapies capable of altering the course of HIV-associated heart disease have not been performed (e.g., intravenous immunoglobulin, nutritional intervention, anti-infective therapy) nor has there been much attention in current ACTG trials to assess changes in cardiac status with experimental therapies or to investigate cardiac complications of therapy. The

effects of HIV infection, and the effects of therapies to combat HIV, on growth and development of the fetal and newborn heart should provide the opportunity to examine the long-term effects of infection and therapy on mechanisms controlling cardiac growth and development.

References

1. Fink L, Reichek N, St John Sutton MG. Cardiac abnormalities in acquired immune deficiency syndrome. Am J Cardiol 1984;54:1161–1163.
2. Francis CK. Cardiac involvement in AIDS. Curr Probl Cardiol 1990;15:571–639.
3. Hecht SR, Berger M, Van Tosh A, Croxson S. Unsuspected cardiac abnormalities in the acquired immune deficiency syndrome: an Echocardiographic study. Chest 1989;96:805–808.
4. Lipshultz SE, Chanock S, Sanders SP, Colan SD, McIntosh K. Cardiovascular manifestations of human immunodeficiency infection in infants and children. Am J Cardiol 1989;63:1489–1497.
5. Marion RW, Wiznia AA, Hutcheon RG, Rubinstein A. Human T-cell lymphotropic virus type III (HTLV-III) embryopathy: A new dysmorphic syndrome associated with intrauterine HTLV-III infection. Am J Dis Child 1986;140:638–640.
6. Iosub S, Bamji M, Stone RK, Gromisch DS, Wasserman E. More on human immunodeficiency virus embryopathy. Pediatrics 1987;80:512–516.
7. Lipshultz SE, Frassica JJ, Orav EJ. Cardiovascular abnormalities in infants prenatally exposed to cocaine. J Pediatr 1991;118:44–52.
8. Vogel RL, Alboliras ET, McSherry GD, Levine OR, Antillon JR. Congenital heart defects in children of human immunodeficiency virus positive mothers [Abstract]. Circulation 1988;78:II-17.
9. Vogel RL. Cardiac manifestations of pediatric acquired immunodeficiency syndrome. In: Yogev R, Connor E, eds. Management of HIV infection in infants and children. St. Louis: Mosby, 1992:357–370.
10. Tripp ME, McKinney RE, Katz SL. Cardiac complications of human immunodeficiency virus (HIV) infection in children [Abstract]. Pediatr Res 1993;33:185A.
11. Craddock C, Pasvol G, Bull R, et al. Cardio-respiratory arrest and autonomic neuropathy in AIDS. Lancet 1987;2:16–18.
12. Lipshultz SE, Luginbuhl LM, Saul JP, McIntosh K. Dysrhythmias, unexpected arrest and sudden death in pediatric HIV infection [Abstract]. Circulation 1991;84:II-660.
13. Luginbuhl LM, Orav EJ, McIntosh K, Lipshultz SE. Cardiac morbidity and related mortality in children with human immunodeficiency virus-1 infection. JAMA 1993;269:2869–2875.
14. Kelly JW, Dooley DP, Lattuada CP, Smith CE. A severe, unusual reaction to trimethoprim-sulfamethoxazole in patients infected with human immunodeficiency virus. Clin Infect Dis 1992;14:1034–1039.

15. Cohen AJ, Weiser B, Afzal Q, Fuhrer J. Ventricular tachycardia in two patients with AIDS receiving ganciclovir (DHPG). AIDS 1990;4: 807–809.

16. Stein KM, Haronian H, Mensah GA, et al. Ventricular tachycardia and torsades de pointes complicating pentamidine therapy of pneumocystis carinii pneumonia in the acquired immunodeficiency syndrome. Am J Cardiol 1990;66: 888–889.

17. Stein KM, Fenton C, Lehany AM, Okin PM, Kligfield P. Incidence of QT interval prolongation during pentamidine therapy of pneumocystis carinii pneumonia. Am J Cardiol 1991;68:1091–1094.

18. Wharton M, Demopulos PA, Goldschlager N. Torsade de pointes during administration of pentamidine isoethionate. Am J Med 1987;83: 571–576.

19. Pollock R, Ames F, Rubio P, et al. Protracted severe immune dysregulation induced by cardiopulmonary bypass: A predisposing etiologic factor in blood transfusion-related AIDS? J Clin Lab Immunol 1987;22:1–5.

20. Schaffer MS, Langendorfer SI, Campbell DN. AIDS-related complex following infant cardiac surgery [Letter]. Pediatr Cardiol 1986;6:335–336.

21. Anonymous. Case records of the Massachusetts General Hospital: Case 8-1987. N Engl J Med 1987;316:466–475.

22. Lemma M, Vanelli P, Beretta L, Botta M, Antinori A, Santoli C. Cardiac surgery in HIV-positive intravenous drug addicts: Influence of cardiopulmonary bypass on the progression to AIDS. Thorac Cardiovasc Surg 1992;40:279–282.

23. Cotton P. AIDS giving rise to cardiac problems. JAMA 1990;263:2149.

24. Anderson DW, Virmani R. Emerging patterns of heart disease in human immunodeficiency virus infection. Human Pathol 1990;21:253–259.

25. Lewis W, Grody WW. AIDS and the heart: Review and consideration of pathogenetic mechanisms. Cardiovasc Pathol 1992;1:53–64.

26. DeCastro S, Miglia UG, Silvestri A, et al. Heart involvement in AIDS: A prospective study during various stages of the disease. Eur Heart J 1992; 12:1452–1459.

27. Hsia J, Adams S, Mohanty N, Ross A. Human immunodeficiency virus-related heart disease during 560 patient-years of follow-up [Abstract]. Circulation 1992;86:I-795.

28. Fong IW, Howard R, Elzawi A, Simbul M, Chiasson D. Cardiac involvement in human immunodeficiency virus-infected patients. J Acquir Immune Defic Syndr 1993;6:380–385.

29. Bestetti RB. Cardiac involvement in the acquired immune deficiency syndrome. Int J Cardiol 1989; 22:143–146.

30. Johnson JE, Slife DM, Anders GT, et al. Cardiac dysfunction in patients seropositive for the human immunodeficiency virus. West J Med 1991;155:373–379.

31. Kaminski HJ, Katzman M, Wiest PM, et al. Cardiomyopathy associated with the acquired immune deficiency syndrome. J Acquir Immune Defic Syndr 1988;1:105–110.

32. Kaul S, Fishbein MC, Siegel RJ. Cardiac manifestations of acquired immune deficiency syndrome: A 1991 update. Am Heart J 1991;122: 535–544.

33. Kavanaugh-McHugh A, Ruff AJ, Rowe SA, Herskowitz A, Modlin JF. Cardiovascular manifestations. In: Pizzo PA, Wilfert CM, eds. Pediatric AIDS: The challenge of HIV infection in infants, children, and adolescents. Baltimore: Williams & Wilkins, 1991:355–372.

34. Kinney EL. Cardiac findings in AIDS. Chest 1988; 94:1113–1114.

35. Reitano J, King M, Cohen H, et al. Cardiac function in patients with acquired immune deficiency syndrome (AIDS) or AIDS prodrome [Abstract]. J Am Coll Cardiol 1984;3:525.

36. Sherron P, Pickoff AS, Ferrer PL, et al. Echocardiographic evaluation of myocardial function in pediatric AIDS patients [Abstract]. Am Heart J 1985;110:710.

37. Scott GB, Hutto C, Makuch RW, et al. Survival in children with perinatally acquired human immunodeficiency virus type 1 infection. N Engl J Med 1989;321:1791–1796.

38. Issenberg HJ, Charytan M, Rubinstein A. Cardiac involvement in children with acquired immune deficiency [Abstract]. Am Heart J 1985;110:710.

39. Kavanaugh-McHugh AL, Hutton N, Holt E, Modlin J, Livingston R, Ruff A. Echocardiographic abnormalities in pediatric HIV infection: Prevalence and serial changes [Abstract]. Pediatr Res 1992;31:166A.

40. Kavanaugh-McHugh AL, Ruff AJ, Rowe S et al. Cardiac abnormalities in a multicenter interventional study of children with symptomatic HIV infection [Abstract]. Pediatr Res 1991;28:1040.

41. Lipshultz SE, Sanders SP, Colan SD, McIntosh K. Enhanced LV function in pediatric human immunodeficiency virus infection [Abstract]. Pediatr Res 1989;25:183A.

42. Lipshultz SE, Chanock S, Sanders SP, Colan SD, McIntosh K. Cardiac manifestations of pediatric HIV infection [Abstract]. Circulation 1987;76: IV–515.

43. Greinier MA, Karr SS, Rakosan TA, Martin GR. Cardiac disease in children with human immunodeficiency virus: Relationship of cardiac disease to virus symptoms [Abstract]. Pediatr Res 1993: 33:21A.

44. Anderson DW, Virmani R, Reilly JM, et al. Prevalent myocarditis at necropsy in the acquired immunodeficiency syndrome. J Am Coll Cardiol 1988;11:792–799.

45. Himelman RB, Chung WS, Chernoff DN, Schiller NB, Hollander H. Cardiac manifestations of human immunodeficiency virus infection: A two-dimensional echocardiographic study. J Am Coll Cardiol 1989; 13:1030–1036.

46. Factor SM. Acquired immune deficiency syndrome: The heart of the matter. J Am Coll Cardiol 1989;13:1037–1038.

47. Lipshultz SE, Sanders SP, Colan SD, Orav EJ, McIntosh K. The use of left ventricular fractional shortening as an index of contractility in HIV-infected children [Abstract]. Am J Cardiol 1990; 66:521.

48. Lipshultz SE, Orav EJ, Sanders SP, Hale AR, McIntosh K, Colan SD. Abnormalities of cardiac structure and function in HIV-infected children treated with zidovudine. N Engl J Med 1992; 327:1260–1265.

49. Lipshultz SE, Sanders SP, Colan SD. Cardiac structure and function in HIV-infected children. N Engl J Med 1993;328:513–514.

50. Stewart JM, Kaul A, Gromisch DS, Reyes E, Woolf PK, Gowitz MH. Symptomatic cardiac dysfunction in children with human immunodeficiency virus infection. Am Heart J 1989;117:140–144.

51. Lipshultz SE, Luginbuhl LM, McIntosh K, Orav EJ. Cardiac morbidity and mortality in children with symptomatic HIV infection [Abstract]. Circulation 1992;86:I-362.

52. Mann J. AIDS in the world 1992. A global epidemic of out control? Global AIDS Policy Coalition News. Jun 3, 1992, p 4.

53. Schocken DD, Arrieta MI, Leaverton PE, Ross EA. Prevalence and mortality rate of congestive heart failure in the United States. J Am Coll Cardiol 1992;20:301–306.

54. Herskowitz A, Willoughby SB, Ansari AA, et al. High risk profile for the development of congestive heart failure in HIV-related cardiomyopathy [Abstract]. Circulation 1991;84:II-3.

55. Joshi VV. Pathology of childhood AIDS. Pediatr Clin North Am 1991;38:97–120.

56. Bharati S, Joshi VV, Connor EM, Oleske JM, Lev M. Conduction system in children with acquired immunodeficiency syndrome. Chest 1989;96: 406–413.

57. Joshi VV, Gadol C, Connor E, et al. Dilated cardiomyopathy in children with acquired immunodeficiency syndrome: A pathologic study of five cases. Human Pathol 1988;19:69–73.

58. Lipshultz SE, Miller TL, Orav EJ, McIntosh K. Exaggerated myocardial hypertrophic responses in pediatric HIV infection [Abstract]. Circulation 1990;82:III-11.

59. Lipshultz SE, Orav EJ, Sanders SP, Rubin A, McIntosh K, Colan SD. Progressive abnormalities of cardiac structure and function in HIV-infected children treated with AZT. [Abstract]. Pediatr Res 1992;31:169A.

60. Lipshultz SE, Sanders SP, Colan SD, et al. Does the increased myocardial mass seen in pediatric human immunodeficiency virus infection result from direct infection of cardiocytes? [Abstract] Circulation 1989;80:II-322.

61. Lipshultz SE, Fox CH, Perez-Atayde AR, et al. Identification of human immunodeficiency virus-1 RNA and DNA in the heart of a child with cardiovascular abnormalities and congenital acquired immune deficiency syndrome. Am J Cardiol 1990;66:246–250.

62. Walsh CA, Better D, Adam HM, Weiss B, Steeg CN. Holter monitor and ECG abnormalities in children with HIV [Abstract]. Am J Dis Child 1990;144:434.

63. Kavanaugh-McHugh AL, Rowe SA, Hutton N, Butz AM, Holt EA, Modlin JF. Prevalence of cardiac involvement in human immunodeficiency virus (HIV) infection [Abstract]. Pediatr Res 1990;27:174A.

64. Frassica JJ, Orav EJ, Walsh EP, Lipshultz SE. Arrhythmias among children prenatally exposed to cocaine [Abstract]. Pediatr Res 1992;31:19A.

65. Bayard PJ, Berger TG, Jacobson MA. Drug hypersensitivity reactions and human immunodeficiency virus disease. J Acquir Immune Defic Syndr 1992;5:1237–1257.

66. Kovacs A, Hinton D, Wong W, Rasheed S, Ono J, Hofman F. HIV infection of myocytes and sudden death in pediatric AIDS [Abstract]. Pediatr Res 1992;31:167A.

67. Brady MT, Reiner CB, Singley C, et al. Unexpected death in an infant with AIDS: Disseminated cytomegalovirus infection. Pediatr Pathol 1988;8:205–214.

68. Raviglione MC, Battan R, Taranta A. Cardiopulmonary resuscitation in patients with the acquired immunodeficiency syndrome. Arch Intern Med 1988;148:2602–2605.

69. Levy WS, Varghese J, Anderson DW, et al. Myocarditis diagnosed by endomyocardial biopsy in human immunodeficiency virus infection with cardiac dysfunction. Am J Cardiol 1988;62:658–659.

70. Monsuez JJ, Kinney EL, Vittecoq, et al. Comparison among acquired immune deficiency syndrome patients with and without clinical evidence of cardiac disease. Am J Cardiol 1988; 62:1311–1313.

71. Cox JN, diDio F, Pizzolato GP, et al. Aspergillus endocarditis and myocarditis in a patient with the acquired immunodeficiency syndrome (AIDS): A review of the literature. Virchows Arch 1990; 417:255–259.

72. Xiu RJ, Jun C, Berglund O. Microcirculatory disturbances in AIDS patients—a first report. Microvasc Res 1991;42:151–159.

73. Joshi VV, Pawel B, Connor E, et al. Arteriopathy in children with acquired immune deficiency syndrome. Pediatr Pathol 1987;7:261–275.

74. Tabib A, Greenland T, Mercier I, Loire R, Mornex JF. Coronary lesions in young HIV-positive subjects at necropsy [Letter]. Lancet 1992;340:730.

75. Lafeuillade A, Alessi MC, Poizot-Martin I, et al. Endothelial cell dysfunction in HIV infection. J Acquir Immune Defic Syndr 1992;5:127–131.

76. Nigro G, Pisano P, Krzysztofiak A. Recurrent Kawasaki disease associated with co-infection with parvovirus B19 and HIV-1. AIDS 1993;7: 288–290.

77. Mast HL, Haller JO, Schiller MS, Anderson VM. Pericardial effusion and its relationship to cardiac disease in children with acquired immunodeficiency syndrome. Pediatr Radiol 1992;22: 548–551.

78. Reynolds MM, Hecht SR, Berger M, Kolokathis A, Horowitz SF. Large pericardial effusion in the acquired immunodeficiency syndrome. Chest 1992;102:1746–1747.

79. Acierno LJ. Cardiac complications in acquired immonodeficiency syndrome (AIDS): A review. J Am Coll Cardiol 1989;13:1144–1154.

80. Cohen IS, Anderson DW, Virmani R, et al. Congestive cardiomyopathy in association with the acquired immunodeficiency syndrome. N Engl J Med 1986;315:628–630.

81. Herskowitz A, Willoughby SB, Beschorner WE, Neumann DA, Baughman KL. Myocarditis associated with severe left ventricular dysfunction in late stage HIV infection [Abstract]. Circulation 1992;86:I-6.

82. Raffanti SP, Chiaramida AJ, Sen P, et al. Assessment of cardiac function in patients with the acquired immunodeficiency syndrome. Chest 1988;93:592–594.

83. Corallo S, Mutinelli MR, Moroni M, et al. Echocardiography detects myocardial damage in AIDS: Prospective study in 102 patients. Eur Heart J 1988;9:887–892.

84. Levy WS, Simon GL, Rios JC, Ross AM. Prevalence of cardiac abnormalities in human immunodeficiency virus infection. Am J Cardiol 1989;63:86–89.

85. Kinney EL, Brafman D, Wright RJ. Echocardiographic findings in patients with acquired immunodeficiency syndrome (AIDS) and AIDS related complex (ARC). Cathet Cardiovasc Diagn 1989;16:182–185.

86. Eisenberg MJ, Gordon AS, Schiller NB. HIV associated pericardial effusions. Chest 1992;102:956–958.

87. Andress JD, Polish LB, Clark DM, et al. Transvenous biopsy diagnosis of cardiac lymphoma in an AIDS patient. Am Heart J 1989;118:421–423.

88. Balasubramanyam A, Waxman M, Kazal HL, et al. Malignant lymphoma of the heart in acquired immune deficiency syndrome. Chest 1986;90:243–246.

89. Gesner M, Pollack H, Lawrence R, Chandwani S, Krasinski K, Borkowsky W. Clinical and laboratory correlates of mycobacterium avium infection (MAI) in HIV-infected children [Abstrtact]. Pediatr Res 1992;31:163A.

90. Ioachim HL, Cooper MC, Hellman GC. Lymphoma in men at high risk for acquired immune deficiency syndrome (AIDS). Cancer 1985;56:2831–2842.

91. Guarner J, Brynes RK, Chan WC, Birdsong G, Hertzler G. Primary non-Hodgkins lymphoma of the heart in two patients with the acquired immunodeficiency syndrome. Arch Pathol Lab Med 1987;111:254–256.

92. Constantino A, West TE, Gupta M, et al. Primary cardiac lymphoma in a patient with acquired immune deficiency syndrome. Cancer 1987;60:2801–2805.

93. Gill PS, Chandraratna AN, Meyer PR, et al. Malignant lymphoma: Cardiac involvement at initial presentation. J Clin Oncol 1987;5:216–224.

94. Kelsey RC, Saker A, Moran M. Cardiac lymphoma in a patient with AIDS. Ann Intern Med 1991;115:370–371.

95. Holladay AO, Siegel RJ, Schwartz DA. Cardiac malignant lymphoma in acquired immune deficiency syndrome. Cancer 1992;70:2203–2207.

96. McDonnell PJ, Mann RB, Bulkley BH. Involvement of the heart by malignant lymphoma: A clinicopathologic study. Cancer 1982;49:944–951.

97. Autran BR, Gorin I, Leibowitch M, et al. AIDS in a Haitian woman with cardiac Kaposi's sarcoma and Whipple's disease. Lancet 1983;1:767–768.

98. Roldan EO, Moskowitz L, Hensley GT. Pathology of the heart in acquired immunodeficiency syndrome. Arch Pathol Lab Med 1987;111:943–946.

99. Cammarosano C, Lewis W. Cardiac lesions in acquired immune deficiency syndrome (AIDS). J Am Coll Cardiol 1985;5:703–706.

100. Stotten JA, Good CB, Downer WR, et al. Pericardial effusion and tamponade due to Kaposi's sarcoma in acquired immunodeficiency syndrome. Chest 1989;951:1359–1361.

101. Steigman CK, Anderson DW, Macher AM, Senner JD, Virmani RL. Fatal cardiac tamponade in acquired immunodeficiency syndrome with epicardial Kaposi's sarcoma. Am Heart J 1988;116:1105–1107.

102. Reilly JM, Cunnion RE, Anderson DW, et al. Frequency of myocarditis, left ventricular dysfunction and ventricular tachycardia in the acquired immune deficiency syndrome. Am J Cardiol 1988;62:789–793.

103. Baroldi G, Corallo S, Moroni M, et al. Focal lymphocytic myocarditis in acquired immunodeficiency syndrome (AIDS): A correlative morphologic and clinical study in 26 consecutive fatal cases. J Am Coll Cardiol 1988;12:463–469.

104. Silver MA, Macher AM, Reichert CM, et al. Cardiac involvement by Kaposi's sarcoma in acquired immmune deficiency syndrome (AIDS). Am J Cardiol 1984;53:983–985.

105. Lewis W, Lipsick J, Cammarosano C. Cryptococcal myocarditis in acquired immune deficiency syndrome. Am J Cardiol 1985;55:1238–1239.

106. Levinson DA, Semple Pd'A. Primary cardiac Kaposi's sarcoma. Thorax 1976;31:595–600.

107. Issenberg HJ, Cho S, Rubinstein A, et al. Cardiac pathology in children with acquired immune deficiency syndrome [Abstract]. Pediatr Res 1986:295A.

108. Niedt GE, Schinella RA. Acquired immunodeficiency syndrome: Clinicopathologic study of 56 autopsies. Arch Pathol Lab Med 1985;109:727–734.

109. Henochowicz S, Mustafa M, Lawinson WE, Pistole M, Lindsay J. Cardiac aspergillosis in acquired immune deficiency syndrome. Am J Cardiol 1985;55:1239–1240.

110. Nahass RG, Weinstein MP, Bartels J, et al. Infective endocarditis in intravenous drug users: A comparison of human immunodeficiency virus type-1 negative and positive patients. J Infect Dis 1990;162:967–970.

111. Hays MD, Wiles HB, Gillette PC. Congenital acquired immunodeficiency syndrome presenting as cor pulmonale in a 10-year-old-girl. Am Heart J 1991;121:929–931.

112. Himelman RB, Dohrmann M, Goodman P, et al. Severe pulmonary hypertension and cor pulmonale in the acquired immunodeficiency syndrome. Am J Cardiol 1989;64:1396–1399.

113. DeCastro S, d'Amati G, Gallo P, et al. Frequency and significance of acute global left ventricular dysfunction (LVD) in human immunodeficiency virus (HIV) infection [Abstract]. J Am Coll Cardiol 1993;21:280A.

114. Jacob AJ, Sutherland GR, Bird AG, et al. Myocardial dysfunction in patients infected with HIV: Prevalence and risk factors. Br Heart J 1992;68:549–553.

115. Blanchard DG, Hagenhoff C, Chow LC, McCann HA, Dittrich HC. Reversibility of cardiac abnormalities in human immunodeficiency virus (HIV)-infected individuals: A serial echocardiographic study. J Am Coll Cardiol 1991;17:1270–1276.

116. Kostianovsky M, Orenstein JM, Schaff Z, et al. Cytomembranous inclusions observed in acquired immunodeficiency syndrome. Arch Pathol Lab Med 1987;111:218–223.

117. Wu T-C, Pizzorno MC, Hayward GS, et al. In situ detection of human cytomegalovirus immediate-early gene transcripts within cardiac myocytes of patients with HIV-associated cardiomyopathy. AIDS 1992;6:777–785.

118. Nathan PE, Arsula EL, Zappi M. Pericarditis with tamponade due to cytomegalovirus in the acquired immunodeficiency syndrome. Chest 1991;99:765–766.

119. Towbin JA, Ni J, Demmler G, Martin A, Kearney D, Bricker JT. Evidence for adenovirus as a common cause of myocarditis in children using polymerase chain reaction (PCR) [Abstract]. Pediatr Res 1993;33:27A.

120. Dittrich H, Chow L, Denaro F, Spector S. Human immunodeficiency virus, coxsackievirus, and cardiomyopathy. Ann Intern Med 1988;108:308–309.

121. Freedberg RS, Gindea AJ, Dieterich D, et al. Herpes simplex pericarditis in AIDS. N Y State J Med 1987;304–306.

122. Eisenstat DDR, Tove B, Gow R, et al. Familial myocarditis associated with human parvovirus B19 infection [Abstract]. Circulation 1990;82:III-390.

123. Odeh M. The role of tumour necrosis factor-alpha in acquired immunodeficiency syndrome. J Intern Med 1990;228:549–556.

124. Ho DD, Pomerantz RJ, Kaplan JC. Pathogenesis of infection with human immunodeficiency virus. N Engl J Med 1986;317:278–286.

125. Grody WW, Cheng L, Lewis W. Infection of the heart by the human immunodeficiency virus. Am J Cardiol 1990;66:203–206.

126. Rodriguez ER, Nasim S, Hsia J, et al. Cardiac myocytes and dendritic cells harbor human immunodeficiency virus in infected patients with and without cardiac dysfunction: Detection by multiplex, nested, polymerase chain reaction in individually microdissected cells from right ventricular endomyocardial biopsy tissue. Am J Cardiol 1991;68:1511–1522.

127. Wu AY-Y, Forouhar F, Cartun RW, et al. Identification of human immunodeficiency virus in the heart of a patient with acquired immunodeficiency syndrome. Mod Pathol 1990;3:625–630.

128. Cenacchi G, Re MC, Furlini G, et al. Human immunodeficiency virus type antigen detection in endomyocardial biopsy: An immunomorphological study. Microbiologica 1990;13:145–149.

129. Calabrese L, Proffitt M, Yen-Lieberman B, et al. Congestive cardiomyopathy and illness related to the acquired immunodeficiency syndrome (AIDS) associated with isolation of retrovirus from myocardium. Ann Intern Med 1987;107:691–692.

130. Flomenbaum M, Soeiro R, Udem SA, Kress Y, Factor SM. Proliferative membranopathy and human immunodeficiency virus in AIDS hearts. J Acquir Immune Defic Syndr 1989;2:129–135.

131. Lafont A, Wolfe M, Marche C, et al. Overwhelming myocarditis due to cryptococcus neoformans in an AIDS patient. Lancet 1987;1:1145–1146.

132. Brivet F, Livertowski J, Herve P, Rain B, Dormont J. Pericardial cryptococcal disease in acquired immune deficiency syndrome [Letter]. Am J Med 1987;821:1273.

133. Schuster M, Valentine F, Holtzman R. Cryptococcal pericarditis in an IVDA. J Infect Dis 1985;152:842.

134. Eng RHK, Bishburg E, Smith SM, et al. Crypotococcal infections in patients with acquired immune deficiency syndrome. Am J Med 1986;81:19–23.

135. Hsia JA. Cardiac complications of HIV infection. Med Aspects Hum Sexual 1990;60–65.

136. Stechel RP, Cooper DJ, Greenspan J, Pizzarello RA, Tenenbaum MS. Staphlococcal percarditis in a homosexual patient with AIDS-related complex. N Y State J Med 1986;68:592–593.

137. D'Cruz IA, Sengupta EE, Abrahams C, Reddy HK, Turlapati RV. Cardiac involvement, including tuberculous pericardial effusion, complicating acquired immune deficiency syndrome. Am Heart J 1986;112:1100–1102.

138. Dalli E, Quesada A, Juan G, et al. Tuberculous pericarditis as the first manifestation of acquired immunodeficiency syndrome. Am Heart J 1987;114:905–906.

139. Sunderam G, McDonald RJ, Maniatis T, et al. Tuberculosis as a manifestation of the acquired immunodeficiency syndrome (AIDS). JAMA 1986;256:362–366.

140. Kinney EL, Monsuez JJ, Kitzis M, et al. Treatment of AIDS-associated heart disease. Angiology 1989:970–976.

141. Hawkins CC, Gold JWM, Whimbey E, et al. Mycobacterium avium complex infections in patients with the acquired immunodeficiency syndrome. Ann Intern Med 1986;105:184–188.

142. Lewis LL, Butler KM, Husson RN, et al. Defining the population of human immunodeficiency virus-infected children at risk for Mycobacterium avium-intracellulare infection. J Pediatr 1992;121:677–683.

143. Woods GL, Goldsmith JC. Fatal pericarditis due to mycobacterium avium-intracellulare in acquired immunodeficiency syndrome. Chest 1989;95:1355–1357.

144. Holtz HA, Lavery DP, Kapila R. Actinomycetales infection in the acquired immunodeficiency syndrome. Ann Intern Med 1985;102:203–205.

145. Medlock MD, Tilleli JT, Pearl GS. Congenital cardiac toxoplasmosis in a newborn with acquired immunodeficiency syndrome. Pediatr Infect Dis J 1990;9:129–132.

146. Grange F, Kinney EL, Monsuez, J-J, et al. Successful therapy for toxoplasma gondii my-

ocarditis in acquired immunodeficiency syndrome. Am Heart J 1990;120;443–444.

147. Adair OV, Randive N, Krashow N. Isolated toxoplasma myocarditis in acquired immune deficiency syndrome. Am Heart J 1989;118:856–857.

148. Guarda LA, Luna MA, Smith LJ, et al. Acquired immune deficiency syndrome: Postmortem findings. Am J Clin Pathol 1984;81:549–557.

149. Klatt EC, Meyer PR. Pathology of the heart in acquired immunodeficiency syndrome (AIDS) [Letter]. Arch Pathol Lab Med 1988;112:114.

150. Dworkin BM, Antonecchia PP, Smith F, et al. Reduced cardiac selenium content in the acquired immunodeficiency syndrome. J Parenter Enter Nutr 1989;13:644–647.

151. Kavanaugh-McHugh AL, Ruff A, Perlman E, Hutton N, Modlin J, Rowe S. Selenium deficiency and cardiomyopathy in acquired immunodeficiency syndrome. J Parenter Enter Nutr 1991;15:347–349.

152. Alden PB, Madoff RD, Stahl TJ, Ring WS, Cerra FB. Cardiac function in malnutrition. In: Watson RR. Nutrition and heart disease. Boca Raton: CRC Press, 1987;2:71–81.

153. Webb JG, Kiess MC, Chan-Yan CC. Malnutrition and the heart. Can Med Assoc J 1986;135:753.

154. Miller TL, Evans SJ, Orav EJ, Morris V, McIntosh K, Winter HS. Growth and body composition in children infected with the human immunodeficiency virus-1. Am J Clin Nutr 1993;57.

155. Parker TG, Schneider MD. Growth factors, protooncogenes, and plasticity of the cardiac phenotype. Annu Rev Physiol 1991;53:179–200.

156. Matsuyama T, Kobayashi N, Yamamoto N. Cytokines and HIV infection: Is AIDS a tumor necrosis factor disease? AIDS 1991;5:1405–1417.

157. Graettinger JS, Parsons RL, Campbell JA. A correlation of clinical and hemodynamic studies in partients with mild and severe anemia with and without congestive failure. Ann Intern Med 1963;58:617.

158. Duke M, Abelmann WH. The hemodynamic response to chronic anemia. Circulation 1969;39:503.

159. Van Vliet PD, Burchell HB, Titus JL. Myocarditis associated with pheochromocytoma. N Engl J Med 1966;274:1102.

160. Szakacs JE, Cannon A. Norepinephrine myocarditis. Am J Clin Pathol 1958;30:425–434.

161. Factor SM, Sonnenblick EH. The pathogenesis of clinical and experimental congestive cardiomyopathies and recent concepts. Prog Cardiovasc Dis 1985;27:395–420.

162. Lewin D, d'Amati G, Lewis W. Hypersensitivity myocarditis: Findings in native and transplanted hearts. Cardiovasc Pathol 1992;1:225–230.

163. Balslev U, Berild D, Nielsen TL. Cardiac arrest during treatment of Pneumocystis carinii pneumonia with intravenous pentamidine isethionate. Scand J Infect Dis 1992;24:111–112.

164. Bibler MR, Chou T, Toltzis RJ, et al. Recurrent ventricular tachycardia due to pentamidine-induced cardiotoxicity. Chest 1988;94:1303–1306.

165. Crogin H, Liem LB. Pentamidine-induced torsades de pointes. Cardiology 1991;2:114–115.

166. Loescher T, Loeschke K, Niebel J. Severe ventricular arrhythmia during pentamidine treatment of AIDS-associated Pneumocystis carinii pneumonia. Infection 1987;15:455.

167. Pujol M, Carratala J, Mauri J, et al. Ventricular tachycardia due to pentamidine isethionate. Am J Med 1988;84:980.

168. Deyton LR, Walker RE, Kovacs JA, et al. Reversible cardiac dysfunction associated with interferon-alpha therapy in AIDS patients with Kaposi's sarcoma. N Engl J Med 1989;321:1246–1249.

169. Werner JC, Sicard RE, Hansen TWR, Solomon E, Cowett RM, Oh W. Hypertrophic cardiomyopathy associated with dexamethasone therapy for bronchopulmonary dysplasia J Pediatr 1992; 120:286–291.

170. Wilkins CE, Sexton DJ, McAllister HA. HIV-associated myocarditis treated with zidovudine (AZT). Tex Heart Inst J 1989;16:44–45.

171. Hsia J, Adams S, Ross AM. National history of human immunodeficiency virus (HIV) associated heart disease [Abstract]. Circulation 1991;84:II-3.

172. Herskowitz A, Willoughby SB, Baughman KL, Schulman SP, Bartlett JD. Cardiomyopathy associated with antiretroviral therapy in patients with HIV infection: A report of six cases. Ann Intern Med 1992;116:311–313.

173. d'Amati G, Kwan W, Lewis W. dilated cardiomyopathy in a zidovudine-treated AIDS patient. Cardiovasc Pathol 1992;1:317–320.

174. Lamperth L, Dalakas MC, Dagani F, Anderson J, Ferrari R. Abnormal skeletal and cardiac muscle mitochondria induced by zidovudine (AZT) in human muscle in vitro and in an animal model. Lab Invest 1991;65:742–751.

175. Lewis W, Gonzalez B, Chomyn A, Papoian T. Zidovudine induces molecular, biochemical, and ultrastructural changes in rat skeletal muscle mitochondria. J Clin Invest 1992;89:1354–1360.

176. Lewis W, Papoian T, Gonzalez B, et al. Mitochondrial ultrastructural and molecular changes induced by zidovudine in rat hearts. Lab Invest 1991;65:228–236.

177. Arnaudo E, Dalakas M, Shanske S, Moraes CT, DiMauro S, Schon EA. Depletion of muscle mitochondrial DNA in AIDS patients with zidovudine-induced myopathy. Lancet 1991;337:508–510.

178. Valentine C, Williams O, Davis A, et al. Case study of zidovudine overdose. AIDS 1993;7:436–437.

179. Beschorner WE, Baughman K, Turnicky RP, et al. HIV-associated myocarditis, pathology and immunopathology. Am J Pathol 1990;137:1365–1371.

180. Fisher LL, Fisher EA. Myocarditis associated wiith human immunodeficiency virus infection. Primary Cardiol 1990;16:49–60.

181. Case records of the Massachusetts General Hospital. Case 44-1992. N Engl J Med 1992; 327:1370–1376.

182. Corboy JR, Fink L, Miller T. Congestive cardiomyopathy in association with AIDS. Radiology 1987;165:139–141.

183. Hensley GT, Moskowitz L. Pathology of the heart in acquired immunodeficiency syndrome (AIDS) [Letter]. Arch Pathol Lab Med 1988;112:114.

184. Klima M, Escudier SM. Pathologic findings in the hearts of patients with acquired immunodeficiency syndrome. Tex Heart Inst J 1991;18:116–121.

185. Lafont A, Marche C, Wolff M, et al. Myocarditis in acquired immunodeficiency syndrome (AIDS): Etiology and prognosis [Abstract]. J Am Coll Cardiol 1988;11:196A.

186. Lewis W. AIDS: Cardiac findings from 115 autopsies. Prog Cardiovasc Dis 1989;3:207–215.

187. Magno J, Margretten W, Cheitlin M. Myocardial involvement in acquired immunodeficiency syndrome: Incidence in a large autopsy series [Abstract]. J Am Coll Cardiol 1988;78:II-459.

188. Cho S, Matano S, Factor SM. Cardiac lesions in 118 autopsied acquired immune deficiency syndrome patients: Intravenous drug abusers and homosexuals [Abstract]. Lab Invest 1989;60:17A.

189. van Hoeven KH, Segal B, Factor SM. AIDS cardiomyopathy: First rule out other myocardial risk factors. Int J Cardiol 1990;29:35–37.

190. Roberts JW, Navarro C, Johnson A, et al. Cardiac involvement is comparable in intravenous drug abusers with and without acquired immunodeficiency syndrome [Abstract]. Circulation 1989; 80:II-322.

191. Turnicky RP, Goodin J, Smialek JE, Herskowitz A, Beschorner WE. Incidental myocarditis with intravenous drug abuse: The pathology, immunopathology, and potential implications for human immunodeficiency virus-associated myocarditis. Hum Pathol 1992;23:138–143.

192. Willoughby SB, Vlahov D, Herskowitz A. Frequency of left ventricular dysfunction and other echocardiographic abnormalities in human immunodeficiency virus seronegative intravenous drug users. Am J Cardiol 1993;71:446–447.

193. Maserati R, Parisi A, Pan A, Lanzarini. Rapidly reversible cardiomyopathy in an AIDS patient. AIDS 1991;5:1145–1146.

194. Hakas JF, Generalovich T. Spontaneous regression of cardiomyopathy in a patient with the acquired immunodeficiency syndrome. Chest 1991; 99:770–772.

195. Kavanaugh-McHugh A, Rowe S, Ruff A, et al. Cardiac involvement in children with human immunodeficiency virus (HIV) infection: Evidence for autoimmunity [Abstract C33]. International Conference on Implications of AIDS for Mothers and Children, 1989.

196. Herskowitz A, Ansari AA, Neumann DA, et al. Cardiomyopathy in acquired immunodeficiency syndrome: Evidence for autoimmunity [Abstract]. Circulation 1989;80:II-322.

197. Gu J, Dische R, Anderson V, et al. Evidence for an autoimmune mechanism of the cardiac pathology in AIDS patients [Abstract]. Circulation 1992;86:I-795.

198. Woodley SL, McMillan M, Shelby J, et al. Myocyte injury and contraction abnormalities produced by cytotoxic T lymphocytes. Circulation 1991;83:1410–1418.

199. Freeman R, Roberts MS, Friedman LS, et al. Autonomic function and human immunodeficiency virus infection. Neurology 1990;40:575–580.

200. Ruttiman S, Hilti P, Spinas GA, Dubach UC. High frequency of human immunodeficiency virus-associated autonomic neuropathy and more severe involvement in advanced stages of human immunodeficiency virus disease. Arch Intern Med 1991;151:2441–2443.

201. Piaggesi A, Ewing DJ. Sequential autonomic function tests in HIV infection. AIDS 1990;4:1279–1281.

202. Villa A, Foresti V. Autonomic nervous system dysfunction associated with HIV infection in intravenous heroin users. AIDS 1992;6:85–89.

203. Cohen J, Laudenslager M. Autonomic nervous system dysfunction in human immunodeficiency virus. Neurology 1989;8:111–112.

204. Miller TL, Winter HS, Orav EJ, Colan SD, McIntosh K, Lipshultz SE. Preservation of cardiac function and mass in pediatric HIV infection accompanied by skeletal muscle wasting and malnutrition [Abstract]. Pediatr Res 1990;27:177A.

205. Luginbuhl LM, Balkaran B, Lipshultz SE, Orav EJ, McIntosh K. Respiratory viral infections in HIV infected children. 31st Interscience Conference on Antimicrobial Agents and Chemotherapy, Chicago, Oct 1991.

206. Ross RD, Bollinger RO, Pinsky WW. Grading the severity of congestive heart failure in infants. Pediatr Cardiol 1992;13:72–75.

207. Johnson JE, Anders GT, Blanton HM, et al. Exercise dysfunction in patients seropositive for the human immunodeficiency virus. Am Rev Respir Dis 1990;141:618–622.

208. Bierman FZ. Guidelines for diagnosis and management of cardiac disease in children with HIV infection. J Pediatr 1991;38A:S53–S56.

209. Lafont A, Darishe H, Sayegh F, et al. At which stage of human immunodeficiency virus infection is echocardiography useful in diagnosing cardiac injury [Abstract]. Circulation 1988;781:II-458.

210. Mugge A, Daniel WG, Frank G, et al. Echocardiography in infective endocarditis: Reassessment of prognostic implications of vegetation size determined by the transthoracic and the transesophageal approach. J Am Coll Cardiol 1989; 14:631–638.

211. Sochowski RA, Chan KL. Transesophageal echocardiography for endocarditis. J Am Coll Cardiol 1993;21:216–221.

212. Hsia J, Colan SD, Adams S, Ross AM. Late potentials and their relation to ventricular function in human immunodeficiency virus infection. Am J Cardiol 1991;68:1216–1220.

213. Chow LH, Radio SJ, Sears TD, McManus BM. Insensitivity of right ventricular endomyocardial biopsy in the diagnosis of myocarditis. J Am Coll Cardiol 1989;14:915–920.

214. Yoshizato T, Edwards WD, Alboliras ET, Hagler DJ, Driscoll DJ. Safety and utility of endomyocardial biopsy in infants, children and adolescents: A review of 66 procedures in 53 patients. J Am Coll Cardiol 1990;15:436–442.

215. Steinherz LJ, Brochstei JA, Robins J. Cardiac involvement in congenital acquired immunodficiency syndrome. Am J Dis Child 1986;140:1241–1244.

216. Newberger JW, Sanders SP, Burns JC, Parness IA, Beiser AS, Colan SD. Left ventricular contractility and function in Kawasaki syndrome: Effect of intravenous gamma-globulin. Circulation 1989; 79:1237–1246.

217. Drucker NA, Colan SD, Wessel DL, et al. Use of intravenous gamma globulin in acute congestive cardiomyopathy [Abstract]. Circulation 1992; 86:I-363.
218. Lipshultz SE, Orav EJ, Sander SP, McIntosh K, Colan SD. Left ventricular structure and function is improved by endogenous and exogenous immunoglobulins in HIV-infected children [Abstract]. Circulation, in press.
219. Viard J-P, Vittecoq D, Lacroix C, Bach J-F. Response of HIV-1 associated polymyositis to intravenous immunoglobulin [Letter]. Am J Med 1992;92:580–581.
220. National Institute of Child Health and Human Development Intravenous Immunoglobulin Study Group. Intravenous immune globulin for the prevention of bacterial infections in children with symptomatic human immunodeficiency virus infection. N Engl J Med 1991;325:73–80.
221. Mofenson LM, Moye J Jr, Bethel J, et al. Prophylactic intravenous immunoglobulin in HIV-infected children with CD4+ counts of 0.20×10^9/L or more: Effect on viral, opportunistic, and bacterial infections. JAMA 1992;268:483–488.
222. Dwyer JM. Manipulating the immune system with immune globulin. N Engl J Med 1992;326:107–116.
223. Chan KY, Iwahara M, Benson LN, Wilson GJ, Freedom RM. Immunosuppressive therapy in the management of acute myocarditis in children: A clinical trial. J Am Coll Cardiol 1991;17:458–460.
224. DeSimone C, Tzantzoglou S, Jirillo E. L-carnitine deficiency in AIDS patients. AIDS 1992;6:203–205.
225. Baruchel S, Wainberg MA. The role of oxidative stress in disease progression in individuals infected by the human immunodeficiency virus. J Leukoc Biol 1992;52:111–114.
226. Oster O, Prellwitz W. Selenium and cardiovascular disease. Biol Trace Element Res 1990;24:91–103.
227. Dworkin BM, Rosenthal WS, Wormwer GP, Weigs L. Selenium deficiency in the acquired immunodeficiency syndrome. J Parenter Enter Nutr 1986; 10:405–407.
228. Lafont A, Zazzo JF, Chappuis P, et al. Are cardiomyopathies in acquired immunodeficiency syndrome dependent on selenium deficiency? [Abstract]. Circulation 1988;78:II-375.
229. Miller TL, Orav EJ, McIntosh K, Lipshultz SE. Is selenium deficiency clinically significant in pediatric HIV infection? [Abstract]. Gastroenterology 1993;104:A746.
230. Waber LJ, Valle D, Neill C, Di Mauro S, Shig A. Carnitine deficiency presenting as familial cardiomyopathy: A treatable defect in carnitine transport. J Pediatr 1982;101:700–705.
231. Maisch B, Schonian U. Elimination of cytomegalovirus DNA by hyperimmunoglobulin therapy in active myocarditis and dilated heart muscle disease [Abstract]. J Am Coll Cardiol 1993;21:21A.
232. Jacob AJ, Boon NA. HIV cardiomyopathy: A dark cloud with a silver lining? Br Heart J 1991;66:1–2.

27

Gastrointestinal and Nutritional Problems in Pediatric HIV Disease

Harland S. Winter and Tracie L. Miller

AIDS in the western world began with reports of *Pneumocystis carinii* pneumonia and Kaposi's sarcoma, whereas in Africa gastrointestinal dysfunction—diarrhea and weight loss—were much more common. The initial reports from Uganda (1) described "slim disease," a syndrome that was distinguished from AIDS and AIDS-related complex (ARC) by extreme wasting and diarrhea. Currently, the gastrointestinal and nutritional manifestations of HIV are recognized as part of the clinical course of human immunodeficiency virus (HIV) infection throughout the world.

The gastrointestinal tract not only is essential for maintaining nutritional status and growth but also is an important determinant of clinical outcome in many chronic diseases including cancer and cystic fibrosis. There are many immunologic similarities between patients with AIDS and those with protein-energy malnutrition. After deterioration of immune function from malnutrition or HIV, enteric pathogens may injure the intestinal mucosa causing malabsorption. Prolonged malabsorption leads to malnutrition that by itself causes immunodeficiency. This cycle of events is depicted in Figure 27.1 and

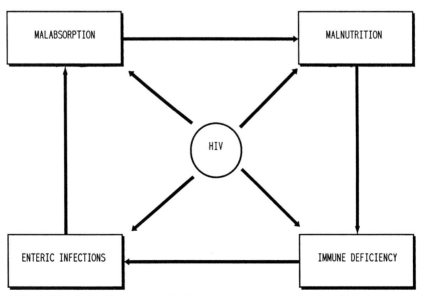

Figure 27.1. Possible relationship between malabsorption, malnutrition, immune deficiency, and enteric infections.

supports the hypothesis that maintenance of appropriate nutrition in the HIV-infected individual may delay decline of immune function and subsequent clinical deterioration.

PATHOGENESIS AND NATURAL HISTORY

The decline in CD4+ lymphocytes consequent to HIV infection results in deficiencies in both cellular and humoral systemic immune function as well as immunoregulatory defects in the mucosal immune system of the gastrointestinal tract. The epithelial surface of the gastrointestinal tract is constantly bathed by potential pathogens and antigens to which it reacts. Antigens are processed by macrophages and follicular dendritic cells and are then presented to T and B cells. Primed lymphocytes migrate to the mesenteric lymph nodes where they are clonally expanded and eventually enter the peripheral circulation via the thoracic duct. These sensitized lymphocytes are recognized by a series of homing proteins on the high endothelial venules and return to the intestine, entering the lamina propria where they act as effector cells. CD4+ lymphocytes comprise the major population in the lamina propria, which could result in HIV infection of the intestinal mucosa. In addition, lamina propria T cells express CD25 (the α-chain of the interleukin-2 receptor), suggesting that these cells are activated. In the epithelium, CD8+ cells predominate and in perinatally infected children as well as in infected adults the ratio of CD8 to CD4 cells is increased (2, 3), possibly owing to decreased numbers of CD4 cells.

In animal models, HIV can be transported across M cells into intestinal lymphoid follicles (4). In humans, HIV RNA has been associated with follicular dendritic cells within lymphoid follicles (Fig. 27.2) (5, 6). There have been a few studies suggesting that epithelial cells can be reservoirs for virus, but most evidence supports the presence of only isolated lamina propria cells expressing HIV RNA (Fig. 27.2) (5–9). These infected cells may be found early in the course of HIV disease, but their relationship with gastrointestinal dysfunction is unknown. The number of intraepithelial lymphocytes are unchanged except when opportunistic infections are identified (10, 11). Mucosal B cell function appears to be modified with an increase in IgM-containing and a decrease in IgA-containing plasma cells (12).

The question of HIV infecting epithelial cells remains unanswered. Studies using isolated epithelial cells and colon cancer cells lines demonstrate that infection can occur even in the absence of demonstrable CD4 on the cell surface (13–15). However, when biopsy material is examined, epithelial cells are rarely infected with HIV (8). Considering the experimental and clinical data, one would conclude that HIV infection of the intestinal epithelium is not a major factor in the pathogenesis of intestinal dysfunction.

Gastrointestinal Disorders

The pathogenesis for the intestinal dysfunction observed in HIV-infected individuals is unknown. It is speculated that abnormalities in epithelial cell function and nutrient absorption may be related to changes in the mucosal immune system. Abnormalities in epithelial cell expression of lactase occur before demonstrable enteric infection or injury to the epithelium (16). This could be related to changes in the immunoregulatory environment of the lamina propria that may, through secondary messengers such as cytokines, alter epithelial cell function. Disruption of the immunologic environment in graft vs. host disease can, for example, result in decreased absorptive surface area (17). Because milk and milk products can be an important source of energy and protein for children, disruption of their absorption may affect a child's growth and well-being.

Opportunistic infections such as cryptosporidium also are involved in the pathogenesis of intestinal dysfunction by injuring the epithelial cells on the villi and causing a compensatory increase in crypt hyperplasia. This decrease in the villus-to-crypt ratio results in less absorptive surface area and loss of nutrients.

Hepatobiliary Disease

Many cells in the liver can become infected with HIV. Although hepatocytes do

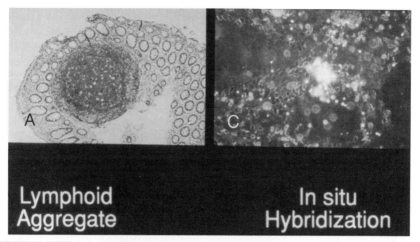

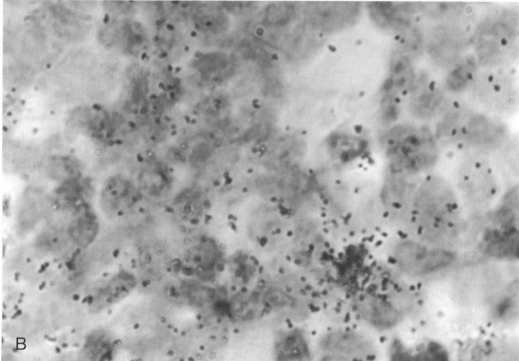

Figure 27.2.   In situ hybridization and immunohistochemical staining of gastrointestinal tract illustrating presence of a lymphoid aggregate with follicular dendritic cells stained with CD21 (red) (**A**), HIV RNA identified by silver grains (black dots) (**B**), and a single HIV-infected cell in lamina propria (**C**). No evidence of HIV-infected epithelial cells could be found. Courtesy of Dr. Cecil Fox, Molecular Histology Laboratory, Gaithersburg, MD. This author also expresses his personal appreciation to Dr. Fox for his major contributions to the pathobiology of HIV disease.

not express CD4, they can become infected with HIV-1 (18, 19). Similarly, hepatoma-derived cell lines can be infected by HIV (20). The increase in idiopathic chronic active hepatitis in HIV-infected children suggests a role for primary HIV infection. Despite clinical and laboratory evidence suggesting that HIV may be involved in the development of hepatic pathology, the role of occult opportunistic infections cannot be eliminated. Although hepatocytes and Kupffer cells can be infected by HIV, there is little clinical evidence to support that HIV itself is an important cause of hepatocellular dysfunction.

Weight Loss

Malnutrition is one of the most common features in the HIV-infected child. Over 95% of children will develop clinically significant malnutrition before their death, and at any one time, 40–60% of HIV-infected infants and children will meet criteria for mild to severe malnutrition. One study examining the effect of zidovudine on symptomatic HIV-infected children documented that 80% had growth abnormalities (21). HIV-infected children with hemophilia have deficits in both height and weight (22). Factors associated with malnutrition include dysfunction of the gastrointestinal tract, including vomiting, diarrhea, and opportunistic infections. However, significant malnutrition may develop in individuals who are otherwise clinically stable and without gastrointestinal symptoms or opportunistic infections. These children may have increased energy expenditure, decreased caloric intake, or psychosocial causes contributing to their malnutrition.

The pathogenesis of malnutrition in HIV infection is unclear. Failure to grow may occur early and precede other clinical manifestations of HIV infection. For most children the causes are multifactorial, including reduced food intake, increased

Table 27.1.   Possible Causes of Malnutrition

Reduction in food intake
    Infection: *Candida*, cytomegaloviral
       esophagitis
    Difficulty in chewing and swallowing: gingival
       and oral ulcers
    Enteropathy/gastritis: nausea, vomiting,
       diarrhea
    Zinc deficiency
    Fever
    Pain
    Dementia
    Depression or despair
Increased nutrient requirements
    Hypermetabolism: fever
    Futile cycling
    Cytokine production
Impaired nutrient absorption
    Opportunistic infection
    Lactose malabsorption
    Pancreatic insufficiency
    Enteropathy

nutrient requirements, and/or impaired nutrient absorption. Poor oral intake is common in symptomatic children with HIV and may be related to many factors (Table 27.1). Inflammation of the upper gastrointestinal tract from peptic ulcerations or infectious agents, such as *Candida*, cytomegalovirus, or herpes simplex, may cause anorexia because of the discomfort of eating. Dental caries and immune deficiency contribute to periodontal disease that causes the child to experience pain when chewing and therefore to avoid eating. Enteropathy associated with a primary or secondary lactose intolerance or generalized malabsorption can result in flatulence, abdominal distention, abdominal pain, and chronic diarrhea. Similarly, pancreatitis causes malabsorption of fat and protein along with abdominal pain. The association of eating with abdominal discomfort, whatever etiology, reinforces the behavior of avoiding food. Specific nutrient deficiencies such as zinc contribute to decreased intake of food because of dysgeusia. Furthermore, fever, pain, dementia, depression, despair, and lack of access to food are factors that cannot be ignored by the clinician trying to determine the pathogenesis for anorexia in an HIV-infected child.

Primary anorexia, which has been described in patients with cancer and other chronic disorders, may also contribute to poor oral intake in HIV-infected children. It is postulated that cytokine production (possibly tumor necorsis factor) may be associated with anorexia. Although some children may not receive adequate calories, many children with altered nutritional status eat sufficient amounts yet do not grow (23). The adult literature in this area is conflicting with reports of suboptimal vs. adequate oral intake (24, 25).

Increased nutrient requirements may also contribute to altered nutritional status of the HIV-infected child. The precise estimation of energy needs in children with HIV infection is unknown but is essential for nutritional rehabilitation. Impaired gastrointestinal function and increased metabolic requirements caused by opportunistic infections may alter caloric requirements. A rise in body temperature of 1° F increases caloric needs by 7%. Because of needs for growth and an increased body surface area-to-weight ratio, baseline caloric requirements per kilogram of body weight are higher in children than in adults. Many current recommendations for average daily energy requirements in healthy infants and children are based largely, although not exclusively, on energy intake (26). The extent to which these recommendations are appropriate for HIV-infected children are uncertain.

In adults with HIV infection, estimates of metabolic requirements have been conflicting (25, 27). Decreased resting energy needs may be a compensatory mechanism to preserve lean body mass in the face of severe malnutrition and malabsorption. In one study, resting energy expenditure as determined by indirect calorimetry was decreased and appropriate for the degree of malnutrition and malabsorption. In other studies, resting energy expenditure was increased (28). Resting metabolic rates are only one component of energy expenditure that contribute to metabolic requirements. Total daily energy expenditure accounts for metabolic requirements in a free living person (i.e., activities of daily living, effects of eating, etc.). To date, there have been no reports of resting or total energy expenditure in HIV-infected children.

Altered nutritional status may occur rapidly or develop gradually over several months. Weight loss may also occur in stepwise fashion so that children lose weight precipitously with intervening stable periods. This pattern has been described in adults. To date, there are limited studies that define growth parameters in children with HIV infection (29). Most of these studies focus on height and weight deficits; very few studies discuss body composition at various stages of HIV infection. Although nutrient intake and body composition were not reported, the weights of Haitian children who were HIV infected were different by 3 months of age compared with HIV-negative, seroreverted and control, HIV-negative children (30).

CLINICAL ASPECTS

The clinical aspects of HIV as they relate to gastrointestinal tract function include upper ghastrointestinal tract problems that are characterized by anorexia, nausea, vomiting, and dysphagia; small bowel and colonic malabsorption manifested by diarrhea, abdominal pain and gastrointestinal bleeding; hepatobiliary tract disease; and malnutrition or growth failure. The epidemiologic aspects, pathogenesis of specific symptoms, clinical presentation, evaluation, and treatment of these problems will be discussed within each symptom complex.

Anorexia, Nausea, and Vomiting

The evaluation of gastrointestinal tract disease begins with a careful history and physical examination. The symptom of vomiting in an HIV-infected child should be taken seriously and is almost always pathologic. Causes of anorexia, nausea, and vomiting in the HIV-infected individual are listed in Table 27.2. Gastrointestinal side effects are caused by many of the drugs children take to control opportunistic infections and HIV replication (Table 27.3).

Oral lesions from *Candida*, which is common in the pediatric population, or hairy leukoplakia (caused by Epstein-Barr virus or human papilloma virus), which is more common in adults with HIV, may cause anorexia related to pain with chewing and/or swallowing. *Candida* can involve the esophageal mucosa as illustrated in Figure 27.3. The use of H_2 antagonists to prevent

Table 27.2. Causes of Anorexia, Nausea, or Vomiting

Complication of pharmacotherapy
    Azidothymidine, ddl, fluconazole, nonsteroidal anti-inflammatory agents, erythromycin,
        metronidazole, ciprofloxacin, dapsone, sulfonamides, clarithromycin, pentamidine, rifampin
Oral candidiasis
Xerostomia: parotid enlargement, ddl
Central nervous system disease: encephalopathy
Upper gastrointestinal tract disease
    Gastritis (cytomegalovirus, idiopathic, *Helicobacter pylori*), splenomegaly, pancreatitis, neoplasms

Table 27.3.   Gastrointestinal and Nutritional Side Effects of Medications Used in Treatment of HIV-infected Children

	Anorexia	Nausea	Vomiting	Diarrhea	Abdominal Pain	Pancreatitis	Dysgeusia	Colitis	Liver Disease	Oral Ulcers	Constipation	Low Vitamin B_{12}
Azidothymidine		+					+		?		+	+
ddC						+			?	+		
ddI						+			?			
Acyclovir		+	+	+			+					
Ganciclovir	+	+	+									
Rifabutin	+						+		+			
Pentamidine		+	+			+						
Spiramycin		+	+	+				+				
Amphotericin B	+	+	+	+								
Ketoconazole		+	+		+							
Nystatin		+	+	+	+							
Trimethoprim-sulfamethoxazole	+					+				+		

acid reflux induced esophagitis may enhance the opportunity for *Candida* to grow in the stomach and esophagus. Xerostomia, or diminished production of saliva, can be related to salivary gland enlargement or to dideoxycytosine (ddC).

Encephalopathy altered mental status or dyscoordinated swallowing mechanism may render the child unable to take oral feedings.

Upper gastrointestinal tract disease and inflammation of the gastric mucosa also are causes of anorexia, nausea, and vomiting. Epigastric pain should alert the clinician to the possibility of gastric or duodenal pathology, but children under age 10 years may not localize abdominal pain. A massively enlarged spleen that impinges on the stomach may cause early satiety, much in the same way that a lesion intrinsic to the stomach, such as a lymphoma, can result in anorexia.

To evaluate anorexia, nausea, and vomiting, the causes listed in Table 27.2 can be assessed by a neurologic examination, mental status, quality of life determination, oral and dental examination, and possible esophagogastroduodenoscopy to look for esophagitis, gastritis, or duodenitis. An upper gastrointestinal radiograph is useful for anatomic abnormalities, but it is not sensitive enough to make a definitive diagnosis or determine the etiology of mucosal disease. In the adult, endoscopic evaluation is necessary because multiple pathogens may be present. In contrast, children usually have one pathogen, but histology and culture of tissue to establish a specific diagnosis can modify therapy.

The treatment for nausea and vomiting depends on the identification of a specific etiology. If no cause can be found, symptomatic therapy may be necessary. Vomiting in the older child can be managed by using various antiemetics. The phenothiazine derivatives (Torecan (triethylperazine maleate), Compazine (prochlorperazine), and Phenergan (promethazine)) are effective but have been associated with extrapyramidal symptoms, drowsiness, hypotension, dizziness, and blurred vision. Additional antiemetics include Emete-con (benzquinamide), Tigan (trimethobenzamide hydrochloride), Vistaril or Atarax (hydroxyzine), Reglan (metoclopramide),

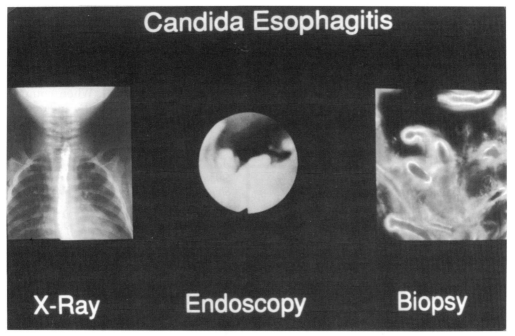

Figure 27.3. Barium swallow illustrating the irregularity of esophageal mucosa from *Candida* esophagitis (*X-ray, left*). Endoscopic photograph of esophageal lumen filled with *Candida* (*Endoscopy, middle*). Photomicrograph of esophageal biopsy demonstrating massive number of hyphae present in esophagus (*Biopsy, right*). Courtesy of Dr. Cecil Fox, Molecular Histology Laboratory, Gaithersburg, MD.

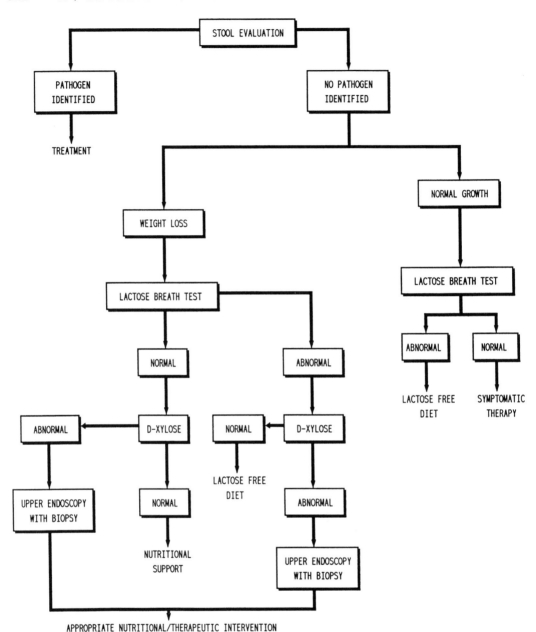

Figure 27.5.   Clinical approach to HIV-infected child with diarrhea.

vety appearance of the duodenal mucosa. Many adults with presumed pathogen-negative diarrhea will be infected with the microsporidium, *Enterocytozoon bienusi* (36), but studies in children are lacking.

If a child continues to defecate after fasting, he or she should be evaluated for a secretory diarrhea. By measuring the electrolyte concentration of the stool water, the difference between secretory and os-

motic diarrhea can be determined. In an osmotic diarrhea, the stool water osmolality is greater than $([Na^+] + [K^+]) \times 2$, because food is incompletely absorbed. The difference between the measured electrolytes and the osmolality may be the result of a nonabsorbed hydrolyzed dietary product such as lactose. If the stool water osmolality is approximately equal to $([Na^+] + [K^+]) \times 2$ and the stool volume is increased, secretory diarrhea is more likely. Secretory diarrhea also can occur if the absorptive villus surface area is severely injured, resulting in crypt secretion without absorption. This may be the cause for secretory diarrhea in the HIV-infected child, but tumors secreting hormones can cause similar symptoms.

In many HIV-infected children with diarrhea in whom no pathogen can be identified, lymphoid hyperplasia may be detected in the gastrointestinal tract. This can be seen endoscopically (Fig. 27.6A) and confirmed by biopsy (Fig. 27.6B). The etiology of this lymphoid expansion of the lamina propria is

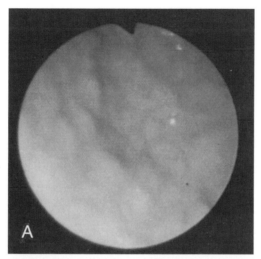

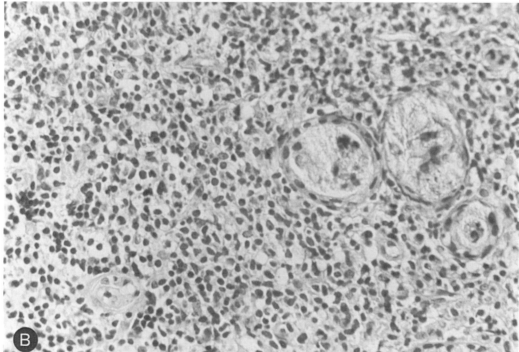

Figure 27.6   **A,** endoscopic view of duodenum of an HIV-infected child with diarrhea. No enteric pathogen could be identified. Note coarse, nodular appearance of mucosa. When biopsied, mucosa was more friable. **B,** photomicrograph of duodenal mucosa in a child with nodules seen at time of endoscopy. Lamina propria is expanded with lymphocytes with areas of lymphoid aggregates.

unknown. It appears to be the gastrointestinal equivalent of lymphocytic interstitial pneumonia, but there are no studies to assess how therapy might alter symptoms.

In the HIV-infected child, lactose intolerance develops earlier than genetically predicted (Fig. 27.7) (37), but evidence for more global brush border enzyme deficiencies is lacking. The mechanism for decreased lactase in the intestinal brush border is unknown, but preliminary observations suggest that the gene for lactase is down-regulated (38).

Therapy for diarrhea depends on the degree of intestinal injury. If a pathogen can be identified, treatment may be available. Unfortunately at this time there is no effective therapy for cryptosporidium, mycobacterium, viral gastroenteritis, or cytomegalovirus colitis. If the villi are severely blunted with marked decrease in brush border enzyme activity, an elemental formula may be required. However, if lactase is deficient, simply restricting lactose or providing lactase in one of the commercially available formulations may cause the stool to become formed. Failing dietary manipulation, there are agents that act nonspecifically or alter motility to decrease stool frequency. Although not used regularly in children, they can be used in the symptomatic child who evades diagnosis and dietary therapy. Cholestyramine, a resin that binds bile acids,

may improve diarrhea. Antimotility agents like Loperamide, Lomotil, or deodorized tincture of opium might decrease crampy pain and slow the frequency of stooling.

Abdominal Pain

The differential diagnosis of abdominal pain in the immunocompromised child can be complicated. Abdominal pain associated with diarrhea may be caused by lactose intolerance or other enteropathies that result in distention of the small intestine with fluid. Children with diarrhea and abdominal pain should be evaluated for enteric pathogens and malabsorption.

Acute pancreatitis usually is manifested by crampy abdominal pain that increases after meals. The association of abdominal pain with eating may result in food avoidance and explain why malnutrition, low CD4 count, and opportunistic infections are associated with pancreatitis. In one study, 17% of children with AIDS had symptoms consistent with pancreatitis as well as elevation of amylase and/or lipase (39). In children, the lipase is often elevated earlier and remains elevated longer than amylase. However, the association of elevated lipase levels to clinical pancreatitis is less well established in children than in adults. Pancreatitis may be due to medications such as dideoxyinosine (ddI) and ddC;

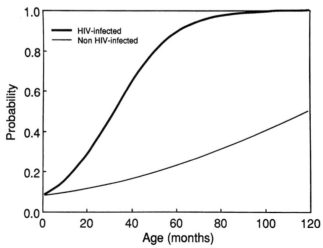

Figure 27.7. Statistical projection of development of lactose intolerance in HIV-infected children. From Miller TM, Orav EJ, Martin SR, Cooper ER, McIntosh K, Winter HS. *Malnutrition and carbohy-* *drate malabsorption in children with vertically transmitted human immunodeficiency virus-1 infection.* Gastroenterology 1991;100:1296–1302.

symptoms from ddI may develop as long as 8 months after starting therapy (40). A recent study from the National Cancer Institute described clinical pancreatitis in seven of 95 children receiving ddI, all at dosages above 360 mg/ml/day. There was a trend suggesting that higher plasma levels (but not cumulative dosage) might be associated with an increased risk for pancreatitis (40a). Pentamidine can cause a fatal acute pancreatitis (41), and children with CD4 counts below 100 cells/mm who are treated with pentamidine are at increased risk for pancreatitis (39). Trimethoprim-sulfamethoxazole and Dapsone may cause pancreatitis as well (42). Infectious agents such as cytomegalovirus and mycobacteria also have been associated with pancreatitis, and there may be pancreatic duct abnormalities identified by endoscopic retrograde cholangiopancreatography. The child with pancreatitis may recover from the acute episode and continue to do well; however, most children have a chronic, relapsing course with progressive nutritional deterioration, abdominal pain, and eventual death. The mean survival of children with pancreatitis was 8 months after onset of disease (39).

Pancreatic disease is defined by the elevation of amylase and lipase, and these biochemical markers are used to follow the course of the disease. Asymptomatic rises in these enzymes may be caused by salivary amylase, intestinal lipase, or macroamylasemia. Thus, biochemical findings must be correlated with symptoms. An ultrasound is important to determine if the pancreatic duct is dilated. In acute pancreatitis, the parenchyma is edematous, but the ducts are of normal caliber. Because ultrasound is not the most sensitive test to determine if an anatomic abnormality exists, injecting contrast into the pancreatic duct may prove useful. Cultures from the duct can be obtained, but it appears that one of the most reliable culture techniques is to place one cup of the forceps into the orifice of the ampulla and obtain a biopsy. Cytomegalovirus can be cultured from pancreatic fluid when other cultures are negative and can be treated with ganciclovir. Although there is no reliable therapy for pancreatitis, stopping suspected medications capable of inducing inflammation, restricting fat and protein intake, and

initiating jejunal feedings or total parenteral nutrition may be of symptomatic benefit.

Gastrointestinal Bleeding

Children with AIDS may develop gastrointestinal bleeding, but it is usually in the clinical setting of a chronically ill, debilitated child. Upper gastrointestinal hemorrhage may arise from the esophagus, stomach, or proximal duodenum. Patients under stress are more likely to develop gastritis or peptic ulceration, but it may be difficult to identify a cause for the bleeding. Cytomegalovirus is a prime suspect when there is bleeding in the gastrointestinal tract. Mucosal biopsies may demonstrate the characteristic intranuclear inclusion with cytoplasmic halo (Fig. 27.8), but frequently cytomegalovirus cannot be identified by biopsy or culture of the tissue. Because of its propensity for endothelial cells, cytomegalovirus should be seriously considered in the child with unexplained chronic gastrointestinal blood loss.

Other agents such as *Clostridium difficile* can cause gastrointestinal bleeding, but it is not as severe as that noted in cytomegalovirus disease. The toxin for *C. difficile* is usually present, but the characteristic pseudomembranes may not be evident by colonoscopy. In adults there are trials starting to use anti-inflammatory agents such as 5-aminosalicylic acid to treat the HIV-infected individual with rectal bleeding from idiopathic colitis. Other less common causes of colitis include: mycobacteria,

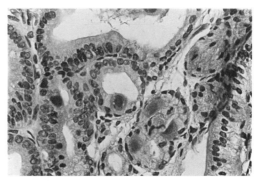

Figure 27.8. Photomicrograph of small bowel biopsy in a child with gastrointestinal bleeding. A cytomegalovirus-infected epithelial cell can be identified by its characteristic intranuclear inclusion.

spirochetosis, Histoplasmosis, *E. histolytica*, *Campylobacter*, and inflammatory bowel disease. As with hepatitis B infection, Crohn's disease activity declines with deterioration of immune function.

Abnormal Liver Function Tests

Hepatic dysfunction is not a common manifestation of HIV disease (43), although over 90% of HIV-infected children will have hepatosplenomegaly (44). Hepatocellular dysfunction characterized by coagulopathy, hypoalbuminemia, ascites, or fulminant hepatic failure as well as hepatic fibrosis resulting in cirrhosis, variceal bleeding, and portal hypertension are unusual in HIV-infected individuals.

Hepatitis B infection may be modified in the HIV-infected individual. Hepatocellular injury from hepatitis B virus (HBV) may be immunologically modulated, and deterioration in immune function results in less hepatocellular damage (see Chapter 20). In adults with HIV and HBV it appears that HBV hepatitis may be milder than in the immunocompetent host (45), but hepatic failure may also be increased in the immunodeficient patient with HBV (46). HBV viral replication may be increased as evidenced by the presence of hepatitis Be antigen and HBV DNA (47). These clinical and serologic findings suggest that decreased antigen-specific cytotoxic T cell function in the HIV-infected host causes increased HBV replication but not a comparable degree of hepatocellular injury. Preservation of cellular immunity early in the course of the HIV-infected child could explain why chronic active hepatitis, presumably associated with HBV, appears to be more common in the pediatric population (48). Other infectious agents that could result in hepatobiliary abnormalities include hepatitis C, hepatitis A, *M. avium intracellulare*, cytomegalovirus, *Cryptosporidium*, *P. carinii*, toxoplasmosis, and histoplasmosis (see Chapter 20).

Many therapeutic agents used to treat children with HIV can cause hepatocellular injury or cholestasis. Some of the more common drugs that can cause damage are listed in Table 27.5. Medications such a trimethoprim-sulfamethoxazole may cause a mixed hepatocellular-cholestatic reaction,

Table 27.5. Hepatotoxic Therapeutic Agents

Acetaminophen
Amphotericin B
Carbenicillin
Clindamycin
Isoniazid
Ketoconazole
Pentamidine
Phenobarbital
Rifampin
Sulfonamides
Dapsone
ddl
Zidovudine

whereas other agents, such as erythromycin, zidovudine, and carbenicillin, produce more of a cholestatic profile. Zidovudine may cause a mixed picture of hepatitis and cholestasis, but most other medications cause a mild hepatitis.

Standard biochemical liver tests provide initial direction for the clinician evaluating the HIV-infected child with suspected liver disease. Elevated transaminases frequently are identified but could be related to HIV, nutritional factors, infectious agents, or medications. Marked elevation of transaminases over four times normal suggests virus or drug-induced hepatitis. Elevation of alkaline phosphatase raises the possibility of *M. avium intracellulare*, hepatic *P. carinii* infection, fungal infection, granulomatous hepatitis, cholangiopathy, or extrahepatic biliary obstruction (49).

Determination of CD4 lymphocyte count helps identify patients at risk for AIDS-related infections and malignancies. To determine the infectious cause of hepatitis as suggested by abnormal liver enzymes, abdominal ultrasound or computed tomography are of little benefit; however, to identify focal lesions that may be associated with increases in alkaline phosphatase, these imaging studies may help to guide the investigation (50). To determine the cause of a dilated extrahepatic biliary tract identified by ultrasound or computed tomography, endoscopic retrograde cholangiopancreatography may be helpful. With the development of smaller instruments, these studies can be performed in infants.

Liver biopsy is the diagnostic test of choice to explain liver function tests that have remained elevated for more than 6 months. In adults infected with HIV, liver biopsy may be helpful in the evaluation of a fever of unknown origin (51). When a liver biopsy is obtained to evaluate a focal hepatic lesion or elevation of alkaline phosphatase, a significant hepatic lesion can be found in about 50% of adults with AIDS and about 25% of adults who are HIV infected but without AIDS (52).

Similar data do not exist for the pediatric population. Treatable disorders such as tuberculosis, fungal disease, *P. carinii* infection, and lymphoma are usually suspected by other clinical features or serologic or imaging studies but can be confirmed by liver biopsy.

There are very few effective therapeutic options for chronic liver disease. Interferon-α, which has been used for the treatment of chronic active hepatitis caused by hepatitis B or C, is least effective in the HIV-infected individual. Except for bacterial disease, infectious complications of the liver do not respond well to therapy.

Malnutrition and Growth Retardation

Clinical Presentation

There is a wide spectrum of nutritional deficits in pediatric HIV disease. Marasmus refers to the nutritional state in which there are inadequate calories and wasting of both fat and muscle stores. Kwashiorkor refers to the nutritional state in which caloric intake is adequate, but protein intake is insufficient (53). Edema is typically the end product of protein deficiency. Cachexia refers to the preferential loss of lean body mass with relative sparing of fat mass. There is considerable evidence from the adult literature and some preliminary observations in children that the cachexia is most commonly found in HIV-infected persons.

Malnutrition may be classified as acute vs. chronic or mild, moderate, or severe. Nutritional status is commonly described as weight for age, yet height for age and weight for height enable the clinician for further classify the degree of malnutrition. In acute malnutrition, weight for age may be below standard with preservation of

height. Consequently, weight for height is below normal standards. In chronic malnutrition, both weight and height for age may be affected because with chronic undernutrition there is compensatory stunting of linear growth. Thus, weight for height may be near normal.

HIV-infected children may be classified with mild, moderate, or severe malnutrition. The most commonly used criteria are those of Waterlow (54) in which malnutrition is expressed as a percentage of normal for age (Table 27.6). The degree of malnutrition correlates with mortality rates in other diseases and seems to be true for pediatric HIV disease as well.

Specific micronutrient deficiencies are often found in children with HIV disease. These include deficiencies of iron, vitamin B_6, selenium, zinc, vitamin A, vitamin E, and albumin. Deficiencies of these nutrients may lead to many clinical symptoms including anemia, neurologic deficits, skin manifestations, and cardiomyopathy.

Diagnostic Considerations

Because nutritional deficits occur early in pediatric HIV disease, evaluation of growth and nutritional status should begin in the child born to a seropositive mother. Dietary history and recall, height, weight, triceps skinfold thickness (measure of fat stores), and arm muscle circumference (measure of lean body mass) should be performed every 3 months to detect subtle changes in growth and altered nutrient intake. In this way, changes in nutritional status as well as body composition may be detected. Dietary intake preferably is obtained through 3-day food records, but a 24-hour recall that is readily accessible in a clinic setting is acceptable. In this way, nutritional advice may be provided on a routine basis, and baseline nutrient intake data will be collected and serve as a basis for future management. If a child has

Table 27.6.   Classification of Malnutrition[a]

	Normal	Mild	Moderate	Severe
Height for age	>95	95–87	87–80	<80
Weight for height	>90	90–80	80–70	<70

[a]Values are percentage of normal.

evidence of malnutrition, an evaluation of nutrient losses should be started. Intestinal function can be assessed in conjunction with the nutritional assessment so that recommendations for refeeding and appropriate modification of the diet can be made.

Micronutrients should also be measured frequently since the HIV-infected child is at risk for deficiencies. Serum albumin and total protein should be monitored but become decreased in advanced stages of disease. Serum levels of iron, selenium, zinc, thiamin, vitamin B_{12}, and vitamin B_6 may be decreased and may be associated with immune dysfunction as well as other pathologic states. Measurements of the serum levels of these vitamins and minerals in moderately to severely malnourished HIV-infected children may enhance the nutritional rehabilitation program.

Accurate evaluation of energy needs by indirect calorimetry or the doubly labeled water technique can help guide nutritional therapy, but each is expensive, time consuming, or impractical in busy clinical settings. The best estimation of energy needs in HIV-infected children is the response to a diet enriched in calories with accurate documentation of caloric intake and type of food or formula. Reevaluation of the nutritional needs will permit each child to be in positive nitrogen balance and maintain appropriate growth.

Treatment

Once diagnosis of malnutrition is established, oral intervention should be started. The family should be involved and a plan developed that matches the child's needs with realistic expectations. Defining goals, explaining specific methods, and reassessing caloric intake help create a partnership between the family and the health care team. Immunodeficient individuals should avoid raw meats, which can harbor *Toxoplasma*, and raw fish, which can contain parasites. Uncooked eggs are a potential source of *Salmonella*. Techniques that increase the caloric density by adding carbohydrate or fat are used most commonly. If the child is taking solid foods, the addition of high fat foods such as margarine and butter might be beneficial. Formulation of the supplement is de-

termined by the absorptive capability of the intestine (Table 27.7). Thus, if the child has significant gastrointestinal malabsorption, a protein hydrolysate formula with medium chain triglyceride may be beneficial. Efforts should be made to increase formula volume, and caloric goals should, in general, be above the recommended daily allowance for age and sex. An initial goal should be 50% above the recommended daily allowance for age and sex, although the child's response to a feeding regimen will determine the need for additional calories. Weight, height, and nutrient intake should be monitored monthly if the nutritional status is deteriorating. If lactose malabsorption is prominent with symptoms of diarrhea, flatulence, and abdominal pain, then a lactose-free diet with lactaid supplementation should be initiated. If a child has a positive lactose hydrogen breath test but has no clinical symptoms of lactose malabsorption, restricting lactose-containing foods may reduce caloric intake since those foods are often most palatable and highest in calories.

Nutritional supplements (Table 27.8) should provide palatable and age- and ethnically appropriate foods that meet the nutritional needs of the child. Children with oral lesions or *Candida* in the mouth or esophagus should avoid acid or spicy food. They often tolerate foods with a softer texture or liquids. In contrast, the child with dysgeusia may eat more if the foods have varied textures and added spices.

If oral interventions are not successful because the child does not meet the caloric goals or appears to have higher caloric needs than can be achieved orally, enteral supplementation should be considered (Fig. 27.9). Nasogastric tube feedings are often the initial approach so that a positive response can be documented. Night feedings are most useful and allow the child to eat normally during the day. Complications related to nasogastric feedings include the possibility of gastroesophageal reflux, sinusitis, and decreased oral intake because of discomfort from the tube. If after 1 or 2 months the need for prolonged nutritional support remains and the nasogastric tube feedings have improved growth, placement of a gastrostomy tube should be considered. The benefits of gastrostomy tube feedings

Table 27.7. Nutritional Supplements Used with Immunocompromised Children[a]

Name	Company	Special Features	cal/ml	CHO g/liter	Protein g/liter	Fat g/liter	OSM
Pregestimel	Mead Johnson	Designed for children birth–1 year 60% fat as MCT	0.66	66	18	36	300
Nutramingen	Mead Johnson	Protein hydrolysate, designed for children birth–1 year	0.68	91	11	27	320
Pediasure	Ross Labs	Lactose free, designed for children 1–6 years	1.0	104	28	47	310
Isocal	Mead Johnson	Isotonic	1.06	135	34	44	270
Osmolyte	Ross Labs	Isotonic, low protein	1.06	137	35	36	300
Newtrition Isofiber	Knight Medical	Fiber enriched	1.2	160	50	37	310
Jevity	Ross Labs	Fiber enriched	1.06	144	44	35	310
Enrich	Ross Labs	Fiber enriched	1.1	153	38	35	480
Ensure	Ross Labs	Lactose free, decreased residue	1.06	137	35	35	470
Ensure plus	Ross Labs	Lactose free, increased calorie	1.5	189	52	50	690
Sustical	Mead Johnson	Lactose free	1.0	140	61	23	650
Sustical Hc	Mead Johnson	Lactose free, decrease residue, increase protein	1.5	190	61	58	670
Sustical with Fiber	Mead Johnson	Fiber enriched	1.06	132	43	33	480
Peptamen	Clintec Nutrition	70% fat as MCT, protein hydrolysate	1.0	127	40	39	260
Carnation Instant Breakfast with Whole Milk	Clintec Nutrition	Lactose containing	1.17	144	56	32	
Portagen	Mead Johnson	86% fat as MCT, lactose free, powder diluted to 20 cal/oz	0.66 cal/oz	74	22	30	233
Polycose	Ross Labs	Glucose polymers	2 cal/ml (liquid) 8 cal/tsp (powder)				
MCT Oil	Mead Johnson		7.7 cal/ml				
Promod	Ross Labs	Protein supplement	20 cal/tbsp				
Casec	Mead Johnson	Protein supplement	16.4 cal/tbsp				

[a]CHO, carbohydrate; OSM, osmolality; MCT, medium chain triglyceride.

include 1) ease of infusion, 2) resumption of routine activity, 3) confidentiality, and 4) avoidance of discomfort and complications of a nasogastric tube. Advances in the techniques of placing gastrostomy tubes endoscopically has greatly simplified the insertion of these tubes and permits their use for nutritional support within 1 day of placement. Replacing the tube with a button permits the patient to be more active.

Parenteral nutrition should be reserved for persistent and recurrent pancreatitis, failure of gastrostomy tube feedings, and severe intractable diarrhea with weight loss. Anecdotal experience suggests that complications associated with central venous catheters are no higher in the HIV-infected individual than that which is reported in the non-HIV-infected patient. Because providing calories through a central venous catheter restricts activity and is costly, all attempts to utilize the gastrointestinal tract should be made before placement of the catheter. In the child with severe weight loss, total parenteral nutrition can restore weight and improve quality of life.

Table 27.8.   Enteral Support for Older Children[a]

Complete Supplement	
Clintec	Nutren, Replete
Mead Johnson	Sustacal, Isocal, Traumacal, Criticar HN
Ross	Promod, Ensure, Ensure with Fiber, Jevity, Osmolite, Promote, Pulmocare
Sandoz Nutrition	Meritene, Citrisource, Resource, Compleat, Fibersource, Stresstein
Low Fat or Medium Chain Triglyceride	
Mead Johnson	Lipisorb
Sandoz Nutrition	Isosource
Elemental	
Metagenics	Opti
Ross	Vital HN
Sandoz Nutrition	Vivonex TEN
Immune Modulating	
McGraw	ImmunAid
Ross	AlitraQ
Sandoz Nutrition	Impact
Parenteral Nutrition Support	
Adult	Aminosyn, FreAmine, Travasol
Pediatric	TrophAmine, Aminosyn-PF
Liver disease	HepatAmine
Renal disease	NephrAmine
Branched-chain amino acids	Aminosyn-HBC

[a]Modified from Cimoch PJ. Current agents for the management of wasting and malnutrition in HIV/AIDS. Nutr HIV/AIDS 1992;1:27–32.

Several pharmacologic agents are under investigation in the adult with HIV disease. Megesterol acetate (Megace), a progesterone derivative, has been shown to increase appetite of cancer patients. Encouraging weight gain has been documented in HIV-infected adults, although much improvement in weight is fat and not lean body mass. Diabetes mellitus and adrenal suppression was been reported with chronic megesterol acetate use. Experience in the pediatric population is limited, and appropriate dosage is unknown. Dronabinol, a tetrahydrocannabinol derivative, is under investigation in HIV-infected adults as an appetite stimulant. Weight gain has been described, but drowsiness, anxiety, poor coordination, and confusion have been observed. Human growth hormone has been used in adults with HIV disease and causes weight gain with increases in lean body mass. There are no reported trials in HIV-infected children.

Early nutritional assessment and intervention for the HIV-infected child is one of the most important aspects of care. Providers should not wait for overt evidence of malnutrition before initiating therapy but should be proactive with respect to the nutritional care of the HIV-infected child. The benefits of this approach are well-known in other chronic illnesses and need not be learned again with HIV.

FUTURE RESEARCH

Little is understood about the role of HIV in the development of malabsorption and malnutrition. Understanding the mechanism by which HIV causes gastrointestinal dysfunction will lead to better therapeutic interventions, and knowledge of the energy and protein requirements at various stages of disease would improve the care of the individual patient. Simple materials such as the development of ethnically and age-appropriate diets for children with malabsorption might enhance their quality of life and longevity. When health care providers begin to view food as an important therapeutic intervention, we will need to understand the pathophysiology of gastrointestinal disease and nutrition along with the feeding, economics, behavior, cultural be-

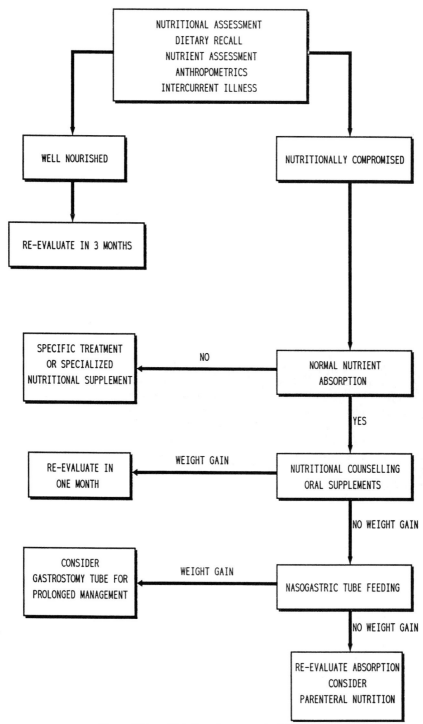

Figure 27.9. Nutritional support decision tree.

liefs, and a commitment to caring for children with a chronic disease.

References

1. Serwadda D, Sewankambo NK, Carswell JW, et al. Slim disease: A new disease in Uganda and its association with HTLV-III infection. Lancet 1985;2: 849–852.
2. Ullrich R, Zeitz M, Heise W, et al. Mucosal atrophy is associated with loss of activated T cells in the duodenal mucosa of human immunodeficiency virus (HIV)-infected patients. Digestion 1990;46(suppl 2):302–307.
3. Rodgers VD, Fassett R, Kagnoff MF. Abnormalities in intestinal mucosal T cells in homosexual populations including those with the lymphadenopathy syndrome and acquired immunodeficiency syndrome. Gastroenterology 1986;90:552–558.
4. Amerongen HM, Weltzin R, Farnet CM. Transepithelial transport of HIV-1 by intestinal M cells: A mechanism for transmission of AIDS. J Acquir Immune Defic Syndr 1991;4:760–765.
5. Jarry A, Cortez A, Rene E. Infected cells and immune cells in the gastrointestinal tract of AIDS patients. An immunohistochemical study of 127 cases. Histopathology 1990;16:133–140.
6. Fox CH, Cottler-Fox M. The pathobiology of HIV infection. Immunol Today 1992;13:353–356.
7. Nelson JA, Wiley CA, Reynolds-Kohler C, Reese CE, Margaretten W, Levy JA. Human immunodeficiency virus detection in bowel epithelium from patients with gastrointestinal symptoms. Lancet 1988;1:259–262.
8. Fox CH, Kotler D, Tierney A, Wilson CS, Fauci AS. Detection of HIV-1 RNA in the lamina propria of patients with AIDS and gastrointestinal disease. J Infect Dis 1989;159:467–471.
9. Heise C, Dandekar S, Kumar P, Duplantier R, Donovan RM, Halsted CH. Human immunodeficiency virus infection of enterocytes and mononuclear cells in human jejunal tissue. Gastroenterology 1991;100:1521–1527.
10. Cummins AG, LaBrooy JT, Stanley DP, Rowland R, Shearmann DJC. Quantitative histological study of enteropathy associated with HIV infection. Gut 1990;31:317–321.
11. Greenson JK, Belitsos PC, Yardley JH, Bartlett JG. AIDS enteropathy: Occult enteric infections and duodenal mucosal alterations in chronic diarrhea. Ann Intern Med 1991;114:366–372.
12. Kotler DP, Scholes JV, Tierney AR. Intestinal plasma cell alterations in the acquired immunodeficiency syndrome. Dig Dis Sci 1987;32:129–138.
13. Adachi A, Koenig S, Gendelmann HE, Daugherty D, Gatton-Celli S, Fauci AS, Martin MA. Productive, persistent infection of human colorectal cell lines with human immunodeficiency virus. J Virol 1987;61:209–213.
14. Moyer MP, Gendelmann HE. HIV replication and persistence in human gastrointestinal cells cultured in vitro. J Leukoc Biol 1991;49:499–504.
15. Fantini J, Yahi N, Chermann JC. Human immunodeficiency virus can infect the apical and basolateral surface of human colonic epithelial cells. Proc Natl Acad Sci USA 1991;88:9297–9301.
16. Miller TM, Orav EJ, Martin SR, Cooper ER, McIntosh K, Winter HS. Malnutrition and carbohydrate malabsorption in children with vertically transmitted human immunodeficiency virus 1 infection. Gastroenterology 1991;100:1296–1302.
17. MacDonald TT, Spencer J. Evidence that activated mucosal T cells play a role in the pathogenesis of enteropathy in human small intestine. J Exp Med 1988;167:1341–1349.
18. Cao Y, Dieterich D, Thomas PA, Huang Y, Mirabile M, Ho DD. Identification and quantitation of HIV-1 in the liver of patients with AIDS. AIDS 1992;6:65–70.
19. Hoda SA, Gerber MA. Immunohistochemical studies of human immunodeficiency virus type 1 in liver tissues of patients with AIDS. Mod Pathol 1991;4:578–581.
20. Cao Y, Friedman-Kein AE, Huang YX, et al. CD4-independent, productive HIV-1 infection of hepatoma cell lines in vitro. J Virol 1990;64:2553–2559.
21. McKinney RE, et al. A multicenter trial of oral zidovudine in children with advanced human immunodeficiency virus disease. N Engl J Med 1991;324:1018–1025.
22. Warrier RP, Kuvibidile S, Suskind D, et al. Nutritional status of hemophillac children with and without human immunodeficiency virus (HIV) antibody [Abstract]. Clin Res 1989;37:833A.
23. Miller TL, Evans S, Morris V, Orav EJ, McIntosh K, Winter HS. Prospective study of the alterations in growth and nutritional requirements in HIV infected children [Abstract]. Gastroenterology 1991;100:A538.
24. Chlebowski RT, Grosvenor MB, Kruger S, Bulcavage L, Beck K, Beall G. Dietary intake of HIV infection: Relative caloric deficiency in patients with AIDS. Fifth International Conference on AIDS, Montreal, Jun 1989:467.
25. Kotler DP, Tierney AR, Brenner SK, Couture S, Wang J, Poerson RN Jr. Preservation of short-term energy balance in clinically stable patients with AIDS. Am J Clin Nutr 1990;51:7–13.
26. FAO/WHO/UNU. Energy and protein requirements: Report of a joint FAO/WHO/UNU expert consultation. World Health Organization, Geneva, 1989;724:206.
27. Hommes MJ, Romijn JA, Endert E, Sauerwein HP. Resting energy expenditure and substrate oxidation in human immunodeficiency virus (HIV)-infected asymptomatic men: HIV affects host metabolism in the early asymptomatic stage. Am J Clin Nutr 1991;54:311–315.
28. Grunfeld C, Feingold K. Metabolic disturbances and wasting in the acquired immunodeficiency syndrome. N Engl J Med 1992;327:329–337.
29. Miller TL, Evans S, Orav EJ, McIntosh K, Winter HS. Growth and body composition in children with human immunodeficiency virus-1 infection. Am J Clin Nutr 1993;57:588–592.
30. Halsey NA, Boulos R, Holt E, et al. Transmission of HIV-1 infection from mothers to infants in Haiti. JAMA 1991;264:2088–2092.
31. Scully C, Laskaris G, Pindborg J, Porter SR, Reichart P. Oral manifestations of HIV infection and their management. I Mopre common lesions. Oral Surg Oral Med Oral Pathol 1991;71:158–166.

32. Edward P, Turner J, Gold J, Cooper DA. Esophageal ulceration induced by zidovudine. Ann Intern Med 1990;112:65–66.
33. Italian Multicentre Study. Epidemiology and clinical features of pediatric HIV infection: Results from an Italian multicentric study on 544 children. Lancet 1988;2:1046–1048.
34. Ullrich R, Heise W, Bergs C, L'age M, Riecken EO, Zeitz M. Gastrointestinal symptoms in patients infected with human immunodeficiency virus: Relevance of infective agents isolated from gastrointestinal tract. Gut 1992;33:1080–1084.
34a. Grohmann GS, Glass RI, Pereira HG, et al. Enteric viruses and diarrhea in HIV-infected patients. N Engl J Med 1993;329:14–20.
35. Yolken RH, Hart W, Oung I, Shiff C, Greenson J, Perman JA. Gastrointestinal dysfunction and disaccharide intolerance in children infected with human immunodeficiency virus. J Pediatr 1991;118:359–363.
36. Orenstein JM, Steinberg W, Chiang J, et al. Intestinal microsporidiosis as a cause of diarrhea in human immunodeficiency virus-infected patients: A report of 20 cases [Abstract WBO 38]. Fifth International Conference on AIDS, Montreal, Jun 1989.
37. Miller TL, Orav EJ, Martin SR, Cooper ER, McIntosh K, Winter HS. Malnutrition and carbohydrate malabsorption in children with vertically transmitted human immunodeficiency virus 1 infection. Gastroenterology 1991;100:1296–1302.
38. Winter HS, Miller TL, Hobson CD, Naim HY. Enteropathy in congenital HIV infection: Histological and molecular evaluation [Abstract]. Gastroenterology 1991;100:A626.
39. Miller TL, Winter HS, Luginbuhl LM, Orav EJ, McIntosh K. Pancreatitis in pediatric human immunodeficiency virus infection. J Pediatr 1992;120:223–227.
40. Yarchoan R, Pluda JM, Thomas RV, et al. Long-term toxicity/activity profile of 2′,3′-dideoxyinosine in AIDS or AIDS-related complex. Lancet 1990;336:526–529.
40a. Butler KM, Venson D, Henry N, et al. Pancreatitis in human immunodeficiency virus-infected children receiving dideoxyinosine. Pediatrics 1993;91:747–751.
41. Zuger A, Wolf BZ, El-Sadr, Simberkoff MS, Rahal JJ. Pentamidine-associated fatal acute pancreatitis. JAMA 1986;256:2282–2385.
42. Mallory A, Kern F. Drug-induced pancreatitis: A critical review. Gastroenterology 1980;78:813–820.
43. Wilcox CM. Hepatic disease associated with human immunodeficiency virus infection. AIDS GI Tract Ser 1991;16:10–19.
44. Shannon KM, Ammann AJ. Acquired immune deficiency syndrome in childhood. J Pediatr 1985;106:332–342.
45. Prufer-Kramer L, Kramer A, Weigel R, et al. Hepatic involvement in patients with human immunodeficiency virus infection: Discrepancies between AIDS patients and those with earlier stages of infection. J Infect Dis 1991;163:866–869.
46. Housset C, Pol S, Carnot F, et al. Interactions between human immunodeficiency virus-1, hepatitis delta virus and hepatitis B virus infections in 260 chronic carriers of hepatitis B virus. Hepatology 1992;15:578–583.
47. Goldin RD, Fish DE, Hay A, et al. Histological and immunohistochemical study of hepatitis B virus in human immunodeficiency virus infection. J Clin Pathol 1990;43:203–205.
48. Thung SN, Gerber MA, Benkov KJ, Guttenberg M, Gordon RE. Chronic active hepatitis in a child with human immunodeficiency virus infection. Arch Pathol Lab Med 1988;112;914–916.
49. Khan SA, Saltzman BR, Klein RS, Mahadevia PS, Friedland GH, Brandt LJ. Hepatic disorders in the acquired immune deficiency syndrome: A clinical and pathological study. Am J Gastroenterol 1986;81:1145–1148.
50. Urbain D, Jeanmart J, Lemone M, et al. Cholestasis in patients with the acquired immune deficiency syndrome: Comparison between ultrasonographic and cholangiographic findings. Am J Gastroenterol 1991;5:574–576.
51. Comer GM, Mukherjee S, Scholes JV, Holness LG, Clain DJ. Liver biopsies in the acquired immune deficiency syndrome: Influence of endemic disease and drug abuse. Am J Gastroenterol 1989;84:1525–1531.
52. Cappell MS. Hepatobiliary manifestations of the acquired immune deficiency syndrome. Am J Gastroenterol 1991;86:1–15.
53. Grant JP, Cluster PB, Thurlow J. Current techniques of nutritional assessment. Surg Clin North Am 1981;61:437–463.
54. Waterlow JC. Classification and definition of protein calorie malnutrition. Br Med J 1972;3:565.

28
Skin Problems

Neil S. Prose

Most children infected with human immunodeficiency virus (HIV) will develop some form of skin disease during their illness. For some, a mucocutaneous disorder is the presenting sign of HIV-related disease. In other cases, skin disease is a manifestation of an important opportunistic infection or is evidence of deterioration in immune status (1). For these reasons, clinicians caring for children who have or who are at risk for HIV infection must become familiar with the wide range of cutaneous diseases that may be manifestations of this disorder (Table 28.1).

Although there is some overlap, the cutaneous manifestations of HIV infection in children are significantly different from those seen in the adult population (2, 3). Some skin disorders, such as chronic varicella-zoster infection, are unique to patients with HIV disease. However, many cutaneous diseases associated with pediatric HIV infection are inflammatory or infectious disorders that are also seen in healthy children. These diseases tend to be more severe and respond less consistently to conventional therapy than in the well child (Table 28.2).

Because skin disorders in children with HIV infection may present in an atypical fashion, an organized diagnostic approach is mandatory. History taking should focus on duration of the cutaneous lesions, presence of pain or pruritus, and association of the skin disease with either systemic symptoms or the use of a new medication. The entire mucocutaneous surface must be examined, and particular attention paid to morphology (e.g., blisters, papules, nodules, plaques)

Table 28.1. Cutaneous Manifestations of HIV Infection in Childhood

Infections
  Bacterial
    Impetigo
    Ecthyma
    Cellulitis
    Folliculitis
  Bacillary angiomatosis
  Fungal
    Thrush
    Monilial diaper rash or intertrigo
    Tinea corporis
    Tinea capitis
    Cryptococcosis
    Sporotrichosis
    Histoplasmosis
  Viral
    Mucocutaneous herpes simplex
    Herpes zoster
    Chronic varicella-zoster infection
    Molluscum contagiosum
    Warts
    Cytomegalovirus
  Scabies
Inflammatory disorders
  Atopic dermatitis
  Seborrheic dermatitis
  Psoriasis
  Drug eruptions
  Vasculitis
  Pyoderma gangrenosum
  Nutritional deficiencies
Neoplasms
  Kaposi's sarcoma
  Leiomyosarcoma

and distribution (e.g., symmetrical, acral, zosteriform) of the lesions. Careful search for a fresh, primary skin lesion may be particularly useful in some cases.

In the child with HIV infection, common skin infections may present with unusual le-

535

Table 28.2.   Common Skin Disorders in Healthy and HIV-infected Child

Disorder	Healthy Child	HIV-infected Child
Impetigo	Discrete areas of erythema with honey-crusting, small blister formation	Lesions similar in appearance but may be extremely widespread or evolve into cellulitis
Oral thrush	Discrete white-yellow patches and plaques on tongue, palate, buccal mucosa; usual rapid response to topical therapy	Lesions may be more extensive, with involvement of entire oral cavity and posterior pharynx; poor response to topical therapy may be noted
Monilial diaper dermatitis	Confluent erythema with satellite pustules; responds to topical imidazole creams	Lesions may be more widespread; rapid recurrence after cessation of therapy
Tinea capitis	Discrete areas of scale and hair loss; responds to 4- to 6-week course of griseofulvin	Area of involvement may extend to face and recur after full course of griseofulvin
Herpes simplex	Primary herpetic gingivostomatitis is sometimes followed by recurrences at vermillion border of lip; lesions on other parts of face or on fingers may also occur	Severe and persistent infection of oral mucosa, fingers, or other skin skin surface may occur
Herpes zoster	Relatively rare; correlates with occurrence of chickenpox during infancy or early childhood	Lesions tend to be more painful and result in scarring; may develop chronic varicella-zoster infection
Warts	Single or multiple lesions on hands and other skin locations common	Lesions may be extremely widespread or persistent; extensive flat warts and giant condyloma acuminata may occur
Scabies	Discrete, intensely pruritic papules or nodules in axilla, diaper area; rapid response to topical therapy	Widespread papular lesions or diffuse eczematous eruption (Norwegian scabies); may recur after course of topical therapy
Molluscum contagiosum	1- to 2-mm umbilicated papules on face, trunk, or extremities	Lesions may be extremely widespread; giant lesions may occur

sions, and unusual organisms or even combinations of organisms may prove to be unexpected pathogens. Depending on the clinical setting, various methods may be used to diagnose cutaneous infection (Table 28.3).

Incisional skin biopsy is an extremely simple and safe procedure that will often lead to diagnosis of either infectious or inflammatory skin disorders. In most cases, a 2- or 3-mm punch biopsy, performed after local infiltration of 2% lidocaine, is adequate. Tissue obtained by this method should be handled with extreme care and appropriately labeled.

HIV EXANTHEM

A generalized cutaneous eruption has been observed in many young adults in association with the infectious mononucleosis-like symptoms of acute HIV infection (4). Lesions are generalized, may be either papulosquamous or morbilliform, and last 2–3 weeks. An acute disease associated with primary intrapartum HIV infection has been observed in several infants (5). In one of these patients, a generalized maculopapular rash was noted.

CUTANEOUS MANIFESTATIONS OF INFECTION

A wide range of cutaneous infections have been described in children with AIDS and less severe forms of HIV disease. These patients may have unusual presentations of common infections or have skin disease caused by combinations of common and uncommon organisms.

Table 28.3. Cutaneous Infection in Child with AIDS

Etiology	Clinical Presentation	Diagnostic Procedure	Treatment
Bacterial			
S. aureus S. pyogenes	Erythematous papules, pustules, plaques, ulcers	Gram stain or culture of blister fluid or tissue aspirate	PO: dicloxacillin 25–50 mg/kg/day Amoxicillin-clavulanate 20–40 mg/kg/day (of amoxicillin) IV: Nafcillin 50–100 mg/kg/day Ceftriaxone 50–100 mg/kg/day
Hemophilus influenzae M. avium-intracellulare M. marinuum M. tuberculosis	Ulcers, nodules, macules	Punch biopsy of skin with special stains; tissue culture	Rifampin, clofazimine, ethambutol ciprofloxacin, amikacin Isoniazid, rifampin, pyrazinamide, ethambutol
Bacillary angiomatosis Rochalimaea henselae	Eruptive angiomatous nodules	Punch biopsy of skin with special stains	Erythromycin 20–50 mg/kg/day
Fungal			
C. albicans	White plaques on oral mucosa; confluent erythema in diaper area and other skin folds; satellite lesions; inflammation of nail folds	Skin swab from involved area; KOH preparation or fungal culture	PO: nystatin 100,000–200,000 units every 6 hr Skin: miconazole, econazole, or clotrimazole cream BID
Dermatophyte (e.g., Trichophyton rubrum, T. tonsurans)	Skin: circular lesions with central clearing Scalp: discrete areas of scale and hair loss Nails: thickening, pitting, loss of nails	KOH preparation or fungal culture of border of lesion	Skin: miconazole, econazole, or clotrimazole cream BID Scalp: griseofulvin 10–20 mg/kg/day
Cryptococcosis Sporotrichosis Histoplasmosis	Papules, nodules, plaques, ulcers, abscesses	Skin biopsy; may require special histologic stains or tissue culture	Amphotericin B 0.5–1.5 mg/kg/day, fluconazole 2–8 mg/kg/day, or amphotericin B + flucytosine Amphotericin B 0.5–1.5 mg/kg/day (disseminated infection) Amphotericin B 0.5–1.5 mg/kg/day or itraconazole 2–5 mg/kg/day
Viral			
Herpes simplex	Clustered vesicles on erythematous base; chronic ulcer	Tzanck smear or viral culture of blister fluid; skin biopsy	Acyclovir 250–500 mg/m^2/dose every 8 hr
Herpes zoster	Clustered vesicles in dermatomal distribution	Tzanck smear or viral culture of blister fluid	Acyclovir 500 mg/m^2/day, every 8 hr
Chronic varicella-zoster infection	Widespread nodules, ulcers, plaques	Skin biopsy; viral culture of tissue from ulcer	Acyclovir 500 mg/m^2/day every 8 hr
Molluscum contagiosum	Small umbilicated papules; larger papules may be present	Histologic examination of lesion	Curettage, tretinoin cream BID
Cytomegalovirus	Ulcerative diaper dermatitis	Histologic examination of lesion; viral culture	Ganciclovir 7.5–15 mg/kg/day
Scabies	Excoriated papules or nodules; widespread eczematous eruption	Examine roof of active lesion with mineral oil; skin biopsy	5% permethrin cream

Bacterial Infections

The profound effect of pediatric HIV infection on humoral immunity has been well documented and accounts for the particularly high incidence of bacterial infection among children with the disease (6). Children with HIV-related disease may develop impetigo, ecthyma, and severe episodes of cellulitis caused by infection with *Staphylococcus aureus* (7). Staphylococcal folliculitis, presenting with papules, pustules, or plaques, and extensive pyoderma of the scalp have also been observed (8–10). Toxic shock syndrome, as a complication of enterotoxin-producing *S. aureus* infection of the skin, has been reported in an adolescent with HIV infection (11).

Other documented bacterial infections of the skin include *Hemophilus influenzae* cellulitis and external otitis caused by *Pseudomonas aeruginosa* (12, 13). Several patients with macular discolored lesions and oral ulcers caused by *Mycobacterium avium-intracellulare*, and with atypical ecthymatous lesions caused by *M. marinuum*, have been described (14–16). Miliary tuberculosis of the skin, presenting with numerous follicular papules, has also been reported (17). A wide range of unusual mixed bacterial, fungal, and viral infections may occur (18).

A single case of fatal, disseminated *Listeria monocytogenes* infection in a neonate born to an HIV-infected woman was reported (19). Diffuse petechiae and pustules were present; biopsy of a lesion showed the presence of the Gram-positive coccobacillus.

In the HIV-infected child with cutaneous infection, the bacterial culture of the lesion, with determination of antibiotic sensitivities, is mandatory. If there is an atypical pyoderma, fungal and/or viral cultures and skin biopsy should be performed to eliminate the possibility of a mixed infection.

In mild cases of localized impetigo, the combination of topical mupirocin ointment and oral therapy with dicloxacillin or amoxicillin-clavulanate (Augmentin) is adequate. Hospitalization and the use of intravenous antibiotics should be strongly considered in children with rapidly worsening bacterial infections or with systemic signs or symptoms (e.g., fever, leukocytosis).

Bacillary Angiomatosis

Bacillary angiomatosis is characterized by the rapid development of multiple purplish red angiomatous papules and nodules over the entire skin surface (20). Severe systemic symptoms, including weight loss and fever, may also occur.

This disorder was originally recognized in adult patients with HIV infection and was attributed to infection with the cat-scratch disease bacillus. The cause of bacillary angiomatosis is now recognized to be *Rochalimaea henselae*, a rickettsia-like organism (21).

Bacillary angiomatosis has not yet been noted to occur in the context of pediatric HIV infection. However, this skin disease was observed in an adolescent undergoing chemotherapy for leukemia (22), and its occurrence should probably be anticipated in children with AIDS. In most cases, treatment with oral erythromycin leads to rapid resolution of skin lesions and systemic symptoms.

Fungal Infections

Candidiasis is the most common mucocutaneous manifestation of HIV infection in children. Most children with AIDS will develop oral candidiasis during their illness. This disorder may present with creamy white or yellowish plaques (thrush), areas of atrophy, or angular cheilitis (23).

Therapy of oral thrush during infancy consists of nystatin solution (100,000 units/ml) in a dose of 1–2 ml four times a day. In older children, clotrimazole troches may prove to be more effective. For infants, these troches may also be inserted into a plastic nipple and used four times a day as a pacifier. Although this topical therapy is almost always successful at first, oral thrush may become less responsive with the progression of immune dysfunction. Children with severe oral involvement should be monitored for development of dysphagia or decreased oral intake, which may be signs of candidal esophagitis. In this situation, treatment with fluconazole may be required. In the event of treatment failure, amphotericin is an alternative therapy.

Cutaneous infection with *Candida* may also occur in the diaper area. Most typically, monilial diaper dermatitis presents as an area of confluent bright red erythema with satellite pustules extending beyond the periphery of the lesion. Simultaneous infection may occur in the axilla or neck folds. Monilial diaper dermatitis must be distinguished from seborrheic dermatitis and psoriasis. Potassium hydroxide preparation, or fungal culture, are recommended for confirmation of this diagnosis.

The therapy for monilial diaper dermatitis consists of an imidazole cream (Monistat-Derm, Lotrimin, Spectazole) or topical nystatin cream applied twice daily. If there is evidence of coexistent seborrheic dermatitis or atopic dermatitis, hydrocortisone cream 1% should be added. Antifungal or anticandidal preparations that contain fluorinated topical steroids (Lotrisone, Mycolog) may cause local cutaneous atrophy, and their use should be avoided in the diaper area. Poor response to topical therapy for a culture-proven monilial dermatitis is sometimes a sign of deteriorating immune function.

We have observed several children with chronic candidal paronychiae and resultant nail dystrophy (Fig. 28.1). Patients with erythema and tenderness of the proximal nail fold should be treated with a topical imidazole lotion after fungal and bacterial cultures have been taken.

Many common dermatophytes may also cause severe cutaneous disease in children with HIV infection. Severe tinea capitis, widespread tinea corporis, and onychomycosis have been observed. Tinea capitis, when confirmed by KOH preparation or fungal culture, requires treatment with griseofulvin (15–20 mg/kg/day) for 4–6 weeks. Infections of the skin in areas other than the scalp may be treated with a topical imidazole cream.

In addition to *C. albicans* and the common dermatophytes, many other fungi infect the skin either locally or as part of a systemic infection. HIV-infected patients with cryptococcosis may develop various cutaneous lesions, including papules, nodules, infiltrated plaques, ulcers, and subcutaneous abscesses. Herpetiform lesions and small umbilicated papules resembling molluscum contagiosum have also been reported (24). Disseminated sporotrichosis, associated with numerous painful ulcers, has been reported in many patients with AIDS (25).

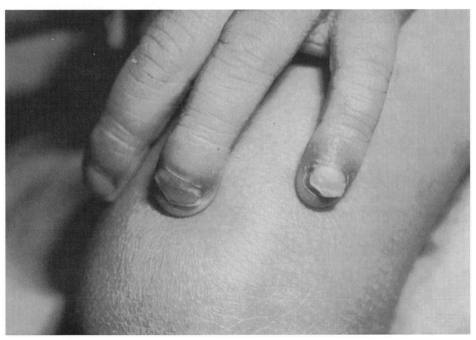

Figure 28.1.   Candidal paronychiae and nail dystrophy in a 4-year girl with AIDS. From Prose NS. HIV infection in childhood: The disease and its cutaneous manifestations. Adv Dermatol 1990;5:113–130.

Finally, disseminated histoplasmosis may lead to several cutaneous lesions. Patients presenting with inflammatory dermatoses, with widespread keratinous papules, and with granulomatous ulcers have been described (24).

Virus Infections

Herpes Simplex

Mucocutaneous infection with herpes simplex may be a significant problem in the child with AIDS. Most commonly, children develop chronic or recurrent herpetic gingivostomatitis (26). Lips, tongue, buccal mucosa, and palate may be involved with painful vesicles and superficial ulcerations. We have also treated several children with severe herpes simplex of the fingers, and chronic herpetic ulcers at other locations have also been observed. Herpes simplex should be suspected as a possible causative agent in any chronic vesicular or ulcerative skin disease, and both Tzanck smear and virus cultures should be performed. Treatment with either oral or intravenous acyclovir (250–500 mg/m^2/dose every 8 hr), depending on the severity of infection, is recommended. The occurrence of herpes simplex resistant to acyclovir has now been reported in patients with AIDS (27). Treatment with foscarnet may be effective in these cases (28).

Cutaneous Cytomegalovirus Infection

A case of diaper dermatitis from cutaneous infection with cytomegalovirus has been reported (29). The patient, a 6-month boy with AIDS, developed an intensely erythematous rash in the perineum, with crusting, erosions, and bullae. Conspicuous viral inclusions were noted on the skin biopsy, and cytomegalovirus was cultured from the skin.

Oral Hairy Leukoplakia

Oral hairy leukoplakia is a form of Epstein-Barr virus infection of the oral mucosa. This disorder, which is common in HIV-infected adults, is characterized by the appearance of corrugated white plaques, which are usually located on the sides of the tongue. Therapy with acyclovir may lead to clinical regression (30).

Oral hairy leukoplakia appears to be uncommon in children with HIV infection. However, a case of this disorder in an 8-year-boy with AIDS has been reported (31).

Herpes Zoster

Herpes zoster, caused by the recurrence of varicella-zoster infection in a dermatomal distribution, is relatively rare in healthy children, with a frequency of 0.15 per 1,000 person-months (32). The occurrence of herpes zoster is now recognized as a presenting sign of HIV infection (33). Herpes zoster in the child with HIV infection tends to be more severe and painful than in the healthy child; the incidence of permanent scarring and recurrence seems to be higher (Fig. 28.2).

Clinical diagnosis is usually made by noting the characteristic clustered vesicles in a dermatomal distribution. This impression should be confirmed by virus culture. Treatment of severe cases consists of intravenous acyclovir (500 mg/m^2/day every 8 hr). In this clinical setting, therapy with oral acyclovir is not an effective alternative. Lesions around the eye or at the tip of the nose may signal the involvement of intraocular structures, and prompt ophthalmologic evaluation is mandatory.

Chronic Varicella-Zoster Infection

A unique form of chronic varicella-zoster infection has been observed in many children and adults with AIDS (34, 35). This disorder may follow the resolution of chicken pox or of herpes zoster. Lesions consist of painful ulcerated nodules or plaques and may be extremely widespread.

In some patients, the lesions of chronic varicella-zoster may be difficult to differentiate from those of pyoderma gangrenosum. Repeated culture of the lesions is sometimes necessary to establish the diagnosis. In addition, the presence of intranuclear inclusion bodies in a skin biopsy indicates virus infection, most frequently caused by herpes simplex.

Treatment of chronic varicella-zoster infection consists of intravenous acyclovir. The

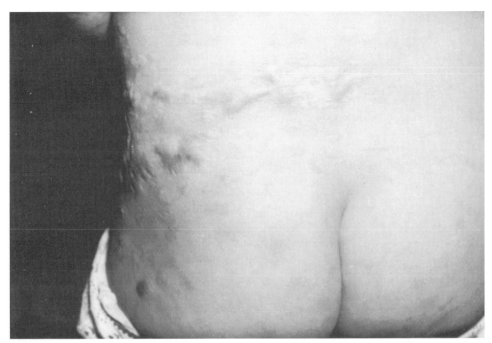

Figure 28.2. Scarring after a severe episode of herpes zoster in a 3-year girl with AIDS. From Weinberg S, Prose N. Color atlas of pediatric dermatology. New York: McGraw-Hill, 1990:162.

continued development of new lesions despite this therapy may indicate the presence of a virus strain that is resistant to this drug. Central nervous system involvement and death resulting from the dissemination of such a strain has been reported (34).

Molluscum Contagiosum

Molluscum contagiosum is a common virus infection of the skin that is caused by a DNA poxvirus. It is characterized by the development of flesh-colored umbilicated papules that are 1–2 mm in diameter. Children with HIV infection may develop severe molluscum contagiosum, with numerous lesions or lesions that are unusually large (Fig. 28.3).

The treatment of molluscum contagiosum must be tailored to the age of the patient and the severity of disease. In a cooperative child with only several lesions, simple removal with a sharp curette is the simplest and most effective approach. More severe cases represent a treatment challenge; liquid nitrogen and topical tretinoin cream are sometimes used. The occurrence of molluscum contagiosum adjacent to or on the eyelids is a particularly difficult management problem, and consultation with an ophthalmologist may be appropriate. Resolution of severe molluscum contagiosum in the course of therapy with zidovudine has been reported (36).

Human Papilloma Virus

Infection with human papilloma virus in the child with HIV infection may result in the evolution of widespread common warts. One treatment modality consists of gentle cryosurgery, and the home application of a salicylic acid preparation.

The occurrence of widespread flat warts on the face, upper back, and upper chest has also been reported (37). In some areas, these subtle lesions may mimic tinea versicolor. Treatment with gentle cryosurgery or with topical tretinoin cream (Retin-A) may be effective.

Children with HIV infection may develop genital or perianal condylomata acuminata (38, 39). Because condylomata acuminata are sometimes associated with sexual abuse, a careful history and investigation for sexual abuse is critical. Small lesions of condy-

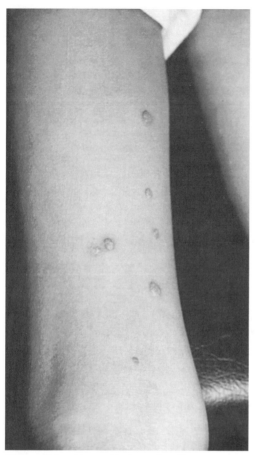

Figure 28.3.   Unusual lesions of molluscum contagiosum on posterior thigh of an 8-year boy with AIDS.

lomata acuminata may respond to the weekly application of 25% podophyllum resin. To avoid severe local irritation, this agent must be carefully washed off 2 hr after application. Occasionally, because of HIV-related immune suppression, the lesions of condylomata acuminata may become quite large. In these cases, surgical removal may be necessary.

Infestations

Atypical forms of scabies are common in patients with immune defects. Among children with AIDS, scabies may present with a generalized papulosquamous eruption or with diffuse areas of crusting and scale (40). Patients with crusted scabies (sometimes termed "Norwegian scabies") are infested

with numerous mites and are highly contagious to family members and health care personnel (41). Diagnosis of scabies may be confirmed by placing a drop of mineral oil on the top of a scalpel blade and scraping the roof of a primary lesion onto a glass slide. Microscopic examination will reveal the presence of mites or eggs.

Treatment of scabies consists of the overnight application of Elimite cream, a 5% permethrin cream. This preparation appears to be as effective as lindane lotion (Kwell) but is not neurotoxic. All clothing and bedding should be laundered at the time of treatment.

It is not unusual for patients to continue to itch for several weeks after the successful completion of antiscabetic therapy. However, scabies may be particularly difficult to eradicate in the child with HIV infection. Therefore, the presence of severe persistent pruritus or of new lesions should prompt the health care provider to repeat scrapings for scabies and to treat again if necessary.

Health care providers who have been unknowingly exposed to children with scabies may elect to be treated with a single overnight application of either lindane lotion or permethrin cream. Simultaneous laundering of clothing and bedding is advised.

Parasitic Infection

Acanthamoeba infection of the skin may rarely occur in patients with HIV infection (42). Lesions are small firm papulonodules, which may ulcerate. Infection with *Naegleria fowleri*, one of the pathogenic species, is responsive to treatment with amphotericin B.

INFLAMMATORY DISORDERS OF THE SKIN

Atopic Dermatitis

The incidence of atopic dermatitis may be increased among children infected with HIV. The onset or worsening of this disorder has been noted particularly among hemophiliacs after seroconversion (43, 44). The management of atopic dermatitis, as in the healthy child, consists of emollients, antihistamines, and topical corticosteroids.

Seborrheic Dermatitis

Severe seborrheic dermatitis has been appreciated as a hallmark of HIV infection among adults. The presentation of this disorder varies markedly with age of the patient. Among infants, seborrheic dermatitis usually begins as a diffuse scaling of the scalp (cradle cap) and may progress to widespread involvement of the intertriginal folds and diaper area. We have also seen several older children with erythema and scaling of the scalp, nasolabial folds, and the postauricular skin. In most cases, seborrheic dermatitis responds to the application twice daily of nonfluorinated topical corticosteroids. Addition of topical ketoconazole cream appears to be helpful in some cases.

Psoriasis

In some patients with HIV infection, severe psoriasis may develop or worsen during their illness (45). This may occasionally occur in children and adolescents. HIV-related psoriasis is sometimes unresponsive to conventional therapy with topical corticosteroids and coal tar preparations. In several patients, this skin disorder has been noted to respond to therapy with zidovudine (46).

Drug Eruptions

Children with HIV infection have a high incidence of drug eruptions, especially from trimethoprim-sulfamethoxazole. In one study, 16% of 50 children with AIDS developed a rash in response to this medication (8). Lesions may be maculopapular or morbilliform; in some children we have noted discrete circular patches of dusky erythema. Diagnosis is usually made by establishing a temporal relationship between the acute eruption and therapy with a particular medication. In cases where the diagnosis is in doubt, skin biopsy may prove helpful.

Most drug eruptions resolve rapidly after discontinuation of the drug. However, severe Stevens-Johnson syndrome and toxic epidermal necrolysis have been seen in HIV-infected children in response to trimethoprim-sulfamethoxazole, antituberculous medications, and phenobarbital (9, 47, 48).

In most cases of drug eruption, discontinuation of the causative medication is necessary. Aerosolized pentamidine may be used as an alternative therapy for *Pneumocystis carinii* prophylaxis.

Vasculitis

Chronic leukocytoclastic vasculitis has been observed in several children with HIV infection (12) (Fig. 28.4). This disorder may be differentiated from infectious diseases, such as chronic varicella-zoster infection, by the presence of a typical inflammation of small dermal vessels on routine skin biopsy. Vasculitis may be caused directly by HIV, by concomitant viral infection, or by a medication. In one child, chronic palpable purpura of the lower extremities was the

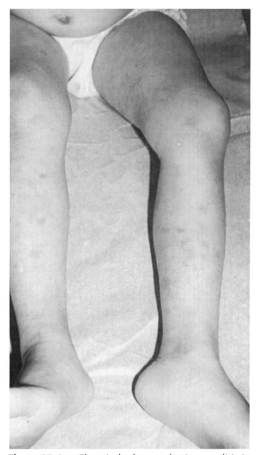

Figure 28.4. Chronic leukocytoclastic vasculitis in a child with AIDS. From Weinberg S, Prose N. Color atlas of pediatric dermatology. New York: McGraw-Hill, 1990:162.

sole manifestation of HIV infection (49). Clinically, this cutaneous manifestation must be differentiated from purpura caused by thrombocytopenia or sepsis and from the common disorder, Henoch-Schlönlein purpura.

Pyoderma Gangrenosum

Pyoderma gangrenosum is an uncommon skin disorder characterized by chronic ulceration of the skin. The ulcer has a mucopurulent base, and the borders are typically violaceous and undermined. The occurrence of pyoderma gangrenosum has been reported in two children with AIDS (50). In one patient, this skin disease responded to treatment with dapsone. Because many bacterial and viral agents may cause chronic cutaneous ulceration in the child with HIV infection, it is extremely important to systematically exclude infection before treating lesions as pyoderma gangrenosum.

Nutritional Deficiencies

Children with chronic HIV infection may develop nutritional deficiencies caused by malabsorption and poor dietary intake. Eruptions with features of kwashiorkor and pellagra have been observed in some children (15). In addition, acrodermatitis enteropathica, the cutaneous manifestation of zinc deficiency, may develop in children with HIV infection (51). This disorder is characterized by erythema and fissuring of periorificial and acral skin. Diarrhea and irritability are associated findings.

NEOPLASM

Kaposi's Sarcoma

Epidemic Kaposi's sarcoma was first described in 1981 (52). This neoplastic disorder is primarily seen in homosexual men with HIV infection. The lesions are plum-colored nodules or plaques that may occur on any skin or mucous membrane surface. Cutaneous Kaposi's sarcoma is extremely unusual in children. To date, only a few such patients have been reported (53–55).

Leiomyosarcoma

Malignant and benign tumors of smooth muscle origin may be a complication of HIV infection in children (56, 57) (see Chapter 33). A case of multiple subcutaneous leiomyosarcomas in a 17-year boy with thalassemia major and HIV infection has recently been reported (56). Lesions presented with local pain, and there was minimal elevation and firmness of the overlying skin.

CONCLUSION

Several other cutaneous disorders have been reported to occur in children with HIV infection. These include cutis marmorata, eruptive dysplastic nevi, vitiligo, and erythema dyschromicum perstans. In addition, marked hypertrichosis of the eyelashes has been reported by several authors and noted by us in many of our patients (59, 60).

To verify these observations, future research should be directed toward determining the incidence and natural history of cutaneous disease in children with HIV infection. Information of this sort will also help the pediatric clinician to appreciate early warning signs of HIV infection and institute antiviral therapy when indicated.

References

1. Lim W, Sadick N, Gupta A, Kaplan M, Pahwa S. Skin diseases in children with HIV infection and their association with degree of immunosuppression. Int J Dermatol 1990;29:24–30.
2. Prose N. Pediatric human immunodeficiency virus infection in childhood; the disease and its cutaneous manifestations. Adv Dermatol 1990;5:113–130.
3. Nance KV, Smith ML, Joshi VV. Cutaneous manifestations of acquired immunodeficiency syndrome in children. Int J Dermatol 1991;30:531–539.
4. Wantzin GRL, Linhard BO, Weisman K, et al. Acute HTLV-III infection associated with exanthema, followed by seroconversion. Br J Dermatol 1986;115:601–606.
5. Luzuriaga K, McQuilken P, Aliment A, et al. Early viremia and immune responses in vertical human immunodeficiency virus type 1 infection. J Infect Dis 1993;167:1008–1013.
6. Bernstein LJ, Ochs HD, Wedgwood RJ, et al. Defective humoral immunity in pediatric acquired immunodeficiency syndrome. J Pediatr 1985;107:352–357.
7. Bernstein LJ, Krieger BZ, Novick B, et al. Bacterial infection in the acquired immunodeficiency syndrome in children. Pediatr Infect Dis J 1985;4:472–475.

8. Straka BF, Whitaker DL, Morrison SH, et al. Cutaneous manifestations of the acquired immunodeficiency syndrome in children. J Am Acad Dermatol 1988;18:1089–1102.

9. Hira SK, Wadhawan D, Kamanga J, et al. Cutaneous manifestations of human immunodeficiency virus in Lusaka, Zambia. J Am Acad Dermatol 1988;19:451–457.

10. Becker BA, Frieden IJ, Odom R, Berger TG. Atypical plaquelike staphylococcal folliculitis in human immunodeficiency virus-infected persons. J Am Acad Dermatol 1989;21:1024–1026.

11. Kline MW, Dunkle LM. Toxic shock syndrome and the acquired immunodeficiency syndrome. Pediatr Infect Dis J 1988;7:736–737.

12. Prose N, Mendez H, Menikoff H, et al. Pediatric human immunodeficiency virus infection and its cutaneous manifestations. Pediatr Dermatol 1987;4:67–74.

13. Centers for Disease Control. Unexplained immunodeficiency and opportunistic infection in infants. New York, New Jersey and California. MMWR 1982;31:665–667.

14. Volpe F, Schwimmer A, Barr C. Oral manifestations of disseminated *Mycobacterium avium-intracellulare* in a patient with AIDS. Oral Surg Oral Med Oral Pathol 1985;60:567–570.

15. Penneys NS, Hick B. Unusual cutaneous lesions associated with acquired immunodeficiency syndrome. J Am Acad Dermatol 1985;13:845–852.

16. Kaplan MH, Sadick N, NcNutt S. Dermatologic findings and manifestations of acquired immunodeficiency syndrome (AIDS). J Am Acad Dermatol 1987;16:485–506.

17. Rohatgi PK, Palazzolo JV, Saini NB. Acute miliary tuberculosis of the skin in acquired immunodeficiency syndrome. J Am Acad Dermatol 1992;26:356–359.

18. Gretzula J, Penneys NS. Complex viral and fungal skin lesions of patients with acquired immunodeficiency syndrome. J Am Acad Dermatol 1987;16:1151–1154.

19. Smith KJ, Skelton III HG, Angritt P, et al. Cutaneous lesions of listeriosis in a newborn. J Cutan Pathol 1991;18:474–476.

20. Cockerell CJ, Whitlow MA, Webster GF, Friedman-Kien AE. Epithelioid angiomatosis: A distinct vascular disorder in patients with acquired immunodeficiency syndrome. Lancet 1987;2:654–656.

21. Welch DF, Pickett DA, Slater LN, et al. *Rochalimaea henselae* sp. nov., a cause of septicemia, bacillary angiomatosis, and parenchymal bacillary peliosis. J Clin Microbiol 1992;30:275–280.

22. Myers SA, Prose NS, Garcia JA, et al. Bacillary angiomatosis in a child undergoing chemotherapy. J Pediatr 1992;121:574–578.

23. Leggott PJ, Robertson P, Greenspan D, et al. Oral manifestations of primary and acquired immunodeficiency diseases in children. Pediatr Dent 1987;9:98–194.

24. Knobler RM. Human immunodeficiency virus infection. Dermatol Clin 1989;7:369–385.

25. Shaw JC, Levinson W, Montanaro A. Sporotrichosis in the acquired immunodeficiency syndrome. J Am Acad Dermatol 1989;21:1145–1147.

26. Scott GB, Buck BE, Leterman JG, et al. Acquired immunodeficiency syndrome in infants. N Engl J Med 1984;310:76–81.

27. Erlich KS, Mills J, Chatis P, et al. Acyclovir-resistant herpes simplex virus infections in patients with the acquired immunodeficiency syndrome. N Engl J Med 1989;320:293–296.

28. Erlich KS, Jacobson MA, Koehler JE, et al. Foscarnet therapy of severe acyclovir-resistant herpes simplex virus infections in patients with acquired immunodeficiency syndrome. Ann Intern Med 1989;110:710–713.

29. Thiboutot DM, Beckford A, Mart CR, Sexton M, Maloney ME. Cytomegalovirus diaper dermatitis. Arch Dermatol 1991;127:396–398.

30. Herbst JS, Morgan J, Raab-Traub N, Resnick L. Comparison of the efficacy of surgery and acyclovir therapy in oral hairy leukoplakia. J Am Acad Dermatol 1989;21:753–756.

31. Greenspan JS, Mastrucci MT, Leggott PJ, et al. Hairy leukoplakia in a child. AIDS 1988;2:143.

32. Baba K, Yabuuchi H, Takahashi M, Ogra PL. Increased incidence of herpes zoster in normal children infected with varicella zoster virus during infancy: Community-based follow-up study. J Pediatr 1986;108:372–377.

33. Friedmann-Kien AE, Lafleur FL, Gendler E, et al. Herpes zoster: A possible early clinical sign for the development of acquired immunodeficiency syndrome in high risk individuals. J Am Acad Dermatol 1986;14:1023–1028.

34. Pahwa S, Biron K, Lim W, et al. Continuous varicella-zoster infection associated with acyclovir resistance in a child with AIDS. JAMA 1988;260:2879–2882.

35. Gilson IH, Barnett JH, Conant MA, et al. Disseminated ecthymatous herpes varicella-zoster infection in patients with acquired immunodeficiency syndrome. J Am Acad Dermatol 1989;20:637–642.

36. Betlloch I, Pinazo I, Mestre F, Altes J. Molluscum contagiosum in human immunodeficiency virus infection: response to zidovudine. Int J Dermatol 1989;28:351–352.

37. Prose NS, von Knebel Doeberitz C, Miller S, Milburn P, Heilman E. Widespread flat warts associated with human papillomavirus type 5: A cutaneous manifestation of human immunodeficiency virus infection. J Am Acad Dermatol 1990;23:978–981.

38. Laraque D. Severe anogenital warts in a child with HIV infection [Letter]. N Engl J Med 1989;320:1220–1221.

39. Forman A, Prendiville J. Association of human immunodeficiency virus seropositivity and extensive perineal condylomata acuminata in a child. Arch Dermatol 1988;124:1010–1011.

40. Sadick N, Kaplan MH, Pahwa SG, et al. Unusual features of scabies complicating human T-lymphotropic virus type III infection. J Am Acad Dermatol 1986;15:482–486.

41. Jucowics P, Ramon ME, Don PC, et al. Norwegian scabies in an infant with acquired immunodeficiency syndrome. Arch Dermatol 1989;125:1670–1672.

42. May LP, Sidhu GS, Buchness MR. Diagnosis of *Acanthamoeba* infection by cutaneous manifesta-

tions in a man seropositive for HIV. J Am Acad Dermatol 1992;26:352–355.

43. Ball LM, Harper JI, et al. Atopic eczema in HIV-seropositive hemophiliacs [Letter]. Lancet 1987;2:627–628.

44. Parkin JM, Eales LJ, Galazka AR, et al. Atopic manifestations in the acquired immune deficiency syndrome: Response to recombinant interferon gamma. Br Med J 1987;294:1185–1186.

45. Johnson TM, Duvic M, Rapini RP, Rios A. AIDS exacerbates psoriasis [Letter]. N Engl J Med 1985;313:1415.

46. Kaplan M, Sadick S, Wieder J, et al. Antipsoriatic effects of zidovudine in human immunodeficiency virus-associated psoriasis. J Am Acad Dermatol 1989;20:76–82.

47. Revuz J. Necrolyse epidermique toxique par les sulfamides au cours du SIDA; a propos de 3 cas [Abstract]. J Dermatol Paris 1986:153.

48. Salomon D, Saurat JH. Erythema multiforme major in a 2-month-old child with human immunodeficiency virus (HIV) infection. Br J Dermatol 1990; 123:797–800.

49. Chren MM, Silverman RA, Sorensen RU, Elmets CA. Leukocytoclastic vasculitis in a patient infected with human immunodeficiency virus. J Am Acad Dermatol 1989;21:1161–1164.

50. Paller AS, Sahn EE, Garen PD, et al. Pyoderma gangrenosum in pediatric acquired immunodeficiency syndrome. J Pediatr 1990;117:63–66.

51. Tong TK, Andrew LR, Albert A, Mickell JJ. Childhood acquired immunodeficiency syndrome manifesting as acrodermatitis enteropathica. J Pediatr 1986;108:426–428.

52. Hymes K, Cheung T, Green JB, et al: Kaposi's sarcoma in homosexual men—report of eight cases. Lancet 1981;2:598–600.

53. Malekzadeh MH, Church J, Siegel SE, et al. Human immunodeficiency virus-associated Kaposi's sarcoma in a pediatric renal transplant recipient. Nephron 1987;42:62–65.

54. Guiterrez-Ortega P, Hierro-Orozoco S, Sanchez-Cisneros R, et al. Kaposi's sarcoma in a 6-day-old infant with human immunodeficiency virus [Letter]. Arch Dermatol 1989;125:432–433.

55. Connor E, Boccon-Gibod L, Joshi V, et al. Cutaneous acquired immunodeficiency syndrome-associated Kaposi's sarcoma in pediatric patients. Arch Dermatol 1990;126:791–793.

56. Chadwick E, Conner EG, Guerra Hanson IC, et al. Tumors of smooth muscle origin in pediatric HIV-infected children: An association of AIDS and cancer. JAMA 1990;263:3182–3185.

57. McLoughlin LC, Nord KS, Joshi JV, et al. Disseminated leiomyosarcomas in a child with acquired immunodeficiency syndrome. Cancer 1991;67:2618–2621.

58. Orlow SJ, Kamino H, Lawrence RL. Multiple subcutaneous leiomyosarcomas in an adolescent with AIDS. Am J Ped Hematol Oncol 1992;14:265–268.

59. Casanova JM, Puig T, Rubio M. Hypertrichosis of the eyelashes in the acquired immunodeficiency syndrome [Letter]. Arch Dermatol 1987;1599–1601.

60. Kaplan MH, Sadick NS, Talmor M. Acquired trichomegaly of the eyelashes: A cutaneous marker of acquired immunodeficiency syndrome. J Am Acad Dermatol 1991;25:801–804.

Delbert R. Wigfall

INITIAL DESCRIPTION: OCCURRENCE IN ADULTS

Since the initial reports of human immunodeficiency virus (HIV) infections, there have been reports of AIDS patients suffering from both acute reversible and chronic irreversible forms of renal failure. In 1983, it was reported that renal disease in AIDS patients progressed in a fulminant manner with uniformly poor survival (1, 2).

Since the initial observations, various renal parenchymal lesions and alterations in kidney function have been described that can be categorized in four groups (1, 2): 1) occurrence of glomerular lesions characterized clinically by proteinuria and histologically most often by focal and segmental glomerulosclerosis (FSGS) (3–5), 2) development of acute tubular dysfunction with electrolyte disturbances, 3) frank renal failure caused by infection (6), or 4) renal injury resultant from nephrotoxic drugs (7).

By convention, the term HIV-associated nephropathy refers to the occurrence of moderate to severe proteinuria accompanied by variable azotemia and FSGS and has been recognized in ~10–20% of patients infected with the HIV virus (8, 9, 10). This lesion histologically bears a striking resemblance to the lesion of heroin-induced nephropathy (11, 12).

The actual incidence of electrolyte disturbance and acute insufficiency is not as well-defined but has been noted in ~50% of hospitalized patients with HIV infection (5). Although HIV-related glomerular abnormalities have received the most attention, acute renal failure from nephrotoxic therapy is probably more common (7).

PREVALENCE OF HIV RENAL COMPLICATIONS IN CHILDREN

The occurrence of renal disease in association with asymptomatic and symptomatic HIV infection has been defined in children, with pathologic studies demonstrating lesions akin to those described in adults (13, 14). Glomerulopathy has been noted to occur in up to 15% of children with HIV infection (13, 9, 15), whereas the occurrence of tubular dysfunction is less well-defined. In our own experience, up to 10% of HIV-infected children will evidence tubular dysfunction, but only 2–5% will develop overt glomerulopathy.

In this chapter, renal manifestations of HIV infection will be reviewed. Evaluation and therapy of these complications will also be discussed.

ETIOLOGIC CONSIDERATIONS
Pathogenesis of Disease

Although the mechanisms leading to expression of renal disease in HIV-infected individuals remains unknown, animal models of disease have given us the opportunity to further explore this question. By using a noninfectious HIV-1 DNA construct, researchers have generated three transgenic mouse lines that develop a syndrome remarkably similar to the human disease. In one such line, proteinuria has been detectable at ~24 days of age, followed by severe nephrotic syndrome and rapid progression to end-stage renal failure. Renal histology shows focal segmental glomerulosclerosis and microcystic tubular dilatation, both characteristic findings in human disease. Northern blot analysis of the total kidney RNA shows expression of virus genes before the appearance of histologic renal disease, with greatly diminished virus gene expression late in the disease. Hence it would appear that the progressive renal dysfunction and glomerulosclerosis demonstrated in these transgenic mice may result from the presence of HIV-1 genes (16, 17).

The actual site of HIV infection within the kidney also remains a mystery, although it has been postulated that the mesangial cells may be pivotal to the sclerosing process. Researchers have been unable to demonstrate infection of mesangial cells in vitro (18), but there has been localization of virus material by Northern analysis in renal epithelial cells (19). It has been postulated that the site of HIV infection within the kidney may be the result of differences in HIV virus strain tropism, rather than differences in susceptibility to infection in specific renal cells (18).

It is most attractive to implicate a direct effect of HIV as the sole cause of nephropathy, but other factors must be considered. Other conditions where glomerular sclerosis may evolve include aging, systemic hypertension, diabetes, sickle cell disease, reflux nephropathy, obesity, unilateral renal agenesis, intravenous drug abuse, and, experimentally, renal ablation (20). Hence, FSGS is a pathologic expression of disease or injury, not a pure entity. Consequently, other factors, such as immunologic injury mediated through immune complexes, opportunistic infections, neoplasms, toxicity of drug therapies, or hemodynamic instability, may contribute to the expression of renal disease (11, 21).

Immune complexes have been routinely observed in the mesangial area of kidney biopsies of HIV-infected individuals (15) and have long been demonstrated to mediate disease in other settings (e.g., postinfectious glomerulonephritis). The significance of these complexes in the pathophysiology of HIV nephropathy is uncertain given the fact that these lesions are present in the mesangium of HIV-infected individuals without renal dysfunction and with normal glomerular pathology (9, 22).

HIV-infected individuals may be predisposed to develop acute renal dysfunction when exposed to one or more nephrotoxic drugs, including pentamidine, aminogylcosides, sulfadiazine, trimethoprim-sulfamethoxazole, the nonsteroidal anti-inflammatory agent meclofenamate, and radiocontrast agents (23, 24, 25). Within the subset of HIV-infected individuals who have evidenced renal dysfunction are intravenous drug, especially heroin, users. Heroin has long been recognized to cause a nephropathy also characterized by glomerulosclerosis but has pathologic features that distinguish it from HIV-associated disease (26).

The presence of disturbances in extracellular fluid volume resulting from vomiting, decreased fluid intake, or chronic diarrhea with bacterial or opportunistic infections may result in hemodynamic abnormalities contributing to renal dysfunction (27). Evidence of other concurrent opportunistic infections and neoplasms has been found on pathologic examination of kidney tissue from HIV-infected individuals. Cytomegalovirus, tuberculosis, *Mycobacterium avium* intracellulare, and *Cryptococcus* have all been localized within the kidney of infected individuals, as have Kaposi sarcoma and non-Hodgkin's lymphoma (28). Infection can result in direct or immune-mediated injury to the kidney.

Vascular lesions have been found during pathologic evaluation of tissues from HIV-infected individuals. These lesions contribute to the observed neurologic, pulmonary, and cardiac dysfunction observed in HIV disease and may also contribute to the observed occurrence of HIV-associated nephropathy (29). Hence, given our current understanding of expression of renal dysfunction in the HIV-infected individual, the etiology remains multifactoral.

Natural History
(Risk Factors, Morbidity, Mortality)

The accepted risk factors for the development of HIV-associated nephropathy are identical to those that identify the person at increased risk of exposure to HIV. In clinical practice, there has been an observed increased incidence of HIV-associated nephropathy in blacks, Haitians, and adults with a history of drug use. Conversely, there is a negligible incidence of nephropathy among homosexual men (9, 30). These differences likely contribute to the reported regional differences in the occurrence of HIV-associated renal disease (increased in Miami and New York but low in San Francisco, Dallas, and Bethesda). HIV-associated nephropathy in children occurs in the absence of any definitive risk factors (31).

The reported incidence of renal disease in the adult population ranges from 3 to 40% (6, 8, 11–13). In children infected by HIV, 30–55% will have renal disease or urinary and electrolyte abnormalities at some time during their illness, with 3–29% having more definite evidence of renal disease (9, 13, 14, 31). In adults, the entity is described as one that progresses fulminantly to end-stage renal disease and death (8, 9). It is recognized in children that HIV-associated renal disease does not carry as grave a prognosis (13), with death more often a consequence of infection or wasting. Therefore renal dysfunction and frank glomerulopathy often complicate the course and therapy but may not greatly contribute to an increased mortality.

Pathologic Lesions

Various lesions have been reported in patients with HIV-associated nephropathy. At autopsy, the renal lesions most commonly encountered are acute tubular necrosis, interstitial nephritis, mesangial hyperplasia, and glomerulosclerosis. The kidney is often the site of silent seeding by opportunistic pathogens (32).

Conversely, renal biopsies in patients with HIV infection (symptomatic or asymptomatic) usually show either focal segmental glomerulosclerosis (see Fig. 29.1) or mesangial hyperplasia (33). HIV-associated nephropathy by convention includes only patients with heavy proteinuria or nephrotic syndrome clinically and glomerulosclerosis histologically (32).

Distinctive microscopic features include 1) a collapsing and predominantly global pattern of glomerulosclerosis, 2) varied degrees of cellular expansion of the mesangium, 3) severe visceral epithelial cell hypertrophy and droplet formation, and 4) dilatation of Bowman's space (26, 32).

Immunofluorescent examination has been positive for IgM, C3, and C1, with segmental to global glomerular staining. In some cases, prominent staining of the visceral epithelial cell droplets has been observed for immunoglobulin and/or albumin in a pattern corresponding to the hyaline droplets seen by light microscopy (26).

The most striking ultrastructural features found have been 1) prominent tubular microcysts and cast formation and 2) numerous tubuloreticular inclusions (see Fig. 29.2) (32). Glomerular electron-dense deposits of possible immune origin are small and focal when present, affecting the mesangium, subendothelial area, subepithelial area, or sometimes a combination (26).

In contrast, children and asymptomatic adult patients often have mesangial hyperplasia on biopsy or autopsy examination of the kidney. This lesion is characterized by moderate glomerular mesangial expansion with mesangial deposits. By electron microscopy, mesangial deposits are present in up to ~70% of cases (9, 26, 32). By immunofluorescent examination, up to 90% of patients will evidence IgM and C3 and occasionally C1q (34, 26, 32).

There have been other lesions defined in the kidneys of HIV-infected individuals including minimal change disease, membranoproliferative disease, postinfectious glomerulnephritis, hemolytic uremic syndrome, membranous nephropathy, and IgA nephropathy (5, 35). Ultimately, lesser occurring lesions may represent random events rather than HIV-related disease.

Clinical Presentation

Renal manifestations of HIV infection are many and range from pathologic abnormalities directly caused by the infection resulting in glomerulopathic lesions to intrarenal infections, interstitial nephritis, and acute tubular necrosis. Disturbances in extracellular fluid volume resulting from vomiting, re-

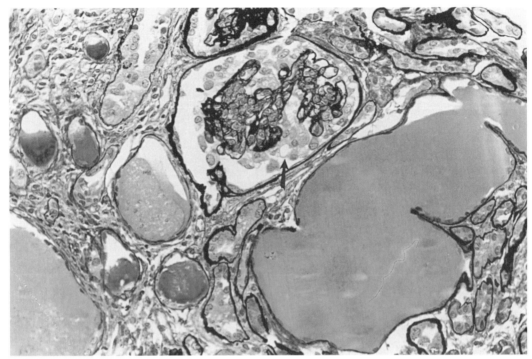

Figure 29.1. Photomicrograph of renal biopsy from a 2-year child with HIV-associated nephropathy. There is glomerular segmental sclerosis in an early stage; note proliferation of visceral epithelial cells (*arrow*), some of which are coarsely vacuolated. Some tubules are considerably dilated and filled with casts of plasma protein. There is also interstitial edema with few leukocytes. Periodic acid-methenamine silver, ×400. Courtesy of Arthur H. Cohen, M.D., Department of Pathology and Laboratory Medicine, Cedars-Sinai Medical Center, Los Angeles, CA.

duced fluid intake, or chronic diarrhea may also contribute to renal dysfunction. Clinical presentation of involvement or dysfunction may be further obscured by the fact that many nephrotoxic drugs are used in the management of opportunistic infections associated with HIV infection. Acid-base and electrolyte abnormalities related to tubular dysfunction are also common (8, 27).

For the following discussion, the clinical spectrum of disease will be categorized as 1) glomerulopathies, 2) acute renal failure, 3) tubular dysfunction and/or electrolyte abnormalities, and 4) urologic manifestations.

Glomerulopathies Associated with HIV Infection

Although other glomerular lesions have been defined in patients with HIV infection (see Table 29.1), FSGS and mesangial hyperplasia are the most common histologic changes detected.

Focal Segmental Glomerulosclerosis

The most commonly reported lesion associated with HIV infection, especially in adults, is that of focal glomerulosclerosis, occurring in an estimated 30–40% of adults who are HIV infected (9). The lesion has been reported to occur twice as frequently in the population of patients who are black (<10% of reported cases in the literature are white (6)) and/or intravenous drug

Table 29.1. Nephropathy in Patients with HIV Infection[a]

Type	% Occurrence in Literature
Glomerulosclerosis	50.8
Mesangial hyperplasia	21.0
Nephrocalcinosis	10.5
Interstitial nephritis	7.6
Acute tubular necrosis	4.8
Other glomerulonephritides	3.8
Minimal change	1.4

[a]Data from lesions found on biopsy or autopsy.

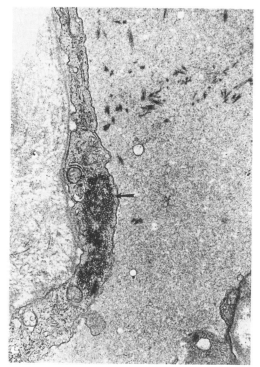

Figure 29.2. Electron micrograph depicting a large tubuloreticular structure (*arrow*) in cytoplasm of a peritubular capillary endothelial cell. ×18,750. Courtesy of Arthur H. Cohen, MD, Department of Pathology and Laboratory Medicine, Cedars-Sinai Medical Center, Los Angeles, CA.

users, in contrast to patients who are heterosexually infected or infected through blood products. In addition, glomerulosclerosis occurs ten times more commonly in intravenous drug users than in homosexuals, regardless of race (8). Given experience in adults and clinical observations of HIV-related illnesses in children followed primarily in large urban areas, it is estimated that 3–10% of children with HIV infection will manifest glomerulopathy (13, 31). These estimates are limited by the fact that tissue is not routinely obtained from all patients (31).

The initial symptoms of HIV-associated glomerulopathy include nephrotic range proteinuria, edema, hypoalbuminemia, and azotemia. Up to 95% of patients are normotensive on presentation and continue despite progressive loss of renal function (6, 12). The clinical course HIV nephropathy in adults has been categorized as rapid loss of function and death (10). Children with

HIV nephropathy tend not to follow the clinical course of adults, because they survive renal failure but succumb to nonrenal complications (13).

Mesangial Hyperplasia

Occasionally adult patients have presented with microscopic or macroscopic hematuria, non-nephrotic range proteinuria, and normal renal function. Although a portion of these less severely affected patients have FSGS, this group is more likely to evidence mesangial hyperplasia or proliferation on biopsy. In children, although FSGS occurs, mesangial hyperplasia represents 50% of biopsy confirmed HIV-associated renal disease (13), whereas in adults, <25% of patients have mesangial hyperplasia (9). The clinical course of these patients is benign, with no development of overt renal insufficiency (13, 9) but continued abnormalities in the urinary sediment.

Acute Renal Failure

Irrespective of etiology, acute renal failure adds significantly to the morbidity and mortality of patients with HIV infection and AIDS. Renal failure may be a terminal event in many who develop sepsis and multiorgan failure (6).

Acute renal failure resulting from acute tubular necrosis is common in hospitalized AIDS patients and results from ischemia secondary to intravascular volume depletion from sepsis and hypotension or depletion from increased losses. Metabolic acidosis, respiratory insufficiency, or nephrotoxins may further contribute to renal failure. Patients may also develop acute renal failure as a hypersensitivity reaction to chosen therapy, such as trimethoprim-sulfamethoxazole, pentamidine, or phenytoin (6, 36).

Acute renal failure is manifested by an azotemic oliguric phase, generally followed by a period of diuresis, with recovery of function if the patient survives the precipitating insult. If the renal failure is the result of allergy, then azotemia may be accompanied by fever, eosinophilia, and skin rash. When suspected, the renal dysfunction is generally reversed by cessation of the offending agent.

Tubular Dysfunction and/or Electrolyte Abnormalities

Several fluid and electrolyte abnormalities may occur in patients with HIV infection. Hyponatremia, the most common electrolyte abnormality, is caused by various pathophysiologic mechanisms including the syndrome of inappropriate antidiuretic hormone secretion, renal or extrarenal wasting of sodium, and adrenal insufficiency (3, 37).

Adrenal dysfunction in AIDS patients (38) has been observed with an abnormal response to Cortrosyn stimulation and adrenal steroid biosynthetic abnormalities. The impact of such abnormalities on sodium balance and response to replacement therapy has yet to be fully explored (3).

Disorders of potassium balance have also been described in patients with HIV disease. Hypokalemia may result from excessive diarrhea or vomiting or in association with amphotericin B therapy. In contrast, hyperkalemia may occur in concert with nephrotoxic therapy (39) or with acute renal failure. These electrolyte abnormalities are best handled by early identification, withdrawal of toxins, judicious administration of corrective fluids, and early intervention with dialysis if indicated (6).

Other acid-base and electrolyte disturbances have been described in HIV-infected individuals. Some disturbances result from nonrenal losses (metabolic alkalosis related to acid losses through vomiting). Other disturbances occur because of renal injury and tubulopathy resulting from nephrotoxic therapy, such as that which results from amphotericin B or foscarnet (3, 6, 33, 40, 44). Regardless of cause, tubulopathy may result in significant renal wasting of sodium, bicarbonate, calcium and magnesium. Hypomagnesemia may further contribute to imbalances of calcium and phosphorus through disturbed vitamin D-parathyroid hormone interactions. Like other electrolyte disturbances, appropriate management includes withdrawal of any offending agents and appropriate replacement.

UROLOGIC MANIFESTATIONS

Two forms of urologic involvement have been described in patients with HIV infections or disease: urinary tract infections and malignancies. Simple pyuria has been described in over 50% of adults with HIV-associated renal abnormalities, with urinary tract infections occurring in 20%. Atypical pathogens including *Candida, Salmonella, Acinetobacter calcoaceticus*, and cytomegalovirus have been encountered (42, 43), but the two most common agents are *Escherichia coli* (33%) and *Pseudomonas* (25%) (27). There are no collected data on the frequency of urinary tract infections in children.

Involvement of the urinary system with malignancy is a known complication of HIV disease. There are case reports of the occurrence of renal cell carcinoma (44) and lymphomas (45) in AIDS patients. Neoplastic or benign retroperitoneal lymphadenopathy may present clinically with urinary obstruction and pain, infection, or renal failure (44, 46).

Other genitourinary tract abnormalities have been identified in AIDS patients by computed tomography and include nephromegaly (40%), hilar adenopathy (35%), bladder wall thickening (22%), medullary hyperattenuation (14%), renal calcifications (8%), hydronephrosis (5%), pyelonephritis (3%), renal abscesses (3%), and solid renal masses (3%). Although these abnormalities are seen on computed tomography scans in many other diseases, in the AIDS patient they likely indicate the presence of an AIDS-related renal disease or involvement of the genitourinary tract by an AIDS-related neoplasm or infection (46). There are no reports of malignancy occurring in the urinary system in children, but primary renal tumors are uncommon in the pediatric age group.

DIAGNOSTIC CONSIDERATIONS

Early recognition of renal dysfunction by routine monitoring and appropriate adjustments in therapy are essential in the management of HIV patients. In so doing, preventable renal complications and added morbidity of therapy can be avoided.

As in any disease, a thorough evaluation must start with a comprehensive history and physical examination. There is often information which can be gathered from the patient and family that will suggest a propensity for renal dysfunction and hence guide the evaluation more specifically. One should question the history relevant to onset of symptoms or the time when the abnormality was first noted. Recent history of ischemia (hypoxia, sepsis, dehydration), exposure to toxins (antibiotic or contrast agents), or edema should be explored in depth (31).

There are several laboratory tests that constitute baseline evaluation. The child should have a urinalysis, complete blood count, creatinine, and blood urea nitrogen. If there is a suspicion of urinary tract anomalies, a urine culture should also be obtained. Glomerular filtration rate may be assessed by timed urine collections in the older child or estimated by the equation:

$$\text{creatinine clearance} = K \times \frac{\text{linear length or height (cm)}}{\text{serum creatinine (mg/dl)}}$$

where K = 0.55 for children older than 1 year and 0.45 for infants (47). This formula gives a value in $ml/min/1.73 \ m^2$ but is useful (and reliable as an estimate of clearance) for children in a steady metabolic state who are not critically ill (48).

A urinalysis that is positive for blood and/or protein would suggest glomerulopathy and warrant further investigation. A recent report describes isolated proteinuria as a first marker of HIV-associated renal disease in children, often occurring in infants lacking other overt clinical manifestations of disease. Proteinuria may occur intermittently, making routine screening critical (49). In children, quantitation of proteinuria may be estimated from the protein-to-creatinine ratio in a random urine sample by the following equation.

$$\text{proteinuria (g/m}^2\text{/day)} = 0.63 \times \frac{\text{urine protein (mg)}}{\text{urine creatinine (mg)}}$$

Subtleties of renal tubular function can be discerned by simple determination of urine specific gravity (concentration ability), fractional excretion of sodium (tubular handling of sodium), and pH (tubular acidification).

Evaluation of the child with suspected HIV-associated glomerulopathy should also include a careful assessment of the renal anatomy. Initial evaluation should include a renal ultrasound with the expectation that gross abnormalities of renal size, parenchymal density, and outflow will be detected. Additionally, ultrasound can be used to evaluate for parenchymal scars and neoplasms and can also evaluate the suprarenal, para-aortic, and pelvic areas. These areas are all potential sites for lymphoid hyperplasia or neoplasms. If further evaluation is indicated by abnormalities on ultrasound and/or laboratory tests, then other specific appropriate studies can be pursued.

For example, if there is dilatation of the collecting system on ultrasound, then the clinical significance of this finding (obstructive vs. nonobstructive dilatation) can be determined by proceeding to more definitive studies. These include excretory urography and radionucleotide renography with or without diuretic augmentation (50, 51, 52).

If there is evidence of tubular dysfunction, then appropriate replacement therapy can be instituted. In addition, dosages of nephrotoxic drugs can be modulated, with more attention to preservation of renal function.

In the patient with overt nephropathy unrelated to prerenal factors or obstruction, renal biopsy may be indicated. The biopsy may help to discern nephrotoxicity as distinct from nephropathy. A biopsy can be useful in evaluation of the patient who develops sediment changes in association with hypocomplementemia, symptoms suggestive of vasculitis, or subsequent to a viral or bacterial illness. In the past, biopsy has generally been recommended with hesitancy, because HIV-associated renal disease is generally unresponsive to therapy and classically accompanied by great morbidity. However, in the patient with nephropathy, a renal biopsy serves to diagnose severity of renal involvement and hence the need for renal replacement therapy.

The complete assessment of renal function in the child with HIV-related disease or seropositivity is presented in Table 29.2.

TREATMENT

Supportive Care and Appropriate Therapy

There are several drugs commonly employed in the therapy of HIV-associated

Table 29.2.   Evaluation of Renal Function in HIV-infected Individual[a]

History
   Family history of renal disease
   Exposure to nephrotoxins (drug, contrast
     agent)
   Recent illness (bacterial, viral, fungal)
   History of volume disturbances (e.g.
     dehydration, hypotension)
Physical examination
   Blood pressure
   Evidence of edema
   Abdominal mass or bruit
Laboratory assessment
   Complete blood count
   Urinalysis and culture
   Electrolytes, creatinine, blood urea nitrogen
   Calcium, phosphorus, magnesium
   Urine collection (for creatinine, protein,
     electrolytes)
   C_3, C_4, ASO, Streptozyme, ANA, circulating
     immune complexes[b]
Radiologic evaluation
   Renal ultrasound
   Voiding cystourethrogram[c]
   Radionuclide scan (^{99m}Tc DTPA), with
     diuretic augmentation[d]
   Computed tomography or magnetic resonance
     imaging[d]

[a]ASO, antistreptolysin O; DTPA, diethylenetriamine pentaacetic acid.
[b]As indicated by presentation.
[c]In patients with urinary tract infections.
[d]In patients with suspected obstruction.

complications that have been reported to precipitate renal failure. The insufficiency has generally been demonstrated to be transient, but severe sustained tubulopathy can result from continued exposure to nephrotoxins such as amphotericin B and aminoglycosides. In addition, there are other agents, inclusive of antiviral agents, that may ultimately be implicated as a source of renal dysfunction (summarized in Table 29.3). When these drugs are included in the therapy of HIV-infected patients, drug levels must be monitored whenever possible, and renal function (creatinine and blood urea nitrogen) followed closely.

For patients who develop tubular dysfunction and acidosis, replacement with alkali (with the dose individualized) and routine monitoring of electrolytes is indicated. Initial dosage of alkali is 1–2 mEq/kg/day, depending on the level of acidosis. Commonly employed alkali solutions include sodium citrate (2 mEq/ml), sodium acetate (1 mEq/ml), and sodium/potassium citrate (2 mEq/ml). Sodium bicarbonate tablets are commercially available in 10-grain tablets (8 mEq/tablet). Selection of tablet vs. solution depends on patient age, dosage requirements, and compliance.

Other electrolyte replacement (calcium, magnesium, phosphate, etc.) should be dosed with the goal of achieving metabolic balance. Magnesium, owing to its impact on normal vitamin D and parathormone secretion, must be normalized before correction of calcium or phosphorus. Replacement of magnesium, calcium, and phosphorus may require parenteral administration of intravenous fluid of appropriate composition before oral maintenance.

For patients who develop urinary tract symptoms, it is important to obtain a culture and sensitivity for identification of the infecting agent. While awaiting the results, the patient can be treated with broad spectrum antibiotics appropriate for likely organisms (*Pseudomonas* and other Gram-negative organisms). Urine should also be evaluated for fungal pathogens in the patient who is more immunologically debilitated.

If a patient is found to have a urinary tract infection, it is also important to evaluate for the presence of anatomical abnormalities (duplications, obstructions, etc.)

Table 29.3.   Drugs Associated with Renal Insufficiency in HIV Patients

Drug	Effect
Pentamidine	Azotemia, hyperkalemia
Amphotericin B	Renal failure, renal tubular acidosis, hypokalemia
Trimethoprim-sulfamethoxazole	Increased creatinine, interstitial nephritis
Foscarnet	Oligoanuria, azotemia
Dapsone	Proteinuria, papillary necrosis
Rifampin	Tubulointerstitial nephritis, renal failure

that might make the patient more susceptible to infection. The evaluation might include ultrasound, intravenous pyelogram, or radionucleotide scan with or withour diuretic. Augmentation of urine flow with a diuretic (commonly Lasix) will help define obstructions or demonstrate nonobstructed dilatation of ureters.

Additional or Adjunctive Therapeutic Modalities

There has been considerable interest in treating the proteinuria of HIV-associated nephropathy with immunosuppressant agents. Children who have biopsy proven minimal change lesions or focal glomerulosclerosis have been treated with prednisone in a conventional protocol (2 mg/kg/day for 1 month followed by alternate day therapy) or low dose cyclosporin (3–6 mg/kg/day) to induce a remission of proteinuria. Unfortunately no clear responsiveness has been demonstrated (14).

In the nephrotic patient with FSGS or glomerulonephritis, supportive therapy includes sodium restriction (assuming no extraordinary gastrointestinal losses) and judicious diuretic use to minimize edema. This management must be balanced with nutritional needs of the patient. There is no specific therapy that improves glomerulopathy in HIV infected individuals.

Renal Replacement Therapy

In the patient who develops renal failure, acute dialysis can be initiated if the process is deemed reversible. Absolute indications for dialysis include hyperkalemia, uremia, and hypervolemia (with resultant hypertension) unresponsive to medical management. Dialysis may also be efficacious in improvement of acidosis, hypocalcemia, and hyperphosphatemia that accompany renal failure.

In general, peritoneal dialysis is chosen in lieu of hemodialysis given ease of access, general stability of clearance of wastes, and adaptability to acute and chronic intervention. In the small child with renal failure, hemodialysis can be technically impossible because of blood volume constraints (extracorporeal blood volume requirements for dialysis) or simply lack of adequate access. Ultimately, given the poor prognosis in HIV-infected children and adults with renal failure (3, 48), an informed decision must be made as to when it is appropriate to institute chronic renal replacement therapy.

The efficacy of renal transplantation in the HIV-infected patient remains controversial. There are limited data on transplant survival in HIV patients (53), but there exists a general acceptance that although HIV infection per se should not preclude transplantation, the presence of symptomatic HIV disease is an absolute contraindication (54). In general, renal transplantation is pursued in a potential recipient who has no other life-threatening medical condition that might be accelerated by the required immunotherapy.

PREVENTION

There are no definitive factors to define the child at risk of developing HIV-associated renal disease. As a result, the goal of monitoring renal function is the early detection of abnormalities. It is hoped that early identification of the child at risk, appropriate intervention with antiviral therapy, along with appropriate management of HIV-associated complications will result in preservation of renal function.

FUTURE RESEARCH

The role of HIV infection in the etiology and evolution of nephropathy continues to be an active area of research. It is hoped that by the use of molecular techniques, we can better define the renal cells most susceptible to viral infection. In so doing, it is hoped that we will come to understand the exact mechanisms that control viral replication on a genetic level. With this knowledge, we will have the tools necessary to prevent and potentially reverse the effects of HIV on the kidney.

References

1. Pardo V, Aldana M, Colton RM, et al. Glomerular lesions in the acquired immunodeficiency syndrome. Ann Intern Med 1984;101:429–434.
2. Rao TKS, Filippone EJ, Nicastri AD, et al. Associated focal and segmental glomerulosclerosis

in the acquired immunodeficiency syndrome. N Engl J Med 1984;310:669–673.

3. Humphreys M, Schoenfield PY. Renal complications in patients with the acquired immune deficiency syndrome (AIDS). Am J Nephrol 1987;7:1–7.

4. Seney FD Jr, Burns DK, Silva FG. Acquired immunodeficiency syndrome and the kidney. Am J Kidney Dis 1990;16:1–13.

5. Glassock RJ. Human immunodeficiency virus (HIV) infection and the kidney. Ann Intern Med 1990;112:35–49.

6. Rao TKS. Human immunodeficiency virus (HIV) associated nephropathy. Annu Rev Med 1991;42:391–401.

7. Berns JS, Cohen RM, Stumacher RJ, Rudnick MR. Renal aspects of therapy for human immunodeficiency virus and associated opportunistic infections. J Am Soc Nephrol 1991;1:1061–1080.

8. Bourgoignie JJ, Meneses R, Ortiz C, Jaffe D, Pardo V. The clinical spectrum of renal disease associated with human immunodeficiency virus. Am J Kidney Dis 1988;12:131–37.

9. Pardo V, Meneses R, Ossa L, et al. AIDS-related glomerulopathy: Occurrence in specific risk groups. Kidney Int 1987;31:1167–1173.

10. Rao TKS, Friedman EA, Nigastri AD. The types of renal disease in the acquired immunodeficiency syndrome. N Engl J Med 1987;316:1062–1168.

11. Bourgoignie JJ, Meneses R, Pardo V. The nephropathy related to acquired immune deficiency syndrome. Adv Nephrol 1988;17:113–126.

12. Rao TKS, Friedman EA. AIDS (HIV)-associated nephropathy; does it exist? Am J Nephrol 1989;9:441–53.

13. Strauss J, Abitbol C, Zilleruelo G, et al. Renal disease in children with the acquired immunodeficiency syndrome. N Engl J Med 1989;321:625–630.

14. Connor E, Gupta S, Joshi V, et al. Acquired immunodeficiency syndrome-associated renal disease in children. J Pediatr 1988;113:39–44.

15. Ingulli E, Tejani A, Fikrig S, Nicastri A, Chen CK, Pomrantz A. Nephrotic syndrome associated with acquired immunodeficiency syndrome in children. J Pediatr 1991;119:710–716.

16. Kopp JB, Klotman ME, Adler SH, et al. Progressive glomerulosclerosis and enhanced renal accumulation of basement membrane components in mice transgenic for human immunodeficiency virus type 1 genes. Proc Natl Acad Sci USA 1992;89:1577–1581.

17. Dickie P, Felser J, Eckhaus M, et al. HIV-associated nephropathy in transgenic mice expressing HIV-1 genes. Virology 1991;185:109–119.

18. Alpers CE, McClure J, Bursten SL. Human mesangial cells are resistant to productive infection by multiple strains of human immunodeficiency virus types 1 and 2. Am J Kidney Dis 1992;19:126–130.

19. Cohen AH, Sun NC, Shapshak P, Imagawa DT. Demonstration of human immunodeficiency virus in renal epithelium in HIV-associated nephropathy. Mod Pathol 1989;Mar:125–128.

20. Goldzer RC, Sweet J, Coltran RS. Focal and segmental glomerulosclerosis. Annu Rev Med 1984;35:429–449.

21. Soni A, Agarwal A, Chander P, et al. Evidence for an HIV-related nephropathy: a clinico-pathological study. Clin Nephrol 1989;31:12–17.

22. Pardo V, Aldana M, Colton RM, et al. Glomerular lesions in the acquired immunodeficiency syndrome. Ann Intern Med 1984;101:429–434.

23. Lachaal M, Venuto RC. Nephrotoxicity and hyperkalemia in patients with acquired immunodeficiency syndrome treated with pentamidine. Am J Med 1989;87:260–263.

24. Carbone LG, Bendixen B, Appel GB. Sulfadiazine-associated obstructive nephropathy occurring in a patient with the acquired immunodeficiency syndrome. Am J Kidney Dis 1988;12:72–75.

25. Sattler FR, Cowan R, Neilsen DM, Ruskin J. Trimethoprim-sulfamethoxazole compared with pentamidine for treatment of *Pneumocystis carinii* pneumonia in the acquired immunodeficiency syndrome. Ann Intern Med 1988;109:280–287.

26. D'Agati V, Suh JI, Carbone L, Cheng JT, Appel G. Pathology of HIV-associated nephropathy: A detailed morphologic and comparative study. Kidney Int 1989;35:1358–1370.

27. O'Regan S, Russo P, Lapointe N, Rousseau E. AIDS and the urinary tract. J Acquir Immune Defic Syndr 1990;3:244–51.

28. Van Der Reijden HJ, Schipper MEI, Danner SA, Arisz L. Glomerular lesions and opportunistic infections of the kidney in AIDS: An autopsy study of 47 cases. In: Amario A, Coatelli P, Campese VM, Massry SG, eds. Drugs, systemic diseases, and the kidney. New York: Plenum, 1989:181–188.

29. Joshi VV, Oleske JM, Connor EM. Morphologic findings in children with acquired immune deficiency syndrome: Pathogenesis and clinical implications. Pediatr Pathol 1990;10:155–165.

30. Mazbar SA, Schoenfeld PY, Humphreys MH. Renal involvement in patients infected with HIV: Experience at San Francisco General Hospital. Kidney Int 1990;37:1325–1332.

31. Tarshish P. Approach to the diagnosis and management of HIV-associated nephropathy. J Pediatr 1991;119:S50–S52.

32. Bourgoignie JJ, Pardo V. The nephropathology in human immunodeficiency virus (HIV-1) infection. Kidney Int 1991;35(suppl):S19–S23.

33. Rao TKS. Clinical features of human immunodeficiency virus associated nephropathy. Kidney Int 1991;35(suppl):S13–S18.

34. Cohen AH, Nast CC. HIV-associated nephropathy. A unique combined glomerular, tubular, and interstitial lesion. Mod Pathol 1988;1:87–97.

35. Trachtman H, Gauthier B, Vinograd A, Valderrama E. IgA nephropathy in a child with human immunodeficiency virus type 1 infection. Pediatr Nephrol 1991;5:724–726.

36. Sattler FR, Cowan R, Nielsen DM, Ruskin J. Trimethoprim-sulfamethoxazole compared with pentamidine for treatment of *Pneumocystis carinii* pneumonia in the acquired immunodeficiency syndrome. A prospective, noncrossover study. Ann Intern Med 1988;109:280–287.

37. Glassock RJ, Cohen AH, Danovitch G, Parsa KP. Human immunodeficiency virus (HIV) infection and the kidney. Ann Intern Med 1990;112:35–49.

38. Greene LW, Cole W, Greene JB, et al. Adrenal Insufficiency as a complication of the acquired immunodeficiency syndrome. Ann Intern Med 1984;100:847–848.
39. Lachaal M, Venuto RC. Nephrotoxicity and hyperkalemia in patients with acquired immunodeficiency syndrome treated with pentamidine. Am J Med 1989;87:260–263.
40. Cacoub P, Deray G, Baumelou A, et al. Acute renal failure induced by foscarnet: 4 cases. Clin Nephrol 1988;29:315–318.
41. Sjovall J, Karlsson A, Ogenstad S, Sandstrom E, Saarimaki M. Pharmacokinetics and absorption of foscarnet after intravenous and oral administration to patients with human immunodeficiency virus. Clin Pharmacol Ther 1988;44:65–73.
42. Kaplan MS, Wechsler M, Benson MC. Urologic manifestations of AIDS. Urology 1987;30:441–443.
43. Benson MC, Kaplan MS, O'Toole K, Romagnoli M. A report of cytomegalovirus cystitis and a review of other genitourinary manifestations of the acquired immune deficiency syndrome. J Urol 1988;140:153–154.
44. Gardenswartz MH, Lerner CW, Seligson GR, et al. Renal disease in patients with AIDS: A clinicopathologic study. Clin Nephrol 1984;21:197–204.
45. Mohler JL, Jarow JP, Marshall FF. Unusual urological presentations of acquired immune deficiency syndrome: Large cell lymphoma. J Urol 1987;138:627–629.
46. Kuhlman JR, Browne D, Shermak M, Hamper UM, Zerhouni EA, Fishman EK. Retroperitoneal and pelvic CT of patients with AIDS: Primary and secondary involvement of the genitourinary tract. Radiographics 1991;11:473–483.
47. Strauss J, Zilleruelo G, Abitbol C, et al. Natural history, clinical presentation and outcome of HIV associated nephropathy in children [Abstract]. J Am Soc Nephrol 1992;2:321.
48. Schwartz GJ, Haycock GB, Edelmann CM Jr, et al. A simple estimate of glomerular filtration rate in children derived from body length and plasma creatinine. Pediatrics 1976;58:259–263.
49. Santos F, Orejas G, Foreman JW, Chan JCM. Diagnostic workup of renal disorders. Curr Probl Pediatr 1991;20:48–74.
50. Kass EJ, Majd M, Belman AB. Comparison of diuretic renogram and the pressure perfusion study in children. J Urol 1985;134:92–96.
51. Keller MS. Renal Doppler sonography in infants and children [Comment]. Radiology 1989;172:603–604.
52. Koff SA, Thrall JH, Keyes JW. Assessment of hydroureteronephrosis in children using diuretic radionucleotide urography. J Urol 1980;123:531–534.
53. Tzakis AG, Cooper MH, Dummer JS, et al. Transplantation in HIV positive patients. Transplantation 1990;49:354–358.
54. Schoenfeld P, Feduska NJ. Aids and renal disease: Report of the National Kidney Foundation—National Institutes of Health Task Force on AIDS and Kidney Disease. Am J Kidney Dis 1990;16:14–25.

30

Myopathies and Neuropathies in HIV-infected Adults and Children

Cheryl Jay and Marinos C. Dalakas

Neuromuscular disorders may develop throughout human immunodeficiency virus (HIV) infection, frequently coexisting with central nervous system (CNS) disease (1–8). Neuropathy or myopathy may accompany seroconversion (9, 10), represent the first clinical manifestation of established but undiagnosed HIV infection (1–8, 11, 12), or complicate full-blown AIDS (1–8, 11–14). These conditions are likely under-recognized during life, since pathologic studies show that subclinical neuromuscular pathology is almost universal (15–18). Neuromuscular disorders can be missed in the setting of serious multisystem disease (1–8, 19), which may account for their wider recognition several years after the CNS syndromes had been well characterized (19, 20). Similar considerations may be even more relevant in pediatric AIDS where nerve and muscle disorders have been considered unusual (5, 21–23). Note, however, that during the last 3 years neuromuscular disorders resembling the adult syndromes have been recognized in HIV-infected children (22, 24–27), suggesting that increased awareness and careful neurological examination may reveal additional cases in the future.

The introduction of nucleoside antiretroviral agents has also increased awareness of neuromuscular disease in HIV-infected patients. Mitochondrial myopathy complicates azidothymidine (AZT) therapy in adults (28–30) and children (5, 24), and peripheral neuropathy is a dose-limiting side effect of dideoxyinosine (ddI) and dideoxycytidine (ddC) in adults (31, 32).

Although the HIV-related neuromuscular disorders are rarely life threatening, they are disabling and potentially treatable, hence the importance for early and accurate diagnosis (1–7, 33). This chapter updates current knowledge of nerve and muscle diseases complicating HIV infection in children and adults. Clinical features, evaluation, and treatment that evolved since edition 1 will be addressed, and suggestions for future research will be made.

MYOPATHIES

Acute HIV seroconversion is frequently accompanied by myalgia and rarely by frank myoglobinuria (1, 10, 34) (Table 30.1). Recurrent myoglobinuria or myalgia, how-

Table 30.1. HIV-related Muscle Disorders in Adults and Children[a]

Seroconversion-related myalgia with or without myoglobinuria
HIV-myopathy with histologic features of inflammation
    necrosis with minimal primary inflammation
    nemaline (rod) bodies
AZT mitochondrial myopathy[b]
Pyomyositis[b]
Subclinical neuromuscular involvement with histologic features of
    inflammation
    denervation
    type II muscle fiber atrophy
    opportunistic organisms

[a]Adapted from Dalakas (5–7).
[b]Described in children.

559

ever, may occur not only acutely but throughout HIV infection (34). Myalgia is also a frequent side effect of several agents used to treat HIV infection such as interferon-α or AZT. In one large treatment trial, 8% of patients treated with AZT experienced myalgia (35).

Patients who are HIV positive may develop a frank myopathy of insidious onset and gradual progression, characterized histologically by endomysial inflammation, muscle fiber necrosis with minimal primary inflammation, and, rarely, nemaline (rod) bodies (1–7, 12). Because these histological features usually coexist in various degrees, we prefer the term "HIV myopathy" (6, 7, 29) as an all-inclusive designation for the morphological spectrum of a clinically homogeneous myopathy in patients with HIV infection (Table 30.1).

HIV myopathy can develop at any stage of the infection and resembles seronegative polymyositis clinically and pathologically (1–7, 36–38). As with all HIV-related neuromuscular syndromes, precise incidence is unknown, but the frequency with which inflammation is seen in autopsy muscle from AIDS patients without known muscle disease (17, 18) suggests that this association is not a mere coincidence. This disorder has not yet been described in children with AIDS, although it should be noted that polymyositis is quite rare in HIV-seronegative children (5). Dermatomyositis, a more common inflammatory myopathy in childhood, has not been seen in HIV-infected children. Two adults with a dermatomyositis-like picture (but not clinicohistologically classic dermatomyositis) have been reported (39, 40), but it is not yet clear if this was a coincidence or a true association.

Pyomyositis, a focal bacterial muscle infection, is not uncommon in HIV-infected children (25, 26) and adults (41, 42), and is often due to *Staphylococcus aureus* or rarely to Gram-negative organisms. Before the AIDS epidemic, pyomyositis was a rarity in the West but frequent in the tropics. Today, HIV infection appears to be emerging as a major risk factor for this disorder in the United States. Because HIV-infected children are more prone to recurrent bacterial infections than adults (43), it is perhaps not surprising that pyomyositis is the best char-

acterized muscle disorder in pediatric AIDS. Infection of the muscle with opportunistic organisms can rarely occur in the course of disseminated infection with *Cryptococcus neoformans* (18), *Toxoplasma gondii* (44), *Mycobacterium tuberculosis* (45, 46), and *M. avium-intracellulare* (18, 47).

A toxic mitochondrial muscle disease related to AZT (AZT-myopathy) (28–30), may develop in up to 17% of adults treated with long-term (>12 month), high-dose (>1200 mg daily) AZT (48). Although cumulative drug dose may be an important determinant (28–30), we have observed the disorder in adults treated exclusively with the newer low-dose regimens for early stage disease (49). We are aware of two pediatric cases of AZT myopathy, one from our personal experience (P. Pizzo and M. Dalakas, unpublished observations, 1989) and another recently reported (24).

Several other myopathies described in HIV-infected adults, but not reported thus far in children, include muscle weakness related to type II muscle fiber atrophy associated with immobilization and malnutrition (1–7, 18) and nemaline rod-body myopathy (1–8, 12, 38, 50).

NEUROPATHIES

Peripheral neuropathies (Table 30.2) usually develop in a stage-specific fashion in HIV-infected adults (1–8, 11, 13–16, 32). Two neuropathies, the Guillain-Barré syndrome (GBS) and the chronic inflammatory demyelinating polyneuropathy (CIDP), both dysimmune demyelinating peripheral nerve disorders, may occur early in the infection or may be the presenting manifestation of unsuspected HIV infection (9, 11). One pedi-

Table 30.2.   HIV-related Peripheral Neuropathies in Adults and Children

Guillain-Barré syndrome[a]
Chronic inflammatory demyelinating
    polyneuropathy[a]
Mononeuritis multiplex
Ganglioneuronitis
Lumbosacral polyradiculoneuropathy, often
    caused by CMV
Painful sensory axonal neuropathy[a]
Nucleosides (ddI, ddC) neuropathy

[a]Described in children.

atric case of HIV-related GBS has recently been reported (27), and we are aware of another HIV-infected child who developed classic features of CIDP (Civitello L, Gilliatt R, Dalakas, unpublished observations, 1991). Other, less common, peripheral neuropathies that may develop in early stage HIV infection include acute ganglioneuronitis coincident with seroconversion (51) and mononeuritis multiplex (1) (Table 30.1).

The most common neuropathy in AIDS patients is a painful sensory axonal neuropathy that affects up to 70% of adults with later stage HIV infection (13, 14). Painful axonal neuropathy can also complicate therapy with ddI or ddC (31, 32) and may represent the cumulative effect on the peripheral nerves of various endogenous or exogenous neurotoxins related to a multisystem disease and dysfunction of many organs (52). Despite the relative lack of motor involvement, severe neuropathic pain in such patients can be disabling. HIV has been cultured from the peripheral nerve (53), but there is no convincing evidence that the neuropathy results from direct infection of the peripheral nerve with the virus. Our own immunocytochemical studies using double-label techniques on sural nerve biopsies have shown that HIV is present only in rare endoneurial macrophages but not within the Schwann cells or the axons (M. C. Dalakas, unpublished observation, 1993). Electrodiagnostic and pathologic studies clearly indicate that peripheral nerve pathology is nearly ubiquitous in AIDS patients, regardless of whether there is clinical evidence of peripheral neuropathy (14–16, 52, 54). Although clinical experience, supported by a small cross-sectional study including electrodiagnostic testing (55), has suggested that axonal neuropathy does not occur in children, Belman (22) recently described two children with a clinical symptomatology consistent with AIDS neuropathy and postulated that primarily sensory neuropathies may be overlooked in young children.

Another neuropathy seen in later stage HIV infection in adults is the lumbosacral polyradiculoneuropathy, affecting roots and sensory ganglia, that is often related to cytomegalovirus (CMV) infection (56–58). CMV polyradiculoneuropathy presents with painful muscle weakness, areflexia, and atrophy mostly of the lower extremities associated with sphincteric dysfunction resembling a cauda equina syndrome. The disease is thought to represent reactivated CMV infection of nerve roots rather than primary infection, which may explain why this neuropathy has not yet been described in pediatric AIDS despite the frequent infection of these children with CMV (43). Recognition is important because anti-CMV therapy may be lifesaving (58).

PREVALENCE OF NEUROMUSCULAR DISORDERS IN HIV-INFECTED CHILDREN

The lower frequency of neuromuscular complications in HIV-infected children could be more apparent than actual. Muscle and nerve diseases are easily missed in a child with serious chronic illness, particularly when there is severe CNS disease (5, 22). In a preverbal child, irritability caused by myalgia or neuropathic pain and motor delay or regression could easily be attributed to encephalopathy. Note that the early adult literature on the neurologic complications of HIV infection focused on CNS abnormalities; as management of these conditions and other AIDS-related conditions improved, awareness of neuromuscular disorders increased. Dideoxynucleoside-related peripheral nerve toxicity appears less prominent in children than in adults, even if the doses used are higher in children (33). Some age-related differences regarding the incidence of neuromuscular disease may be due to biological differences or to differences in susceptibility to nerve and muscle injury between adults and children. For example, AIDS dementia and pediatric AIDS encephalopathy are clinically and pathologically similar but not identical (20, 23). Myelopathy appears to be far more frequent in adults than children, both clinically and pathologically (59). Drugs and alcohol, which cause significant neuromuscular toxicity, may be additional factors that increase the risk for neuromuscular diseases in HIV-infected adults compared with children.

PATHOGENESIS AND NATURAL HISTORY

Possible mechanisms of the HIV-related neuromuscular disorders include 1) direct viral infection, 2) immune alterations triggered by the viral illness, 3) complications of antiretroviral therapy, and 4) sequelae of chronic illness.

Direct Virus Infection

Five retroviruses have been associated with inflammatory myopathy in humans and primates (39, 61, 62): HIV (1–4), human T cell lymphotropic virus-I (60, 61), human foamy retrovirus (62), simian retrovirus-I (63, 64), and simian immunodeficiency virus (M. Dalakas and N. Gravell, unpublished observations, 1991). Ultrastructural, immunocytochemical, molecular biological, and tissue culture studies that we have performed on muscle biopsies from HIV-infected patients have not revealed evidence of direct infection of the muscle by the virus. Virus particles have not been seen by electron microscopy within the muscle fibers (1–7, 65). With immunocytochemistry using specific antibodies to HIV and with in situ hybridization using specific HIV RNA probes, we could localize HIV antigens and detect HIV RNA signals only in occasional endomysial lymphoid cells in proximity to muscle fibers but not within the muscle fibers (1–7, 36, 66, 67). With the polymerase chain reaction, we found virus genome in only two of 12 biopsies and in up to two 4-μm serial consecutive sections (68). Because 4 μm correspond to the size of a lymphoid cell, we have interpreted this finding as being consistent with the presence of nucleic acid within the infiltrating lymphoid cells rather than the muscle fibers (68). Human muscle and tissue cultures were also resistant to infection by HIV alone, to transfection with HIV proviral DNA construct, or to infection with HIV-infected and HIV-stimulated autologous lymphocytes (69). Taken together, our data suggest that human muscle is resistant to infection with the virus and that HIV-related myopathy is not associated with persistent retroviral infection of the muscle fiber. Similar studies that we performed in nerve biopsies have shown HIV gp41 antigen in rare endoneurial cells identified with double immunocytochemistry as macrophages (M. C. Dalakas, I. Illa, and M. L. Monzon, unpublished observation, 1993).

Immunologic Abnormalities

Our immunocytochemical studies on muscle biopsies from HIV-positive patients with inflammatory myopathies and patients with seronegative polymyositis have shown that CD8+ cells and macrophages are the main subpopulations of cells that surround and invade healthy muscle fibers that also express the major histocompatibility complex-I antigen (36). B cells and natural killer cells are rare in endomysial infiltrates and interferon is not immunolocalized. Based on these observations, we have proposed that HIV myopathy, like the seronegative polymyositis, is due to a T cell-mediated and major histocompatibility complex-I restricted cytotoxic process probably triggered by the virus (37, 70). This cell-mediated attack on muscle can occur in the face of marked immunosuppression, because HIV-myopathy may develop in all stages of HIV infection. Whether similar mechanisms also operate in inflammatory demyelinating neuropathies, which tend to occur in the early stages of HIV infection, is unclear. Of interest, the endoneurial infiltrates in the sural nerve biopsies from such patients consist mostly of macrophages and very few CD8+ cells (M. C. Dalakas, unpublished observations, 1993). The muscle or nerve antigen(s) recognized by these sensitized endomysial or endoneurial cells are unknown (6, 7, 37, 70). The systemic virus infection or the rare HIV-infected endomysial or endoneurial lymphoid cells may release lymphokines and cytokines that expose new antigens against which there is no self-tolerance, generating a tissue-specific autoimmune attack (6, 7). Molecular antigenic mimicry may be another cause of self-sensitization because of sequence homologies between polypeptides coded for by retroviral *gag* and *pol* genes and muscle proteins (71, 72).

As HIV infection progresses, immune dysregulation gives way to frank immunosuppression, setting the stage for direct muscle infection by opportunistic pathogens. Although very rare, *M. avium-intracellularae* (18, 47) and *Cryptococcus* (18) have been identified in autopsy muscle of patients dying with disseminated infection. Whether these patients had myopathic signs or symptoms antemortem is uncertain, and hence the clinical significance of these findings is unknown. Symptomatic tuberculous muscle infection, both focal (46) and diffuse (49), has been seen in two patients who responded to antibiotic therapy. Similarly, five patients developed myopathy coincident with cerebral toxoplasmosis with cysts identified in the muscle fibers. Antitoxoplasma therapy improved the myopathy in two patients (44).

The pathogenesis of pyomyositis complicating HIV infection is incompletely understood (25, 26, 41, 42). Antecedent muscle trauma or bacteremia (although variably present) and the common colonization of HIV-positive patients by *S. aureus*, the major pathogen in this disorder, have been implicated. HIV-infected children may be at particular risk for this disorder since they are less likely than adults to have antibodies to common pathogens and thus are more vulnerable to bacterial infection (43).

Complications of Therapy

AZT Myopathy

Although muscle biopsies from patients who develop myopathy during long-term AZT therapy may show inflammation similar to that seen in HIV myopathy, the distinguishing histologic feature of AZT myopathy is the "ragged red fiber," a morphological sign of abnormal muscle mitochondria (28–30). By electron microscopy, muscle biopsies from patients with AZT myopathy show mitochondrial proliferation and structural changes characterized by variation in size and shape, vacuolization, abnormal cristae, and, rarely, paracrystalline inclusions (65). With molecular and DNA immunocytochemical studies we have found depletion of muscle mitochondrial DNA only in the muscle biopsies of AZT-treated patients but not of patients with HIV myopathy (73). This is consistent with the known properties of AZT to inhibit mitochondrial γ-DNA polymerase, an enzyme found solely in the mitochondrial matrix, causing DNA chain termination (74). In AZT myopathy, muscle mitochondria are also functionally abnormal because they are deficient in cytochrome *c* oxidase (75). AZT causes a DNA-depleting mitochondrial my-

opathy (29) not only in the setting of HIV infection but also in healthy experimental animals. Two studies have convincingly shown that AZT-treated rats accumulate the drug in the heart and skeletal muscle and develop a myopathy that has the clinical, histological, and biochemical features of AZT-myopathy (76, 77). Finally, magnetic resonance spectroscopy, a noninvasive in vivo method for assessing muscle metabolism, shows marked phosphocreatine depletion with slow recovery, consistent with mitochondrial dysfunction (78, 79). Of interest, ddC in vitro does not inhibit γ-polymerase as efficiently as AZT (74), perhaps accounting for the apparent lack of myotoxicity of ddC (M. C. Dalakis, unpublished observations, 1991–1993).

Nucleoside Neuropathy

Clinical data suggest that ddC and ddI cause a dose-dependent reversible axonal painful sensory neuropathy (30–32). Animal studies, however, suggest that ddC may be primarily toxic to the myelin sheath, whereas the axonal damage is secondary (80). The major feature that distinguishes a ddI- or ddC-related painful neuropathy from the painful sensory axonal neuropathy of AIDS is that the latter tends to be progressive, whereas the nucleoside peripheral neuropathies tend to improve when the drugs are discontinued (32–32). Another clinical feature of nucleoside neuropathy is "coasting" or worsening of symptoms for a period after the drug is discontinued, followed by clinical improvement (81, 82). Of interest, epidemiologic studies and clinical experience have not implicated AZT as a peripheral neurotoxin (83). Whether specific structure-function relationships dictate nucleoside neuro- or myotoxicity is uncertain but would have obvious implications for developing new antiretroviral agents without neuromuscular toxicity.

Sequelae of Chronic Illness

Biopsy and autopsy tissues from HIV-infected patients show type II muscle fiber atrophy (1–7) in isolation or coexisting with other muscle pathology, especially a smoldering mild endomysial inflammation (17,

18) (Table 30.1). Type II fiber atrophy is not specific to HIV infection. It is often related to immobilization or malnutrition, both of which are common complications in late-stage HIV infection. This probably accounts for the AIDS-wasting syndrome whose histologic correlate is type II muscle fiber atrophy and is not, as has been suggested, a true myopathy (84).

Peripheral nerve, likewise, is sensitive to the effects of systemic illness and toxins. Antibiotics, particularly antimycobacterial agents, and chemotherapeutic agents are known peripheral neurotoxins. If multiple medical insults contribute to the cause of AIDS-related painful sensory neuropathy (52), the rarity of the neuropathy in pediatric AIDS might be explained by the shorter incubation for HIV infection in children compared with adults (43).

CLINICAL PRESENTATION AND DIFFERENTIAL DIAGNOSIS

Myopathies

HIV-myopathy is clinically similar to AZT myopathy. Without specialized diagnostic testing such as muscle biopsy (5–7, 28, 30) or magnetic resonance spectroscopy (78, 79), the only clinical means to distinguish AZT myopathy from HIV myopathy is by stopping AZT and monitoring for clinical improvement on the basis of increased strength, decreased muscle pain, and reduction in serum creatine kinase. These myopathies present with subacute, symmetric, proximal muscle wasting, weakness, and myalgia that develop over weeks to months, and they are often accompanied by elevation of creatine kinase (Table 30.3). In patients who are taking AZT, the duration of therapy can often help distinguish between HIV myopathy and AZT myopathy. AZT myopathy typically develops after at least 12 months of AZT therapy (5–7, 28). Although rare cases with earlier onset can occur, duration of AZT therapy can be, in general, a useful clinical guide in predicting cause of the myopathy. HIV positive patients who present with myopathy and have been on AZT for fewer than 4–6 months are more likely to have HIV-related rather than AZT-related muscle disease. Exertional myalgia and fatigue, more prominent in legs than

arms, are frequent signs in AZT myopathy. Whether similar symptomatology occurs in children is uncertain. In one child treated with intravenous AZT on protocol at the National Cancer Institute, intense crying with passive movement of muscles and creatine kinase elevation raised concern for AZT-myopathy, prompting confirmation of the diagnosis with muscle biopsy that showed the classic histological signs of AZT myotoxicity (P. Pizzo and M. Dalakas, unpublished observations, 1989). However, creatine kinase may be elevated in the absence of symptomatic myopathy. For example, of 87 children receiving AZT, 72 had at least one creatine kinase greater than 65 IU; 18 (20%) had one value above 260 IU, and three patients had levels exceeding 520 IU. None had symptoms of myopathy, and no dosage adjustments of AZT were made (24).

Although creatine kinase elevations usually accompany both HIV and AZT myopathy, we have seen patients with histologically severe AZT myopathy who have repeatedly normal creatine kinase measurements (5–7, 49). Serum creatine kinase alone, therefore, is not a reliable screening test for AZT myopathy. Similarly, electromyography cannot distinguish between the two because myopathic changes characterized by low amplitude, short-duration polyphasic voluntary motor units accompanied by various degrees of spontaneous activity are common to AZT myopathy and HIV myopathy. Nerve conduction studies, however, are helpful to detect clinical or subclinical peripheral neuropathy that may account for some of the patients symptomatology.

Muscle biopsy is the only definitive laboratory means to distinguish HIV myopathy from AZT myopathy. In HIV myopathy the biopsy shows primary inflammation with lymphocytes and macrophages invading healthy muscle fibers, muscle fiber degeneration, necrosis, and increased endomysial connective tissue (Fig. 30.1). In contrast, AZT myopathy shows ragged-red fibers indicating abnormal mitochondria, along with red-rimmed cracks and neutral fat accumulation (Fig. 30.2A, 2B) (5–7, 28). These morphological features, in conjunction with the associated depletion of muscle mitochondrial DNA and the apparent dysfunction of the remaining mitochondria within

Table 30.3. Clinical and Diagnostic Characteristics of Myopathies in HIV-positive Patients[a]

	HIV Myopathy	AZT Myopathy	Pyomyositis
Clinical symptoms and signs			
Proximal muscle weakness	+	+	Localized to one muscle
Myalgia	+	++	Localized to one muscle
Myopathic EMG	+	+	?
Elevated creatine kinase	+	+	?
Clinical setting	Any stage of HIV infection	After 12 months of AZT therapy	Any stage of HIV infection
Onset	Subacute	Insidious	Subacute or acute
Risk factors	?	Long-term AZT therapy	Trauma, bacteremia
Muscle biopsy findings			
Inflammation	++	+	?
Rods	Rare	+++	?
AZT fibers	Absent	+++	?
Myopathic features	++	+++	?
Muscle imaging (MRI, CT, ultrasound)	?	?	Muscle abscess
Muscle immunocytochemistry			
Main endomysial cell subsets	CD8+ cells and macrophages	CD8+ cells and macrophages	?
MHC-1 antigen in muscle fibers	++	++	?
Muscle virology			
HIV antigens within muscle fibers	Absent	Absent	?
HIV antigens in endomysial lymphoid cells	+	+	?
Molecular studies and DNA immunocytochemistry			
Muscle mitochondrial DNA	Normal	Depletion	?
Immunostainable mitochondrial DNA	Normal	Reduced	?
MRS spectroscopy	Normal	Abnormal energy metabolism	?
Therapy	Prednisone, IVIG	NSAID; discontinuation of AZT; can start ddl, ddC	Antibiotics

[a]Conditions are present (+) in increasing degree (++, +++), or presence is uncertain (?). EMG, electromyography; MRI, magnetic resonance imaging; CT, computerized tomography; MHC, major histocompatibility complex; NSAID, nonsteroidal anti-inflammatory drug; IVIG, intravenous immunoglobulin. Adapted from Dalakas (5–7, 29).

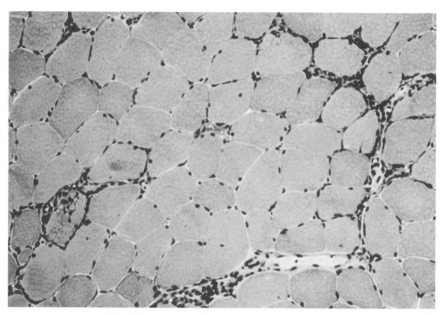

Figure 30.1. Cross-section of fresh-frozen muscle biopsy from a patient with primary HIV inflammatory myopathy demonstrates interstitial inflammatory cells surrounding or invading healthy muscle fibers. Trichrome stain; ×320.

the fiber (as described earlier), comprise what we now call "AZT-fibers" (5–7, 29). Other histological features seen in AZT myopathy include rods, increased connective tissue, and various degrees of endomysial inflammation from sparse to moderate (5–7, 28–30). The patchy nature of histopathology and sampling errors inherent to biopsy of a large organ such as muscle should be considered if these features are not seen in a given biopsy (5–7).

In a child with proximal weakness and creatine kinase elevation, myopathy can be diagnosed with reasonable confidence, if trauma (including recent electromyography) and intramuscular injections can be excluded as causes for creatine kinase elevation. Medications should be reviewed for other myotoxic exposures, and thyroid function should be assessed. Muscle biopsy with muscle enzyme histochemistry should be performed whenever possible to confirm the type of myopathy, because accurate diagnosis is critical for rational treatment. HIV positive patients presenting with myoglobinuria as an isolated clinical event should be screened for metabolic and enzymatic defects known to cause muscle necrosis (29).

Although the HIV infected child with weakness and normal creatine kinase may still have myopathy, other neurologic disorders should be excluded. Upper motor neuron causes of weakness are often accompanied by other symptoms and signs such as language delay in encephalopathy, sensory level and sphincter disturbances in myelopathy, and spasticity and Babinski signs in both. Weakness from neuropathy is typically distal rather than proximal and is accompanied by early loss of reflexes. Because abnormalities may be present at multiple levels of the neuraxis in HIV-infected patients, neurological consultation may be necessary to assist in localizing the major pathology.

Pyomyositis

Pyomyositis presents with fever, local muscle pain, and swelling of 1–2 weeks duration (25, 26, 41, 42). A history of local trauma may be elicited, and a source of bacteremia may be evident by history or examination. The affected area is usually indurated without the presence of typical fluctuance. Peripheral leukocytosis is not uniformly present and creatine kinase is usually normal; blood cultures may be posi-

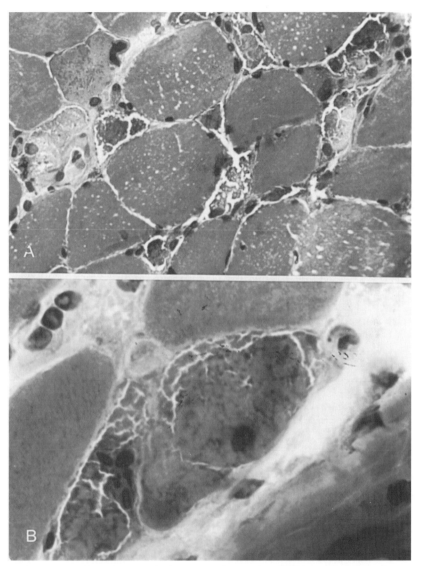

Figure 30.2.   A, cross-section of a muscle biopsy from a patient with AZT myopathy shows typical "AZT fibers" characterized by red-rimmed cracks, increased connective tissue, degenerating and "ragged-red" fibers. Tiny vacuoles correspond to lipid droplets. **B,** typical ragged-red fiber with subsarcolemmal accumulation of mitochondria. Trichrome stain.

tive. Ultrasound, computerized tomography, or magnetic resonance imaging of the affected extremity is the diagnostic method of choice to document the presence of a muscle abscess and distinguish it from other similar conditions caused by muscle contusion, hematoma, venous thrombosis, osteomyelitis, cellulitis, or neoplasm. A high index of suspicion is essential and leads to appropriate imaging studies that typically demonstrate a muscle abscess that spares

the subcutaneous tissues (85). Technetium bone scan or gallium scan may also detect clinically unapparent secondary sites of infection especially since 30–40% of these patients may have multiple abscesses.

Neuropathies

Older children with neuropathy may complain of pain, numbness, and distal weakness. The diagnostic approach is similar to myopathy and should begin with a careful review to exclude exposure to peripheral neurotoxins. Common neurotoxic exposures in the setting of HIV infection include isoniazid, pyridoxine, ethambutol, metronidazole, and vincristine, in addition to ddI and ddC. Serum vitamin B_{12} should be checked. Electromyography with nerve conduction studies that include late responses (F waves and H reflexes) is essential to determine whether the neuropathy is demyelinating or axonal because this will determine therapy. It is the demyelinating and not the axonal neuropathies that respond to immunomodulating agents such as intravenous immunoglobulin or plasmapheresis (1, 11). Cerebrospinal fluid examination is helpful in the evaluation of neuropathies. In painful axonal neuropathy, cerebrospinal fluid shows nonspecific changes, whereas in demyelinating neuropathies the cerebrospinal fluid protein is markedly elevated and often accompanied by lymphocytic pleocytosis (1, 11, 86, 87). The clinical dogma of albuminocytologic dissociation classically associated with acute demyelinating neuropathies

does not apply in HIV-related GBS (1, 11). Polymorphonuclear pleocytosis in late stage patients with rapidly progressive axonal neuropathy affecting the legs may suggest infection with CMV and hence the need for virus cultures and virus isolation studies (56, 57). Syphilis should also be considered in appropriate clinical settings (88). When clinical and electrodiagnostic evaluation has not elucidated whether the neuropathy is axonal or demyelinating, nerve biopsy with teased fiber preparation is indicated. In painful sensory neuropathy, the nerve biopsy shows axonal dropout degeneration. By contrast, in chronic or acute demyelinating neuropathies the biopsy shows segmental demyelination with possible secondary axonal changes. Sparse or prominent perivascular inflammation be seen in either.

TREATMENT

All HIV-infected patients with neuromuscular complications should be assessed for adequate nutrition and receive physical therapy.

Table 30.4. Clinical Features of HIV-related Peripheral Neuropathies[a]

	Guillain-Barré	CIDP	Polyradiculitis	PSN
Disease stage	Early	Early	Late	Late
Onset	Acute	Subacute	Subacute	Subacute
Course	Resolution (spontaneous or with treatment)	May be relapsing	Progressive	Progressive
Pain	Rare	Rare	Occasional	Marked
Weakness	Marked	Moderate to marked	Marked	Mild or absent
CSF protein	Markedly elevated	Markedly elevated	Elevated	Mild or mildly elevated
Pleocytosis	Lymphocytic	Lymphocytic	Polymorphonuclear	Mild or absent
EMG/NCS	Demyelinating features	Demyelinating features	Polyradiculoneuropathy	Axonal features
Other	Respiratory compromise		Sphincters involved	
Treatment	Plasmapheresis, IVIG, steroids	Same as Guillain-Barré	Gancyclovir	Symptomatic

[a]CIDP, chronic inflammatory demyelinating polyneuropathy; PSN, painful sensory neuropathy; CSF, cerebrospinal fluid; EMG, electromyography; IVIG, intravenous immunoglobulin.

Myopathies

Patients with mild myopathic symptoms and signs that are not functionally limiting can be monitored with serial examinations and creatine kinase determinations. In our experience, many of these patients will remain stable and not require specific therapy. Nonsteroidal anti-inflammatory drugs may be useful in managing myalgia.

Patients with HIV myopathy not taking AZT may benefit from AZT, although the drug has worsened myopathy in a recent report (89). In patients already on AZT or who do not improve with AZT, 1 mg/kg/day prednisone may be tried with slow taper following the regimen described in seronegative polymyositis (37). In these cases, however, we favor treatment with high dose intravenous immunoglobulin at 2 g/kg divided over 2–4 days, a regimen we have used successfully in seronegative inflammatory myopathies (90). Although it has not been studied prospectively in HIV myopathy, intravenous immunoglobulin is an attractive therapy because it avoids steroid side-effects or further immunosuppression. Intravenous immunoglobulin is our recommended treatment of choice for HIV myopathy.

AZT myopathy will often improve if the dose of AZT is reduced, with or without a drug holiday. Improvement generally begins within 1–2 months and may be incomplete, even when the drug is stopped permanently (28, 91). Alternative antiretroviral therapy with ddI or ddC may be other options. Two of our patients with clinically suspected AZT myopathy improved clinically on ddI, and two others with histologically proven AZT myopathy improved clinically and histologically, one after change to ddI and the other after change to ddC (90).

In patients taking AZT who are unable or unwilling to undergo biopsy, a nonsteroidal anti-inflammatory drug with or without reduction of AZT is suggested. If disabling myopathy persists, AZT should be held and another antiretroviral agent substituted if possible. If functionally significant myopathy persists after 4–8 weeks off AZT, the myopathy is probably a primary inflammatory myopathy requiring either a short course of prednisone or intravenous immunoglobulin. Such clinical guesswork can be avoided if the diagnostic work-up includes a muscle biopsy, a procedure we recommend for all HIV-infected patients whose clinical picture suggests myopathy. If biopsy is unavailable, it is advisable to intervene in a stepwise fashion whenever possible so that therapeutic responses can be clearly determined.

Patients with histological signs of type II muscle fiber atrophy should receive supportive care, with particular attention to physical therapy and mobilization. In all patients with myopathy, it is important to remember that creatine kinase is a marker for muscle disease and not a clinical end point. Thus, it is essential to monitor strength as well as creatine kinase. Normal creatine kinase, although comforting to the physician, means little if significant weakness persists (37).

Pyomyositis

There is general agreement on the management of pyomyositis in adults and children (25, 26, 41, 42). All patients should receive intravenous antibiotics active against *S. aureus* (anti-staphylococcal penicillin or vancomycin) pending results of blood and abscess cultures. While most patients will recover with antibiotics alone, surgical incision and drainage may be required, particularly for later stage infection. A high index of suspicion for secondary abscesses must be maintained because these may also require surgical intervention. Patients should be closely monitored for evidence of sepsis. HIV-infected patients with pyomyositis reported in the literature have received 1–2 weeks intravenous antibiotics followed by 1–8 weeks oral therapy.

Neuropathy

Demyelinating neuropathies improve with immunomodulatory therapies such as intravenous immunoglobulin or plasmapheresis. Steroids may be considered for CIDP (1, 11). Intravenous immunoglobulin is our treatment of choice because it augments rather than suppresses immune function and has been effective in seronegative GBS or CIDP in both children and adults. In GBS, respiratory function may require monitoring in an intensive care unit setting, with mechanical ventilatory support considered for vital capacity below 15–20 ml/kg (93).

Ganciclovir appears to be effective in CMV-related polyradiculitis (58). The role of foscarnet, recently approved for CMV retinitis, in this disorder remains to be delineated. Foscarnet was also successful in one such patient that we treated (C. A. Jay, unpublished observations, 1992). Painful sensory neuropathy can be quite disabling because of intractable pain even though muscle weakness may be minimal. Tricyclic antidepressants, nonsteroidal anti-inflammatory drugs, anticonvulsants (carbamazepine and phenytoin), narcotic analgesics, and topical capsaicin in various combinations provide some relief from neuropathic pain, though symptomatic management of this condition is notoriously difficult.

PREVENTION

There are no interventions proven to prevent the neuromuscular complications of HIV infection. Although we have observed AZT myopathy on low-dose regimens, lower doses are probably less likely to cause clinically disabling myopathy. As with bone marrow suppression, the lower limits of effective therapy may be defined by the doses needed to manage cerebral HIV infection (94). To follow AZT-treated patients for myotoxicity, a baseline assessment of muscle strength and bulk and creatine kinase determination before starting therapy would seem reasonable. These should be monitored 2 to 3 times per year in asymptomatic patients and more frequently in children with neuromuscular symptoms. Analogous follow-up recommendations apply to treatment with ddI or ddC, but in these cases tendon reflexes, sensory examination, and, if possible, nerve conduction studies should additionally be obtained before treatment begins and periodically thereafter. As mentioned in regard to therapy, adequate nutrition and physical activity are important.

We are frequently asked about administering AZT to patients with a preexisting active or inactive muscle disease or ddI or ddC to patients with a preexisting neuropathy. These decisions must be made on an individual basis with assessment of the severity of the preexisting neuromuscular disease and feasibility of other therapies. There may be cross-toxicity between ddI and ddC (82). Serial nerve conduction studies may be helpful for following neuropathies, since electrical evidence of nerve damage may precede clinical symptoms and signs. Whenever possible, the lowest possible doses should be used, since neuromuscular toxicity of these agents is dose dependent (30–32). Whether combination regimens of antiretrovirals, which seem to be a particularly promising strategy in controlling HIV infection (95), have the additional benefit of avoiding neuromuscular toxicity is uncertain.

FUTURE RESEARCH

The frequency of neuromuscular disease in HIV-infected adults and children is not precisely known (1–7). As children with HIV infection live longer, it seems likely that nerve and muscle disease will become more common, if not from the underlying disease, then from the antiretroviral drugs used to treat it. Prospective studies utilizing serial examinations, blood tests, and electrodiagnosis to precisely determine the incidence of these disorders is needed. Increased awareness and careful clinical observation will also be important to identify the subtle signs of myopathy and neuropathy and to recognize new syndromes as they evolve.

As the immunopathogenesis of HIV-related inflammatory myopathies and demyelinating neuropathies is better understood it may become possible to develop effective therapies with fewer side effects. Delineation at the molecular level of the mitochondrial abnormalities resulting from AZT therapy may allow identification of patients at particularly high-risk or institution of myoprotective therapy to avoid muscle disease. Studies using animal models for AZT myopathy should be replicated with ddI and ddC to confirm the clinical impression that these agents are not myotoxic. ^{31}P-magnetic resonance spectroscopy appears to be a useful noninvasive method for monitoring AZT mitochondrial toxicity in adults (78, 79). These studies should be expanded and repeated in children. Better noninvasive methods for monitoring and diagnosing nucleoside-related neuromuscular disease would help clinicians caring for HIV-infected children in settings where sophisticated muscle pathology is unavailable.

References

1. Dalakas MC, Pezeshkpour GH. Neuromuscular diseases associated with human immunodeficiency virus infection. Ann Neurol 1988;23(suppl):S38–S48.
2. Dalakas MC, Pezeshkpour GH. Neuromuscular complications of AIDS. Muscle Nerve 1986; 9:1992.
3. Dalakas MC, Pezeshkpour GH, Gravell M, Sever JL. Polymyositis in patients with AIDS retrovirus. JAMA 1986;256:2381–2383.
4. Dalakas MC, Wichman A, Sever JL. AIDS and the nervous system. JAMA 1989;261:2396–2399.
5. Dalakas MC, Illa I. HIV-associated myopathies. In Pizzo P, Wilfert CM, eds. Pediatric AIDS: The Challenge of HIV Infection in Infants, Children, and Adolescents. Baltimore: Williams & Wilkins, 1991:420–429.
6. Dalakas MC. Retroviruses and inflammatory myopathies. Bailliere's Clin Neurol 1993;2:659–691.
7. Dalakas MC. Retroviral myopathies. In: Engel AG, ed. Myology. New York: McGraw-Hill, in press.
8. Lange DL, Britton CB, Younger DS, Hays AP. The neuromuscular manifestations of human immunodeficiency virus infections. Arch Neurol 1988;45:1084–1088.
9. Piette AM, Tusseau F, Vignon D, et al. Acute neuropathy coincident with seroconversion for anti-LAV/HTLV-III. Lancet 1986;1:852.
10. Mahe A, Bruet A, Chabin E, Fendler J-P. Acute rhabdomyolysis coincident with primary HIV-1 infection. Lancet 1989;2:1454–1455.
11. Cornblath DR, McArthur JC, Kennedy PGE, Witte AS, Griffin JW. Inflammatory demyelinating peripheral neuropathies associated with human T-cell lymphotropic virus type III infection. Ann Neurol 1987;21:32–40.
12. Dalakas MC, Pezeshkpour GH, Flaherty M. Progressive nemaline (rod) myopathy associated with HIV infection. N Engl J Med 1987;317:1602–1603.
13. Cornblath DR, McArthur JC. Predominantly sensory neuropathy in patients with AIDS and AIDS-related complex. Neurology 1988;38:794–796.
14. So YT, Holtzman DM, Abrams DI, Olney RK. Peripheral neuropathy associated with acquired immunodeficiency syndrome: Prevalence and clinical features from a population-based survey. Arch Neurol 1988;45:945–948.
15. Mah V, Vartavarian LM, Akers M-A, Vinters HV. Abnormalities of peripheral nerve in patients with human immunodeficiency virus infection. Ann Neurol 1988;24:713–717.
16. de la Monte SM, Gabuzda DH, Ho DD, et al. Peripheral neuropathy in the acquired immunodeficiency syndrome. Ann Neurol 1988;23:485–492.
17. Gebbai AA, Schmidt B, Castelo, Oliveira ASB, Lima JGC. Muscle biopsy in AIDS and ARC: Analysis of 50 patients. Muscle Nerve 1990;13:541–544.
18. Wrzolek MA, Sher JH, Kozlowski PB, Rao C. Skeletal muscle pathology in AIDS: An autopsy study. Muscle Nerve 1990;13:508–513.
19. Snider WD, Simpson DM, Nielsen S, Gold JWM, Metroka CE, Posner JE. Neurological complications of acquired immune deficiency syndrome: Analysis of 50 patients. Ann Neurol 1983;14:403–418.
20. Levy RM, Bredesen DE, Rosenblum ML. Neurological manifestations of the acquired immunodeficiency syndrome (AIDS): Experience at UCSF and review of the literature. J Neurosurg 1985;62:475–495.
21. Johnson RT, McArthur JC, Narayan O. The neurobiology of human immunodeficiency virus infections. FASEB J 1988;2:2970–2981.
22. Belman AL. AIDS and pediatric neurology. Neurol Clin 1990;8:571–603.
23. Ianetti P, Falconieri P, Imperato C. Acquired immune deficiency syndrome in childhood: Neurological aspects. Child Nerv Syst 1989;5:281–282.
24. Walter EB, Drucker RP, McKinney RE, Wilfert CM. Myopathy in human immunodeficiency virus-infected children receiving long-term zidovudine therapy. J Pediatr 1991;119:152–155.
25. Raphael SA, Wolfson BJ, Parker P, Lischner HW, Faerber EN. Pyomyositis in a child with acquired immunodeficiency syndrome. Am J Dis Child 1989;143:779–781.
26. Gardiner JS, Zauk AM, Minnefor AB, Boyd LC, Avella DG, McInerney VK. Pyomyositis in an HIV-positive premature infant: Case report and review of the literature. J Pediatr Orthop 1990;10:791–793.
27. Raphael SA, Price ML, Lischner HW, Griffin JW, Grover WD, Bagasra O. Inflammatory demyelinating polyneuropathy in a child with symptomatic human immunodeficiency virus infection. J Pediatr 1991;118:242–245.
28. Dalakas MC, Illa I, Pezeshkpour GH, Laukaitis JP, Cohen B, Griffin JL. Mitochondrial myopathy caused by long-term zidovudine therapy. N Engl J Med 1990;322:1098–1105.
29. Dalakas MC. Inflammatory and toxic myopathies. Curr Opin Neurol Neurosurg 1992;5:645–654.
30. Mhiri C, Baudrimont M, Bonne G, et al. Zidovudine myopathy: A distinctive disorder associated with mitochondrial dysfunction. Ann Neurol 1991;29:606–614.
31. Lambert JS, Seidlin M, Reichman RC, et al. 2',3'-Dideoxyinosine (ddI) in patients with the acquired immunodeficiency syndrome or AIDS-related complex: A phase I trial. N Engl J Med 1990;322:1333–1340.
32. Dubinsky RM, Yarchoan R, Dalakas M, Broder S. Reversible axonal neuropathy from the treatment of AIDS and related disorders with 2',3'-dideoxycytidine (ddC). Muscle Nerve 1989;12:856–860.
33. Pizzo PA. Treatment of human immunodeficiency virus-infected infants and young children with dideoxynucleosides. Am J Med 1988;88(suppl 5B):16S–19S.

34. Younger DS, Hays AP, Uncini A, Lange DJ, Lovelace RE, DiMauro S. Recurrent myoglobinuria and HIV seropositivity: Incidental or pathogenic association? Muscle Nerve 1989;12:842–843.

35. Richman DD, Fischl MA, Grieco MH, et al. The toxicity of azidothymidine (AZT) in the treatment of patients with AIDS and AIDS-related complex. N Engl J Med 1987;317:192–197.

36. Illa I, Nath A, Dalakas M. Immunocytochemical and virological characteristics of HIV-associated inflammatory myopathies: Similarities with seronegative polymyositis. Ann Neurol 1991;29:474–481.

37. Dalakas MC. Polymyositis, dermatomyositis and inclusion body myositis. N Engl J Med 1991;325:1487–1498.

38. Simpson DM, Bender AN. Human immunodeficiency virus-associated myopathy: Analysis of 11 patients. Ann Neurol 1988;24:79–84.

39. Baguley E, Wolfe C, Hughes GRV. Dermatomyositis in HIV infection. Br J Rheumatol 1988;27:493–494.

40. Gresh JP, Aguilar JL, Espinoza LR. Human immunodeficiency virus (HIV) infection-associated dermatomyositis. J Rheumatol 1989;16:1397–1398.

41. Schwartzman WA, Lambertus MW, Kennedy CA, Goetz MB. Staphylococcal pyomyositis in patients infected by the human immunodeficiency virus. Am J Med 1991;90:595–600.

42. Widrow CA, Kellie SM, Saltzman BR, Mathur-Wagh U. Pyomyositis in patients with the human immunodeficiency virus: An unusual form of disseminated bacterial infection. Am J Med 1991;91:129–136.

43. Falloon J, Eddy J, Wiener L, Pizzo PA. Human immunodeficiency virus infection in children. J Pediatr 1989;114:1–30.

44. Gherardi R, Baudrimont M, Lionnet F, et al. Skeletal muscle toxoplasmosis in patients with acquired immunodeficiency syndrome: A clinical and pathological study. Ann Neurol 1992;32:535–542.

45. Pouchot J, Vinceneux P, Barge J, Laparre F, Boussougant Y, Michon C. Tuberculous polymyositis in HIV infection. Am J Med 1990;89:250–251.

46. Johnson SC, Stamm CP, Hicks CB. Tuberculous psoas muscle abscess following chemoprophylaxis with isoniazid in a patient with human immunodeficiency virus infection. Rev Infect Dis 1990;12:754–756.

47. Wrzolek MA, Rao C, Kozlowski PB, Sher JH. Muscle and nerve involvement in AIDS patient with disseminated *Mycobacterium avium intracellulare* infection. Muscle Nerve 1989;12:247–249.

48. Peters BS, Winer J, Landon DN, et al. Mitochondrial myopathy associated with chronic zidovudine therapy in AIDS. Q J Med 1993;86:5–15.

49. Jay C, Ropka M, Hench K, Grady C, Dalakas M. Prospective study of myopathy during prolonged low-dose AZT: Clinical correlates of AZT mitochondrial myopathy (AZT-MM) and HIV-associated inflammatory myopathy (HIV-IM) [Abstract]. Neurology 1992;42(suppl 3):145.

50. Gonzales MF, Olney RK, So YT, et al. Subacute structural myopathy associated with human immunodeficiency virus infection. Arch Neurol 1988;45:585–587.

51. Elder G, Dalakas M, Pezeshkpour G, Sever G. Ataxic neuropathy due to ganglioneuritis after probable acute human immunodeficiency virus infection. Lancet 1986;2:1275–1276.

52. Fuller GN, Jacobs JM, Guiloff RJ. Subclinical peripheral nerve involvement in AIDS: An electrophysiological and pathological study. J Neurol Neurosurg Psychiatry 1991;54:318–324.

53. Ho DD, Rota TR, Schooley RT, et al. Isolation of HTLV-III from cerebrospinal fluid and neural tissues of patients with neurologic syndromes related to the acquired immunodeficiency syndrome. N Engl J Med 1985;313:1493–1497.

54. Chavanet P, Solary E, Giroud M, et al. Infra-clinical neuropathies related to immunodeficiency virus infection associated with higher T-helper cell count. J Acquir Immune Defic Syndr 1989;2:564–569.

55. Koch TK, Koerper MA, Wesley AM, Lewis EM, Weintrub PS, Bredesen DE. Absence of an AIDS-related peripheral neuropathy in children and young adult hemophiliacs [Abstract]. Ann Neurol 1989;26:476–477.

56. Eidelberg D, Sotrel A, Vogel H, Walker P, Kleefield J, Crumpacker CS. Progressive polyradiculopathy in acquired immune deficiency syndrome. Neurology 1986;36:912–916.

57. Behar R, Wiley C, McCutchan A. Cytomegalovirus polyradiculoneuropathy in acquired immune deficiency syndrome. Neurology 1987;37:557–561.

58. Miller RG, Storey JR, Greco CM. Ganciclovir in the treatment of progressive AIDS-related polyradiculopathy. Neurology 1990;40:569–574.

59. Dickson DW, Belman AK, Kim TS, Horoupian DS, Rubinstein A. Spinal cord pathology in pediatric acquired immunodeficiency syndrome. Neurology 1989;39:227–235.

60. Morgan OS, Rodgers-Johnson P, Mora C, Char G. HTLV-1 and polymyositis in Jamaica. Lancet 1989;2:1184–1187.

61. Wiley CA, Nerenberg M, Cros D, Soto-Aguilar M. HTLV-1 polymyositis in a patient also infected with the human immunodeficiency virus. N Engl J Med 1989;320:992–995.

62. Bothe K, Aguzzi A, Lassmann H, Rethwilm A, Horak I. Progressive encephalopathy and myopathy in transgenic mice expressing human foamy virus genes. Science 1991;253:555–557.

63. Dalakas MC, London WT, Gravell M, Sever JL. Polymyositis in an immunodeficiency disease in monkeys induced by a type D retrovirus. Neurology 1986;36:569–572.

64. Dalakas MC, Gravell M, London WT, Cunningham GC, Sever JT. Morphological changes of an inflammatory myopathy in rhesus monkeys with simian acquired immunodeficiency syndrome. Proc Soc Exp Biol Med 1987;185:369–376.

65. Pezeshkpour G, Illa I, Dalakas MC. Ultrastructural characteristics and DNA immunocytochemistry in human immunodeficiency virus and

zidovudine-associated myopathies. Hum Pathol 1991;22:1281–1288.

66. Lamperth L, Illa I, Dalakas M. In situ hybridization in muscle biopsies from patients with HIV-associated polymyositis (HIV-PM) using labeled HIV-RNA probes [Abstract]. Neurology 1990;40(suppl 1):121.

67. Chad DA, Smith TW, Blumenfeld, Fairchild PG, DeGirolami U. Human immunodeficiency virus (HIV)-associated myopathy: Immunocytochemical identification of an HIV antigen (gp41) in muscle macrophages. Ann Neurol 1990;28:579–582.

68. Leon-Monzon MEL, Lamperth L, Dalakas MC. Search for HIV proviral DNA and amplified sequences in the muscle biopsies of patients with HIV-polymyositis. Muscle Nerve 1993;16:408–413.

69. Lamperth L, Vicenzi E, Dalakas M. Infection and transfection of human muscle by HIV or HIV proviral-DNA construct [Abstract]. Neurology 1991;41(suppl 1):211.

70. Dalakas MC. Inflammatory myopathies: Pathogenesis and treatment. Clin Neuropharmacol 1992;15:327–351.

71. Illa I, Leon-Monzon M, Dalakas M. Retroviral sequences in patients with polymyositis (PM), dermatomyositis (DM), and inclusion body myositis (IBM). [Abstract]. Neurology 1992;42(suppl 3):302.

72. Rucheton M, Graafland H, Fanton H, Ursule L, Ferrier P, Larsen CJ. Presence of circulating antibodies against *gag* gene MuLV proteins in patients with autoimmune connective tissue disorders. Virology 1985;144:468–480.

73. Arnaudo E, Dalakas M, Shanske S, Moraes CT, DiMauro S, Schon EA. Depletion of muscle mitochondrial DNA in AIDS patients with zidovudine-induced myopathy. Lancet 1991;337:508–510.

74. Simpson MV, Chin CD, Keilbaugh SA, Lin T, Prusoff WH. Studies on the inhibition of mitochondrial DNA replication by 3'-azido-3'-deoxythymidine and other dideoxynucleoside analogs which inhibit HIV-1 replication. Biochem Pharmacol 1989;38:1033–1036.

75. Chariot P, Gherardi R. Partial cytochrome c oxidase deficiency and cytoplasmic bodies in patients with zidovudine myopathy. Neuromuscul Disord 1991;1:357–363.

76. Lamperth L, Dalakas MC, Dagani F, Anderson J, Ferrari R. Abnormal skeletal and cardiac muscle mitochondria induced by zidovudine (AZT) in human muscle *in vitro* and in an animal model. Lab Invest 1991;65:742–751.

77. Lewis W, Gonzalez, Chomyn A, Papoian T. Zidovudine induces molecular, biochemical, and ultrastructural changes in rat skeletal muscle mitochondria. J Clin Invest 1992;89:1354–1360.

78. Weissman JD, Constantinitis I, Hudgins P, Wallace DC. ^{31}P magnetic resonance spectroscopy suggests impaired mitochondrial function in AZT-treated HIV-infected patients [Abstract]. Neurology 1991;41:619–623.

79. Soueidan S, Sinnwell T, Jay C, Frank J, McLaughlin A, Dalakas M. Impaired muscle energy metabolism in patients with AZT-myopathy: A blinded comparative study of exercise ^{31}P mag-

netic resonance spectroscopy with muscle biopsy [Abstract]. Neurology 1992;42(suppl 3):146.

80. Feldman D, Brosnan C, Anderson TD. Ultrastructure of peripheral neuropathy induced in rabbits by 2',3'-dideoxycytidine. Lab Invest 1992;66:75–85.

81. Kieburtz KD, Seidlin M, Lambert JS, Dolin R, Reichman R, Valentine F. Extended follow-up of peripheral neuropathy in patients with AIDS and AIDS-related complex treated with dideoxyinosine. J Acquir Immune Defic Syndr 1992;5:60–64.

82. LeLacheur SF, Simon GL. Exacerbation of dideoxycytidine-induced neuropathy with dideoxyinosine. J Acquir Immune Defic Syndr 1991;4:538–539.

83. Bozzette SA, Santangelo J, Villasana D, et al. Peripheral nerve function in persons with asymptomatic or minimally symptomatic HIV disease: Absence of zidovudine neurotoxicity. J Acquir Immune Defic Syndr 1991;4:851–855.

84. Simpson DM, Bender AN, Farraye J, Mendelson SG, Wolfe DE. Human immunodeficiency virus wasting syndrome may represent a treatable myopathy. Neurology 1990;40:535–538.

85. Fleckenstein JL, Burns DK, Murphy FK, Jayson HT, Bonte FJ. Differential diagnosis of bacterial myositis in AIDS: Evaluation with MR imaging. Radiology 1991;179:653–658.

86. Chaunu M-P, Ratinahirana H, Raphael M, et al. The spectrum of changes on 20 nerve biopsies in patients with HIV infection. Muscle Nerve 1989;12:452–459.

87. Miller RG, Parry GJ, Pfaeffl W, Lang W, Lippert R, Kiprov D. The spectrum of peripheral neuropathy associated with ARC and AIDS. Muscle Nerve 1988;11:857–863.

88. Lanska MJ, Lanska DJ, Schmidley JW. Syphilitic polyradiculopathy in an HIV-positive man. Neurology 1988;38:1297–1301.

89. Berger JR, Shebert, Gregorios JB. Exacerbation of HIV-associated myopathy by zidovudine. AIDS 1991;5:229–230.

90. Dalakas MC, McCrosky S, D'Ambrosia JM, et al. High-dose intravenous immunoglobulin (IVIg) in the treatment of dermatomyositis (DM): A double-blind placebo-controlled trial. Neurology 1993;43:356–357.

91. Chalmers AC, Greco CM, Miller RG. Prognosis in AZT-myopathy. Neurology 1991;41:1181–1184.

92. Jay CA, Hench K, Ropka M, et al. Improvement of AZT myopathy after change to dideoxyinosine (ddI) or dideoxycytidine (ddC) [Abstract]. Neurology 1993;43(suppl 2):A374–A375.

93. Ropper AH. ICU management of acute inflammatory-postinfectious polyneuropathy (Landry-Guillain-Barré-Strohl syndrome). In Ropper AH, Kennedy SF, eds. Neurological and neurosurgical intensive care. Rockville, MD: Aspen, 1988:259–262.

94. Fischl MA. State of antiretroviral therapy with zidovudine. AIDS 1989;3(suppl 1):S137–S143.

95. Pizzo PA, Butler K, Balis F, Brouwers E, Hawkins M, Eddy J, et al. Dideoxycytidine alone and in an alternating schedule with zidovudine in children with symptomatic human immunodeficiency virus infection. J Pediatr 1990;117:799–808.

31
Abnormalities in Growth and Development

Louisa Laue and Gordon B. Cutler Jr.

AIDS in children is frequently associated with failure to thrive (FTT), defined as a subnormal rate of growth and weight gain for age. The incidence of FTT ranges from 20 to 80% of symptomatic human immunodeficiency virus (HIV)-infected children (1–7), and weight loss or growth failure is included in the Centers for Disease Control and World Health Organization clinical case definition of AIDS. Evaluation of all children with HIV infection should include accurate serial measurements of height and weight plotted on a growth chart. Normal growth velocity varies considerably throughout childhood and adolescence, from 12 cm/year during the first year of life to 5–6 cm/year between age 4 and 10 years. In a similar fashion, weight velocity varies from 7 kg/year during the first year of life to 2–3 kg/year between age 3 and 10 years. The correlation among FTT, compromised immunologic function, and increased incidence of opportunistic infections intensifies ongoing efforts to restore normal growth and nutrition. This review summarizes current knowledge of the etiological factors, pathogenesis, and natural history of growth failure and suggests an approach for the evaluation, treatment, and prevention of FTT in HIV-infected children.

OVERVIEW OF ABNORMALITIES IN GROWTH AND DEVELOPMENT

The time of acquisition of HIV infection has significant implications for the degree and pattern of growth failure occurring in infants and children with AIDS. Thus, children with FTT and AIDS must be evaluated in an age-appropriate manner and with regard to whether HIV infection was acquired vertically from the mother or from transfusion of blood products.

Infants with HIV infection are heterogeneous, comprised of those with HIV infection acquired vertically before, during, or after delivery and those with HIV infection acquired postnatally from transfusions. A prospective study of height and weight in 44 HIV-seropositive children born to HIV-infected women revealed that height and weight percentiles were comparable with those of uninfected children at birth and during the first 3 months of life. By 3–6 months, however, the HIV-infected infants were smaller in height and weight percentiles (8). Other retrospective studies report that one-quarter to one-half of infants with vertically acquired HIV infection were small for gestational age and remained smaller in height and weight percentiles (2, 4, 6, 9–12). These discrepancies in birth weight and growth pattern most likely reflect the heterogeneity of the infant population with vertically acquired HIV infection. Furthermore, other factors, such as malnutrition, drug abuse, and social/environmental factors, that are present in infants with vertically acquired HIV infection also affect birth weight and postnatal growth.

Children with blood product-related HIV infection may show growth failure as one of the first presenting signs, often coincident with the onset of opportunistic infections. In one study the growth failure preceded the diagnosis of AIDS or AIDS-related complex by a median of 24 months. With progression of the disease, the growth retardation becomes more profound and often evolves into a wasting state. A positive correlation has been shown between height and weight for age and helper-to-suppressor T cell ratios. Jason et al. (13) compared hemophiliac children who were asymptomatic carriers of HIV with uninfected controls. The seropositive asymptomatic children <11 years old (or before pubertal growth spurt) had a decline of 25 percentiles in height for age over 3-year. This was associated with a decline in helper-to-suppressor T cell ratio. These findings in boys with hemophilia were confirmed by Brettler et al. (14) who suggested that a decline of >15 percentiles in height or weight for age on two successive measurements may predict the development of other HIV-related symptoms. Growth failure in HIV-infected children is also associated with delayed onset of puberty.

ETIOLOGIC CONSIDERATIONS

Whether the route of HIV infection affects the severity or rate of progression of growth failure is unknown. Although severity of illness is associated with greater degrees of growth and skeletal retardation, it is unclear whether this is due to the severity of the HIV infection itself or to concurrent opportunistic infections such as cytomegalovirus, *Pneumocystis carinii*, or hepatitis. Whether there is a critical time in fetal maturation when growth and development are more susceptible to HIV and whether other factors during pregnancy may obviate or promote growth retardation are unknown.

The magnitude of the growth retardation and pubertal delay observed in children with HIV infection is similar to that observed in protein and calorie malnutrition and in chronic illness involving the bowel, kidney, heart, and lung. In the course of AIDS, part of the loss of body weight can be attributed to acute catabolic states related to fever or evolving infections. However,

many children fail to thrive even in periods free of opportunistic infections. For this reason, the nutritional aspects of AIDS have received much attention. Oral and esophageal infections may limit caloric intake. Central nervous system manifestations may impair appetite or deglutition. However, even when intake is adequate growth failure often persists. This raises the possibility that accelerated losses from the gastrointestinal tract, in conjunction with a hypermetabolic state, may be etiologic factors in FTT (Fig. 31.1).

PATHOGENESIS AND NATURAL HISTORY OF GROWTH FAILURE

Subtle and varied abnormalities of the endocrine axes have been reported in HIV-infected children. However, none of the three major endocrine causes of growth failure in children, namely, growth hormone deficiency, thyroid hormone deficiency, or adrenal dysfunction, have been observed consistently in children with FTT and AIDS. Conversely, gastrointestinal abnormalities that result in malabsorption and malnutrition occur frequently in children with AIDS. However, efforts to augment caloric intake, through parenteral or enteral feedings, or to treat opportunistic infections of the gastrointestinal tract have not consistently improved growth.

An increase in resting energy expenditure (REE) has been reported in adults with AIDS who are clinically stable but malnourished (15). The normal metabolic response to malnutrition is weight loss associated with a decrease in REE. Many malnourished AIDS patients demonstrate the opposite change in REE. Although the cause of this HIV-associated hypermetabolic-catabolic state is unknown, we hypothesize that it may impair the physical development of HIV-infected children. The following three sections will review current knowledge of neuroendocrine, gastrointestinal-nutritional, and metabolic dysfunction in children with HIV infection and FTT.

Neuroendocrine Dysfunction in AIDS

Many hormones, growth factors, their receptors, and their intracellular signaling

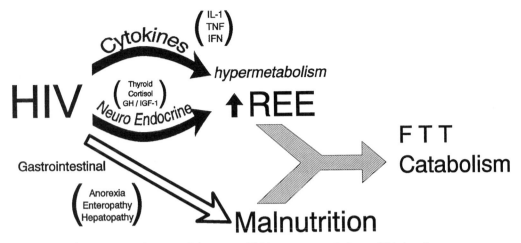

Figure 31.1.   *GH*, growth hormone; *TNF*, tumor necrosis factor; IFN, interferon.

cascades are involved in directing cells to enter the cell cycle, replicate, and grow. The brain regulates the secretion of many of these hormones and growth factors through neurogenic input to the hypothalamus and pituitary. Infection of higher cortical centers by HIV may affect hypothalamic and pituitary function by altering production of neural transmitters (i.e., GABA, serotonin, norepinephrine) that inhibit or facilitate release of hypothalamic and pituitary hormones (i.e., corticotropin-releasing hormone (CRH), adrenocorticotropic hormone (ACTH), and arginine vasopressin. Because AIDS encephalopathy is more prevalent in children than in adults, central nervous system-mediated endocrine deficiency associated with hypothalamic dysfunction may be more common in the pediatric AIDS population. To date, neither autopsy studies of the pituitary gland or hypothalamus nor clinical hypopituitarism have been reported in children with AIDS. However, abnormalities in diurnal thyroid-stimulating hormone levels in children (which indicate early hypothalamic-pituitary dysfunction) and delayed puberty in adolescents with AIDS are suggestive of hypothalamic-pituitary dysfunction (16, 17).

Neuroendocrine dysfunction involving the hypothalamic-pituitary-thyroid, -adrenal, -gonadal axis and growth hormone-insulin-like growth factor (IGF)-1 axis has been observed in HIV-infected children, but the findings are heterogeneous (Table 31.1).

Subtle degrees of biochemical hypothyroidism have been observed in children with HIV infection, and further study is needed to determine whether overt clinical hypothyroidism will ensue (16, 18). Frank adrenal insufficiency has not been observed in children with AIDS, although minor defects in steroidogenesis as well as abnormalities in the regulation of the hypothalamic-pituitary-adrenal axis have been noted (16). Delayed maturation of the hypothalamic-pituitary-gonadal axis is manifest clinically as delayed puberty and retarded skeletal maturation in HIV-infected adolescents. Growth hormone and IGF-1 levels range from normal to low in children with AIDS (16, 17).

Although these endocrine abnormalities may contribute to FTT in some HIV-infected children, neither the prevalence nor severity of the endocrine dysfunction can explain the profound wasting observed in so many children. Therefore additional etiologies for FTT, which may involve gastrointestinal and/or metabolic dysfunction, must be sought.

Gastrointestinal Dysfunction in AIDS

Acute and chronic diarrhea, weight loss, abdominal pain, esophagitis and other gastrointestinal symptoms have been observed frequently in adults with HIV infection. These symptoms are most often due to infections of the gastrointestinal tract. Many pathogens have been implicated, including

Table 31.1. Summary of Endocrine Findings in Adults and Children with AIDS[a]

Endocrine Axis	Adults	Children
Thyroid	↑T4, ↑TBG ↑T3 ↓rT3, ↓rT3/T4 TSH unknown	N or ↑T4, ↑TBG N or ↓T3 rT3, rT3/T4 unknown N or ↑TSH N or ↓ nocturnal TSH rise
Adrenal	N or ↑basal ACTH N or ↑basal cortisol ↓ Cortisol response to ACTH ↓ 17-Deoxysteroid response to ACTH N renin, aldosterone CRH testing: 1° adrenal failure and pituitary failure	N basal ACTH N, ↑, or ↓ basal cortisol N cortisol response to ACTH Precursors unknown N or ↑ renin, N or ↓ aldosterone CRH testing not done
Gonad	↓ Testosterone	↓ testosterone
Hypothalamus-pituitary	Abnormal CRH response TRH response unknown Prolactin unknown ↓ Gonadotropins	CRH response unknown TRH response unknown N prolactin ↓ Gonadotropins
Growth hormone	Unknown	N or ↓ GH on provocative testing
IGF-1	Unknown	N or ↓ IGF-1 in preadolescents ↓ IGF-1 in adolescents

[a]N, normal; ↑, increased; ↓, decreased; TBG, thyroid binding globulin; TRH, thyroid releasing hormone.

HIV enteropathy (19–22). The growth failure in children with HIV infection has been postulated to result in part from altered gastrointestinal function, which can produce diarrhea, abdominal distension, pain, and malabsorption. Although enteric infection with *Giardia lamblia*, *Cryptosporidium*, *Shigella*, *Salmonella*, *Campylobacter*, *Yersinia*, and other pathogens may contribute to impaired gastrointestinal function, the frequency of these infections in children with HIV infection is substantially less than in adults. Several studies have shown that HIV disease in children is often associated with gastrointestinal dysfunction despite the absence of infection by recognized enteropathogens (20, 23).

Diarrhea and malabsorption are two additional factors that distinguish gastrointestinal dysfunction in adults and children with HIV infection. First, diarrhea occurs more frequently in adults than children. Diarrhea occurs in more than half of the adult patients with AIDS in the United States and in 95% of adult Haitian and African patients (22, 24–26). By contrast, in one series of 36 children with AIDS, 39% of the children had diarrhea (6), whereas 94% had FTT. Most children with diarrhea did not have an identifiable enteric pathogen as a cause.

Second, the malabsorption in children with HIV infection appears primarily to affect carbohydrate absorption, suggesting an intestinal brush border defect, whereas the malabsorption in adults is less selective and suggests a more generalized mucosal injury. Up to 40% of HIV-infected children demonstrate disaccharide malabsorption, although the mechanism involved in the development of this malabsorption is unknown. Studies suggest that it may be caused by direct mucosal injury since intestinal villous blunting has been demonstrated in some children with lactose malabsorption (25–27). However, other children show malabsorption of both lactose and sucrose, suggesting a nonspecific effect on the intestinal brush border rather than an isolated enzyme deficiency. Regardless of the cause, the loss of calories from malabsorbed dietary sugars, combined with the osmotic diarrheal state that leads to reduced dietary intake, may contribute to growth retardation.

The hypothesis that malnutrition results in the wasting state leading to demise in adults with AIDS has been examined (28). Although deficiency of both macro- and micronutrients undeniably contributes to morbidity and mortality in AIDS, it is not in itself the sole cause. Because of the interrelationship among growth, development, and nutritional status in children, many attempts have been made to ensure that HIV-infected children receive a diet adequate in protein, calories, and other essential nutrients either by supplemental enteral or parenteral alimentation. Unfortunately, despite these measures to optimize nutritional status, little improvement in the growth or body composition of these children has been observed.

In summary, the gastrointestinal mechanisms contributing to FTT in children with AIDS are multifactorial. They include decreased caloric intake caused by anorexia or odynophagia, malabsorption resulting from opportunistic infections, carbohydrate malabsorption or other enteropathies, and fluid-electrolyte and nutrient losses from diarrhea. However, all these factors may be absent in some children who remain clinically stable and nevertheless have progressive FTT. Therefore, other factors, including alterations in metabolic rate, must be considered as potential causes of FTT.

Metabolic Dysfunction in AIDS

The progressive wasting observed in adult patients with AIDS has been shown to result from hypermetabolism and/or alterations in basal energy expenditure (15, 29, 30). The normal metabolic response to malnutrition is weight loss associated with a decrease in REE. Many malnourished AIDS patients do not demonstrate this phenomenon. In fact, Hommes et al. (29) demonstrated a 9% increase in resting metabolic rate in patients losing weight with AIDS-related complex and AIDS compared with that in control subjects. Similarly, Melchoir et al. (31) showed a 12% increase in REE in HIV-infected adults compared with controls. However, both of these studies included patients with lymphoma or Kaposi's sarcoma, which may have influenced the results since malignancy is known to increase REE. Because of this variable, recent studies have been performed in asymptomatic HIV-infected patients, without either AIDS, AIDS-related complex, malignancy, or weight loss, that have also demonstrated increased REE (30). This suggests two possi-

bilities: 1) that HIV infection affects metabolic rate independent of other associated illnesses (i.e., infection, malignancy) and 2) that other factors, such as inadequate caloric intake or malabsorption coupled with an increase in REE, must be present to cause weight loss.

The physiologic response to illness involves secretion of catabolic hormones and cytokines that modulate metabolic rate and energy expenditure. Specific hormones that may contribute to a catabolic state include triiodothyronine, thyroxine, and cortisol. Additionally, increased production of cytokines, such as tumor necrosis factor and interleukin-1, have been proposed as possible mediators of cachexia (32). These cytokines may alter metabolism either directly or indirectly through modulation of hormone secretion and action. To date, studies examining levels of cortisol, cortisol precursors, thyroid hormones, catecholamines, and cytokines in AIDS have not yielded consistent findings, perhaps because of the heterogeneity of the patient population studied and the degree of disease activity in these patients.

We hypothesize that HIV infection in children leads to a hypermetabolic state, which, in conjunction with malnutrition, causes catabolism and progressive deterioration in physical and mental health. The hypermetabolic state may result from HIV-induced secretion of cytokines that alter energy expenditure either directly or indirectly (Fig. 31.1). Reversing this hypermetabolic-catabolic state and restoring normal growth in HIV-infected children may be feasible by hormonal therapy (ie., IGF-1) to divert energy expenditure from a catabolic into an anabolic pathway.

CLINICAL PRESENTATION AND DIFFERENTIAL DIAGNOSIS

To assess growth failure in children with congenital or acquired HIV infection, one should begin by constructing growth charts for height and weight, determining growth velocity and pattern of growth, and assessing body proportions and bone age. Children with vertically acquired HIV infection show persistently subnormal rates of growth and weight gain from as early as 3 months of age and continue to deviate from the normal height and weight curves. Children with acquired HIV infection follow a normal growth pattern until the onset of infection and then show declining height and weight velocities.

Determination of body proportions, such as upper-to-lower segment ratio and arm span, provides additional information about the diagnosis of growth failure. Children with osteochondrodystrophies have short extremities leading to disproportionate short stature. Almost all other causes of growth failure, including HIV infection, have normal body proportions.

The major mechanism of statural growth is endochondral ossification. When epiphyseal chondrocyte multiplication stops, the epiphyseal plate ossifies, the metaphysis and epiphysis fuse, and growth ceases. Growth potential can be assessed radiographically by measuring the degree of ossification within the epiphysis. The standards of Greulich and Pyle (33) are commonly used to determine skeletal maturation (33). Epiphyseal maturation is delayed in systemic diseases (including AIDS), in endocrine disorders that cause growth failure, and in constitutional delay of growth.

Once it is determined that a child with AIDS is growing at a suboptimal rate, the differential diagnosis includes constitutional delay of growth and development, intrauterine growth retardation, neuroendocrine, metabolic, and gastrointestinal dysfunction, and psychosocial factors. The workup for these causes of FTT are discussed in the following sections.

Children with vertically or blood product acquired HIV infection frequently have both growth failure and pubertal delay. The onset of puberty is heralded by an increase in testicular volume in boys and breast budding in girls. These events should occur by age 14 in boys and 13 in girls. The pubertal growth spurt is often significantly delayed or may not occur in children with AIDS, which further exacerbates growth failure. Skeletal maturity, which correlates with pubertal development, is usually delayed. This bone age delay may allow time for some catch-up growth to occur and improve adult height. Differential diagnosis of pubertal

delay includes primary gonadal failure and delayed maturation of the hypothalamic-pituitary-gonadal axis.

DIAGNOSTIC CONSIDERATIONS
Neuroendocrine Evaluation

Endocrine dysfunction in AIDS can be either primary in which there is dysfunction of a specific gland (i.e., thyroid, adrenal) or secondary in which there is dysfunction of the hypothalamic-pituitary unit. Children with HIV infection and FTT should undergo screening endocrine evaluations to exclude abnormalities in the hypothalamic-pituitary-adrenal, -thyroid, and growth hormone-IGF-1 axes. Boys older than 14 years and girls older than 13 years who do not show signs of puberty should undergo evaluation of their hypothalamic-pituitary-gonadal axis.

Thyroid Axis

Thyroid hormone regulates body metabolism throughout life and is critical in normal growth and development. Although congenital hypothyroidism produces irreversible damage to the central nervous system, hypothyroidism acquired after age 2–3 years has reversible effects. Signs and symptoms of congenital hypothyroidism include prolonged jaundice, lethargy, constipation, poor suck, hypotonia, hoarse cry, macroglossia, dry skin, large fontanelles, and umbilical hernia. If diagnosis and treatment of hypothyroidism is delayed, postnatal growth rate is subnormal, and developmental milestones are delayed.

Signs and symptoms of acquired hypothyroidism include constipation, anorexia, cold intolerance, dry skin, myxedema, goiter, and delay of growth, skeletal maturation, and puberty. The onset of this disorder is often insidious, and the most common presenting abnormality is a decrease in growth rate, which may be accompanied by a goiter. If hypothyroidism persists long enough, all classic signs and symptoms may evolve.

Diagnosis of primary hypothyroidism is confirmed by finding a low serum T4, free T4, T3, and an elevated serum TSH concentration, whereas the diagnosis of secondary hypothyroidism is confirmed by finding a low serum T4, free T4, and T3 in the face of a normal or low TSH. Thyroid binding globulin deficiency is associated with a low T4 and normal free T4, T3, and TSH levels. The thyroid axis in children with HIV infection should be screened by measuring free T4 and TSH. A more detailed evaluation to monitor early HIV-related changes would include T3, reverse T3, reverse T3-to-T4 ratio, and thyroid binding globulin. Thyroid releasing hormone testing and measurement of diurnal TSH are indicated only in specific cases (Table 31.2).

Serial sampling of TSH hourly from 1400 to 1800 hours and from 2200 to 0200 hours reveals a nocturnal increase in TSH secretion of at least 50% over basal levels in normal children. Patients with secondary hypothyroidism demonstrate an absence of this nocturnal TSH increase, which may be the first abnormality observed at the onset of hypothyroidism. Children with HIV infection generally demonstrate normal T4 and free T4, T3, and TSH but may have absent diurnal variation in TSH (16). Whether these children will eventually develop overt biochemical and/or clinical evidence of hypothyroidism remains to be determined. We recommend that diurnal TSH sampling be considered as a research procedure in the prospective evaluation of children with HIV infection who have normal basal thyroid function studies (Table 31.2)

Adrenal Axis

Many signs and symptoms of HIV infection, such as nausea, vomiting, anorexia, weight loss, fever, diarrhea, fatigue, and orthostatic hypotension, are also manifestations of adrenal insufficiency. Adrenal insufficiency is divided pathophysiologically into two types: primary, in which the adrenal glands are destroyed, and secondary, in which either the pituitary gland or hypothalamus fails. Clinical manifestations, which may be gradual or acute, include weakness and fatigue, weight loss, anorexia, hyperpigmentation (caused by increased ACTH levels in primary adrenal insufficiency), abdominal pain, vomiting (occasionally with diarrhea), and hypotension. Laboratory tests reveal diminished serum

sodium, increased serum potassium, hypoglycemia, a low morning cortisol, and an elevated serum ACTH. To confirm the diagnosis, one should administer 0.25 mg synthetic ACTH (cosyntropin) i.v. or i.m. and obtain a serum cortisol 60 min later. Failure of the serum cortisol to rise above 500 nmol/liter (18 µg/dl) indicates primary or secondary adrenal insufficiency. In primary adrenal insufficiency plasma aldosterone levels are low, whereas renin levels are high. In secondary adrenal insufficiency, plasma ACTH and cortisol levels are low in conjunction with normal plasma renin and aldosterone levels.

Primary and secondary adrenal insufficiency can also be distinguished by infusing synthetic ACTH i.v. for 48 hr (Rose test). Patients with primary adrenal insufficiency do not respond to ACTH even with prolonged administration, whereas adult patients with secondary adrenal insufficiency will elevate urinary 17-hydroxycorticosteroids to 10–40 mg/day during the second day of ACTH.

CRH can also be used to evaluate the hypothalamic-pituitary-adrenal axis. Administration of CRH to patients with primary adrenal insufficiency results in low cortisol levels and marked stimulation of ACTH levels. Patients with secondary adrenal insufficiency also have low cortisol levels in response to CRH; however, ACTH responses are either absent or are similar to those of normal subjects. The patients with no ACTH response to CRH appear to represent those with corticotroph failure (pituitary destruction), whereas those patients with normal ACTH responses are thought to have CRH deficiency (adrenal insufficiency of hypothalamic origin). CRH testing has been used to diagnose both primary and secondary adrenal insufficiency (caused by pituitary failure) in patients with AIDS.

An initial screen of the hypothalamic-pituitary-adrenal axis in HIV-infected children with FTT should include measurements of morning plasma cortisol and ACTH. A cortrosyn test should be performed if adrenal insufficiency is suspected. Plasma renin activity, CRH testing, and/or a 48-hr cosyntropin infusion are indicated only in cases where the site of origin of the adrenal insufficiency is controversial.

Table 31.2. Evaluation of Neuroendocrine, Gastrointestinal and Nutritional, and Metabolic Dysfunction in Children with HIV Infection and FTT[a]

Neuroendocrine Evaluation	Gastrointestinal and Nutritional Evaluation	Metabolic Evaluation (Research Studies)
Thyroid Free T4, TSH (initial screen) Free T4, TSH, rT3, TBG, T3:T4 (for comprehensive evaluation) Diurnal TSH (only in selected cases) **Adrenal** ACTH, cortisol (0900 hr) Plasma renin activity (0900 hr) Cortrosyn test (if adrenal insufficiency suspected) **Growth hormone-IGF-1** Bone age Growth hormone stimulation test (if GHD suspected) IGF-1 IGF-binding protein 3, GHBP (research studies) **Gonadal** Tanner staging Basal testosterone (boys), estradiol (girls), SHBG, LH, FSH LHRH stimulation test (in select cases)	**Anthropometric measurements/body composition** Standing height × 10 by Harpenden stadiometer Sitting height × 10 Weight Body mass index Body surface area Head circumference Mid upper arm circumference Caliper measurements of triceps and subscapular skinfold thickness **Caloric intake and nutritional status** 3-day calorie count to assess nutrient intake Chemistry panel (sodium, potassium, chloride, serum bicarbonate, blood urea nitrogen, creatinine, glucose, total protein, albumin, cholesterol/LDL/VLDL, triglyceride, calcium, magnesium, zinc, folate, iron, and ferritin levels) **Malabsorption and infection** Albumin Vitamin A Stool studies for measurement of pH, reducing substances guaiac, random spot fat, random trypsin, culture, ova and parasites, and *Cryptosporidium* smear Xylose challenge test (if malabsorption is suspected) Hydrogen breath test (if malabsorption is suspected) 72-hr Van Gen Kramer fat assay (if three random fecal fats are positive) **Hepatic function** Total and direct bilirubin, SGOT, SGPT, GGT, alkaline phosphatase Ultrasonography (if biliary tract disease suspected) Liver biopsy (if undiagnosed hepatopathy found)	**REE** Calcium and bond metabolism Bone resorption Parathormone (intact) Urinary pyridinium Urinary hydroxyproline **Bone formation** 1,25-dihydroxyvitamin D_3 Bone alkaline phosphatase, total and ionized calcium, phosphorus, magnesium Osteocalcin (bone gla protein) **Lipid metabolism** Total cholesterol LDL/VLDL cholesterol Triglycerides Free fatty acids Lipoprotein lipase **Protein metabolism** Total serum protein Total urinary nitrogen Serum amino acids Urine amino acids Urinary polyamines **Muscle mass and energy metabolism** ^{31}P-NMR spectroscopy

[a]LDL, low density lipoprotein; VLDL, very low density lipoprotein; GHBP, growth hormone binding protein; SHBG, sex hormone binding globulin; LH, luteinizing hormone; FSH, follicle stimulating hormone; LHRH, luteinizing hormone-releasing hormone; NMR, nuclear magnetic resonance; SGOT, serum glutamic-oxaloacetic transaminase; SGPT, serum glutamic-pyruvic transaminase; GGT, γ-glutamyltranspeptidase.

Growth Hormone/IGF-1 Axis

Children with growth hormone deficiency (GHD) have subnormal rates of growth and show progressive deviation away from the normal growth curve. Children with congenital GHD from panhypopituitarism usually develop growth failure at age 12–18 months, but early manifestations in infancy include microphallus, hypoglycemia, cyanosis, and shock. Acquired GHD may be isolated or be associated with other endocrine, visual, and neurologic impairments attributable to a hypothalamic or pituitary lesion.

To determine whether a child is growth hormone-deficient requires measurement of growth hormone levels. However, growth hormone is secreted in a pulsatile fashion, and levels in the plasma are therefore often undetectable. Consequently, growth hormone release must be stimulated by agents such as arginine, L-dopa, insulin, clonidine, propranolol, glucagon, or exercise. If a growth hormone level in excess of 7 µg/l is achieved in at least one of three tests, the child is considered to have normal growth hormone reserve. If the level is <7 µg/l in all three tests, the child is considered to have GHD. GHD may also be demonstrated by a mean growth hormone night level of < 1.2 µg/l when blood is sampled for 12 hr at 20-min intervals (34).

A binding protein for growth hormone has recently been identified and is presumed to be a portion of the growth hormone receptor. This growth hormone binding protein is undetectable in states where the growth hormone receptor is absent on a genetic basis (Laron dwarfism). Growth hormone acts by binding to its receptor. Subsequent intracellular events cause the synthesis and release of IGF-1. IGF-1 is carried in the circulation by binding proteins and stimulates cells through specific receptors. IGF-1 directly stimulates longitudinal bone growth and lymphocyte proliferation, acts on the central nervous system and Leydig cells, and plays a role in muscle and nerve regeneration.

In the child with HIV infection and growth failure we recommend obtaining a bone age. Growth hormone deficiency may be excluded by measurement of IGF-1 levels and/or growth hormone stimulation testing with clonidine, L-dopa, and/or arginine (Table 31.2).

Gonadal Axis

In adolescents with pubertal delay, Tanner staging, a bone age, and measurement of basal gonadotropin (luteinizing hormone and follicle stimulating hormone) and sex steroid levels (testosterone in boys and estrogen in girls) should be performed (Table 31.2). In primary gonadal failure sex steroids are low and follicle stimulating hormone levels are high, whereas in constitutional delay both sex steroids and gonadotropin levels are low. A luteinizing hormone-releasing hormone stimulation test may be useful to assess hypothalamic-pituitary-gonadal axis activity. This test involves injecting 100 µg luteinizing hormone-releasing hormone (Factrel) i.v. and measuring luteinizing hormone and follicle stimulating hormone levels at 0, 15, 30, 45, 60, and 90 min relative to the bolus injection of luteinizing hormone-releasing hormone. In girls a pubertal response is characterized by a peak luteinizing hormone of >15 mIU/ml or a ratio of peak luteinizing hormone to peak follicle stimulating hormone of >0.66 and in boys by a difference of >25.5 mIU/ml between peak and basal luteinizing hormone (35).

Gastrointestinal and Nutritional Evaluation

In children with HIV infection and FTT we divide the gastrointestinal and nutritional workup into two parts. The first part is an assessment of body composition and nutritional status through anthropometric measurements, records of caloric/nutrient intake, and measurement of biochemical indexes of nutritional and hydration status. The second part is an assessment of gastrointestinal function. Stool and blood specimens are examined to exclude malabsorption and/or enteric infection. Stool pH, random fat, α_1-antitrypsin, trypsin, culture, leukocyte, and ova and parasite examination are recommended. A stool with pH of <6.0 suggests either intestinal bacterial activity or malabsorbed carbohydrates. Malabsorption of sugars such as glucose and lactose can be detected by testing for reducing substances. Conditions that produce osmotic diarrhea will require breath hydrogen measurements and tolerance tests for diagnosis. A 72-hr VanGen Kramer fat assay is also recommended if three fecal fats are positive. Liver function can be assessed by measuring liver enzymes, bile acid, albumin, prealbumin, direct and total bilirubin, prothrombin time, and partial thromboplastin time. Ultrasonography is recommended in suspected cases of biliary tract dysfunction (Table 31.2).

Metabolic Evaluation

No consistent metabolic derangement has been described in patients with AIDS. Because we hypothesize that a hypermetabolic state contributes to FTT in HIV-infected children, we quantitate REE and screen for abnormalities in calcium and bone, protein, lipid, and muscle metabolism (Table 31.2).

TREATMENT

Despite the fact that the etiology of FTT is unknown, several possible therapeutic interventions exist (Fig. 31.2). First, all attempts should be made to optimize nutritional status and treat opportunistic infections of the gastrointestinal tract that may lead to malabsorption and malnutrition. Nutritional status, growth, immune function, and resistance to opportunistic infections are interdependent in children with AIDS. Guidelines for nutritional support were recently summarized in a review that included clinical and laboratory parameters for nutritional assessment, as well as formulas to calculate adequate caloric intake (36). If caloric intake requires supplementation, oral high caloric feedings should be tried first. Megestrol acetate has been used to increase appetite, intake, and weight gain in adults with AIDS (37). Our experience using this agent is limited, but some children have shown temporary gains, especially when combined with high caloric oral supplements. Children with disrupted oral and esophageal integrity or oromotor function may benefit from enteral tube feedings. Nasogastric and gastrostomy tube

feedings have been efficacious in adults and some children with AIDS (38). Total parenteral nutrition is also effective but should be reserved as a last resort (24, 39). Finally, vitamin supplementation may benefit, particularly supplemental vitamin D in infants to prevent rickets.

Second, treatment with reverse transcriptase inhibitors in combination with nutritional intervention has improved growth and cellular and humoral immune responses in some children with AIDS. Which antiviral agents, either alone or in combination, are most efficacious and whether earlier vs. later treatment will improve growth and maintain anabolism is unknown. Some suggest that growth failure is significantly ominous to prompt administration of antiretroviral therapy even in the absence of other symptoms.

Third, aggressive treatment of concurrent opportunistic infections may lead to improved growth and weight gain (40).

Fourth, psychosocial factors and family social background influence the health, growth, and development of children with HIV infection. Many of these children come from families in which drug and alcohol abuse is common and where the parent or primary caretaker may also have HIV infection. Poverty and economic instability negatively affect parental nurturing behavior. Improvement in the home environment or transfer to foster homes has resulted in resolution of FTT in some children.

Fifth, although endocrine dysfunction is seldom if ever the sole cause for FTT in these children, its presence will contribute to their overall morbidity and should therefore not go unrecognized or untreated. A high index of suspicion and appropriate endocrine studies are needed to diagnose hypothyroidism, adrenal insufficiency, and growth hormone deficiency.

Treatment of hypothyroidism in children with AIDS consists of daily replacement with oral levothyroxine. Thyroid function tests should be monitored to ensure appropriate individualization of dosage, because thyroid hormone metabolism may be altered by the disease process or by other drugs.

Treatment of both types of adrenal insufficiency requires daily replacement with

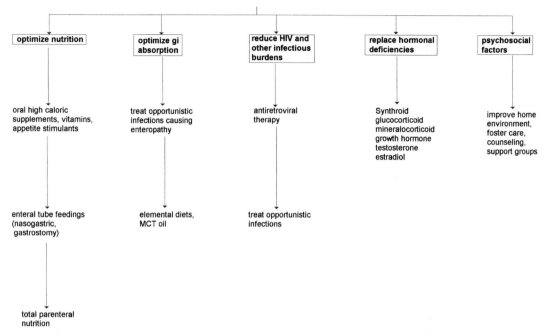

Figure 31.2.   Treatment of HIV-infected children with FTT. *MCT,* medium chain triglycerides.

oral glucocorticoid. Whereas secondary adrenal insufficiency requires only glucocorticoid replacement, primary adrenal insufficiency requires treatment with both glucocorticoid and mineralocorticoid. We use hydrocortisone (12–15 mg/m^2/day) and florinef (0.1–0.2 mg daily) to replace the deficient adrenal cortical hormones. Prednisone in equivalent dosage can also be used as an alternative to hydrocortisone. Adequacy of treatment should be monitored clinically by the absence of signs and symptoms of adrenal insufficiency or glucocorticoid excess. Adequate florinef dosage in primary adrenal insufficiency is confirmed by showing restoration of normal plasma renin activity. During times of stress, such as acute febrile illness, the dosage of glucocorticoid should be doubled to prevent development of adrenal crisis. Treatment of acute adrenal crisis involves expanding the blood volume with intravenous saline and replacing the deficient adrenal hormones with intravenous cortisol (100 mg/m^2, every 4–6 hr) and intramuscular desoxycorticosterone acetate (2–3 mg every 24 hr) until normal electrolytes and cardiovascular function are restored and standard oral steroid replacement can be resumed.

Treatment of growth hormone deficiency consists of administration of recombinant human growth hormone. However, because of the concern that growth hormone might promote viral replication, and the normal growth hormone levels in most patients, children with HIV infection have not received treatment with growth hormone. Aside from the linear growth-promoting effects, growth hormone is an anabolic agent and has been used to counteract catabolic states and restore positive nitrogen balance in children with burns and other chronic systemic illnesses. These anabolic effects may theoretically be beneficial for children with AIDS, and clinical trials of growth hormone therapy in these children should help resolve these issues. Until that time, however, parents inquiring about the use of growth hormone for children with AIDS and normal growth hormone levels should be told that the use of growth hormone remains experimental and without proven benefit.

Children with pubertal delay who have retarded maturation of the hypothalamic-pituitary-gonadal axis can be treated with exogenous sex steroids. We are treating adolescent boys with transfusion acquired

HIV infection with intramuscular testosterone enanthate. The starting dose is 50 mg every month for the first 6 months. The dose is increased to 100 mg every month for the next 6 months. This has resulted in the development of secondary sexual characteristics, an increase in muscularity, weight, and height velocity (without excessive advancement of the bone age), and an improvement in self-image. Although we have not yet treated any girls with exogenous sex steroids, our recommendation would be to administer ethinyl estradiol at an initial dose of 5 μg/day. This dose can be gradually increased over 3–4 years to a full replacement dose of 20 μg/day. At this point a progestin (Provera) should be added to induce withdrawal bleeding and prevent buildup of the endometrial lining.

PREVENTION

There is no definitive way to prevent FTT in children with HIV infection. However, with a more aggressive approach to diagnosis and therapy the incidence of growth failure appears to be declining. This may be related to optimizing nutrition, aggressive treatment of opportunistic infections, administration of antiretroviral agents, and intense supportive care to families. Until the etiologies of FTT are defined, all children should have their growth, development, and nutritional status closely monitored at regular intervals. Anthropometric measurements, coupled with determination of REE, body composition, and IGF-1 levels (which reflect nutritional state), may be able to detect when a child is becoming catabolic before clinical signs are evident. This may allow therapy to be modified or caloric intake to be supplemented to meet increased metabolic demands. Thyroid function tests should be performed every 6 months to diagnose subclinical hypothyroidism, and children with suspected endocrinopathies should undergo appropriate hormonal testing.

FUTURE RESEARCH

Normal growth is a complex process involving many interacting hormonal and nonhormonal factors. The mechanisms of action of growth factors are still incompletely understood, and, as in many endocrine systems, there are both stimulatory and inhibitory factors that modulate the actions of each other. Factors such as IGF-2, epidermal growth factor, fibroblast growth factor, transforming growth factor-β, and cytokines may modulate the growth-promoting actions of growth hormone, thyroid hormone, and IGF-1. Studies are needed to define the role of these growth factors and cytokines in children with HIV infection and to determine whether a state of resistance to growth factors is associated with HIV infection.

Recombinant human growth hormone has been used to enhance growth in children with growth hormone deficiency. Additionally, metabolic studies have shown that growth hormone has an anabolic effect on protein and muscle. Specifically, muscle mass increases, fat mass decreases, and adipose tissue is redistributed from a gynecoid to a more android pattern during growth hormone treatment.

Both growth hormone and IGF-1 appear to modulate the immune system, although the results of available studies are conflicting. Growth hormone treatment of growth hormone-deficient children was observed to decrease T helper to suppressor cell ratios, B cell fractions, phytohemagglutinin responsiveness, and natural killer activity (41–43). In contrast, other studies have shown growth hormone to have either no effect on the immune system (44–46) or to increase lymphocyte proliferation (47, 48) and natural killer cell activity (49, 50). In mice with severe combined immunodeficiency, growth hormone stimulates proliferation of T lymphocytes.

In vitro studies have shown growth hormone to have diverse effects on immune function, ranging from decreased lymphocyte and B cell proliferation (48) to augmented colony formation by human T cell lymphotropic virus-1 or human T cell lymphotropic virus-II transformed human T lymphocytes (51, 52). Administration of growth hormone to HIV-positive adults improved body composition, functional capacity, and reversed weight loss. However, immunologic enhancement in this group of patients has not been demonstrated.

Recombinant human IGF-1 has become available for diagnostic and therapeutic study. Studies in healthy adults established that doses up to 24 µg/kg/hr administered as a subcutaneous infusion does not cause hypoglycemia (53). In this study, IGF-1 increased glomerular filtration rate, renal plasma flow, creatinine clearance, and decreased urea nitrogen levels. Adults that were rendered catabolic through starvation tolerated a dose of 12 µg/kg/hr before experiencing hypoglycemia. Children with Laron-type dwarfism (growth hormone insensitivity syndrome) (54, 55), Mendenhall's syndrome (insulin-resistant diabetes mellitus caused by mutation of the insulin receptor) (56), insulin-dependent diabetes mellitus, and normal children have been treated with recombinant human IGF-1 without significant adverse effects. Current studies are underway to examine the long-term growth-promoting and metabolic effects of IGF-1 in Laron dwarfism and children with idiopathic short stature.

The in vivo and in vitro effects of IGF-1 on immune function are being studied. Administration of IGF-1 to diabetic rats reverses thymic atrophy (57) and increases thymic and splenic weights in hypophysectomized rats (58). Lymphocytes have receptors for IGF-1 and show proliferation and augmentation of colony formation in response to IGF-1. Other cell types, such as monocytes, hematopoietic precursor cells, and transformed or tumorigenic cells are also responsive to IGF-1. IGF-1 has been shown to stimulate replication of HIV; however, this action can be inhibited in vitro by addition of the antiretroviral agents zidovudine or dideoxyinosine.

Studies to determine whether children with HIV infection and FTT will benefit from addition of growth hormone or IGF-1 to antiretroviral therapy and nutritional support have been initiated by the National Cancer Institute Pediatric Branch.

References

1. Arico M, Azzini M, Caselli D, et al. AIDS: Outcome of children born to HTLV-III/LAV infected mothers. Helv Paediatr Acta 1986;41:477–486.
2. Rubinstein A, Sicklick M, Gupta A, et al. Acquired immunodeficiency with reversed T4/T8 ratios in infants born to promiscuous and drug-addicted mothers. JAMA 1983;249:2350–2356.
3. Rubinstein A. Acquired immunodeficiency syndrome in infants. Am J Dis Child 1983;137:815–817.
4. Scott GB, Buck BE, Leterman JG, et al. Acquired immuno-deficiency syndrome in infants. N Engl J Med 1984;310:76–80.
5. Shannon KM, Ammann AJ. Acquired immune deficiency syndrome in childhood. J Pediatr 1985;106:332–342.
6. Minkoff H, Nanda D, Menez R, Fikrig S. Pregnancies resulting in infants with acquired immunodeficiency syndrome or AIDS-related complex. Obstet Gynecol 1987;69:285–287.
7. Oleske JM, Minnefore A, Cooper R, et al. Immune deficiency syndrome in children. JAMA 1983;249:2345–2349.
8. McKinney RE Jr, Wilfert CM, Katz SL. The effect of human immunodeficiency virus (HIV) infection on the growth of children less than 24 months old. Pediatr Res 1992;31:170A.
9. Cowan M, Hellmann D, Chudwin D, et al. Maternal transmission of AIDS. Pediatrics 1984;73:382–386.
10. Lapointe N, Michand J, Pecovic D, et al. Transplacental transmission of HTLV III virus. N Engl J Med 1985;312:1325–1326.
11. Scott GG, Fischl MA, Klimas N, et al. Mothers of infants with the acquired immunodeficiency and asymptomatic carriers. JAMA 1985;256:363–366.
12. Rubinstein A. Pediatric AIDS. Curr Probl Pediatr 1986;16:361–409.
13. Jason, J, Gomperts E, Lawrence DN, et al. HIV and hemophiliac children's growth. J Acquir Immune Defic Syndr 1989;2:277–282.
14. Brettler DB, Forsberg A, Boliver E, Brewster F, Sullivan J. Growth failure as a prognostic indicator for progression to acquired immunodeficiency syndrome in children with hemophilia. J Pediatr 1990;117:584–588.
15. Melchior J, Salmon D, Rigaud D, et al. Resting energy expenditure is increased in stable, malnourished HIV-infected patients. Am J Clin Nutr 1991;53:437–441.
16. Laue L, Pizzo PA, Butler K, Cutler GB Jr. Growth and neuroendocrine dysfunction in children with acquired immunodeficiency syndrome. J Pediatr 1990;117:541–545.
17. Laue L, Pizzo PA, Cutler GB Jr. Mechanism of delayed puberty in adolescents with HIV infection. Pediatr Res 1992;30:79A.
18. Rapaport R, McSherry G, Connor E, et al. Growth and hormonal parameters in symptomatic human immunodeficiency virus (HIV) infected children [Abstract]. Pediatr Res 1989;25:187A.
19. Nelson JA, Wiley CA, Reynolds-Kohler C, et al. Human immunodeficiency virus detected from patients with gastrointestinal symptoms. Lancet 1988;1:259–262.
20. Ullrich R, Zeitz M, Heise W, L'age M, Höffken G, Riecken EO. Small intestinal structure and function in patients infected with human immunodeficiency virus (HIV): Evidence for HIV-induced enteropathy. Ann Intern Med 1989;111:15–21.

21. Smith PD, Lane HC, Gill JV, et al. Intestinal infections in patients with the acquired immunodeficiency syndrome (AIDS): Etiology and response to therapy. Ann Intern Med 1988;108:328–333.

22. Kotler DP, Gaetz HP, Lange M, Klein EB, Holt PR. Enteropathy associated with the acquired immunodeficiency syndrome. Ann Intern Med 1984;101:421–428.

23. Singer P, Katz DP, Dillon L, Kirvela O, Lazarus T, Askanazi J. Nutritional aspects of the acquired immunodeficiency syndrome. Am J Gastroenterol 1992;87:265–273.

24. Lane GP, Lucas CR, Smallwood RA. The gastrointestinal and hepatic manifestations of the acquired immunodeficiency syndrome. Med J Aust 1989;150:139–143.

25. Dworkin B, Wormser GP, Rosenthal WS, et al. Gastrointestinal manifestations of the acquired immunodeficiency syndrome: A review of 22 cases. Am J Gastroenterol 1985;80:774–778.

26. Garcia ME, Collins CL, Mansell PA. The acquired immune deficiency syndrome: Nutritional complications and assessment of body weight status. Nutr Clin Pract 1987;2:108–111.

27. Miller TL, Orav EJ, Martin SR, Cooper ER, McIntosh K, Winter HS. Malnutrition and carbohydrate malabsorption in children with vertically transmitted human immuno-deficiency virus 1 infection. Gastroenterology 1991;100:1296–1302.

28. Chlebowski RT, Grosvenor MB, Bernard NK, et al. Nutritional status, gastrointestinal dysfunction and survival in patients with AIDS. Am J Gastroenterol 1989;84:1288–1292.

29. Hommes MJT, Romijn JA, Godried MH, et al. Increased resting energy expenditure in HIV-infected men. Metabolism 1990;39:1186–1190.

30. Hommes MJT, Romijn JA, Endert E, Sauerwein HP. Resting energy expenditure and substrate oxidation in human immunodeficiency virus (HIV)-infected asymptomatic men: HIV affects host metabolism in the early asymptomatic stage. Am J Clin Nutr 1991;54:311–315.

31. Melchoir JC, Salmon D, Rigaud D, et al. Resting energy expenditure is increased in stable, malnourished HIV-infected patients. Am J Clin Nutr 1991;53:437–441.

32. Mintz M, Rapaport R, Oleske JM, et al. Elevated serum levels of tumor necrosis factor are associated with progressive encephalopathy in children with acquired immunodeficiency syndrome. Am J Dis Child 1989;143:771–774.

33. Greulich WW, Pyle SI. Radiographic atlas of skeletal development of the hand and wrist. 2nd ed. Stanford: Stanford University Press, 1959.

34. Rose SR, Ross JL, Uriarte M, et al. The advantage of measuring stimulated as compared with spontaneous growth hormone levels in the diagnosis of growth hormone deficiency. N Engl J Med 1988;319:201–207.

35. Oerter KE, Manasco P, Barnes KM, Jones J, Hill S, Cutler GB Jr. Adult height in precocious puberty after long-term treatment with Deslorelin. J Clin Endocrinol Metab 1991;73:1235–1240.

36. Nicholas SW, Leung J, Fennoy I. Guidelines for nutritional support of HIV-infected children. J Pediatr 1991;119:S59–S62.

37. Von Roenn JH, Murphy RL, Weber KM, Williams LM, Weitzman SA. Megestrol acetate for treatment of cachexia associated with human immunodeficiency virus (HIV) infection. Ann Intern Med 1988;109:840–841.

38. Kotler DP, Tierney AR, Ferraro R, et al. Enteral alimentation and repletion of body cell mass in malnourished patients with acquired immunodeficiency syndrome. Am J Clin Nutr 1991;53:149–154.

39. Kotler DP, Tierney AR, Culpepper-Morgan JA, Wang J, Peirson RN. Effect of home total parenteral nutrition on body composition in patients with acquired immunodeficiency syndrome. J Parenter Enter Nutr 1990;14:454–458.

40. Kotler DP, Tienrey AR, Altilio D, Want J, Pierson RN. Body mass repletion during ganciclovir treatment of cytomegalovirus infections in patients with acquired immunodeficiency syndrome. Arch Intern Med 1989;149:901–905.

41. Rapaport R, Oleska J, Ahdieh H, Solomon S, Delfaus C, Denny T. Suppression of immune function in growth hormone-deficient children during treatment with human growth hormone. J Pediatr 1986;109:434–439.

42. Kiess W, Doers H, Cutenandt O, Celohradsky BH. Lymphocyte subsets and natural killer activity in growth hormone deficiency. N Engl J Med 1986;314:321–322.

43. Petersen BH, Rapaport R, Henry DP, Huseman C, Moore WV. Effect of treatment with biosynthetic human growth hormone (GH) on peripheral blood lymphocyte populations and function in growth hormone-deficient children. J Clin Endocrinol Metab 1990;70:1756–1760.

44. Bozzola M, Maccario R, Cisternino M, et al. Immunological and endocrinological response to growth hormone therapy in short children. Acta Paediatr Scand 1988;77:675–680.

45. Etzioni A, Pollack S, Hochberg Z. Immune function in growth hormone-deficient children treated with biosynthetic growth hormone. Acta Paediatr Scand 1988;77:169–170.

46. Bozzola M, Cisternino M, Valtorta A, et al. Effect of biosynthetic methionyl growth hormone (GH) therapy on the immune function in GH-deficient children. Horm Res 1989;31:153–156.

47. Rapaport R, Oleske J, Ahdieh H, et al. Effects of human growth hormone on immune functions: In vitro studies on cells of normal and growth hormone-deficient children. Life Sci 1987;41:2319–2324.

48. Abbassi V, Bellanti JA. Humoral and cell-mediated immunity in growth hormone deficient children. Effect of therapy with human growth hormone. Pediatr Res 1985;19:299–301.

49. Bozzola M, Valtarta A, Moretta A, et al. In vitro and in vivo effect of growth hormone on cytotoxic activity. J Pediatr 1990;117:596–599.

50. Crist DM, Kraner JC. Supplemental growth hormone increases the tumor cytotoxic activity of natural killer cells in healthy adults with normal growth hormone secretion. Metabolism 1990;39:1320–1324.

51. Geffner ME, Golde DW, Lippe BM, Kaplan SA, Bersch N, Li CH. Tissues of the Laron dwarf are sensitive to insulin-like growth factor 1 but not to

growth hormone. J Clin Endocrinol Metab 1987; 64:1041–1046.

52. Geffner ME, Kaplan SA, Bersch N, et al. Leprechaunism: *In vitro* insulin action despite genetic insulin resistance. Pediatr Res 1987;22: 286–291.

53. Guler HP, Zapf J, Schmid C, Froesch ER. Effects of recombinant insulin-like growth factor 1 on insulin secretion and renal function in normal human subjects. Proc Natl Acad Sci USA 1989;86:2868–2872.

54. Laron Z, Klinger B, Silbergeld A, Lewin R, Erster B, Gil-Ad I. Intravenous administration of recombinant IGF-1 lowers serum GHRH and TSH. Acta Endocrinol (Copenh) 1990;123:378–382.

55. Walker JL, Ginalska-Malinowska M, Romer TE, Pucilowska JB, Underwood LE. Effects of the infusion of insulin-like growth factor 1 in a child with growth hormone insensitivity syndrome (Laron dwarfism). N Engl J Med 1990;324:1483–1488.

56. Quin J, Fisher BM, Paterson KR, Inoue A, Beastall GH. Acute response to recombinant insulin-like growth factor 1 in a patient with Mendenhall's syndrome. N Engl J Med 1990;323:1425–1426.

57. Binz K, Joller P, Frosesch P, Binz H, Zapf J, Froesch ER. Repopulation of the atrophied thymic in diabetic rats by insulin-like growth factor 1. Proc Natl Acad Sci USA 1990;87:3690–3694.

58. Guler HP, Zapf J, Scheiwiller E, Froesch ER. Recombinant human insulin-like growth factor 1 stimulates growth and has distinct effects on organ size in hypophysectomized rats. Proc Natl Acad Sci USA, 1988;85:4889–4893.

Hematological Problems and Their Management in Children with HIV Infection

Brigitta U. Mueller

Hematological abnormalities are found in many adult and pediatric patients with human immunodeficiency virus (HIV) infection. Involvement of the hematopoietic system tends to be more severe in advanced stages of the disease. Not only does this seriously worsen the clinical situation, but it can complicate the ability to administer therapy for HIV disease, opportunistic infections, and malignancies. It is difficult to distinguish primary HIV-related events and drug-associated toxicities. In some patients, only one hematopoietic cell line may be involved, but in other cases multilineage failure and even myelodysplasia may be found. The etiology of hematological problems in the HIV-infected patient includes the direct effect of HIV-1, opportunistic infections, drug toxicities, and, albeit rare in children, malignancies. Peripheral blood is an easily accessible source for diagnosis of the nutritional, infectious, and therapy-related problems that can directly affect the hematopoietic system. In some children a more extended evaluation, including bone marrow examination, may be necessary.

BONE MARROW ABNORMALITIES

Incidence

Morphologic changes are found in most bone marrow aspirates and biopsies obtained from adult patients with HIV infection (1–7). The most common abnormality is myelodysplasia, usually affecting the megakaryocytic and erythroid cell lines.

Dysplastic granulocytes, a maturation arrest, and abnormal and irregular nuclei can also be observed.

Etiology

Infection of early myeloid progenitor cells and megakaryocytes with HIV-1 has been demonstrated (8–10). Macrophages, which are an important component of the bone marrow microenvironment, and stromal fibroblasts that are derived from human bone marrow also have been shown to be infected with HIV in vitro and thus can transmit the virus to myeloid and lymphoid cell lines (11). An impaired in vitro growth of bone marrow cultures from HIV-infected patients has been described, as measured by significantly fewer colonies than derived from bone marrow cultures from uninfected controls (12–14). It has been postulated that this altered growth may be related to an antibody-mediated suppression or a defective modulation of progenitor cell growth that is normally conducted by helper cells (13, 14). Recent data have also implicated growth factors and hematopoietic cytokines in the development of bone marrow failure. In particular, elevated levels of transforming growth factor-β and tumor necrosis factor-α may have an inhibitory effect on the formation of hematopoietic progenitor cells (15).

Drug-induced bone marrow suppression can also be a problem for HIV-infected children. The dideoxynucleosides (azidothymidine (AZT), dideoxyinosine (ddI), and dideoxycytosine) can inhibit colony formation of erythroid and granulocyte-macrophage progenitor cells and stem cell colonies (16). Acyclovir, ganciclovir, or trimethoprim-sulfamethoxazole, used for the prevention or treatment of opportunistic infections, can also contribute to bone marrow suppression as can concomitant infections with *Mycobacterium avium-intracellulare* (MAI) or cytomegalovirus (CMV). Furthermore, when bone marrow suppression is observed, the possibility of an HIV-associated malignancy must also be considered (5).

Diagnosis

Bone marrow suppression should be considered in a child with a low reticulocyte count, persistent leukopenia, or thrombocytopenia and especially if more than one cell line is affected. The decision to further investigate these abnormalities is not so much dependent on absolute numbers than on clinical and laboratory findings combined. Evaluation of a child with bone marrow suppression requires a bone marrow examination. Both an aspirate and biopsy should be performed and the marrow should be cultured for mycobacteria and fungi.

ABNORMALITIES OF ERYTHROPOIESIS
Incidence

Anemia is the most common hematologic disorder observed in HIV-infected children. The reported incidence ranges between 16 and 94% and is related to the severity of HIV disease, the age group, and the use of antiretroviral therapy (17–22). It has been postulated that children with a hematocrit of <25% have a poor prognosis (20). The reticulocyte count is disproportionately low, and unlike in adults, where the anemia is typically normochromic and normocytic, children are more likely to have microcytosis (56%) and hypochromia (40%), possibly because of concurrent iron deficiency (20, 23–25). Macrocytosis, conversely, is most frequently associated with the use of AZT, and some centers use the degree of macrocytosis as a marker for drug compliance (26, 27).

Rouleaux formation and an elevated sedimentation rate are frequently observed. A positive direct (Coombs) antibody test is found in 18–100% of patients with AIDS, but is usually not associated with a significant degree of hemolysis (17, 20, 24, 28–30). Cold agglutinins, most often of anti-I specificity, are increased and can be correlated with elevated IgM levels, albeit independent of the overall disease state (28, 31, 32). We have recently cared for an infant who acquired a warm autoantibody causing life-threatening hemolytic transfusion reactions.

Etiology

Anemias observed in children with HIV infection are multifactorial, and hereditary conditions like sickle cell disease or the thalassemia syndromes must be considered. Treatable disorders of erythrocyte production include iron deficiency, which can be aggravated by repeated phlebotomy, occult intestinal blood loss, or nutritional deficiencies that accompany HIV infection in children. This is often difficult to differentiate from the so-called anemia of chronic disease.

Anemia with iron deficiency occurs in three stages: 1) low serum ferritin (iron stores decreased); 2) high iron binding capacity, low serum iron (loss of circulating iron); 3) low red cell indexes (MCV, MCH), low transferrin saturation, low hemoglobin (hemoglobin production decreased). Anemia that occurs with chronic infection is characterized by

- serum ferritin normal or elevated
- normal or decreased iron binding capacity
- red cell indexes usually normal
- low serum iron, low transferrin saturation, low hemoglobin.

In addition to iron, vitamin B_{12} (cobalamin) deficiency should be considered. This can present as a megaloblastic anemia with evidence of hypersegmented neutrophils. Subnormal serum vitamin B_{12} levels have been found in 20% of adult patients with AIDS; the association of this finding with hematologic disease is unclear

(33). Serum folate levels have not been studied extensively, but preliminary data in adult patients suggest that they may be within the normal range (33).

Pure red cell aplasia secondary to acute or persistent B19 parvovirus infection has been observed in some HIV-infected children and adults and should be considered when the red blood cell production rate is less than expected for the degree of anemia (34–36). Other myelosuppressive pathogens, such as MAI or CMV, usually cause neutropenia before the onset of clinically significant anemia. Impaired erythropoietin production can be found in patients with chronic inflammatory diseases or protein malnutrition. However, even very high levels of erythropoietin do not necessarily stimulate red cell production in children with HIV infection (37).

Hemoglobin levels below 7.5 g/dl have been observed in 24% of adult patients who received AZT at a dosage of 1500 mg/day (38). Even lower dosages of AZT (600 mg/day) have been associated with anemia in more than 25% of patients (39). Similarly, anemia has been found in 18–67% of children receiving AZT, and the degree and severity may be dose dependent (21, 26, 40).

Clinically significant hemolysis in patients with HIV infection appears to be quite rare (41). We have recently treated a child whose course of AIDS was complicated by a fatal hemolytic uremic syndrome. It is, however, important to remember that drug-induced hemolysis in patients with G6PD deficiency can occur with agents such as dapsone and other sulfonamides that are commonly used as a prophylaxis for *Pneumocystis carinii* pneumonia in HIV-positive patients.

Treatment

Treatment of iron deficiency anemia with ferrous sulfate (6 mg/kg/day) will result in a reticulocytosis after 1–2 weeks, and the hemoglobin will correct over 4–8 weeks. Patients with chronic anemia may require periodic packed red blood cell transfusions to maintain their hemoglobin level above 8 g/dl. Although the irradiation of blood products has not been recommended for HIV-infected patients, many centers administer CMV negative blood products to patients who are still CMV negative. Alternatively, erythropoietin (150 U/kg given 3 days per week s.c.) can be tried. Although data in children are limited, studies in adult HIV-infected patients have shown a significant decrease in transfusion requirement and an increase in mean hematocrit levels when the patient's baseline endogenous erythropoietin level was <500 IU/liter (42) (Tables 32.1).

ABNORMALITIES OF MYELOPOIESIS
Incidence

A white blood cell count of <3000 cells/mm³ has been observed in 26–38% of untreated pediatric patients, 19–41% of adults with AIDS-related complex, and in 57–76% of patients with AIDS (2, 19, 21, 24). A decrease in the total white blood cell

Table 32.1. Practical Guidelines for Diagnosis and Treatment of Anemia

Diagnosis
  Complete blood count with red blood cell indexes, description of morphology
  Reticulocyte count
  Serum iron, transferrin, ferritin
  Eliminate hereditary diseases (thalassemia syndromes, sickle cell disease)
  Optional: lactate dehydrogenase, haptoglobin, bone marrow aspirate or biopsy, erythropoietin level
Treatment
  Treat iron deficiency if present (6 mg elemental Fe/kg/day divided TID p.o. for at least 3 months)
  If patient is symptomatic or has a hemoglobin of <8 g/dl transfuse with 10–15 ml/kg packed red blood cells
  In the case of recurrent transfusion requirement (more than 2 per month) or if transfusion not possible (e.g., for religious reasons): if on AZT, consider dose reduction to 120 mg/m² every 6 hr p.o., switch to another antiretroviral agent, or treat with erythropoietin 150–600 units/kg s.c. 3 days/week

count may be restricted to one cell line or may occur simultaneously with anemia and thrombocytopenia (43).

Neutropenia, defined as an absolute neutrophil count (ANC) of <1500 cells/mm^3, has been observed in 43% of previously untreated children with HIV infection (21). This can increase with progression of HIV disease or as a consequence of concurrent opportunistic infections. In a study of 100 HIV-infected children, neutropenia was observed in 34% of patients without an opportunistic infection and in 65% of those with opportunistic infections (20). Hyposegmentation of neutrophils, and a left shift with appearance of early myeloid precursors (i.e., promyelocytes, myelocytes, metamyelocytes) in the peripheral blood, is common. Monocytes can have cytoplasmic vacuoles and marked nuclear alterations, and monocytopenia is not infrequent. Several functional defects of the myeloid phagocytes have been described, including impaired bacterial killing, decreased chemotaxis, and decreased phagocytosis of *Candida albicans* (44, 45).

Lymphopenia (<800 cells/mm^3) occurs in 18% of adult patients with AIDS-related complex, but in 70% of patients with AIDS (46). Progressive depletion of CD4-positive T lymphocytes is one hallmark of HIV infection. Both total number of lymphocytes and absolute CD4 counts are age dependent, and infants and young children have higher numbers than adults (47). Both the absolute number and percentage of the CD4 cell counts are used to monitor progression of HIV disease, as indications for the initiation of antiretroviral therapy and *P. carinii* pneumonia prophylaxis, and to assess the risk for development of certain opportunistic infections such as MAI (48, 49) (see Chapter 16B).

Etiology

Although the dideoxynucleosides can improve the CD4 cell number and function (see Chapter 35), these drugs can also have myelotoxicity. The currently recommended AZT dose for children of 180 mg/m^2 every 6 hr orally has been associated with neutropenia (ANC < 750 cells/mm^3) in 48% of the children (40). When neutropenia develops, it is generally recommended that the dosage of AZT be reduced to 120 mg/m^2 or even 90 mg/m^2 every 6 hr. However, it must be cautioned that lower doses of AZT may prove suboptimal for children who have evidence of, or who are at risk for, encephalopathy. In one study of oral AZT given at a dosage of 100 mg/m^2 every 6 hr, neutropenia was still a major side effect. A dose modification was necessary in 52% of the children, and 83% of those were for an ANC between 500 and 1000 cells/mm^3 (26). Myelosuppression is infrequent with dideoxycytidine or ddI. Other commonly prescribed drugs in children with HIV infection can have a myelosuppressive effect, most notably including trimethoprim-sulfamethoxazole, acyclovir, and ganciclovir. Finally, antineutrophil antibodies have been described in 10% of the patients with AIDS-related complex and in 35% of patients with AIDS; they may result in an increased peripheral destruction of white blood cells (50, 51).

Treatment

Although a neutrophil count of <500 cells/mm^3 is commonly associated with an increased risk for infectious complications in children and adults with cancer, this association is not clearly defined for HIV-infected children. Nonetheless, when a fever occurs in a neutropenic HIV-infected child it is still prudent to promptly initiate empirical broad spectrum antibiotics. A study in HIV-positive adult patients treated with AZT did not find a statistically significant difference in the incidence of bacterial infections with an ANC between 500 and 1000 cells/mm^3 or greater than 1000 cells/mm^3. However, with an ANC of <500 cells/mm^3, the incidence of bacterial infections was significantly higher ($P = 0.016$) (52).

Recently, cytokines have been used to treat neutropenia in patients with HIV infection. Both granulocyte-macrophage colony-stimulating factor (GM-CSF) and granulocyte-colony-stimulating factor (G-CSF) can partially correct the bactericidal defect of neutrophil function (44, 53). Although effective in rising the neutrophil count, there is concern that GM-CSF, when used in patients with HIV infection, will enhance viral replication as measured by serum p24 antigen levels. However, there is also evidence that the combination of AZT and GM-CSF is more effective than AZT alone in preventing the transfer and amplification of HIV in the target lymphocytes (54, 55). At the National Cancer Institute Pediatric Branch, we have evaluated the effect of subcutaneous G-CSF in 19 children who developed neutropenia, with an ANC of <800 cells/mm³, while receiving AZT despite dosage reductions to 120 mg/m² every 6 hr. We demonstrated that daily subcutaneous doses of recombinant G-CSF enabled children with AZT-related bone marrow suppression to continue to receive higher therapeutic doses of AZT. Median white blood cell counts increased from 2000 cells/mm³ before treatment to 4140 cells/mm³ after adding G-CSF ($P = 0.004$). ANC increased from a median of 1020 to 2960 cells/mm³ ($P = 0.0006$). There was marked individual variation in both the dose of G-CSF required to overcome neutropenia and the dose of AZT that was tolerated. With doses of G-CSF between 1 and 20 μg/kg/day, 17 of 19 patients could tolerate 120–180 mg/m² AZT every 6 hr. The only side effects were the development of a hematoma at the site of the injection in one hemophiliac, and a burning sensation with the injection in another child (56). However, the cost effectiveness and activity in patients with other causes of bone marrow suppression (e.g., MAI infection), as well as the potential for unanticipated side effects require further evaluation. In addition, the long-term effects of a chronic stimulation of hematopoietic progenitor cells with cytokines are unknown. We have observed one child with HIV infection and a concurrent severe myelodysplastic syndrome who developed bone marrow abnormalities resembling acute myeloid leukemia, with up to 30% blasts, during treatment with AZT and G-CSF. Of interest, this was completely reversible upon stopping G-CSF (Table 32.2).

ABNORMALITIES OF THROMBOPOIESIS
Incidence

The association of thrombocytopenia with HIV infection was established in 1982 and has since been observed in both children and adults as either an initial manifestation of AIDS or during the infection (57–63). A transient form of thrombocytopenia associated with the acute retroviral syndrome has been described in adults (64). Although there is no correlation between the severity of the thrombocytopenia and progression to AIDS, the incidence of thrombocytopenia is higher in more advanced stages of HIV infection. Studies show that it is a major complication in at least 10% of HIV-infected adults, and in our patient population at the National Cancer Institute we have found a platelet count of <50,000 cells/mm³ in 19% of the children (24, 43, 46, 61, 65). Thrombocytopenia has also been described in HIV-infected infants (59, 66–68).

The risk for severe bleeding appears to be higher in patients with HIV infection and thrombocytopenia, especially if the patient also suffers from hemophilia. In one study, 81% of the patients had clinically significant but not life-threatening bleeding episodes (62). The gravest risk of severe thrombocytopenia is intracranial hemorrhage. Although this has been observed in <1% of patients with non-HIV-associated thrombocytopenia, in the HIV-infected

Table 32.2. Practical Guidelines for Diagnosis and Treatment of Neutropenia

Diagnosis
  Complete blood count with differential, description of morphology
  Cultures for mycobacterial and viral infections
  Optional: bone marrow aspirate or biopsy for morphology and mycobacterial cultures
Treatment
  ANC 800–1500 cells/mm³: follow closely, stop, if possible, myelotoxic drugs other than AZT (e.g., trimethoprim-sulfamethoxazole, cephalosporins, acyclovir, ganciclovir, etc.)
  ANC <800 cells/mm³: if on AZT, consider dose reduction to 120 mg/m² every 6 hr p.o., switch to another antiretroviral agent, or treat with G-CSF (1–20 mg/kg/day s.c.)

hemophiliac the risk may be as high as 15–36% (62, 63, 66, 69, 70).

Etiology

Pathophysiology of the thrombocytopenia that occurs in children with HIV infection is not well understood. Increased destruction of platelets by immune-mediated mechanisms, similar to that observed in classical immune thrombocytopenic purpura (ITP), may be an explanation. ITP is characterized by severe thrombocytopenia, in which the bone marrow aspirate shows abundant megakaryocytes, usually without other symptoms (63). There is evidence that increased levels of antibody and complement can be found on platelets of HIV-infected patients with and without thrombocytopenia (71–73). At least a portion of these platelet associated IgG antibodies appear to be HIV-1 specific (74). The presence of platelet associated IgG and complement may accelerate platelet destruction by facilitating the recognition of platelets by the reticuloendothelial system. Although studies of platelet life span have been limited, the fact that high dose intravenous immunoglobulins can temporarily overcome the thrombocytopenia may be attributed to Fc receptor blockade of binding sites in the reticuloendothelial system.

In some patients with thrombocytopenia there may be a decreased production of platelets or megakaryocytes. Because megakaryocytes express the CD4 receptor, their infection with HIV is possible, and in situ hybridization has demonstrated viral RNA in megakaryocytes of HIV-infected patients with thrombocytopenia (9, 10, 75). There have also been reports of structural changes of megakaryocytes, and a lack of compensatory megakaryopoiesis in vitro, possibly caused by an inadequately low local GM-CSF production (76, 77).

Thrombotic thrombocytopenic purpura, characterized by thrombocytopenia, microangiopathic anemia, renal abnormalities, neurological signs, and fever, has been described in a few HIV-infected patients, mainly adults. At present, the significance of the association between thrombotic thrombocytopenic purpura and HIV infection remains to be determined (78, 79).

Finally, thrombocytopenia can be observed during episodes of acute illness (e.g., sepsis with disseminated intravascular coagulopathy) that can accompany HIV infection or in association with the frequent use of heparin to flush central venous catheters. These latter processes usually resolve once the problem is recognized and treated (80).

Treatment

Treatment of HIV-associated thrombocytopenia in children has not been adequately studied. Several reports indicate that ~50–60% of adult patients with HIV-associated thrombocytopenia will have an initial response to treatment with AZT, but the time to response may be prolonged and highly variable (81–84). In the National Cancer Institute study of ddI, a sustained improvement of the platelet count in three children with refractory thrombocytopenia was observed (19).

Corticosteroids, commonly used in the treatment of classic ITP, have a 40–60% initial response rate in HIV-infected individuals, but relapses are common after tapering (70). Although there is appropriate concern regarding further immunosuppression with steroids in an already vulnerable host, a recent study did not demonstrate any deleterious side effects when a short course of corticosteroids was given to children with HIV infection (85).

Although splenectomy can result in an immediate rise of platelets postoperatively in all patients, a long-term elevation is sustained in only 40–60% of the patients. At the same time, splenectomy is associated with a substantial risk for overwhelming sepsis with encapsulated bacterial organisms (61, 86).

Intravenous immunoglobulins achieve a rapid response in most thrombocytopenic patients, but the duration may only be transient (70, 87). Doses between 0.4 and 2 g/kg/dose have been given over 2–5 days with comparable results. Although well suited for emergency situations, this treatment is also expensive when given on a chronic basis.

Another approach is the use of anti-D preparations, which contain a larger proportion of aggregated IgG than intravenous immunoglobulins, and have a greater inhibitory effect on Fc receptors (88). Oksenhendler et al. (89) used a commercially available intravenous preparation of anti-D immunoglobulin in 14 Rh+ patients with HIV-related thrombocytopenia. All patients had mild evidence for hemolysis, and one patient experienced severe hemolysis with a drop of the hemoglobin from 12.4 to 7.4 g/dl. Bussel et al. (90) reported the successful treatment of 43 patients with ITP, including 20 children, with an anti-D product prepared for intravenous use (Winrho). This study included three children and 14 adults who were HIV-positive. A study evaluating the efficacy of antiretroviral therapy with or without anti-D for the treatment of thrombocytopenia in HIV-infected children is underway at the National Cancer Institute (Table 32.3).

ABNORMALITIES OF COAGULATION

Incidence

Circulating anticoagulants are frequently observed in HIV-infected patients but are rarely of clinical relevance. A lupus anticoagulant, as seen in other immune disorders, neoplasms, chronic infections, and several drug therapies, has been described in up to 70% of adult patients with HIV infection and presents as a prolonged partial thromboplastin time and an increased dilute Russell's viper venom clotting time assay (91–93). Another group of anticoagulants are the anticardiolipin antibodies that, like lupus anticoagulants, occur more frequently in patients with concurrent opportunistic infections (94). In the absence of other defects of the coagulation system, it is rare to see hemorrhagic problems associated with lupus anticoagulants and anticardiolipin antibodies, but thrombotic events have been described in HIV-negative individuals. Note that there have been two reports of a heparin-like anticoagulant leading to severe bleeding (95, 96). In one case the prolonged prothrombin time and partial thromboplastin time were corrected by the administration of protamine sulfate. In the other case, which was associated with vasculitis, the heparin-like anticoagulant was resistant to protamine sulfate, and the patient was successfully treated with methyl prednisolone and aminocaproic acid.

Although hemophiliacs constitute only 4% of the children younger than 13 years with AIDS, they comprise 35% of all adolescents between ages 13 and 19 years reported to the Centers for Disease Control through December 1992 (97). The HIV-infected child with hemophilia does not seem to be at an increased risk for bleeding in the absence of thrombocytopenia, but intracranial hemorrhages are more frequent in the thrombocytopenic hemophiliac patient (62). In addition it has recently been recognized that bleeding tendency and platelet function can be markedly abnormal in hemophiliacs who are treated with AZT and ibuprofen simultaneously (98).

Etiology

Deficiency of the vitamin K dependent factors II, VII, IX, and X is relatively common and most often caused by enteropathy, including that associated with antibiotics. This can easily be corrected with oral or parenteral vitamin K.

Table 32.3. Practical Guidelines for Diagnosis and Treatment of Thrombocytopenia

Diagnosis
    Complete blood count with platelet count
    Bone marrow aspirate and biopsy
Treatment
    Platelet count >50,000 cells/mm^3: follow closely
    Platelet count 20,000–50,000 cells/mm^3: follow closely, if on AZT consider switch to ddI, if
        hemophiliac treat as if platelet count was lower (see below)
    Platelet count <20,000 cells/mm^3: treat with intravenous immunoglobulin for 1–5 days
        (0.4–1 g/kg/day)
    If unsuccessful or if hemorrhagic complications occur: consider treatment with anti-D infusion or treat
        with steroids for 3 weeks (1–2 mg/kg day) or consider splenectomy in a child older than 5 years

Disseminated intravascular coagulopathy has been described as a complication of fulminant infectious conditions, but there are no data to indicate that this complication occurs more frequently in HIV-infected individuals. However, we have recently documented two cases of low grade disseminated intravascular coagulopathy in association with the use of G-CSF that were reversible upon stopping the cytokine.

An iatrogenic coagulopathy is the hyperviscosity syndrome associated with the use of intravenous immunoglobulins, which has in one case resulted in temporary neurological symptoms (99). It is therefore recommended to use a slower infusion rate of intravenous immunoglobulin in children with very high levels of serum IgG (Table 32.4). Finally, there has been an isolated report of protein S deficiency found in 31% of 71 HIV-positive men. Two of these patients presented with extensive vascular thrombosis (100).

HEMATOLOGIC MALIGNANCIES

Only 2.1% of the 4249 children younger than 13 years who met the criteria for AIDS as of December 1992 had a malignancy as their AIDS-defining illness. Several case reports of malignancies associated with HIV infection in children have been published, with the most common cancer described being non-Hodgkin's lymphoma, either as a systemic disease or primary central nervous system tumor. In addition there have been a few case reports describing hematologic malignancies, mostly acute B cell lymphoblastic leukemias (101). A consensus in regard to treatment has not yet been reached, but intensive chemotherapy should be considered and, when indicated, be given in combination with cytokines (G-CSF, erythropoietin). For a more extensive discussion of malignancies in HIV-infected children see Chapter 32.

FUTURE RESEARCH

The pathophysiologic mechanisms of hematologic problems in the HIV-infected patient are still only partially understood. The question of whether bone marrow precursor cells are directly infected by HIV-1 or whether they are involved as innocent bystanders and are influenced by an altered microenvironment is the subject of intensive investigation. The dosing of potentially myelosuppressive drugs (AZT, ganciclovir, etc.) and the development of equally effective, but less toxic, drugs is being studied. Other cytokines, especially for the treatment of thrombocytopenia or in form of a stem cell factor that stimulates the growth of several cell lines, will hopefully soon be available for clinical trials (for more information see Chapter 36). Hematological problems must be studied in children because some adult manifestations of HIV infection may be irrelevant to children and because the pediatric patient may have age-specific findings and a different response to treatments.

Table 32.4.   Practical Guidelines for Diagnosis and Treatment of Coagulopathy

Diagnosis
    Platelet count, PT, PTT, TT, fibrinogen
    Optional: full coagulation profile, fibrin split
        products, bleeding time, bone marrow
        aspirate or biopsy
Treatment
    Eliminate iatrogenic causes (heparin
        contamination from central line)
    Vitamin K deficiency: treat with oral
        or parenteral vitamin K
    Lupus anticoagulant present: no intervention
        necessary
    Disseminated intravascular coagulopathy
        present: exclude iatrogenic cause (e.g., G-
        CSF), treat underlying disease (e.g., sepsis)

References

1. Harris CE, Biggs JC, Concannon AJ, Dodds AJ. Peripheral blood and bone marrow findings in patients with acquired immune deficiency syndrome. Pathology 1990;22:206–211.
2. Castella A, Croxson TS, Mildvan D, Witt DH, Zalusky R. The bone marrow in AIDS. A histologic, hematologic, and microbiologic study. Am J Clin Pathol 1985;84:425–432.
3. Geller SA, Muller R, Greenberg ML, Siegal FP. Acquired immunodeficiency syndrome. Distinctive features of bone marrow biopsies. Arch Pathol Lab Med 1985;109:138–141.
4. Gluckman RJ, Rosner F, Guarneri JJ. The diagnostic utility of bone marrow aspiration and biopsy in patients with acquired immunodeficiency syndrome. J Natl Med Assoc 1989;81:119–125.
5. Karcher DS, Frost AR. The bone marrow in human immunodeficiency virus (HIV)-related disease. Am J Clin Pathol 1991;95:63–71.

6. Osborne BM, Guarda LA, Butler JJ. Bone marrow biopsies in patients with the acquired immunodeficiency syndrome. Hum Pathol 1984;15:1048–1053.

7. Duggan MJ, Weisenburger DD, Sun NC, Purtilo DT. Bone marrow findings in immunodeficiency syndromes. Hematol Oncol Clin North Am 1988; 2:637–656.

8. Folks TM, Kessler SW, Orenstein JM, Justement JS, Jaffe ES, Fauci AS. Infection and replication of HIV-1 in purified progenitor cells of normal human bone marrow. Science 1988;242:919–922.

9. Zucker-Franklin D, Cao Y. Megakaryocytes of human immunodeficiency virus-infected individuals express viral RNA. Proc Natl Acad Sci USA 1989;86:5595–5599.

10. Louache F, Bettaieb A, Henri A, et al. Infection of megakaryocytes by human immunodeficiency virus in seropositive patients with immune thrombocytopenic purpura. Blood 1991;78:1697–1705.

11. Scadden DT, Zeira M, Woon A, et al. Human immunodeficiency virus infection of human bone marrow stromal fibroblasts. Blood 1990;76:317–322.

12. Leiderman IZ, Greenberg ML, Adelsberg BR, Siegal FP. Defective myelopoiesis in acquired immunodeficiency syndrome (AIDS). In: Acquired immunedeficiency syndrome. New York: Alan R. Liss, 1984:281–289.

13. Stella CC, Ganser A, Hoelzer D. Defective in vitro growth of the hematopoietic progenitor cells in the acquired immunodeficiency syndrome. J Clin Invest 1987;80:286–293.

14. Donahue RE, Johnson MM, Zon LI, Clark SC, Groopman JE. Suppression of in vitro haematopoiesis following human immunodeficiency virus infection. Nature 1987;326:280–283.

15. Geissler RG, Ottmann OG, Eder M, Kojouharoff G, Hoelzer D, Ganser A. Effect of recombinant human transforming growth factor beta and tumor necrosis factor alpha on bone marrow progenitor cells of HIV-infected persons. Ann Hematol 1991;62:151–155.

16. Ganser A, Greher J, Völkers B, Staszewsli S, Hoelzer D. Inhibitory effect of azidothymidine, 2'-3'-dideoxyadenosine, and 2'-3'-dideoxycytidine on in vitro growth of hematopoietic progenitor cells from normal persons and from patients with AIDS. Exp Hematol 1989;17:321–325.

17. Scott GB, Buck BE, Leterman JG, Bloom FL, Parks WP. Acquired immunodeficiency syndrome in infants. N Engl J Med 1984;310:76–81.

18. McKinney RE, Pizzo PA, Scott GB, et al. Safety and tolerance of intermittent intravenous and oral zidovudine therapy in human immunodeficiency virus-infected pediatric patients. J Pediatr 1990; 116:640–647.

19. Butler KM, Husson RN, Balis FM, et al. Dideoxyinosine in children with symptomatic human immunodeficiency virus infection. N Engl J Med 1991;324:137–144.

20. Ellaurie M, Burns ER, Rubinstein A. Hematologic manifestations in pediatric HIV infection: Severe anemia as a prognostic factor. Am J Pediatr Hematol Oncol 1990;12:449–453.

21. Pizzo PA, Eddy J, Falloon J, et al. Effect of continuous intravenous infusion of zidovudine (AZT) in children with symptomatic HIV infection. N Engl J Med 1988;319:889–896.

22. Tovo PA, De Martino M, Gabiano C, et al. Prognostic factors and survival in children with perinatal HIV-1 infection. Lancet 1992;339: 1249–1253.

23. Schneider DR, Picker LJ. Myelodysplasia in the acquired immune deficiency syndrome. Am J Clin Pathol 1985;84:144–152.

24. Perkocha LA, Rodgers GM. Hematologic aspects of human immunodeficiency virus infection: Laboratory and clinical considerations. Am J Hematol 1988;29:94–105.

25. Treacy M, Lai L, Costello C, Clark A. Peripheral blood and bone marrow abnormalities in patients with HIV related disease. Br J Haematol 1987;65:289–294.

26. Blanche S, Duliege A-M, Navarette MS, et al. Low-dose zidovudine in children with an human immunodeficiency virus type 1 infection acquired in the perinatal period. Pediatrics 1991;88:364–370.

27. Fischl MA, Richman DD, Hansen N, et al. The safety and efficacy of zidovudine (AZT) in the treatment of subjects with mildly symptomatic human immunodeficiency virus type 1 (HIV) infection. Ann Intern Med 1990;112:727–737.

28. Sandhaus LM, Scudder R. Hematologic and bone marrow abnormalities in pediatric patients with human immunodeficiency virus (HIV) infection. Pediatr Pathol 1989;9:277–288.

29. Toy PTCY, Reid ME, Burns M. Positive direct antiglobulin test associated with hyperglobulinemia in acquired immunodeficiency syndrome (AIDS). Acta Haematol 1985;19:145–150.

30. McGinniss MH, Macher AM, Rook AH, Alter HJ. Red cell autoantibodies in patients with acquired immune deficiency syndrome. Transfusion 1986; 26:405–409.

31. Pruzanski W, Roelcke D, Donnelly E, Lui L-C. Persistent cold agglutinins in AIDS and related disorders. Acta Haematol 1986;75:171–173.

32. Bolton-Maggs PHB, Rogan PD, Duguid JKM, Mutton KJ, Ball LM. Cold agglutinins in haemophiliac boys infected with HIV. Arch Dis Child 1991;66:732–733.

33. Burkes RL, Cohen H, Krailo M, Sinow RM, Carmel R. Low serum cobalamin levels occur frequently in the acquired immune deficiency syndrome and related disorders. Eur J Haematol 1987;38:141–147.

34. Griffin TC, Squires JE, Timmons CF, Buchanan GR. Chronic human parvovirus B19-induced erythroid hypoplasia as the initial manifestation of human immunodeficiency virus infection. J Pediatr 1991;118:899–901.

35. Parmentier L, Boucary D, Salmon D. Pure red cell aplasia in an HIV-infected patient. AIDS 1992; 6:234–235.

36. Frickhofen N, Abkowitz JL, Safford M, et al. Persistent B19 parvovirus infection in patients infected with human immunodeficiency virus type 1 (HIV-1): A treatable cause of anemia in AIDS. Ann Intern Med 1990;113:926–933.

37. Spivak JL, Barnes DC, Fuchs E, Quinn TC. Serum immunoreactive erythropoietin in HIV-infected patients. JAMA 1989;261:3104–3107.

38. Richman DD, Fischl MA, Grieco MH, et al. The toxicity of azidothymidine (AZT) in the treatment of patients with AIDS and AIDS-related complex. A double-blind, placebo-controlled trial. N Engl J Med 1987;317:192–197.

39. Fischl MA, Parker CB, Pettinelli C, et al. A randomized controlled trial of a reduced daily dose of zidovudine in patients with the acquired immunodeficiency syndrome. N Engl J Med 1990; 323:1009–1014.

40. McKinney RE, Maha MA, Connor EM, et al. A multicenter trial of oral zidovudine in children with advanced human immunodeficiency virus disease. N Engl J Med 1991;324:1018–1025.

41. Rapaport AP, Rowe JM, McMican A. Life-threatening autoimmune hemolytic anemia in a patient with the acquired immune deficiency syndrome. Transfusion 1988;28:190–191.

42. Fischl MA, Galpin JE, Levine JD, et al. Recombinant human erythropoietin for patients with AIDS treated with zidovudine. N Engl J Med 1990;322:1488–1493.

43. Rossi G, Gorla R, Stellini R, et al. Prevalence, clinical, and laboratory features of thrombocytopenia among HIV-infected individuals. AIDS Res Hum Retroviruses 1990;6:261–269.

44. Roilides E, Mertins S, Eddy J, Walsh TJ, Pizzo PA, Rubin M. Impairment of neutrophil chemotactic and bactericidal function in children infected with human immunodeficiency virus type 1 and partial reversal after in vitro exposure to granulocyte-macrophage colony-stimulating factor. J Pediatr 1990;117:531–540.

45. Ellis M, Gupta S, Galant S, et al. Impaired neutrophil function in patients with AIDS or AIDS-related complex: A comprehensive evaluation. J Infect Dis 1988;158:1268–1276.

46. Zon LI, Arkin C, Groopman JE. Haematologic manifestations of the human immune deficiency virus (HIV). Br J Haematol 1987;66:251–256.

47. Erkeller-Yuksel FM, Deneys V, Hannet I, et al. Age-related changes in human blood lymphocyte subpopulations. J Pediatr 1992;120:216–222.

48. McKinney RE, Wilfert CM. Lymphocyte subsets in children younger than 2 years old: Normal values in a population at risk for human immunodeficiency virus infection and diagnostic and prognostic application to infected children. Pediatr Infect Dis J 1992;11:639–644.

49. Denny T, Yogev R, Gelman R, et al. Lymphocyte subsets in healthy children during the first 5 years of life. JAMA 1992;267:1484–1488.

50. Ganser A. Abnormalities of hematopoiesis in the acquired immunodeficiency syndrome. Blut 1988;56:49–53.

51. McCance-Katz EF, Hoecker JL, Vitale NB. Severe neutropenia associated with anti-neutrophil antibody in a patient with acquired immunodeficiency syndrome-related complex. Pediatr Infect Dis J 1987;6:417–418.

52. Shaunak S, Bartlett JA. Zidovudine-induced neutropenia: Are we too cautious? Lancet 1989;2:91–92.

53. Roilides E, Walsh TJ, Pizzo PA, Rubin M. Granulocyte colony-stimulating factor enhances the phagocytic and bactericidal activity of normal and defective human neutrophils. J Infect Dis 1991;163:579–583.

54. Pluda JM, Yarchoan R, Smith PD, et al. Subcutaneous recombinant granulocyte-macrophage colony-stimulating factor used as a single agent and in an alternating regimen with azidothymidine in leukopenic patients with severe human immunodeficiency virus infection. Blood 1990;76:463–472.

55. Hammer SM, Gillis JM, Pinkston P, Rose RM. Effect of zidovudine and granulocyte-macrophage colony-stimulating factor on human immunodeficiency virus replication in alveolar macrophages. Blood 1990;75:1215–1219.

56. Mueller BU, Jacobsen F, Butler KM, Husson RN, Lewis LL, Pizzo PA. Combination treatment with azidothymidine and granulocyte colony-stimulating factor in children with human immunodeficiency virus infection. J Pediatr 1992;121:797–802.

57. Walsh CM, Nardi MA, Karpatkin S. On the mechanism of thrombocytopenic purpura in sexually active homosexual men. N Engl J Med 1984;311:635–639.

58. Morris L, Distenfeld A, Amorosi E, Karpatkin S. Autoimmune thrombocytopenic purpura in homosexual men. Ann Intern Med 1982;96:714–717.

59. Labrune P, Blanche S, Catherine N, Maier-Redelsperger M, Delfraissy JF, Tchernia G. Human immunodeficiency virus-associated thrombocytopenia in infants. Acta Paediatr Scand 1989;78:811–814.

60. Hollak CEM, Kersten MJ, van der Lelie J, Lange JMA. Thrombocytopenic purpura as first manifestation of human immunodeficiency virus type 1 (HIV-1) infection. Neth J Med 1990;37:63–68.

61. Landonio G, Galli M, Nosari A, et al. HIV-related severe thrombocytopenia in intravenous drug users: Prevalence, response to therapy in a medium-term follow-up, and pathogenic evaluation. AIDS 1990;4:29–34.

62. Ragni MV, Bontempo FA, Myers DJ, Kiss JE, Oral A. Hemorrhagic sequelae of immune thrombocytopenic purpura in human immunodeficiency virus-infected hemophiliacs. Blood 1990;75:1267–1272.

63. Ellaurie M, Burns ER, Bernstein LJ, Shah K, Rubinstein A. Thrombocytopenia and human immunodeficiency virus in children. Pediatrics 1988;82:905–908.

64. Karpatkin S. HIV-1-related thrombocytopenia. Hematol Oncol Clin North Am 1990;4:193–218.

65. Peltier J-Y, Lambin P, Doinel C, Couroucé A-M, Rouger P, Lefrere J-J. Frequency and prognostic importance of thrombocytopenia in symptom-free HIV-infected individuals: A 5-year prospective study. AIDS 1991;5:381–384.

66. Stuart MJ, Kelton JG. The platelet: Quantitative and qualitative abnormalities. In: Nathan DG, Oski FA, ed. Hematology of infancy and childhood. Philadelphia: WB Saunders, 1987:1343–1478.

67. Weinblatt ME, Scimeca PG, James-Herry AG, Pahwa S. Thrombocytopenia in an infant with AIDS [Letter]. Am J Dis Child 1987;141:15.

68. Rigaud M, Leibovitz E, Sin Quee C, et al. Thrombocytopenia in children infected with

human immunodeficiency virus: Long term follow-up and therapeutic considerations. J Acquir Immune Defic Syndr 1992;5:450–455.

69. Brusamolino E, Malfitano A, Pagnucco G, et al. HIV-related thrombocytopenic purpura: A study of 24 cases. Haematologica 1989;74:51–56.

70. Oksenhendler E, Bierling P, Farcet J-P, Rabian C, Seligmann M, Clauvel J-P. Response to therapy in 37 patients with HIV-related thrombocytopenic purpura. Br J Haematol 1987;66:491–495.

71. Ellaurie M, Burns ER, Rubinstein A. Platelet-associated IgG in pediatric HIV infection. Pediatr Hematol Oncol 1991;8:179–185.

72. Karpatkin S, Nardi M, Lennette ET, Byrne B, Poiesz B. Anti-human immunodeficiency virus type 1 antibody complexes on platelets of seropositive thrombocytopenic homosexuals and narcotic addicts. Proc Natl Acad Sci USA 1988;85:9763–9767.

73. Sthoeger D, Nardi M, Travis S, Karpatkin M, Karpatkin S. Micromethod for demonstrating increased platelet surface immunoglobulin G: Findings in acute, chronic, and human immunodeficiency virus-1-related immunologic thrombocytopenias. Am J Hematol 1990;34:275–282.

74. Karpatkin S. Autoimmune thrombocytopenia and AIDS-related thrombocytopenia. Curr Opin Immunol 1990;2:625–632.

75. Sakaguchi M, Sato T, Groopman JE. Human immunodeficiency virus infection of megakaryocytic cells. Blood 1991;77:481–485.

76. Zauli G, Re MC, Gugliotta L, et al. Lack of compensatory megakaryocytopoiesis in HIV-1-seropositive thrombocytopenic individuals compared with immune thrombocytopenic purpura patients. AIDS 1991;5:1345–1350.

77. Zucker-Franklin D, Termin CS, Cooper MC. Structural changes in the megakaryocytes of patients infected with the human immunodeficiency virus (HIV-1). Am J Pathol 1989;134:1295–1303.

78. Nair JMG, Bellevue R, Bertoni M, Dosik H. Thrombotic thrombocytopenic purpura in patients with the acquired immunodeficiency syndrome (AIDS)-related complex. Ann Intern Med 1988;109:209–212.

79. Leaf AN, Laubenstein LJ, Raphael B, Hochster H, Baez L, Karpatkin S. Thrombotic thrombocytopenic purpura associated with human immunodeficiency virus type 1 (HIV-1) infection. Ann Intern Med 1988;109:194–197.

80. Potter C, Cox J, Scott P, McFarland JG. Heparin-induced thrombocytopenia in a child. J Pediatr 1992;121:135–138.

81. Oksenhendler E, Bierling P, Ferchal F, Clauvel J-P, Seligmann M. Zidovudine for thrombocytopenic purpura related to human immunodeficiency virus (HIV) infection. Ann Intern Med 1989;110:365–368.

82. Swiss Group for Clinical Studies on the Acquired Immunodeficiency Syndrome (AIDS). Zidovudine for the treatment of thrombocytopenia associated with human immunodeficiency virus (HIV). Ann Intern Med 1988;109:718–721.

83. Hymes KB, Greene JB, Karpatkin S. The effect of azidothymidine on HIV-related thrombocytopenia. N Engl J Med 1988;318:516–517.

84. Rarick MU, Espina B, Montgomery T, Easley A, Allen J, Levine AM. The long-term use of zidovudine in patients with severe immune-related thrombocytopenia secondary to infection with HIV. AIDS 1991;5:1357–1361.

85. Saulsbury FT, Bringelsen KA, Normansell DE. Effects of prednisone on human immunodeficiency virus infection. South Med J 1991;84:431–435.

86. Ferguson CM. Splenectomy for immune thrombocytopenia related to human immunodeficiency virus. Surg Gynecol Obstet 1988;167:300–302.

87. Pollak AN, Janinis J, Green D. Successful intravenous immune globulin therapy for human immunodeficiency virus-associated thrombocytopenia. Arch Intern Med 1988;148:695–697.

88. Boughton BJ, Chakraverty RK, Simpson A, Amith N. The effect of anti-Rho (D) and non-specific immunoglobulins on monocyte Fc receptor function: The role of high molecular weight IgG polymers and IgG subclasses. Clin Lab Haematol 1990;12:17–23.

89. Oksenhendler E, Bierling P, Brossard Y, et al. Anti-Rh immunoglobulin therapy for human immuno-deficiency virus-related immune thrombocytopenic purpura. Blood 1988;71:1499–1502.

90. Bussel JB, Graziano JN, Kimberly RP, Pahwa S, Aledort LM. Intravenous anti-D treatment of immune thrombocytopenic purpura: Analysis of efficacy, toxicity, and mechanism of effect. Blood 1991;77:1884–1893.

91. Bloom EJ, Abrams DI, Rodgers G. Lupus anticoagulant in the acquired immunodeficiency syndrome. JAMA 1986;256:491–493.

92. Cohen H, Mackie IJ, Anagnostopoulos N, Savage GF. Lupus anticoagulant, anticardiolipin antibodies, and human immunodeficiency virus in haemophilia. J Clin Pathol 1989;42:629–633.

93. Burns ER, Krieger B-Z, Bernstein L, Rubinstein A. Acquired circulating anticoagulants in children with acquired immunodeficiency syndrome. Pediatrics 1988;82:763–765.

94. Canoso RT, Zon LI, Groopman JE. Anticardiolipin antibodies associated with HTLV-III infection. Br J Haematol 1987;65:495–498.

95. Bernard E. Dellamonica P, Michiels JF, et al. Heparin-like anticoagulant vasculitis associated with severe primary infection by HIV. AIDS 1990; 4:932–933.

96. de Prost D, Katlama C, Pialoux G, Karsenty-Mathonnet F, Wolff M. Heparin-like anticoagulant associated with AIDS [Letter]. Thromb Haemost 1987;57:239.

97. Centers for Disease Control. HIV/AIDS Surveillance Rep 1993;Jan:1–22.

98. Ragni MV, Miller BJ, Whalen R, Ptachcinski R. Bleeding tendency, platelet function, and pharmacokinetics of ibuprofen and zidovudine in HIV (+) hemophilic men. Am J Hematol 1992;450: 176–182.

99. Hague RA, Eden OB, Yap PL, Mok JYQ, Rae P. Hyperviscosity in HIV infected children—a potential hazard during intravenous immunoglobulin therapy. Blut 1990;61:66–67.

100. Lafeuillade A, Alessi M-C, Poizot-Martin I, et al. Protein S deficiency and HIV infection [Letter]. N Engl J Med 1991;324:1220.

101. Montalvo FW, Casanova R, Clavell LA. Treatment outcome in children with malignancies associated with human immunodeficiency virus infection. J Pediatr 1990;116:735–738.

33

Malignancies in Children with HIV Infection

Brigitta U. Mueller, Aziza T. Shad, Ian T. Magrath, and Marc E. Horowitz

Although cancer is a rare disorder in childhood, it still constitutes the second leading cause of death in children beyond infancy in the United States. The annual incidence of all malignant tumors in children younger than 15 years is ~130/million, the most common of which are acute leukemias and brain tumors (1). Although the cause for most pediatric malignancies is unknown, immunodeficiency increases the risk for cancer, as has been well demonstrated in hereditary disorders such as Wiskott-Aldrich syndrome and ataxia-telangiectasia and the iatrogenic immunosuppression after organ transplantation (2, 3). This association between immunodeficiency and the risk for cancer has been defined in adults with AIDS, both by the high incidence of Kaposi's sarcomas in young homosexual men as well as an unusual number of high grade non-Hodgkin's lymphomas (NHL) that have been observed (4, 5). Indeed, it has been postulated that up to 40% of adult human immunodeficiency virus (HIV)-infected patients will develop a malignancy at some point (6). However, estimates of cancer incidence vary widely, possibly because the studies have described different subgroups of the HIV-infected population (7, 9). For example, Kaposi's sarcoma occurs in >20% of homosexual men but only in 1% of hemophiliacs with HIV infection and is rare in children and women (10). About 13–15% of the adult HIV-infected patients have a malignancy (i.e., NHL or Kaposi's sarcoma) as their AIDS indicator disease (11).

Of the 4249 children under the age of 13 years who met the criteria for AIDS as of

December 1992, 88 or 2.1% had a malignancy as their AIDS-defining illness; 21 children were reported to have Kaposi's sarcoma and 67 NHL (CDC, verbal communication, 1993). A multicenter study from Italy reported seven malignancies, four cases of NHL, one case each of Kaposi's sarcoma, hepatoblastoma, and acute B cell lymphoblastic leukemia among 1321 children with HIV infection (13). Since the first report of Kaposi's sarcoma in two infants with AIDS in 1983, several case reports of malignancies associated with HIV infection in children have been published (14). The most common cancer described is NHL, either as a systemic disease or as a primary central nervous system (CNS) tumor (13, 15–23). Kaposi's sarcoma remains rare in children, but an increased incidence of soft tissue tumors, a cancer that is rarely associated with immunodeficiency (except after organ transplantation), has been observed (24, 25).

Several possible mechanisms by which HIV infection predisposes patients to neoplastic diseases are being investigated. Suppression or loss of immune surveillance presumably is crucial, and the constant stimulation by virus or other infections may be a cofactor. Patients with HIV infection have not only profound cellular and humoral immune suppression and dysfunction but tend to be infected with other potentially oncogenic viruses such as human T cell lymphotropic virus types 1 and 2, cytomegalovirus, Epstein-Barr virus (EBV), human papilloma virus (HPV), and hepatitis B virus (26, 27). HIV-induced production of growth factors like interleukin-1, interleukin-6, and tumor necrosis factor may also sustain uncontrolled proliferation of malignant cells (28). Retroviruses can introduce activated proto-oncogenes or insert inactivational pieces of tumor suppressor genes, or they may insert a viral promoter near normal cellular genes, which leads to amplification of a normal cellular product and to transformation (29).

This chapter summarizes current understanding of the clinical and biologic features of lymphoid malignancies, Kaposi's sarcoma, and soft tissue tumors in patients with HIV infection and will discuss the occurrence of some other tumors that may be associated with AIDS. However, just as cancer in the non-HIV-infected child differs significantly from cancer in the adult, and the clinical manifestations of HIV infection differ between children and adults, one can be certain that this will also be true for cancer and perhaps the tolerance of cancer treatment in the HIV-infected child. Investigators involved in the care of children with HIV infection must develop specific protocols to evaluate and treat cancer with the goal of characterizing the problems and learning how they can be most effectively managed.

LYMPHOID MALIGNANCIES
Clinical Manifestations

An increased incidence of malignant lymphomas in HIV-infected patients was first noted in 1984 (5). In 1985 primary lymphomas of the brain and Burkitt's or immunoblastic lymphomas were included as AIDS indicator diagnoses in the revised definition for AIDS (30, 31). In 1992 NHL was the AIDS indicator disease in 3.4% of the adults and in 0.8% of the children reported to the CDC (11). This number underestimates the true incidence, because NHL often occurs after the diagnosis of AIDS has been made and is therefore not reported.

Adults

It is estimated that the incidence of NHL in adults is about 60 times greater in persons with AIDS than in the general population. However, primary lymphoma of the brain and Burkitt's lymphoma, rare in

adults, are at least 1000 times more frequent in people with AIDS than in non-HIV-infected people (32). Between 8 and 27% of all cases of NHL that occur per year in the United States are thought to arise as a consequence of HIV infection (33). In a group of patients with symptomatic HIV disease enrolled on antiretroviral treatment protocols, Pluda and coworkers (8) found an estimated probability of developing a lymphoma of 28.6% by 30 months of therapy and 46.4% by 36 months. An additional study of 1030 patients showed an incidence of 2.3% after 2 years of azidothymidine therapy and a stable hazard of developing NHL of 0.8% for each additional 6 months on therapy (34). Risk for the development of a lymphoid malignancy is inversely related to the number of circulating CD4 cells, and in adults a marked increase was noted in the National Cancer Institute study once the CD4 count falls below 50 cells/mm^3 (8).

Hodgkin's disease shows a bimodal distribution with an early peak during young adulthood, when HIV disease is also most prevalent. Until recently it has been unclear whether the incidence of Hodgkin's disease is increased in HIV-infected adults. In a recent study of HIV-infected homosexual men an excess incidence of 19.3 cases/100,000 person-years was documented (35). The ratio of NHL to Hodgkin's disease appears to be influenced by the route of acquisition of HIV disease, with a ratio of 2:1 for intravenous drug users and a ratio of 12.4:1 in homosexual men (35, 36).

Children

Recently, a 360-fold increase of NHL in HIV-infected children younger than 19 years has been reported (32). However, in the United States 97% of the NHL in the non-HIV-infected population are diagnosed in patients older than 20 years, and the incidence rate shows a steady increase with age. This pattern is also seen in HIV-infected patients, as shown by Beral et al. (32). Hodgkin's disease, however, is rare in children younger than 15 years. Because over 85% of infected children acquired HIV disease perinatally and their course of progression to death is usually fairly rapid, this may explain the relatively small number of lymphoid malignancies observed in HIV-infected children. However, as children survive for longer periods because of antiretroviral and supportive therapy, an increase number of NHL cases may well be observed.

Non-Hodgkin's Lymphoma

HIV-associated NHLs are predominantly high grade B cell tumors, have a high frequency of extranodular site involvement, and behave clinically aggressively (Table 33.1). They can present as a systemic process that often exhibits secondary subarachnoid CNS involvement or as an isolated primary intraparenchymal CNS lymphoma without systemic spread.

Systemic NHL

Approximately 57% of HIV-infected adult patients diagnosed with NHL already have AIDS (37). Extranodal sites are involved in most patients (87%), and ~34% have bone marrow infiltration at the time of diagnosis (5, 37). Other commonly involved extranodal sites are the gastrointestinal tract, liver, CNS, lungs, and bone, but almost any organ can be affected (5, 37, 38). NS involvement, seen in one autopsy series in 66%, is generally leptomeningeal (38). Fever, drenching night sweats, and weight loss of at least 10% of body weight ("B symptoms") have been described in 45–82% of the patients (39, 40).

The spectrum of histologic appearances of these lesions is very different from that usually seen in non-HIV-infected adults with NHL and resembles that common to children with NHL. For example, high grade malignant tumors comprise ~65% of these cases, intermediate grade 30%, and low grade tumors only 7% of HIV-associated NHL (5, 37). Most are histologically and immunophenotypically consistent with B cell origin (37, 41). Diffuse NHL with small noncleaved cell, large cell immunoblastic, or diffuse large cell histologies account for almost 80% of the tumors (5). Although most NHLs in the HIV-infected adult are of B cell origin, there have been a few case reports of T cell tumors, one of them a Ki-1+ anaplastic large cell lymphoma (42–45). Pediatric system NHL in the context of HIV infection has been documented in several case reports (13, 15–18, 46). All tumors were of B cell origin, and several presented as leukemias with extensive bone marrow involvement.

Therapy of adults with HIV infection and systemic NHL has had a poor rate of success. HIV-associated NHL is highly aggressive, with short survival after diagnosis despite intervention. Most chemotherapy protocols used have been relatively intensive, using modified COMP-regimens (cyclophosphamide, vincristine, methotrexate, and prednisone), PROMACE-MOPP (prednisone, methotrexate, doxorubicin, cyclophosphamide, etoposide-mechlorethamine, vincristine, prednisone, and procarbazine) or M-BACOD (methotrexate, bleomycin, adriamycin, cyclophosphamide, vincristine, and dexamethasone) (37, 39). Most regimens resulted in a median survival of only 5–6 months, with death often caused by intercurrent opportunistic infections (5, 37, 47). In fact, the more intensive protocols were associated with worse outcome (48). Survival rate clearly depends on several HIV-related factors: performance status, history of AIDS before diagnosis of lymphoma, and CD4 cell count. A Karnofsky perfor-

Table 33.1.   NHL in Immunocompetent vs. HIV-infected Patient

Immunocompetent	HIV Infected
CNS primary rare	CNS primary common
Low to intermediate grade in adults	High grade in adults
High grade in children	High grade in children
Extranodal sites uncommon	Extranodal sites common
T or B cell origin	B cell origin
14;18 translocations most frequent	8;14 translocations most frequent

mance status of <70% and a CD4 count of <100 cells/mm³ independently predict a worse prognosis (39, 40, 49). Bone marrow involvement at presentation is also associated with poor outcome (39). Because of the high incidence of opportunistic infections, low dose chemotherapy regimens in conjunction with bone marrow stimulating cytokines have recently been initiated. Levine et al. (50) reported a complete response rate of 46% with a median survival of 15 months in patients treated with a low dose modification of the M-BACOD regimen in combination with CNS prophylaxis and zidovudine maintenance therapy. Opportunistic infections occurred in 21% of the treated patients.

We and others have cared for HIV-infected children with NHL who tolerated chemotherapy (including most commonly cytoxan, methotrexate, vincristine, and prednisone) fairly well and who survived for up to 2 years and longer (18, 20, 46, 51). The National Cancer Institute Pediatric Branch is investigating a protocol that includes three cycles of cyclophosphamide and methotrexate, as well as intrathecal methotrexate and cytarabin for the treatment of NHL in HIV-infected children.

This protocol also includes granulocyte-colony stimulating factor to shorten neutropenia as well as concurrent antiretroviral therapy with zidovudine and didanosine.

CNS Lymphoma

Primary CNS lymphomas account for 4–40% of the NHL in HIV-infected adults (32, 38). Patients with primary CNS lymphoma commonly are symptomatic for several weeks before diagnosis. Confusion, lethargy, memory loss, seizures, hemiparesis, or other focal neurologic signs are described (23, 52–55). Computed tomographic brain scanning demonstrates an isodense or hypodense single lesion that enhances with contrast, although multiple lesions may be present (21, 22, 56). Magnetic resonance imaging is equally sensitive for diagnosing these lesions. Representative computed tomography and magnetic resonance imaging images of a CNS lymphoma are illustrated in Figure 33.1. Differential diagnosis of a parenchymal brain lesion in a patient with HIV infection includes neoplasm (usually lymphoma), infection (usually toxoplasmosis), and hemorrhage. Primary malignant lymphomas of the brain

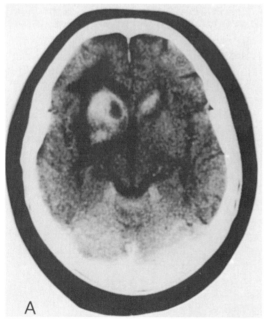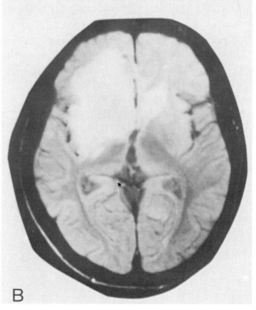

Figure 33.1. NHL of CNS (right frontoparietal region) in an HIV-infected child. **A**, contrast-enhanced computed tomography scan. **B**, T2 weighted magnetic resonance imaging scan.

have been described in children with AIDS, and through December 1992 the CDC documented 14 cases of primary CNS lymphoma listed as AIDS indicator disease in children younger than 13 years (12, 19, 22, 23, 56). Clinical, histological, and radiographic findings are similar to the adult population. However, in children in the United States, where CNS toxoplasmosis is very rare, the most likely diagnosis of a intraparenchymal brain lesion is lymphoma. Abnormalities of cerebrospinal fluid examinations with mild mononuclear pleocytosis, slightly elevated protein, and sometimes decreased glucose have been described (53, 55). Malignant cells were found in ~25% of the patients in whom it was considered safe to perform a lumbar puncture.

The CNS lymphomas in HIV-infected patients are intracranial intraparenchymal tumors characterized by frequent histological multifocality, indistinct borders, and often an angiocentric arrangement (52, 53). They are generally high grade tumors, mostly large cell immunoblastic lymphomas (in 45%), and small noncleaved lymphomas (in 36%) (19, 48). Most tumors are of B cell origin, and there is a strong association with EBV infection, as discussed below.

HIV-infected patients with primary NHL of the CNS have a poor prognosis, and often diagnosis is only made at the time of autopsy (38). Treatment of CNS lymphoma, unsuccessful in most cases arising in the general population, is similarly ineffective in patients with HIV infection. In a series of eight patients treated with cranial irradiation, six patients that received at least 4000 rad responded completely and one partially (52). Two of the complete responders were free of recurrence 8 and 14 months from treatment, two relapsed at 7 and 16 months, and two died of opportunistic infections. Other reports confirm the poor prognosis of patients with CNS lymphoma, with most dying of either progressive lymphoma or opportunistic infections. The median survival after onset of symptoms is between 1.7 and 5.5 months (52, 53). As many of these patients have multifocal disease histologically, whole brain irradiation should be considered. There is little published experience with the use of systemic chemotherapy for the treatment of CNS lymphoma. In a recent report,

a retrospective review of 35 patients with CNS lymphoma (only one had HIV infection) demonstrated no survival advantage for the patients who received chemotherapy in addition to radiotherapy (55).

Hodgkin's Disease

The natural history of Hodgkin's disease in HIV-infected patients is notable for several features: there is a high incidence of B symptoms, which occur in 81% of the cases (36). Often the patients present with an advanced stage, 90% of the patients have stage III or IV disease at the time of diagnosis. Bone marrow invasion is common (in 50%), and cytopenias are often seen before treatment. Other extranodal sites may also be involved, such as liver, skin, or lung (57–59). Histology shows a mixed cellularity or a nodular sclerosing pattern in most tumors, histologies that are considered to be aggressive.

Serrano and coworkers (36) reported a decreased response to chemotherapy and a significant decrease in survival in patients with HIV-associated HD. Twelve of 21 patients who received chemotherapy had a complete response, four achieved a partial remission, and five had progressive disease. The average survival was 18 months for the whole group, but patients with AIDS survived only for an average duration of 13 months, a significantly shorter period ($P = 0.05$). Another negative prognostic factor was the presence of cytopenia before treatment.

Hodgkin's disease is rare in children before adolescence; however, Montalvo and coworkers (46) reported a 4.5-year boy with HIV infection and nodular sclerosing Hodgkin's disease. This child underwent a complete remission with systemic chemotherapy MOPP (mechlorethamine, vincristine [Oncovin], procarbazine, prednisone), ABVD (doxorubicin, bleomycin, vinblastine, dacarbazine) that has been maintained for 20 months after chemotherapy was stopped.

Pathogenesis

Despite a recent increase in the number of reported cases of NHL in children with

HIV infection, definitive comments on pathogenesis cannot be made; however the considerable volume of data available on the development of NHL in patients with inherited and acquired immunodeficiency disorders, including adults with HIV infection, provides a firm foundation on which to construct a probable scenario (60–63). Because there is minimal evidence available to indicate an increase in the frequency of T cell neoplasias in adult patients with HIV infection, the discussion that follows will focus primarily on lymphomas of the B cell lineage (43).

Preneoplastic Proliferation

It has become clear that NHL is a consequence of multiple molecular and cytogenetic aberrations that occur in a somatic cell. In familial forms of cancer, this aberration may be superimposed on a predisposing, inherited genetic abnormality or a mutation associated with gametogenesis. Because somatic genetic changes may be associated with "active" genes and because only particular subsets of genes are active in specific tissues and at specific stages of cellular differentiation, it follows that the molecular genetic abnormalities that give rise to different types of cancer can only arise in specific cell types (64). Such cells can be targets for the specific molecular changes that define individual cancers. Inherent in the concept of target cells is the concept that the risk of the development of NHL is dependent on the size of the target cell pool—simply because of the numerically greater likelihood that at least one target cell will undergo the one or more genetic changes necessary to induce neoplasia, even if such changes are random. Although in normal children evidence of hyperplasia of a target cell lymphoid population is largely confined to increased γ-globulin levels and sometimes the presence of splenomegaly, in children with immunodeficiency (and a correspondingly greater degree of lymphoid hyperplasia) there is often overt, chronic lymphadenopathy.

Lymphadenopathy accompanied by hypergammaglobulinemia is well described in both adults and children with HIV infection; furthermore, as is also the case in the lymphadenopathy associated with inherited immunodeficiency syndromes (e.g., Wiskott-Aldrich syndrome), it is frequently associated with the predominant proliferation of a small subset of clones (63, 65). Although the stage of differentiation of the cell in which neoplastic transformation occurs remains unknown, it seems highly probable that such transformational events are made more likely by both the numerical increase in potential target cells and by the increased rate of proliferation itself (genetic changes are more likely to arise in proliferating cells, i.e., those replicating their DNA).

Mechanism of Lymphomagenesis in HIV-infected Patients

The mechanisms of lymphomagenesis in the setting of HIV infection are probably multiple.

Role of HIV. The general consensus is that HIV per se is not directly involved in the malignant transformation of B lymphocytes, and the lack of integration of HIV genomic sequences into the hyperplastic lymphoid tissue of patients with AIDS-related complex or into tumor cells of those patients with NHL is in favor of this view (37). The results of polymerase chain reaction analysis of AIDS lymphoma tissue is consistent with the presence of HIV in infiltrating T cells within these tissues as opposed to actual HIV infection of the B lymphoma cells (18, 65–67). More recently, HIV expression in clonal cell lines derived from two AIDS-related lymphomas has been reported, as well as the ability to infect nonimmortalized peripheral B lymphocytes from EBV-seropositive, HIV-seronegative donors with HIV (68, 69). Further studies of larger numbers of cases are needed to confirm the above data, which are somewhat inconsistent with the bulk of existing data. However, it seems that HIV is not a prerequisite for the development of these lymphomas.

HIV may, however, participate indirectly in the evolution of lymphomatous disease in several different ways, one of them being cytokine release. Interleukin-1, -2, -6, -7, and -10 as well as interferon-γ, tumor necrosis factor, and B cell growth factor 25 are among the stimuli responsible for proliferating and differentiating B cells and ultimately increasing, therefore, the likelihood of genetic changes resulting in neoplasia (40, 70–76). An example is interleukin-6, which has been classified as a differentiating factor for B lymphocytes and has been shown to function as an autocrine growth factor in tumor cell lines derived from non-HIV- and non-EBV-related malignant lymphomas (77). Pluda et al. (78) have shown that elevated interleukin-6 levels in the serum of patients with symptomatic HIV infection may be predictive for the development of lymphoma (78). It has also been demonstrated that some EBV-positive cell lines from patients with AIDS-associated Burkitt's lymphomas express large amounts of interleukin-10, suggesting a role for interleukin-10 in the immortalization and growth of B cells in HIV-infected individuals (79).

Thus HIV may be responsible for the release of many cytokines, some of which may increase the replication of HIV, whereas others may be responsible for producing a state of B cell growth, activation, and differentiation (40). It has also been suggested that direct polyclonal activation of B cells by HIV along with cytokine release may be the cause of ongoing B cell proliferation, which could very well explain the B cell hyperplasia seen in reactive lymphadenopathy as well as the polyclonal hypergammaglobulinemia seen in patients with HIV infection (80, 81).

Nonrandom Chromosomal Translocation in HIV-associated NHL. Although the increased size of the target cell pool for transformational events is probably the primary reason for the increased frequency of NHLs in HIV-infected individuals, most high grade lymphomas that occur in adults with HIV infection have been associated with chromosomal translocations—and specifically those same translocations (8;14, 8;22, and 2;8) that occur in the small noncleaved lymphomas—indicating that an intrinsic genetic abnormality is necessary for actual neoplastic transformation (82). These same translocations have been observed in a proportion of large cell lymphomas arising in non-HIV-infected individuals and are also present in the large cell lymphomas arising in HIV-infected individuals (83).

The likelihood of the development of a chromosomal translocation could be increased in HIV-infected individuals owing to the probable accumulation of a significant number of mutations in tumor suppressor genes that occur because of the continued proliferation of B cells secondary to immunosuppression. It has been shown, for example, that failure of p53 controlled pausing in the cell cycle to permit DNA repair will allow mutations to persist in successive cell generations. Progression from oligoclonality to monoclonality, associated with the occurrence of chromosomal abnormalities in immunodeficient individuals, has been shown by Pelicci et al. (65) and Hanto et al. (84) who demonstrated the presence of multiple clonal B cell expansions in reactive lymphadenopathy as multiple immunoglobulin gene rearrangements. However, only one of these clones has been found to have a c-*myc* rearrangement, suggesting that only one clone carries the genetic abnormality associated with a B cell lymphoma, whereas the other B cell expansions only represent precursor lesions.

Much is known of the biochemical consequences of the nonrandom chromosomal translocations associated with the small noncleaved cell lymphomas. It appears likely that the translocations occur in cells in which the recombinases necessary for physiologic immunoglobulin gene recombination are present and that sequences similar to the recognition sequences to which such recombinases bind to DNA (or occasionally the signal sequences themselves) mediate the translocational events. The translocations invariably result in the juxtaposition of immunoglobulin sequences (derived from either heavy or light chain loci) to the c-*myc* gene, normally situated on chromosome 8. In 8;14 translocations, c-*myc* is translocated to chromosome 14, whereas in 8;22 or 2;8 translocations, light chain sequences are translocated to a site distal to c-*myc* on chromosome 8. Alterations in the regulatory region of c-*myc*, probably coupled to the influence of regulatory signals from the juxtaposed immunoglobulin locus, result in the inappropriate expression of the c-*myc* protein, which in turn drives the cell to proliferate.

The frequency and specific mechanism of c-*myc* dysregulation and activation in HIV-associated lymphomas remains controversial. Ballerini et al. (85) describe c-*myc* rearrangements in 12 of 16 small noncleaved cell lymphomas, whereas Meeker and Shiramizu (86) find a much smaller number of c-*myc* rearrangements (4 of 9 and 5 of 25, respectively) in the peripheral lymphomas analyzed by them (45). However, despite this discrepancy, it appears that c-*myc* dysregulation is involved in the pathogenesis of HIV-associated lymphomas, although by itself the abnormality is not sufficient for neoplastic growth.

EBV-induced Lymphoproliferation. EBV has been found to be associated with various distinct forms of human lymphoid malignancies, including the sporadic and endemic forms of Burkitt's lymphoma, various congenital and acquired immunodeficiency states, and transplant-associated lymphomas (87–89). It has been speculated that EBV is at least a cofactor in the oncogenesis of HIV-associated lymphomas, where ~40% of the cases have been found to contain EBV sequences (83).

Although it is not possible to provide a detailed review of the biology of EBV infection here, those aspects that are particularly relevant are discussed. Table 33.2 lists the nomenclature used to describe the commonly measured EBV antigens. EBV can transform normal B lymphocytes into continuously proliferating cell lines in vitro. Such lines produce little or no virus, since virus replication results in cell death and the virus

information persists as circular DNA episomes located in the cell nucleus. Cells nonproductive of virus are said to be latently infected, and in this state a limited number (probably 10) of EBV genes, referred to as "latent genes," are expressed (90). Thus, cell transformation is necessarily the result of the expression of latent EBV genes, and at least two of them (EBV nuclear antigen 2 and the latent membrane protein) have been shown to be essential in this process (82, 91, 92). The latent EBV antigens, including EBV nuclear antigens 2 and 3 and latent membrane protein, have also been shown to provide targets for immune recognition by EBV-specific T cells (82, 93). Although nuclear antigens, they are processed by the cell and expressed at the cell surface in the context of human lymphocyte antigen class I molecules. Thus, the EBV latent genes both induce transformation and ensure that transformed cells will be destroyed by the normal immune system. This is the basis of the self-limitation of EBV infection in the normal host (94). In immunodeficient individuals unable to mount an immune response against EBV epitopes, EBV-transformed cells, which may be cytogenetically quite normal, can undergo indefinite and therefore life-threatening proliferation, as occurs in vitro (60). Although the clinical consequences may be very similar, such processes clearly differ pathogenically from what might be referred to as true neoplasia, in which an intrinsic cellular abnormality, genetically induced, results in uncontrolled proliferation even in the presence of a normal immune system.

Table 33.2.   EBV Latent Gene Expression in Lymphoproliferative States[a]

Gene	Function	Expression in monoclonal tumors	Expression in polyclonal lymphoproliferation	Immunogenicity
EBNA-1	Plasmid replication Enhancement of latent gene expression	+	+	−
EBNA-2	Cell transformation Induction of LMP and CD23	−	+	+
EBNA-3	Cell transformation	−	+	+
EBNA-4	?	−	+	?
EBNA-5	?	−	+	?
EBNA-6	?	−	+	?
LMP	Cell transformation	−	+	+
EBER-1	?	+	+	−
EBER-2	?	+	+	−

[a]EBNA, EBV nuclear antigen; LMP, latent membrane protein; EBER, EBV-encoded RNA. + Expression; − reduced (compared with transformed B cells) or absent expression.

In vivo there are four consequences of EBV infection: 1) persistent antibody titers to virus antigens, 2) intermittent virus shedding from the oropharynx, 3) establishment of a viral latent state in circulating B lymphocytes, and 4) T cell dependent cellular immunity, directed to virus-infected B lymphocytes (95). Thus, any disease, including HIV infection, that affects the immune system may result in changes of these parameters. In patients with HIV infection, for example, there is an increase in anti-EBV antibody titers, polyclonal B cell activation, and impaired T cell-mediated control of EBV carrying lymphocytes (96–98).

The precise role of EBV in the development of HIV-associated lymphomas is still not very well understood. In a recent study of 21 cases of primary CNS lymphomas in patients with AIDS, evidence of latent EBV infection was provided by the detection of the Epstein-Barr virus-encoded RNA (EBER) transcripts in all the lymphomas (99). Forty-five percent of these lymphomas also showed evidence of latent membrane protein, which is known to have oncogenic potential (82). However, in direct contrast, only 42% of the systemic AIDS-associated lymphomas expressed the EBER transcript. The latter findings were also reinforced by Subar et al. (83) who only found EBV sequences in 38% of the cases and Levine et al. (100) who found EBV in 68% of the cases demonstrated by Southern blot analysis or indirect immunofluorescence. Nonetheless, it appears that when EBV is present, it enters the cell before or during tumorigenesis, not after. Neri et al. (101), in an analysis of 10 HIV-associated lymphomas, showed that the EBV termini are uniformly clonal in AIDS-associated NHL, strongly suggesting that EBV infection probably precedes and most likely contributes to clonal expansion in these malignancies.

The relationship of EBV to lymphoproliferative disorders in patients with HIV infection has also been examined extensively. Lymphocytic interstitial pneumonitis usually presents as a subacute pneumonitis in children with HIV infection. EBV DNA has been associated with at least 80% of these lesions, usually in the absence of other pathogens. Many children show clearly deranged EBV serology with very high early antigen titers, indicating that primary EBV infection may contribute to this disorder (102).

In a recent study done by Shibata et al. (103) on 35 biopsies taken from patients with progressive generalized lymphadenopathy and HIV infection, using polymerase chain reaction and in situ hybridization, a positive correlation was seen between EBV positivity (35%) and the development of EBV positive NHLs at another site or the subsequent development of a lymphoma. No patient whose biopsy was negative for EBV went on to develop lymphomas.

These findings support the hypothesis that EBV may be involved in the development of at least some HIV-associated lymphomas. In conclusion, it appears that the etiology of HIV-associated lymphomas is multifactorial. In the setting of immunodeficiency, there is ongoing B cell proliferation caused by viruses such as HIV and EBV, which could result in mutations in important oncogenes and/or tumor suppressor genes, and chromosomal translocations, leading to c-*myc* activation and dysregulation (although the role of c-*myc* dysregulation in HIV-associated lymphomas is unclear), clonal selection, and the eventual development of a monoclonal B cell lymphoma (40).

KAPOSI'S SARCOMA

The association of malignancy with HIV infection was made in 1981, with the observation of an outbreak of a rare cancer, Kaposi's sarcoma, in young homosexual men in New York City and California (4). These patients developed a fulminant malignancy that was clinically and biologically distinct from the Kaposi's sarcoma typically seen in elderly men of European heritage but not unlike some forms of African Kaposi's sarcoma. More than 24,000 cases of HIV-associated Kaposi's sarcoma have been reported to the CDC (104). In the early stages of the AIDS epidemic 35–40% of patients had Kaposi's sarcoma; this has decreased to 12%. This change in incidence is a reflection of the following facts: Kaposi's sarcoma, although seen in all HIV risk groups, predominantly afflicts homosexual or bisexual men (95% of reported cases); the incidence of Kaposi's sarcoma in homosexual or bisexual men has decreased from 40 to 20%; and homosexual or bisexual men constitute a decreasing proportion of the HIV-infected population (104–106). Kaposi's sarcoma remains relatively rare in the pediatric HIV-infected population with 21 cases reported as the AIDS-defining illness among the 4249 children with AIDS registered by the CDC (12). The Italian Register for HIV infection in children, which has information on 1321 patients, reported seven cases of malignant tumor, one of which was Kaposi's sarcoma in an 11-year-old (13).

Clinical Manifestations

The "classic" form of Kaposi's sarcoma is typically indolent and, despite local or distant cutaneous progression, manifests visceral involvement in only 10% of patients (107). A second form of Kaposi's sarcoma, termed African, was noted in eastern equatorial Africa in the 1950s. Classified into four subtypes on the basis of clinical features, African Kaposi's sarcoma encompasses nodular, florid, infiltrative, and lymphadenopathic variants (108). The nodular variant is very similar to the classic form seen in North America and Europe, with lower extremity nodules or plaques and an indolent course. Florid Kaposi's sarcoma demonstrates locally invasive fungating masses arising at previous nodules or de novo and rarely metastasizes. Infiltrative Kaposi's sarcoma invades subdermal structures and is frequently associated with a fibroblastic reaction and diffuse swelling of the affected hand or foot. The lymphadenopathic variant, which occurs predominantly in children, demonstrates a fulminant course with cervical, inguinal, and other node groups involved as well as progressive visceral invasion and is often fatal. Kaposi's sarcoma has been reported in association with immunosuppressive therapy postorgan transplant with agents such as cyclosporine, corticosteroids, and azathioprine (109, 110). Cutaneous and mucosal lesions are common, and pulmonary and gastrointestinal diseases occur in 25% of patients; however, lymphatic involvement is rare in this form of Kaposi's sarcoma.

HIV-associated Kaposi's sarcoma in adults is usually an aggressive disseminated disease with involvement of lymph nodes, skin, mucosal surfaces, and visceral organs, particularly the gastrointestinal tract. The latter occurs in ~50% of patients, although it generally does not produce obvious symptoms. Advanced gastrointestinal involvement can be associated with diarrhea, weight loss, obstruction, or abdominal pain. Lymphadenopathy is common in patients with HIV-associated Kaposi's sarcoma. Cutaneous lesions appear as pink or purple nodules and plaques of variable size and number situated on most skin surfaces, without concentration at a specific site. Disruption of the epidermis can occur, with consequent drainage and secondary infection. Severe pitting edema, particularly in the lower extremities, may also be seen, as well as periorbital edema secondary to facial lesions. Mucosal surfaces may be involved and can compromise respiration if allowed to progress without intervention.

Several children with HIV-associated Kaposi's sarcoma have been reported in detail. One child with transfusion acquired HIV infection was also 5 years from cadaveric kidney transplantation (111). His primary manifestation was the appearance of multiple subcutaneous nodules on the head and trunk. He had no visceral involvement. Two infants with perinatally acquired HIV infection born to Haitian mothers died of pneumonia at age 7 and 8 months. At autopsy each was found to have Kaposi's sarcoma involving lymph nodes, spleen, and thymus (14). An HIV-infected infant born with hypertrichosis of the lanugo type and hepatomegaly manifested red-purple hard facial skin lesions on the sixth day of life that were confirmed by biopsy as being Kaposi's sarcoma. The child died of infection at age 4 weeks; an autopsy was refused (112). A 6-year child with vertically acquired HIV infection, who died from sepsis, was found at autopsy to have lymphadenopathic Kaposi's sarcoma with involvement of mesenteric, pericolic, and iliac lymph nodes (113). Two children, ages 5 and 8 years, have been reported with dermatopathic Kaposi's sarcoma manifested as diffuse nodular skin lesions. Both had a progressive course, one despite interferon-α therapy

(24). In summary, the pediatric patients for whom details are available have been manifestations spanning the clinical spectrum of Kaposi's sarcoma, and no patterns are identifiable.

Pathogenesis

The pathogenesis of AIDS-associated Kaposi's sarcoma is not completely understood; however, pieces of the puzzle are falling into place, primarily from work at the National Cancer Institute by Ensoli et al. (114). They question whether Kaposi's sarcoma is a true neoplasm based on the following: 1) strong male predominance implying a hormone-responsive factor in its pathogenesis; 2) multifocal nature of the tumor rather than a primary tumor with metastases; 3) rarity of cytogenetic abnormalities; 4) observation of spontaneous regression in some patients; and 5) inflammatory nature of early lesions. The authors hypothesize that factors released by activated T cells and the HIV TAT protein released by infected T cells initiate the Kaposi's sarcoma lesion by stimulating the growth of a mesenchymal cell, the Kaposi's sarcoma spindle cell. These spindle cells then produce a multitude of growth factors such as fibroblast growth factor, interleukin-1, interleukin-6, platelet-derived growth factor, granulocyte-macrophage colony-stimulating factor, and transforming growth factor-β. Most recently, oncostatin, which stimulates neoangiogenesis, spindle cell proliferation, endothelial cell proliferation, and inflammatory cell infiltration was also found to be important (115). Laboratory findings supporting this hypothesis arise from their work with cultured Kaposi's sarcoma spindle cells as well as with a transgenic mice model bearing the *tat* gene (116–118).

Treatment

The Oncology Committee of the AIDS Clinical Trials Group (ACTG) has specified criteria for the evaluation, staging, and response determination in AIDS Kaposi's sarcoma (119). Initial evaluation includes a physical exam, a biopsy confirming the diagnosis, chest X-ray, and routine laboratory studies. Further studies are dictated by the findings. All lesions are carefully recorded, and three to five indicator lesions are identified to follow for response. The staging system proposed by the ACTG considers extent of the tumor, immune status (CD4 count), and signs of systemic illness to categorize patients into good and poor risk groups.

A detailed review of the treatment of AIDS Kaposi's sarcoma is beyond the scope of this chapter. There is no useful information about the treatment of children with AIDS Kaposi's sarcoma. In adults radiation therapy is used to control localized lesions. Other local therapies include liquid nitrogen, intralesional vinblastine, and surgery. Interferon-α alone and in combination with zidovudine has been extensively studied in patients with AIDS Kaposi's sarcoma (120). It is active in patients with more limited disease, especially those with CD4 counts above 200 cells/mm^3 (121). Trials of systemic chemotherapy resulted in the demonstration of activity for vinblastine, etoposide, and doxorubicin (121). A child responded completely to etoposide for 1 year. Regimens with multiple drugs such as doxorubicin, bleomycin, and vincristine have yielded a higher response rate (84%) but have also resulted in increased opportunistic infections (122). Unfortunately, although chemotherapy can clearly produce tumor regression, increases in survival are rarely achieved because of the morbidity and mortality of opportunistic infections (123).

OTHER MALIGNANCIES

Only 5–10% of malignancies in HIV-infected adults are neither Kaposi's sarcoma nor NHL. They include seminomas, lung cancer, brain tumors, epithelial and mucosal malignancies, and germ cell tumors (124–127). The incidence of these tumors is difficult to assess because they are not diagnostic of AIDS, and estimates rely heavily on case reports. In children it is even more difficult to discern trends in the incidence of cancer, because the number of HIV-infected children is small in comparison with the adult population; HIV disease is often rapidly progressing, and the overall incidence of cancer in childhood is much lower than in adults. However, two important observations may represent the emergence of a new problem in childhood AIDS, an increased incidence of soft tissue tumors, as well as the occurrence of cervical and anal neoplasias.

Soft Tissue Tumors

Recently there have been several reports of soft tissue tumors in pediatric patients with AIDS. One child with a fibrosarcoma of the liver, one with a rhabdomyosarcoma of the gallbladder, and eight children with smooth muscle tumors have been reported, and we are aware of four additional children with leiomyomatous tumors (Table 33.3) (25, 128–132).

Smooth muscle tumors are very rare in the pediatric population, accounting for <2% of the soft tissue sarcomas (133). The retroperitoneum and gastrointestinal tract are the most common primary sites of smooth muscle tumors in children without evidence of HIV infection (134–136). However, in children with HIV infection unusual localizations, like spleen, liver, or lung, appear to be common. Although leiomyomatous tumors have not been described with increased frequency in children with congenital immunodeficiency disorders or after immunosuppression for bone marrow or organ transplantation, it appears that leiomyomas and leiomyosarcomas occur with increased frequency in children with HIV infection (137). The annual incidence of soft tissue tumors in the general pediatric population is ~8.4 cases per million, but at least 13 cases (12 leiomyomas/leiomyosarcomas and one rhabdomyosarcoma) have been reported in association with pediatric HIV infection (1). As of December 1992, 4249 children with AIDS have been reported to the CDC (11). In a population this size not more than one case would be expected to have occurred over the last 10 years.

Kaposi's sarcoma, which, like leiomyoma, has a spindle cell component, is uncommon in children and does not have a clear association with the degree of immunosuppression. However, recently published data indicate a relationship of cultured Kaposi's

sarcoma cells to leiomyoblasts (138). Another intriguing fact is that insulin-like growth factor genes have recently been shown to be important in the pathogenesis of smooth muscle tumors. IGF-I is expressed at high levels in leiomyomas, whereas IGF-II is predominant in leiomyosarcomas and other sarcomas (139–141). Both growth factors are markedly influenced by nutritional status and caloric intake (142).

Treatment for leiomyomas consists of surgery alone, an approach that is often chosen for leiomyosarcomas as well. The role of chemotherapy and radiation therapy is unknown, but both have been used by some centers. Unfortunately, leiomyosarcomas that cannot be completely resected tend to be rather treatment resistant and often recur with pulmonary metastasis (133). A localized leiomyosarcoma in the HIV-infected child should be surgically removed and local radiotherapy considered. In more widespread disease there are no clear guidelines for treatment. Prolonged chemotherapy regimens may not be tolerated, and there is only very limited experience with the use of interferon-α (because of similarities with Kaposi's sarcoma) in this setting.

Cervical and Anal Neoplasias

Recent reports have suggested an association between HIV infection and cervical disease in women. In one study the incidence of squamous intraepithelial lesions was 40% in HIV-positive women vs. 9% in HIV-negative women (143). Cervical neoplasia often has a more rapid course and is associated with early and widespread metastatic disease in HIV-infected women (144, 145). There is a clear association between concurrent infection with human papillomavirus (HPV), especially with types 16 and 18, and the development of intraepithelial cervical neoplasias (146). HPV is more strongly associated with intraepithelial lesions in symptomatic HIV-infected women (odds ratio 29.3) and asymptomatic HIV-positive women (odds ratio 8.8.) than in HIV-negative women (odds ratio 2.3) (147). Infection with HPV is a sexually acquired disease, and adolescents start to be sexually active already in their early teens. In fact one published case of invasive cervical carcinoma occurred in a 16-year girl (145). Thus, the pediatrician must be prepared for the evaluation of urogenital infections and cervical epithelial abnormalities in adolescent girls; the recommendation that a sexually active woman should be followed with at least annual Papanicolaou smears and pelvic examinations is even more important in the HIV-infected teenager.

A similar association with HPV infection has been observed in anal epithelial abnormalities. In one study of homosexual men from Washington DC and New York City 53% of the HIV-positive men compared with 29% of the HIV-negative men had anal swabs positive for HPV. Anal epithelial abnormalities were found in 14% and were again strongly associated with certain HPV genotypes ($P = 0.001$) (148). Low CD4 counts are associated with higher prevalence rates for HPV (148, 149).

HPV is one of the most common infectious agents in pediatrics, causing nonvenereal warts, condylomata acuminata, and rarely recurrent respiratory papillomatosis, probably caused by neonatal aspiration of virus shed from maternal condylomata at delivery (150). Although malignant degeneration has not yet been observed, children with HIV infection have been described with either widespread cutaneous flat warts or severe and extensive perineal condylomata acuminata (151–153).

GENERAL CONSIDERATIONS

With the advent of better antiretroviral treatment, many children (and adults) with HIV infection live longer and remain relatively asymptomatic for a prolonged time. The decision to treat a malignancy has become an accepted therapeutic intervention, although it will always be guided by stage of the cancer as well as overall performance status of the child. Concomitant antiretroviral therapy is an important part of cancer treatment protocols, because therapy for cancer will only be of benefit to the child if the clinical manifestations of HIV infection can be controlled and disease progression during times of added iatrogenic immunosuppression is avoided. The hematopoietic growth factor granulocyte colony-stimulating factor diminishes problems with neutropenia and may allow delivery of the dose intensity of chemotherapy that is necessary for cure. Aggressive supportive care combined with prophylaxis during chemotherapy is of great importance, because many children will be at risk for opportunistic infections like *Pneumocystis carinii* pneumonia or fungal infections. Another mainstay of successful chemotherapy in the HIV-infected child with cancer is the preservation of an adequate nutritional status, if necessary with temporary parenteral nutrition.

Not every child with AIDS and cancer will be a candidate for intensive therapy. Some will be too ill from AIDS to benefit from cancer treatment. However, if treatment is initiated it should always be with an intent to cure the child of the malignancy even though the prospect for cure of AIDS remains unlikely.

Progress in the treatment of pediatric cancers has been made in large part through the willingness of pediatric oncologists to collaborate in the systematic study of these relatively rare diseases. A better understanding of incidence, etiology and course of malignant diseases in this immunocompromised population can only be gained by a nationwide or even worldwide coordinated effort. If a cancer has a relatively high incidence in a certain population, like Hodgkin's lymphoma in young adults, it is imperative to compare the frequency of occurrence with data from established surveillance programs, like the Surveillance, Epidemiology, and End Results Program (154). A nationwide registry to assess incidence, risk factors, biologic features, and outcome of neoplastic diseases in HIV-infected children and adolescents has recently been initiated in a collaboration of the ACTG and the Pediatric Oncology Group. Patients can be registered through the Pediatric Oncology Group Statistical Office in Gainesville, Florida (telephone 904-375-6838). Estimates are based on the assumption of a similar incidence for cancer of 5–40% in the HIV-infected child as seen in adults. Clearly, progress in the treatment of HIV-related malignancies will require such a collaborative effort, because most single institutions will not have a patient base large enough to address the relevant questions.

Table 33.3.   Leiomyomas and Leiomyosarcomas in HIV-infected Children[a]

Age	Sex	Acquisition	History	Location	Outcome	Ref.
yr 4	F	V	LIP CD4 count 43 cells/mm³	Multiple leiomyosarcomas (grade I) in stomach, duodenum, ileum, cecum, small bowels, appendix At autopsy: metastases in lungs, brain, throughout gastrointestinal tract	Surgery, increasing O_2 requirement, died 4 months after laparotomy of respiratory arrest	128
5	M	T	CD4 count 6 cells/mm³, p24 antigen 527 pg/ml Lung culture positive for *Mycobacterium scrofulaceum*	Multiple leiomyomas in lungs	Died 2 months after diagnosis	128
8	F	T	CD4 count 67 cells/mm³ Bronchoalveolar lavage and blood culture positive for *M. kansasii* On AZT	Leiomyoma in endobronchial tree, later leiomyosarcoma in colon with multiple pulmonary as well as mediastinal and peribronchial node involvement	Alive with disease 6 months after treatment with adriamycin	128
17	M	T	CD4 count <100 cells/mm³ *M. avium* complex On AZT, then switched to ddC	Multiple painful, subcutaneous leiomyosarcomas Later masses in spinal cord at C7, T2, and T10; autopsy declined	Surgical excision of some subcutaneous nodules Paralysis of lower extremities, radiation therapy of spine and high dose corticosteroids without response; died 10 months after initial diagnosis	129
4	F	V		Multiple leiomyomas of gut	Treated with interferon-α, limited response	K. Belani, personal communication, 1992
7	F	V	CD4 count 160 cells/mm³ On AZT LIP	Leiomyoma of trachea and leiomyosarcoma of left mainstem bronchus	Partial resection of tracheal and left mainstem mass Persistent left lower lobe atelectasis, O_2 dependent, died later	130

Table 33.3.—*continued*

Age yr	Sex	Acquisition	History	Location	Outcome	Ref.
9	F	T	s/p AZT, then ddI, now AZT/ddI *M. avium* complex	Leiomyosarcoma of the spleen (encapsulated)	Partial splenectomy, 8 months later no evidence of disease	J. Goldsmith, personal communication, 1992
6	M	V	CD4 count 250, then dropped to 70 cells/mm³ Severe LIP On AZT	Bilateral pulmonary nodules (leiomyosarcomas, biopsy proven), tumor in small bowel area	Treated with interferon-α, radiotherapy to lungs (800 rad) for severe LIP, died, autopsy pending	D. Johnson, personal communication, 1992
9	F	V	On AZT Cardiomyopathy, fungal infections, pancreatitis	Leiomyosarcoma (3×4 cm) of lower back area, no metastasis	Local radiotherapy	B. Sison, personal communication, 1992
7	F	V	CD4 count 0 cells/mm³ On ddC/AZT, later on ddI	Leiomyoma of liver	Resection of lobectomy, died later of PCP, no evidence of malignancy	25
5	M	V	CD4 count 45 cells/mm³ Cryptosporidiosis On AZT, later on ddI	Leiomyomas in colon and ileum	Incidental finding at autopsy	25
3	M	V	CD4 count 14 cells/mm³ *M. avium* complex On AZT	Leiomyoma in liver	Incidental finding at autopsy	25

ªV, vertical; T, transfusion; LIP, lymphocytic interstitial pneumonitis; AZT, azidothymidine; ddI, dideoxyinosine; ddC, dideoxycytosine; PCP, *P. carinii* pneumonia.

References

1. Robison LL. General principles of the epidemiology of childhood cancer. In: Pizzo PA, Poplack DG, eds. Principles and practice of pediatric oncology. 2nd ed. Philadelphia: JB Lippincott, 1993:3–10.
2. Penn I. Occurrence of cancer in immune deficiencies. Cancer 1974;34:858–866.
3. Groopman JE, Broder S. Cancers in AIDS and other immunodeficiency states. In: DeVita VT, Hellman S, Rosenberg SA, eds. Cancer: Principles and practice of oncology. 3rd ed. Philadelphia: JB Lippincott, 1989: 1953–1970.
4. Friedman-Kien AE, Laubenstein LJ, Rubinstein P, et al. Disseminated Kaposi's sarcoma in homosexual men. Ann Intern Med 1982;96:693–700.
5. Ziegler JL, Beckstead JA, Volberding PA, et al. Non-Hodgkin's lymphoma in 90 homosexual men. Relation to generalized lymphadenopathy and the acquired immunodeficiency syndrome. N Engl J Med 1984;311:565–570.
6. Fauci AS, Macher AM, Longo DL, et al. Acquired immunodeficiency syndrome: Epidemiologic, clinical, immunologic, and therapeutic considerations. Ann Intern Med 1984;100:92–106.
7. Rabkin CS, Biggar RJ, Horm JW. Increasing incidence of cancers associated with the human immunodeficiency virus epidemic. Int J Cancer 1991;47:692–696.
8. Pluda JM, Yarchoan R, Jaffe ES, et al. Development of non-Hodgkin lymphoma in a cohort of patients with severe human immunodeficiency virus (HIV) infection on long-term antiretroviral therapy. Ann Intern Med 1990;113:276–282.
9. Monfardini S, Vaccher E, Lazzarin A, et al. Characterization of AIDS-associated tumors in Italy: Report of 435 cases of an IVDA-based series. Cancer Detect Prev 1990;14:391–393.
10. Beral V, Peterman TA, Berkelman RL, Jaffe HW. Kaposi's sarcoma among persons with AIDS: A sexually transmitted infection? Lancet 1990;335:123–128.
11. Centers for Disease Control and Prevention. HIV/AIDS Surveillance Rep 1993;Feb:1–23.
12. Centers for Disease Control and Prevention. Cumulative number of malignancies as an AIDS-indicative disease in children. AIDS Public Information Data Set, 1993.
13. Arico M, Caselli D, D'Argenio P, et al. Malignancies in children with human immunodeficiency virus type 1 infection. Cancer 1991;68:2473–2477.
14. Buck BE, Scott GB, Valdes-Dapena M, Parks WP. Kaposi sarcoma in two infants with acquired immune deficiency syndrome. J Pediatr 1983;103:911–913.
15. Gordon EM, Berkowitz RJ, Strandjord SE, Kurczynski EM, Goldberg JS, Coccia PF. Burkitt lymphoma in a patient with classic hemophilia receiving factor VIII concentrates. J Pediatr 1983;103:75–77.
16. Andiman WA, Martin K, Rubinstein A, et al. Opportunistic lymphoproliferations associated with Epstein-Barr viral DNA in infants and children with AIDS. Lancet 1985;2:1390–1393.

17. Honda NS, Sun NC, Heiner DC. Isolated IgG4 subclass deficiency and malignant lymphoma in a child with acquired immunodeficiency syndrome. M J Dis Child 1987;141:398–399.
18. Rechavi G, Ben-Bassat I, Berkowicz M, et al. Molecular analysis of Burkitt's leukemia in two hemophilic brothers with AIDS. Blood 1987;70:1713–1717.
19. DiCarlo FJ, Joshi VV, Oleske JM, Connor EM. Neoplastic diseases in children with acquired immunodeficiency syndrome. Prog AIDS Pathol 1990;2:163–185.
20. Katz BZ, Andiman WA, Eastman R, Martin K, Miller G. Infection with two genotypes of Epstein-Barr virus in an infant with AIDS and lymphoma of the central nervous system. J Infect Dis 1986;153:601–604.
21. Goldstein J, Dickson DW, Rubinstein A, et al. Primary central nervous system lymphoma in a pediatric patient with acquired immune deficiency syndrome. Cancer 1990;66:2503–2508.
22. Douek P, Bertrand Y, Tran-Minh VA, Patet JD, Souillet G, Philippe N. Primary lymphoma of the CNS in an infant with AIDS: Imaging findings. Am J Radiol 1991;156:1037–1038.
23. Epstein LG, DiCarlo FJ, Joshi VV, et al. Primary lymphoma of the central nervous system in children with acquired immunodeficiency syndrome. Pediatrics 1988;82:355–363.
24. Connor E, Boccon-Gibod L, Joshi V, et al. Cutaneous acquired immunodeficiency syndrome-associated Kaposi's sarcoma in pediatric patients. Arch Dermatol 1990;126:791–793.
25. Mueller BU, Butler KM, Feuerstein IM, et al. Smooth muscle tumors in children with human immunodeficiency virus infection. Pediatrics 1992;90:460–463.
26. Broder S, Karp JE. The expanding challenge of HIV-associated malignancies. CA-A Cancer J Clin 1992;42:69–73.
27. Cremer KJ, Spring SB, Gruber J. Role of human immunodeficiency virus type 1 and other viruses in malignancies associated with acquired immunodeficiency disease syndrome. J Natl Cancer Inst 1990;82:1016–1024.
28. Matsuyama T, Kobayashi N, Yamamoto N. Cytokines and HIV infection: Is AIDS a tumor necrosis factor disease? AIDS 1991;5:1405–1417.
29. Levy JA. The multifaceted retrovirus. Cancer Res 1986;46:5457–5468.
30. Centers for Disease Control. Classification system for human immunodeficiency virus (HIV) infection in children under 13 years of age. MMWR 1987;36:225–236.
31. Centers for Disease Control. Revision of the CDC surveillance case definition for acquired immunodeficiency syndrome. MMWR 1987;36(suppl 1s):1S–15S.
32. Beral V, Peterman T, Berkelman R, Jaffe H. AIDS-associated non-Hodgkin lymphoma. Lancet 1991;337:805–809.
33. Gail MH, Pluda JM, Rabkin CS, et al. Projections of the incidence of non-Hodgkin's lymphoma related to acquired immunodeficiency syndrome. J Natl Cancer Inst 1991;83:695–701.

34. Moore RD, Kessler H, Richman DD, Flexner C, Chaisson RE. Non-Hodgkin's lymphoma in patients with advanced HIV infection treated with zidovudine. JAMA 1991;265:2208–2211.

35. Hessol NA, Katz MH, Liu JY, Buchbinder SP, Rubino CJ, Holmberg SD. Increased incidence of Hodgkin disease in homosexual men with HIV infection. Ann Intern Med 1992;117:309–311.

36. Serrano M, Bellas C, Campo E, et al. Hodgkin's disease in patients with antibodies to human immunodeficiency virus. A study of 22 patients. Cancer 1990;65:2248–2254.

37. Knowles DM, Chamulak GA, Subar M, et al. Lymphoid neoplasia associated with the acquired immunodeficiency syndrome (AIDS). Ann Intern Med 1988;108:744–753.

38. Loureiro C, Gill PS, Meyer PR, Rhodes R, Rarick MU, Levine AM. Autopsy findings in AIDS-associated lymphoma. Cancer 1988;62:735–739.

39. Gill PS, Levine AM, Krailo M, et al. AIDS-related malignant lymphoma: Results of prospective treatment trials. J Clin Oncol 1987;5:1322–1328.

40. Levine AM. Acquired immunodeficiency syndrome-related lymphoma. Blood 1992;80:8–20.

41. Hamilton-Dutoit SJ, Pallesen G, Franzmann MB, et al. AIDS-related lymphoma. Histopathology, immunophenotype, and association with Epstein-Barr virus as demonstrated by in situ nucleic acid hybridization. Am J Pathol 1991;138:149–163.

42. Gold JE, Ghali V, Gold S, Brown JC, Zalusky R. Angiocentric immunoproliferative lesion/T-cell non-Hodgkin's lymphoma and the acquired immune deficiency syndrome: A case report and review of the literature. Cancer 1990;66:2407–2413.

43. Ruff P, Bagg A, Papadopoulos K. Precursor T-cell lymphoma associated with human immunodeficiency virus type 1 (HIV-1) infection. Cancer 1989;64:39–42.

44. Gonzalez-Clemente JM, Ribera JM, Campo E, Bosch X, Montserrat E, Grau JM. Ki-1+ anaplastic large-cell lymphoma of T-cell origin in an HIV-infected patient. AIDS 1991;5:751–755.

45. Shiramizu B, Herdier B, Meeker T, Kaplan L, McGrath M. Molecular and immunophenotypic characterization of AIDS-associated, Epstein-Barr virus-negative, polyclonal lymphoma. J Clin Oncol 1992;10:383–389.

46. Montalvo FW, Casanova R, Clavell LA. Treatment outcome in children with malignancies associated with human immunodeficiency virus infection. J Pediatr 1990;116:735–738.

47. Ioachim HL, Cooper MC, Hellman GC. Lymphomas in men at high risk for acquired immune deficiency syndrome (AIDS). Cancer 1985;56:2831–2842.

48. Levine AM. Epidemiology, clinical characteristics, and management of AIDS-related lymphoma. Hematol/Oncol Clin North Am 1991;5:331–342.

49. Kaplan DL. AIDS-associated lymphomas. In: Volberding P, Jacobsen HA, eds. AIDS Clinical Review New York: Marcel Dekker, 1989:193–205.

50. Levine AM, Wernz JC, Kaplan L, et al. Low-dose chemotherapy with central nervous system prophylaxis and zidovudine maintenance in AIDS-related lymphoma. A prospective multi-institutional trial. JAMA 1991;266:84–88.

51. Nadal D, Brändle B, Frey E, deRoche B, Caduff R, Seger RA. Lymphome beim Kind mit AIDS: Wie behandeln? [Abstract 27]. Schweiz Med Wochenschr 1992;122(suppl 47):11.

52. Formenti SC, Gill PS, Lean E, et al. Primary central nervous system lymphoma in AIDS. Results of radiation therapy. Cancer 1989;63:1101–1107.

53. So YT, Beckstaed JH, Davis RL. Primary central nervous system lymphoma in acquired immune deficiency syndrome: A clinical and pathological study. Ann Neurol 1986;20:566–572.

54. Gill PS, Levine AM, Meyer PR, et al. Primary central nervous system lymphoma in homosexual men. Clinical, immunologic, and pathologic features. Am J Med 1985;78:742–748.

55. Socié G, Piprot-Chauffat C, Schlienger M, et al. Primary lymphoma of the central nervous system. An unresolved therapeutic problem. Cancer 1990;65:322–326.

56. Anderson DW, Macher AM, Shanks D, et al. AIDS. Case for diagnosis series. Milit Med 1987;152:M34–M40.

57. Schoeppel SL, Hoppe RT, Dorfman RF, et al. Hodgkin's disease in homosexual men with generalized lymphadenopathy. Ann Intern Med 1985;102:68–70.

58. Scheib RG, Siegel RS. Atypical Hodgkin's disease and the acquired immunodeficiency syndrome [Letter]. Ann Intern Med 1985;102:554.

59. Gongora RA, Gonzales-Martinez P, Bastarrachea-Ortiz J. Hodgkin disease as the initial manifestation of acquired immunodeficiency syndrome [Letter]. Ann Intern Med 1987;107:112.

60. Magrath IT. Infectious mononucleosis and malignant neoplasia. In: Schlossberg D, ed. Infectious mononucleosis. New York: Springer Verlag, 1989:142–171.

61. Filipovich A. Lymphoproliferative disorders associated with immunodeficiency. In: Magrath IT, ed. The non-Hodgkin's lymphomas. London: Edward Arnold, 1990:135–154.

62. Ziegler JL, McGrath MS. Lymphomas in HIV-positive individuals. In: Magrath IT, ed. The non-Hodgkin's lymphomas. London: Edward Arnold, 1990:155–159.

63. Levine AM. Reactive and neoplastic lymphoproliferative disorders and other miscellaneous cancers associated with HIV infection. In: Broder S, ed. AIDS. New York: Marcel Dekker, 1987:263–275.

64. Magrath IT. Lymphocyte differentiation: An essential basis for the comprehension of lymphoid neoplasia. J Natl Cancer Inst 1981;67:501–514.

65. Pelicci P-G, Knowles DM, Arlin ZA, et al. Multiple monoclonal B cell expansions and c-myc oncogene rearrangements in acquired immune deficiency syndrome-related lymphoproliferative disorders. Implications for lymphomagenesis. J Exp Med 1986;164:2049–2076.

66. Groopman JE, Sullivan JL, Ginsburg D, et al. Pathogenesis of B cell lymphoma in a patient with AIDS. Blood 1986;67:612–616.

67. Shibata D, Brynes RK, Nathwani B, Kwoks S, Shinsky J, Arnheim N. Human immunodeficiency viral DNA is readily found in lymph node biopsies from seropositive individuals. Am J Pathol 1989;135:697–702.

68. Ford RJ, Goodacre A, Bohannon B, Donehower L. Identification of human retrovirus(es) in lymphoma cells from AIDS patients. AIDS Res Hum Retroviruses 1990;6:142–148.

69. Laurence J, Astrin SM. Human immunodeficiency virus induction of malignant transformation in human B lymphocytes. Proc Natl Acad Sci USA 1991;88:7635–7639.

70. Paul WE. Interleukin 4/ B cell stimulatory factor 1: One lymphokine, many functions. FASEB J 1987;1:456–460.

71. Jelinek DF, Spawski JB, Lipsky PE. The roles of interleukin-2 and interferon-gamma in human B-cell activation, growth and differentiation. Eur J Immunol 1986;16:925–928.

72. Jelinek DF, Lipsky PE. Enhancement of human B cell proliferation and differentiation by tumor necrosis factor-alpha and interleukin 1. J Immunol 1987;139:2970–2972.

73. Hirano T, Yasukawa K, Harada H, et al. Complementary DNA for a novel human interleukin (BSF-2) that induces B lymphocytes to produce immunoglobulin. Nature 1986;324:73–76.

74. Sharma S, Mehta S, Morgan J, Maizel A. Molecular cloning and expression of a human B-cell growth factor gene in *Escherichia coli*. Science 1987;235:1489–1492.

75. Saeland S, Duvert V, Pandrau D, et al. Interleukin-7 induces the proliferation of normal human B cell precursors. Blood 1991;78:2229–2238.

76. Zlotnik A, Morre KW. Interleukin 10. Cytokine 1991;3:366–371.

77. Yee C, Biondi A, Wang XH, et al. A possible autocrine role of IL-6 in two lymphoma cell lines. Blood 1989;74:789–793.

78. Pluda JM, Venzon D, Tosato G, et al. Factors which predict for the development of non-Hodgkin's lymphoma in patients with HIV infection receiving antiretroviral therapy [Abstract]. Blood 1991;78:285a.

79. Benjamin D, Knobloch TJ, Abrams J, Dayton MA. Human B cell IL-10: B cell lines derived from patients with AIDS and Burkitt's lymphoma constitutively secrete large quantities of IL-10 [Abstract]. Blood 1991;78:384a.

80. Schnittman SM, Lane HC, Higgins SE, Folks T, Fauci AS. Direct polyclonal activation of human B lymphocytes by the AIDS virus. Science 1986;233:1084–1086.

81. Levine AM. Reactive and neoplastic lymphoproliferative disorders and other miscellaneous cancers associated with HIV infection. In: DeVita VT Jr, Hellman S, Rosenberg SA, eds. AIDS. Etiology, diagnosis, treatment, and prevention. 2nd ed. Philadelphia: Lippincott, 1989:263–275.

82. Wang D, Liebewitz D, Keiff E. An EBV membrane protein expressed in immortalized lymphocytes transforms established rodent cells. Cell 1985;43:659–665.

83. Subar M, Neri A, Inghirami G, Knowles DM, Dalla-Favera R. Frequent c-myc activation and infrequent presence of Epstein-Barr virus genome in AIDS-associated lymphoma. Blood 1988;72:667–671.

84. Hanto DW, Frizzera G, Gajl-Peczalska, et al. Epstein-Barr virus induced B-cell lymphoma after renal transplantation: Acyclovir therapy and transition from polyclonal to monoclonal B-cell proliferation. N Engl J Med 1982;306:913–918.

85. Ballerini P, Gaidano G, Gong J, et al. Multiple genetic lesions in acquired immunodeficiency syndrome-related non-Hodgkin's lymphoma. Blood 1993;81:166–176.

86. Meeker TC, Shiramizu B, Kaplan L, et al. Evidence for molecular subtypes of HIB-associated lymphoma: Division into peripheral monoclonal, polyclonal and central nervous system lymphoma. AIDS 1991;5:669–674.

87. Epstein MA, Achong BG. The relationship of the virus to Burkitt's lymphoma. In: Epstein MA, Achong BG, ed. The Epstein-Barr Virus. New York: Springer-Verlag, 1979:321–337.

88. Saemundsen AK, Purtilo DT, Sakamoto K, et al. Documentation of Epstein-Barr virus infection in immunodeficient patients with life-threatening lymphoproliferative disease by Epstein-Barr virus complementary RNA/DNA and viral DNA/DNA hybridization. Cancer Res 1981;41:4237–4242.

89. Hanto DW, Frizzera G, Gail-Peczalska KJ, Simmons RL. Epstein-Barr virus, immunodeficiency, and B-cell proliferation. Transplantation 1985;39:461–472.

90. Damburgh T, Henessy K, Fennewald S, Kieff E. The virus genome and its expression in latent infection. In: Epstein MA, Achong BG, ed. The Epstein-Barr virus. Recent advances. New York: Wiley, 1986:13–15.

91. Magrath IT. The pathogenesis of Burkitt's lymphoma. Adv Cancer Res 1990;55:133–270.

92. Dillner J, Kallin B. The Epstein-Barr virus proteins. Adv Cancer Res 1988;50:95–157.

93. Moss DJ, Misko IS, Burrows SR, Burman K, McCarthy R, Scully TB. Cytotoxic T-cell clones discriminate between A- and B-type Epstein-Barr virus transformants. Nature 1988;331:719–721.

94. Tosato G. Cell mediated immunity. In: Schlossberg D, ed. Infectious mononucleosis. New York: Springer-Verlag, 1989:100–116.

95. Ernberg I. Epstein-Barr virus and acquired immunodeficiency syndrome. Adv Viral Oncol 1989;8:203–217.

96. Birx DL, Redfield RR, Tosato G. Defective regulation of Epstein-Barr virus infection in patients with acquired immunodeficiency syndrome (AIDS) or AIDS-related disorders. N Engl J Med 1986;314:874–879.

97. Ragona G, Sirianni M, Soddu S, Vercelli B, Piccoli M, Aiuti F. Evidence for dysregulation in the control of Epstein-Barr virus latency in patients with AIDS-related complex. Clin Exp Immunol 1986;66:17–24.

98. Lane CH, Masur H, Edgar LC, Whalen G, Rook AH, Fauci AS. Abnormalities of B-cell activation and immunoregulation in patients with the acquired immunodeficiency syndrome. N Engl J Med 1983;309:453–458.

99. MacMahon EME, Glass JD, Hayward SD, et al. Epstein-Barr virus in AIDS-related primary central nervous system lymphoma. Lancet 1991;338:969–973.

100. Levine AM, Shibata D, Sullivan-Halley J, et al. Case control study of HIV-positive and HIV-negative lymphoma in Los Angeles County [Abstract]. Am Soc Clin Oncol 1992;11:333.

101. Neri A, Barriga F, Inghirami G, et al. Epstein-Barr virus infection precedes clonal expansion in Burkitt's and acquired immunodeficiency syndrome-associated lymphoma. Blood 1991;77:1092–1095.

102. Levine AM. Non-Hodgkin's lymphomas and other malignancies in the acquired immune deficiency syndrome. Semin Oncol 1987;14(suppl 3):34–39.

103. Shibata D, Weiss LM, Nathwani BN, Brynes RK, Levine AM. Epstein-Barr virus in benign lymph node biopsies from individuals infected with the human immunodeficiency virus is associated with concurrent or subsequent development of non-Hodgkin's lymphoma. Blood 1991;77:1527–1533.

104. Safai B, Diaz B, Schwartz J. Malignant neoplasms associated with human immunodeficiency virus infection. CA-A Cancer J Clin 1992;42:74–95.

105. Rutherford GW, Payne SF, Lemp GF. The epidemiology of AIDS-related Kaposi's sarcoma in San Francisco. J Acquir Immun Defic Syndr 1990;3(suppl 1):S4–S7.

106. Dalgleish AG. Kaposi's sarcoma. Br J Cancer 1991;64:3–6.

107. Safai B, Mike V, Giraldo G, Beth E, Good RA. Association of Kaposi's sarcoma with secondary primary malignancies. Possible etiopathogenic implications. Cancer 1980;45:1472–1479.

108. Taylor JF, Templeton AC, Vogel CL, Ziegler JL, Kyalwazi SK. Kaposi's sarcoma in Uganda: A clinico-pathological study. Int J Cancer 1971;8:122–135.

109. Penn I. Kaposi's sarcoma in organ transplant recipients. Report of 20 cases. Transplantation 1979;27:8–11.

110. Siegel JH, Janis R, Alpor JC, Schutte H, Robbins L, Blaufox MD. Disseminated visceral Kaposi's sarcoma. Appearance after human renal homograft operation. JAMA 1969;207:1493–1496.

111. Malekzadeh MH, Church JA, Mitchell WG, Opas L, Lieberman E. Human immunodeficiency virus-associated Kaposi's sarcoma in a pediatric renal transplant recipient. Nephron 1987;42:62–65.

112. Gutierrez-Ortega P, Hierro-Orozco S, Sanchez-Cisneros R, Montana LF. Kaposi's sarcoma in a 6-day-old infant with human immunodeficiency virus. Arch Dermatol 1989;125:432–433.

113. Baum LG, Vinters HV. Lymphadenopathic Kaposi's sarcoma in a pediatric patient with acquired immune deficiency syndrome. Pediatr Pathol 1989;9:459–465.

114. Ensoli B, Barillari G, Gallo RC. Pathogenesis of AIDS-associated Kaposi's sarcoma. Hematol Oncol Clin North Am 1991;5:281–296.

115. Lusso P, Gallo RC. Pathogenesis of AIDS. J Pharm Pharmacol 1992;44(suppl 1):160–164.

116. Ensoli B, Barillari G, Salahuddin SZ, Gallo RC, Wong-Staal F. Tat protein of HIV-1 stimulates growth of cells derived from Kaposi's sarcoma lesions of AIDS patients. Nature 1990;345:84–86.

117. Salahuddin SZ, Nakamura S, Biberfeld P, et al. Angiogenic properties of Kaposi's sarcoma-derived cells after long-term culture in vitro. Science 1988;242:430–433.

118. Vogel J, Hinrichs SH, Reynolds RK, Luciw PA, Jay G. The HIV tat gene induces dermal lesions resembling Kaposi's sarcoma in transgenic mice. Nature 1988;335:606–611.

119. Krown SE, Metroka C, Wernz JC, AIDS Clinical Trials Group Oncology Committee. Kaposi's sarcoma in the acquired immune deficiency syndrome: A proposal for uniform evaluation, response, and staging criteria. J Clin Oncol 1989;7:1201–1207.

120. Krown SE, Gold JWM, Niedziecki D, et al. Interferon-α with zidovudine: Safety, tolerance, and clinical and virologic effects in patients with Kaposi sarcoma associated with the acquired immunodeficiency syndrome (AIDS). Ann Intern Med 1990;112:812–821.

121. Kahn J, Northfelt D, Volberding P. Chemotherapy for AIDS-associated Kaposi's sarcoma. Oncology 1991;5:57–63.

122. Laubenstein LJ, Krigel RL, Odajnyk CM, et al. Treatment of epidemic Kaposi's sarcoma with etoposide or a combination of doxorubicin, bleomycin and vinblastine. J Clin Oncol 1984;2:1115–1120.

123. Volberding PA. The role of chemotherapy for epidemic Kaposi's sarcoma. Semin Oncol 1987;14(suppl 3):23–26.

124. Monfardini S, Vaccher E, Pizzocaro G, et al. Unusual malignant tumours in 49 patients with HIV infection. AIDS 1989;3:449–452.

125. Cohen P. Miscellaneous cancers associated with AIDS. Curr Opin Oncol 1989;1:68–71.

126. Tirelli U, Vaccher E, Zagonel V, et al. Malignant tumors other than lymphoma and Kaposi's sarcoma in association with HIV infection. Cancer Detect Prev 1988;12:267–272.

127. Ravalli S, Chabon AB, Khan AA. Gastrointestinal neoplasia in young HIV antibody-positive patients. Am J Clin Pathol 1989;91:458–461.

128. Chadwick EG, Connor EJ, Guerra Hanson IC, et al. Tumors of smooth muscle origin in HIV-infected children. JAMA 1990;263:3182–3184.

129. Orlow SJ, Kamino H, Lawrence RL. Multiple subcutaneous leiomyosarcomas in an adolescent with AIDS. Am J Pediatr Hematol Oncol 1992;14:265–268.

130. Sabatino D, Martinez S, Young R, Balbi H, Ciminera P, Frieri M. Simultaneous pulmonary leiomyosarcoma and leiomyoma in pediatric HIV infection. Pediatr Hematol Oncol 1991;8:355–359.

131. Ninane J, Moulin D, Latinne D, et al. AIDS in two African children—one with fibrosarcoma of the liver. Eur J Pediatr 1985;144:385–390.

132. Scully RE, Mark RE, McNeely BU. Case records of the Massachusetts General Hospital. N Engl J Med 1986;314:629–640.

133. Miser JS, Triche TJ, Pritchard DJ, Kinsella TJ. The other soft tissue sarcomas of childhood. In: Pizzo PA, Poplack DG, ed. Principles and practice of pediatric oncology. 2nd ed. Philadelphia: JB Lippincott, 1993:823–840.

134. Lack EE. Leiomyosarcomas in childhood: A clinical and pathological study of 10 cases. Pediatr Pathol 1986;6:181–197.

135. Delucchi MA, Latorre JJ, Guiraldes E, Oddo D. Intestinal leiomyosarcoma in childhood: Report of two cases. J Pediatr Surg 1988;23:377–379.

136. Cohen SR, Thompson JW, Sherman NJ. Congenital stenosis of the lower esophagus associated with leiomyoma and leiomyosarcoma of the gastrointestinal tract. Ann Otol Rhinol Laryngol 1988;97:454–459.

137. Penn I. Tumors of the immunocompromised patient. Ann Rev Med 1988;39:63–73.

138. Wittek AE, Mitchell CD, Armstrong GR, et al. Propagation and properties of Kaposi's sarcoma-derived cell lines obtained from patients with AIDS: Similarity of cultured cells to smooth muscle cells. AIDS 1991;5:1485–1493.

139. Höppener JWM, Mosselman S, Roholl PJM, et al. Expression of insulin-like growth factor-I and -II genes in human smooth muscle tumours. EMBO J 1988;7:1379–1385.

140. Gloudemans T, Prinsen I, Van Unnik JAM, Lips CJM, Otter WD, Sussenbach JS. Insulin-like growth factor gene expression in human smooth muscle tumors. Cancer Res 1990;50:6689–6695.

141. Tricoli JV, Rall LB, Karakousis CP, et al. Enhanced levels of insulin-like growth factor messenger RNA in human colon carcinomas and liposarcomas. Cancer Res 1986;46:6169–6173.

142. Philipps A, Drakenberg K, Persson B, et al. The effects of altered nutritional status upon insulin-like growth factors and their binding proteins in neonatal rats. Pediatr Res 1989;26:128–134.

143. Feingold AR, Vermund SH, Burk RD, et al. Cervical cytologic abnormalities and papillomavirus in women infected with human immunodeficiency virus. J Acquir Immune Defic Syndr 1990;3:896–903.

144. Rellihan MA, Dooley DP, Burke TW, Berkland ME, Longfield RN. Rapidly progressing cervical cancer in a patient with human immunodeficiency virus infection. Gynecol Oncol 1990;36:435–438.

145. Maiman M, Fruchter RG, Serur E, Remy JC, Feuer G, Boyce J. Human immunodeficiency virus infection and cervical neoplasia. Gynecol Oncol 1990;38:377–382.

146. Winkler B, Richart RM. Human papillomavirus and gynecologic neoplasia. Curr Probl Obstet Gynecol Fertil 1987;10:49–90.

147. Centers for Disease Control. AIDS in women—United States. MMWR 1990;39:845–849.

148. Caussy D, Goedert JJ, Palefsky J, et al. Interaction of human immunodeficiency and papilloma viruses: Association with anal epithelial abnormality in homosexual men. Int J Cancer 1990;46:214–219.

149. Melbye M, Palefsky J, Gonzales J, et al. Immune status as a determinant of human papillomavirus detection and its association with anal epithelial abnormalities. Int J Cancer 1990;46:203–206.

150. Cripe TP. Human papillomavirus: Pediatric perspectives on a family of multifaceted tumorigenic pathogens. Pediatr Infect Dis J 1990;9:836–844.

151. Prose NS, von Knebel-Doeberitz C, Miller S, Milburn PB, Heilman E. Widespread flat warts associated with human papillomavirus type 5: A cutaneous manifestation of human immunodeficiency virus infection. J Am Acad Dermatol 1990;23:978–981.

152. Forman A, Prendiville J. Association of human immunodeficiency virus seropositivity and extensive perineal condylomata acuminata in a child. Arch Dermatol 1988;124:1010–1011.

153. Laraque D. Severe anogenital warts in a child with HIV infection. N Engl J Med 1989;320:1220–1221.

154. Biggar RJ, Horm J, Lubin JH, Goedert JJ, Greene MH, Fraumeni JF. Cancer trends in a population at risk of acquired immunodeficiency syndrome. J Natl Cancer Inst 1985;74:793–797.

SECTION V

Medical Management and Treatment

General Principles of Care

Case Management

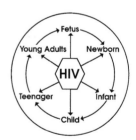

34
Drug Development and Clinical Pharmacology of Antiretroviral Drugs

Frank M. Balis and David G. Poplack

The rapid spread of AIDS and its uniformly fatal outcome underscore the urgency to develop effective therapies to treat and prevent this modern-day plague. Before the etiology of AIDS was defined, treatment was limited to supportive care measures, such as the treatment of opportunistic infections. With the discovery and characterization of human immunodeficiency virus (HIV), the retrovirus that is the etiologic agent in AIDS, new therapies that specifically inhibit this virus are being rapidly developed (1–3).

From a pharmacologic and therapeutic perspective the pathogenesis of HIV infection (Chapters 7 and 8) has several implications. There appears to be little hope of eradicating the latent HIV infection with agents currently under development, short of destroying all infected cells (2). Therefore, lifelong therapy may be required. The progressive immunologic, neurologic, and growth impairment in patients infected with HIV appears to be directly related to virus replication. Therefore, the current goal of antiretroviral therapy is to control or eliminate virus replication, diminishing spread of the virus to uninfected cells (1).

The complex and highly regulated nature of HIV replication (Chapter 7) provides many targets for pharmacologic intervention. Ideally, compounds being considered as potential antiretroviral agents should selectively inhibit virus encoded events in the HIV life cycle (1, 2). Targeting host cell mechanisms used by the virus, such as RNA polymerase or the enzymes responsible for post-translational glycosylation or myristylation of proteins, would also interfere with normal host cell function, resulting in toxicity and a lower therapeutic index.

In addition to the site of action in the virus life cycle, other pharmacologic properties must also be considered in the design and development of new antiretroviral agents (2). The need for lifelong therapy requires that potential agents have a high therapeutic index and that they be inexpensive, easy to administer (preferably orally bioavailable), and free of long-term toxicities. Even toxicities that are considered minor when associated with a short course of therapy can become intolerable when therapy is administered over a long period. To effectively control all manifestations of HIV in vivo, a drug must be active in all infected cell types and be able to penetrate the blood-brain barrier to control central nervous system infection. From a societal perspective, an effective agent also should block virus excretion and transmission to prevent spread of the disease.

The principles established for the development and use of anticancer drugs appear to be applicable to the discovery, development, and eventual use of antiretroviral agents. The National Cancer Institute drug development program has served as a model for the screening and preclinical development of potential new antiretroviral drugs. The design of initial antiretroviral agent clinical trials to establish the optimal dose, define toxicities, and establish efficacy is based on the strategy employed for phase I and phase II trials of new anticancer drugs in refractory cancer patients. Other principles of cancer therapy that may have application for the treatment of HIV infection include the use of therapy earlier in infection and the use of drugs in combination

There is a potentially compelling rationale for initiating treatment for HIV early in infection, although this must be balanced with the risk for the emergence of virus resistance. In treating the patient with AIDS, the clinician frequently must contend with controlling HIV replication; treating opportunistic infections, secondary tumors, and various other complications; as well as reconstituting normal immunologic function. However, by initiating antiretroviral therapy in the incubation period before the patient becomes symptomatic, the focus is limited to adequately controlling HIV replication, which, if successful, might permit preservation of normal immunologic and neurologic function and the delay or prevention of progressive disease. Some clinical trials of zidovudine in asymptomatic HIV-infected adult patients with CD4 counts of $<500/mm^3$ support this approach (4, 5), although other recent studies (e.g., Concorde trial) have failed to demonstrate that early intervention with zidovudine conveys a significant survival advantage or delay in the onset of AIDS-related events (see also Chapter 35). Similar data are not available for children.

The use of combination antiretroviral regimens offers the potential for additive or synergistic anti-HIV effects, while delaying or preventing the development of drug-resistant strains of the virus. Ideally agents incorporated into combination regimens should inhibit different phases of the virus life cycle, be non-cross-resistant, and have nonoverlapping toxicity spectra (6, 7). Combination antiretroviral therapy is being intensively investigated, and initial results with the combination of zidovudine and zalcitabine are promising (8–10).

The first portion of this chapter describes the drug development process as it applies to antiretroviral agents, highlighting the important steps in the process that range from drug acquisition and screening to clinical trials in humans. In the later sections, the clinical pharmacology of the dideoxynucleosides is discussed.

DEVELOPMENT OF ANTIRETROVIRAL DRUGS

The urgency to identify effective antiretroviral drugs has stimulated an unprecedented drug development initiative (11). This national AIDS drug development effort is coordinated at the National Institutes of Health by the National Institute of Allergy and Infectious Diseases (NIAID) and the National Cancer Institute (NCI). The comprehensive Drug Development Program of the NCI, which has been at the forefront of anticancer drug development for the last 30 years, is now also committed to the discovery and development of new antiretroviral agents. A large AIDS drug development program focused on the acquisition and screening of novel compounds has been incorporated into this existing drug development structure, which has considerable resources in place for the preclinical and clinical development of new drugs. The application of an already functioning drug development effort to testing antiretroviral agents should markedly facilitate AIDS drug development.

To encourage the cooperation and collaboration of academic investigators and private industry, the NIAID has established the National Cooperative Drug Discovery Program for the Treatment of AIDS with the goal of stimulating, supporting, and coordinating an integrated national multidisciplinary drug development effort. Investigators from different institutions with similar research interests are encouraged to form collaborative groups. To expedite the eventual clinical development of potential new agents arising from this collaborative effort, the groups will frequently include an industrial partner such as a pharmaceutical company (12). The NIAID also sponsors the AIDS Clinical Trials Group, a cooperative network of institutions that conducts collaborative, multidisciplinary clinical trials of antiretroviral agents. Pooling clinical resources into multi-institutional groups allows even large clinical trials to be conducted rapidly and efficiently.

Drug Development Process

The steps in the AIDS drug development process are shown in Figure 34.1. Preclinical development includes acquisition of potential agents from various sources (Table 34.1), screening for biologic effects and anti-HIV activity, chemical synthesis and bulk production of the compound for the preclinical studies and clinical trials, evaluation of the toxicology and pharmacology in animals to establish a safe dose and schedule for clinical trials in humans, and development of a practical clinical formulation (preferably an oral formulation). Issues involving synthesis, production, and formulation of a drug are beyond the scope of this chapter, but the remaining steps in this process are described below.

Acquisition

Two basic strategies are employed for identifying potential new agents: random

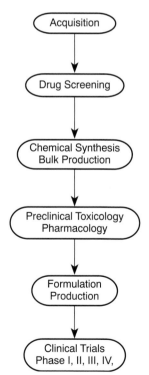

Figure 34.1.   Steps in antiretroviral drug development process.

Table 34.1.   Sources of New Antiretroviral Compounds[a]

NCI synthetics and natural products repositories
NCI congener and prodrug synthesis programs
NIAID National Cooperative Drug Screening
  Groups
National Institutes of Health intramural laboratories
NIAID Clinical Drug Development Committee
Other government laboratories
National Institutes of Health grantees and
  contractors
Private research institutes and foundations
Individual investigators
Universities and other academic institutions
Pharmaceutical, chemical, and biotechnological
  industries
International collaborations.

[a]Adapted with permission from Boyd MR. Strategies for the identification of new agents for the treatment of AIDS: A national program to facilitate the discovery and preclinical development of new drug candidates for clinical evaluation. In DeVita VT, Helman S, Rosenberg SA, eds. AIDS, etiology, diagnosis, treatment, and prevention. Philadelphia: Lippincott, 1988:305–319.

drug screening and rational drug design (12). The random drug screening program targets compounds with unique chemical structures or properties. Along with numerous extramural sources (Table 34.1), the NCI repositories of natural and synthetic compounds have provided an abundant supply of potential agents to be screened for anti-HIV activity. Particular emphasis has been placed on the investigation of natural products, and an international effort has been mounted to acquire extracts from a wide variety of both plant and marine organisms for random screening.

Rational drug design targets specific steps in the HIV life cycle, which has been largely delineated and is extraordinarily complex (1, 13). Once comprehensive biochemical and molecular biologic studies of the enzymes, cofactors, and regulatory proteins involved in a specific step have been performed, the chemical structures of specific inhibitors are predicted, synthesized, and tested. The most promising viral targets for pharmacologic intervention include reverse transcriptase that synthesizes proviral DNA from the viral RNA template, the viral protease that cleaves viral polyproteins into functional units, and the family of at least six virally encoded regulatory proteins, such as the *tat* gene product (1, 2, 13). Several selective reverse transcriptase inhibitors have already been developed and are in various phases of preclinical or clinical testing.

Screening

There are several approaches to screening for anti-HIV activity. Most compounds are screened in in vitro cell culture systems in which the ability of the potential agent to protect an HIV-susceptible cell line against the cytopathic effects of the virus is used to assess antiretroviral activity. These in vitro assay systems have the advantage of being rapid and relatively inexpensive, making them ideal for large-scale screening. Animal models used to study the pathogenesis of retroviral infections are also useful in assessing the antiretroviral activity of compounds in vivo and, at the same time, in defining the optimal dose and schedule of the drug. In addition, the activity of rationally synthesized compounds can be tested against specific virus components. For example, the cloning of the gene that encodes for reverse transcriptase has made sufficient quantities of reverse transcriptase available for direct testing of potential reverse transcriptase inhibitors. Potential viral protease inhibitors are also initially being screened directly against the enzyme. These cell- and virus-free systems have the advantage of not exposing investigators to HIV.

In Vitro Drug Screen. Various in vitro assays have been developed to assess antiretroviral activity. One of the first assays, described by Mitsuya and coworkers (14), uses an immortalized T cell line that can be infected by HIV. In culture, these cells are exposed to HIV both in the presence and absence of the compound being screened. At the end of a 5- to 7-day incubation, the number of viable cells remaining is assessed as a measure of the degree of protection from the cytopathic effects of HIV infection. This assay system, which has also been modified to assess the degree of inhibition of viral DNA synthesis and RNA expression in susceptible T cells, has been instrumental in the development of zidovudine, didanosine, and zalcitabine (14) (Fig. 34.2). Other in vitro assays directly quantitate HIV-1-induced cytopathic effects by measuring virus plaque formation or syncytium formation (15–17), but these assays are more time consuming and

are not as applicable for screening large numbers of potential antiretroviral agents.

The NCI has developed and implemented an automated microculture assay capable of rapidly screening many compounds for anti-HIV activity (18). In this assay infected and uninfected CEM-SS-T

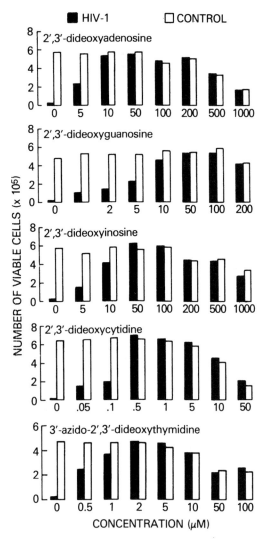

Figure 34.2. Inhibition of cytopathic effect of HIV by 2',3'-dideoxynucleosides against ATH8 cells. ATH8 cells (2×10^5) were infected with HIV and cultured in presence of varying concentrations of 2',3'-dideoxynucleosides. *Solid bars,* infected cell cultures exposed to drug. *Open bars,* control cells treated similarly but not exposed to virus. From Mitsuya H, Matsukura M, Broder S. Rapid in vitro systems for assessing activity of agents against HTLV-III/LAV. In: Broder S, ed. AIDS modern concepts and therapeutic challenges. New York: Marcel Dekker, 1987:303–334.

lymphoid target cells are exposed to serial dilutions of the test compound. After a 6-day incubation in microtiter plates, the colorless XTT tetrazolium salt (2,3-bis[2-methoxy-4-nitro-5-sulfophenyl]-5-[(phenylamino)carbonyl]-2H-tetrazolium hydroxide) is added, and cell viability is assessed colorimetrically by measuring the formation of the orange dye XTT formazan in viable cells (Fig. 34.3). This in vitro assay can screen ~50,000 compounds per year, making it practical for random drug screening. Despite this tremendous capacity, however, very few potentially clinically useful compounds have been identified.

Animal Models. Animal models have a potential role in the study of the pathogenesis of lentivirus infection and AIDS, in the development and testing of vaccines for HIV, and in the assessment of the antiretroviral activity of potential anti-HIV drugs. Although retrovirus-infected animals (especially primates) are not as practical for large-scale drug screening as the in vitro assays described above, they offer the opportunity of studying a potentially active drug's effect in vivo as well as identifying an effective dose, schedule, and route of administration for new antiviral agents (19).

The ideal animal model—one in which HIV-1 infects an inexpensive and readily available laboratory animal and produces a disease analogous to AIDS—has yet to be discovered (20). HIV has been experimentally transmitted to chimpanzees and gibbons resulting in a specific antibody response, but these animals do not develop signs of disease and are not practical as a research model because of their endangered status and prohibitive cost. Attempts at producing HIV infection in numerous small animal species have been unsuccessful (21).

Lentivirus infections in sheep, goats, horses, cattle, and cats are analogous to HIV infection in humans. These viruses are genetically similar to HIV (contain *gag, pol,* and *env* genes) and share many clinical and immunologic features (20, 22). The naturally occurring lentivirus infection with the most striking similarities to HIV is the simian immunodeficiency virus (SIV) of macaques. Infected monkeys become deficient in CD4+ cells, and most experience weight loss, opportunistic infections (including *Pneumocystis carinii* pneumonia, disseminated CMV, and mycobacterial infections), and primary simian immunodeficiency virus encephalitis (20). Considerable

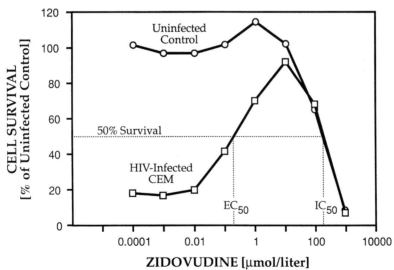

Figure 34.3. Quantitation of anti-HIV activity of zidovudine in NCI soluble-formazan drug screening assay. Infected and uninfected CEM-SS target cells (10^4/well) are incubated with varying concentrations of zidovudine, and cell survival is expressed as a percentage of an untreated and uninfected control. Comparison of the EC_{50} (protection in infected cells) to the IC_{50} (cytotoxicity in uninfected cells) allows calculation of an in vitro therapeutic index (IC_{50}/EC_{50}), which for zidovudine is 1027. This colorimetric test is rapid, accurate, and suitable for high-flux in vitro antiretroviral drug screening. Adapted from Ref. 18.

effort is being expended to develop this simian immunodeficiency virus model as a research tool.

A novel approach to the development of a small animal model of HIV infection involves the xenogeneic transplantation of human peripheral blood lymphocytes into the severe combined immunodeficient mouse. This chimeric model permits the study of HIV infection in human T cells in an in vivo setting (23, 24). Although these animals do not develop clinical signs of AIDS, the human cells can be reliably infected with HIV, and the infection can be quantitated. Therefore, the model may have application in the screening of drugs for antiretroviral activity (23). From a pharmacologic perspective, studying the pharmacodynamics of anti-HIV drugs in human cells in this model eliminates potential interspecies differences in the intracellular metabolism of a drug in the target cell. For example, the rate and degree of metabolic activation (phosphorylation) of zidovudine and zalcitabine are highly dependent on the cell species (25).

Murine retroviruses, like the CAS-Br-E neurotropic virus and the LP-BM5 leukemia virus, may also have application in the study of new drugs. The CAS-Br-E retrovirus infects the lymphocytes and central nervous system of fetal or newborn mice and produces neuropathologic changes similar to HIV infection in humans. Zidovudine has been shown to be therapeutically beneficial in this model (26). The LP-BM5 retrovirus infection results in an immunodeficiency state similar to AIDS and causes neurologic changes. Similarities between the clinical and immunologic changes that occur in this model and those seen early in HIV infection in humans are striking, making LP-BM5 a potential model for drug evaluation (27).

Toxicology and Pharmacology

Antiretroviral agents identified as active against HIV in the screen and available in sufficient amounts undergo preclinical toxicology and pharmacology studies in animals (usually rodents and dogs). Toxicology studies describe the type of side effects produced by a drug and define its maximally tolerated dose, which in turn is used to determine an appropiate and safe starting dose for initial clinical studies in humans. Pharmacokinetic studies in animals elucidate the plasma concentration profile of the drug and other relevant parameters like its route of elimination, oral bioavailability, and degree of central nervous system penetration. A rhesus monkey model developed at the NCI has been useful in assessing the central nervous system pharmacology of antiretroviral agents (see below) (28). These pharmacokinetic parameters contribute to the selection of the optimal dose, route, and schedule of administration in humans. Establishing a relationship between plasma drug concentration and the dose-limiting toxicity in the animal toxicology and pharmacology studies may allow more rapid dose escalation in the human trials. Once the pharmacokinetic profile of the drug is defined in initial patients treated at a safe starting dose, the dose and schedule in humans required to achieve this toxic level from the animal studies can be calculated. This approach is being tested wtih new anti-cancer drugs (29).

Clinical Trials

New investigational drugs traditionally proceed through three phases of clinical investigation in humans to establish their safety and efficacy before being either approved for routine use and marketed or dropped from further consideration. However, with the current emphasis on expediting the drug approval process for anti-retroviral agents, the clinical phase of drug development is often compressed by combining objectives from different phases into a single trial (e.g., phase I/II). In addition, new anti-HIV drugs are being considered for approval by the Food and Drug Administration (FDA) before completing all phases of the clinical investigation process. As a result, a greater emphasis must be placed on continued clinical investigation of agents after approval and marketing to refine the optimal dose and schedule, establish indications for use of the drug, and determine its efficacy compared with standard therapy. With zidovudine, for example, continued clinical investigations have demonstrated that a considerably lower daily dose (500 mg/day) is as effective and less toxic in adults than the dose that received FDA approval (1500 mg/day). In addition, there has been an expansion of the patient population for which zidovudine is indicated to include asymptomatic HIV-positive patients with CD4 cell counts of $< 500/mm^3$.

Clinical Trial Design. In the initial or phase I trial, the new agent is administered to patients whose disease is refractory to conventional therapy with the primary objectives of 1) determining the maximum tolerated dose on a clinically useful schedule, 2) defining the spectrum and reversibility of toxicities, and 3) performing detailed pharmacokinetic studies. The starting dose on the phase I trial is derived from animal toxicology studies. If tolerated, the dose is then escalated in subsequent cohorts of patients (usually three to six per dose level) until dose-limiting toxicity is consistently observed and a safe dose for subsequent trials is defined. Phase I trials enroll patients who are intolerant of standard therapy, have refractory disease, or are asymptomatic and for whom standard antiretroviral therapy is not indicated. Careful baseline evaluation and follow-up of the status and function of all organ systems are essential to define the incidence and severity of both expected and unexpected toxicities of new phase I agents. Despite the fact that phase I trials of anti-HIV drugs are principally designed to define the toxicities and determine the tolerable dose of a new agent, these trials are performed with therapeutic intent, and drug activity is usually assessed in the patients treated.

Once a safe and tolerable dose has been defined, a phase II trial is performed to define the degree of clinical activity of the new agent. In these trials the degree of activity is generally measured by changes in surrogate markers of the disease over the course of treatment compared with pretherapy measurements as a control (30). Unfortunately, an ideal clinical or laboratory marker of virus replication or disease progression in HIV infection has not been identified. Parameters that have been monitored in children include clinical manifestations of HIV infection such as growth velocity and neuropsychological status, laboratory markers of damage to the immune system such as CD4+ cell count and percentage of CD4+ cells, and laboratory measures of virus replication and virus load such as p24 antigen level and quantitative viral culture. Other clinical manifestations of HIV infection such as opportunistic infections and cancers are also a result of the immunosuppression, but occur sporadically and unpredictably and do not always clearly denote disease progression. Since most phase I trials of new antiretroviral agents in children also incorporate these phase II end points, these studies would be more appropriately classified as phase I/II trials.

Finally, drugs found to be safe and active proceed to phase III trials, where they are compared in a randomized fashion to existing standard therapy (standard vs. new) or are added to standard therapy as a combination regimen (standard plus new vs. standard). Phase III trials have usually been performed in previously untreated patients, and efficacy (benefit to the patient) is the primary end point. Subjects must therefore be closely followed for evidence of disease improvements or prgression. The clinical and laboratory surrogate markers of response discussed above are usually monitored, but the experience with surrogate markers to date does not allow them to completely replace clinical end points, such as survival and new opportunistic infections, in phase III trials (30). This situation creates a dilemma, because trials are now enrolling asymptomatic HIV-infected subjects who have a lower incidence of these clinical events, requiring larger sample sizes or longer observation periods to evaluate the agent. To establish the validity and predictive ability of potential surrogate markers as true measures of therapeutic efficacy, ongoing and future phase III trials should continue to monitor both clinical outcomes as well as clinical laboratory surrogate markers to evaluate the predictive ability of the markers. The number of patients required to complete a phase III trial depends on the magnitude of the difference between the regimens being compared. For example, if standard therapy yields a 50% response rate, to detect a 20% improvement (response rate of 70%) with the new or experimental treatment at a significance level of $P < 0.05$ would require that 124 patients be entered on each arm of a randomized trial (31). Attempting to show equivalency between regimens can require enormous numbers of patients.

Clinical Trials in Children.   As in cancer therapy where many modern principles of treatment are based on early success in treating children with cancer, the clinical investigation of new therapies for HIV infection in children may benefit all patients with the disease. In fact, the novel and apparently efficacious approach of continuously infusing dideoxynucleosides like zidovudine was initially tested by pediatric investigators in children (32).

Traditionally, there has been a reluctance to perform initial clinical trials of investigational agents in children. As a result, drugs are frequently approved by the FDA and marketed without being fully tested in infants and children. Even though the FDA is responsible for assuring the safety and efficacy of drugs marketed in this country, there is no regulatory requirement that new agents be tested in children before approval, despite the fact that once on the market drugs can be legally prescribed to infants and children. Approximately 75% of the drugs prescribed by office pediatricians are not approved for pediatric use, and most have labeling cautions regarding use in children.

If clinical trials of any type of new drug are not performed in children, because of ethical or regulatory concerns, the optimal dose and schedule, toxicity spectrum, clinical pharmacology, and efficacy will not be determined for the pediatric age group, raising the possibility that children may ultimately be treated under unsafe conditions (i. e., based only on adult data). Current regulations that allow approval of new agents without testing in children are being revised to ensure that drugs are tested in all age groups, and a new attitude toward testing promising investigational agents early in children is being increasingly fostered to ensure that active drugs can be made available and administered safely to children.

Separate phase I trials of new antiretroviral agents are being conducted in HIV-infected children and adults, because of the presumed age-related physiologic differences in body composition and excretory organ function that lead to differences in drug disposition (absorption, distribution, and excretion or metabolism) and sensitivity to toxicity. In the past, the starting dose for phase I trials of new agents in children was based on the maximum tolerated dose identified in phase I trials in adults, which necessitated significant delays in the drug development process in children until adult trials were completed. In a uniformly fatal disease such as AIDS for which no alternative curative therapy is available, delaying pediatric phase I trials of potentially beneficial agents has been challenged (33), and there are signs that this policy, like many other regulatory directives regarding new drug development, may change.

This new approach to drug development has included more and earlier clinical trials of investigational agents in infants and children. Pediatric phase I/II trials of didanosine were initiated before the completion of adult trials without serious consequences, and didanosine received unprecedented simultaneous FDA approval in children and adults, making this agent available to pediatric patients earlier and at a dose and schedule that was found to be safe and efficacious in children. If these pediatric trials had been delayed until after the agents had received expedited approval for use in adults, accruing HIV-infected children to the trials would have been very difficult beause the drug would have been available on the open market.

The limitations of performing clinical trials of investigational agents in HIV-infected children include 1) limited patient population available for study, 2) difficulty in establishing the diagnosis of HIV infection in an infant, 3) need to evaluate several age groups (neonate, infant, child, and adolescent), 4) difficulty in obtaining informed consent because of the often formidable social situation, 5) lack of a satisfactory drug formulation (e. g., oral suspension), 6) lack of support from pharmaceutical sponsors who shy away from studies in children, because of legal issues, cost, and a limited sales market, and 7) ethical issues involved in using investigational agents in children. These disadvantages, however, are far outweighed by the advantages outlined above, and because of the need to rapidly develop new agents for the treatment of HIV disease in children, every attempt should be made to place eligible children into ongoing clinical trials of investigational agents rather than treat them with second-line therapy in a nonresearch setting.

Regulatory Issues

Role of FDA

The development of new drugs is regulated by the FDA, which is responsible for ensuring that new agents are safe and effective for their proposed indications before they are approved for marketing. After preclinical testing of a potential new drug is completed (see above) and before clinical trials in humans can begin, the sponsor of the new drug (pharmaceutical company, government, or private research institution) must file an Investigational New Drug (IND) application with the FDA. This document contains results of the preclinical testing, manufacturing information, and a protocol for the initial phase I clinical trial. The holder of the IND then conducts or sponsors clinical trials that are closely monitored by the FDA.

If the clinical trials demonstrate that the new drug is safe and efficacious, a New Drug Application (NDA) is submitted by the sponsor to the FDA for review and approval. The NDA contains detailed chemistry and manufacturing information, results of preclinical and clinical testing, and proposed labeling for the new agent with indications for its use and appropriate warnings. The NDA is reviewed by a primary FDA review team and in many cases by an advisory panel of outside experts. Traditionally, the FDA has required substantial evidence of efficacy from adequate, well controlled investigations (including clinical investigations) before a new drug could be licensed for marketing.

The sponsor can also apply for a treatment IND, a protocol to provide for wide distribution of a promising investigational agent, before FDA approval. The agent must be intended to treat a serious or life-threatening illness, there must be no comparable or satisfactory alternative therapy,

the drug must be under investigation (or controlled clinical trials must have been completed), and the sponsor must be actively pursuing marketing approval.

The FDA can encourage but not require that a sponsor perform studies to support a pediatric indication for their drug. Regulations only require that statements addressing pediatric use of a new drug be supported by substantial evidence derived from adequate and well controlled studies even for an indication approved for adults. If such evidence is unavailable the label must state that "safety and effectiveness in children have not been established."

Criteria for final approval for the use of anti-HIV drugs in children have not been firmly established. Once the efficacy of zidovudine was demonstrated in adults in the placebo-controlled trial, the drug was rapidly approved by the FDA for adults with AIDS. However, approval for the use of zidovudine in children was delayed, in part because similar placebo-controlled efficacy data were unavailable in pediatric AIDS patients. Since the pathogenesis of HIV infection is the same in children and adults (even though the clinical manifestations are strikingly different), a more logical and ethical approach to assess drugs that have demonstrated efficacy in adult phase II and phase III trials would be to require only safety (toxicity) and pharmacokinetic data in children before approval. This approach would avoid a long delay in the approval of an active agent for use in children, as occurred with zidovudine.

Impact of AIDS on Drug Development

The urgency to find effective drugs to treat HIV infection has not only stimulated the scientific community to alter research priorities but has also compelled the FDA and other regulatory agencies to reassess regulations governing new drug development and approval (34). Public and political pressure have mandated fundamental changes in the previously accepted model of clinical testing of new agents, placing a greater emphasis on accelerating or expediting the process (33). The FDA is taking a more proactive role in the development of drugs, working with the new drug's sponsor from the earliest stages to design the most efficient preclinical and clinical studies to demonstrate safety and efficacy.

This expedited review process leads to approval of new agents based on an incomplete data base. Didanosine approval, for example, was based primarily on uncontrolled phase I trials and limited data from the expanded access program, although a preliminary review of a controlled trial in adults was also utilized. Therefore, postmarketing studies take increasing importance in better defining the drug's optimal dose and schedule and indications for its use.

In addition to the establishment of fast track criteria for regulatory approval of new drugs, the FDA has adopted an expanded compassionate release program for investigational agents (expanded access), which permits promising investigational AIDS drugs to be distributed to patients whose disease is immediately life threatening and who are not otherwise eligible for ongoing clinical trials, after initial phase I testing and before completion of phase II and phase III trials (35). This expanded access or parallel track mechanism provides access to new agents much earlier for patients with AIDS who are willing to accept the potential risks associated with receiving an investigational (incompletely tested) drug.

This new policy has also raised concern among some clinical investigators who fear that reducing patients' incentive to participate in clinical studies could limit the eventual ability to successfully conduct phase II and phase III trials. For didanosine, the ratio of patient enrollment on the expanded access protocol to open clinical trials of the drug was 5 to 1 at the San Francisco General Hospital (36). To ensure the timely completion of pediatric drug trials, an attempt should be made to enter every HIV-infected child into an ongoing clinical trial if the child is eligible and the family is willing to participate and comply with the protocol requirements. The effect of expanded access drug distribution on pediatric trials is unclear, but the expanded access mechanism should be reserved only for children who do not meet the eligibility criteria of the ongoing studies, who are unwilling to participate in the trial, or for whom the trials are inaccessible.

An additional challenge posed to regulatory agencies by pediatric AIDS relates to the need for testing of new agents in infants and newborns. Perinatally acquired infection has become the dominant mode of transmission of HIV to children, and the increasing numbers of infected newborns and infants underscores the need both to identify new agents that can prevent perinatal transmission and to develop drugs to effectively treat children in this age group.

CLINICAL PHARMACOLOGY OF ANTIRETROVIRAL DRUGS

The only antiretroviral drugs currently approved for treatment of HIV infection are the deoxynucleoside analogs zidovudine (azidothymidine), didanosine (dideoxyinosine), and zalcitabine (dideoxycytidine) (Fig. 34.4). All three agents have undergone phase I/II clinical trials in children (see Chapter 35) and have demonstrated activity, but each drug also produces significant toxicities (9, 32, 37, 38).

To ensure that these antiretroviral drugs are used safely and effectively, the clinician must have an in-depth knowledge of the clinical pharmacology of the agents, including their mechanism of action, pharmacokinetics, spectrum of toxicities, potential drug interactions, and mechanism of virus drug resistance. Ongoing clinical trials should further define the optimal dose and schedule and role for each of these agents in the treatment of HIV-infected children (39).

Mechanism of Action

The dideoxynucleosides are structurally related compounds that inhibit the critical virus enzyme reverse transcriptase, which synthesizes proviral double-stranded DNA from a virus RNA template. As shown in Figure 34.5, these agents are prodrugs that require intracellular conversion by host cell kinases to their 5'-triphosphate form before expressing their antiretroviral activity. The active dideoxynucleotide triphosphates compete with their endogenous deoxynucleotide triphosphate counterpart for incorporation into the proviral DNA by reverse transcriptase. Once incorporated, the absence of a hydroxyl group at the 3'-position

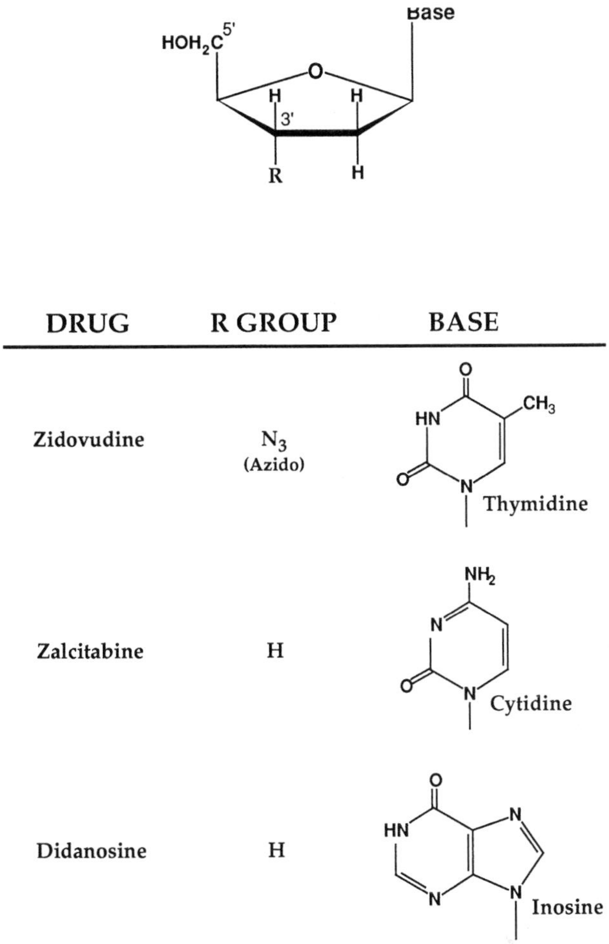

Figure 34.4.   Chemical structure of dideoxynucleosides. R group at the 3' position of endogenous deoxynucleosides in a hydroxyl group.

on the sugar moiety prevents further elongation of the DNA chain.

The selectivity of these agents for incorporation into proviral DNA is related to the greater affinity of HIV reverse transcriptase for the dideoxynucleotide triphosphates compared with host cell DNA polymerases. For example, the K_i (in μmol/liter) of zidovudine triphosphate for HIV reverse transcriptase is 0.01 and for human DNA polymerases-α and -β it is 230 and 73, respectively (40).

With prodrugs like the dideoxynucleosides, where an additional cell or tissue dependent step of drug activation is required, intracellular levels of the active form of the drug may vary in different cell types based on the activity of kinases, the enzymes responsible for phosphorylation of these

agents. For example, in vitro studies have demonstrated that zidovudine triphosphate formation in cells of the monocyte-macrophage lineage is limited compared with the degree of drug activation in T cells (41).

Pharmacokinetics

The discipline of pharmacokinetics deals with quantitative aspects of drug disposition in the body, including drug absorption, distribution, metabolism, and excretion. Pharmacokinetics is important in the clinical development of new antiretroviral compounds and in the daily management of children receiving these agents. Detailed pharmacokinetic monitoring of plasma drug concentrations performed on patients treated on initial phase I and II trials is used

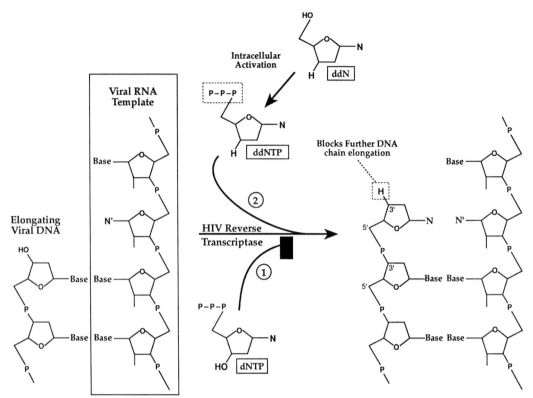

Figure 34.5. Mechanism of action of dideoxynucleosides (*ddN*). After intracellular activation by enzymatic conversion to triphosphate dideoxynucleotide form (*ddNTP*), these agents inhibit reverse transcriptase by 1) competing with endogenous deoxynucleotide triphosphates (*dNTP*) for binding to reverse transcriptase and 2) becoming incorporated into elongating proviral DNA and acting as a chain terminator because of the absence of the 3'-hydroxyl group required to form 3',5'-phosphodiester bridge between nucleotides.

to define the rate of drug elimination (clearance and half-life) as well as the route of elimination (metabolism vs. renal or biliary excretion). In addition, for drugs that are administered by nonintravenous routes (e.g., orally), the rate and extent of absorption are also determined. Because antiretroviral therapy must be administered for prolonged intervals, and possibly lifelong, the oral route is clearly most feasible provided an oral formulation of the drug is bioavailable.

Because of the severe consequences of HIV encephalopathy, the ability of potential antiretroviral agents to penetrate the blood-brain barrier and effectively reverse this complication is an important consideration in antiretroviral pharmacology. Measurement of cerebrospinal fluid (CSF) drug concentration is an indicator of the degree of penetration of drug into the central nervous system and thus a potentially useful guide in the selection of appropriate antiretroviral therapy.

The pharmacokinetic parameters noted above are used to determine the optimal drug dose, schedule, and route of administration and any adjustments in the dose and schedule required for excretory organ dysfunction. The latter is a common problem in children with symptomatic HIV infection. An HIV-associated nephropathy has been described in both children and adults with AIDS and is characterized by proteinuria and renal failure requiring dosage modification (42, 43). In addition, children with AIDS are often receiving many potentially hepatotoxic or nephrotoxic drugs. The fact that some opportunistic infections or other complications of AIDS can adversely affect renal and hepatic function must also be considered.

In addition, if a relationship can be established between these pharmacokinetic parameters and toxicity or drug response, further dose adjustments in individual patients could be based on plasma drug concentrations (therapeutic drug monitoring). Individualizing therapy based on drug levels can enhance the safety and effectiveness of the therapy.

Developmental Pharmacology

A particular concern in treating children relates to the age-dependent disposition of many drugs. Maturational changes in body composition, size of body compartments, and excretory organ function occur during childhood and are responsible for the differences in drug distribution and elimination between children and adults. Many of these physiologic changes in body water and fat content, extracellular fluid volume, glomerular filtration rate, renal tubular secretory mechanisms, and levels of hepatic drug metabolizing enzymes actually occur in the first days to months of life (44). Table 34.2 summarizes some of these maturational changes in body composition and organ function that can influence drug disposition. The pharmacokinetic data collected during the initial trials of a new

agent are useful in establishing relationships between drug disposition and age both by correlating the parameters to age in newborns, infants, children, and adolescents and by comparing pharmacokinetic parameters in children to those in adults.

An understanding of development pharmacology is particularly relevant for clinicians treating children with HIV infection. Perinatal acquisition now accounts for more than 90% of new cases of HIV infection in children, and with the trend toward earlier intervention with antiretroviral therapy, it is likely that neonates and infants will become the focus of treatment. In fact, consideration is being given to in utero therapy to prevent the spread of HIV from mother to fetus.

Therapeutic Drug Monitoring

Administering a standard fixed dose (normalized to body weight or surface area) to a group of patients will not result in a uniform response or equivalent degrees of toxicity. This variability in the pharmacologic effect of a drug may be due to various factors, such as individual variation in the sensitivity of the host and virus to the effects of the

Table 34.2.   Physiological Differences between Children and Adults That May Influence Drug Disposition[a]

Characteristic	Value at Birth	Age Adult Values Are Reached	Effect on Drug Disposition
Body composition			
Total body water	↑	6 mo	↑ Distribution volume
Extracellular fluid	↑	6 mo	↑ Distribution volume
Fat	↓	Adolescence	↓ Distribution volume of lipophilic drugs
Protein binding	↓	1 yr	↑ Free drug levels
Kidney			
Size[c]	↑		
Renal blood flow	↓	1 yr	↓ Renal excretion
Glomerular filtration	↓	6 mo	↓ Renal excretion
Tubular function	↓	1 yr	↓ Tubular secretion
Liver			
Size[c]	↑		
Oxidative metabolism	↓	6 mo	↓ Metabolic clearance
Glucuronidation	↓	2–3 yr	↓ Metabolic clearance
Biliary excretion	↓	6 mo	↓ Biliary excretion
Gastrointestinal			
Acid secretion	↓	3 mo	Altered drug absorption
Motility	↓	6 mo	Delayed absorption

[a]Modified from Balis FM, Holcenberg JS, Poplack DG. General principles of chemotherapy. In: Pizzo PA, Poplack DG, eds. Principles and practice of pediatric oncology. Philadelphia: Lippincott, 1989;165–205. ↓ decreased; ↑ increased.
[b]Compared with adult values and relative to body surface area.
[c]Organ weight as a percent of total body weight.

drug (pharmacodynamics) and individual variation in drug disposition (pharmacokinetics). The concentration of drug achieved in the body after a standard dose is a function of the developmental factors noted above, the status of excretory organs, and individual differences in drug absorption, distribution, metabolism, and excretion. These individual differences in otherwise healthy subjects can explain considerable variability in the systemic level of a drug that is achieved. For example, in children without clinical evidence of organ dysfunction, the clearance of zidovudine ranges from 280 to 950 ml/min/m^2 (45). This variation in systemic drug level can be regulated with the use of therapeutic drug monitoring. Plasma concentrations of the drug or its active metabolites are measured following a standard starting dose, and then the dose and schedule of the drug are adjusted to bring the systemic drug concentrations within a predefined, desired range.

The basic assumption underlying therapeutic drug monitoring is that the concentration of drug at the site of action (and, in the case of prodrugs like zidovudine, the amount of activated metabolites formed) is proportional to the plasma concentration of the drug. If this relationship exists, then it should theoretically be possible to define a therapeutic and toxic plasma concentration of the drug. Plasma concentration is then maintained in this therapeutic window between the therapeutic and toxic concentrations. Therapeutic drug monitoring is only practical if this window has been defined in the initial clinical trials.

The other requirement for making therapeutic drug monitoring practical in the daily management of patients receiving the drug is the availability of a simple monitoring schedule. For drugs with a long half-life and a relatively short dosing interval (e.g., dilantin), a single sample drawn at a defined time after the dose is usually sufficient. With drugs that are more rapidly eliminated, like many antibiotics, peak and trough levels are sufficient to describe the disposition of the drug. Studies are under way to devise a simple monitoring scheme for the dideoxynucleosides zidovudine and didanosine with the use of a limited sampling strategy approach (46).

Toxicity

Despite similarity in the chemical structure of the dideoxynucleosides (Figure 34.4), their toxicity profiles are quite different. In the initial clinical trials in children, the dose-limiting toxicities of zidovudine, didanosine, and zalcitabine were myelosuppression, pancreatitis, and rash/mucositis, respectively. These nonoverlapping toxicity spectra may be useful in the design of dideoxynucleoside combination regimens, since the lack of addictive toxic effects may allow each agent to be administered at its optimal dose.

Drug intolerance is a significant problem with the dideoxynucleosides and a major reason for discontinuation of therapy. In addition to the dose-limiting toxicities listed above, other toxicities like headache and nausea that would be considered minor if associated with a short course of therapy can become intolerable when therapy is administered over a long period. However, considering the limited number of treatment alternatives, the clinician and patient may be forced to either tolerate toxicity or in some instances to institute supportive care measures to reverse the toxicity rather than changing or discontinuing a therapy.

Manifestations of the underlying HIV infection and its complications may be difficult to distinguish from drug toxicity in symptomatic patients. HIV can cause nonspecific symptoms like headache, fever, and malaise, and its later stage can suppress bone marrow function leading to anemia and neutropenia. Because of the difficulty at times in differentiating between an adverse drug effect and manifestations of the underlying HIV infection in symptomatic patients, baseline measurements of the parameters to be monitored must be obtained before start of antiretroviral therapy.

Drug Interactions

Treatment of children with symptomatic HIV infection often involves the use of many drugs in addition to specific antiretroviral therapy, such as *Pneumocystis* prophylaxis, antibacterial and antifungal chemotherapy, intravenous γ-globulin, and colony stimulating factors (granulocyte colony-stimulating factor, erythropoietin). In addition, the use of combination antiretroviral therapy is now under study. With this degree of polypharmacy the probability for an interaction between two drugs is increased. Drug interactions can lead to unexpected or severe toxicities or antagonism that can diminish a drug's antiretroviral effect.

One drug can potentially interfere with or enhance the pharmacologic effects of another drug at a pharmacokinetic level or a pharmacodynamic level. At a pharmacokinetic level, absorption, protein binding, metabolism, or excretion can be altered, leading to an increase or decrease in the concentration of the affected drug in the body. At a pharmacodynamic level one drug can biochemically antagonize or potentiate the effect of a second drug on a target cell or tissue level.

To recognize and circumvent this potential problem, clinicians must have a firm understanding of the pharmacology of the drugs being administered and anticipate potential drug interactions. Because most significant interactions occur at the level of drug metabolism (either activation or degradation) or excretion, knowledge of the metabolism and route of elimination of these agents is the most critical. In addition, an adverse drug interaction should be suspected when unexpected or severe side effects are observed.

Drug Resistance

Virus isolates from patients receiving prolonged therapy with dideoxynucleosides have been shown to have decreased drug sensitivity in vitro (47–50). This is consistent with the clinical observation that most HIV-infected patients who were initially responsive to single agent dideoxynucleoside therapy will eventually experience progression of disease despite being maintained on long-term therapy with the same agent. The emergence of these drug-resistant HIV strains is the result of underlying mutations in the *pol* gene of the viral genome that render the gene product, reverse transcriptase, less susceptible to the inhibitory effects of the antiretroviral drugs. In addition, with isolates taken over from the same patient there is often a progressive stepwise increase in the

in vitro drug resistance that is associated with the accumulation of multiple mutations that appear to act additively or synergistically.

Clinical implications of these in vitro observations are under intensive investigation. Drug resistance has been a major obstacle in the treatment of other virus and bacteria (including mycobacterial) infections, as well as the treatment of cancer, and strategies used to overcome resistance in these diseases, such as the use of drug combinations, may be applicable to the treatment of HIV infection (49).

Zidovudine

Zidovudine, a deoxythymidine analogue (Figure 34.4), was the first antiretroviral agent to be approved for use in HIV-infected adults and children and is the standard of frontline therapy for the disease. Zidovudine has been administered to children orally and intravenously (including by long-term continuous infusion). Oral dosage forms include a 100-mg capsule and a 10 mg/ml syrup, and the recommended oral dose is 180 mg/m^2/dose every 6 hr in children >3 months old. In newborns <2 weeks old, 2 mg/kg every 6 hr is well tolerated and achieves comparable plasma zidovidine concentrations (50a). The dose can be safely increased to 3 mg/kg every 6 hr in infants >14 days old.

Zidovudine was initially approved in adults under the accelerated approval process at a dose of 250 mg every 4 hr based on the randomized placebo-controlled trial demonstrating its safety and efficacy (51, 52). However, because of significant hematologic toxicities, subsequent studies evaluated lower dose regimens (500 mg/day) that have proved to be equally efficacious and less toxic (53). Similar dose comparison studies are ongoing in children, but care must be taken to ensure that neuropsychometric end points are included in any evaluation of a lower dosage regimen of the drug, since drug exposure in the central nervous system is lower than that achieved systemically.

Pharmacokinetics

Intravenously administered zidovudine is rapidly eliminated from plasma with a terminal half-life of 1.5 hr and a clearance of 650 ml/min/m^2 in children aged 12 months to 13 years (Table 34.3) (45, 54). Disposition of the drug in this age group was very similar to that reported in adults (Table 34.3) (54). The primary route of drug elimination is hepatic metabolism to the 5'-glucuronide conjugate that is then excreted in the urine (55). The glucuronide of zidovudine is detectable in plasma but has no anti-HIV activity. Approximately one-fourth of a zidovudine dose is excreted in the urine unchanged, and the renal clearance of zidovudine actually exceeds the rate of creatinine clearance, suggesting that the drug undergoes both glomerular filtration and renal tubular secretion (45, 55).

When administered by continuous infusion, steady state plasma concentrations of zidovudine exceeding 1.0 μmol/liter can be achieved with a daily dose of 360 mg/m^2 (45). Maintaining a trough level of 1.0 μmol/liter on an intermittent 6-hr schedule would require a 10-fold higher daily dose.

Organ Dysfunction.   In one study in patients with renal failure, plasma zidovudine concentrations after an oral dose were 2-fold higher than in normal subjects, and both renal clearance and urinary excretion were markedly reduced (56). Plasma concentrations of the glucuronide conjugate of zidovudine were increased more than 15-fold in patients with renal dysfunction. Although the recommendation from this single-dose study was that no zidovudine dose adjustment is necessary in patients with severe renal dysfunction (creatinine clearance between 10 and 30 ml/min), with chronic administration, a 2-fold increase in plasma concentrations for a drug with a low therapeutic index could be significant, and dose adjustments may become necessary.

In patients with end-stage renal disease undergoing hemodialysis, a chronic oral dosing regimen of 100 mg three times a day maintained trough zidovudine concentrations in the target range and was well tolerated by the patients (57).

Bioavailability.   In children zidovudine is rapidly absorbed when administered orally with a mean time to peak < 1 hr (Fig. 34.6) (54). The absolute bioavailability in ten children monitored after both an intravenous and oral dose was 68%, and eight of the ten absorbed more than 50% of the oral dose (54). Since over 90% of the dose can be recovered from urine as either parent drug or the 5'-glucuronide, the remaining drug probably undergoes first pass metabolism to glucuronide conjugate before reaching the systemic circulation (55).

Administration of zidovudine with a high-fat meal resulted in delayed absorption and a substanitally reduced peak drug concentration (58).

Central Nervous System Pharmacology. Penetration of zidovudine into the CSF in adults treated on an intermittent oral dosing schedule has been reported to be 60%

Table 34.3.   Mean Pharmacokinetic Parameters for Dideoxynucleosides in Children and Adults[a]

Subjects	Ref.	Intravenous Dose			Oral Dose		
		Clearance	Half-life	Volume of Distribution	Peak	Half-life	Absorption
		ml/min/m^2	hr	liter/m^2	μmol/liter	hr	%
Zidovudine							
Children (n =12)	54	640	1.5	45	8.8[b]	1.5	68
Adults (n = 9)	59	650	1.1	42			63
Didanosine							
Children (n = 48)	46	510	1.0	24	1.8[c]	1.0	19
Adults (n = 20)	75	500	0.6	30	9.2[d]		38
Zalcitabine							
Children (n = 5)	9	150	0.8	9.3	0.17[e]	0.9	54
Adults (n = 10)	87	230	1.2	16			88

[a]Data extracted from the references cited. Adult parameters reported per kilogram were converted to body surface area using a factor of 30.
[b]Peak level at a dose of 180 mg/m^2 (n = 7).
[c]Peak level at a dose of 90 mg/m^2 (n = 8).
[d]Peak level at a dose of 6.4 mg/kg (n = 3–4).
[e]Peak level at a dose of 0.03 mg/kg (n = 3).

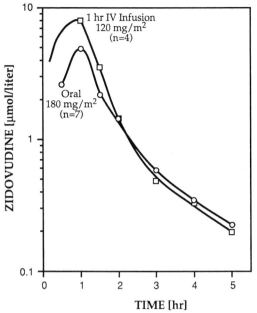

Figure 34.6. Plasma disappearance curve for zidovudine after an intravenous dose of 120 mg/m² over 1 hr in four patients and after an oral dose of 180 mg/m² in seven patients.

(13). This ratio is based on a single CSF sample taken 2–4 hr after the dose, and ratios calculated under these non-steady state conditions range from 15 to 135% and are highly dependent on the sample timing (59). A more accurate measure of the CSF penetration of zidovudine was obtained in 21 children treated on the continuous intravenous infusion schedule of zidovudine. The ratio of steady state CSF and plasma concentrations in this study was 24% (45).

The CSF penetration of zidovudine was compared with several structurally related pyrimidine deoxynucleoside analogues in a nonhuman primate model that is highly predictive of human CSF drug disposition to define factors that influence a drug's ability to penetrate the blood-brain barrier (28) (Table 34.4). Zidovudine penetration into the CSF was 21% compared with only 3% for zalcitabine. The CSF penetration of the complementary nucleoside analogues dideoxythymidine and azidodideoxycytidine was 30 and 1%, respectively. Despite the 3- to 5-fold increase in the lipophilicity conferred by the addition of the azido group to the dideoxyribose moiety, it is the nucleobase (thymine, cytosine) that deter-

mines the degree of CSF penetration of these compounds (Table 34.4). This structural specificity, unrelated to lipophilicity, suggests that a carrier-mediated process is involved in zidovudine entry into CSF (28).

Developmental Pharmacology Zidovudine elimination in newborns is delayed relative to older children and adults (50a, 60–62), an observation that has been confirmed in studies of newborn rhesus monkeys (63). Delayed elimination is probably the result of a decreased capacity for glucuronide conjugation and renal excretion, the two major routes of elimination for zidovudine. The clearance of zidovudine in infants <14 days old is 11 ml/min/kg compared with 19 ml/min/kg in infants >14 days old (50a). The half-life was also more prolonged in the younger age group. The bioavailability of oral ziduvudine was 89% in infants younger than 14 days and 61% in those older than 14 days, consistent with the observation that first pass metabolism was also decreased in the younger infants (50a). The use of zidovudine in this age group is discussed in Chapter 38.

When administered during pregnancy, zidovudine readily crosses the placenta, apparently by passive diffusion, so that drug concentrations in the fetus are equivalent to those achieved in the mother (61, 62, 64).

With continuous infusion of zidovudine in children older than 1 year, the rate of zidovudine clearance, normalized to body weight, was age dependent, with younger patients showing more rapid clearance (45). This resulted in lower steady state plasma concentrations in the children who were 1–3 years old when they were dosed according to body weight. If zidovudine

Table 34.4. CSF Penetration of Zidovudine and Related Pyrimidine Dideoxyribonucleosides[a]

Nucleobase	CSF Penetration[b]	
	2',3',-Dideoxy	3'-Azido-2',3'-dideoxy
	%	
Thymidine	30	21[c]
Cytidine	3[d]	1
Uridine	15	18

[a]From Collins JM, Klecker RW, Kelley JA, et al. Pyrimidines dideoxyribonucleosides: Selectivity of penetration into cerebrospinal fluid. J Pharmacol Exp Ther 1988;245:466–470.
[b]Ratio of area under concentration-time curve in CSF to that in plasma.
[c]Zidovudine.
[d]Zalcitabine.

clearance is normalized to body surface area, this age dependency is much less significant, indicating that more uniform plasma drug levels would be achieved by basing the dose on body surface area rather than body weight. This difference reflects the fact that hepatic and renal function are more closely correlated with body surface area than with body weight. In treating children, and especially newborns and infants, the maturational and physiologic changes that are occurring as the child grows must be considered along with the clinical pharmacology of the drug in determining the appropriate dose and schedule.

Therapeutic Drug Monitoring   Neutropenia is the dose-limiting toxicity of zidovudine on both the intermittent oral and continuous infusion schedules and is a serious complication in patients who are already severely immunosuppressed. In addition, children with AIDS have a greater incidence of serious bacterial infections that could be exacerbated by depletion of neutrophils. In the continuous infusion trial noted above, the occurrence of severe neutropenia (neutrophil count below $500/mm^3$) correlated with the steady state plasma zidovudine concentration (45). Six of the eight patients with severe neutropenia had steady state plasma zidovudine concentrations above 3.0 μmol/liter, whereas nine of 13 who maintained a neutrophil count above 500 had zidovudine levels below 3.0 μmol/liter. Although further studies are in progress to confirm these findings, 3.0 μmol/liter appears to be a toxic level on the continuous infusion schedule.

Toxicity

Although zidovudine has been well tolerated by HIV-infected children, a significant proportion experience hematologic toxicity from the drug (32, 38). In a multicenter phase II trial of zidovudine (180 mg/m² every 6 hr) nearly 50% of subjects developed neutropenia (<750/mm³) and 25% developed a macrocytic anemia (hemoglobin <7.5 mg/dl) (38). One-third of the children receiving zidovudine required a transfusion or a modification in the dose of zidovudine as a result of hematologic toxicity, but <5% needed the zidovudine discon-

tinued. The erythrocyte mean corpuscular volume increased gradually over time from 80 fl at entry to 96 fl at 6 months and 99 fl by 1 year. Monitoring of mean corpuscular volume has been used to assess compliance on oral zidovudine regimens (38).

Other toxicities of zidovudine noted in a small fraction of children include nausea and vomiting, insomnia, and headache (38). These side effects are often self-limited and rarely result in dose modifications or discontinuation of the drug. Long-term zidovudine use has also rarely been associated with the development of myopathy characterized clinically by muscle weakness and marked elevation of serum creatine kinase (65, 66). Although HIV can also produce a myopathy, zidovudine-associated myopathy can be distinguished from HIV-associated myopathy histologically (67).

Zidovudine at doses ranging from 300 to 1200 mg/day was well tolerated in 43 pregnant women including 12 treated during the first trimester. All infants exposed to zidovudine in utero were born alive, and there was no evidence of teratogenicity, no apparent increased risk of premature births or perinatal problems, and no obvious pattern of hematologic toxicity (68).

Drug Interactions

Probenicid is a uricosuric and renal tubular blocking agent that, like zidovudine, undergoes glucuronide conjugation. When the drugs are coadministered, probenicid blocks the catabolism of zidovudine to a glucuronide conjugate, resulting in a 2-fold increase in total plasma zidovudine exposure and an increase in the half-life of zidovudine from 1 to 1.5 hr (69). This interaction between probenicid and zidovudine could be exploited to allow for a lower dose or a less frequent administration schedule of oral zidovudine.

Acetaminophen, another drug that is cleared by glucuronidation, caused enhanced hematologic toxicity when administered in combination with zidovudine (52), presumably by interfering with metabolic elimination of zidovudine similar to probenicid.

The interaction between ribavirin, another nucleoside analogue, and zidovudine occurs at a pharmacodynamic level. Ribavirin has been shown to antagonize the anti-HIV activity of zidovudine in vitro by inhibiting the conversion of zidovudine to its activated triphosphate form (70).

Drug Resistance

The emergence of zidovudine-resistant isolates of HIV appears to be related to the duration of zidovudine therapy but not the dose (48). Isolates from patients treated for more than 6 months showed reduced susceptibility to zidovudine when tested in vitro compared with those from untreated patients. In addition, patients with advanced HIV infection develop resistance more rapidly than those with early-stage disease. After 12 months of zidovudine therapy, 90% of patients with AIDS or advanced AIDS-related complex had resistant isolates compared with 30% from early-stage patients (48). For the most part, zidovudine-resistant strains of HIV have not been cross-resistant to zalcitabine and didanosine.

The clinical significance of isolating zidovudine-resistant HIV strains has been difficult to establish in adults (50). However, in children zidovudine resistance seemed to precede disease progression. However, the CD4 count was decreased in most patients, and it is not possible to determine if disease progression was due to virus resistance (71). The concentration of zidovudine required to inhibit HIV strains from patients who subsequently deteriorated or died was 7-fold higher than the concentration required to inhibit strains from patients with stable disease.

Didanosine

Didanosine is a purine (inosine) deoxynucleoside analog (Figure 34.4) that has also recently been approved for use in children and adults after undergoing an accelerated approval process. Approval was based on uncontrolled phase I trials and data from the expanded access program that demonstrated a significant effect of didanosine on surrogate markers. Because of this limited clinical experience, further clinical studies will be required to better define the long-term efficacy, indications, and optimal dose and schedule of didanosine (72).

Unlike zidovudine, approval for the use of didanosine in children was granted simultaneously with approval in adults. The pediatric phase I/II trial of didanosine in HIV-infected children was conducted concurrently with the adult trials, and data from the pediatric study had a significant impact on the FDA decision to release the drug for use in all age groups. This agent serves as a model for the optimal approach to drug development in children.

In acid conditions didanosine rapidly undergoes spontaneous hydrolysis of the glycosidic bond to yield hypoxanthine and dideoxyribose, thereby inactivating the drug. This has necessitated administering the drug after antacids or in a buffered formulation to neutralize gastric acids and stabilize the drug. Oral formulations include chewable-dispersible buffered tablets (25, 50, 100, or 150 mg), single dose buffered powder packets (100, 167, 250, and 375 mg) that are taken up in water before administration, and a pediatric oral solution that is mixed with an equal volume of antacid (10 mg/ml). Gastric acid secretion can be detected within hours of birth and approaches the lower limit of adult values by age 3 months. Therefore, in small children and patients receiving a reduced dose of the pediatric formulation of didanosine, a supplemental dose of antacid may be necessary to completely neutralize gastric acid.

The current recommended pediatric dose is 100 mg/m^2 twice daily. Despite its rapid elimination and short half-life (see below), didanosine is administered on a twice daily schedule based primarily on in vitro studies demonstrating a prolonged half-life (>12 hr) of the active intracellular metabolite, ddATP (73).

Pharmacokinetics

After an intravenous dose the elimination of didanosine in children is rapid with a plasma half-life of 1.0 hr and a clearance of 500 ml/min/m^2 (Table 34.3) (46). Peak plasma concentration and area under the plasma concentration-time curve increase linearly with the dose over a 9-fold dosage range. The pharmacokinetic behavior of didanosine in adults is similar with a total clearance of 650–750 ml/min/m^2 (74, 75) and a half-life ranging from 0.6 to 1.7 hr (74–76).

Renal clearance of didanosine in adults accounts for 35–50% of total clearance and exceeds the glomerular filtration rate, indicating that the drug undergoes tubular secretion (74, 75). In patients with impaired renal function the plasma concentration and half-life of didanosine are increased (77). The drug was dialyzable in the uremic patients undergoing hemodialysis.

Bioavailability.   Orally administered didanosine is rapidly absorbed, and bioavailability in adults appears to be ~40% (74–76). However, in two of these trials, bioavailability was only 23% in patients treated at the higher dose levels (74, 76), and in the other, significant interpatient variability was observed (75). The bioavailability of the "sachet" (citrate/phosphate buffered) formulation is comparable with that of the oral solution preceded by an antacid (74, 78). The chewable-dispersible buffered tablet appears to be 20–25% more bioavailable. Administration of didanosine with food significantly impairs its absorption, and it is therefore recommended that oral didanosine be administered in a fasting condition (79).

In children the plasma didanosine concentrations achieved with an oral dose were considerably lower than with an equivalent intravenous dose (Fig. 34.7A), and overall only about 20% of the oral dose was absorbed. In a small subgroup of children plasma didanosine concentrations were undetectable for the 8 hr after an oral dose (46). There was also considerable interpatient variability in the fraction of the dose absorbed (range 2–89%) and in the actual plasma concentrations achieved (Fig. 34.7B). At the 120 mg/m^2 dose level the area under the plasma concentration-time curve in the 13 patients ranged from 0.8 to 9.1 μmol•hr/liter. The fraction of the didanosine dose absorbed also tended to be lower at the higher dose levels in children (46). Acid lability of the drug may be, in part, responsible for the limited and variable bioavailability.

Central Nervous System Pharmacology. Didanosine was not detectable (<0.1 μmol/liter) in 17 of 20 CSF samples obtained from children 2 hr after an oral dose. Two patients receiving 180 mg/m^2 had CSF didanosine concentrations of 0.40 and 0.35 μmol/liter, and one patient receiving 9 mg/m^2 had a CSF concentration of 0.15 μmol/liter (46). These low CSF levels are consistent with the 5% CSF penetration of didanosine observed in a primate model (unpublished data). Although the

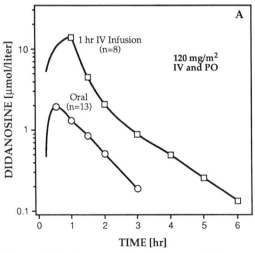

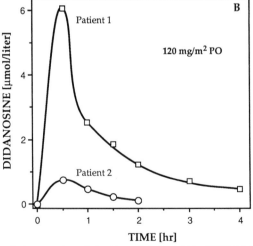

Figure 34.7.   **A,** plasma disappearance of didanosine after an intravenous dose of 120 mg/m^2 over 1 hr, in eight patients and after an oral dose of 120 mg/m2 in 13 patients. From Balis FM, Pizzo PA, Butler KM, et al. Clinical pharmacology of 2',3'-dideoxyinosine in children with human immunodeficiency virus infection. J Infect Dis 1992;165:99–104. **B,** plasma didanosine concentrations in two patients treated with an identical dose of 120 mg/m2 by mouth demonstrating variability in didanosine levels with oral dosing.

CSF-to-plasma ratio in adults is reported to be 20% (75), this value is based on the ratio of a single CSF and plasma time point and therefore may not accurately represent total drug exposure in the central nervous system over time relative to systemic exposure.

Developmental Pharmacology. Didanosine appears to cross the placental barrier, although fetal blood drug concentrations were only 15% of maternal plasma concentrations in two subjects who received a single oral dose of didanosine before planned abortions in the second trimester (80). The experience with didanosine in newborns and infants is very limited; however, over the age range of 8 months to 18 years, there was no evidence of age dependence in didanosine clearance (46).

Therapeutic Drug Monitoring. In the initial pediatric phase I trial a relationship was observed between plasma didanosine concentration and both decline in serum p24 antigen and improvement in neuropsychometric tests (46). Area under the plasma concentration-time curve of didanosine was significantly higher (1.9 vs. 0.8 μmol · hr/liter) in the group of patients judged to have responded to therapy by a fall in p24 antigen from levels exceeding 100 pg/ml to undetectable levels. Similarly, plasma didanosine concentrations correlated with change in full scale IQ score after 6 months of therapy. A relationship between didanosine plasma drug exposure and suppression of p24 antigen was also observed in adult phase I trials (81).

A limited sampling strategy developed for didanosine allows the accurate estimation of area under the plasma concentration-time curve using only one to three plasma samples (46). At a dose of 120 mg/m^2 the plasma concentrations at 0.5 hrs ($C_{0.5}$) and 1.5 hrs. ($C_{1.5}$) after an oral dose were predictive of the area under the plasma concentration-time curve (AUC) with an r^2 of 0.98 using the equation AUC = 0.44 · $C_{0.5}$ + 2.78 · $C_{1.5}$ – 0.26.

Toxicity

The most significant toxicity from didanosine in the pediatric trial was pancreatitis, which developed in seven of 95 patients treated at the highest dose levels

($\geq$360 mg/m^2/day). Clinical pancreatitis was characterized by abdominal pain, nausea, and elevations of serum amylase and lipase (82) The pancreatitis resolved in all patients after discontinuation of the drug. Pancreatitis occurred in 9% of patients on the adult phase I trials and 5% of patients treated on the expanded access program (72). However, estimating the incidence of pancreatitis from didanosine in uncontrolled trials is difficult because it may have multiple etiologies. For example, the incidence of pancreatitis in a group of HIV-infected children not receiving didanosine was 17% (83).

A painful peripheral neuropathy of the lower extremities was the most frequent dose-limiting toxicity on the adult trials (76, 84). The neuropathy was related to both higher daily doses of the drug and to the cumulative dose (76). Symptoms usually developed after 12–20 weeks of continuous didanosine therapy and then resolved over 1–2 months after discontinuation of the drug. Neuropathy was not reported on the pediatric trial (37).

Peripheral atrophy of the retinal pigment epithelium was observed in three of 43 patients prospectively monitored with ocular exams on the pediatric phase I trial, including two patients treated at the highest dose level (85). Retinal atrophy was not observed in adults on didanosine.

Other toxicities of didanosine include diarrhea (related to antacid or citrate buffer), nausea and vomiting, headache, insomnia, rash, elevated uric acid (metabolite of inosine), and transient elevations of hepatic transaminases. Hematologic toxicity was not prominent.

Zalcitabine

Zalcitabine was the second dideoxynucleoside to enter human trials propelled by its potent anti-HIV activity in in vitro screening assays. In these systems zalcitabine is about 10-fold more potent than zidovudine on a molar basis (86). The experience with zalcitabine, particularly its long-term use, is limited in children. In the initial pediatric phase I trial its use was limited to 8 consecutive weeks because of concerns about neurotoxicity observed in the adult trial. Up to

0.03 mg/kg orally every 6 hr was well toler-ated by children for this limited duration of therapy (9). Current studies are evaluating long-term administration of lower doses of zalcitabine and the use of zalcitabine in combination with zidovudine (see Chapter 35).

Commercial formulations of zalcitabine include a 0.375-mg tablet of a 0.75-mg tablet. The drug company also supplies a syrup (0.1 mg/ml) for clinical trials.

Pharmacokinetics

Because of the relatively low doses of zal-citabine studied in children, plasma con-centrations of the drug were difficult to quantitate, and only limited pharmacoki-netic data are available (9). The mean val-ues of pharmacokinetic parameters after the intravenous dose in five children treated with 0.03 or 0.04 mg/kg (Table 34.3) include a total clearance of 150 ml/min/m² and a half-life of 0.8 hr. Comparable results have been reported in adults receiving zalcitabine at doses ranging from 0.03 to 0.5 mg/kg (Table 34.3) (87).

In adults urinary excretion of the parent drug accounted for 75% of total drug elimi-nation. This route of elimination contrasts with naturally occurring cytidine and other cytidine analogs like cytarabine that are eliminated by enzymatic deamination to uridine or uridine analogs. Dose adjust-ments of zalcitabine may be necessary in patients with renal dysfunction. The pedi-atric patient with the lowest clearance (58 ml/min/m²) in the phase I trial had evidence of a nephropathy with protein-uria, hematuria, and casts present on uri-nalysis (9).

The mean bioavailability of zalcitabine in adults was 88% with a range of 72–121% (87, 88). In children the bioavailability was lower (54%) and ranged from 29 to 100% in the small sample (9).

As noted above, the CSF penetration of dideoxycytidine in primates was limited with a CSF-to-plasma ratio of only 3% (Table 34.4) (28). Zalcitabine was detected in the CSF of several adults 2 hr after a dose at concentrations between 0.03 and 0.05 µmol/liter (87).

Toxicity

In the pediatric phase I trial, there was no evidence of either hematologic toxicity or neurotoxicity. Stomatitis consisting of ulcers on the tongue and lips developed in over half the patients usually after 2–3 weeks of continuous therapy. These lesions were generally not painful but resulted in discon-tinuation of therapy in one patient. An ery-thematous, maculopapular rash involving the trunk and extremities (including the palms) developed in three of the six pa-tients treated with 0.04 mg/kg zalcitabine and resolved when the dose was lowered (9).

In adults zalcitabine has been associated with skin rashes, fever, malaise, stomatitis, and a dose-related, painful peripheral neu-ropathy. The neuropathy was a dose-limit-ing toxicity on the adult phase I trial and was both dose and schedule dependent. It usually developed after 6–14 weeks of ther-apy and was more common with higher doses and shorter dosing intervals (10, 88). Patients usually presented with painful dysethesias of the feet but also developed loss of sensation, numbness, and weakness. The neuropathy worsened for up to 1 month after discontinuation of zalcitabine and then gradually improved (10).

Less common side effects in adults in-cluded arthalgias, nail changes, and diar-rhea. Thrombocytopenia and neutropenia were dose limiting at doses of 0.09 mg/kg every 4 hr and 0.25 mg/kg every 8 hr (10, 88).

CONCLUSIONS

Clinical pharmacology, and specifically pharmacokinetics, are critical in the devel-opment of new antiretroviral compounds. Preclinical and clinical studies evaluating the absorption, distribution (including central nervous system penetration), me-tabolism, and excretion of a new drug help define the optimal dose, schedule, and route of administration. In addition, know-ing the route of elimination of an agent alerts the clinician to the need for possible dose adjustments in patients with excretory organ dysfunction and in very young chil-dren with immature organ function.

Correlating pharmacokinetic parameters with measures of drug toxicity and efficacy enables therapeutic and toxic concentrations to be determined and subsequently used in the daily management of patients receiving the agent. With the application of therapeutic drug monitoring, each patient's dose can be adjusted to maintain a therapeutic, nontoxic level and ensure that the patient receives maximal benefit from the drug while minimizing the chance for a toxic reaction.

References

1. Haseltine WA. Development of antiviral drugs for the treatment of AIDS: Strategies and prospects. J Acquir Immune Defic Syndr 1989;2:311–334.
2. Jeffries DJ. Targets for antiviral therapy of human immunodeficiency virus infection. J Infect 1989; 18 (suppl 1):5–13.
3. Broder S. The life-cycle of human immunodeficiency virus as a guide to the design of new therapies for AIDS. In: DeVita VT, Rosenberg S, Helman S, eds. AIDS: Etiology, diagnosis, treatment, and prevention. 2nd ed. Philadelphia: Lippincott, 1988:79–86.
4. Volberding PA, Lagakos SW, Koch MA, et al. Zidovudine in asymptomatic human immunodeficiency infection: A controlled trial in persons with fewer than 500 CD4-positive cells per cubic millimeter. N Engl J Med 1990;322:941–949.
5. Hamilton JD, Hartigan PM, Simberkoff MS, et al. A controlled trial of early versus late treatment with zidovudine in symptomatic human immunodeficiency virus infection: Results of the Veterans Affairs Cooperative Study. N Engl J Med 1992;326:437–443.
6. Fauci AS. Combination therapy for HIV infection: Getting closer. Ann Intern Med 1992;116:85-86.
7. Merigan TC. Treatment of AIDS with combinations of antiretroviral agents. Am J Med 1991;90 (suppl 4A):8–17.
8. Meng T-C, Fischl MA, Boota AM, et al. Combination therapy with zidovudine and dideoxycytidine in patients with advanced human immunodeficiency virus infection. Ann Intern Med 1992;116:13–20.
9. Pizzo PA, Butler K, Balis FM, et al. Dideoxycytidine alone and in an alternating schedule with zidovudine in children with symptomatic human immunodeficiency virus infection. J Pediatr 1990;117: 799–808.
10. Yarchoan R, Perno CF, Thomas RV, et al. Phase I studies of 2',3'-dideoxycytidine in severe human immunodeficiency virus infection as a single agent and alternating with zidovudine (AZT). Lancet 1988;1:76–81.
11. Fox JL. Federal AIDS drug development program: Advice and innovation. Am Soc Microbiol News 1989;55:183–188.
12. McGowan J, Hoth D. AIDS drug discovery and development. J Acquir Immune Defic Syndr 1989;2:335–343.
13. Yarchoan R, Mitsuya H, Myers CE, Broder S. Clinical pharmacology of 3'-azido-2',3'-dideoxythymidine (zidovudine) and related dideoxynucleosides. N Engl J Med 1989;321: 726–738.
14. Mitsuya H, Matsukura M, Broder S. rapid in vitro systems of assessing activity of agents against HTLV-III/LAV. In: Broder S, ed. AIDS modern concepts and therapeutic challenges. New York: Marcel Dekker, 1987:303–334.
15. Harada S, Koyanagi Y, Yamamoto N. Infection of HTLV-III/LAV in HTLV-1-carrying cells MT-2 and MT-4 and application in a plaque assay. Science 1985;229:563–566.
16. Dalgleish AG, Beverley PCL, Clapham PR, Crawford DH, Greaves MF, Weiss RA. The CD4 (T4) antigen is an essential component of the receptor for the AIDS retrovirus. Nature 1984;312: 763–767.
17. Nara PL, Hatch WC, Dunlop NM, et al. Simple, rapid, quantitative, syncytium-forming microassay for the detection of human immunodeficiency virus neutralizing antibody. AIDS Res Hum Retroviruses 1987;3:283–302.
18. Weislow OS, Kiser R, Fine DL, Bader J, Shoemaker RH, Boyd MR. New soluble-formazan assay for HIV-1 cytopathic effects: Application to high-flux screening of synthetic and natural products for AIDS-antiviral activity. J Natl Cancer Inst 1989;81:577–586.
19. Watson RR. Murine models for acquired immune deficiency syndrome. Life Sci 1989;44:3–15.
20. Letvin NL. Animal models for AIDS. Immunol Today 1990;11:322–326.
21. Spertzel RO, Public Health Service Animal Models Committee. Animal models of human immunodeficiency virus infection. Antiviral Res 1989;12:223–230.
22. Letvin NL, King NW. Naturally occuring animal models of the acquired immune deficiency syndrome. Am J Physiol Imaging 1991;6:1–15.
23. McCune J, Kaneshima H, Krowka J, et al. The SCID-hu mouse: A small animal model for HIV infeciton and pathogenesis. Annu Rev Immunol 1991;9:399–429.
24. Mosier DE, Gulizia RJ, Baird SM, Wilson DB. Transfer of a functional human immune system to mice with severe combined immunodeficiency. Nature 1988;335:256–259.
25. Balzarini J, Pauwels R, Baba M, et al. The in vitro and in vivo anti-retrovirus activity and intracellular metabolism of 3'-azido-2',3'-dideoxythymidine and 2',3'-dideoxycytidine are highly dependent on the cell species. Biochem Pharmacol 1988;37:897–903.
26. Sharpe AH, Jaenisch R, Ruprecht RM. Retroviruses and mouse embryos: A rapid model for neurovirulence and transplacental antiviral therapy. Science 1987;236:1671–1674.
27. Mosier DE. Animal models for retrovirus-induced immunodeficiency disease. Immunol Invest 1986;15:233–261.
28. Collins JM, Klecker RW, Kelley JA, et al. Pyrimidine dideoxyribonucleosides: Selectivity of penetration into cerebrospinal fluid. J Pharmacol Exp Ther 1988;245:466–470.

29. Collins JM, Zaharko DS, Dedrick RL, Chabner BA. Potential roles for preclinical pharmacology in Phase I clinical trials. Cancer Treat Rep 1986; 70:73–80.

30. Lagakos SW, Hoth DF. Surrogate markers in AIDS: Where are we? Where are we going? Ann Intern Med 1992;116:599–601.

31. Ellenberg SS. Determining sample sizes for clinical trials. Oncology 1989;3:39–46.

32. Pizzo PA, Eddy J, Falloon J, et al. Effect of continuous intravenous infusion of zidovudine (AZT) in children with symptomatic HIV infection. N Engl J Med 1988;319:889–896.

33. Chabner B. Approval of cancer and AIDS drugs: The question of time. Am Soc Microbiol News 1989;55:170–171.

34. Merigan TC. You can teach an old dog new tricks: How AIDS trials are pioneering new strategies. N Engl J Med 1990;323:1341–1343.

35. Cohen C, Shevitz A, Mayer K. Expanding access to investigational new therapies. Prim Care 1992; 19:87–96.

36. Coleman R, Kahn J, Gumbley-Smith D, Woodring H, Mills J, Volberding P. Enrollment in parallel tract studies of dideoxyinosine (ddI) vs. AIDS clinical treatment group (ACTG) trials at San Francisco General Hospital, an ACTG site [Abstract SD 789]. Sixth International Conference on AIDS, San Francisco, Jun 1990.

37. Butler KM, Husson RN, Balis FM, et al. Dideoxyinosine in children with symptomatic human immunodeficiency virus infection. N Engl J Med 1991;324:137–144.

38. McKinney RE, Maha MA, Connor EM, et al. A multicenter trial of oral zidovudine in children with advanced human immunodeficiency virus disease. N Engl J Med 1991;324:1018–1025.

39. Krasinski K. Retroviral therapy and clinical trials for HIV-infected children. J Pediatr 1991;119 (suppl):S63–S68.

40. Furman PA, Barry DW. Spectrum of antiviral activity and mechanism of action of zidovudine. Am J Med 1988;85 (suppl 2A):176–181.

41. Perno C-F, Yarchoan R, Cooney DA, et al. Inhibition of human immunodeficiency virus (HIV-1/HTLV-IIIBa-L) replication in fresh and cultured human peripheral blood monocytes/macrophages by azidothymidine and related 2',3'-dideoxynucleosides. J Exp Med 1988;168:1111–1125.

42. Bourgoignie JJ, Meneses R, Ortiz C, Jaffe D, Pardo V. The clinical spectrum of renal disease associated with human immunodeficiency virus. Am J Kidney Dis 1988;12:131–137.

43. Strauss J, Abitbol C, Zilleruelo G, et al. Renal disease in children with the acquired immunodeficiency syndrome. N Engl J Med 1989;321:625–630.

44. Reed MD, Besunder JB. Developmental pharmacology: Ontogenic basis of drug disposition. Pediatr Clin North Am 1989;36:1053–1074.

45. Balis FM, Pizzo PA, Murphy RF, et al. The pharmacokinetics of zidovudine administered by continuous infusion in children. Ann Intern Med 1989;110:279–285.

46. Balis FM, Pizzo PA, Butler KM, et al. Clinical pharmacology of 2',3'-dideoxyinosine in human immunodeficiency virus-infected children. J Infect Dis 1992;165:99–104.

47. Darby G, Larder BA. The clinical significance of antiviral drug resistance. Res Virol 1992;143:116–120.

48. Richman DD. AZT resistance in isolates of HIV. Immunodefic Rev 1991;2:315–318.

49. Richman DD. Selection of zidovudine-resistant variants of human immunodeficiency virus by therapy. Curr Top Microbiol Immunol 1992;176:131–142.

50. Richman DD. The clinical significance of drug-resistant mutants of human immunodeficiency virus. Res Virol 1992;143:130–131.

50a. Boucher FD, Modlin JF, Wellers, et al. Phase I evaluation of zidovudine administered to infants exposed at birth to the human immunodeficiency virus. J Pediatr 1993;122:137–144.

51. Fischl MA, Richman DD, Grieco MH, et al. The efficacy of azidothymidine (AZT) in the treatment of patients with AIDS and AIDS-related complex: A double-blind, placebo-controlled trial. N Engl J Med 1987;317:185–191.

52. Richman DD, Fischl MA, Grieco MH, et al. The toxicity of azidothymidine (AZT) in the treatment of patients with AIDS and AIDS-related complex: A double-blind, placebo-controlled trial. N Engl J Med 1987;317:192–197.

53. Fischl MA, Parker CB, Pettinelli C, et al. A randomized controlled trial of a reduced daily dose of zidovudine in patients with the acquired immunodeficiency syndrome. N Engl J Med 1990;323:1009–1014.

54. Balis FM, Pizzo PA, Eddy J, et al. Pharmacokinetics of zidovudine administered intravenously and orally in children with human immunodeficiency virus infection. J Pediatr 1989;114:880–884.

55. Blum MR, Liao SHT, Good SS, de Miranda P. Pharmacokinetics and bioavailability of zidovudine in humans. 1988;85 (suppl 2A):189–194.

56. Singlas E, Pioger J-P, Taburet A-M, Colin J-N, Fillastre J-P. Zidovudine disposition in patients with severe renal impairment: Influence of hemodialysis. Clin Pharmacol Ther 1989;46:190–197.

57. Paoli I, Dave M, Cohen BD. Pharmacodynamics of zidovudine in patients with endstage renal disease. N Engl J Med 1992;326:839–840.

58. Collins JM, Unadkat JD. Clinical pharmacokinetics of zidovudine: An overview of current data. Clin Pharmacokinet 1989;17:1–9.

59. Klecker RW, Collins JM, Yarchoan R, et al. Plasma and cerebrospinal fluid pharmacokinetics of 3'-azido-3'-deoxythymidine: A novel pyrimidine analog with potential application for the treatment of patients with AIDS and related diseases. Clin Pharmacol Ther 1987;41:407–412.

60. Barry DW, Blum MR. Pharmacokinetics of zidovudine in adults and children [Abstract Thb 050]. Fifth International Conference of AIDS, Montreal, Jun 1989.

61. Chavanet P, Diquet B, Waldner A, Portier H. Perinatal pharmacokinetics of zidovudine. N Engl J Med 1989;321:1548–1549.

62. Watts DH, Brown ZA, Tartaglion T, et al. Pharmacokinetic disposition of zidovudine during pregnancy. J Infect Dis 1991;163:226–232.

63. Lopez-Anaya A, Unadkat JD, Schumann LA, Smith AL. Pharmacokinetics of zidovudine (azidothymidine). II. Development of metabolic and renal clearance pathways in the neonate. J Acquir Immune Defic Syndr 1990;3:1052–1058.

64. Schenker S, Johnson RF, King TS, Schenken RS, Henderson GI. Azidothymidine (zidovudine) transport by the human placenta. Am J Med Sci 1990;299:16–20.

65. Gertner E, Thurn JR, Williams DN, et al. Zidovudine-associated myopathy. Am J Med 1989;86:814–818.

66. Walter EB, Drucker RP, McKinney RE, Wilfert CM. Myopathy in human immunodeficiency virus-infected children receiving long-term zidovudine therapy. J Pediatr 1991;119:152–155.

67. Dalakas MC, Illa I, Pezeshkpour GH, Laukaitis JP, Cohen B, Griffin JL. Mitochondrial myopathy caused by long-term zidovudine therapy. N Engl J Med 1990;322:1098–1105.

68. Sperling RS, Stratton P, O'Sullivan MJ, et al. A survey of zidovudine use in pregnant women with human immunodeficiency virus infection. N Engl J Med 1992;326:857–861.

69. de Miranda P, Good SS, Yarchoan R, et al. Alteration of zidovudine pharmacokinetics by probenicid in patients with AIDS or AIDS-related complex. Clin Pharmacol Ther 1989;46:494–500.

70. Vogt MW, Hartshorn KL, Furman PA, et al. Ribavirin antagonizes the effect of azidothymidine on HIV replication. Science 1987;235:1376–1379.

71. Tudor-Williams G, Clair MHS, McKinney RE, et al. HIV-1 sensitivity to zidovudine and clinical outcome in children. Lancet 1992;339:15–19.

72. Shelton MJ, O'Donnell AM, Morse GD. Didanosine. Ann Pharmacother 1992;26:660–669.

73. Ahluwalia G, Johnson MA, Fridland A, Cooney DA, Broder S, Johns DG. Cellular pharmacology of the anti-HIV agent 2',3'-dideoxyadenosine [Abstract A1388]. Proc Annu Meet Am Assoc Cancer Res 1988;29:349.

74. Knupp CA, Shyu WC, Dolin R, et al. Pharmacokinetics of didanosine in patients with acquired immunodeficiency syndrome or acquired immunodeficiency syndrome-related complex. Clin Pharmacol Ther 1991;49:523–535.

75. Hartman NR, Yarchoan R, Pluda JM, et al. Pharmacokinetics of 2',3'-dideoxyadenosine and 2',3'-dideoxyinosine in patients with severe human immunodeficiency virus infection. Clin Pharmacol Ther 1990;47:647–654.

76. Lambert JS, Seidlin M, Reichman RC, et al. 2',3'-Dideoxyinosine (ddI) in patients with the acquired immunodeficiency syndrome or AIDS-related complex. N Engl J Med 1990;322:1333–1340.

77. Singlas E, Parent O, Borsa-Lebas F, Taburet A-M, Humbert G. Pharmacokinetics of dideoxyinosine (ddI) in patients with normal and impaired renal function; influence of haemodialysis [Abstract 1352]. 31st Interscience Conference on Antimicrobial Agents and Chemotherapy, Chicago, 1991.

78. Hartman NR, Yarchoan R, Pluda JM, et al. Pharmacokinetics of 2',3'-dideoxyinosine in patients with severe human immunodeficiency infection. II The effects of different oral formulations and the presence of other medications. Clin Pharmacol Ther 1991;50:278–285.

79. Shyu WC, Knupp CA, Pittman KA, Dunkle L, Barbhaiya RH. Food-induced reduction in bioavailability of didanosine. Clin Pharmacol Ther 1991;50:503–507.

80. Pons JC, Boubon MC, Taburet AM, et al. Fetoplacental passage of 2',3'-dideoxyinosine [Letter]. Lancet 1991;337:732.

81. Drusano GL, Yuen GJ, Lambert JS, Seidlin M, Dolin R, Valentine FT. Relationship between dideoxyinosine exposure, CD4 counts, and p24 antigen levels in human immunodeficiency virus infection. Ann Intern Med 1992;116:562–566.

82. Butler KM, Venzon D, Henry N, et al. Pancreatitis in HIV-infected children receiving dideoxyinosine. Pediatrics 1993;91:747–751.

83. Miller TL, Winter HS, Luginbuhl LM, Orav EJ, McIntosh K. Pancreatitis in pediatric human immunodeficiency virus infection. J Pediatr 1992;120:223–237.

84. Cooley TP, Kunches LM, Saunders CA, et al. Once-daily administration of 2',3'-dideoxyinosine (ddI) in patients with the acquired immunodeficiency syndrome or AIDS-related complex. N Engl J Med 1990;322:1340–1345.

85. Whitcup SM, Butler KM, Caruso R, et al. Retinal toxicity in human immunodeficiency virus-infected children treated with 2',3'-dideoxyinosine. Am J Ophthalmol 1992;113:1–7.

86. Mitsuya H, Broder S. Inhibition of the in vitro infectivity and cytopathic effect of human T-lymphotrophic virus type III/lymphadenopathy-associated virus (HTLV-III/LAV) by 2',3'-dideoxynucleosides. Proc Natl Acad Sci USA 1986;83:911–915.

87. Klecker RW, Collins JM, Yarchoan RC, et al. Pharmacokinetics of 2',3'-dideoxycytidine in patients with AIDS and related disorders. J Clin Pharmacol 1988;28:837–842.

88. Broder S, Yarchoan R. Dideoxycytidine: Current clinical experience and future prospects. Am J Med 1990;88 (suppl 5B):31–33.

35
Antiretroviral Treatment for Children with HIV Infection

Philip A. Pizzo and Catherine M. Wilfert

Although antiretroviral therapy is still in its infancy, considerable progress has been made during the past several years in developing treatment strategies that have improved the quality and duration of life of infants and children with symptomatic human immunodeficiency virus (HIV) or AIDS. Even though curative therapy remains an elusive goal, several drugs have entered the clinic that can impact HIV and that will hopefully help pave the way for future treatment advances. This progress has emanated from a better understanding of the life cycle and pathogenesis of HIV, the evolving concepts of drug development for children, and the configuration of a national network of pediatric investigators and health care providers committed to developing more effective approaches for the treatment and prevention of HIV-infected infants, children, and adolescents (see also Chapters 7, 34, 38–40, 45–47) .

The cornerstone of the effective treatment of HIV infection will be agents that can eliminate or suppress virus replication. Antiretroviral therapy must be coupled with comprehensive multidisciplinary supportive care that includes treatment and prevention of both the infectious and noninfectious complications that arise during HIV infection as well as the nutritional, pain, and psychosocial support. Assuring that the benefits of current therapies are available to all infected children will help optimize future progress.

HIV infection in children differs in many ways from adults in its clinical presentation and rate of disease progression. The shorter period of clinical latency and more rapid course of disease progression that characterizes HIV infection in infants and children can, however, make the responses to treatment more dramatic and clinically measurable (1–3). For example, the devastating impact of HIV infection on the linear growth, weight gain, and neurocognitive development of infants and children provides disease-specific measures to assess the activity and efficacy of antiretroviral agents (see Chapters 23 and 31). Similarly, the fact that the immune system is normally maturing in infants complicates the measurement of immune recovery and response. Conversely, the potential for immune recovery may be greater in young children, and thus measurement of the magnitude of immune response to intervention may be greater than in HIV-infected adults. Furthermore, because drug dosages in infants and children must be delivered on a body weight or surface area basis, careful pharmacokinetic monitoring can permit clinical-pharmacological correlations that can help to validate the activity or toxicity of new antiretroviral agents. Indeed, such clinical-pharmacological correlations were important in the evaluation and licensure of dideoxyinosine (ddI), not only for children but also for adults (see Chapter 34). Therapeutic drug monitoring is essential for treatment of children and can provide unique data that are also relevant to HIV-infected adults. A realignment of priorities is necessary to assure that suitable pediatric formulations of new agents are available early in the development of new drugs so that they can be assessed in pediatric AIDS patients (4–9). For example, the pharmaceutical industry must be prepared, and expected, to have a plan for developing new agents for pediatric usage, and, at the same time, the pediatric community must be proactive in assuring that new agents are promptly studied in infants and children. The phase I study of most new agents can begin either simultaneously with those in adults or follow closely after their initiation so that promising new agents can be available to infants and children. Fortunately, the regulatory community, especially at the federal level, shares our concerns and has become increasingly proactive for early drug development in children with catastrophic diseases. We should anticipate and applaud their continued leadership to assure that this progress continues.

In this chapter, we will review the current status of antiretroviral therapy for children. In so doing, we will convey both the current clinical standard of practice as well as the areas of ongoing investigation, uncertainty, or controversy. Clearly, in this rapidly evolving area of medicine it is presumptive to define any therapy as standard. Yet it is important that standards of care be established, both to serve as benchmarks to monitor future progress and as a means for assuring that children at risk receive the best current therapy.

CURRENT APPROACHES TO TREATMENT OF CHILDREN WITH HIV INFECTION

Antiviral Armamentarium: Agents Currently Available or in Active Development

Efforts have been directed to developing agents that impact on different features of the HIV-life cycle (see Fig. 35.1). An essential goal has been to develop agents singly and in combination that have a high therapeutic index and that are selective for HIV compared with host cellular functions. Ideally agents should be highly bioavailable, with long serum and tissue half-lives and a

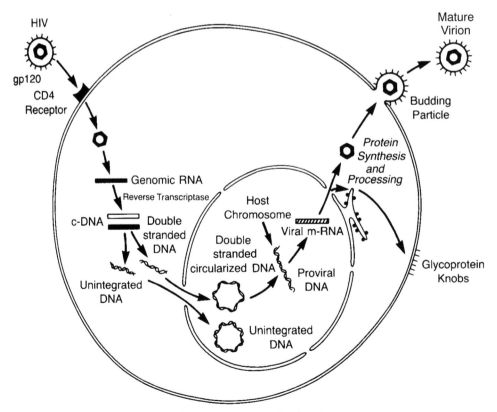

Figure 35.1. Life cycle of HIV.

high plasma-to-CSF ratio (this being especially important in infants and children), and effective in different target cells (e.g., macrophages and lymphocytes) and have antiretroviral activity against both HIV-1 and -2 as well as wild type virus representing different clades (4–9). Other desirable properties include a slow emergence of drug resistance and low rate of toxicity so that treatment can be maintained for long periods. Because lifelong therapy may be necessary for patients with HIV infection, low cost is also important as is compatibility with the many other drugs that may be required during HIV disease. Moreover, it is desirable to have antiretroviral agents that can be used in combination with additive or synergistic antiretroviral activity that require distinct virus mutations to confer resistance and do not have additive toxicity.

Agents That Decrease HIV Replication or Interfere with Its Life Cycle

Reverse Transcriptase Inhibitors

Dideoxynucleosides. Zidovudine or 2′,3′-azidothymidine (AZT) is the most extensively studied antiretroviral agent in adults and children. Although it was licensed for adults with AIDS in March 1987, it was not approved for use in children with symptomatic HIV infection or severe immunological compromise until May 1990 (10–17). After the efficacy trial in adults had been completed, clinical trials with AZT in children began in the fall of 1986 (18–20). These initial studies were limited in size and scope, but they provided the pharmacokinetic, safety, and tolerance data that eventuated in the Food and Drug Administration approval of this drug for infants and children.

AZT is highly bioavailable (oral absorption is ~65%) and has the best plasma-to-CSF ratio of the dideoxynucleosides. However, it has a short plasma half-life (~1 hr), necessitating multiple daily dosages (generally every 6 hr in children). The pharmacokinetics of AZT in children older than several months are similar to those in adults, (21–25, 26a). Pharmacokinetics were evaluated in infants younger than 3 months. As expected, significant differences were observed in the infants younger than 2

weeks. Glucuronide conjugation of AZT was decreased so that the serum half-life was longer, bioavailability was greater, and clearance was less in infants younger than 14 days. AZT is administered orally at doses of 2 mg/kg every 6 hr to infants younger than 2 weeks and at 3 mg/kg every 6 hr to infants older than 6 weeks.

AZT crosses the placenta (it can be detected in amniotic fluid, fetal tissues, and cord blood), making it theoretically possible to use this agent for fetal treatment or the prevention of vertical transmission (26, 27). Although data are limited, infants born to mothers who received AZT during pregnancy appear to have a prolonged clearance and half-life (in one report the serum half-life was 14.4 ± 7.5 hr during the first 24–36 hr of life), consistent with the pharmacokinetics observed in infants younger than 14 days.

AZT has clear benefits in infants and children, even though the degree and duration of these benefits are variable. The most notable clinical effects of AZT include improvements in activity, weight gain, linear growth velocity, and, perhaps most notably in children, improvements in neurocognitive function (6, 18–20, 28). Static or progressive encephalopathy can be found in many untreated HIV-infected children so that the observed improvements in cognitive function (as measured by IQ scores) or reduction of the degree of structural deficits (as reflected by decreased brain-to-ventricular ratios or improved positron emission tomography scanning) and excitatory amino acids (e.g., quinolinic acid) in encephalopathic children receiving AZT are notable (29–37). Coupled with these findings is the fact that children receiving AZT also have reductions in p24 antigenemia and at least transient elevations of their CD4 counts. When children die of progressive AIDS despite antiretroviral therapy, extensive amounts of HIV are still present in several tissues (most notably lymph nodes, spleen, colon, central nervous system (CNS) (38–45). This documents the enormous virus burden and reminds us that the measurement of HIV in blood is an incomplete assessment of the total body burden of infection.

AZT administered to children with advanced disease also improved their growth and decreased the level of hypergammaglob-ulinemia, and, 4 years after the conclusion of this trial, the median survival of these perin-tally infected children was 7.2 years, which is longer than that for children reported be-fore the availability of antiretroviral therapy.

In general AZT is well tolerated in infants and children. The major side effects of treatment include myelosuppression (espe-cially anemia and neutropenia) and, to a lesser extent, nausea, headache, hepatic transaminase elevations, and myositis (19, 20, 46–48). Of these, the hematological tox-icity is the most likely to be dose limiting (see below).

An increasing problem with AZT is the development of resistant virus. Mutations in the reverse transcriptase gene have resulted in amino acid changes at positions 41, 67, 70, 215, and 219 (49–51). Virus resistance occurs as the CD4 count falls and the virus burden increases. Clinical failure has been associated with virus resistance and these markers of disease progression. Recent con-firmation that AZT-resistant HIV can be transmitted horizontally, coupled with its increasing prevalence, is troubling and has serious implications for infants whose moth-ers may transmit an AZT-resistant virus.

AZT has been employed in many clinical studies in children, both as a single agent and in combination with other antiretrovi-ral agents or biologicals (52–55). Although more is known about AZT than any other dideoxynucleoside, questions arise regard-ing its optimal use in infants and children. For example, the optimal dose and sched-ule of AZT remain uncertain (7–28). Studies in adults have demonstrated that low daily doses of AZT (300–500 mg/day) are as effective and less toxic than higher doses (e.g., 800–1200 mg/day), except that patients with encephalopathy appear to benefit from higher doses. The more fre-quent occurrence of encephalopathy in children compared with adults has prompted the recommendation that higher doses of AZT (e.g., 180 mg/m^2/day) should be used in this patient population. Whether lower doses (i.e., 90 mg/m^2/day) can be used in asymptomatic or minimally sympto-matic children is being assessed in a ran-domized clinical trial; the results should be available within the next 2 years.

Also uncertain is whether the intermit-tent dosage schedule of administration (i.e., divided daily dosage) that is employed is op-timal for children with encephalopathy. In one of the first clinical studies, AZT was given to children by a continuous intra-venous delivery to maintain steady state drug concentrations in the plasma and cerebrospinal fluid. This schedule was asso-ciated with an unexpected degree of im-provement of impaired neurological func-tion in children with overt or subclinical neuroencephalopathy (18, 19, 29). To fur-ther assess the value of steady state AZT in children, a study is being conducted by the National Cancer Institute (NCI) in which patients who have received the standard dose of AZT (180 mg/m^2 every 6 hr) for a minimum of 24 weeks and who have devel-oped evidence of encephalopathy or failed to improve on therapy are switched to steady state administration of AZT at daily dosages of 480 mg/m^2/day. Clearly these are extremely high risk and complicated pa-tients, and if objective improvements can be shown in this patient population, it will have significant implications for other pa-tient populations. Of the 22 enrolled to date, a complete or partial response has been observed in nine (50%). These data suggest that continuous infusion AZT can, in some patients, improve an encephalopa-thy that occurred or progresses despite full dose oral AZT therapy. These data have po-tential implications for the management of children with encephalopathy and may also have implications for adults, in particular those with neurological problems.

The optimal time to initiate antiretroviral therapy in children is unknown. It is possi-ble that early therapy, before the onset of symptoms, could prevent the neurodevelop-mental deficits that occur when the CNS is developing. In fact, there is a suggestion that CNS complications may be less frequent since children began receiving antiretroviral therapy. For example, the baseline neu-ropsychological examinations of sympto-matic children who began antiretroviral therapy in 1986 and 1987 had a greater pro-portion of developmental deficits than chil-dren entering clinical trials in 1993. This may reflect the earlier initiation of treat-ment. Indeed, it is plausible that if children begin therapy during the first months of life that both the rate of progression of disease and survival may be improved. Currently, AIDS Clinical Trials Group (ACTG) 182 is enrolling patients to address this question.

Like AZT, ddI has a short plasma half-life but, in contrast, has a poor oral bioavailablity ($\sim$19 ± 17%), with significant interpatient variability and relatively poor penetration into the CNS (56, 57). Because it is acid labile, ddI must be taken with antacids and the variable amount of antacid necessary to neutralize the gastric acids may impact on its absorption. Studies with ddI began at the NCI in January 1989, just months after the initiation of the phase I clinical trials in adults. A milestone for pediatrics was the simultaneous approval of ddI by the Food and Drug Administration in October 1991 for children and adults. It was especially noteworthy that the pediatric data were important for the approval of ddI for adults because of the clinical pharmacological correlations that were made in the pediatric study. For example, in patients with a pretreatment p24 antigenemia exceeding 100 pg/ml, a significant reduction was observed in patients whose area under the plasma concentration time curve exceeded 1.0 μM · hr compared with patients with lower ddI levels who did not clear p24 antigen. Furthermore, a significant plasma concentration response relationship of ddI was observed with neuropsychometric responses.

ddI has also been shown to have a significant impact on the CD4 count and T helper function. Three-year follow-up data from the NCI study demonstrate that the CD4 count can be maintained for years in some patients, although this effect is more notable in those who begin treatment while their CD4 count was greater than 100/mm^3. In addition, ddI can improve both neutrophil function as well as T helper function; the latter is associated with a significant reduction in the incidence of opportunistic or bacterial infections. Even though the penetration of ddI into the cerebrospinal fluid is poor and most children do not show improvements in neurocognitive scores, a small number of patients with encephalopathy treated with ddI show significant improvements, despite this apparently unfavorable pharmacokinetic profile.

Although it is generally well tolerated, toxicity to ddI in children can include pancreatitis, peripheral neuropathy, and retinal depigmentation (56–58). These side effects appear to be dose related, occurring at levels above 270 mg/m^2/day. More than 100 children have been treated with ddI at the NCI, and follow-up exceeds 3 years. Pancreatitis has been observed in 7% of these children but has not been life threatening. Hyperamylasemia, without symptoms of pancreatitis, can be observed in children receiving ddI and is not a reason to either reduce the dose or discontinue therapy. Peripheral neuropathy associated with ddI appears to be exceedingly rare in children, occurring in <3% of patients. A peripheral depigmentation, albeit without a loss of vision, has been observed in <5% of patients and appears to improve when the ddI is discontinued. In contrast to AZT, however, ddI is rarely associated with hematological toxicity and, in fact, is beneficial in some patients with HIV-associated thrombocytopenia.

As with AZT, long-term clinical and laboratory benefits with ddI are observed in some patients, but over time most appear to show signs of disease progression. A drug resistance mutation has been observed at position 74 and has been observed in many of these patients but is not clearly associated with high level resistance (50). Nonetheless, these findings add realistic concerns regarding the likelihood for long-term benefits from ddI or any single antiretroviral agent.

Clearly, ddI is an important addition to the antiretroviral armamentarium. Although its formulation and pharmacokinetic properties are suboptimal, it has clear antiretroviral activity and exerts a beneficial effect on T helper number and function (59). Its limited CNS penetration makes it less desirable for children with encephalopathy, although benefits can still be observed in some of these patients. If early intervention with antiretroviral therapy decreases the occurrence of neurodevelopmental delays, ddI may be less optimal as a single agent. It can be safely used in patients with hematological toxicity and is a good candidate for combination regimens.

Zalcitabine or 2′,3′-dideoxycytidine (ddC) is the most potent of the dideoxynucleosides in vitro. Its initial use as a single agent in the clinic, however, was marred by toxicity, especially mouth sores, rash, and, most notably, a painful peripheral neuropathy. Like the other dideoxynucleosides, ddC has a short plasma half-life (0.8 hr) and has a bioavailability of 54%. ddC penetrates into the cerebrospinal fluid poorly, and in the initial study performed at the NCI, children appeared to have CNS deterioration while receiving ddC monotherapy (55). In 1992, ddC was approved for use in combination with AZT for adults. Similar experience with ddC in children is limited, although it was successfully employed in a small number of children in an alternating sequence with AZT. In addition, two low doses of ddC have been compared as a salvage regimen in children treated on ACTG protocol 138. To date, both doses have been safe in children. Preliminary data suggest that ddC can also be a useful agent albeit it has been most appropriately employed in combination with AZT. Currently ACTG 190 is accruing patients randomized to receive AZT and ddC or AZT alone and should provide additional safety, pharmacological, and activity data of this combination in children.

Lamivudine or 2'-deoxy-3'-thiacytidine (3TC) is an analog of ddC, the negative enantiomer that entered clinical testing in children in April 1992. This new nucleoside analog exhibits less cytotoxicity in vitro than either ddC or AZT while retaining good antiviral activity. To date, over 70 children have been enrolled at doses ranging from 0.5 to 20 mg/kg (60). Preliminary analysis for the first three dose levels reveals linear pharmacokinetics with a mean bioavailability of 62% (range 37–92%). The CSF-to-serum ratio ranges from 0.09 to 0.46, with a mean of 0.20, although it is important to underscore that these are not steady state values. Encouragingly, 3TC seems to produce a significant improved sense of well-being and increased appetite and weight gain in children. Whether this is due to the antiretroviral activity of 3TC or to a nonspecific effect remains to be determined. Declines in p24 and plasma virus RNA (as measured by a quantitative polymerase chain reaction (PCR) assay) have been observed in patients receiving 3TC, suggesting that this agent has antireroviral activity.

Moreover, 3TC appears to be very well tolerated in children, and a pilot study investigating a combination regimen using 3TC and AZT and/or ddI is being initiated, based on the prospect that the different clinical and laboratory effects of these agents may provide additive patient benefits. For example, AZT has important effects on the CNS involvement but only a transient impact on the CD4 count; ddI, conversely, appears to have more impressive effects on preservation of immune function and CD4 counts but less effect on the CNS; and 3TC has shown benefit in improving appetite and weight gain and general sense of well-being. These differences underscore the need for comprehensive assessments during clinical trials since different effects may be observed despite the similarities in drug action. To date, no single drug prolongs life in a clearly superior manner to others currently available. These three agents may have complementary activities or when used in combination will provide more effective inhibition of virus replication.

Stavudine or 2',3'-didehydro-2',3'-dideoxythymidine (D4T) is another member of the dideoxynucleoside reverse transcriptase inhibitor group of antiretroviral agents and is being used in the Parallel Tract in adults (61, 62). D4T appears to have a good bioavailability and penetration into the CNS. The clinical experience recently published from a phase I/II study of D4T in adults demonstrates increases in weight, increases or stabilization in CD4 counts, and drops in P24 antigen. The dose limiting toxicity is peripheral neuropathy. Clinical experience with D4T in children is limited to date to a phase I trial performed at the Los Angeles Children's Hospital and Baylor School of Medicine where ~16 patients were evaluated at the time of this writing. In vitro, it is notable that AZT appears to inhibit formation of D4T phosphates, suggesting that these two agents should probably not be used in combination. Although a similar adverse biochemical interaction with ddI has not been observed, the possibility of additive neurotoxicity with a ddI and D4T combination must be considered. A comparative trial of AZT and D4T in children (ACTG 240) will begin accrual in late 1993.

Non-nucleoside Reverse Transcriptase Inhibitors. The non-nucleoside reverse transcriptase inhibitors belong to different chemically distinct groups but have in common a high degree of antiretroviral activity and minimal toxicity (63–73). Included in this group are agents such as Nevirapine (BI-RG-587), a diplyridodiazepinone developed by Boehringer-Ingelheim; L-661, a member of a pyridinone class of drugs produced by Merck; U-87 and U-90, BHAP compounds produced by Upjohn, which not only serve as non-nucleoside reverse transcriptase inhibitors, but virus does not appear to be cross resistant to L-661 and nevirapine; and the TIBO compounds such as R86,183 produced by Janssen Pharmaceutica. The initial introduction of these agents was heralded with excitement, because P24 antigen levels fell and CD4 counts increased with the initiation of therapy. Enthusiasm about their therapeutic promise was diminished when the rapid emergence of high level drug-resistant mutations occurred within weeks after the start of therapy. The presence of resistant virus was correlated with an increase in P24 antigen and a decrease in CD4 counts to their pretreatment values, suggesting that virus levels may precede changes in surrogate markers and subsequent clinical deterioration. Recently, however, interest has been renewed because of the observation that the use of three reverse transcriptase inhibitors in vitro can inhibit virus replication and that if the virus becomes resistant to all three agents it is not replication competent. This has been reported with the combination of nevirapine (or to a lesser degree with L-661) with AZT and ddI. These data suggested that such combinations may have beneficial effects for patients who have advanced disease with virus that has become resistant to AZT and ddI (74, 75). Unfortunately, the proposed convergent resistance therapy could not be reproduced with additional experiments (75a, 75b), although several clinical trials are still assessing the possible benefits of these combination regimens.

As a single agent, nevirapine has potent inhibitory activity against the reverse transcriptase of HIV-1 but not against the reverse transcriptases of HIV-2 or other common retroviruses. When used alone, a resistant HIV-1 mutant, characterized by the substitution of cysteine for tyrosine at position 181 of the reverse transcriptase, rapidly emerges in cell cultures and has been observed in the clinic. Nevirapine trials were initiated simultaneously in children and adults and appears to be safe and well tolerated (64, 65, 67–70, 73, 76). When doses of nevirapine ranging from 2.5 to 400 mg were administered to HIV-infected adults, the drug was rapidly absorbed, with a primary peak level observed at 90 min and secondary peaks between 2 and 12 hr or 24 and 28 hr. The major side effect was mild headache and a sedative effect that occurred in some patients who were receiving high dose levels. Rashes were observed in 50–60% of adults and children who received higher doses initially (more than 200 mg/day or 12/mg/m^2/day in children). This could be avoided by starting with lower doses and then escalating upward. Unfortunately, resistance was demonstrated in virus isolates within 4–6 weeks after initiating therapy, making nevirapine of limited utility for monotherapy. Studies with L-661 showed a similar pattern of rapid emergence of resistance and is also being studied in combination regimens. Similarly, U-87 and U-90 are non-nucleoside agents currently in phase I/II clinial trials in adults and children in combination with AZT or AZT + ddI.

In vitro studies performed by Chow et al. (74) attempted to exploit the mutational interactions that occur when dideoxynucleosides and non-nucleoside reverse transcriptase inhibitors are used in combination. As noted above, mutations to AZT associated with resistance have been observed at positions 41, 67, 70, 215, and 219. The most prevalent form of resistance to ddI occurs at position 74. Nevirapine resistance is expressed by a mutation at position 181. Chow's studies suggested that when these agents (AZT, ddI, and nevirapine) were used in combination, mutations occurred that were incompatible with virus replication. Indeed, when clinically achievable drug concentrations (0.3 µM AZT, 10 µM ddI, and 0.09 µM nevirapine) were incubated in vitro, only minimal HIV-DNA was detectable 24–72 hr after infection, and no

HIV-DNA could be detected by PCR 21 days after infection. It was hypothesized that HIV has a finite ability to mutate successfully. Administration of these three drugs either induces virus mutation, producing a replication incompetent virus, or does not induce mutation, and the virus remains susceptible to the inhibitory effect(s) of the drug(s). Although the basis for these in vitro observations cannot be attributed to convergent resistance per se (75a, 75b) the ultimate clinical utility of these regimens awaits the outcome of clinical trials currently underway in both adults and children.

Blockers of Virus Attachment

Once it was demonstrated that the major route of virus entry into target cells was through binding to the CD4 receptor, several investigators purified this receptor, and ultimately a recombinant soluble CD4 molecule was derived (77–82). It was hoped that this molecule would bind circulating HIV and thus prevent the infection of cells bearing the CD4 receptor. Indeed, initial in vitro studies were highly encouraging. This strategy had particular relevance to pediatric AIDS since it could be theorized that such a product might be used to block the vertical transmission of virus from mother to fetus or child. Two preparations were introduced sequentially into clinical testing. The first was recombinant soluble rsCD4, and the second was an IgG-CD4 chimera that had a much longer half-life.

A phase I study was conducted at the NCI to determine the safety and pharmacokinetics of rsCD4 administered by continuous intravenous infusion to children with symptomatic HIV infection (52). Three dose levels of rsCD4 were evaluated: 100, 300, and 1000 μg/kg/day. After an initial 12 weeks of treatment with rsCD4 alone, ddI at a dose of 90 mg/m^2 every 8 hr was added, and patients were observed for an additional 12 weeks. Combination therapy was continued in patients in whom it was well tolerated. In addition to toxicity and pharmacokinetic monitoring, surrogate markers of antiviral activity were also evaluated. Eleven children were enrolled in this study. During the initial 12 weeks of rsCD4 alone

and the subsequent 12 weeks of combined rsCD4 and ddI, no significant toxicity was observed. Low level anti-CD4 antibodies developed in two patients. Steady state rsCD4 levels increased proportionately at higher doses. Changes in the CD4 cell counts and serum p24 antigen levels did not occur in a manner that suggested antiviral activity. Thus, although tolerable, this regimen did not appear to offer promise of antiretroviral activity. In addition, an overall trend suggesting a decline in cognitive function was noted particularly in younger children.

In addition, an ACTG phase I study of rsCD4 administered by intermittent injection was conducted in children aged between 3 and 17 years (83). Although the drug was well tolerated, no clinical or immunological benefits were accrued during the 10 weeks of study.

These disappointing findings appear to be explained, in part, by the observations that rsCD4 was more active against laboratory strains but failed to effectively bind or neutralize wild-type or clinical isolates of HIV. These data provided two lessons: the first is the importance of testing new agents or strategies on clinical HIV virus isolates (in addition to laboratory strains that may have surface changes) before proceeding to patient studies; the second is that even a carefully designed strategy, elegantly executed and effective in vitro, may not be effective in the human host.

Although discouraging, future strategies will try to employ refinements of this selective blocking. If effective and if agents in this category are developed, prevention of perinatal transmission would be an important goal. Use of such an agent in conjunction with agents that work on other components of the HIV virus life cycle might also provide greater therapeutic benefits than either approach alone.

Interference with Regulatory Genes and Proteins

Tat, rev, and *nef* are among the regulatory genes that appear to impact HIV replication. *Tat* serves as transactivator and impacts the transcription of genes that are under the control of the HIV LTR (long terminal repeat). Although the precise mechanism of *Tat* action is still undefined, it appears to exert its activity through its interaction with the *Tat*-responsive element known as TAR that permits *Tat* to initiate HIV transcription (84–87). Accordingly, Tat is a potential target for antiretroviral activity, especially because inhibition of this regulatory protein might affect the chronically infected cells that are not impacted by the reverse transcriptase inhibitors. Through a methodical screening program by scientists at the Roche Institute and its collaborators, Ro 5-3335, a benzodiazepine, was discovered that has anti-Tat activity in chronically infected cells. This agent has a high bioavailability (~85%), albeit it has minimal CNS penetration. Currently, Ro 5-3335 has been studied in adults as a single agent and in combination with AZT or ddI through the ACTG. To date, however, demonstrable decreases in P24 antigen or increases in CD4 counts have not been demonstrated.

Interference with Virus Assembly

A promising area for intervention is the virus encoded protease that is critical in the assembly of the virus protein coat. Blocking the protease could interfere with the production of infectious virions in chronically infected cells. The protease gene has been purified, and the HIV protease has been chemically synthesized (88, 89). Many protease inhibitors have been either discovered by screening or by specific synthesis based on computer modeling (90–100). Several of these agents are under active development, have shown impressive in vitro activity, and are in phase I testing in adults. It is anticipated that phase I testing in children with one or more protease inhibitors will be initiated before the end of 1993 (101). Although it is hoped that these agents will be clinically active alone, their greatest benefit will likely accrue from their combination with agents that work on other components of the HIV life cycle.

Agents That Decrease Stimulation of HIV

It is now clear that virus replication is continuous (and not latent) in the HIV-infected patient, and that the level of virus replication in vitro can be up-regulated by various growth factors, cytokines, and antigenic stimuli (102–107). This has particular relevance to the growing infant and child, for whom many of these factors are necessary for normal growth and development. It is plausible that the presence of such growth factors contributes to the more accelerated course of HIV infection in children compared with adults. Further, the usual sequential exposure to new foreign antigens during infancy and childhood normally results in nonspecific activation of the immune system, which could theoretically heighten HIV activation. These are normal concomitants of developing immunity. Treatment approaches that could interfere with stimulation or activation of the immune system might offer another component of multidimensional antiretroviral strategy, but the potential for adverse consequences also requires evaluation.

Antioxidants

An abundance of in vitro data suggests that the balance between cellular oxidants and antioxidants can impact HIV replication, presumably mediated via cellular cytokines. Among the most important antioxidants is glutathione, a moiety that may be deficient in HIV-infected individuals. Kalebic et al. (107) previously reported that in chronically infected cells in vitro glutathione, glutathione ester, and *N*-acetyl cysteine suppressed the expression of HIV induced by transcriptional inducers tumor-necrosis factor, (TNF)-α and PMA, or a posttranscriptionally active cytokine interleukin-6. A decreased level of acid soluble thiols such as GSH and cysteine have been found in plasma, peripheral blood monocytes and lymphocytes, and pleural fluid of HIV-seropositive individuals. In animal models, the decrease of GSH in plasma may be one of the earliest detectable changes caused by infection with simian immunodeficiency virus. An alteration in cellular antioxidant status, due to relative glutathione deficiency, may be associated with overproduction of HIV-inducing cytokines and may thus be important in progression of HIV infection. This provides a rationale for the evaluation of antioxidants as a component of antiretroviral therapy. GSH provides cells with their reducing environment and serves as the major cellular antioxidant. The transport of GSH into cells, however, is not efficient due to its degradation by a membrane bound GSH transpeptidase. Alternative pathways to restore a physiologic intracellular redox environment in HIV-infected cells were therefore examined. Recently, administration of *N*-acetyl cysteine (NAC) was attempted in adults to achieve this objective. Oral doses of NAC between 600 and 9600 mg/day were administered, and although dose limiting toxicities were not observed, the bioavailability was low (2.6%) and no appreciable changes in virologic, immunologic, or biochemical changes of HIV disease were observed (108).

Because of these results, alternatives to NAC are being pursued. A family of antioxidants includes amifostine and its analogs, including WR 151327, an organic thiophosphate with antioxidant and free radical scavenging activities (106). In in vitro models of HIV latency, WR 151327 suppressed, in dose dependent fashion, the induction of HIV mediated by TNF-α, GM-CSF, and PMA. Another possible approach is L-2-oxothiazolidine-4-carboxylic acid, an analog of 5-oxo-L-proline, which is metabolized to L-cysteine intracellularly with the promotion of glutathione synthesis. This agent, Procysteine, is being investigated in HIV-infected adults. It is rapidly absorbed and achieves peak blood levels in 40–60 min. Procysteine appears able to influence glutathione and cysteine concentrations. No data are yet available to indicate whether a measurable effect on virus burden or clinical disease occurs with this therapy. Evaluation of this or related agents is being pursued as a means for decreasing the stimulation of HIV.

Agents to Decrease Antigenic Stimulation

Infants and children are constantly exposed to new antigenic stimuli, many involving exposure to common infectious agents. The role that these events play on the course of HIV infection is unclear, but it is not illogical to assume that the immune activation that accompanies many of these infectious challenges contributes to some increase of HIV replication. How this relates to the accelerated course of HIV infection in many children is also unclear. It is, therefore, intriguing that studies by Mofenson et al. (109, 110) suggest that children receiving routine passive immunization with intravenous immunoglobulin may slow the decline in the loss of CD4 cells. Whether this observation was due to the effect of the passive immunization on the incidence or impact of intercurrent infections or due to a direct impact on HIV per se, is unknown at this time. If these data are confirmed they would suggest that modalities designed to decrease the antigenic stimulation accompanying common infections may also be of some benefit. Clearly this is an area requiring additional research, especially since the preliminary evaluation of ACTG 051 (comparing intravenous immunoglobulin with placebo therapy in children receiving AZT) does not appear to demonstrate a similar effect of passive immunization on the CD4 count.

Blocking Cytokines or Other Mediators That Might Stimulate HIV Infection

TNF-α concentrations are elevated in HIV-infected adults and children and may be an important cause of the cachexia (or the wasting syndrome) that occurs in these patients. Importantly, in vitro, TNF-α also enhances HIV-1 replication and appears to inhibit the effectiveness of AZT. Studies have correlated elevated serum TNF-α concentrations with HIV-associated encephalopathy in children. Pentoxifylline (Trental) has been shown to reduce the levels of TNF-α and other proinflammatory cytokines. Studies of this agent, along with other blockers of interleukin-1 or TNF, are essential to demonstrate whether such modalities will contribute to reductions of HIV stimulation (as measured by markers of virus burden) in HIV-infected children.

Agents That Improve or Stimulate Immune System
Hormones and Growth Factors

Many hormones and growth factors can impact the immune system. Most notable are growth hormone and its cellular substrates. Studies in rodents suggest that growth hormone and insulin-like growth factor-1 (IGF-1) can result in regeneration of both humoral and cellular immunity. Whether this is also true in humans is unknown, but the prospect for recruiting immune progenitors that might not be infected with HIV is a notable goal. At the same time, it must be recognized that growth hormone and IGF-1, like cytokines and immunomodulators, can also stimulate HIV replication, so that their administration without effective antiretroviral agents would be contraindicated.

Based on observations that some HIV-infected children with growth failure have deficiency in plasma IGF-1 levels, a pilot study has been initiated in 1993 by the Pediatric Branch of the NCI to assesses the safety, effect on growth, and immunologic effects of recombinant human IGF-I and recombinant human growth hormone in children with HIV infection and growth failure. The purpose of the study is to establish the feasibility and safety of administering recombinant human IGF-I and recombinant human growth hormone in this population, and to establish clinical and laboratory parameters that would be required for subsequent efficacy studies.

Use of Cytokines and Immunomodulators

Both cytokines and immunomodulators are important in immune development and regulation (see Chapter 9) but can also result in the stimulation of HIV replication (see Chapter 8). Although high doses of interleukin-2 are associated with considerable toxicity, recent studies in adults suggest that low doses of interleukin-2, administered with antiretroviral therapy, might recruit or sustain the CD4 count over time. Similar studies in children have not yet been performed. This is an area worthy of future research.

Active Immunization

Initial studies by Redfield et al. (110a) suggested that active immunization of HIV-infected adults might favorably impact the immune status, as indicated by development of antibody to envelope epitopes and lymphocyte proliferation to gp160. In these early studies, a recombinant gp160 vaccine was administered on a repetitive basis to HIV-infected adult patients with Walter Reed stage 1 or 2 (CD4 >400, normal delayed-type hypersensitivity) with promising results (110a). If these observations can be confirmed, and beneficial effects on virus burden or clinical progression can be convincingly demonstrated, then strategies designed to boost or stimulate the immune response to HIV infection with active immunization may also become a component of current therapeutic strategies. The validity of this concept must be assessed.

Pilot studies assessing the currently available rgp 120 MN based envelope vaccines (i.e., Genetech, Chiron) and rgp 160 IIIB vaccine (MicroGeneSys) are being tested in HIV-infected children and P-0 children born to HIV-infected mothers. Studies will test the immunogenicity of these vaccines in infected and uninfected children as well as their impact on plasma viremia, CD4 number, and Th cell function.

Bone Marrow Transplantation and Gene Therapy

The use of syngeneic bone marrow transplantation (i.e., from an uninfected twin to his identical HIV-infected sibling) proved unsuccessful perhaps because current antiretroviral agents are insufficient in eradicating the residual nonhematogenous tissue burden of HIV (111). The prospect for modifying stem cells with gene therapy to make them resistant to HIV infection looms on the horizon. By using retroviral or other vectors, it may be possible to insert genes (e.g., ribosymes or antisense) that interfere with key steps in the virus life cycle. Although exploratory clinical trials are just getting started in adults, it seems likely that this will be a very fruitful area for clinical investigations in children. Nonetheless, even successful gene therapy of stem cells still leaves the problem of HIV infection in tissues such as the central nervous system.

Development of Multidimensional Combination Antiretroviral Strategies

It has become increasingly clear that combination regimens will be necessary to optimize clinical efficacy, decrease the emergence of drug resistance, and address the various clinical symptoms and disease manifestations that complicate HIV infection in infants and children. Several current studies are combining antiretroviral agents that work on different aspects of the virus life cycle. These studies are designed to either employ agents that might provide additive or synergistic activity against the same virus target (e.g., reverse transcriptase) or that work on different components of the virus life cycle (e.g., attachment, intranuclear regulation, virus assembly). For example, if agents that inhibit either regulatory genes (e.g., *tat*) or structural genes (e.g., protease inhibitors) prove to be active and nontoxic, regimens incorporating them into the antiretroviral repertoire will be likely.

Note that enhanced benefit has already been observed from simply combining agents that work against the reverse transcriptase enzyme. For example, combinations of AZT and ddI are being assessed not only because of their in vitro synergy but also because they have complementary clinical benefits (53). AZT, for example, has clear activity in improving neurocognitive function but may have only a transient benefit on the CD4 count. Didanosine, in contrast, has a more sustaining effect on maintaining the numbers and function of the CD4 compartment but has only a limited penetration into the CNS. Preliminary data from pilot studies in adults and children demonstrate that these agents can be combined without additive toxicity and that they provide benefits that appear to exceed those achieved with monotherapy. Comparative clinical trials are underway in children and adults to fully substantiate the benefits of combining AZT with ddI, both for primary treatment and for salvage therapy.

Furthermore, as noted above, new combination regimens are being evaluated with AZT, ddI, and nevirapine in both adults and children. Other combination regimens (e.g., AZT + ddI + 3TC) are also being pursued. So too are studies with other nucleoside and non-nucleoside reverse transcriptase inhibitors. These include combinations of L-661 with AZT and U-87 or U-90 with AZT or with AZT and ddI. Although it is hoped that each of these combinations may

provide important insights and advances, they are still largely focused on a single virus target, its reverse transcriptase. Accordingly, the emerging availability of agents that act on other portions of the HIV life cycle (e.g., *tat* and protease inhibitors) offer an exciting prospect for combining agents that can impact both acutely and chronically infected cells. Studies of the *tat* and protease inhibitors are in progress in adults and children, and it is anticipated that regimens combining them with reverse transcriptase inhibitors will soon be underway.

In addition to combining drugs that work on different features of the HIV life cycle per se, utilizing agents that either inhibit stimulation of the virus or that might stimulate or improve the host's defense against the virus should also be considered part of the approach to therapy. Indeed, until a truly curative modality is available, such multidimensional combination therapy might prove useful in controlling the impact of this virus on the host. Certainly this provides a blueprint by which to approach future intervention regimens for adults and children with HIV infection or AIDS (see Fig. 35.2).

CURRENT STANDARDS OF ANTIRETROVIRAL THERAPY FOR CHILDREN WITH HIV OR AIDS

It is certainly hoped and expected that, in the years ahead, improvements and refinements of current antiretroviral agents coupled with the discovery of new more potent drugs will make the treatment of infants and children more successful. Although treatment guidelines will be constantly evolving over time, it is still important to define the current state-of-the-art therapy for the pediatric community. To assist with this goal, the National Pediatric HIV Resource Center recently convened a group of health care providers and parents to define what constitutes the best current optimal therapy for HIV-infected children (112). Although such guidelines have limitations and flaws, they represent an opportunity to develop standards and offer practitioners an opportunity to assure that their patients are receiving the best possible therapies available.

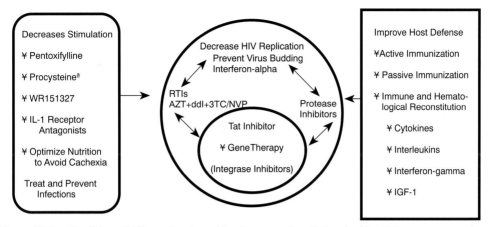

Figure 35.2. Possible multidimensional combination strategies. *IL,* interleukin; *RTI,* reverse transcriptase inhibitor; *NVP,* nevirapine.

When Should Antiretroviral Therapy Be Initiated?

To optimize patient care, the patient's primary health care provider should decide when to begin antiretroviral therapy in collaboration with a physician conversant with the management of HIV infection in children. Whenever possible, children should be enrolled in clinical trials: access and information can be obtained by calling 1-800-TRIALS-A (ACTG) or 301-402-0696 (Pediatric Branch, NCI).

Currently, antiretroviral therapy is recommended for children who either have evidence of significant immunodeficiency or who have defined HIV-associated symptoms. Although therapy is recommended for asymptomatic infants and children who have evidence of immunodeficiency, there are no data to guide therapeutic recommendations for asymptomatic infants with normal immune status, and thus antiretroviral therapy cannot be recommended for this group of children. In particular, this has implications for infants who have been shown to be infected but who lack clinical evidence of HIV and immunological deterioration. The risk-to-benefit ratio for these infants can only be determined from the prospective clinical trials that are being initiated. Children with lymphadenopathy, hepatomegaly, or hypergammaglobulinemia as their only manifestations of HIV infection are considered "asymptomatic" because these findings alone have not been associated with adverse outcome.

Defining Immunodeficiency Criteria for Initiation of Antiretroviral Therapy

There are a broad array of cellular and humoral immunological abnormalities in HIV-infected infants and children (see Chapters 8 and 9). Which of these should be used to guide the initiation of antiretroviral therapy, to monitor the response to intervention, or to define when to stop or switch therapy are matters of controversy. The CD4 count has become a standard guide for assessing the HIV-infected adult and for initiating either prophylactic therapies (e.g., *Pneumocystis carinii* pneumonia (PCP) prophylaxis) or antiretroviral treatment. Data in adults and children confirm that the risk for opportunistic infections (e.g., PCP and *Mycobacterium avium-intracellulare* (MAI)), as well as survival, are closely associated with CD4 count. From a strategic perspective, treatments that either increase or maintain the CD4 count as high above the danger levels as possible may delay the onset of AIDS-related events and prolong survival. Nonetheless, it is also clear that there are other variables (many still undefined) that also impact the risk for AIDS-related events or survival. Even patients with very low CD4 counts can have long durations of survival. Antiretroviral therapy has been recommended for adults whose CD4 count has fallen below 500/mm^3, but recent reports of the European Concorde study, which failed to confirm a benefit from the initiation of AZT in asymptomatic patients, have raised questions about the overall value of early intervention. Because of the age-related differences in CD4 numbers in infants and children (see Chapter 9), a different set of guidelines is appropriate for the pediatric population. The level for beginning antiretroviral therapy in adults is set at a CD4 number that is higher than that used to guide PCP prophylaxis (currently ≤200 CD4 cells/mm^3). Because it seems rational to commence antiretroviral therapy before the risk for opportunistic infections is heightened, the recommended starting points for children have been set at age-specific levels that are 2–300 CD4 cells higher than that indicated for PCP prophylaxis (112). Accordingly, the CD4 based criteria for initiating either or both antiretroviral therapy and PCP prophylaxis based on the age of the infant or child are shown in Table 35.1. It must be underscored that one CD4 determination should not be used for therapeutic decision making. Indeed, because of the variations observed when measuring CD4 number, at least two determinations should be used to validate a result and establish a baseline. However, a child with a presumptively diagnosed HIV infection who otherwise meets the criteria for intervention should have antiretroviral therapy initiated while the confirmatory CD4 count results are pending.

Clinical Criteria For Initiating Antiretroviral Therapy

Independent of their CD4 count, antiretroviral treatment is recommended for

Table 35.1.   CD4 Lymphocyte Counts for Initiation of Antiretroviral Therapy and PCP Prophylaxis[a]

	Criteria for Antiretroviral Therapy	Criteria for PCP Prophylaxis
CD4 (%)		
<1 yr	<30	<20
1–2 yr	<25	<20
>2 yr	<20	<20
CD4 (cells/mm^3)		
<1 yr	<1750	<1500
1–2 yr	<1000	<750
2–6 yr	<750	<500
>6 yr	<500	<200

[a]Data based on recommendations of Working Group on Antiretroviral Therapy, National Pediatric HIV Resource Center.

HIV-infected infants and children who develop any AIDS-identifying disease manifestations. Those clinical conditions that clearly warrant the initiation of therapy are listed in Table 35.2. There is also a wide array of other symptoms that may, depending on the patient's overall status and the analysis of the care team, also indicate the need for initiating antiretroviral therapy. These presumably less severe clinical symptoms are also listed in Table 35.2.

Which Antiretroviral Agent or Agents Should Be Chosen for Initial Treatment and What Dosages Should Be Employed

The drug of choice for initial treatment of the HIV-infected child should be AZT. This is based on the demonstrable impact of this drug on improving neurodevelopmental deficits, weight gain, and survival. In the immediate future, this recommendation may change for one or more reasons. Indeed combination regimens (e.g., AZT + ddI) may prove superior to monotherapy both in their clinical and immunological impact and in reducing the likelihood of the emergence of resistant mutants. Second, as the prevalence of AZT resistance increases, it is plausible that infants may acquire an HIV strain from their mothers that is already AZT resistant. In fact, data already exist that an AZT-resistant virus can be transmissible, but it remains to be determined whether this will become the more dominant transmissible virus in vertical transmission. Clearly, if this is true, it will become necessary to initiate antiretroviral therapy with another agent. At this time, however, it is still the consensus that the starting agent should be AZT.

The dosage(s) of AZT that are recommended are also subject to change as more data become available. Presently, for children aged between 4 weeks and 13 years, dosage of 180 mg/m^2 administered every 6 hr is recommended (7, 9, 20). This dosage, which is higher than that used in adults, is based on the increased frequency of CNS symptoms that occur in HIV-infected children. Should ongoing studies (e.g., ACTG 128) demonstrate that lower dosages of AZT (e.g., 90 mg/m^2 every 6 hr) are satisfactory in asymptomatic or minimally symptomatic

Table 35.2.   Clinical Criteria for Instituting Antiretroviral Therapy[a]

Clinical conditions that definitely warrant initiating antiretroviral therapy regardless of CD4 count
- AIDS-defining opportunistic infection
- Wasting syndrome or failure to thrive (defined as crossing two percentiles over time or being below the fifth percentile for age and falling from the growth curve) despite oral alimentation
- Progressive encephalopathy attributable to HIV
- HIV-associated malignancy
- Recurrent septicemia or meningitis (i.e., two or more episodes)
- Thrombocytopenia (platelet count < 75,000 /mm^3 on two or more occasions)
- Hypogammaglobulinemia (total IgG/IgM/IgA < 250/mm^3)

Clinical conditions that may warrant initiating antiretroviral therapy, independent of CD4 count, based on overall clinical profile and judgment of health care provider
- Lymphoid interstitial pneumonitis and/or parotitis
- Splenomegaly
- Oral candidiasis that persists for more than 1 month or that is recurrent despite appropriate therapy
- Diarrhea that is otherwise unexplained and either persistent (defined as three or more loose stools per day for 2 weeks or longer) or recurrent (defined as two or more episodes of diarrhea accompanied by dehydration within 2 months)
- Symptomatic HIV-associated cardiomyopathy that requires specific intervention
- Nephrotic syndrome (not associated with non-HIV etiologies)
- Hepatic transaminase more than five times normal, not associated with non-HIV etiologies
- Chronic bacterial infections (e.g., sinusitis or pneumonia)
- Recurrent or persistent herpes simplex or varicella zoster infections (i.e., two or more episodes within 1 year)
- Neutropenia (< 750/mm^3) or age-corrected anemia on at least two occasions over 1 week

[a]Data based on recommendations of Working Group on Antiretroviral Therapy, National Pediatric HIV Resource Center.

children, these dosage recommendations may be changed. If a patient receiving full dose AZT is restriced from oral intake for more than 48 hr because of an intercurrent event or illness, it is recommended that the child receive intravenous AZT at a dosage of 120 mg/m^2 every 6 hr (i.e., two-thirds of the oral dose to approximate the oral bioequivalence) (112). If a child who is eligible for AZT has pre-existing hematological compromise, a lower starting dose (i.e., 120 mg/m^2 every 6 hr) should be employed with the plan to increase the dosage as tolerated.

For infants younger than 4 weeks, in whom the clearance and half-life of AZT are prolonged, a modified dosing schedule is recommended. During the first 2 weeks of life, the dose of AZT should be 2 mg/kg/dose every 6 hr, and for infants aged 2–4 weeks the dose should be increased to 3 mg/kg/dose every 6 hr. Therapeutic dose monitoring is important in infants because of developmental changes in clearance during the first month of life.

For adolescents, the currently recommended adult dosage (i.e., 500 mg/day) seems most appropriate, although specific data in this age group are lacking. Indeed, higher doses of AZT may well be needed for adolescents who have evidence of CNS symptoms related to HIV.

How Should Antiretroviral Therapy Be Monitored?

Three features should be considered in monitoring of antiretroviral therapy in children: 1) whether the therapy has evidence of activity; 2) whether it is safe and tolerable; 3) maintenance of activity as indicated by virus and immunological markers and clinical progression.

Both clinical and laboratory parameters can be used to determine whether an antiretroviral agent has activity. Note that even agents that are in the same pharmacological class (e.g., dideoxynucleosides) may have different effects on the clinical or laboratory profile of HIV infection, making it important to assess several of these measures with each drug being evaluated. Some of these effects may be related to the clinical pharmacology of the drug itself (e.g., differential penetration across the blood-brain barrier), whereas other effects may reflect intrinsic differences in the activity of the drug per se (e.g., effect on appetite (with 3TC) or CD4 preservation (with ddI)) (5, 6, 8, 9, 112). Ideally, a palette of different clinical and laboratory features should be selected to evaluate whether a drug is working in a child.

Clinical Measures of Antiretroviral Activity

The most reliable clinical assessment of the activity of an antiretroviral agent includes either an improvement or reversal of the AIDS-identifying illness that led to the initiation of therapy or the improvement or reversal of HIV-related manifestations that are commonly associated with symptomatic infection. Of these, changes in physical growth and development (e.g., weight gain, growth velocity), improvements in neurocognitive function (e.g., improved IQ score, motor or neurological function), reduction in the incidence of infections (e.g., PCP, bacterial infections) have been the most studied. It is important to recognize that a child who is receiving therapy may not develop these symptoms and that the absence of progression (or maintenance of stable disease) can also be a measure of response to an antiretroviral regimen.

Assessment of Physical Growth. HIV-infected children are significantly smaller than uninfected children in their weight-for-age and length-for-age. However, because both linear growth and weight gain may have decreased, impairment of weight-for-length may be less apparent (20). Moreover, because children are normally growing, before a gain in weight or height can be attributed to a specific antiretroviral therapy, it must be clear that other factors are not contributing to the clinical improvements or serving as confounding variables. Further, it is important to accurately assess small-for-age HIV-infected infants and children by using a z score to explain that the patient being assessed may be below the standard deviation for the population. In general, growth failure consequent to social deprivation is initially characterized by a decrease in the z scores for weight-for-age and weight-for-length, followed by a decline in length-for-age. If a child with symptomatic HIV infection, whose preantiretroviral growth parameters were abnormal, was placed on a new therapy but simultaneously also took part in a comprehensive program of nutritional intervention, it could be difficult to assure that observed changes in weight, weight-for height, or height for-weight were directly related to the antiretroviral therapy per se compared with changes consequent to improved nutrition or other supportive care modalities. Clearly, it is important to standardize, as much as possible, the nutritional features of supportive care, ideally coupling them with a comprehensive nutritional history.

Current Recommendations. An approach to assessing growth failure is being developed through the ACTG. To meet the definition of growth failure, the child's weight or weight-for-height must be below the 25th percentile on standard National Center of Health Standards growth charts. The weight growth velocity is calculated 24 weeks after the baseline measurement and then every 12 weeks thereafter. Growth failure is defined when the 24-week weight-growth velocity is below the third percentile for age and gender. A minimum interval of 161 days between measurements is required for growth-velocity calculations. During the 24 week interval, there should be no acute illnesses or other explainable causes of growth failure that could confound the accurate measurement of weight-growth velocity.

Assessment of Neurodevelopmental Function. Serial psychometric evaluation as well as structural changes described by brain imaging studies (e.g., computerized tomography, magnetic resonance scan), changes in cytokine concentrations, or other neurochemical correlates of CNS activity (e.g., quinolonic acid levels) can be used to monitor the impact of an antiretroviral agent on neurodevelopmental function (29, 30, 32–34, 113, 114). A methodological problem with psychometric tests is the potential for a practice effect (or learning effect) that might occur if the testing intervals are too close in time (see Chapter

23). Based on the observations in children with HIV disease or other chronic disorders, an age-appropriate battery has been developed that permits evaluation of patients at approximately 12-week intervals. The tests that are more vulnerable to a practice effect are administered at 24-week intervals.

Changes in the full-scale IQ score can be used to quantify changes in cognitive function as a consequence of the HIV disease per se or treatment with antiretroviral agents. It would be predicted that agents that cross the blood-brain barrier would be more likely to demonstrate a significant impact on the neurodevelopmental problems associated with HIV disease. To date, this appears to be true, since AZT has more consistent and superior CNS activity than agents that cross more poorly into the CNS (e.g., ddI, ddC) (7, 8, 19, 56). In general, a response is defined as an increase in the IQ score of 10 points over the baseline value. However, also note that to assess whether an agent has an effect on neurocognitive function of this magnitude, there must be room for improvement. That is, a child whose baseline IQ score is in the normal range (i.e., 90–110) will be less likely to reflect a change in IQ score of 10 or more points compared with the child whose IQ score had declined to subnormal values and who might improve to the normal range. Accordingly, a stratified analysis of the population being evaluated is appropriate, so that the more impaired group of children can be assessed independently from the group that may have had less neurocognitive deterioration (and thus less likelihood to show an effect). It is still notable, however, that we have also observed children whose baseline IQ scores placed them in the normal to high-normal range who improved to the superior range after AZT therapy. In these children, the degree of cognitive impairment was masked by their residual level of function. Furthermore, maintenance of "normal" cognitive function may also be a measurement of successful therapy.

In assessing IQ scores and psychometric tests, it is also important to assure that the tests being administered are culturally as well as age appropriate, and that the patients were not ill or otherwise impaired at the time of the testing session. Considerable expertise is necessary to assure that the test results are accurate and reproducible (see Chapter 23).

In addition to cognitive function, CNS responsiveness to antiretroviral therapy can also be assessed by improvements or changes in brain structure. It has been demonstrated that 79% of children with symptomatic HIV infection referred for treatment have abnormalities on their preantiretroviral scans, including alterations in ventricular dilatation, subarachnoid enlargment, periventricular enhancement, and the presence of calcifications in the basal ganglia and frontal lobes (37). The presence of calcifications appeared to be associated with vertical transmission and a lower level of intellectual functioning. Interestingly, even when there are improvements in the child's cognitive function as a consequence of antiretroviral therapy, concomitant alterations in brain calcifications have not been observed (35). In contrast, although the degree of abnormalities of other computerized tomography-related findings based on an analogue rating scale can also be inversely associated with the level of intellectual function (as measured by the IQ score), it is possible to demonstrate improvements in the ventricular-to-brain ratios with antiretroviral therapy that improve neurocognitive function (7, 18, 19, 29, 35, 112). Such correlations provide powerful measures of the activity of an antiretroviral agent since they reflect improvements in HIV-related organ-specific abnormalities.

A third means to assess the impact of antiretroviral activity on CNS function is to determine whether chemical markers of infection are altered with therapy. It has been demonstrated in adults that quinolinic acid, a metabolite of L-tryptophan, is elevated in the cerebrospinal fluid of adults with encephalopathy. Significant elevations of quinolinic acid have been observed in the cerebrospinal fluid of HIV-infected children, particularly those with evidence of encephalopathy, compared with children receiving cancer chemotherapy (36). Of note, after antiretroviral therapy, a significant decline in the cerebrospinal fluid quinolinic acid levels have been observed in tandem with clinical improvements of the encephalopathy and significant increases in IQ score. Even though no clear etiologic association of quinolinic acid and HIV-related encephalopathy can be drawn from these data, the baseline and follow-up measure of quinolinic acid provides another method to assess the activity of the antiretroviral activity on the CNS.

Current Recommendations. As shown in Table 35.3, serial assessment of CNS function (both cognitive and neurological) and imaging should be performed before beginning antiretroviral therapy (or up to 6 weeks after beginning therapy). A monitoring battery that is based on an evaluation of clinical and neurological changes is administered 3 months after initiation of treatment and is repeated at 6-month intervals. A more comprehensive examination that includes the detailed age-appropriate psychometric testing, motor and neurological evaluation, and neuroimaging studies performed at baseline should be repeated 6 months after the initiation of treatment and then at 6-month intervals thereafter. This alternating monitoring and comprehensive assessment permits careful follow-up of children receiving antiretroviral therapy, providing both a measure of its success and an early warning of its failure (see Table 35.4).

Assessment on Risk or Frequency of Infectious Complications. When AZT was first introduced into adult clinical trials, deaths and opportunistic infections occurred less frequently in the treated compared with placebo group of patients and provided strong evidence that this antiretroviral agent had a specific activity on the course of HIV infection. Because the infectious complications that arise secondary to profound immunosuppression can dominate the clinical picture of AIDS, it seems obvious that an effective antiretroviral agent might decrease the prevalence and severity of such infectious complications (115–121). Other appropriate supportive care modalities can also affect these infectious complications (122–140). For example, the routine use of prophylaxis with trimethoprim-sulfamethoxazole, pentamidine, or dapsone has reduced the frequency of PCP to the point where it cannot serve as a reliable end point to assess the efficacy of a new antiretroviral agent in most clinical studies (see Chapter 21).

Similarly, bacterial infections (especially with encapsulated organisms such as *Streptococcus pneumoniae*) were common in children with HIV infection in the 1980s and were initially employed as end points by which to assess the efficacy of intervention strategies. Indeed studies have demonstrated that intravenous immunoglobulin can reduce the frequency of bacterial infections in HIV-infected children who have CD4 counts above $200/mm^3$ (110, 116, 141, 142). Other recent studies suggest that AZT, when given in conjunction with trimethoprim-sulfamethoxazole for PCP prophylaxis, also reduces the frequency of bacterial infections in HIV-infected children and that the role of intravenous immunoglobulin or other antibiotic prophylaxis is less clearly defined. As AZT, trimethoprim-sulfamethoxazole and/or IVIG become routinely used in HIV-infected children, the ability to assess a further reduction in the frequency of bacterial infections may be more difficult (118). Thus measureable clinical end points may shift effective interventions after the asessment of disease progression.

Current Recommendations. Although a reduction in the frequency or severity of in-

Table 35.3. Suggested Schedule for Neurodevelopmental Evaluation in Symptomatic HIV-infected Children Who Do Not Have Evidence of CNS Abnormalities[a]

Yr	Base	3 Months	6 Months	9 Months	12 Months	15 Months	18 Months	24 Months	30 Months	36 Months	48 Months
<2.5	Co	Mo	Co	Mo	Co	Mo	Co	Co	Mo	Co	Co
2.5–6	Co		Mo		Co		Mo	Co		Mo	Co
>6	Co		Mo		Co			Co			Co

[a]Monitoring battery (Mo) can be based on both evaluation of clinical events (loss or prolonged plateau of milestones by local physicians or other health care providers or on more formal assessment using a subpart of comprehensive examination (Co). Comprehensive examination should at least include an age-appropriate standardized test of general cognitive functioning with which psychologist is familiar (such as Bayley, McCarthy, WISC, etc.). In addition the monitoring battery should be repeated at these times. On an annual basis the comprehensive examination should include a standardized neurologic and motor examination. Data based on the recommendations of the Working Group on Antiretroviral Therapy, National Pediatric HIV Resource Center.

Table 35.4.   Neurodevelopmental Criteria for Evidence of CNS Disease Progression[a]

Impairment of brain growth
  Abnormal head growth rate
- For infants aged <1 year this is defined as a no increase in head circumference or crossing two percentiles in 2 months
- For infants aged >1 year this is defined as a loss of 1 SD from baseline on National Center for Human Statistics growth curve.
- For children aged >2 years neuroimaging is necessary to confirm atrophy

Progressive loss of cerebral parenchymal volume demonstrated on serial neuroimaging studies at least 2 months apart

Decline of cognitive function
- For infants from birth to 30 months, a fall of 2 SD (32 points) on Mental Developmental Index or a fall of 1 SD from baseline maintained over two assessments separated by at least 1 month
- For children >30 months, a fall of ≥1 SD on McCarthy GCI or Wechsler (WISC-R and WAIS) Full Scale IQ

Clinical neurologic dysfunction: progressive over at least 2 months or, in youngest infants, persistent in two exams over 1 month
- Loss or deterioration of previously attained motor skills
- Significant changes in neurobehavioral status in children aged <6 including significant changes in range of regulation of arousal and attention that is sustained over 1 month without alternative explanation
- Diffuse symmetric loss or decrease in power or strength that is not result of a systemic, nutritional, or metabolic complication
- Diffuse, symmetric, and pathologically increased deep tendon reflexes
- Diffuse and symmetric abnormalities of tone, including, but not limited to, hypotonia or hypertonia

[a]Data based on recommendations of the Working Group on Antiretroviral Therapy, National Pediatric HIV Resource Center.

fectious complications can be a powerful end point by which to assess the activity of an antiretroviral agent, the current prophylactic and early intervention strategies that characterize care of the HIV-infected patient make these impractical end points for clinical assessment. Unless the impact is likely to be of enormous magnitude, large numbers of patients would be required to validate a benefit. This is even more challenging with studies designed to show equivalence, wherein extremely large numbers of patients would be necessary to compare one regimen with another—a costly and largely impractical study approach.

Assessment of Other Clinical Measures of HIV Disease. In addition to altered growth and neurodevelopment, many organ systems are affected by HIV disease and might serve as indicators to measure response to therapy. Included might be changes in the degree and size of lymphadenopathy, hepatosplenomegaly, or altered organ functions (e.g., respiratory distress secondary to lymphoid interstitial pneumonia, cardiac dysfunction related to

cardiomyopathy, nephritis or nephrosis related to renal involvement). Reduction in lymphadenopathy and organomegaly have been shown in many studies of antiretroviral therapies (e.g., with AZT and ddI), but these responses are variable and difficult to quantify and therefore serve as only imperfect measures by which to assess or monitor an antiretroviral agent.

It is also notable that other putative HIV-associated organ abnormalities may not improve with current antiretroviral therapy(ies) or may progress despite other indications of successful therapy. Included is the cardiomyopathy and renal complications associated with HIV disease (see Chapters 26 and 29) that, although responding to specific supportive care modalities, do not appear to improve with currently available antiretroviral agents. The reasons for these discordant organ responses whereby certain organ systems (e.g., CNS, growth) appear to respond to intervention and others do not remains unclear but must be considered when assessing whether an antiretroviral agent works and, equally importantly, whether it is failing. Thus, certain organ-specific abnormalities, even though representing an important manifestation of HIV infection, should not be used to guide or alter current antiretroviral therapies.

Survival as a Measure of Antiretroviral Activity. The initial placebo-controlled trial of AZT in adults with AIDS demonstrated a significant survival advantage for treated vs. nontreated patients (143). Clearly, placebo-controlled trials can no longer be performed for symptomatic patients with this disease. Using survival as an end point to evaluate an antiretroviral agent or regimen is not realistic because of the length of study and multifactorial contributions. Moreover, it is important to have more immediate and time-relevant methods to assess the activity of an antiretroviral agent rather than its impact on survival per se. At the same time, it is relevant, whenever possible, to assess the impact of evolving state-of-the-art treatment on the quality and duration of life.

Laboratory Measures of Antiretroviral Activity

Although clinical end points constitute the clearest measures of altered disease progression impacted by an antiretroviral agent, they take time to evolve and become evaluable. Furthermore, many of these clinical measurements can also be influenced by changes in supportive care and other therapeutic or prophylactic interventions. Other measures of disease that might precede changes in the clinical course, and that could be rapidly assessed and quantitated, are highly desirable, especially if they could be correlated with the patient's eventual clinical outcome. Virologic, immunologic, and other surrogate markers of disease activity have been explored in both adults and children to monitor disease activity and assess its response or progression to therapeutic interventions. Several of these surrogate markers (e.g., CD4 count) have been the topics of intense debate and controversy, and although no one of these laboratory measures provides a consistently reliable end point, collectively they may portray a depiction of the child's disease status and the impact of therapy. Intuitively,

it would seem that if a therapy is no longer effective, increased virus burden or virulence would precede immunological deterioration and clinical disease progression.

Virologic Measures of Disease Activity. The ability to quantify the level of HIV as a measure of disease activity and response to therapy would seem straightforward. However, reliable, predictive, technically feasible, and cost-effective measures to assess virus burden remain an obstacle (144–147). Although it seems clear that the level of virus in plasma and circulating cells varies during different stages of the patient's disease, it is also clear that the level of virus in the blood does not completely portray the true virus burden in the body (38–43, 45, 148, 149). For example, several investigators have demonstrated that after acute infection, the level of plasma viremia rises over several weeks (see Chapters 7 and 8) and then falls and remains low until the time that the patient's CD4 declines and symptoms of AIDS appear, at which time the level of circulating virus rises once again (145, 147). In adults, the period of clinical latency, during which the level of plasma viremia is low, can be as long as 8–10 years, whereas in infants and children, this asymptomatic period may be as short as months to 2 years or less. Throughout this apparent clinical latency, however, in both adults and children, virus replication is active in body tissues, particularly lymph nodes and related tissues (e.g., adenoids and tonsils) (40, 41, 43, 45). Thus, measurement of virus activity in the peripheral blood represents only a relative portrayal of the overall state of virus activity.

The current methods to detect or quantify HIV include measurement of P24 antigen (including the recently introduced immune complex dissociated methodology), quantitation of plasma viremia using end point dilutions and virus culture, and determination of the level of cell-associated virus DNA or RNA or plasma RNA using quantitative PCR techniques. Each of these techniques has advantages and disadvantages for the diagnosis and monitoring of either disease progression or the response to therapeutic interventions (144, 150–163). P24 antigen determination, for example, can be helpful in establishing the diagnosis of HIV infection, especially in infants in whom the presence of maternal antibody represents a confounding variable for establishing a diagnosis. P24 can also be used to provide evidence that an antiretroviral agent has biologic activity, since the levels of P24 can be demonstrated to decline with various reverse transcriptase inhibitors and can be correlated with the level of the drug (e.g., ddI) achieved in the plasma. However, P24 antigenemia has not been shown to be a reliable prognostic indicator in either adults or children and even when measurable levels are high or rising, it is unclear that it serves as a useful marker of true disease activity (150, 151, 154). Measures of virus burden by culture or PCR in the peripheral blood can also be shown to decrease with the antiretroviral agents. Despite drops in plasma viremia, the body burden of virus can still be notable. For example, Sei and colleagues (personal communication, 1993) demonstrated that both children and adults who died with AIDS still had high levels of HIV that were detectable by PCR in lymph nodes, spleen, colon, and other body tissues, even though they had received antiretroviral therapy for varying periods. These observations raise the question of whether monitoring the burden of disease in certain body organs (e.g., lymph nodes) as well as in the peripheral blood should be performed as part of the evaluation of certain antiretroviral strategies.

In addition to measuring the level of virus burden in the peripheral blood and tissues, an assessment of virus virulence and drug resistance may also be useful. Emerging data suggest that the phenotype of the virus may change during infection. Early in the disease, the virus is more likely to be monocytotropic. It has been proposed that the lymphotropic strains that dominate the latter stages of illness are more virulent.

Furthermore, whether the virus in the host is sensitive or resistant to the drugs being employed may also be an important determinant in the assessment of antiretroviral activity. Drug-resistant mutants have been described with all of the nucleoside and non-nucleoside reverse transcriptase inhibitors, and, in some cases, cross-resistance has also been demonstrated (49, 65, 75, 164, 165). Transmission of HIV that is resistant to AZT has been described and may have clear implications for whether a patient will respond to intervention with this or other drugs. Indeed, the prospect that the dominant virus transmitted vertically from mother to fetus or child might be drug resistant has ominous implications. Presently, it is not routine to assess drug resistance before beginning an antiretroviral therapy, even with new agents. In the future, it is likely that as the prevalence of drug resistance becomes more common and correlations of virus resistance with outcome are more established, the sensitivity pattern of the patient's virus(es) will become a component of the initial evaluation and the monitoring of patients receiving antiretroviral therapy.

Current Recommendations. Although the detection of HIV, by various techniques, can be useful diagnostically (see Chapter 12) and can provide evidence for the activity of an antiretroviral agent, it is not yet clear that these techniques provide a means to assess either clinical progression or a failure of response. However, as better correlations are drawn between the level of plasma RNA and tissue burdens of HIV (e.g., in lymph nodes) these measurements may take on greater utility. We hope to have markers that precede evidence of clinical progression so that alterations in therapy can be implemented before disease progression ensues. Moreover, although it is not currently routine practice to measure the virus phenotype or determine its sensitivity pattern, this also might become more standard as correlations with clinical end points and disease progression are more sharply defined.

Immunological Measures of Disease Activity. Assessment of the patient's cellular and humoral immune systems provides potential measures of disease activity and of the response to therapeutic or prophylactic interventions. The most common laboratory measures that have been explored include the patient's CD4 number and percentage, the CD8 number and percentage, and the CD4-to-CD8 ratio (127, 135, 139, 149, 154, 166–172). Other measures of immune function (e.g., antibody-dependent cell-mediated cytotoxicity, NK cells, cytotoxic lymphocytes, serum immunoglobulin levels, and the presence of neutralizing antibody titers) and various nonspecific measures (e.g., β_2-microglobulin, interferon-α, neopterin levels) have been evaluated as markers of disease progression and of therapeutic response (173–177). These measures are a consequence of HIV infection and might be expected to precede evidence of clinical progression later than changes in virus parameters.

The CD4 count has perhaps received the greatest level of attention. There is no doubt that strong correlations can be made with the CD4 count and the risk for progression to AIDS. In particular, the risk for opportunistic infections (e.g., PCP, MAI) can be closely correlated with the level of the CD4 count in adults and children. In addition, the depth of the CD4 count also serves as a predictor of survival. For example, when the CD4 count falls below 50 cells/mm^3 in adults, the likelihood for a fatal outcome within the next year is heightened. Similarly, if the age-associated differences in CD4 count are adjusted to approximate this level of 50 CD4 cells (i.e., by taking <21% of the lower limit of normal for age), a highly significant correlation with survival can be made in children as well (154). Clearly, children with CD4 counts below this level, even when receiving antiretroviral therapy, are more likely to die than those with higher CD4 numbers. At the same time, the median survival for children with low CD4 counts is ~22 months, and the fact that children can survive this long, despite such immunological compromise, suggests that other host and viral factors likely affect disease progression. Determining what these factors are will have significant implications for both disease monitoring and future therapeutic interventions.

In addition to measuring the number of CD4 cells, assessing T helper function can provide another measure of disease activity and a parameter for assessing antiretroviral activity (178). As noted above, deficits in T helper function can precede drops in the CD4 count. Importantly, it has been shown that certain dideoxynucleosides (e.g., ddI) can improve phagocyte chemotaxis and bactericidal activity as well as improve T helper function in response to recall and alloantigens (59). That these immunological enhancements can be correlated with a reduction in the frequency of bacterial and opportunistic infections, independent of changes in CD4 number, thus provides another important measure of antiretroviral activity and, potentially, a means for both screening promising agents as well as defining which ones to use in combination regimens.

Changes in humoral immunity can also be correlated with disease progression and can provide another marker for assessing antiretroviral interventions (110, 116, 141, 179). For example, children with HIV disease have a polyclonal hypergammaglobulinemia, although no specific subtype pattern of IgG characterizes this profile. When dideoxynucleoside therapy is administered to HIV-infected children, significant drops in the IgG level can be observed but have no specific correlation with clinical end points. The precise mechanism for this change is unkown, but it might represent improved B cell regulation and could be used as a means to assess antiretroviral activity. Measurement of changes in IgG levels cannot, however, be used to assess prognosis or to serve as a basis for defining a treatment failure.

The prospect that neutralizing antibody against various HIV epitopes might modify the disease course would provide another measure of disease activity as well as an end point for therapeutic monitoring. Several studies have suggested that either antibody against the V3 hypervariable loop, syncytia-forming elements, or against total neutralizing antibody can be correlated with alterations of the rate of progression of AIDS. For example, a recent study from the NCI has shown that patients with higher levels of neutralizing antibody (but not with antibody against linear epitopes on V3) who also had some preservation of cellular immunity had fewer AIDS related events compared with patients with lower levels of neutralizing antibody (180). Such data have implications for monitoring disease progression as well as for configuring treatment approaches that might either passively or actively elevate antibody titers against HIV (see Chapters 45 and 47).

Several nonspecific measures of immune function have also been used as indicators of disease progression or for monitoring a therapeutic response (175, 177, 181–183).

Although these have demonstrated some correlations with clinical manifestations, these nonspecific markers will have less clinical relevance as more specific virus markers of disease activity are defined.

Current Recommendations. The CD4 count has become a common laboratory parameter for assessing the state of disease, monitoring the point at which to initiate antiretroviral therapy, measuring the response to therapy, and providing a criterion for potentially changing or modifying the therapeutic regimen. However, many problems must be noted. First, there can be considerable variation in the CD4 number between laboratories and even within the same patient depending on the time of day the sample was collected, the presence of intercurrent illnesses, and other variables. Quality control is critically important and laboratories should conform to established standards (such as those recommended through the ACTG). It is important, therefore, not to base a therapeutic decision on a single determinant but rather to have at least two CD4 measures at least 2 weeks apart when a major decision is imminent. Responses in CD4 have also been variably defined and in adults have included either the 10/10 or 50/50 rule, i.e, an increase in the CD4 count by 10% over baseline and at least 10 cells or by 50% over baseline and at least 50 cells. The patient's CD4 count before initiation of therapy has a considerable impact on the degree of the antiretroviral effect. Patients with low CD4 counts, especially those with a baseline value below 100 cells/mm^3, are unlikely to have either a large rise or a sustained effect with an antiretroviral agent (e.g., ddI) compared with patients with higher baseline values. Furthermore, the duration of the CD4 response can be transient and not necessarily correlated with the continuum of clinical improvement. This can also vary with the dideoxynucleoside being administered.

Assessment of Toxicity of Antiretroviral Agents

Although the patterns of toxicity related to antiretroviral agents are generally similar in children compared with those observed in adults, there are differences in the frequency and severity of these complications of therapy. It is, of course, imperative that children receiving antiretroviral therapy be closely monitored for toxicity and that health care providers be cognizant of the known side effects of therapy. In the development of new agents for children, careful consideration must be given to the risks vs. benefits as part of their evaluation.

The nucleosides are the most studied antiretroviral agents to date, and more information about toxicity exists for these agents compared with other drugs. Even though some of these agents (e.g., AZT) have been extensively used, it is still important to remember that the overall experience with these agents is limited when compared with agents used in hundreds of thousands of children. A rare complication previously unrecognized could occur as experience expands. The predominant side effects vary among the dideoxynucleosides, so that the monitoring schemes must be modified according to which agent is being administered. However, as more patients receive combination therapy regimes, the panoply of potential side effects is broadened and the potential for additive or overlapping side effects must also be considered.

The monitoring battery suggested by the National HIV Resource Center consensus report that is shown in Table 35.5 permits the serial assessment of several measures of both drug activity and toxicity. Depending on the agent being used, several other measures of toxicity must be included. The major side effects of the antiretroviral agents in current clinical trials in pediatrics and suggested frequency with which they should be monitored are shown in Table 35.6. Based on current clinical experience, the following comments can be offered with regard to the major side effects associated with antiretroviral therapy.

Hematological Toxicity

Hematological side effects are most commonly associated with AZT and include predominantly anemia and neutropenia. Drug-related thrombocytopenia is less common. The bone marrow suppression associated with dideoxynucleosides is dose related and tends to emerge with chronic therapy. Over

Table 35.5.   Monitoring Schedule for Children Receiving Antiretroviral Therapy (e.g., AZT)[a]

	Pre	0 wk	2 wk	4 wk	8 wk	12 wk	16 wk	20 wk	24 wk	28 wk	32 wk	36 wk	40 wk	44 wk	48 wk	52 wk
History and PE	X	X		X	X	X	X	X	X	X	X	X	X	X	X	X
CBC, diff, retics	X	X	X	X	X	X	X	X	X	X	X	X	X	X	X	X
Chemistries/LFT	X			X		X			X			X			X	
Urinalysis	X								X			X			X	
IgG, IgA, IgM	X								X						X	
Lymphocyte subsets	X			X		X			X			X			X	
p24 antigen	X			X		X			X			X			X	
CXR[b]	X											X				
ECG[b]	X															
CT or MRI[c]	X															

[a]After 52 weeks patients should be monitored as per second 6 months of the first year. Neurodevelopmental testing should be performed as per neuropsychologic testing schedule in Table 35.3. PE, physical examination; CBC, complete blood count; diff, differential; retics, reticulocytes; LFT, liver function test; CXR, chest x-ray; ECG, electrocardiogram; CT, computerized tomography; MRI, magnetic resonance imaging. Data based on recommendations of Working Group on Antiretroviral Therapy, National Pediatric HIV Resource Center.
[b]Repeat as needed to monitor cardiac symptoms.
[c]Repeat as needed to monitor CNS disease.

Table 35.6. Major Side Effects of Antiretroviral Agents in Current Clinical Practice

Agent	Side Effects
AZT	Anemia, neutropenia, myositis. Less serious: headache, nausea, hepatic transaminitis
ddI	Pancreatitis, peripheral neuropathy, retinal depigmentation
ddC	Peripheral neuropathy, pancreatitis, mouth sores, rash

time, 20–40% of children receiving AZT will develop evidence of bone marrow suppression that may become dose limiting. Bone marrow suppression is relatively rarely observed with ddI, ddC, 3TC, or the non-nucleoside reverse transcriptase inhibitors.

When hematological toxicity is observed, the potential for additive myelosuppression from other agents used as part of the overall regimen must also be considered. The most notable is trimethoprim-sulfamethoxazole used for antipneumocystis prophylaxis. Even the three times per week schedule of trimethoprim-sulfamethoxazole prophylaxis can result in bone marrow suppression, especially in children with advanced disease or those with other chronic infections than can also suppress the bone marrow (e.g., MAI, cytomegalovirus). Patients with hematological toxic-

ity should, whenever possible, be switched to either pentamidine or dapsone for PCP prophylaxis.

If a child has evidence of bone marrow suppression and is receiving AZT, the decision to modify the antiretroviral therapy depends on the perceived value of the drug, the nature of the complications and supportive care modalities, and the availability of alternative antiretroviral agents. Figure 35.3 delineates the recommendations of the consensus statement of the National HIV Resource Center (112). In practice, if the patient's hemoglobin falls to below 8 g/dl, the dosage of AZT should be reduced by 25–30% (i.e., from 180 to 120 mg/m² every 6 hr). If the patient continues to remain anemic despite the dose reduction and transfusions are necessary to maintain the hemoglobin above 8 g/dl, then either ery-

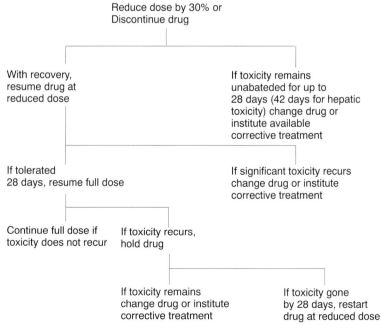

Figure 35.3. Algorithm for management of hematological toxicity related to zidovudine based on recommendations of Working Group on Antiretroviral Therapy, National Pediatric HIV Resource Center.

progression of such organ specific manifestations of HIV infection cannot constitute a basis for changing therapy. Clearly, such a decision must be based on the patient's overall clinical status, duration of therapy, and the available therapeutic options. Certainly, intensive supportive care (e.g., antimicrobial therapy, prophylaxis, or organ specific treatments) should be employed in tandem with continuing antiretroviral therapy.

Current Recommendations. Although the development of new AIDS-related manifestations in a child receiving antiretroviral therapy is disturbing, most infectious and noninfectious events (except for growth failure and neurodevelopmental deterioration as noted above) should not, at this time, be used as criteria for changing antiretroviral therapy. If a symptom is part of an overall picture of clinical deterioration, strong consideration should be given to changing antiretroviral therapy. Again, this also is strongly dependent on the available alternatives. As new drugs enter the clinic, earlier changes in therapy may become more appropriate.

Laboratory Criteria for Therapeutic Failure

Both virological and immunological criteria have been used to determine the extent and prognosis of HIV disease, but, to date, neither can be definitive without concomitant clinical findings to delineate treatment failure or a need to change antiretroviral therapy. It is likely, however, that as these laboratory measures become more specific, sensitive, and coordinated with clinical disease progression, that they will be used as early indicators of the need to change therapy.

Virological Measures. As noted above, measures of the virus burden in plasma, cells, and tissues can be used to define the extent of HIV disease and its response to an antiretroviral agent. However, neither the level of virus by culture, measurement of P24 antigen (including by immune complex dissociated), or quantitative DNA or RNA PCR assays can be used to clearly indicate a need for changing antiretroviral therapies. For example, changes in P24 antigen (including measurement of rising values over time) cannot be used to define disease progression or treatment failure. However, the newer and more sensitive measures of virus burden (e.g., quantitative PCR) may eventually prove useful in defining treatment failure, and it is anticipated that their perturbations will antedate clinical disease progression.

Similarly, although measures of virus virulence can be correlated with the stage of disease and serve as a potential marker for disease progression, insufficient data exist to use these as indicators for a change in therapy. More perplexing is how to interpret the measurement of antiretroviral resistance in relation to therapeutic change. It is increasingly clear that the emergence of a resistant phenotype can be correlated with disease progression. At the same time, nearly a quarter of patients with laboratory evidence of AZT resistance will not show any concurrent evidence of disease progression. Whether antiretroviral therapy should be changed on the basis of drug resistance alone, or whether this needs to be correlated with clinical or other laboratory evidence of disease progression, is a matter of debate and controversy. Clearly, if effective therapeutic alternatives to which HIV was sensitive were in abundance, it would be an easy decision. In the absence of these, changing therapy on the basis of laboratory evidence of drug resistance alone is not recommended at this time.

Current Recommendations. Although measures of virus burden and virulence, including drug resistance, should not be used as sole determinants for changing therapy, it is probable that they will assume an ever increasing level of importance. Presently, if a patient is doing well, continued close monitoring would seem appropriate. If there are also signs of clinical progression of the infection, a change in therapy or the addition of another agent is appropriate. This recommendation may change as more therapies become available.

Immunological Measures of Disease Activity. As with the virologic markers, considerable data now exist demonstrating that the CD4 count and T helper function can be correlated with disease progression and can serve as measures of the therapeutic response. Although the CD4 number, in particular, is used as a guide for beginning either antiretroviral therapy (see above) or various antimicrobial prophylactic agents, it is less clearly established that drops in the CD4 count alone, without other clinical evidence of disease progression, should be used as criteria to change the antiretroviral therapy. Thus, for the present, the Working Group of the National HIV Resource Center recommended that alterations in therapy not be made on the basis of changes in CD4 count alone. Note, however, that in studies in adults and some trials in children, therapeutic changes based on a 50% drop in the CD4 count or a fall below a threshold (e.g., an absolute count of 200 CD4 cells/mm^3) on two or more occassions at least 4 weeks apart are being used to guide therapy. At the same time, it is important to underscore that the CD4 count remains a controversial marker of therapeutic improvement, although as more data emerge, modifications of its role and usefulness may unfold.

THE FUTURE OF ANTIRETROVIRAL TREATMENT

It seems clear that progress in the immediate future will come from combination regimens that enhance and expand the activity of currently available antiretroviral agents, ideally impacting various components of the HIV life cycle and that overcome or avoid the emergence of drug resistance. As noted earlier, strategies that inhibit or prevent HIV replication (in both acute and chronically infected cells) should be combined with regimens that decrease or limit HIV stimulation and enhance or expand the immune defense and that might recruit uninfected immune cells. The recognition that the body burden of virus is significant suggests that intervention might need to begin as soon after infection as possible. Clearly, early therapy will always need to be balanced against the prospect for the early emergence of drug resistance. Because children with vertically acquired HIV become infected either during gestation or during the intrapartum period, the initiation of therapy as soon as HIV infection can be confirmed (i.e., during the first 3–6 months of life) may ultimately prove to

be most optimal. Such intervention will need to consider the impact of early treatment on the developing child and must place such therapy within the psychosocial setting of the child and family. It will be important for the pediatric community to continue to take bold steps to assure that infants and children benefit from treatment advances as rapidly as possible and to continue to advocate that drug development proceeds in children on pace with that in adults. Not only is this important for the children who might derive benefit from current and future therapies, but it remains likely that insights gained from studies in children will continue to have ramifications for all HIV-infected people.

As important as treatment programs are for HIV-infected children, there is no doubt that the most successful strategy will come from preventing the infection of the fetus or infant. This will necessitate the treatment of HIV-infected pregnant women with either antiretroviral agents, immune interventions, or both. Studies assessing these approaches are underway (see Chapters 45 and 47). Clearly, the challenges are significant and mandate that all involved in the care and treatment of HIV-infected children and families be knowledgeable not only about drug development but also about the legal, ethical, and psychosocial issues affecting children and families. Moreover, pediatricians and health care providers must be advocates for progress.

References

1. Scott GB, Hutto C, Makuch RW, et al. Survival in children with perinatally acquired human immunodeficiency virus type 1 infection. N Engl J Med 1989;321:1791–1796.
2. Tovo PA, De Martino M, Gabiano C, et al. Prognostic factors and survival in children with perinatal HIV-1 infection. Lancet 1992;339:1249–1253.
3. Krasinski K, Barkowsky W, Holzman RS. Prognosis of human immunodeficiency virus infection in children and adolescents. Pediatr Infect Dis J 1989;8:216–220.
4. Mueller BU, Pizzo PA. Medical treatment of children with HIV infection. In: Crocker AC, Cohen HJ, Kastner TA, eds. HIV infection and developmental disabilities. Baltimore: Paul H. Brookes, 1992:63–74.
5. Pizzo PA. Considerations for the evaluation of antiretroviral agents in infants and children infected with human immunodeficiency virus: A perspective from the National Cancer Institute. Rev Infect Dis 1990;12(suppl 5):S561–S569.

6. Pizzo P. Emerging concepts in the treatment of HIV infection in children. JAMA 1989;26: 1989–1992.

7. Pizzo PA. Pediatric AIDS: Problems within problems. J Infect Dis 1990;161:316–325.

8. Pizzo PA. Practical issues and considerations in the design of clinical trials for HIV-infected infants and children. J Acquir Immune Defic Syndr 1990;3 (suppl 2):S61–S63.

9. Pizzo PA, Wilfert C. Treatment considerations for children with HIV infection. In: Pizzo PA, Wilfert CM, eds. Pediatric AIDS. The challenge of HIV infection in infants, children, and adolescents. Baltimore: Williams & Wilkins, 1991:478–494.

10. Yarchoan R, Mitsuya H, Myers CE, Broder S. Clinical pharmacology of 3′-azido-2′,3′-dideoxythymidine (zidovudine) and related dideoxynucleosides. N Engl J Med 1989;321: 726–738.

11. Fischl MA, Parker CB, Pettinelli C, et al. A randomized controlled trial of a reduced daily dose of zidovudine in patients with the acquired immunodeficiency syndrome. N Engl J Med 1990;323:1009–1014.

12. Fischl MA, Richman DD, Hansen N, et al. The safety and efficacy of zidovudine (AZT) in the treatment of subjects with mildly symptomatic human immunodeficiency virus type 1 (HIV) infection. Ann Intern Med 1990; 112:727–737.

13. Fischl MA. Zidovudine: Clinical experience in symptomatic HIV disease. AIDS Clin Rev 1989:221–242.

14. National Institutes of Health. State-of-the-art conference on azidothymidine therapy for early HIV infection. Am J Med 1990;89:335–344.

15. Ayers KM. Preclinical toxicology of zidovudine. Am J Med 1988;85(suppl 2A):186–188.

16. Swiss Group for Clinical Studies on the Acquired Immunodeficiency Syndrome (AIDS). Zidovudine for the treatment of thrombocytopenia associated with human immunodeficiency virus (HIV). Ann Intern Med 1988;109:718–721.

17. Richman DD, Fischl MA, Grieco MH, et al. The toxicity of azidothymidine (AZT) in the treatment of patients with AIDS and AIDS-related complex. A double-blind, placebo-controlled trial. N Engl J Med 1987;317:192–197.

18. Brouwers P, Moss H, Wolters P, et al. Effect of continuous-infusion zidovudine therapy on neuropsychologic functioning in children with symptomatic human immunodeficiency virus infection. J Pediatr 1990;117:980–985.

19. Pizzo PA, Eddy J, Falloon J, et al. Effect of continuous intravenous infusion of zidovudine (AZT) in children with symptomatic HIV infection. N Engl J Med 1988;319:889–896.

20. McKinney RE, Maha MA, Connor EM, et al. A multicenter trial of oral zidovudine in children with advanced human immunodeficiency virus disease. N Engl J Med 1991;324:1018–1025.

21. Balis FM, Pizzo PA, Murphy RF, et al. The pharmacokinetics of zidovudine administered by continuous infusion in children. Ann Intern Med 1989;110:279–285.

22. Klecker RW, Collins JM, Yarchoan R, et al. Plasma and cerebrospinal fluid pharmacokinetics of 3′-azido-3′-deoxythymidine: A novel pyrimidine analog with potential application for the treatment of patients with AIDS and related diseases. Clin Pharmacol Ther 1987;41:407–412.

23. Cretton EM, Schinazi RF, McClure HM, Anderson DC, Sommadossi J-P. Pharmacokinetics of 3′-azido-3′-deoxythymidine and its catabolites and interactions with probenecid in rhesus monkeys. Antimicrob Agents Chemother 1991;35:801–807.

24. Collins JM, Unadkat JD. Clinical pharmacokinetics of zidovudine. An overview of current data. Clin Pharmacokinet 1989;17:1–9.

25. Balis FM, Pizzo PA, Eddy J, et al. Pharmacokinetics of zidovudine administered intravenously and orally in children with human immunodeficiency virus infection. J Pediatr 1989; 114:880–884.

26. Watts DH, Brown ZA, Tartaglione T, et al. Pharmacokinetic disposition of zidovudine during pregnancy. J Infect Dis 1991;163:226–232.

26a. Boucher FD, Modlin, JF, Weller, S et al. Phase I evaluation of zidovudine administered to infants exposed at birth to the human immunodeficiency virus. J Pediatr 1993;122:137–144.

27. Sperling RS, Roboz J, Dische R, Silides D, Holzman I, Jew E. Zidovudine pharmacokinetics during pregnancy. Am J Perinatol 1992;9:247–249.

28. Blanche S, Duliege A-M, Navarette MS, et al. Low-dose zidovudine in children with an human immunodeficiency virus type 1 infection acquired in the perinatal period. Pediatrics 1991;88: 364–370.

29. DeCarli C, Fugate L, Falloon J, et al. Brain growth and cognitive improvement in children with human immunodeficiency virus-induced encephalopathy after 6 months of continuous infusion zidovudine therapy. J Acquir Immune Defic Syndr 1991;4:585–592.

30. Pert CB, Smith CC, Ruff MR, Hill JD. AIDS and its dementia as a neuropeptide disorder: Role of VIP receptor blockade by human immunodeficiency virus envelope. Ann Neurol 1988;23(suppl): S71–S73.

31. Epstein LG, Goudsmit J, Paul DA, et al. Expression of human immunodeficiency virus in cerebrospinal fluid of children with progressive encephalopathy. Ann Neurol 1987;21:397–401.

32. European Collaborative Study. Neurologic signs in young children with human immunodeficiency virus infection. Pediatr Infect Dis J 1990;9: 402–406.

33. Kleihues P, Leib SL, Strittmatter C, Wiestler OD, Lang W. HIV encephalopathy: Incidence, definition and pathogenesis. Results of a Swiss Collaborative Study. Acta Pathol Jpn 1991;41: 197–205.

34. Brunetti A, Berg G, Di Chiro G, et al. Reversal of brain metabolic abnormalities following treatment of AIDS dementia complex with 3′-azido-2′,3′-dideoxythymidine (AZT, zidovudine): A PET-FDG study. J Nucl Med 1989;30:581–590.

35. Brouwers P, DeCarli C, Civitello L, Moss H, Wolters P, Pizzo, PA. Correlations between CT-brain scan abnormality and neuropsychological function in children with symptomatic HIV disease. Ann Neurol, in press.

36. Brouwers P, Heyes M, Moss H, et al. Quinolinic acid in the cerebrospinal fluid of children with symptomatic HIV disease: Correlations with clinical status and therapeutic response. J Infect Dis, in press.

37. DeCarli C, Civitell LA, Brouwers P, Pizzo, PA. The prevalence of computed axial tomographic abnormalities of the cerebrum in 100 consecutive children with symptomatic HIV infection. J Neurol, in press.

38. Fauci AS, Schnittman SM, Poli G, Koenig S, Pantaleo G. Immunopathogenic mechanisms in human immunodeficiency virus (HIV) infection. Ann Intern Med 1991;114:678–693.

39. Fox CH, Kotler D, Tierney A, Wilson CS, Fauci AS. Detection of HIV-1 RNA in the lamina propria of patients with AIDS and gastrointestinal disease. J Infect Dis 1989;159:467–471.

40. Fox CH, Tenner-Racz K, Racz P, Firpo A, Pizzo PA, Fauci AS. Lymphoid germinal centers are reservoirs in human immunodeficiency virus type 1 RNA. J Infect Dis 1991;164:1051–1057.

41. Pantaleo G, Graziosi C, Butini L, et al. Lymphoid organs function as major reservoirs for human immunodeficiency virus. Proc Natl Acad Sci USA 1991;88:9838–9842.

42. Rosenberg ZF, Fauci AS. Activation of latent HIV infection. J NIH Res 1990;2:41–45.

43. Pantaleo G, Graziosi C, Fauci AS. The immunopathogenesis of human immunodeficiency virus infection. N Engl J Med 1993;328:327–335.

44. Temin HM, Bolognesi DP. Where has HIV been hiding? Nature 1993;362:292–293.

45. Pantaleo G, Graziosi C, Demarest JF, et al. HIV infection is active and progressive in lymphoid tissue during the clinically latent stage of disease. Nature 1993;362:355–358.

46. Dalakas MC, Illa I, Pezeshkpour GH, Laukaitis JP, Cohen B, Griffin JL. Mitochondrial myopathy caused by long-term zidovudine therapy. N Engl J Med 1990;322: 1098– 1105.

47. McKinney RE, Pizzo PA, Scott GB, et al. Safety and tolerance of intermittent intravenous and oral zidovudine therapy in human immunodeficiency virus-infected pediatric patients. J Pediatr 1990;116:640–647.

48. Till M, MacDonell KB. Myopathy with human immunodeficiency virus type 1 (HIV-1) infection: HIV-1 or zidovudine? Ann Intern Med 1990; 113:492–493.

49. Tudor-Williams G, StClair M, McKinney RE, et al. HIV-1 sensitivity to zidovudine and clinical outcome in children. Lancet 1992;339:15–19.

50. Husson R, Shirasaka T, Butler KM, Pizzo PA, Mitsuya, H. High level resistance to zidovudine but not zalcitabine or didanosine in human immunodeficiency virus from children receiving antiretroviral therapy. J Pediatr, in press.

51. Larder B, Kemp SC. Multiple mutations in HIV-1 reverse transcriptase confer high-level resistance to zidovudine (AZT). Science 1989;246:1155–1158.

52. Husson RN, Chung Y, Mordenti J, et al. Phase I study of continuous-infusion soluble CD4 as a single agent and in combination with oral dideoxyinosine therapy in children with symptomatic human immunodeficiency virus infection. J Pediatr 1992;121:627–633.

53. Husson RN, Mueller BU, Farley M, et al. Zidovudine and didanosine combination therapy in children with human immunodeficiency virus infection. Pediatrics, in press.

54. Mueller BU, Jacobsen F, Butler KM, Husson RN, Lewis LL, Pizzo PA. Combination treatment with azidothymidine and granulocyte colony-stimulating factor in children with human immunodeficiency virus infection. J Pediatr 1992;121: 797–802.

55. Pizzo PA, Butler K, Balis F, et al. Dideoxycytidine alone and in an alternating schedule with zidovudine in children with symptomatic human immunodeficiency virus infection. J Pediatr 1990; 117:799–808.

56. Butler KM, Husson RN, Balis FM, et al. Dideoxyinosine in children with symptomatic human immunodeficiency virus infection. N Engl J Med1991;324:137–144.

57. Balis FM, Pizzo PA, Butler KM, et al. Clinical pharmacology of 2′,3′-dideoxyinosine in human immunodeficiency virus-infected children. J Infect Dis 1992;165:99–104.

58. Butler K, Venzon D, Henry N, et al. Pancreatitis in children receiving dideoxyinosine. Pediatrics 1993;747–751.

59. Clerici M, Roilides E, Butler KM, DePalma L, Shearer GM, Pizzo PA. Changes in T-helper cell function in human immunodeficiency virus-infected children during didanosine therapy as a measure of antiretroviral activity. Blood 1992; 80:2196–2202.

60. Lewis L, Wells M, Church S, et al. A phase I/II study of 3TC (GR109714X) in children with HIV infection [Abstract POB 262059]. Ninth International Conference on AIDS, Berlin, Jun 1993.

61. Russell JW, Whiterock VJ, Marrero D, Klunk LJ. Pharmacokinetics of a new anti-HIV agent: 2′,3′-dideoxy-2′,3′-didehydrothymidine (d4T). Nucleosides Nucleotides 1989;8:845–848.

62. Browne MJ, Mayer KH, Chafee SBD, et al. 2′,3′-didehydro-3′-deoxythymidine (d4T) in patients with acquired immunodeficiency syndrome or AIDS-related complex: A phase I trial. J Infect Dis 1993;167:21–29.

63. Romero DL, Busso M, Tan C-K, et al. Nonnucleoside reverse transcriptase inhibitors that potently and specifically block human immunodeficiency virus type 1 replication. Proc Natl Acad Sci USA 1991;88:8806–8810.

64. Merluzzi VJ, Hargrave KD, Labadia M, et al. Inhibition of HIV-1 replication by a nonnucleoside reverse transcriptase inhibitor. Science 1990;250:1411–1413.

65. Richman D, Rosenthal AS, Skoog M, et al. BI-RG-587 is active against zidovudine-resistant human immunodeficiency virus type 1 and synergistic with zidovudine. Antimicrob Agents Chemother 1991;35:305–308.

66. Grob PM, Wu JC, Cohen KA, et al. Nonnucleoside inhibitors of HIV-1 reverse transcriptase: Nevirapine as a prototype drug. AIDS Res Hum Retroviruses 1992;8:145–152.

67. Cheeseman SH, Hattox SE, McLaughlin MM, et al. Pharmacokinetics of nevirapine: Initial single-

rising dose study in humans. Antimicrob Agents Chemother 1993;37:178–182.

68. Norris SH, Silverstein HH, St. George RL, Johnstone JN. Nevirapine, an HIV-1 reverse transcriptase inhibitor: Absorption, distribution, and excretion in rats [Abstract]. Pharmaceut Res 1992;9:S263).

69. Norris SH, Pav JW, Erickson DA, Silverstein HH, Daly DJ, Hattox SE. Nevirapine and hydroxymethylnevirapine plasma levels and in vitro nevirapine metabolism in rats [Abstract]. Pharmaceut Res 1992;9:S 263.

70. Hargrave KD, Proudfoot JR, Grozinger KG, et al. Novel non-nucleoside inhibitors of HIV-1 reverse transcriptase. 1. Tricyclic pyridobenzo-and dipyridodiazepinones. J Med Chem 1991;34: 2231–2241.

71. Skoog MT, Hargrave KD, Miglietta JJ, Kopp EB, Merluzzi VJ. Inhibition of HIV-1 reverse transcriptase and virus replication by a non-nucleoside dipyridodiazepinone BI-RG-587 (nevirapine). Med Res Rev 1992;12:27–40.

72. Klunder JM, Hragrave KD, West MA, et al. Novel non-nucleoside inhibitors of HIV-1 reverse transcriptase. 2. Tryciclic pyridobenzoxazepinones and dibenzoxazepinones. J Med Chem 1992;35: 1887–1897.

73. Goldman ME, Nunberg JH, O'Brien J, et al. Pyridinone derivatives: Specific human immunodeficiency virus type 1 reverse transcriptase inhibitors with antiviral activity. Proc Natl Acad Sci USA 1991;88:6863–6867.

74. Chow Y-K, Hirsch MS, Merrill DP, et al. Use of evolutionary limitations of HIV-l multidrug resistance to optimize therapy. Nature 1993;361: 650–654.

75. Richman DD. Playing chess with reverse transcriptase. Nature 1993;361:588–589.

75a. Chow Y-K, Hirsch MS, Kaplan JC, DiAquila RT. HIV-1 error revealed [Letter]. Nature 1993; 364:679.

75b. Emini EA, Graham DJ, Gotlib L, Condra JH, Byrnes JW, Schleif WA. HIV and multidrug resistance [Letter]. Nature 1993;364:679.

76. Hattox S, Cohn D, Norris S, et al. Single and multiple dose pharmacokinetics of nevirapine, a non nucleoside HIV-1 reverse transcriptase inhibitor, in chimpanzees [Abstract]. Pharmaceut Res 1992;9:S268.

77. Schooley RT, Merigan TC, Gaut P, et al. Recombinant soluble CD4 therapy in patients with the acquired immunodeficiency syndrome (AIDS) and AIDS-related complex. A phase I-II escalating dosage trial. Ann Intern Med 1990; 112:247–253.

78. Kahn JO, Allan JD, Hodges TL, et al. The safety and pharmacokinetics of recombinant soluble CD4 (rCD4) in subjects with the acquired immunodeficiency syndrome (AIDS) and AIDS-related complex. A phase I study. Ann Intern Med 1990;112:254–261.

79. Johnson VA, Barlow MA, Merrill DP, Chou T-C, Hirsch MS. Three-drug synergistic inhibition of HIV-1 replication in vitro by zidovudine, recombinant soluble CD4, and recombinant interferon-alpha A. J Infect Dis 1990;161:1059–1067.

80. Johnson VA, Barlow MA, Chou T-C, et al. Synergistic inhibition of human immunodeficiency virus type 1 (HIV-1) replication in vitro by recombinant soluble CD4 and 3'-azido-3'-deoxythymidine. J Infect Dis 1989;159:837–844.

81. Gerety RJ, Hanson DG, Thomas DW. Human recombinant soluble CD4 therapy [Letter]. Lancet 1989;2:1521.

82. Hodges TL, Kahn JO, Kaplan LD, et al. Phase I study of recombinant human CD4-immunoglobulin G therapy of patients with AIDS and AIDS-related complex. Antimicrob Agents Chemother 1991;35:2580–2586.

83. Weintraub P, Yogev R, Connor E, Wilfert C, Mordenti J, Ammann AJ. Safety and pharmacokinetics of recombinant CD4 in children with HIV infection [Abstract FB 23]. Sixth International Conference on AIDS, San Francisco, Jun 1990.

84. Muesing M, Smith DW, Capon DJ. Regulation of mRNA accumulation by a human immunodeficiency virus transactivator protein. Cell 1987;48: 691–701.

85. Laspia M, Rice AP, Matthews MB. HIV–1 Tat protein increases transcriptional initiation and stabilizes elongation. Cell 1989;59:283–292.

86. Fisher AG, Aldovini A, Debouck C, et al. The transactivator gene of HTLV II is essential for virus replication. Nature 1986;120:367.

87. Dayton A, Sodroski J, Rosen CA, et al. The transactivator gene of the human T cell lymphotropic virus type III is required for replication. Cell 1986;44:941–947.

88. Debouck C, Gorniak JG, Strickler JE, Meek TD, Metcalf BW, Rosenberg M. Human immunodeficiency virus protease expressed in *Escherichia coli* exhibits autoprocessing and specific maturation of the gag precursor. Proc Natl Acad Sci USA 1987;84:8903–8906.

89. Nutt RF, Brady SF, Darke PL, et al. Chemical synthesis and enzymatic activity of a 99-residue peptide with a sequence proposed for the human immunodeficiency virus protease. Proc Natl Acad Sci USA 1988;85:7129–7133.

90. Erickson J, Neidhart DJ, VanDrie J, et al. Design, activity, and 2.8 Å crystal structure of a C2 symmetric inhibitor complexed to HIV-1 protease. Science 1990;249:527–533.

91. Fitzgerald PMD, McKeevert BM, VanMiddlesworth JF, et al. Crystallographic analysis of a complex between human immunodeficiency virus type 1 protease and acetyl-pepstatin at 2.0-Å resolution. J Biol Chem 1990;265:14209–14219.

92. Heimbach JC, Garsky VM, Michelson SR, Dixon RAF, Sigal IS, Darke PL. Affinity purification of the HIV-1 protease. Biochem Biophys Res Commun 1989;164:955–960.

93. Kotler M, Katz RA, Danho W, Leis J, Skalka AM. Synthetic peptides as substrates and inhibitors of a retroviral protease. Proc Natl Acad Sci USA 1988;85:4185–4189.

94. McQuade TJ, Tomasselli AG, Liu L, et al. A synthetic HIV-1 protease inhibitor with antiviral activity arrests HIV-like particle maturation. Science 1990;247:454–456.

95. Meek TD, Lambert DM, Dreyer GB, et al. Inhibition of HIV-1 protease in infected T-lym-

phocytes by synthetic peptide analogues. Nature 1990;343:90–92.

96. Navia MA, Fitzgerald PMD, McKeever BM, et al. Three-dimensional structure of aspartyl protease from human immunodeficiency virus HIV-1. Nature 1989;337:615–620.

97. Miller M, Jaskolski M, Rao JKM, Leis J, Wlodawer A. Crystal structure of a retroviral protease proves relationship to aspartic protease family. Nature 1989;337:576–579.

98. Miller M, Schneider J, Sathyanarayana BK, et al. Structure of complex of synthetic HIV-1 protease with a substrate-based inhibitor at 2.3 Å resolution. Science 1989;246:1149–1152.

99. Tomasselli AG, Hui JO, Sawyer TK, et al. Proteases from human immunodeficiency virus and avian myeloblastosis virus show distinct specificities in hydrolysis of multidomain protein substrates. J Virol 1990;64:3157–3161.

100. von der Helm K, Gürtler L, Eberle J, Deinhardt F. Inhibition of HIV replication in cell culture by the specific aspartic protease inhibitor pepstatin A. FEBS Lett 1989;247:349–352.

101. Kempf DJ, Marsh KC, Paul DA, et al. Antiviral and pharmacokinetic properties of C2 symmetric inhibitors of the human immunodeficiency virus type 1 protease. Antimicrob Agents Chemother 1991;35:2209–2214.

102. Buhl R, Holroyd K, Mastrangeli A, et al. Systemic glutathione deficiency in symptom-free HIV-seropositive individuals. Lancet 1989;2:1294–1298.

103. Mihm S, Ennen J, Pessara U, Kurth R, Dröge W. Inhibition of HIV-1 replication and NF-κB activity by cysteine and cysteine derivatives. AIDS 1991;5:497–503.

104. Roederer M, Staal FJT, Raju PA, Ela SW, Herzenberg LA, Herzenberg LA. Cytokine-stimulated human immunodeficiency virus replication is inhibited by N-acetyl-L-cysteine. Proc Natl Acad Sci USA 1990;87:4884–4888.

105. Roederer M, Raju PA, Staal FJT, Herzenberg LA, Herzenberg LA. N-acetylcysteine inhibits latent HIV expression in chronically infected cells. AIDS Res Hum Retroviruses 1991;7:563–567.

106. Kalebic T, Schein PS, Pizzo PA. Suppression of induction of HIV expression in chronically infected promonocytic cells by an organic thiophosphate WR 151327 [Abstract]. J Cell Biochem 1992:Q529a.

107. Kalebic T, Kinter A, Poli G, Anderson ME, Meister A, Fauci AS. Suppression of human immunodeficiency virus expression in chronically infected monocytic cells by glutathione, glutathione ester, and N-acetyl cysteine. Proc Natl Acad Sci USA 1991;88:986–990.

108. Walker R, Boenning C, Murphy G, et al. The safety, pharmacokinetics, and antiviral activity of N-acetylcysteine in HIV-infected individuals [Abstract]. Am Rev Respir Dis Int Conf Suppl 1993;147:A1004.

109. Mofenson LM, Burns DN. Passive immunization to prevent mother-infant transmission of human immunodeficiency virus: Current issues and future directions. Pediatr Infect Dis J 1991;10:456–462.

110. Mofenson LM, Moye J Jr, Bethel J, et al. Prophylactic intravenous immunoglobulin in HIV-infected children with CD4- counts of $0.02 \times 10^9/L$ or more. Effect on viral, opportunistic, and bacterial infections. JAMA 1992;268:483–488.

110a. Redfield, RR, Birx, DL, Ketter, N, et al. A phase I evaluation of the safety and immunogenicity of vaccination with recombinant gp160 in patients with early human immunodeficieny virus infection. N Engl J Med 1991;324:1677–1684.

111. Lane HC, Zunich KM, Wilson W, et al. Syngeneic bone marrow transplantation and adoptive transfer of peripheral blood lymphocytes combined with zidovudine in human immunodeficiency virus (HIV) infection. Ann Intern Med 1990;113: 512–519.

112. Working Group on Antiretroviral Therapy: National Pediatric HIV Resource Center. Antiretroviral therapy and medical management of the human immunodeficiency virus-infected child. Pediatr Infect Dis J 1993;12:513–522.

113. Mitchell WG, Gomperts E, Ross LA, Nelson M, Gonzalez-Gomez I. Progressive encephalopathy in a young man with AIDS. AIDS Reader l991; May/Jun:77–81.

114. Price RW, Sidtis J, Rosenblum M. The AIDS dementia complex: Some current questions. Ann Neurol 1988;23(suppl):S27–S33.

115. Tirard V, Niel G, Rosenheim M, et al. Diagnosis of toxoplasmosis in patients with AIDS by isolation of the parasite from the blood [Letter]. N Engl J Med 1991;324:634.

116. National Institute of Child Health and Human Development Intravenous Immunoglobulin Study Group. Intravenous immune globulin for the prevention of bacterial infections in children with symptomatic human immunodeficiency virus infection. N Engl J Med 1991;325:73–80.

117. Roilides E, Butler KM, Husson RN, Mueller BU, Lewis LL, Pizzo PA. *Pseudomonas* infections in children with human immunodeficiency virus infection. Pediatr Infect Dis J 1992;11:547–553.

118. Roilides E, Marshall D, Venzon D, Butler K, Husson R, Pizzo PA. Bacterial infections in human immunodeficiency virus type 1-infected children: The impact of central venous catheters and antiretroviral agents. Pediatr Infect Dis J 1991;10:813–819.

119. Janoff EN, Breiman RF, Daley CL, Hopewell PC. Pneumococcal disease during HIV infection. Epidemiology, clinical, and immunologic perspectives. Ann Intern Med 1992;117:314–324.

120. Krasinski K, Borkowsky W, Bonk S, Lawrence R, Chandwani S. Bacterial infections in human immunodeficiency virus-infected children. Pediatr Infect Dis J 1988;7:323–328.

121. Adamson PC, Wu TC, Meade BD, Rubin M, Manclark CR, Pizzo PA. Pertussis in a previously immunized child with human immunodeficiency virus infection. J Pediatr 1989;115:598–592.

122. Bartlett MS, Smith JW. *Pneumocystis carinii*, an opportunist in immunocompromised patients. Clin Microbiol Rev 1991;4:137–149.

123. Berger TG, Tappero JW, Leoung GS, Jacobson MA. Aerosolized pentamidine and cutaneous eruptions. Ann Intern Med 1989;110:1035–1036.

124. Blum RN, Miller LA, Gaggini LC, Cohn DL. Comparative trial of dapsone versus trimetho-

prim/sulfamethoxazole for primary prophylaxis of *Pneumocystis carinii* pneumonia. J Acquir Immune Defic Syndr 1992;5:341–347.

125. Bozzette SA, Sattler FR, Chiu J, et al. A controlled trial of early adjunctive treatment with corticosteroids for *Pneumocystis carinii* pneumonia in the acquired immunodeficiency syndrome. N Engl J Med 1990;1323:1451–1457.

126. Bye MR, Bernstein LJ, Glaser J, Kleid D. *Pneumocystis carinii* pneumonia in young children with AIDS. Pediatr Pulmonol 1990;9: 251–253.

127. Centers for Disease Control. Guidelines for prophylaxis against *Pneumocystis carinii* pneumonia for children infected with human immunodeficiency virus. MMWR 1991;40:1–13.

128. Centers for Disease Control. Recommendations for prophylaxis against *Pneumocystis carinii* pneumonia for adults and adolescents infected with human immunodeficiency virus. MMWR 1992;41: 1–11.

129. Conte JE, Chernoff D, Feigal DW, Joseph P, McDonald C, Golden JA. Intravenous or inhaled pentamidine for treating *Pneumocystis carinii* pneumonia in AIDS. Ann Intern Med 1990;113: 203–209.

130. Falloon J, Kovacs J, Hughes W, et al. A preliminary evaluation of 566C80 for the treatment of *Pneumocystis* pneumonia in patients with the acquired immunodeficiency syndrome. N Engl J Med 1991;325:1534–1538.

131. Fischl MA. Treatment and prophylaxis of *Pneumocystis carinii* pneumonia. AIDS 1988;2 (suppl 1):S 143–S150.

132. Hughes WT, Rivera GK, Schell MJ, Thornton D, Lott L. Successful intermittent chemoprophylaxis for *Pneumocystis carinii* pneumonitis. N Engl J Med 1987;316:1627–1632.

133. Hughes WT. *Pneumocystis carinii* pneumonia. In: Pizzo PA, Wilfert CA, eds. Pediatric AIDS: The challenge of HIV infection in infants, children, and adolescents. Baltimore: Williams & Wilkins, 1991:288–298.

134. Kovacs JA, Ng VL, Masur H, et al. Diagnosis of *Pneumocystis carinii* pneumonia: Improved detection in sputum with use of monoclonal antibodies. N Engl J Med 1988;318:589–593.

135. Kovacs A, Frederick T, Church J, Eller A, Oxtoby M, Mascola L. CD4 T-lymphocyte counts and *Pneumocystis carinii* pneumonia in pediatric HIV infection. JAMA 1991;265:1698–1703.

136. Masur H. Prevention of *Pneumocystis carinii* pneumonia. Rev Infect Dis 1989;11(suppl 7):S1664–S1668.

137. Mueller BU, Butler KM, Husson RN, Pizzo PA. *Pneumocystis carinii* pneumonia despite prophylaxis in children with human immunodeficiency virus infection. J Pediatr 1991;119:992–994.

138. Mueller BU, Pizzo PA, Steinberg S. Failure of intravenous pentamidine prophylaxis for *Pneumocystis carinii* pneumonia [Reply]. J Pediatr 1993;122: 163–164.

139. Phair J, Munoz A, Detels R, et al. The risk of *Pneumocystis carinii* pneumonia among men infected with human immunodeficiency virus type 1. N Engl J Med 1990;322:161–165.

140. National Institutes of Health-University of Califomia Expert Panel for Corticosteroids as Adjunctive Therapy for *Pneumocystis* Pneumonia. Consensus statement on the use of corticosteroids as adjunctive therapy for *Pneumocystis* pneumonia in the acquired immunodeficiency syndrome. N Engl J Med 1990;323:1500–1504.

141. Stiehm ER. New uses for intravenous immune globulin. N Engl J Med 1991;325:123–125.

142. Yap PL, Todd AAM, Williams PE, et al. Use of intravenous immunoglobulin in acquired immune deficiency syndrome. Cancer 1991;68:1440–1450.

143. Fischl MA, Richman DD, Grieco MH, et al. The efficacy of azidothymidine (AZT) in the treatment of patients with AIDS and AIDS-related complex. N Engl J Med1987;317:185–191.

144. Alimenti A, Luzuriaga K, Stechenberg B, Sullivan JL. Quantitation of human immunodeficiency virus in vertically infected infants and children. J Pediatr 1991;119:225–229.

145. Daar ES, Moudgil T, Meyer RD, Ho DD. Transient high levels of viremia in patients with primary human immunodeficiency virus type 1 infection. N Engl J Med 1991;324:961–964.

146. Ho DD, Moudgil T, Alam M. Quantitation of human immunodeficiency virus type 1 in the blood of infected persons. N Engl J Med 1989;321:1621–1625.

147. Coombs RW, Collier AC, Allain J-P, et al. Plasma viremia in human immunodeficiency virus infection. N Engl J Med 1989;321:1626–1631.

148. Folks TM, Kessler SW, Orenstein JM, Justement JS, Jaffe ES, Fauci AS. Infection and replication of HIV-1 in purified progenitor cells of normal human bone marrow. Science 1988;242:919–922.

149. Schnittman SM, Greenhouse JJ, Psallidopoulos MC, et al. Increasing viral burden in CD4+ T cells from patients with human immunodeficiency virus (HIV) infection reflects rapidly progressive immunosuppression and clinical disease. Ann Intern Med 1990;113:438–443.

150. Merigan TC, Skowron G, Bozzette SA, et al. Circulating p24 antigen levels and responses to dideoxycytidine in human immunodeficiency virus (HIV) infections. Ann Intern Med 1989;110:189–194.

151. Mulder JW, Goudsmit J, Schattenkerk JKME, Reiss P, Lange JMA. HIV-1 p24 antigenemia does not predict time of survival in AIDS patients. Genitourin Med 1990;66:138–141.

152. Borkowsky W, Krasinski K, Paul D, et al. Human immunodeficiency virus type 1 antigenemia in children. J Pediatr 1989;114:940–945.

153. Nishanian P, Huskins KR, Stehn S, Detels R, Fahey JL. A simple method for improved assay demonstrates that HIV p24 antigen is present as immune complexes in most sera from HIV-infected individuals. J Infect Dis 1990;162:21–28.

154. Butler KM, Husson RN, Lewis LL, Mueller BU, Venzon D, Pizzo PA. CD4 status and p24 antigenemia. Are they useful predictors of survival in HIV-infected children receiving antiretroviral therapy? Am J Dis Child 1992;146:932–936.

155. Drusano GL, Yuen GJ, Lambert JS, Seidlin M, Dolin R, Valentine FT. Relationship between dideoxyinosine exposure, CD4 counts, and p24 antigen levels in human immunodeficiiency virus infection. Ann Intern Med 1992;116:562–566.

156. Bollinger RC, Kline RL, Francis HL, Moss MW, Bartlett JG, Quinn TC. Acid dissociation increases the sensitivity of p24 antigen detection for the evaluation of antiviral therapy and disease progression in asymptomatic human immunodeficiency virus-infected persons. J Infect Dis 1992;165:913–916.

157. Tudor-Williams G, Mueller BU, Stocker V, et al. Serum p24 antigen levels and disease progression in HIV-1 infected children [Abstract]. Keystone Symposium on Pathogenesis of HIV Infection, Albuquerque, NM, Apr 1993.

158. Williams P, Simmonds P, Yap PL, et al. The polymerase chain reaction in the diagnosis of vertically transmitted HIV infection. AIDS 1990;4:393–398.

159. Horsburgh CR, Ou CY, Jason J, et al. Concordance of polymerase chain reaction with human immunodeficiency virus antibody detection. J Infect Dis 1990;162:542–545.

160. Scarlatti G, Lombardi V, Plebani A, et al. Polymerase chain reaction, virus isolation and antigen assay in HIV-1-antibody-positive mothers and their children. AIDS 1991;5:1173–1178.

161. Piatak M Jr, Saag MS, Yang LC, et al. High levels of HIV-1 in plasma during all stages of infection determined by competitive PCR. Science 1993;259:1749–1754.

162. Embretson J, Zupancic M, Beneke J, et al. Analysis of human immunodeficiency virus-infected tissues by amplification and in situ hybridization reveals latent and permissive infections at single-cell resolution. Proc Natl Acad Sci USA 1993;90:357–361.

163. Bagasra O, Hauptman SP, Lischner HW, Sachs M, Pomerantz RJ. Detection of human immunodeficiency virus type 1 provirus in mononuclear cells by in situ polymerase chain reaction. N Engl J Med 1992;326:1385–1391.

164. Richman D, Shih C-K, Lowy I, et al. Human immunodeficiency virus type 1 mutants resistant to nonnucleoside inhibitors of reverse transcriptase arise in tissue culture. Proc Natl Acad Sci USA 1991;88:11241–11245.

165. Larder BA. 3'-Azido-3'deoxythymidine resistance suppressed by a mutation conferring human immunodeficiency virus type 1 resistance to nonnucleoside reverse transcriptase inhibitors. Antimicrob Agents Chemother 1992;36:2664–2669.

166. Yanase Y, Tango T, Okumura K, Tada T, Kawasaki T. Lymphocyte subsets identified by monoclonal antibodies in healthy children. Pediatr Res 1986;20:1147–1151.

167. Leibovitz E, Rigaud M, Pollack H, et al. *Pneumocystis carinii* pneumonia in infants infected with the human immunodeficiency virus with more than 450 CD4 T lymphocytes per cubic millimeter. N Engl J Med 1990;323:531–533.

168. Erkeller-Yuksel FM, Deneys V, Hannet I, et al. Age-related changes in human blood lymphocyte subpopulations. J Pediatr 1992;120:216–222.

169. McKinney RE, Wilfert CM. Lymphocyte subsets in children younger than 2 years old: Normal values in a population at risk for human immunodeficiency virus infection and diagnostic and prognostic application to infected children. Pediatr Infect Dis J 1992;11:639–644.

170. Stein DS, Korvick JA, Vermund SH. CD4+ lymphocyte cell enumeration for prediction of clinical course of human immunodeficiency virus disease: A review. J Infect Dis 1992;165:352–363.

171. Shearer GM, Clerici M. Early T-helper cell defects in HIV infection. AIDS 1991;5:245–253.

172. Phillips AN, Lee CA, Elford J, et al. Serial CD4 lymphocyte counts and development of AIDS. Lancet 1991;337:389–392.

173. Ljunggren K, Moschese V, Broliden P-A, et al. Antibodies mediating cellular cytotoxicity and neutralization correlate with a better clinical stage in children born to human immunodeficiency virus-infected mothers. J Infect Dis 1990;161:198–202.

174. Blumberg RS, Paradis T, Hartshorn K L, et al. Antibody-dependent cell-mediated cytotoxicity against cells infected with the human immunodeficiency virus. J Infect Dis 1987;156:878–884.

175. Chan MM, Campos JM, Josephs S, Rifai N. β_2-Microglobulin and neopterin: Predictive markers for human immunodeficiency virus type 1 infection in children? J Clin Microbiol 1990;28:2215–2219.

176. Tyler DS, Lyerly HK, Weinhold KJ. Minireview. Anti-HIV-1 ADCC. AIDS Res Hum Retroviruses 1989;5:557–563.

177. Ellaurie M, Calvelli T, Rubinstein A. Neopterin concentrations in pediatric human immunodeficiency virus infection as predictor of disease activity. Pediatr Infect Dis J 1992;11:286–289.

178. Roilides E, Clerici M, DePalma L, Rubin M, Pizzo PA, Shearer GM. Helper T-cell responses in children infected with human immunodeficiency virus type 1. J Pediatr 1991;118:724–730.

179. Roilides E, Black C, Reimer C, Rubin M, Venzon D, Pizzo PA. Serum immunoglobulin G subclasses in children infected with human immunodeficiency virus type 1. Pediatr Infect Dis J 1991;10:134–139.

180. Robert-Guroff M, Roilides E, Muldoon R, et al. HIV-1$_{MN}$ neutralizing antibody in HIV-infected children: Correlation with clinical status and prognostic value. J Infect Dis 1993;167:538–546.

181. Matsuyama T, Kobayashi N, Yamamoto N. Cytokines and HIV infection: Is AIDS a tumor necrosis factor disease? AIDS 1991;5:1405–1417.

182. Rautonen J, Rautonen N, Martin NL, Philip R, Wara DW. Serum interleukin-6 concentrations are elevated and associated with elevated tumor necrosis factor-α and immunoglobulin G and A concentrations in children with HIV infection. AIDS 1991;5:1319–1325.

183. Hessol NA, Lifson AR. Predictors of HIV disease progression. AIDS Clin Rev 1990:63–79.

184. Whitcup S, Butler K, Pizzo P, Nussenblatt R. Retinal lesions in children treated with dideoxyinosine. N Engl J Med 1992;326:1226–1227.

185. Whitcup SM, Butler KM, Caruso R, et al. Retinal toxicity in human immunodeficiency virus-infected children treated with 2',3'-dideoxyinosine. Am J Ophthalmol 1992;113:1–7.

36

Biologic and Immunomodulating Factors in Treatment of Pediatric AIDS

Arthur J. Ammann and Anne-Marie S. Duliège

Rapid biotechnical advances over the past decade have resulted in the availability of many potent biologic factors that have entered clinical trials. In this chapter, only those biologic and immunomodulating factors are discussed which have been shown to be of benefit in HIV infection and its complications or which have potential for altering the course of the disease based on preclinical or early clinical evaluation. These factors include agents that may alter the immune system (interferons, interleukins), stimulate the hematopoietic system (erythropoietin, colony-stimulating factors), participate in control of human immunodeficiency virus (HIV) replication (passive antibody, interferons, tumor necrosis factor), and reverse the wasting syndrome (growth hormone, insulin-like growth factor.)

Biologic factors have been available as therapeutic agents for many decades. Their initial clinical use was relegated to impure or partially purified preparations that were felt to have specific biologic effects. For example, mixtures of bacteria were injected into patients to cause tumor regression as early as 1891. The factor responsible for this effect (tumor necrosis factor) was not purified until 1975 (1). It took an additional decade to be able to distinguish tumor necrosis factor from lymphotoxin, a closely related molecule.

Immunomodulators were also difficult to isolate. In the mid 1970s Hooper et al. (2) discovered that extracts of the thymus could affect immunologic function in vitro.

Based on in vitro studies, this compound, initially believed to be a single agent, entered limited clinical trials in 1975 in immunodeficient patients (3). Subsequently it was discovered that thymosin fraction V consisted of not one but at least 20 different polypeptides.

The ability to make significant advances in identifying and evaluating specific biologic factors during the 1970s was hampered by many difficulties. New factors that were discovered were available only in small amounts, which made purification and in vitro testing difficult. However, in the late 1970s and early 1980s, advances in techniques included the production of monoclonal antibodies, sensitive immunoassays, recombinant DNA technology, and specific bioassays for the evaluation of in vitro biologic activity.

Once limited amounts of a highly purified biologic reagent became available, the structural sequence of that molecule could be determined. By means of recombinant DNA techniques, large amounts of a factor could be produced, purified, and assayed by monoclonal antibodies or other methods. The availability of significant amounts (grams) of a specific factor permitted extensive evaluation of biologic and toxic effects in animal models. The availability of even larger amounts of material (kilograms) permitted extensive clinical evaluation of the safety and efficacy of a factor in humans and ultimate documentation of a beneficial effect in human diseases.

The process described above often resulted in the discovery of new biologic activities of a specific compound and clarification of the identity of certain biologics. For example, interferon-γ (IFN-γ) and macrophage activation factor, described by two separate investigators, were found to be identical (4). Diverse investigators, working in seemingly unrelated areas, discovered identical compounds but named them differently because the biologic assays that were used suggested different activities. Tumor necrosis factor, which had been evaluated in animal models as early as 1975, but only cloned and produced by recombinant DNA technology in 1984, was found to be identical to cachectin, a factor discovered by Kawakami and coworkers (5) to result in a wasting syndrome in animals. Unfortunately, many names assigned to biologic factors on their initial discovery failed to be consistent with the diverse biologic activities subsequently discovered. The antiviral activity of IFN-γ constitutes only a small portion of its overall biologic activity, which also includes activation of immune cells, induction of pulmonary surfactant, macrophage activation, induction of diverse cytokines, and antitumor cell activity.

STEPS LEADING TO CLINICAL EVALUATION OF BIOLOGIC FACTORS

In vivo testing of a new biologic factor is necessary to confirm its in vitro biologic activities, evaluate the safety, and determine dose ranges for initial studies in humans. Initial studies of tumor necrosis factor (TNF) in animals confirmed the in vitro antitumor activity but also suggested that TNF might have significant effects on cardiovascular dynamics and be involved in endotoxin shock. The pharmacokinetics of biologic factors in animals are usually predictive of the pharmacokinetics in humans and therefore provide data for minimum and maximum doses in designing clinical studies.

After completion of animal safety and efficacy testing, all developmental and preclinical testing data, including data on methods of production and purification, are submitted to the Food and Drug Administration (FDA) as an Investigational New Drug application (see also Chapters 33 and 43) (6). If

approved, then phase I human testing can proceed. Phase I testing is usually performed on limited numbers of subjects (normal controls and patients with target disease). The study is designed to answer safety and pharmacokinetic issues rather than efficacy. Phase II and III studies are expanded safety studies that include larger numbers of subjects and may assess activity. Phase IV studies are definitive efficacy studies that, if positive, result in drug approval. After drug approval, the drug is marketed, but surveillance of drug safety continues. This process is referred to as "post-marketing survey." The average time from drug discovery to drug approval is 9 years.

The urgency of AIDS has resulted in some modifications of the drug approval process. Depending on the agent under study, phase I and II studies may be combined, and if efficacy is shown during the phase II/III evaluation a drug may be approved. An accelerated approval occurred with the evaluation of azidothymidine (AZT). For children with AIDS the drug approval process remained unnecessarily slower than that for adults. In the past, a misunderstanding of the normal developmental biology of children resulted in the requirement that drugs first be evaluated in older children before they could be tested in infants. Many now feel that the biologic differences between older children and adults are insignificant, and therefore drug safety and pharmacokinetic testing in children should be performed only in infants younger than 3 months, where developmental biologic differences are known to exist. Accelerated testing would be particularly important when a life-threatening disease such as AIDS exists in infants. The FDA has recently proposed guidelines that would permit new drugs to be approved for use in children based on limited safety studies providing that the targeted disease is similar to that of adults. Once approved, this should result in more rapid drug approval for children with life-threatening diseases and reimbursement for drug use by third party carriers.

PASSIVE THERAPY OF HIV INFECTION

Passive intervention is aimed at providing temporary protection against microbial agents by either preventing infection, reducing the infectious load, or attenuating the course of an illness, and has been shown to be at least partially effective in several virus diseases (7–10). In the case of HIV, passive intervention includes immunoglobulins rich in HIV-specific antibodies (HIV immunoglobulin (HIVIG)), monoclonal antibodies, and analogues of the CD4 receptor cells, mainly soluble CD4 (sCD4) or recombinant CD4-IgG (rCD4-IgG).

HIV Immunoglobulin

Currently available HIVIG preparations are purified and concentrated plasma from HIV-infected asymptomatic donors. A future safer alternative might be plasmapheresis from non-HIV-infected volunteers immunized with an HIV vaccine, an easier and larger source of HIVIG. There is some evidence that high titers of antibodies to HIV (HIVIG) can either prevent infection in a chimpanzee experiment (see Chapter 45) or reduce virus burden (11). In this chapter, we focus on this latter concept, which was initially supported by results of studies looking at the natural progression of the disease in HIV-infected adults. Adults with low HIV antibody titers, especially antibodies directed to the core p24 and to the envelope (such as neutralizing antibodies), progress more rapidly than adults with high antibody titers, but this may be a result of more advanced disease with greater virus burden. Three clinical trials in a limited number of adults with advanced AIDS suggest that infusion of hyperimmune plasma from asymptomatic HIV-infected donors was associated with signs of clinical improvement along with decreases in p24 antigenemia and, in some cases, appearance of neutralizing antibodies (12–14). Controlled trials are needed to confirm the potential benefit of HIVIG as an immunomodulator. No trials have been performed in children to date. A study of HIVIG in HIV-infected pregnant women began in September 1993 (see Chapter 45).

Monoclonal Antibodies

Observations of the natural history of HIV disease as well as results from animal experiments have shown that the level and specificity of antibodies may be crucial in trans-

mission. Recent studies suggested that HIV-infected pregnant women with high titers of antibodies to certain epitopes of the gp120 envelope protein, including the third hypervariable loop (V3), had a lower rate of HIV transmission to their infants (15–17), but other studies have not been able to replicate this strong association. Emini and colleagues (18) used a preparation of mouse/human chimeric Ig1 antibodies specific for the principal neutralizing domain of HIV-1 IIIB gp120 in a chimpanzee model. Twenty-four hours after injection of this monoclonal antibody, the chimpanzee was challenged (75 chimpanzee infectious doses of an HIV-1 IIIB isolate) and was protected from infection, whereas the control animal rapidly became infected. These data provide evidence for the in vivo protective effect of anti-principal neutralizing domain antibodies. Most studies looking at the effect of passive or active intervention to protect chimpanzees from infection have confirmed the strong correlation between high titers of neutralizing antibodies and antibodies to the V3 domain with protection (19).

Human monoclonal antibodies have been developed that neutralize HIV-1. They recognize either the V3 domain of gp120 conformational determinants or the CD4 binding domain of gp120. In vitro neutralization assays have shown a strong synergistic interaction between these types of monoclonal antibodies, suggesting that their appropriate combinations may provide a broad spectrum of protection, an essential factor in the development of passive immunization therapies (20). Clinical trials of monoclonal antibodies in HIV-infected adults are under consideration. Because of the specificity of these monoclonal antibodies, the design of such clinical trials should include testing them in combination.

CD4 Receptor Analogues

The CD4 receptor, whose natural ligand is class II major histocompatibility complex antigen, is the receptor for HIV on both CD4+ lymphocytes and monocytes (21). The normal function of the CD4 receptor is to bring into apposition antigen-presenting cells and T cells to facilitate the immune response. The gp120 of HIV binds to the first (amino terminal) of four domains on the extramembrane portion of the CD4 receptor with an affinity of ~10^{-9} M (22).

Biologic Activities

Various CD4 molecules have been produced by recombinant DNA technology. Recombinant or soluble CD4 consists of a truncated part of the native molecule containing only the extramembrane soluble domain (22). In human studies the serum half-life of CD4 is ~60 min. Hybrid molecules of CD4 consisting of the extramembrane portion of the CD4 and the Fc region of human IgG have been produced that combine the gp120 binding capacity of CD4 with the biologic functions of IgG-Fc. This results in a molecule (referred to as immunoadhesin) of rCD4 IgG with diverse biologic effects, including an extended half-life (35–70 hr), Fc receptor binding, complement fixation, antibody-dependent cytotoxicity, and potentially the ability to cross from the maternal circulation into the fetal circulation in pregnant women. In vitro sCD4 and rCD4 IgG can block HIV infection of T cells and monocytes and prevent syncytia formation. In addition, these molecules might neutralize free circulating gp120 in HIV-infected individuals and result in either recovery of immunologic function or prevention of further loss of immunity. HIV infection with laboratory isolates (IIIB) can be blocked in vitro using very low concentrations of sCD4 or rCD4 IgG (<1 μg/ml). It has been recently shown that much higher concentrations of these molecules are required to block HIV infection with field isolates (23). Their 50% inhibitory concentration for field isolates ranges between 5 and 100 μg/ml. This difference in sensitivity between laboratory and field isolates is the result of several mechanisms, involving among others the tissue tropism of HIV strains (24). sCD4 and rCD4 IgG have been tested in several animal species, including Rhesus monkeys and chimpanzees. Both molecules were safe and nonimmunogenic; sCD4 did not cross the placenta of pregnant Rhesus monkeys, whereas rCD4 IgG did. When injected 8 hr before and up to 9 weeks after an HIV-IIIB challenge, rCD4 IgG also protected two chimpanzees from HIV infection (25).

CD4 has also been conjugated to potent immunotoxins such as ricin A chain, *Pseudomonas* toxin, and *Pseudomonas* exotoxin A (26). In vitro studies evaluating the ability of these immunotoxins to destroy HIV-infected cells indicate that there is selective destruction of HIV-infected cells (those bearing surface gp120), with a sparing of uninfected cells. A potential difficulty with the use of immunotoxins relates to the high degree of immunogenicity of the toxin portion of the conjugate.

Clinical Trials

Phase I trials with sCD4 showed that this molecule is safe and nonimmunogenic in adults and children. However, no evidence of in vivo antiviral activity was observed (27). The interest in sCD4 clinical development has rapidly decreased, because of the availability and advantages of rCD4 IgG. Recombinant CD4 IgG is safe and nonimmunogenic in adults and children and crosses the placenta in pregnant women. Preliminary assessment of efficacy of this molecule in adults showed that at high dose, rCD4 IgG can increase the platelet counts in HIV-infected patients with immune thrombocytopenia (28). The mechanism involved (direct antiviral action or IgG-mediated effect) is unclear. In some cases, rCD4 IgG has also been associated with a temporary decrease in p24 antigenemia and plasma viremia. However, this effect was not observed consistently, even when using high doses of rCD4 IgG. Because of the lack of consistent antiviral effect in these adult phase I trials, further clinical trials are not anticipated unless more effective molecules can be developed.

INTERFERONS

Interferons were first discovered by Isaacs and Lindenmann in 1957 after investigations of virus interference. The association of virus interference by a putative factor resulted in the adoption of the term interferon. After several decades of research it became apparent that there was more than one interferon and that these interferons had multiple biologic effects beyond the ability to interfere with viral replication.

Interferons are now known to belong to a regulatory network of cytokines (29). (Cytokine is a general term often used to refer to a factor produced by cells that acts on cells within or outside the immune system, e.g., interferons, TNF, interleukins.) Interferons exert homeostatic control over various cellular functions and replication and become active regulators of host defense when stimulated by infection or other cytokines (Fig. 36.1). The regulatory network of interferons is complex and consists of both endocrine and autocrine effects.

Inital attention to interferons concentrated on their antiviral activity but later focused on their control of cell replication, with particular emphasis on effects on tumor cells in vitro and in vivo (30). Subsequently the interaction of interferon and the immune system, particularly IFN-γ, received emphasis. Most recently it has been found that interferons also regulate gene expression and can increase the expression of cellular antigens such as human leukocyte class I and II surface antigens (HLA) (31). Three

major categories of interferons exist (Table 36.1). In contrast to other cytokines, some interferons such as interferon-α (IFN-α) and interferon-β (IFN-β) are produced by most nucleated cells. Agents that activate interferons are diverse and include mitogens, antigens, various microbial agents, cytokines (interleukin-2, tumor necrosis factor), and colony-stimulating factors (32). The interactions between interferons and other cytokines amplify the effects of a specific interferon and complicate the clinical evaluation of interferon when used for the treatment of specific diseases. IFN-α, IFN-β, and IFN-γ are all in clinical trials for the treatment of HIV-related disorders. IFN-α has received FDA approval as a therapeutic agent for the control of hairy cell leukemia, Kaposi's sarcoma, and chronic viral hepatitis.

Interferon-α

Biologic Activities

IFN-α is one of three major subclasses of interferon (Table 36.1). There are more

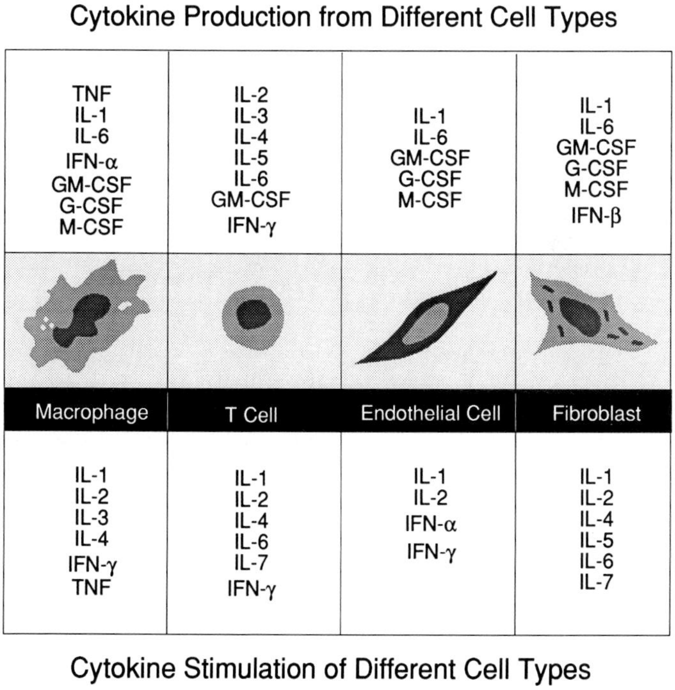

Cytokine Production from Different Cell Types

TNF IL-1 IL-6 IFN-α GM-CSF G-CSF M-CSF	IL-2 IL-3 IL-4 IL-5 IL-6 GM-CSF IFN-γ	IL-1 IL-6 GM-CSF G-CSF M-CSF	IL-1 IL-6 GM-CSF G-CSF M-CSF IFN-β
Macrophage	T Cell	Endothelial Cell	Fibroblast
IL-1 IL-2 IL-3 IL-4 IFN-γ TNF	IL-1 IL-2 IL-4 IL-6 IL-7 IFN-γ	IL-1 IL-2 IFN-α IFN-γ	IL-1 IL-2 IL-4 IL-5 IL-6 IL-7

Cytokine Stimulation of Different Cell Types

Figure 36.1. Cytokine production from different cell types and cytokine stimulation of different cell types. *Upper panels,* cytokines that are produced by specific cells when stimulated by various agents such as antigen, mitogens, and endotoxin; *middle panels,* major cell types involved in cytokine production; *lower panels,* cytokines that are stimulatory to specific cells. It is apparent that there are both endocrine and autocrine loops, that multiple cytokines are produced by a single cell, and that a single cytokine can act on multiple cells.

Table 36.1.   Interferons

Interferon Type	Other Designations	Primary Biologic Activities
Interferon-α (18 subtypes)	Lymphoblastoid type I	Antiviral Antiproliferative Enhances NK cell activity, monocyte tumor toxicity, and HLA class I and II antigen expression Inhibits HIV replication
Interferon-β (two types)	Fibroblast type I	Antiviral Antiproliferative Inhibits HIV replication
Interferon-γ	Immune type II	Antiviral Antiproliferation Stimulates macrophages, lymphocytes, interleukin-2, TNF, HLA class I and II antigens, Fc-gamma receptors, and antibody formation Inhibits HIV replication

than 14 subtypes of IFN-α. Recombinant IFN-α is produced in *Escherichia coli* and contains DNA encoding for the human protein IFN-α-2a with an approximate molecular mass of 19,000 daltons. The biologic activity of IFN-α is restricted to humans. Pharmacokinetic studies indicate an elimination half-life of 5 hr. Neutralizing antibodies occur in a high proportion of patients treated with recombinant IFN-α.

The cellular mechanism of action of IFN-α is unknown, but it has a wide range of biologic activities, including antiviral effects mediated by inhibition of transcription and translation of virus messenger RNA, protein synthesis, or assembly of the final virion. In addition, IFN-α is antiproliferative, augments NK cell activity, increases monocyte tumor toxicity, and increases cell membrane expression of HLA class I and II antigens (33). Recent studies indicate that the antiretroviral effect of IFN-α on HIV-1 is a result of interference with the release of mature virions from infected cells (34).

Clinical Studies

The first clinical trials of IFN-α in AIDS used human lymphoblastoid IFN-α, whereas subsequent trials have evaluated recombinant interferon. Although initial trials provided somewhat confusing results, more recent clinical trials provide convincing data that IFN-α has an effect on both HIV and Kaposi's sarcoma, which occurs in ~40% of adult patients with HIV infection (35, 36). The negative results of early trials of IFN-α

on Kaposi's sarcoma may have been a result of the interferon used (lymphoblastoid) or the total dose used. When doses between 15 and 20 million units/m² were used, some tumor responses were observed. Patients who responded tended to have higher total CD4 cells. Additional studies used recombinant IFN-α-2a in doses ranging from 1 to 50 million units/m² given daily for varying periods. Clinical responses were seen at low and high doses. The response rate correlated with stage of disease; patients with milder disease and no opportunistic infection had a higher response rate (37–40).

Several investigators have demonstrated an anti-HIV effect of IFN-α in vitro (41). Some reports indicated that IFN-α and IFN-β but not IFN-γ suppressed replication of several HIV isolates at the time of peak virus production. The results for IFN-α and IFN-β were confirmed by others, but some investigators found that IFN-γ could suppress virus replication when HIV-infected monocyte-macrophage cell lines were used. Subsequent studies evaluated IFN-α in combination with AZT in vitro and found that the two agents were synergistic. These encouraging in vitro results led to several clinical trials of combined AZT and IFN-α treatment of AIDS patients with Kaposi's sarcoma. Results of these studies suggest that there is both a high tumor response rate and a possible antiviral effect. It is difficult to interpret the results of many combination therapy trials because an anti-HIV-1 effect of AZT is expected. Thus, some trials report an immediate effect on virus (decreased plasma p24, virus isolation), whereas other studies indicate that the effects are transient (42–46). The ability to tolerate IFN-α was related to the dose of AZT administered. Further controlled trials will be necessary to determine if combined AZT and IFN-α will alter clinical disease and long-term prognosis. Experimental protocols include the evaluation of IFN-α combined with AZT or interleukin-2 or granulocyte-macrophage colony-stimulating factor (GM-CSF). IFN-α may be used to treat other viral infections that occur in HIV-1 infected patients. Clinical trials demonstrate that IFN-α is effective topically in preventing rhinovirus infection and systemically in treating chronic hepatitis B and C infections. It has also been used effectively for papillomavirus warts of the larynx, skin, and anogenital region (47–49). Other uses of IFN-α may include treatment of HIV-associated thrombocytopenia (50).

Treatment Regimens

Treatment regimens for IFN-α have varied considerably (1–20 million units/day), but a common approach is to use daily subcutaneous or intramuscular IFN-α in doses of 10 million units each day for 12–18 weeks. This is followed by a maintenance schedule three times per week. Two forms of recombinant IFN-α are in use that differ in one amino acid (IFN-α-2a, lysine at position 23; IFN-α-2b, arginine at position 23).

Side Effects

Side effects of recombinant IFN-α appear to be fewer and less severe than those observed using leukocyte IFN-α. Common side effects include a flu-like syndrome, fevers, chills, malaise, nausea, diarrhea, leukopenia, hepatic toxicity, and some mental status alterations. Neutralizing antibody to recombinant IFN-α has been described and may interfere with the biologic response (51). The addition of other chemotherapeutic agents to IFN-α does not appear to increase the therapeutic response but may increase toxicity.

Use in Pediatric HIV Infection

IFN-α has had limited evaluation in pediatric HIV infection. There is only one published study with limited results. A study

combining AZT and IFN-α has been initiated by the AIDS Clinical Trials Group to assess safety and tolerance.

Interferon-β

Biologic Activities

In vitro studies indicate that IFN-β has antiviral, antiproliferative, and immunomodulatory activities similar to IFN-α and IFN-γ (52, 53). Recombinant IFN-β in vitro has been shown to inhibit HIV replication, prevent syncytium formation of HIV-infected cells, and function synergistically along with AZT in inhibition of virus replication (54).

Clinical Studies and Treatment Regimens

Based on the in vitro biologic effects of IFN-β, several clinical trials have been initiated to determine if IFN-β may be of use in patients with AIDS-related complex or AIDS with or without Kaposi's sarcoma. Doses of IFN-β range from 15 to 150 million units daily, administered subcutaneously. Although some patients with Kaposi's sarcoma responded and some anti-HIV-1 effects were observed, these were minimal, and in one study a suggestion of progression was observed when combined with IFN-γ (55). There are no clinical trials of IFN-β in children with HIV infection.

Side Effects

Side effects of IFN-β are similar to those of other interferons and include a flu-like syndrome, hematologic suppression, elevated liver function tests, and mild proteinuria. Exacerbation of Kaposi's sarcoma has been reported in patients with AIDS treated with a combination of interleukin-2 or IFN-γ and IFN-β.

Interferon-γ

Biologic Activities

IFN-γ was first identified as an antiviral biologic factor in 1965 and was subsequently shown to be distinct from IFN-α and IFN-β. Because the source of IFN-γ was primarily from T cells, the name immune interferon was suggested (Table 36.1). However, detailed studies over the past decade indicate that IFN-γ has diverse antimicrobial and immunomodulating effects that distinguish it as a more broadly based biologic agent than either IFN-α or IFN-β (56, 57).

IFN-γ, like other interferons, has antiproliferative effects on several tumor cells and acts synergistically with TNF in vitro (Fig. 35.1). IFN-γ inhibits the replication of various microbial agents, including *Toxoplasma, Chlamydia,* malaria, and a significant number of viruses, including HIV (58). The immunomodulatory effects of IFN-γ are also broadly based. In vitro it has the capability of inducing HLA class I and II surface antigens and pulmonary surfactant. It also stimulates antibody formation, activates macrophages, and induces oxidative metabolism in granulocytes. Many biologic effects of IFN-γ may be mediated by other cytokines; for example, it is known that IFN-γ stimulates the in vitro production of interleukin-2, lymphotoxin, and other cytokines (58).

Recent investigations using IFN-γ have focused on its immunomodulatory effects in vitro and in vivo. IFN-γ has been shown to be the major cytokine that activates monocytes and macrophages to inhibit the replication and growth of such diverse intracellular pathogens as *Toxoplasma, Leishmania donovani,* and *Chlamydia.* The phagocytic respiratory burst, which is stimulated by IFN-γ, is most likely critical in the control of intracellular organisms. The effect of IFN-γ on various microbial agents is not universal; *Mycobacterium avium-intracellulare* is resistant to the effects of IFN-γ. The in vitro antimicrobial effects of IFN-γ have also been evaluated in animal models, primarily in the mouse. Because IFN-γ is strictly species specific, the availability of murine recombinant IFN-γ made the in vivo evaluation of IFN-γ more efficient and rapid. Beneficial effects have been shown for *Toxoplasma, Salmonella typhimurium, L. donovani,* and certain stages of *Plasmodium* in experimental malaria (58). In some instances, such as in experimental cytomegalovirus infection, IFN-γ is effective only when given before, or at the same time as, virus inoculation.

Clinical Studies

Many in vitro biologic activities of IFN-γ have been confirmed in animal and human studies, but the most extensive experience has been obtained in patients wilh malignancies (59). These studies have progressed to phase III evaluations. Although there have been few tumor responses in these studies, many biologic activities, such as induction of HLA class II antigens, increased NK cell activity, and stimulation of oxidative metabolism, were confirmed. IFN-γ is approved for prophylactic use in chronic granulomatous disease to reduce bacterial and fungal infections.

IFN-γ may act synergistically with other cytokines. IFN-γ and TNF are synergistic in controlling tumor cell proliferation and HIV replication in vitro. However, several recent studies show that TNF alone enhances HIV-1 replication in vitro (60, 61). These initial in vitro observations have been the basis of several clinical trials using IFN-γ in AIDS-related disorders either alone or in combination with TNF or AZT.

Treatment Regimens

The IFN-γ used in clinical trials is produced by recombinant DNA technology in *Escherichia coli* (57). The molecular mass of IFN-γ is ~20,000 daltons. Pharmacokinetic studies indicate that IFN-γ has a half-life of <1 hr. IFN-γ is species specific. IFN-γ has not been immunogenic in humans.

Despite the pronounced biologic effects of IFN-γ and the demonstration of decreased IFN-γ production in patients with HIV infection, trials of recombinant IFN-γ in patients with Kaposi's sarcoma and AIDS have not shown significant responses. Doses of IFN-γ have ranged from 1 to 10 million units/m²/day by continuous infusion or by daily injection. However, the beneficial effects of IFN-γ in chronic granulomatous disease is achieved using three injections per week (62). Side effects of IFN-γ administration include a flu-like syndrome, malaise, fever, and alteration of mental status.

Use in Pediatric HIV Infection

Early results of clinical trials of IFN-γ in patients with chronic granulomatous disease and the observation of decreased IFN-γ production of mononuclear cells from patients with AIDS suggest that IFN-γ may be of benefit in reducing various opportunistic infections found in patients with AIDS. Although IFN-γ is approved for the prevention of infections in chronic granulomatous disease, further clinical trials are needed to determine its value in either the prevention or treatment of infection in AIDS. The low dose required for a beneficial effect and the broad antimicrobial activity make IFN-γ an attractive potential prophylactic agent.

INTERLEUKINS

Interleukins are a group of polypeptide factors that belong to the general category of cytokines. The term "interleukin" was devised to simplify the terminology and classification of a growing list of factors that were discovered and named primarily for their biologic effects, for example, T cell growth factor (interleukin-2). The term interleukin refers to a factor, derived from white blood cells, that acts between cells. Whether this classification scheme will survive with time remains to be seen, because there are already problems associated with the original definition. Interleukin-1, for example, is produced by monocytes and macrophages and stimulates T cells but also activates endothelial cells and acts on the cells of the central nervous system (Fig. 36.1). Additional interleukins are produced by cells other than white blood cells such as hepatic and endothelial cells. In addition, it may be somewhat arbitrary whether a factor is called an interleukin or some other name. For example, interleukin-6 is the same as IFN-β-2.

There are at least twelve characterized interleukins, several newly described interleukins, but only six that are defined in any detail (Table 36.2). Of these, only interleukin-2 has had extensive clinical evaluation in HIV infection. However, other interleukins may be evaluated in HIV infection, especially those that have the ability to acti-

Table 36.2.   Interleukins

Designation	Previous Designations	Major Activities
Interleukin-1 (IL-1α; IL-1β)	Endogenous pyrogen Leukocyte activation factor B cell activating factor B cell differentiating factor	Fever; bone resorption; activates T cells, B cells, NK cells; increases interleukin-2, interleukin-3, interleukin-6, colony-stimulating factor
Interleukin-2	T cell growth factor Thymocyte mitogenic factor Thymocyte stimulating factor Killer cell helper factor	Stimulates cytokine production by T cells; increases NK cells, LAK cells, monocyte cytotoxicity; stimulates growth of T cells, differentiation of B cells
Interleukin-3	Burst promoting activity Multicolony-stimulating factor Pan-specific hemopoietin Mast cell growth factor CFU stimulating activity	Differentiation to granulocytes, macrophages, lymphocytes, megakaryocytes, mast cell; stimulates histamine, phagocytosis; synergy with erythropoietin and CSF-1
Interleukin-4	B cell growth factor B cell stimulating factor	Stimulates B cells, IgE, IgG1, IgE receptor, HLA-Dr expression, resting T cells, granulocytes, macrophages, mast cells, megakaryocytes; synergy with G-CSF, erythropoietin; inhibits NK LAK; antagonized by IFN-γ
Interleukin-5	B cell growth factor II Eosinophil differentiation factor	Enhances eosinophil differentiation, B cell growth, IgA production
Interleukin-6	B cell stimulating factor 2 B₂ interferon Hepatocyte stimulating factor Plasmacytoma growth factor	Stimulates T cells, interleukin-2 receptor, megakaryocytes, acute phase reactants, immunoglobulin; induced by virus, TNF, platelet-derived growth factor, interleukin-1, GM-CSF.
Interleukin-7	None	Stimulates growth of B cell precursors, interleukin-2 receptors, thymocytes, CD4 cells, CD8 cells
Interleukin-8	None	

vate immune cells and increase T cell, B cell, and phagocyte immunity. Interleukin-3 (multicolony-stimulating factor), is particularly attractive since it has the ability to differentiate cells of multiple lineages and to act synergistically with erythropoietin and colony-stimulating factor-I.

Interleukin-6 may be involved in the pathogenesis of some clinical and laboratory manifestations of HIV-1 infection. Interleukin-6 can be induced by HIV-1 in vitro. Interleukin-6 stimulates B cells to produce immunoglobulin and has been found to be a growth factor for Kaposi's sarcoma cells. Evaluation of adults with HIV-1 infection, with or without Kaposi's sarcoma, has shown an elevation of serum interleukin-6 in patients with Kaposi's sarcoma (63). An elevation of serum interleukin-6 in association with hypergammaglobulinemia has also been observed in children with HIV-1 infection (64).

Much remains to be learned about the biology of interleukins. Their effects on cells and organs outside the imumune system complicate their clinical application, because many biologic effects such as fever, mental confusion, and the "capillary leak" syndrome make clinical trials difficult. In addition, the dose required for a biologic effect, the pharmacokinetics, and the best means of administering interleukins are not fully understood. Nevertheless, much progress has been made, and the availability of recombinant interleukins should greatly accelerate our understanding of these potent molecules.

INTERLEUKIN-2

Biologic Activities

In 1976 Morgan and coworkers described a soluble factor produced by phytohemagglutinin-stimulated mononuclear cells that could support the growth of T cells in culture. Significant amounts of this factor, initially called T cell replacing factor and subsequently renamed interleukin-2, was derived from T cell leukemia cell line (Jurkat). This permitted biochemical definition of the factor as a 15- to 17-kilodalton sialic-rich glycoprotein and allowed for the development of monoclonal antibodies,

cloning of the cDNA and genomic DNA, and identification of interleukin-2 receptors on cells of the immune system. The eventual availability of large amounts of recombinant interleukin-2, and the lack of species specificity, permitted rapid advances of the understanding of the in vivo biologic effects of this cytokine (65).

Before evaluating the effect of interleukin-2 in humans, extensive animal preclinical studies were performed. These confirmed many in vitro biologic observations. Specifically, interleukin-2 increased the primary immune response after immunization of mice, restored T cell responsiveness in athymic mice, induced lymphokine activated killer cell (LAK cell) activity, generated NK cell activity, and increased the alloreactive T cell response. Although interleukin-2 alone has some therapeutic activity toward malignant cells in vivo (pulmonary, hepatic, and subcutaneous tumors in mice), the primary effects of interleukin-2 appear to be mediated through LAK cells.

There are marked differences between the in vitro concentrations of interleukin-2 required to generate an immune response (100–1000 units/ml) vs. the relative lack of in vivo effects with as much as 1000 units interleukin-2/g mouse. This differential was felt to be a consequence of the 3- to 5-min half-life of a single dose of intravenous interleukin-2. Interleukin-2 is rapidly distributed extravascularly and metabolized by the kidney. Subcutaneous injection prolongs the half-time and favors cellular activation, because in vitro studies indicate that lymphocytes are better activated by interleukin-2 if interleukin-2 remains in contact with interleukin-2 receptors for several hours.

Continued administration of high doses of interleukin-2 to mice resulted in significant toxicity to the animals. Wasting, diarrhea, fluid retention, pulmonary edema, and ascites were observed. Experiments were performed to enhance the antitumor effect of interleukin-2 without enhancing toxicity. This was accomplished initially in mice by treating tumor-bearing animals with interleukin-2 and injecting in vitro interleukin-2-activated LAK cells (66). These studies subsequently led to similar approaches in humans. Initially interleukin-2 was infused separately to evaluate safety of the recombinant material in humans. Efficacy studies demonstrated partial responses in patients with melanoma or renal cell carcinoma treated with interleukin-2 and LAK cells. Response rates in various clinical trials varied from 20 to 40% (67). Despite initial excitement, the toxicity of interleukin-2 has limited its application. Patients treated with high doses of interleukin-2 experience malaise, weight gain, and fever, and most patients develop hepatic and renal failure. Severe pulmonary edema requiring oxygen supplementation and ventilation has occurred. Many systemic side effects of interleukin-2 have been explained on the basis of a capillary leak syndrome. Side effects are rapidly reversible after cessation of treatment.

Clinical Trials

In vivo effects of interleukin-2 in humans are variable and depend to a great extent on the timing of studies in relation to interleukin-2 administration. During interleukin-2 administration, profound lymphopenia develops and is associated with decreased proliferative responses of mononuclear cells to interleukin-2 in vitro and decreased NK cell activity. In contrast, 24 hr following the discontinuation of interleukin-2, there is a rebound lymphocytosis associated with an increased mononuclear cell proliferative response to interleukin-2 and increased NK and LAK cell activity.

Interleukin-2 was first used in clinical trials to treat patients with primary or acquired immunodeficiency syndrome. Initial doses used were low relative to the amounts given to patients with cancer. The use of interleukin-2 was approached cautiously, not only because the potential side effects could further compromise the clinical status of patients but also because interleukin-2 might enhance HIV proliferation. In vitro studies had shown that interleukin-2 in culture media favored the growth of HIV in T cells. Nevertheless, studies of mononuclear cells from patients with AIDS demonstrated that they were deficient in interleukin-2 production and interleukin-2 receptor expression, suggesting a therapeutic role of interleukin-2 in AIDS in correcting lymphocyte, NK cell, LAK cell, and antibody formation.

Treatment Regimens

Clinical trials of interleukin-2 in HIV-infected patients were first begun in 1983. Initial phase I studies in limited numbers indicated that transient improvement in immunologic function could be achieved. The results of a larger study were published in 1987 (68). Patients with or without Kaposi's sarcoma were treated with recombinant interleukin-2 at dose levels of 1000–10 million units/m². Early toxicity at high doses necessitated modification of the doses of 1000–2 million units/m² intravenously three times per week. Only three of 55 patients with Kaposi's sarcoma were judged to have responded to interleukin-2. The remainder were felt to have progressed during the study. Despite the large doses of interleukin-2 given, with significant serum levels (>200 units/ml), no effects were seen on the immune parameters assays. These included total T cells, CD4 cells, CD8 cells, helper-suppressor cell ratios, mitogenic responses, antigen responses, and delayed hypersensitivity reactions. The failure to respond may have been a result of many factors, including a short serum half-life of < 20 min.

Current clinical trials of interleukin-2 in AIDS patients emphasize combined treatment with interleukin-2 and AZT. Combination therapy of an immunologic modulator and an antiretroviral agent is scientifically more sound than the use of interleukin-2 alone, because there is abundant information indicating that interleukin-2 in vitro will facilitate HIV replication. Results of recent studies, using interleukin-2 in combination with AZT, showed a transient increase in total CD4 cells associated with a decrease in quantitative virus in a limited number of patients (69).

Side Effects

Low doses of interleukin-2 are tolerated without any apparent toxicity. As doses increase to over 1 million units/m² several toxicities are observed. These include decreased granulocytes, increased serum transaminase, lethargy, gastrointestinal tract symptoms, rigors, and hypotension. A capillary leak syndrome, observed in clinical trials of interleukin-2 in cancer patients, has not been observed in patients with HIV infection. This may be related to the lower doses used in AIDS clinical trials. One study has reported an increased incidence of bacterial infections in patients with HIV infection receiving interleukin-2 therapy (70).

Use in Pediatric HIV Infection

Interleukin-2 has been used in children with primary immunodeficiency disease and malignancy and after bone marrow transplantation. Trials combining interleukin-2 with antiretroviral therapy are planned by the National Cancer Institute Pediatric Branch.

COLONY-STIMULATING FACTORS

Colony-stimulating factors are fibroblast-produced glycoprotein growth factors necessary for the proliferation of progenitor cells and for stimulating certain functional activities of more mature cells (Table 36.3). They may also respond to acute and chronic demands for increased cell production. The term colony-stimulating factor is derived from the observation that these compounds stimulate progenitor cells of different hematopoietic lineage to form individual colonies of recognizable maturing cells. Although originally defined as reliably specific factors for certain cell lineages, such as granulocytes and macrophages, it has become clear that some colony-stimulating factors may have multiple biological effects. For instance, multiple potential colony-stimulat-

ing factors have B cell and mast cell stimulatory activity as well as the ability to stimulate erythroid and megakaryocyte colony-forming units (CFU). Because of its diverse biologic effects on the immune system, it has also been termed interleukin-3. Erythropoietin, a specific colony-stimulating factor, has retained its original name.

Most colony-stimulating factors have now become available in sufficiently purified quantities to permit in vivo evaluation in animals and humans (71). GM-CSF, G-CSF, and erythropoietin have been extensively evaluated in clinical trials, and their use in humans has been approved by the FDA. A phase I trial of human stem cell factor (Hu-SCF) is under consideration. Undoubtedly, the remaining colony-stimulating factors will be evaluated clinically once they become available in highly purified quantities sufficient to define their biologic properties and safety profiles in animals and humans.

HIV infection is associated with multiple defects in immune regulation and hematopoiesis, including decreased proliferation of hematopoietic progenitor cells, increased destruction of mature cells, and disturbances of regulatory cytokines. The use of hematopoietic growth factors might be a successful approach in this disease.

Granulocyte-Macrophage Colony-Stimulating Factor
Biologic Activities

GM-CSF was purified to homogeneity from conditioned medium obtained from

Table 36.3.   Colony-stimulating Factors[a]

Designation	Major Target Cells	Major Biologic Activities
GM-CSF	CFU-EO CFU-GEMM CFU-GM BFU-E	Stimulates granulocyte, macrophage, and eosinophil colonies and, with EPO, stimulates BFU-E and CFU-MIX
	CFU-MEG Granulocytes Monocytes	Stimulates megakaryocytopoiesis, ADCC, phagocytosis, oxidative metabolism, ADCC to HIV-infected cells
G-CSF	CFU-G Granulocytes	Stimulates granulocyte colonies, granulocyte oxidative metabolism; produced by macrophages; increased production by TNF and interleukin-1; stimulates ADCC
M-CSF	CFU-M Monocytes	Stimulates macrophages precursors and macrophage colonies
Erythropoietin	BFU-E CFU-E	Stimulates proliferation and maturation of erythroid precursors; increases red cell production

[a]G, granulocytes; E, erythroid; MEG, megakaryocytes; M, macrophage; EO, eosinophils; BFU, burst forming units.

cell cultures of an HTLV-II infected T lymphoblastic cell line. The molecular mass of GM-CSF is 14,000–35,000 daltons, the variability of which may be accounted for by variable degrees of glycosylation. GM-CSF has been localized to chromosome 5q2l-5q32. In vitro studies indicate that GM-CSF stimulates granulocyte-macrophage and eosinophil colony formation but that the in vitro effects are not limited to these colonies when erythropoietin is added to GM-CSF (Fig. 36.2). Under the latter conditions erythroid burst forming units (BFU-E) and CFU-MIX (erythroid and granulocyte

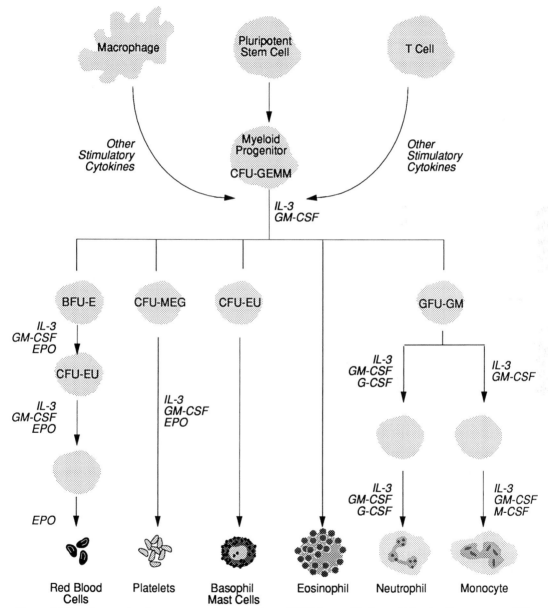

Figure 36.2. Interaction between cytokines and various progenitor cells. Macrophages and T cells produce both cytokines and colony-stimulating factors, which result in differentiation of progenitor cells. Certain cytokines such as interleukin-3 have activity toward multiple cells, while erythropoietin (*EPO*) is specific for red blood cell precursors. GM-CSF results in differentiation of precursors of granulocytes and monocytes but also has activities that result in differentiation to eosinophils, platelets, and red blood cells.

and/or monocyte colony forming unit) are stimulated. Megakaryocytopoiesis is also stimulated. Other effects of GM-CSF include inhibition of neutrophil migration in vitro, stimulation of antibody-dependent cell-mediated cytotoxicity (ADCC), enhancement of neutrophil phagocytosis (including increased expression of cell adhesion molecules and stimulation of oxidative metabolism), and enhanced monocyte TNF production. Recent studies show that GM-CSF also increases neutrophil-mediated ADCC to HIV-infected target cells. An effect of GM-CSF that raises concern for its use in clinical disorders associated with malignancy is the ability to support the growth of leukemic cells in vitro.

The usefulness of GM-CSF in stimulating granulocyte and monocyte precursors as well as mature cells has been largely documented in leukopenic patients. Regarding HIV infection, the in vitro effects of GM-CSF on HIV-infected cells have been variable. In vitro studies indicate that some but not all HIV isolates replicate in response to GM-CSF (72). However, when added before infection, and with continued presence of the cytokine, GM-CSF reduced reverse transcriptase activity of persistently infected cell cultures as well as acutely infected cells (see Chapter 6). In combination with AZT, GM-CSF acts as a potentiator of the antiviral effects of AZT (73).

Clinical Studies

Several clinical trials in HIV-infected patients have shown that GM-CSF increased the number of neutrophils, eosinophils, and monocytes and enhanced in vivo neutrophil ADCC and oxidative metabolism of these patients (74, 75). These effects were dose dependent and were not maintained after GM-CSF was discontinued.

Other clinical trials have looked at the effect of GM-CSF in combination with therapy for HIV infection such as AZT. The pharmacologic basis for this combination is provided by the finding that inhibition of HIV by AZT may be augmented by GM-CSF. Phase I controlled trials have shown that patients with severe leukopenia and intolerance to AZT can have reconstitution of effective myelopoiesis with low doses of subcutaneously self-adminis-

tered GM-CSF and become hematologically tolerant of AZT at 1200 mg/day (76–78). GM-CSF has no effect on the pharmacokinetics of AZT (79).

GM-CSF at the dose of 0.6–1.25 μg/kg/day also prevented neutropenia secondary to combination therapy with IFN-α and AZT in HIV-infected patients and Kaposi's sarcoma and induced no adverse effects on immune function or HIV activity (80, 81). Treatment was not associated with tumor response, CD4 count improvement, or change in hemoglobin concentration or p24 antigenemia levels (82). In a phase I trial of patients treated for HIV-associated non-Hodgkin's lymphoma, GM-CSF, given subcutaneously from day 4 to day 13 of each chemotherapy cycle, was associated with higher neutrophil counts, fewer chemotherapy cycles complicated by neutropenia, and fewer reductions in chemotherapy dosages. No differences in response rates to chemotherapy or survival were detected (83). Additional studies of GM-CSF in patients treated with ganciclovir for HIV-related cytomegalovirus retinitis showed a trend toward a decrease in intensity and incidence of neutropenia. No consistent proliferative effect of this agent on HIV and cytomegalovirus infections was observed (84, 85).

Doses of GM-CSF used in these studies varied between 0.25 and 20 μg/kg/day and were either subcutaneous injection or continuous infusions. Although there is concern that GM-CSF administration may increase HIV replication in myeloid cells, this effect has not been observed in clinical studies. The major side effects of GM-CSF are usually mild to moderate. They are dose dependent constitutional cytokine-like symptoms that include malaise, transient skin rash, anorexia, fever, fatigue, and anemia that, in some patients, are dose-limiting and always resolve when therapy is discontinued (80, 81).

A study of GM-CSF in children was initiated at the National Cancer Institute but was terminated early because of excessive toxicity.

In conclusion, these studies have shown that GM-CSF can improve myelopoiesis and abrogate the myelotoxicity of chemotherapeutic agents in HIV-infected patients, but no clinical improvement was observed. Additional data are necessary to assess whether the use of this hematopoietic growth factor will ultimately bring clinical benefits in terms of opportunistic infection, mortality, or quality of life.

Granulocyte Colony-Stimulating Factor

Biologic Activities

G-CSF consists of 177 amino acids with a predicted molecular mass of 19,000 daltons. G-CSF can stimulate granulocyte progenitors as well as BFU-E and CFU-MIX (Fig. 36.2). G-CSF also stimulates ADCC of neutrophils.

Clinical Studies and Treatment Regimens

Like GM-CSF, G-CSF corrects leukopenia, neutropenia, and neutrophil defects in patients with AIDS in a dose dependent fashion without altering HIV expression (78, 86, 87). G-CSF alone, by increasing the number of circulating BFU-E, also induces reticulocytosis and increases hemoglobin levels. This effect is both time and dose dependent, is correlated with the magnitude of increase in neutrophils, and is most marked in severely anemic patients with elevated pretreatment erythropoietin levels (88).

In a phase I trial of AIDS patients, the combination of G-CSF and recombinant human erythropoietin completely reversed the AZT-induced neutropenia and anemia; all 22 volunteers had a mean 10-fold increase in neutrophils occurring in less than 2 weeks, and all 20 evaluable patients had an increase in hemoglobin within 8 weeks. The reinstitution of AZT at 1–1.5 g/day resulted, however, in a decline in neutrophil counts to 5,000 cells/mm^3; this was still a significant increase over baseline counts, and enabled previously intolerant patients to tolerate AZT. It also resulted in a decline in hemoglobin to ~10 g/dl and the reappearance of transfusion requirements in eight of the 20 patients, six of whom had the study medications stopped. No change in plasma and lymphocytes cocultured for HIV and p24 antigenemia was attributed to G-CSF or erythropoietin (89, 75). In these studies, no significant G-CSF related toxicity was reported, including no flu-like symptoms.

A study of G-CSF in HIV-infected children intolerant to AZT, performed by the National Cancer Institute, indicates that G-CSF is well tolerated in this population and has a beneficial effect on neutrophil counts, similar to the one observed in adults, enabling children with AZT-related neutropenia to receive therapeutic doses of AZT (90).

Erythropoietin

Biologic Activities

Erythropoietin is a glycoprotein produced primarily in the kidneys and to some extent the liver. Mature erythropoietin consists of 166 amino acids with a molecular mass of ~35,000 daltons. The gene for erythropoietin has been localized to chromosome 7q11-q22. Recombinant erythropoietin has properties identical to natural erythropoietin and results in vitro in the proliferation and maturation of erythroid CFU and a subset of presumably mature BFU-E into red-blood cells (91). Interleukin-3 and GM-CSF control only early precursors of erythrocytes.

Increases in erythropoietin levels are associated with tissue hypoxia and anemia, whereas decreases are found in patients with certain forms of end-stage renal disease (91).

Clinical Studies

In randomized, placebo-controlled trials, erythropoietin treatment, regardless of dose and route of administration used, was associated with an increase in hematocrit level and a decrease in the transfusion requirements of patients receiving AZT (78). This beneficial effect was initially thought to occur mainly in volunteers with endogenous erythropoietic levels less or equal to 500 IU per liter at baseline (92). Recent observations suggested that erythropoietin might also be helpful in patients with higher levels of endogenous erythropoietin (93). However, as many as 25–50% of patients with severe HIV infection who receive erythropoietin do not achieve a significant increase in hemoglobin while receiving AZT (89). In these trials, the dose of erythropoietin was 100–200 units/kg three times a week given by intravenous subcutaneous injection with no drug-related toxicity observed. Erythropoietin has now been tested in larger HIV-infected populations. In a recent study of 1943 subjects, erythropoietin therapy (4000 units SC for 6 days each week) corrected anemia and was well tolerated, both in patients with or without AZT (94). Combination therapy with G-CSF and erythropoietin can ameliorate the neutropenia and anemia of AIDS, as described above (see G-CSF). Erythropoietin is now approved by the FDA for treatment of HIV-related anemias. It is under evaluation in HIV-infected children at the National Cancer Institute.

HUMAN STEM CELL FACTOR
Biologic Activities

HuSCF is a glycosylated cytokine produced by bone marrow stroma and other cells, which directly stimulates primitive pluripotent human bone marrow progenitor cells (95). When used in conjunction with erythropoietin in vitro, HuSCF results in a marked increase in BFU-E formation. Preliminary in vivo studies of HuSCF in primates suggest that the increase in BFU-E formation observed in vitro is responsible for the increase in hemoglobin that was observed. The pluripotent nature of the progenitor cell proliferation may explain the increases seen in other lineages as well (CFU-GM and CFU-MIX).

HuSCF also decreases the sensitivity of BFU-E to inhibition by AZT without altering HIV replication in lymphocytes or monocytes, peripheral blood mononuclear cell proliferation to phytohemagglutinin and interleukin-2, or altering the effectiveness of AZT or dideoxyinosine in inhibiting HIV replication in lymphocytes or monocytes (95). When HuSCF was used with erythropoietin and GM-CSF in vitro, synergistic increases in early red blood cell, white blood cell, and mixed blood cell proliferation were observed. Hu-CSF has no effect on HIV replication in vitro. Clinical studies of HuSCF alone and in combination with erythropoietin and G-CSF are planned.

Conclusion

The hematopoietic effect of these factors may allow the continued administration of full doses of antiviral or other myelosuppressive medications in previously hematologically intolerant patients with AIDS. Investigations of the hematopoietic, virologic, and immunologic effects of these agents alone and in combination with other hematopoietins, cytokines, and chemotherapeutic agents will ultimately define the clinical utility of individual agents or combination therapy in patients with HIV infection.

TUMOR NECROSIS FACTOR

The existence of a tumor necrosing factor was suspected as early as 1931, when Gratia and Linz observed that bacterial filtrates or endotoxins could induce hemorrhagic necrosis in transplanted tumors in animals. A specific tumor necrosis factor was identified in 1975 by Carswell and coworkers. As in earlier reports, the TNF was induced by endotoxin. Production of sufficient amounts of TNF for animal studies was initially accomplished by inoculating animals with Bacillus Calmette-Guérin and subsequently treating with endotoxin. The initial emphasis on the biologic role of TNF centered on control of tumor growth. However, with the availability of specific assays for TNF, increased TNF levels were demonstrated in individuals experiencing endotoxin shock and in chronically infected patients. These studies, along with intensive in vitro evaluation of TNF, indicated a more complex role of TNF in homeostasis (96, 97).

Biologic Activities

With the availability of recombinant TNF in vivo and in vitro the biology of TNF could be elucidated. Two closely related molecules were found to exist: TNF and lymphotoxin (TNF-β) (97). Lymphotoxin was found to bind to the same receptor as TNF. Lymphotoxin was found to be produced primarily by B cells in contrast to TNF, which is produced by monocytes and macrophages. Although homology exists between murine and human TNF, the biologic activity of human TNF in mice is significantly reduced. The availability of recombinant murine TNF provided a valuable tool for examining the biology of TNF in a small animal model before its evaluation in humans.

TNF inhibits the proliferation of various tumor cells in vitro, and TNF in combination with certain cytokines such as IFN-γ acts synergistically to inhibit tumor cell proliferation. Regression of tumors in animal models in vivo can be accomplished by either injecting TNF intralesionally or administering TNF systemically (96). After intralesional administration of TNF, tumor necrosis occurs within 24 hr. The mechanism of tumor necrosis is not understood and may relate either to direct cytotoxic effects of TNF or effects of TNF on other cells that elaborate additional cytokines, resulting in compromised blood flow to the tumor. The systemic administration of TNF in animals is often accompanied by toxic effects in other organs.

TNF has been studied extensively in cachexia. Kawakami and coworkers (5) isolated an endotoxin-induced factor, which they termed cachectin and which was subsequently shown to be TNF (96). In vitro TNF causes decreased lipoprotein lipase activity, increased triglycerides, and hypoglycemia. Many of these metabolic effects are those observed in endotoxin shock. Cerami and Beutler (97) postulated that TNF was a major mediator of endotoxin shock. Indeed, it has been shown that antibodies to TNF resulted in increased survival of animals who are treated with lethal doses of endotoxin. However, it is probable that TNF is not the sole mediator of endotoxin shock and may act in conjunction with interleukin-1 as well as other cytokines such as IFN-γ and platelet activating factor.

TNF may also have an important biologic function in the control of infection (98–101). In vitro, TNF was found to be cytotoxic to herpes-infected cells. TNF alone or in combination with IFN-γ has been shown to inhibit HIV replication in vitro (102). Mitogen-stimulated mononuclear cells from patients with AIDS and AIDS-related complex were found to produce significantly less TNF in vitro than controls, although several studies report increased TNF serum and cerebrospinal fluid levels in vivo.

Clinical Trials

Initial clinical trials of TNF were conducted in patients with advanced malignancy (100). In these phase I trials, escalation of TNF doses was limited by toxicity of TNF. Additional trials of TNF in humans with malignancy included combinations of IFN-γ and TNF in an attempt to reduce the dose of TNF and take advantage of the synergy between IFN-γ and TNF that had been observed in vitro. Although individual tumor responses have been observed with the administration of TNF alone or in combination with IFN-γ, the overall antitumor effects have been disappointing.

Based on in vitro observations of an antiretroviral effect of TNF alone or in combination with IFN-γ, clinical trials with TNF and IFN-γ in combination have been initiated. A limited number of patients have been enrolled in these studies, which are proceeding with caution because of the observed toxicity of TNF in animal models. Results of studies evaluating the use of TNF and IFN-γ in Kaposi's sarcoma are discussed in "Interferon-γ." A single study has been performed using the direct inoculation of TNF into Kaposi's sarcoma skin lesions (103). Although control of Kaposi's sarcoma lesions was demonstrated using this technique, the method is tedious and does not result in control of lesions distant from the skin sites injected or lesions not accessible to direct injection. There are no clinical trials of TNF in children with HIV infection.

Side Effects

Increasing doses of TNF result in increasing fever, muscle pain, central nervous system effects, hypotension and endotoxin-like reactions. Because a significant number of TNF side effects are seen spontaneously in AIDS, including a wasting syndrome, and because TNF levels are elevated in many patients, studies are being performed to determine if inhibition of TNF may have a beneficial effect. The physiologic effects of TNF can be inhibited by monoclonal antibodies or pentoxifylline, both of which are in early clinical trials in adults.

HUMAN GROWTH HORMONE AND INSULIN-LIKE GROWTH FACTOR

There is emerging evidence that both human growth hormone and insulin-like growth factor-1 (IGF) have potent in vitro and in vivo effects on the immune system. IGF, which mediates the action of growth hormone, appears to be the more potent of the two factors (104–106). An association between growth hormone and the immune system was first suggested in 1967 when it was observed that the hereditary recessive pituitary dwarf mouse had reduced thymus and lymphoid tissue. More recently it has been shown that growth hormone treatment of mice with severe combined immunodeficiency results in an increase in CD4 and CD8 cells. When thymus was used to reconstitute these mice, administration of growth hormone resulted in the acceleration of the appearance of immune tissue (104).

In addition to the effects of growth hormone on the immune system, IGF has been shown to result in an expansion of the thymus gland (105). Functional receptors for growth hormone and IGF have been found on immune cells, and both hormones increase the proliferation of immune cells (106). In vivo treatment of hypophysectomized rats infused with IGF increases the size of the thymus to a greater extent than other organs (105).

Extensive studies of growth hormone and IGF in HIV-infected subjects have not been performed. However, there are individual reports of growth hormone and/or IGF-1 deficiencies in HIV-infected patients (107, 108).

Preliminary studies were performed to evaluate the safety of recombinant growth hormone in HIV-infected adults. The intent of these early studies was to determine if the known anabolic effects of growth hormone occur in HIV-infected subjects with the wasting syndrome. To date, the trials have been uncontrolled but suggest that growth hormone may result in increased muscle mass, nitrogen retention, and weight gain (109). No effects of growth hormone have been observed on the immune system, but studies have thus far been performed only in patients with severe immunodeficiency and advanced AIDS. Studies are in progress in adults using recombinant IGF-1 alone, or in combination with recombinant growth hormone. Growth hormone and/or IGF are under consideration in the pediatric population with HIV infection. Growth and development is easier to assess in children and there is a long history of evaluating and treating children with recombinant growth hormone.

FUTURE DIRECTIONS IN DEVELOPMENT OF BIOLOGIC AND IMMUNOREGULATORY AGENTS

Over the next several years, the availability of new biologic and immunoregulatory agents will increase significantly as a result of new discoveries, improved technology, and more rapid production of specific factors by recombinant DNA technology. The number of new molecules already in clinical trials is significant, and the challenges that face the clinicians who must evaluate these factors are multiple. HIV infection results in disruption of the immune system as well as other biologic systems. The treatment of AIDS must be directed toward control of HIV infection and opportunistic infection and the restoration of normal immunity. We are at the point of effectively evaluating the effects of only single agents in HIV-infected individuals. As the pharmacokinetics and biologic properties of single agents are understood, the individual agents will undoubtedly be evaluated in combinations of two or more simultaneously or sequentially. Future challenges require us to understand more about how cytokines interact with one another and how the various endocrine and autocrine pathways function. Although treating HIV infection with antiviral agents is the most direct approach to controlling disease, it would appear logical to use immunoregulatory agents to stimulate recovery of the immune system. This goal has not yet been achieved and illustrates the need for more intensive investigation.

The challenge before us is to rapidly evaluate the multiple biologic reagents already available as well as those that will be available in the near future. There are many obstacles that will need to be overcome to achieve these goals in a timely manner. Many pharmaceutical companies are reluctant to perform clinical studies in infants and children (see Chapter 33). This may be a consequence of the perception that clinical trials are more difficult in infants and children, that there are greater liability risks in performing studies in infants and children, or that approval of drugs for diseases in infants and children may not represent a significant financial advantage. The federal government, by means of the Orphan Drug

Act and vaccine liability legislation, has addressed some of these issues. However, additional difficulties relate to current perceptions about how drugs should be evaluated in infants and children. Although current guidelines for the evaluation of drugs in children reflect concern regarding the safety of drug evaluation, they should not be viewed as inflexible regulations. For example, in diseases such as HIV infection, where the causative agent is identical in infants and adults and where one is dealing with a life-threatening illness, it does not seem reasonable to require a separate demonstration of efficacy of antiretroviral agents in clinical trials in children. Rather, emphasis should be placed on the unique pharmacokinetics and safety of drugs in very young infants compared with those in adults. These studies can be performed rapidly, address unique issues in infants, and should be the only studies required if efficacy has already been proved in adults. The FDA has recently issued new guidelines to address some of these issues. It should also be possible to approve a drug based on efficacy trials in children in the absence of such trials in adults. For example, if an antiretroviral agent were found to rapidly reverse the central nervous system abnormalities in infants with HIV infection, this could be the basis of approval. Also, since it is highly likely that certain drugs will be used to treat life-threatening illnesses in pregnant women, drugs should be evaluated for safety in the pregnant woman and the fetus early in drug development rather than in the final stages. Because the population of infants and children infected with HIV is smaller than that of adults, the evaluation of the efficacy of an agent becomes more difficult. Clinical trials of biologic agents and immunoregulatory molecules in infants and children should therefore be performed judiciously, and, where questions to be answered are not unique to infants and children, the study should be performed in adults.

References

1. Carswell S. Changes in aerobic power in patients undergoing elective surgery. J Physiol (Lond) 1975;215:42–43.
2. Hooper JA, McDaniel MC, Thurman GB, Cohen GH, Schulof RS, Goldstein AL. Purification and properties of bovine thymosin. Ann NY Acad Sci 1975;249:125–144.
3. Wara DW, Goldstein AL, Doyle NE, Ammann AJ. Thymosin activity in patients with cellular immunodeficiency. N Engl J Med 1975;292:70–74.
4. Talmadge KW, Gallati H, Sinigaglia F, Walz A, Garotta G. Identity between human interferon-gamma and "macrophage-activating factor" produced by human T lymphocytes. Eur J Immunol 1986;16:1471–1477.
5. Kawakami M, Watanabe N, Ogawa H, et al. Cachectin/TNF kills or inhibits the differentiation of 3T3-L1 cells according to developmental stage. J Cell Physiol 1989;138:1–7.
6. Kessler DA. The regulation of investigational new drugs. N Engl J Med 1989;320:281–288.
7. Stiehm ER. Immunodeficiency disorders: General considerations in immunologic disorders in infants and children. In: Stiehm ER, Fulginitti VA, eds. Immunodeficiency disorders in infants and children. Philadelphia: WB Saunders, 1973: 145–167.
8. Ammann AJ, Schiffman G, Abrams D, Volberding P, Ziegler J, Conant M. B-cell immunodeficiency in acquired immune deficiency syndrome. JAMA 1984;251:1447–1449.
9. Hague RA, Yap PK, Mok JY, et al. Intravenous immunoglobulin in HIV infection: Evidence for the efficacy of treatment. Arch Dis Child 1989;64:1146–1150.
10. Yap PK, Williams PE. Immunoglobulin preparations for HIV-infected patients [Review]. Vox Sang 1988;44:65–74.
11. Zolla-Pazner S, Gorny MK. Passive immunization for the prevention and treatment of HIV infection. AIDS 1992;6:1235–1247.
12. Jackson GG, Perkins JT, Rubenis M, et al. Passive immunoneutralization of human immunodeficiency virus in patients with advanced AIDS. Lancet 1988;2:647–652.
13. Karpas A, Hill F, Youle M, et al. Effects of passive immunization in patients with the acquired immunodeficiency complex and acquired immunodeficiency syndrome. Proc Natl Acad Sci USA 1988;85:9234–9237.
14. Vittecoq D, Mattlinger B, Barre-Sinoussi AM, et al. Passive immunotherapy in AIDS: A randomized trial of serial human immunodeficiency virus-positive transfusions of plasma rich in p24 antibodies versus transfusions of seronegative plasma. J Infect Dis 1992;165:364–368.
15. Rossi P, Moschese V, Broliden PA, et al. Presence of maternal antibodies to human immunodeficiency virus 1 envelope glycoprotein gp120 epitopes correlates with the uninfected status of children born to seropositive mothers. Proc Natl Acad Sci USA 1989;86:8055–8058.
16. Goedert JJ, Mendez H, Drummond JE, et al. Mother-to-infant transmission of human immunodeficiency virus type 1: Association with prematurity or low anti-gp120. Lancet 1989;2:1351–1354.
17. Devash Y, Calvelli TA, Wood DG, et al. Vertical transmission of human immunodeficiency virus is correlated with the absence of high-affinity/avidity maternal antibodies to the gp120 principal neutralizing domain. Proc Natl Acad Sci USA 1990;87:3445–3449.

18. Emini EA, Nara PK, Schleif WA, et al. Antibody-mediated in vitro neutralization of human immunodeficiency virus type 1 abolishes infectivity for chimpanzees. J Virol 1990;64:3674–3678.

19. Berman PW, Gregory TJ, Riddle L. Protection of chimpanzees from infection by HIV-1 after vaccination with recombinant glycoprotein gp120 but not gp160. Nature 1990;345:622–625.

20. Karwowska S, Zolla-Paznser S. Passive immunization for the treatment and prevention of HIV infection. Biotechnol Ther l991;2:31–48.

21. Lasky LA, Nakamura G, Smith DH, et al. Delineation of a region of the human immunodeficiency virus type 1 gp120 glycoprotein critical for interaction with the CD4 receptor. Cell 1987;50:975–985.

22. Smith DH, Byrn RA, Marsters SA, et al. Blocking of HIV-1 infectivity by a soluble, secreted form of the CD4 antigen. Science 1987;238:1704–1707.

23. Daar ES, Li XL, Moudgil T, Ho DD. High concentrations of recombinant soluble CD4 are required to neutralize primary human immunodeficiency virus type 1 isolates. Proc Natl Acad Sci USA 1990;87:6574–6578.

24. Hwang SS, Boyle TJ, Lyerly K, Cullen BR. Identification of envelope V3 loop as the major determinant of CD4 neutralization sensitivity of HIV-1. Science 1992;257:535–537.

25. Ward RHR, Capon DJ, Jett CM, et al. Prevention of HIV-1 IIIB infection in chimpanzees by CD4 immunoadhesion. Nature 1991;352:434–436.

26. Till MA, Ghetie V, Gregory T, et al. HIV-infected cells are killed by rCD4-ricin A chain. Science 1988;240:1166–1168.

27. Husson RN, Chung Y, Mordenti J, et al. A phase I study of continuous infusion soluble CD4 as a single agent and in combination with oral dideoxyinosine in children with symptomatic human immunodeficiency virus infection. J Pediatr 1992;921:627–633.

28. Kahn J, Hassner C, Arri R, et al. A phase I study of recombinant human CD4 immunoglobulin (rCD4-IgG) in patients with HIV-associated thrombocytopenic purpura [Abstract WB 2156]. Seventh International Conference on AIDS, Florence, Jun 1992.

29. DeMaeyer E, DeMaeyer-Guignard J, eds. Interferon and other regulatory cytokines. New York: Wiley, 1988.

30. Adolf GR. Structure and effects of interferon-gamma. Oncology 1985;42:33–40.

31. Maio M, Gulwani B, Morgano A, Ferrone, S. Differential modulation by tumor necrosis factor and immune interferon of HLA class-II antigens expressed by melanoma cells. Int J Cancer 1989;44:554–559.

32. Vilcek J, Henriksen-DeStefano D, Siegel D. IFN-γ induction in peripheral blood leukocytes by interleukin 2: Role of monocytes, interleukin 1 and IFN-γ in the interferon system. In: Dianzani F, Rossi GB, eds. The interferon system. International Ares-Serono Symposium on Interferon System, Rome, May 1985. New York: Raven, 1985;24:43–47.

33. Krown SE, Real FX, Cunningham-Rundles S, et al. Preliminary observations on the effects of recombinant leukocyte A interferon in homosexual men with Kaposi's sarcoma. N Engl J Med 1983;308:1071–1076.

34. Finter NB, Chapman S, Dowd P, et al. The use of interferon-alpha in virus infections. Drugs 1991;42:749–765.

35. Volberding PA, Mitsuyasu RT, Golando JP, Siegel RJ. Treatment of Kaposi's sarcoma with interferon alpha-2b (IntronA). Cancer 1987; 59(suppl 3):620–625.

36. De Wit R. AIDS-associated Kaposi's sarcoma and the mechanisms of interferon alpha's activity; a riddle within a puzzle. J Intern Med 1992;231:321–325.

37. Mitsuyasu RT. Use of recombinant interferons and hematopoietic growth factors in patients infected with human immunodeficiency virus. Rev Infect Dis 1991;13:979–984.

38. Krown SE. Interferon and other biologic agents for the treatment of Kaposi's sarcoma. Hematol Oncol Clin North Am 1991;5:311–322.

39. De Wit R, Danner SA, Bakker PJ, et al. Combined zidovudine and interferon-alpha treatment in patients with AIDS-associated Kaposi's sarcoma. J Intern Med 1991;229:35–40.

40. Fischl MA, Uttamchandani RB, Resnick L, et al. A phase I study of recombinant human interferon-alpha 2a or human lymphoblastoid interferon-alpha n1 and concomitant zidovudine in patients with AIDS-related Kaposi's sarcoma. J Acquir Immune Defic Syndr 1991;4:1–10.

41. Hartshoarn KL, Vogt MW, Chou TC, et al. Synergistic inhibition of human immunodeficiency virus in vitro by azidothymidine and recombinant alpha A interferon. Antimicrob Agents Chemother 1987;31:168–172.

42. Pan XZ, Qiu ZD, Baron PA, et al. Three-drug synergistic inhibition of HIV-1 replication in vitro by 3'-fluoro-3'-deoxythymidine, recombinant soluble CD4, and recombinant interferon-alpha. AIDS Res Hum Retroviruses 1992;8:589–595.

43. Pan XZ, Qiu ZD, Baron PA, et al. Three-drug synergistic inhibition of HIV-1 replication in vitro by 3'-fluoro-3'-deoxythymidine, recombinant soluble CD4, and recombinant interferon-alpha. AIDS Res Hum Retroviruses 1992;8:589–595.

44. Edlin BR, Weinstein RA, Whaling SM, et al. Zidovudine-interferon-alpha combination therapy in patients with advanced human immunodeficiency virus type 1 infection: Biphasic response of p24 antigen and quantitative polymerase chain reaction. J Infect Dis 1992;165:793–798

45. Gill PS. Phase I/II trials of alpha-interferon alone or in combination with zidovudine as maintenance therapy following induction chemotherapy in the treatment of acquired immunodeficiency syndrome-related Kaposi's sarcoma. Semin Oncol 1991;18:53–57.

46. Lai PK, Tamura Y, Bradley WG, et al. Cytokine regulation of the human immunodeficiency virus (HIV). Int J Immunopharmacol 1991;13:55–61.

47. Handley JM, Horner T, Maw RD, et al. Subcutaneous interferon alpha 2a combined with cryotherapy vs. cryotherapy alone in the treat-

ment of primary anogenital warts: A randomised observer blind placebo controlled study. Genitourin Med 1991;67:297–302.

48. Gwaltney JM Jr. Combined antiviral and antimediator treatment of rhinovirus colds. J Infect Dis 1992;166:776–782.

49. Finter NB, Chapman S, Dowd P, et al. The use of interferon-alpha in virus infections. Drugs 1991;42:749–765.

50. Northfelt DW, Kaplan LD, Abrams DI. Continuous, low-dose therapy with interferon-alpha for human immunodeficiency virus (HIV)-related immune thrombocytopenic purpura. Am J Hematol 1991;38:238–239.

51. Ronnblom LE, Janson ET, Perers A, et al. Characterization of anti-interferon-alpha antibodies appearing during recombinant interferon-alpha 2a treatment. Clin Exp Immunol 1992;89:330–335.

52. Miles SA, Wang HJ, Cortes E, et al. Beta-interferon therapy in patients with poor-prognosis Kaposi's sarcoma related to the acquired immunodeficiency syndrome (AIDS). A phase II trial with preliminary evidence of antiviral activity and low incidence of opportunistic infections. Ann Intern Med 1990;112:582–589.

53. Sehgal PB, May LT. Human interferon-beta 2. J Interferon Res 1987;7:521–527.

54. Borack MJ, Pollard RB. An open label study of the safety and efficacy of co-administration of zidovudine and recombinant IFN-beta [Abstract 405]. Fifth International Conference on AIDS, Montreal, Jun 1987.

55. Brockmeyer NH, Mertins L, Goos M. Progression of Kaposi's sarcoma under a combined interferon-beta and interferon-gamma therapy in AIDS patients. Klin Wochenschr 1990;68:1229.

56. Cerami A. Inflammatory cytokines. Clin Immunol Immunopathol 1992;62:S3–S10.

57. Gray PW, Goeddel DV. Molecular biology of interferon-gamma. Lymphokines 1987;13:151–162.

58. Murray HW. Interferon-gamma, the activated macrophage, and host defense against microbial challenge. Ann Intern Med 1988;108;595–608.

59. Kurzrock R, Feinberg B, Talpaz M, Saks S, Gutterman JU. Phase I study of a combination of recombinant tumor necrosis factor-alpha and recombinant interferon-gamma in cancer patients. J Interferon Res 1989;9:435–444.

60. Vesanen M, Wessman M, Salminen M, et al. Activation of integrated human immunodeficiency virus type 1 in human neuroblastoma cells by the cytokines tumour necrosis factor-alpha and interleukin-6. J Gen Virol 1992;73:1753–1760.

61. Swingler S, Easton A, Morris A. Cytokine augmentation of HIV-1 LTR-driven gene expression in neural cells. AIDS Res Hum Retroviruses 1992;8:487–493.

62. Dinauer MC, Orkin SH. Chronic granulomatous disease. Annu Rev Med 1992;43:117–124.

63. De Wit R, Raasveld MH, Ten Berge RJ, et al. Interleukin-6 concentrations in the serum of patients with AIDS-associated Kaposi's sarcoma during treatment with interferon alpha. J Intern Med 1991;229:539–542.

64. Rautonen J, Rautonen N, Martin NL, et al. Serum interleukin-6 concentrations are elevated and associated with elevated tumor necrosis factor-alpha and immunoglobulin G and A concentrations in children with HIV infection. AIDS 1991;5:1319–1325.

65. Malkovsky M, Sondel PM, Strober W, et al. The interleukins in acquired disease [Review]. Clin Exp Immunol 1988;74:151–161.

66. Chang AE, Hyatt CL, Rosenberg SA. Systemic administration of recombinant human interleukin-2 in mice. J Biol Response Mod 1984;3:561–566.

67. Rosenberg SA. Adoptive immunotherapy of cancer using LAK cells and recombinant IL-2. In: DeVita VT, Hellman SA, Rosenberg SA, eds. Important advances in oncology. Philadelphia: JB Lippincott, 1986:55.

68. Volberding P, Moody DJ, Beardslee D, et al. Therapy of acquired immune deficiency syndrome with recombinant interleukin-2. AIDS Res Hum Retroviruses 1987;3:115–124.

69. Clark AG, Holodniy M, Schwartz DH, et al. Decrease in HIV provirus in peripheral blood mononuclear cells during zidovudine and human rIL-2 administration. J Acquir Immune Defic Syndr 1992;5:52–59.

70. Murphy PM, Lnae C, Gallin JI, et al. Marked disparity in incidence of bacterial infections in patients with the acquired immunodeficiency syndrome receiving interleukin-2 or interferon-α. Ann Intern Med 1988;108:36–41.

71. Sieff CA. Hematopoietic growth factors. J Clin Invest 1987;79:1549–1557.

72. Hammer SM, Gillis JM, Pinkston P, Rose RM. Effect of zidovudine and granulocyte-macrophage colony-stimulating factor on human immunodeficiency virus replication in alveolar macrophages. Blood 1990;75:1215–1219.

73. Perno CF, Yarchoan R, Cooney DA, et al. Replication of human immunodeficiency virus in monocytes. Granulocyte/macrophage colony-stimulating factor (GM-CSF) potentiates viral replication yet enhances the antiviral effect mediated by 3'-azido-2'3'-dideoxythymidine (AZT) and other dideoxynucleoside congeners of thymidine. J Exp Med 1989;169:933–951.

74. Groopman JE, Mitsuyasu RT, DeLeo MF, et al. Effect of recombinant human granulocyte macrophage colony-stimulating factor on myelopoieis in the acquired immunodeficiency syndrome. N Engl J Med 1987;317:593–598.

75. Mitsuyasu RT. Use of recombinant interferons and hematopoietic growth factors in patients infected with human immunodeficiency virus. Rev Infect Dis 1991;13:979–984.

76. Groopman JE. Granulocyte-macrophage colony-stimulating factor in human immunodeficiency virus disease. Semin Hematol 1990; 27:8–14.

77. Levine JD, Allan JD, Tessitore, JH, et al. Recombinant human granulocyte-macrophage colony-stimulating factor ameliorates zidovudine-induced neutropenia in patients with acquired immunodeficiency syndrome (AIDS)/AIDS-related complex. Blood 1991;78:3148–3154.

78. Miles SA. The use of hematopoietic growth factors in HIV infection and AIDS-related malignancies. Cancer Invest 1991;9:229–238.

79. Aweeka F, Mak M, Al-Uzri A, et al. Effects of GM-CSF (SCH39300) on the pharmacokinetics (PK) of zidovudine (Z) in subjects with HIV infection [Abstract PoB 3727]. Eighth International Conference on AIDS, Amsterdam, Jul 1992.

80. Davey RT Jr, Davey VJ, Metcalf JA, et al. A phase I/II trial of zidovudine, interferon-alpha, and granulocyte-macrophage colony-stimulating factor in the treatment of human immunodeficiency virus type 1 infection. J Infect Dis 1991;164:43–52.

81. Krown SE, Paredes J, Bundow D, et al. Inteferon-α, zidovudine and granulocyte-macrophage colony-stimulating factor: A phase I AIDS clinical trials group study in patients with Kaposi's sarcoma associated with AIDS. J Clin Oncol 1992;10:1344–1351.

82. Scadden DT, Bering HA, Levine JD, et al. GM-CSF as an alternative to dose modification of the combination zidovudine and interferon-alpha in the treatment of AIDS-associated Kaposi's sarcoma. Am J Clin Oncol 1991;14:S40–S44.

83. Kaplan LD, Kahn JO, Crowe S, et al. Clinical and virologic effects of recombinant human granulocyte-macrophage colony-stimulating factor in patients receiving chemotherapy for human immunodeficiency virus-associated non-Hodgkin's lymphoma: Results of a randomized trial. J Clin Oncol 1991;9:929–940.

84. Grossberg HS, Bonnen EM, Buhles WC Jr. GM-CSF with ganciclovir for the treatment of cytomegalovirus retinitis in acquired immune deficiency syndrome [Letter]. N Engl J Med 1989; 320:1560.

85. Hardy WD. Combined ganciclovir and recombinant human granulocyte-macrophage colony-stimulating factor in the treatment of cytomegalovirus retinitis in AIDS patients. J Acquir Immune Defic Syndr 1991;4:S22–S228.

86. Kimura S, Matsuda J, Ikematsu S, et al. Efficacy of recombinant human granulocyte colony-stimulating factor on neutropenia in patients with AIDS. AIDS 1990;4:1251–1255.

87. Mitsuyasu RT, Miles SA, Golde DW. The use of myeloid hematopoietic growth factors in patients with HIV infection. Int J Cell Cloning 1990;8: 347–355.

88. Miles SA, Mitsuyasu RT, Lee K, et al. Recombinant human granulocyte colony-stimulating factor increases circulating burst forming unit-erythron and red blood cell production in patients with severe human immunodeficiency virus infection. Blood 1990;75:2137–2142.

89. Miles SA, Mitsuyasu RT, Moreno J, et al. Combined therapy with recombinant granulocyte colony-stimulating factor and erythropoietin decreases hematologic toxicity from zidovudine. Blood 1991;77:2109–2117.

90. Mueller BU, Jacobsen F, Butler KM, et al. Combined treatment with azidothymidine and granulocyte colony-stimulating factor in children with HIV infection. J Pediatr 1992;121:797–802.

91. Spivak JL. Erythropoietin. Blood Rev 1989;3: 130–135.

92. Fischl M, Galpin JE, Levine JD, et al. Recombinant human erythropoietin for patients with AIDS treated with AZT. N Engl J Med 1990;322:1488–1493.

93. DaCosta NA, Hultin MB. Effective therapy of human immunodeficiency virus-associated anemia with recombinant human erythropoietin despite high endogenous erythropoietin. Am J Hematol 1991;36:71–72.

94. Phair J, Abels R. Recombinant human erythropoietin (r-HuEPO) treatment IND protocol for the anemia of AIDS—overall results and AZT subgroup analysis [Abstract, MoA 0008]. Eighth International Conference on AIDS, Amsterdam, Jul 1992.

95. Miles SA, Lee K, Hutlin L, et al. Potential use of human stem cell factor as adjunctive therapy for human immunodeficiency virus-related cytopenias. Blood 1991;78:3200–3208.

96. Beutler B, Cerami A. The biology of cachectin/TNF—a primary mediator of the host response. Annu Rev Immunol 1989;7:625–655.

97. Cerami A, Beutler B. The role of cachectin/TNF in endotoxic shock and cachexia. Immunol Today 1988;9:28–31.

98. Shalaby MR, Espevik T, Rice GC, et al. The involvement of human tumor necrosis factors-alpha and -beta in the mixed lymphocyte reaction. J Immunol 1988;141:499–503.

99. Ammann AJ, Palladino MA. Biologic effects of tumor necrosis factors alpha and beta. In: Ranson JH, Ortadlo JR, eds. Leukolysins and cancer. Clifton, NJ: Humana, 1988:303–311.

100. Palladino MA, Ammann AJ. Tumor necrosis factors-alpha and -beta. A family of biochemically related cytokines. In: Ransom JH, Ortaldo JR, eds. Leucolysins and cancer. Clifton, NJ: Humana, 1988:235–244.

101. Sugarman BJ, Lewis GD, Eessalu TE, et al. Effects of growth factors on the antiproliferative activity of tumor necrosis factors. Cancer Res 1987; 47:780–786.

102. Wong GHW, Krowka JF, Stites DP, et al. In vitro anti-human immunodeficiency virus activities of tumor necrosis factor-alpha and interferon-gamma. J Immunol 1988;140:120–124.

103. Kahn JO, Kaplan LD, Volberding PA, et al. Intralesional recombinant tumor necrosis factor-alpha for AIDS-associated Kaposi's sarcoma: A randomized double-blind trial. J Acquir Immune Defic Syndr 1989;2:217–223.

104. Murphy WJ, Durum SK, Longo DL. Growth hormone accelerates peripheral T cell reconstitution in mice with severe combined immune deficiency (SCID) [Abstract]. FASEB, Atlanta, Apr 1991.

105. Binz K, Joller P, Froesch P, et al. Repopulation of the atrophied thymus in diabetic rats by insulin-like growth factor I. Proc Natl Acad Sci USA 1990;87:3690–3694.

106. Verland S, Gammeltoft S. Functional receptors for insulin-like growth factors I and II in rat thymocytes and mouse thymona cells. Mol Cell Endocrinol 1989;67:207–216.

107. Laue L, Pizzo PA, Butler K, et al. Growth and neuroendocrine dysfunction in children with ac-

quired immunodeficiency syndrome. J Pediatr 1990;117:541–545.

108. Dluhy RG. The growing spectrum of HIV related endocrine disorders. J Clin Endocrinol 1990;70: 563–565.

109. Krenz AJ, Kaster FT, Crest DM, et al. Beneficial effects of recombinant growth hormone in the treatment of AIDS [Abstract]. 31st Interscience Conference on Antimicrobial Agents and Chemotherapy, Chicago, Oct 1991.

37
Ethical Issues Surrounding Care of HIV-infected Children

John G. Twomey Jr. and John C. Fletcher

Health care professionals and others are radically rethinking their approaches to AIDS because of its threat to world health. Traditional models of care, research, and prevention have been challenged by the deadly and spreading epidemic of the human immunodeficiency virus (HIV). Infectious disease specialists cope with a transmissible organism that in adults may now respond to treatment before symptoms occur (1), a finding that is being studied in children (2). Public health officials face a sexually transmitted disease in which partner notification has been challenged because of the stigmatization linked to AIDS and the possible inadequacy of early, one-time screening (3). Societies reflect this scientific and social dissonance by reactions that vary from shifting funds from study of other diseases to address AIDS to inhibitions on a patient's ability to travel, work, attend school, or purchase adequate health insurance. HIV infection has caused great divisiveness in society because of its modes of transmission, its victims, and disagreements over who ought to be in the vanguard of the fight against the illness.

CHALLENGES OF AIDS TO BIOETHICS

Bioethics, a new branch of ethics addressing ethical issues in health care and research, has also been stressed by the AIDS epidemic (4). We first discuss the impact of AIDS on bioethical theory and the concept of a right to health care before reviewing some specific ethical issues surrounding the medical care of HIV-infected children.

The ethical problems associated with AIDS provide a rationale for vigorous evaluation of the cogency of the main theories and interpretations of bioethics. "Principlism", which may be the dominant perspective in bioethics (5), has drawn criticism from clinicians (6) and philosophers (7). Moral principles and rules are valuable and familiar tools of the moral life. However, these elements do not of themselves supply the traits of character and strength of community to carry out the claims and imperatives of rules and principles in everyday life. Something more is needed, as our examination of pediatric ethics in the AIDS epidemic will show. We argue for additional resources for ethical inquiry into the needs of children and families directly affected by AIDS and the practices of those who provide health care and do research in their midst. Also, the sheer magnitude of inadequate access to health care revealed by the AIDS epidemic questions whether health care is a right of each person in the society, including children.

Principlism and Its Influence

The principlist perspective in ethics proceeds from sets of principles to analyze various problems in the light of arguments drawn from the claims of such principles. Principlists are primarily concerned with describing and defending the rights of various parties in ethical conflicts. This approach has shaped the framework within which ethical issues in clinical research and medical care are examined in the United States. A seminal report of a national commission on research involving children (8) and the "Belmont report" describe the key ethical principles (9) governing research. The Belmont report significantly influenced subsequent federal guidelines for research with human subjects (10). Basic ethical principles are also the framework of ethical codes for most health care professionals (11, 12), except for a recent code adopted by genetic counselors (13) that is set forth in a framework of relationships. Our view is that an ethical perspective based on principles and rights is crucial. Apart from actual communities of motivated persons who care deeply about persons and their rights, an ethics of rights tends to hover over real problems and lacks power to inspire action to resolve them. AIDS has caused the essential humanity and value of persons with AIDS to be questioned so that a rights-based ethics must be strengthened by an ethics of caring. The next section sketches ways to broaden this ethical perspective to include themes more responsive to the needs of children, families, and those who provide clinical care and do research in pediatric AIDS.

An Ethic of Caring

A strong challenger to principlism is an ethical theory based on caring. Drawing on writings of philosopher David Hume (14), and advanced by psychologist and educational theorist Carol Gilligan (15), this view finds that principlism's rights-based language tends to neglect crucial relationships. It can be too abstract and often fails to recognize the human needs that also underlie conflicts of ethical principles. In bioethics, those who argue from an ethics of care presume that ethical reasoning is not only for "ethics emergencies" in health care decision making but is also to guide those involved in such decisions about how to act to strengthen relationships in daily clinical care. In this light, bioethics is concerned less with dramatic confrontations by "ethical dilemmas" and more with restoration and strengthening of bonds between professionals, patients, and families. Such bonds are necessary to shared decision making in ethical dilemmas. Principlism and caring, as ethical positions, share a common point of departure in their respect for persons and their autonomous choices. However, an ethics of caring emphasizes responsibilities to others and preserves the web of relations necessary for community. The principlist influence on the ethics of research arose at a time of great concern about protecting individuals from risks and dangers of research. Continuing this protective emphasis today can be criticized in pediatric populations when health care resources are scarce and many children are poor. Children are not empowered to enroll themselves. An ethics of caring compensates by supporting inclusion of children in research activities that have acceptable risks and that bring them within the margins of adequate health care.

HIV Infection and Rights in Health Care

An ethics of principles and rights is problematic because of the difficulty in establishing health care as a basic right in this society. A national commission studying access to health care in 1983 preferred to use a framework of the "societal obligation" to secure adequate access rather than argue that health care is a right (16). There are several proposals to reform the delivery of basic health care services to the American people. Embedded in the debate about these proposals is the question of whether health care will be considered a right or an interest. The distinction between concepts of patient interests and patient rights tends to be blurred. Rights are justified claims upon others or society for action due a person or group of people simply because of their membership in a group. Claims of rights, however, are often an attempt by a minority to establish a nonmoral good as so important that is must be granted status as a right for the few who have interests. Few people are eligible for organ transplantation, and it is not a basic right of a citizen. Should organ transplantation be seen as an actionable right or a gift to the needy patient that is not a mandated resource but a luxury that society can occasionally grant? Clearly, HIV-infected persons have interests in treatment, but claims to a right to treatment are debatable.

Health care rights in this society are vague and often are specified only in relationship to one's access to medical care payment plans. Such access is negotiated usually at the local level, and one's rights hinge on the limits of an employer's negotiations with insurance carriers. Health care interests are just as nebulous and often develop only in relationship to one's state of health. Historically, AIDS activists have argued that the interests of seropositive people should be defined as the basic right to access such goods as research drugs. AIDS has exposed the wide differences in access to basic health care that are tolerated in this society. Addressing these inequities requires an understanding of adequate access to health care not only as a right due individuals but as the care due all members of a community where health is among the greatest goods. It makes little sense to claim a right to health care without the reality of commitment and the means to act upon such claims.

CONTEXTUAL FACTORS IN ETHICS OF PEDIATRIC HIV DISEASE
Pediatric HIV as a Unique Chronic Illness

Care of the child with a chronic illness is recognized as a task with special imperatives. Whether the affliction is genetic, as in cystic fibrosis, or possibly curable, as in an oncological disease, tenets of pediatric care demand recognition of the special personhood of the child that is dependent on his or her developmental stage and how the illness impacts the growth process through which all children proceed.

General ethical concepts that pediatric health care providers consider when engaged in chronic pediatric care include 1) respect for parental involvement in caretaking and treatment decisions (17); 2) protection of confidentiality of patients and families (17); 3) respect for the moral authority of parents to accept or refuse experimental treament for their children does not apply to refusals of proven treatments, based on religious or other reasons, that would be harmful to withhold from children (17).

Additionally, society considers chronic illness in children to be of such a burden to the family that added provisions are made for the care of the ill child that imply added ethical considerations. Specifically, the care of chronic illnesses is considered to be so complex that health care specialties develop around the individual disease, such as juvenile-onset diabetes mellitus. Society mandates guaranteed access to these specialists treating the illness.

Pediatric HIV poses special challenges as a chronic illness for several reasons. It is a communicable disease with deadly consequences. Like juvenile-onset diabetes, treatment at this time is palliative, but the life span of children afflicted with HIV appears much shorter than that of diabetic children. And unlike other pediatric chronic illnesses, the population infected is predominantly minority families with limited financial and health care resources. (Table 37.1).

Special Factors in Pediatric HIV Illness

Adults who are infected with HIV tend to have progression to AIDS with a median time of 8–10 years. The progression of pediatric HIV disease is more rapid than in adults, with most children developing symptoms within the first two years of life.

All children born to seropositive women will be at least transiently seropositive themselves. The inability to distinguish these temporarily seropositive but uninfected children from those who are seropositive and are truly infected presents a major

Table 37.1.   Contextual Issues in Pediatric HIV Ethics

Theoretical Concepts
Patient interests vs. patient rights
Communal interests vs. societal investment
Individualism vs. community
Operational Concepts
Transmission factors
Seropositivity status
Ability of patient to participate in decisions
Needs of patient re counseling, therapy, prevention
Available resources in research and clinical care
Age of child and developmental status
Family status and abilities of caretakers

problem in early diagnosis and management. This problem may be ameliorated by the availability of several specific virus sensitive diagnostic tests (e.g., virus culture, polymerase chain reaction, P24 antigen assay) that may permit diagnosis of truly infected infants within the first months of life. Treating the symptomatic seropositive infant requires a commitment to research drug protocols that are ethically straight forward, in the attempt to bring some relief for an ill child. Treating the asymptomatic or seropositive infant whose infection status is undetermined raises large ethical questions.

Another factor in ethical analysis of children with HIV is that data continue to mount indicating that in the United States a child's status in a minority race or economically deprived group directly affects his or her chances of being born to a seropositive mother. Rates of generational transmission in minority populations are remarkably consistent: African-American and Hispanic children represented 85% of vertically transmitted AIDS in 1992 (18) and constitute 84% of this exposure group in this country in 1993 (19).

Families of these minority populations are typically poor, with little or no health insurance, and because of the disease in the adults in the family, care of the children may be compromised. Indeed, a significant number of seropositive children do not live in the homes of their birth parents. Because the best interests of the child involve living in an intact family that responds to the needs of the child, absence of such a protective system places the child in a very vulnerable position, one that demands that society occasionally assume the parental role in some fashion (Table 37.2).

Table 37.2.   Primary Ethical Issues in Pediatric HIV

Methods of surveillance
Counseling parents on options
  (including the pregnant woman)
Decision making about investigational drugs
Effects of involvement on clinical care
Involvement of children in foster care in
  clinical research
Confidentiality and disclosure issues
Rights and obligations of providers

PREBIRTH ISSUES

Counseling the Woman Who Is of Childbearing Age about HIV

Two primary ethical issues arise related to HIV when women of childbearing age enter the obstetrical setting. The first involves surveillance policies for HIV in pregnancy. The second concerns how counseling should be conducted with seropositive women about their options if pregnant.

Ethics of HIV Antibody Testing in Pregnancy

Should HIV testing in the obstetrical setting be compulsory? The alternative is to offer it to each pregnant woman. Testing that is compulsory, defined as done without either the permission or sometimes the knowledge of the woman, can also be blinded or "unlinked" so that the results are not traceable to those tested. Although strong utilitarian arguments can and have been made for the value of epidemiologic data compiled from such methods, obtaining data about a disease with such significance for the individual donor without prior notification violates the position that communal interests ought not to be furthered by abusing the rights of individuals (20). Therefore, as the epidemic has expanded, and retroviral therapy and other supportive care measures become important for the health of the woman and infant, recommendations to offer HIV testing to all pregnant women are deemed reasonable.

Some obstetrical settings may mandate total compulsory HIV screening of their patients under the guise of staff protection or to obtain further health data on the women. This is often done in conjunction with the many blood tests collected from women in pregnancy. However, the practice of universal precautions would seem to preclude the need-to-know argument for compulsory testing. The argument for caretaker knowledge of HIV status to better care for the pregnant woman may be more justified but only with some analysis.

Pregnancy is not defined as a potentiator of HIV disease in the seropositive woman, but the status of her HIV disease may necessitate therapy. The knowledge of serum status is an aid to the current care of the pregnant women to that of planning for the care of the woman and infant. We discuss later treatment and research options in seropositive pregnant women. Suffice to say such care requires involvement of the woman in the decision about care, and therefore universal anonymous and compulsory testing must be eliminated as a routine part of screening in childbearing women for the lack of benefit it offers either party in this setting.

Having eliminated testing that is not consented to by all women in the obstetrical setting, what of selective, anonymous testing based on risk factors? It can be argued that strong epidemiologic data have identified those women in certain geographic, racial, and demographic groups that are at high risk for HIV seropositivity (21). Screening women by acknowledged risk factors has failed to identify nearly half of those who are infected. As heterosexual transmission continues to increase, pregnancy can be used to define a woman who has had unprotected sex and who might be at risk of infection. Accordingly, HIV testing should be offered to pregnant women.

Women at risk for HIV live in worlds that can be quite unsupportive. Partners may still be injecting drugs, and physical abuse may exist that forces the woman to continue a life-style that further exposes her to HIV. The health care system can be a lifeline to such persons to access services that can help them escape some unhealthy risk factors through education and other services. By not soliciting consent from women at risk for HIV on a selective basis, health care professionals may increase the feelings of discrimination many people feel about the health care system, and they will not attempt to enter the system at a time when health care is essential. An optimal approach is to offer HIV testing and counseling to every woman of childbearing age. If this cannot be achieved, HIV testing and counseling should certainly be offered to each pregnant woman as part of the informed consent process of voluntary testing.

Directive and Nondirective Counseling

What ought to be done when a pregnant woman is found to be seropositive? It has been noted that the seropositive woman in our society has been an object of scorn, rather than of compassion (22). Along these lines of contempt, the seropositive woman who becomes pregnant may face derision about her decision about whether to continue her pregnancy.

Health care providers obviously must show extreme respect for any decision made by a seropositive woman about her childbearing options. At issue is whether providers should show preferences for either option in counseling, since refraining from bearing children is an absolute means of avoiding the transmission of the virus to another generation and a morally desirable goal.

In any ethical theory it is immoral to cause harm to others that is unjustifiable. Although there is some commentary in ethics and law that knowingly to transmit harm (by genetic means) to children ought to carry moral blame and legal penalties, this view has little effect on actual practice (23). Bearing children in circumstances in which there is a probable risk of harm has not been widely regarded as morally blameworthy or legally proscribed in this society. Genetics counselors in many nations have widely adopted a "nondirective" criterion for their work with pregnant patients before and after prenatal diagnosis. Their position is that education about the disorder, the options posed, and discussion with the woman (or couple) about their choices in the light of their own values is the preferred practice (24). If society permits parents with a genetic risk as high as 50% or even more to enjoy reproductive freedom, it is difficult to find ethical grounds to conduct a different approach to counseling HIV-infected pregnant women.

The range of transmission rates from seropositive women to their offspring is in the range of ~25% (25). What moral burden does this place upon the seropositive woman contemplating pregnancy and motherhood? It means that she must fully consider the hardships she assumes with the decision. These include rearing a child, possibly a chronically sick one, while she herself is ill. She must become informed about the modes of treatment available for herself and her planned child. Most importantly, she must consider her own mortality and decide how her child will be raised when she becomes incapacitated or dies.

These concerns occur in the lives of many parents and impose various burdens. Nolan (26) has argued that the autonomy of the woman in any circumstance should not be a paramount moral factor in the decision to bear children if she does not consider the prospective child's best interests. Such a position is difficult to apply to the seropositive woman, for it is not apparent in our society that any other women are held to this ethical standard.

Care of Seropositive Pregnant Woman and Her Unborn Child

Inclusion of the Seropositive Woman in Investigational Drug Trials: An Ethical Decision?

Three issues deserve attention under this topic. Should pregnancy itself exclude a seropositive woman from entering an early clinical trial involving drugs to treat her own HIV disease? Second, should unborn and newborn infants who are nonsymptomatic be enrolled into clinical research trials (or be treated with) anti-HIV drugs? Finally, are placebo controlled trials ethically justified in nonsymptomatic populations enrolled in HIV clinical research?

Minkoff and Moreno (27) argued in 1990 that the availability of HIV agents, specifically pentamidine prophylaxis, ought to be made known to pregnant women who were infected with HIV, asymptomatic, and whose CD4 counts would warrant prophylaxis. At the time, they discussed azidothmidine (AZT) but did not recommend that it be presented as an option in the informed consent process. Out of respect for autonomous choices of women, investigators ought not regard pregnancy as an exclusionary factor for informed consent. The decision to recommend drugs on or off trial to a seropositive pregnant woman depends on considerations for her own condition, in a context in which considerations of potential effects for the fetus are also revealed. The most dependable source of caring for the fetus' interest is also the pregnant woman.

A current clinical trial (28) that involves administration of AZT or placebo to pregnant women and their children pre- and postnatally offers AZT to asymptomatic women with CD4 counts of >200. Participation cannot begin before 14 weeks of gestation or after 34 weeks. The purpose of the trial is to study whether AZT prevents transmission of HIV from mother to fetus or infant. The consent document makes two statements regarding benefits to the HIV-infected woman who receives AZT and whose CD4 count is between 200 and 500: 1) that she may benefit from the trial, because of the action of AZT in slowing the replication of HIV in infected adults and 2) that she and her baby may not benefit directly from the study. Daily doses of AZT (500 mg daily to the mother and intravenous doses during labor until the umbilical cord is clamped) are recommended. A complex message regarding unknowns and potential benefit or nonbenefit to the HIV-infected woman is involved in this trial that focuses primarily on prevention of vertical transmission from mother to child. Without significant attention in the consent process, this message could easily be misunderstood or mislead.

The administration of AZT to unborn infants posed difficult ethical issues that were addressed both in a review by the Food and Drug Administration and the Office of Protection from Research Risks of the National Institutes of Health. It was feared that AZT carried risks of fetal bone marrow suppression and possibly other harms. Two encouraging reports have appeared while the trial continues. One, required by Office of Protection from Research Risks, resulted from data from the first 30 mother-infant pairs to complete the trial. No differences in adverse events were found in either arm of the trial (P. Stratton, personal communication, 1992). In a second, Sperling and others (29) reported on a survey of AZT use in 43 pregnant women, 24 of whom took it for two trimesters. They found AZT well tolerated in the women, not associated with fetal malformations or hematologic toxicity, but possibly linked to anemia and growth retardation in a few infants.

Ethics of Methodologies

The methodology of this placebo trial also raises ethical questions. Ethicists describe the use of placebo controlled trials as acceptable in HIV disease (30), but some questions remain about why this research design to study the question of infant transmission was chosen. From an analytical standpoint, the efficacy of the treatment will be determined by the incidence of infection in the infants. The variations in transmission rates preclude the ability to carry this type of study by using historical controls, although some have suggested this approach (31).

Promoting the autonomy of the mother provides the most robust case for this trial. Historically, excluding women from opportunities to be research subjects has prevented them from reaping the benefits that come from the increase in scientific knowledge about their health (32). However, from a care perspective, there is a danger that entering women into trials of dubious value will cause them to lose trust in the community of caretakers who are necessary to their health.

CARE OF SEROPOSITIVE CHILDREN FROM BIRTH THROUGH LIFE SPAN OF CHILD

Surveillance

From an ethical perspective, the results of any use of data obtained from a research subject must be accessible to that person if such information would contribute to his or her health. Indisputably, knowledge of HIV antibody status could have a significant impact on a person's health. However, it is evident that some maternal transmission surveillance data that HIV epidemiologists use have been obtained through unlinked testing of infants whose parents were not notified that the testing was being done. The results could not be related to patient and therefore were not available to these parents (31).

Other surveillance studies have limited the scope of their investigations and provide parents with diagnostic findings and the offer of follow-up studies. The Woman-Infant Transmission Study is a multicenter, National Institutes of Health-sponsored surveillance study that enrolls seropositive women during pregnancy, follows them through the pregnancy, and then asks to test the infant for HIV and follow seropositive children. The goal is to collect data on transmission and progression of HIV in pregnant women and seropositive infants.

Surveillance studies of any type must meet several criteria to meet standards of ethical propriety. A baseline consideration is that the information be scientifically useful. Another factor is that such studies must serve to directly help both those screened and society at large by protecting citizens from the spread of the screened disease. Finally the integrity of the individual tested must be protected not only by involving them in the decision to be tested, but by also protecting their privacy.

Surveillance studies may, on occasion, perform weakly on the point of maintaining confidentiality. Isaacman (33) has indicated that many maternal transmission studies routinely violate the spirit of laws intended to protect patients' privacy by releasing personal information linked to serum status to disparate domains of epidemiological researchers. One of us (JGT) has reported that even in the Woman-Infant Transmission Study program, there is a concern that too many people even well-meaning clinicians have access to the identities of subjects and the privacy of the seropositive families is jeopardized (31).

In summary, any surveillance studies must have as their first goal to provide useful information for those tested. Parents who are to be tested must be counseled about the reasons for testing and how results will be shared and what follow-up services are available. Similar conditions should be included in the proposals for neonatal surveillance. The mandatory precondition for any surveillance should be subject/parental consent and the right to refuse.

Parental Involvement and Paternal Professionals

It has been observed that when children with HIV enter the health care sphere the authority of parents was questioned regarding their ability to make the health care choices (31). Sometimes the parents' abilities to adequately care for their ill children was challenged (31). Should enrolling a child in an HIV clinical care setting cause a parent to be measured by a higher standard when parenting skills are assessed? Because much of the treatment of seropositive children occurs in conjunction with clinical research these areas of concern will be discussed concomitantly with the ethics of research in pediatric HIV drug investigations.

Treatment and Research

Because of the nature of HIV in the pediatric population, defining the numbers of afflicted children as well as addressing the problem of treatment, is crucial (34). Probably the most confounding phenomenon is that the natural progression of the disease is variable in individual children so that it makes predictive intervention strategies somewhat presumptive. It means that clinicians and researchers must deal with the questions of when and whom to treat. Guidelines for medical management of antiretroviral therapy have recently been reported by a consensus group sponsored by the National HIV Resource Center (35).

Autonomy and Pediatric HIV Research

The moral framework of informed consent for children built around parental responsibility and rights has weaknesses when applied to pediatric HIV research. Parents may be absent, ill themselves, or simply assumed to be incompetent to give informed consent.

In families in which the children are cared for by their birth parents the informed consent process seems to work well to educate parents about the nature of clinical research and its differences in goals with clinical care. This situation is likely due to the efforts of the research teams during the consent process and the oversight of the Institutional Review Boards that must approve consent forms. However one specific issue that remains is who should give consent when birth parents are absent and the child is in foster care (see Chapter 49). The current practice in most study sites is for the research teams to negotiate with the local agency and the foster or adoptive parents charged with the responsibility for caring for the child to allow the child to enter into a research protocol.

There are several drawbacks to this system, for foster parents may be excluded from this process, eliminating those individuals that are most involved in the child's care. Additionally, regulations are often written to require the foster agency to search for absent but still living birth parents to get their signatures on consent forms. This process does little to promote the involvement of caregivers in the consent process and may serve only to delay entry of seropositive children into necessary protocols.

Risk-Benefit Assessment in Pediatric HIV Research

Because of the major morbidities seen in children with HIV, it would seem that a higher degree of risk would be justified in research with infected children. Currently, virus culture or polymerase chain reaction can establish the diagnosis of HIV infection in 95–100% of infected infants by the time they are 3–6 months old. Nonetheless, the decision not to investigate in this age group when the diagnosis is unclear means that the significant number of asymptomatic children who progress to have AIDS and deteriorate quickly may suffer from lack of clinical drug and diagnostic knowledge.

Another ethical issue regarding risks and benefits has been the decision, in the past, by some investigators to use placebo controls in trials with children with HIV (36). Because these trials are phase III trials involving drugs that were believed to have some efficacy in the treatment of HIV, some commentators have claimed that administration of a placebo to symptomatic children placed them at risk because of the withholding of a possibly therapeutic drug for the sake of fastidious methodology (31).

Justice Issues and Pediatric HIV

Because of the added burden of poverty and belonging to racial minority groups, most children with HIV may be placed in positions of vulnerability that recruited into trials. Several specific justice issues have stood out in pediatric HIV trials.

One large trial included in its informed consent procedure the incentive that enrollment would guarantee that the subjects would receive better care from the clinician-investigators (36). The implication was that nonenrollment would mean that resultant care would be suboptimal. Such a message can be powerfully coercive for poor parents seeking treatment for their child. Current pediatric AIDS clinical treatment units that specialize in HIV research usually construct systems of inter-related care and research so that parents can refuse a research protocol and not have to face leaving the HIV health care organization. This approach is to be supported and encouraged.

A significant question of equity arises regarding access of foster children into research protocols. A significant number of people involved in pediatric HIV research were interviewed and stated that their local child protective agencies required that researchers attest to benefits of investigational drugs before children would be allowed to enroll in the proposed studies (31). Although this requisite worked well when applied to an acutely ill child who was judged in need of a "salvage" therapy, it often excluded mildly ill children who were needed to fill the samples of protocols investigating outcomes such as efficacy and safety. Perhaps allowing consent regulations to include inputs of foster caretakers will provide for more equitable recruitment of seropositive children who are not in the care of their birth parents.

SPECIAL ISSUES
Developmental Issues
Entrance into School and Day Care

The early days of the HIV pandemic saw much confusion and cruelty directed toward people with HIV, including children. Although educational efforts have increased the sensitivity of society toward seropositive people, it is still apparent that ignorance about factors such as transmission exist and that resultant discrimination can hamper the family with HIV as it attempts to live a meaningful life.

Entry into school or day care represents a significant step in the developmental growth of any child, well or ill. The stimulation provided in such settings as Head Start can provide essential elements to the seropositive child's neurodevelopmental status and overall happiness. School attendance also symbolizes to parents that their child is progressing in life and that his or her existence consists of more than visits to the doctor and blood sticks. Therefore care must be taken to see that protocol visits and medication administrations do not pose more than minimal disruptions to the child's participation in these normal daily childhood activities.

Additionally, pediatric health care providers with seropositive patients can provide guidance to teachers and day care providers who seek to learn more about HIV disease in children and who are responsible for writing guidelines about allowing chronically ill children in the classroom setting (see chapter 48). Such efforts serve to strengthen the rights of seropositive children to participate in the normal developmental events in a child's life.

Disclosure Issues

The classroom represents one of the early areas where families must face the issue of sharing the seropositive child's diagnosis with outsiders. Several factors deserve discussion on this topic that has ethical impact on children's rights and parental responsibility.

First, there are some restrictions placed on foster parents' abilities to share the diagnosis of their wards to outsiders, such as teachers. Child protective agencies with overall responsibility for the seropositive child should be consulted to find out how much information foster parents can share.

Another consideration is how much information about a child's condition must be shared with outsiders? The concept of a nonfamily member's need to know about a child centers on how much disclosure of seropositivity will aid the person to help the child and how it will enable the person to protect him or herself. The former consideration must be left to the parent, for few people outside the health care sphere can claim to add to the health of the child if they are privy to the diagnosis. Parents are the best judge of what church elder, teacher, or community member may help the family with emotional support. The latter issue is moot if educators learn to use universal precautions around body waste and fluids.

The asymptomatic seropositive child probably will stand out little from his or her schoolmates. Exceptions to nondisclosure may include parents sharing the diagnosis with teachers when their toddler tends to bite or if a child's condition will necessitate frequent disruptions in daily classroom activities. Parents should be counseled by health care providers to question any agency that mandates unconditional disclosure of HIV status of their children, for the necessity of such a requirement is dubious.

A more recent enigma that is challenging parents and the health care providers involves the right of the child to know his or her HIV infection status. Several health care providers have described that as survivors of early childhood HIV disease enter late school age and early adolescence, they quite normally develop more interest in the etiology of their illness (31). An anecdote told to one of the authors described how one seropositive school aged child compared the news reports that he heard about Magic Johnson testing HIV positive and asked his mother if he had the same illness as Magic. The mother refused to reveal his diagnosis, explaining to his research nurse that she feared he would despair and give up hope if he knew he had HIV.

Fletcher et al. (17) summarized the arguments for and against disclosure of diagnosis of cancer to children and concludes that the usual ethical imperative urges the inclusion of the child in early meetings with parents to discuss diagnosis and treatment. Inclusion helps to reinforce the child's developing personhood and prepares them to assume more responsibility for their illness as they grow. This position assumes particular importance as the adolescent matures sexually and begins to engage in behaviors that might endanger partners.

There are several counterarguments to disclosure. One parental concern could be that a younger seropositive child with knowledge of the diagnosis may share this information with outsiders and thereby make him or her and the family targets of discrimination. Other parents could believe that their symptomatic son or daughter may be so close to the end of their life that such information is not useful to the child. Although this is bleak and may signal the health care provider that the parents are projecting their emotions onto the child, maintaining the integrity of the family may mean that sharing of the child's seropositive status might have to be a slow process as the child becomes more aware of his or her condition gradually.

Rights and Obligations of Providers

The HIV pandemic has caused some reconsideration of the ethical imperatives and status accorded to individuals given their membership in the health care professions. Examinations of professional codes and discussions among groups of physicians, nurses, and others involved in the care of people with HIV reveal that although arguments can be made that professional status does not legally mandate that one care for seropositive people, the needs of such an ill population require strong moral commitments to care, rather than withdraw (37).

The traditional pediatric juxtaposition of providers to children places the health care professional in a special relation. Pediatricians, nurses, physical therapists, and others assume a paternalistic role with their patients. In the special case of pediatric HIV, with the frequent family dysfunction that providers see, this substitute parental role becomes especially poignant.

Furthermore, the cadre of professionals who are specially equipped to care for seropositive children comes from several small subspecialties, such as pediatric infectious disease and hematology/oncology. Therefore limits exist on the numbers of capable people to care for these children.

Ethical rights and responsibilities of individuals in this area of health care are probably best described from the caring perspective. Such a viewpoint emphasizes the relationships that develop between professionals, parents, and children and deemphasizes principles such as autonomy and justice that often can seem to oppose each other, such as when protection of the child seems incompatible with enrollment in research protocols.

The caring ethic stresses interdependence. It recognizes that although children have no inherent right to investigational drugs, it is in society's interest to provide resources to develop such drugs. This validates the decisions of physicians and nurses who devote their careers to such research. Although principled ethics tend to obscure the moral tie between caretakers and researchers, the caring ethic embraces the concept of the combination of both in pediatric HIV care, for separation of the two would lead to such fragmentation of inquiry and care as to make either meaningless.

Just as the interests of families with HIV have been accepted by society as substantial enough to commit resources such as research money, this commitment must be made also to the researchers and caretakers who have devoted their careers to seropositive children. Researchers have described inordinate pressure to produce results, and they feel that this may compromise the quality of their efforts by influencing enrollment procedures. Realization by granting agencies that the pediatric HIV research program is necessarily tied into care and labors under unique constraints may decrease such pressure.

CONCLUSION

The HIV epidemic has strained the traditional bioethical theoretical framework by forcing examination of old questions from new perspectives. This has resulted in a reconsideration of the dominant status once accorded principle-based approaches in bioethics. These approaches are being supplemented with ethical reflection based upon caring and other virtue-oriented concepts to enrich the moral analysis of the care of HIV-seropositive children.

Any such analysis must recognize the special factors of pediatric HIV. These involve transmission modes, the natural history of pediatric HIV, and the conundrums it poses for caretakers and researchers. Of particular concern must be the special status of children with HIV who most often come from disadvantaged groups in our society and must be accorded special protection as they are involved in care and research.

References

1. Volberding, PA, Lagakos SW, Koch MA, et al. Zidovudine in asymptomatic human immunodeficiency virus infection: A controlled trial in persons with fewer than 500 CD4-positive cells per cubic millimeter. N Engl J Med 1990;322:941–949.
2. Gibb D, Newell M. HIV infection in children. Arch Dis Child 1992;67:138–141.
3. Schoeman F. AIDS and privacy. In: Reamer F, ed. AIDS and ethics. New York: Columbia University Press, 1991:240–276.
4. Fost N. Ethical issues in pediatric AIDS. In: Pizzo P, Wilfert C, eds. Pediatric AIDS: The challenge of HIV infection in infants, children, and adolescents, Baltimore: Williams & Wilkins, 1991: 595–604.
5. Beauchamp T, Childress J. Principles of biomedical ethics. 3rd ed. New York: Oxford University Press, 1989.
6. Sider R, Clements CD. The new medical ethics: A second opinion. Arch Intern Med 1985;145: 2169–2173.
7. Clauser KD, Gert B. A critique of principlism. J Med Philos 1990;15:219–236.
8. National Commission for the Protection of Human Subjects of Biomedical and Behavioral Research. Research involving children: Report and recommendations. (DHEW (OS)77–0004 Appendix, DHEW (OS) 77–0005), Washington DC: US Government Printing Office, 1977.
9. National Commission for the Protection of Human Subjects of Biomedical and Behavioral Research. Belmont report: Ethical principles and guidelines for the protection of human subjects of research. (DHEW (OS) 78–0012 Appendix I, DHEW (OS) 78–0013, Appendix II, DHEW 78–0014), Washington DC: US Government Printing Office, 1978.
10. Department of Health and Human Services. Basic HHS policy for protection of human research subjects. Fed Register 1983a;48(46), Mar 8: §46.101–§46.124.
11. Anonymous. Code for nurses with interpretive statements. Kansas City, MO: American Nurse's Association, 1985.
12. American Medical Association Council on Ethical and Judicial Affairs, Current Opinions, Chicago: American Medical Association, 1986.
13. National Society of Genetic Counselors Code of Ethics. J Genet Counselling 1992;1:1.
14. Baier A. Hume, the women's moral theorist? In: Kittay E, Meyers D, eds. Women and moral theory. Savage, MD: Rowman & Littlefield, 1987:37–55.
15. Gilligan C. In a different voice. Cambridge: Harvard University Press, 1982.
16. President's Commission for the Study of Ethical Problems in Medicine and Biomedical and Behavioral Research. Securing access to health care. Washington DC: US Government Printing Office, 1983.
17. Fletcher JC, van Eys J, Dorn L. Ethical considerations in pediatric oncology. In: Pizzo P, Poplack G, eds. Practices and principles in pediatric oncology. 2nd ed. Philadelphia: JB Lippincott, 1993: 1179–1191.

18. Centers for Disease Control. HIV/AIDS Surveillance Report. 1992;Jul:1–18.

19. Centers for Disease Control. HIV/AIDS Surveillance Report. 1993;May:1–19.

20. Bayer R. AIDS public health and civil liberties: Consensus and conflict in policy. In: Reamer F, ed. AIDS and ethics. New York: Columbia University Press, 1991:26–49.

21. Gwinn M, Pappaionou M, George J, et al. Prevalence of HIV infection on childbearing women in the United States: Surveillance using newborn blood samples. JAMA 1991;265:1704–1708.

22. Shayne V, Kaplan B. Double victims: Poor women and AIDS. Women Health 1991;17:21–37.

23. Shaw M. Preconception and prenatal torts. In: Milunsky A, Annas GJ, ed. Genetics and the law. 2nd ed. New York: Plenum,1980:225–232.

24. Wertz DC, Fletcher JC. An international survey of attitudes of medical geneticists toward mass screening and access to results. Public Health Rep 1989;104:35–44.

25. Bremer J, Hollinger F. Pediatric HIV infection and AIDS: Diagnostic tests. Semin Pediatr Infect Dis 1990;1:27–30.

26. Nolan K. Ethical issues in caring for pregnant women and newborns at risk for human immunodeficiency virus infection. Semin Perinatol 1989;13:55–65.

27. Minkoff HL, Moreno JD. Drug prophylaxis for human immunodeficiency virus infected pregnant women: Ethical considerations. Am J Obstet Gynecol 1990;163:1111–1114.

28. AIDS Clinical Trials Group 076. A phase III randomized placebo-controlled trial to evaluate the efficacy, safety and tolerance of zidovudine for the prevention of maternal-fetal HIV transmission.

Bethesda, MD: National Institute of Allergy and Infectious Diseases, 1992.

29. Sperling RS, Stratton P, O'Sullivan MJ, et al. A survey of zidovudine use in pregnant women with human immunodeficiency virs infection. N Engl J Med 1992;326:857–861.

30. Levine C, Dubler N, Levine R. Building a new consensus: Ethical principles and policies for clinical research on HIV/AIDS. IRB Rev Human Subjects Res 1991;13:1–17.

31. Twomey J. Pediatric HIV infection and clinical research ethics, [Thesis] Charlottesville: University of Virginia, 1992.

32. Levine C. Women and HIV/AIDS research: The barriers to equity. IRB Rev Human Subjects Res 1991;13:18–22.

33. Isaacman S. Neonatal HIV testing: Governmental inspection of the baby factory. John Marshall Law Rev 1991;24:571–624.

34. Oxtoby M. Perinatally acquired HIV infection. In: Pizzo P, Wilfert C, eds. Pediatric Aids: The challenge of HIV infection in infants, children, and adolescents, Baltimore: Williams & Wilkins, 1991:3–21.

35. Working Group on Antiretroviral Therapy; National Pediatric HIV Resource Center, Antiretroviral therapy and medical management of the human immunodeficiency virus-infected child. Pediatric Infect Dis J 1993;12:513–522.

36. Anonymous. Clinical trial of the efficacy of intravenous gamma-globulin in the treatment of symptomatic children infected with human immunodeficiency virus. Bethesda, MD: National Institute of Child Health and Human Development, 1988.

37. Zuger A. AIDS and the obligations of health care professionals. In: Reamer F, ed. AIDS and ethics. New York: Columbia University Press, 1991:215–276.

Medical Management and Care of Newborns and Infants Born to HIV-seropositive Mothers

Andrea Kovacs and James Oleske

Since 1985, essentially all new cases of human immunodeficiency virus (HIV) infection among infants and children have been perinatally acquired. Because the mothers of these infants are also infected, it is imperative for the clinician to have a basic understanding of those issues related to maternal HIV infection that impact mother to infant transmission and timing of infection, because these in turn affect early diagnosis, treatment, and daily management of the infant. This chapter will briefly review the impact of the changing epidemiology of perinatal HIV infection on care of the infant and will discuss diagnostic dilemmas encountered in newborns exposed to HIV and the surrogate immune markers that are used in anticipating clinical progression in infants that become HIV infected. Other laboratory evaluations, especially those that assess the presence of other congenital infections, will be briefly discussed. The major portion of this chapter will review the medical management of the newborn and infant at risk for HIV infection. Suggested guidelines were derived from a review of the literature as well as clinical experience and will include a discussion of prenatal care and its effect on the newborn, the immediate care of the newborn, and the care required for both infants of unknown HIV infection status as well as those with proven HIV infection. Prophylaxis of both common and opportunistic infections seen in HIV-infected infants, recommended immunization sched-

ules, supportive care (including nutritional assessment, intervention strategies, and pain management), antiretroviral therapy in infants, and nosocomial infections that threaten the health of HIV-infected infants are all considered. The applicability and limitation of these suggestions outside the United States will be summarized. We will try to place these clinical management suggestions into the context of the family caring for the HIV-infected infant and will suggest some challenges and questions that will require further study.

IMPACT OF CHANGING EPIDEMIOLOGY, TRANSMISSION AND NATURAL HISTORY OF PERINATAL HIV INFECTION ON MEDICAL MANAGEMENT AND CARE

Epidemiology

Since the initial descriptions of infants and children with symptoms similar to those described in adults with AIDS, the number of children thought to be infected with HIV has risen at an alarming rate worldwide. In the United States alone there have been more than 3500 case of AIDS among children, and it is estimated that at least 1800 perinatally infected infants are born each year (1, 2) Although the seroprevalence of HIV infection in women of childbearing age has been estimated to be 0.15% nationally in the United States, many inner cites with large intravenous drug using populations have rates of HIV infection among childbearing women as high 2–3% (2, 3). There has been an increase in HIV infection in rural areas as well. Thus, the identification and care of these mothers and infants will greatly impact the national health policy for children over several decades (4, 5).

Perinatal HIV Transmission

Studies evaluating the rates of transmission from mother to infant have varied throughout the world. Early studies from Africa reported mother to infant transmission rates as high as 40–60% (6). However, more recent studies from the United States and Europe have reported rates of transmission ranging from 12 to 30% of infants born to infected women (7–11). Women who are recently infected or those who have AIDS probably have higher virus loads, less HIV-specific immune responses, and as a result may have increased maternal to infant transmission (8, 9). Since the United States is earlier in the epidemic than Africa, there may be more asymptomatic HIV-infected women becoming pregnant. As more women with AIDS deliver babies, an increase in the transmission rate may be seen in the United States and Europe.

Although there is very little information concerning the mechanism of maternal to infant transmission, it appears that HIV infection can occur in utero, at delivery, and through breast feeding (12–18). A recent study demonstrates that there is an increased incidence of HIV infection in the firstborn of twins as well as discordant infection among twins (18). Factors that affect the timing of infection and rates of infection among newborn infants are unknown. There are conflicting reports as to the importance of maternal neutralizing antibodies to the hypervariable region of the major envelope protein gpl20 of HIV (19–22). Other factors such as maternal immune status and coinfections with other agents may impact maternal virus load or cause a disruption in the placental barrier (8, 9). Although complete information is unavailable, the timing of infection most probably affects infant outcome. Those infected early in pregnancy may have severely impaired immunity and high virus load at birth, with other organ involvement such as the brain. Those infected late in pregnancy or at birth would probably be asymptomatic with a stable immune system at birth and into the first year of life.

Natural History of Perinatal HIV

Most cases of pediatric AIDS have been reported in the first 24 months of life with a large peak in the first 6 months of life representing HIV infected infants with early onset of *Pneumocystis carinii* pneumonia (PCP) (10, 23–30). Infants and children with HIV infection progress more rapidly than adults. However, prospective natural history and epidemiologic studies have shown that the progression to AIDS among infants and children infected perinatally with HIV is indeed quite variable (10, 24, 26–27). Current information suggests that 80% of HIV-infected infants have some symptoms before one year of age, and 17–30% have rapidly progressive disease with the development of AIDS before the age of one year (10, 23–27). Many older children with HIV infection are now being identified, and some cohorts report that most infected children are still alive at age 6 years (27). Over the last 2 years there have been great strides in the development of new diagnostic techniques for early identification of infected infants and new prophylactic and treatment modalities resulting in improved quality of life and a prolonged life span for infants and children.

DILEMMAS IN DIAGNOSIS OF HIV INFECTION IN INFANTS BORN TO INFECTED WOMEN THAT AFFECT MANAGEMENT AND CARE
Screening for HIV

The first step in the early diagnosis of HIV infection is to identify those who are at risk. Although universal testing and counseling for HIV infection of pregnant women or their infants is unavailable nationally, it is recommended by AIDS specialists in the field of pediatrics and obstetrics. Since many unidentified infected women and their newborns or their older infected infants will manifest signs of HIV infection in the years to come, both obstetricians and pediatricians must be aware of the relative prevalence of HIV infection in their community and the signs and symptoms of HIV infection in women and their infants and children. It has become imperative to encourage HIV testing and counseling of pregnant women or newborns in areas of high HIV prevalence because prophylaxis for infections and new treatment modalities are available that can alter the course of disease and prolong survival (31). Pediatricians and obstetricians must be aware that although women using drugs are the largest at risk group of women on a national basis, there is also a dramatic increase in HIV infection among women infected through heterosexual contact. In fact, substance abusing women are also at risk for HIV infection from heterosexual activity, although they may be repeated as a consequence of drug abuse. Indeed, many HIV infected women are unaware that they are infected and claim no risk factors (32).

CDC Diagnostic Criteria

The diagnosis of HIV infection in infants born to infected women has been difficult. Infants were diagnosed to be HIV infected only when symptomatic with a constellation of symptoms or as outlined by the Centers for Disease Control (CDC) (see Chapter 12) and/or wlth persistently positive HIV specific antibody in a child older than 15 months with culture (33, 34). However, over the last few years there have been tremendous advances in the early diagnosis of HIV infection. By using a combination of laboratory tests listed in Table 38.1, it is now possible to identify the majority of infected children before age 6 months (11, 12, 35–62). In areas of the country where the prevalence of HIV infection is high the clinician must include HIV in the differential diagnosis and workup of many infants or children. Table 38.2 lists those children who should be offered HIV testing, and Figure 38.1 outlines the steps to be taken in the workup of a child suspected to have HIV infection.

Physical Signs and Symptoms of Perinatal HIV Infection

Along with laboratory evaluations careful longitudinal evaluation of the infant with a thorough physical exam can lead to the pre-

Table 38.1.   Laboratory Diagnosis of HIV

Definitive diagnosis
  ELISA with Western blot in child aged >18 months
  Culture positive
  PCR positive
  P24 antigen positive
  IgA antibody detectable
  In vitro antibody production
Highly suspicious with positive ELISA and Western blot in infant or child aged <18 months
  Reduced CD4 count
  Increased CD8 count
  Reduced CD4-to-CD8 ratio
  Hypergammaglobulinemia
  Hypogammaglobulinemia
  Diminished lymphocyte proliferative response to mitogens and antigens
  Anemia
  Thrombocytopenia
  Leukopenia
  High globulin fraction
  Low albumin
  Increased alanine amino transferase, aspartate amino transferase
  Proteinuria

sumptive diagnosis of HIV infection. Special attention must be focused on early clinical signs of HIV infection in the first year of life. Most HIV-infected children have very mild clinical abnormalities in the first few months of life (7, 10, 11, 27, 63–66). The earliest symptoms seen in the first 2–4 months of age that may indicate HIV infection are an increasing size of the liver and spleen, development of diffuse adenopathy, most notably in the axilla and groin, and oral candidiasis, which is resistant to standard therapy. Perhaps the most sensitive sign is the presence of splenomegaly because this would not routinely be seen in uninfected children. However, one must remember that other congenital and perinatal infections such as cytomegalovirus (CMV), toxoplasmosis, or syphilis may also present with signs and symptoms similar to HIV. After 3–6 months of age, children may show signs of developmental delays and poor weight gain and growth. Some infants and children may present with sepsis, meningitis, pneumonia, frequent and unusual bacterial infections, abscesses, or nonspecific rashes. Newborns who are severely immunocompromised may present with sig-

Table 38.2. Children Who Should Be Tested

HIV-positive mother
Mother with risk factor (drug use, prostitution, multiple sex partners, husband or partner with risk factor, transfusion before 1985 in United States or anytime in developing country, or artificial insemination)
Mother symptomatic
High prevalence area: all newborns and women
Infant or child with following signs or symptoms in high prevalence area (1/1000 HIV-infected pregnant women)
    Any AIDS indicator disease
    Suspected congenital infection (toxoplasmosis, syphilis, CMV)
    Hepatomegaly, splenomegaly
    Axillary and inguinal adenopathy
    Massive or diffuse adenopathy
    Unusual tumors
    Chronic sinusitis or otitis
    Development delay, speech delay
    Spasticity or unusual neurologic findings
    Failure to thrive
    Petechiae
    Positive tuberculin test or active tuberculosis
    Recurrent, severe, or unusual infections
    Sepsis with unusual organisms
    Chronic interstitial pneumonia
    Cardiomyopathy of unknown etiology
    Recurrent pneumonia
    Persistent oral *Candida*
    Recurrent oral gingivostomatitis
    Severe varicella or recurrent varicella
    Congenital syphilis
    Chronic diarrhea
    Parotitis
    Clubbing
    Recurrent or unusual skin rashes
    Night sweats
    Recurrent fever
    Renal disease of unknown etiology

nificant AIDS defining infections in the first few months of life, supporting the observation of in utero infection (10, 27).

HIV Serology

Infants born to HIV infected women have passively acquired maternal IgG antibody. Thus, the standard diagnostic technique using enzyme-linked immunosorbent assay (ELISA) to detect HIV specific antibody followed by Western blot can only be useful if done sequentially in the first 2 years of life (65). At birth the western blot of the infant is generally identical to the mothers. Infants who are infected will usually remain positive to Western blot but may show changing banding patterns over the first year of life. Those who are uninfected will gradually lose maternal antibody, which on Western blot is seen as a gradual disappearance of bands. Although 75% of uninfected infants born to infected women will lose maternal antibody by 12 months of age (67), it has been estimated that 10% of uninfected infants born to infected women will lose antibody after 15 months and 2% after 18 months (10). Infected infants will begin making their own antibody and will thus remain antibody positive. Some infected infants will not mount an immune response and will be antibody negative despite HIV infection (7, 35, 68). However, these children are usually symptomatic and have other immunologic abnormalities. Because most IgG is actively transported through the placenta after 28–32 weeks gestational age, there may be low or no maternal HIV spe-

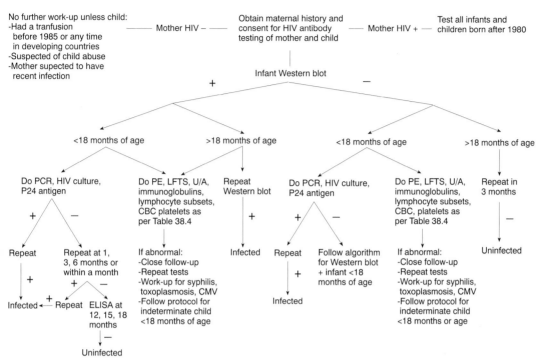

Figure 38.1. Assessment of infants suspected to have HIV infection. PE, physical exam; LFTS, liver function tests; U/A, urinalysis; CBC, complete blood count.

cific IgG present when some premature infants born before the third trimester are later tested. Thus, one must remember that they may actually be infected with a negative ELISA.

Since maternal IgG confounds early diagnosis in the infant, many groups have sought to identify HIV specific antibody made by the infant. Neither IgM nor IgA cross the placenta. IgM assays have lacked sensitivity; however, several groups have developed sensitive assays to detect HIV specific IgA antibody (58–60). Although this test has a sensitivity and specificity of >95% after 3–6 months of life, IgA assays have had variable sensitivity in the first few months (49, 52, 58, 59). Another method of detecting infant antibody is in vitro antibody production assays (57, 61, 62). These methods utilize the infant lymphocytes that are cultured and observed for specific HIV antibody production by Western blot or ELISA. Alternatively, lymphocytes stimulated to produce HIV specific antibodies will form plaques that can be detected in the ELISPOT assay (69, 70). Since infants who are infected at birth may not produce anti-body for weeks to months, these assays will undoubtedly be less sensitive than those that detect virus or viral genome. In addition, these in vitro antibody assays are not readily available.

HIV Detection Assays (HIV Culture, P-24 Antigen, and Polymerase Reaction)

Definitive diagnosis of HIV infection is based on isolation of the virus, virus protein or antigen, or virus genome. The timing of HIV infection, whether in utero or at birth, may affect the sensitivity of each test in the first 6 months of life. Those infected in utero may be identified at birth or in the first month of life by the tests that either isolate virus or virus genome, whereas those infected at birth may only show evidence of infection several weeks or months after delivery depending on the initial infecting virus load. Thus the need for prospective evaluations of infants and repeated testing is paramount.

Culture for HIV has been the gold standard for laboratory diagnosis of HIV infection. Over the last few years the sensitivity and specificity of culture in infants by the age of 6 months has approached 100% (40, 46, 53, 11). However, in the first 6 months of life sensitivity has varied with reports of 38–50% at birth and increasing thereafter (46, 53). The standard p24 antigen has been shown to be less sensitive than culture with a sensitivity of ~20% at birth increasing to 50% at 2 months and >80% after that (46, 53, 54). A recent modification using acid hydrolysis has been reported to greatly increase sensitivity (45, 48, 50, 55). There is, however, the potential for false positive results at birth or in the first few days of life because of passive transfer of maternal p24 antigen but not virus. Further studies are needed to verify these initial promising results. Since this test is relatively inexpensive and easily performed with minimal technology, it is useful in combination with the other tests and may be important for the developing world.

The most sensitive test reported to date is the polymerase chain reaction (PCR) (35–44, 47, 51–53, 56). By using PCR, proviral DNA extracted from white cells or RNA from plasma can be amplified a million-to a billion-fold, thus making it possible to detect HIV infection even with low virus load. PCR has been reported to be more sensitive than p24 antigen detection, and results are more rapidly available than culture. Sensitivity ranges from 40 to 55% at birth and rapidly increases to >95% (37, 44, 47, 51–53, 56). Because of the high sensitivity and specificity even in the first 6 months of life and the rapidity of performing the test, PCR will most probably become the test of choice for the diagnosis of HIV infection in infants as standardized commercially available kits are marketed (36).

Other Laboratory Tests Appropriate in Infants Born to HIV-infected Women

Evaluation of routine laboratory tests, such as complete blood counts, chemistry panel, and urinalysis, may reveal leukopenia, anemia, thrombocytopenia, elevated transaminase or proteinuria (27, 71, 72). Although these nonspecific findings can also be seen in HIV-uninfected children who may have other congenital or perinatal infections such as CMV, toxoplasmosis, or syphilis, they may be useful to alert the physician that the child may be infected with HIV.

IMMUNE SURROGATE MARKERS IN HIV-INFECTED INFANTS THAT INFLUENCE MEDICAL MANAGEMENT AND CARE

Although immunologic evaluations are not diagnostic for HIV infection, they are useful as guidelines for differentiating children who are at risk for HIV infection and its complicating infections from those who are uninfected. Although children have been found to have various immunologic abnormalities, the most useful laboratory tests for diagnosing and evaluating immunodeficiency in an infant or child suspected to be HIV infected are immunoglobulin levels and CD4 counts (10, 11, 28, 63, 73–81). One of the earliest clues for HIV infection could be seen on a routine chemistry panel that may show an increased globulin fraction. Although hypogammaglobulinemia has been reported in some very ill children, most have hypergammaglobulinemia, with extremely high levels of IgG, IgM, and especially IgA (10, 27, 68).

Children with HIV infection have been shown to have decreased CD4 lymphocyte numbers as well as percent of total lymphocytes and CD4 to CD8 ratios (10, 28, 73, 75–77, 79). These values decline as illness progresses (73, 77, 79). Healthy children younger than 6 years have significantly higher lymphocytes and CD4 numbers than adults with levels decreasing with age (Fig. 38.2) (74). Infants with PCP and other opportunistic infections have been shown to have significantly reduced CD4 numbers when compared with age appropriate values obtained in uninfected children born to infected women or serorevertors (79) (Table 38.3) or normal children born to HIV negative women. Children who serorevert have significantly higher CD4 numbers than those who are infected or have AIDS. Those who are younger than 1 year and have CD4 counts that are below 1500 cell/mm³ are more likely to develop PCP and other AIDS defining conditions (73, 79). Although there is some overlap in CD4 numbers in infected and uninfected children born to infected

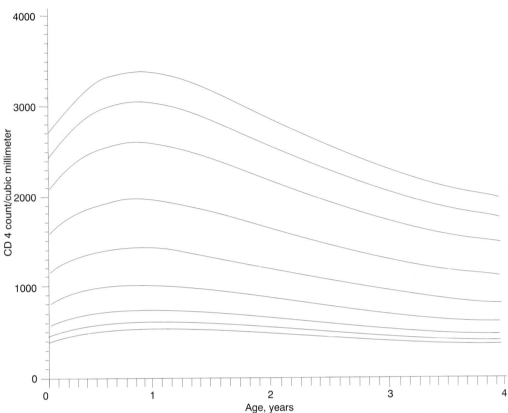

Figure 38.2. CD4 lymphocyte counts for uninfected children born to HIV-1-infected women. Adapted from European Collaborative Study. Age-related standards for T lymphocyte subsets based on uninfected children born to human immunodeficiency virus 1-infected women. Pediatr Infect Dis J 1992;11:1018–1026.

Table 38.3. CD4 Lymphocyte Count by Age and Classification of Pediatric HIV Surveillance Population in Los Angeles County from June 1982 through June 1990[a]

CDC Classification Group	Total	≤1 yr		13 mo-4 yr		>4 yr	
		n	CD4	n	CD4	n	CD4
P-2 (total 170)							
PCP	39	20	702 ± 615	4	156 ± 98	15	104 ± 100
Other AIDS[b]	39	8	847 ± 934	19	636 ± 657	12	207 ± 279
Not AIDS	92	4	2643 ± 1186	25	1017 ± 635	63	512 ± 443
P-1	31	6	2796 ± 753	4	1699 ± 1076	21	831 ± 518
P-0	33	30	3147 ± 1679	3	2725 ± 949		
Seroreverters	32	8	3719 ± 1776	24	2673 ± 1492		
Total	266	76	2267 ± 1757	79	1484 ± 1334	111	484 ± 469
P^c			<0.0001		<0.0001		<0.0001

[a]Values are means ± SD. Adapted from Ref. 73.
[b]Pulmonary and esophageal *Candida*, CMV, lymphoid interstitial pneumonia, encephalopathy, and bacterial infections.
[c]Overall analysis of variance F test for each age group.

women, rarely do unifected infants younger than 1 year have CD4 counts below 1500 cell/mm³ (78). After 1 year of age, the discepancy between CD4 counts in uninfected and infected children becomes larger.

MEDICAL MANAGEMENT AND CARE OF INFANT SUSPECTED OF HIV INFECTION
Prenatal Care Issues

Universal counseling and offering of HIV testing is now recommended as standard of care for all pregnant women and their infants. However, since this has not yet been implemented , if a pregnant woman is in a known high risk area or has indicated that she may be at risk for HIV infection because of high risk practices by herself or her spouse, (intravenous drug use, prostitution, multiple sex partners, transfusion before 1985 in the United States or at any time in a developing country, or artificial insemination or a transplantation before routine HIV testing) she should be encouraged to have HIV testing (31, 82, 83) for her benefit and for the care of the infant. If found to have antibody to HIV she should be considered infected and at risk to transmit the infection to her newborn infant. If the mother refuses HIV testing or has no prenatal care, testing should be requested for the newborn infant. Although, a positive HIV test by standard techniques should identify the majority of infected women, there has been the rare report of newly infected women who are transiently seronegative but can transmit HIV to the newborn infant (84). Since there would be no maternal transmission of HIV specific antibody the infant would be seronegative as well. If there is strong suspicion of HIV infection, repeat testing should be performed in 6 weeks to 3 months. If available more definitive testing, such as culture or PCR, should be performed.

Because many HIV-infected women are also infected with CMV, herpes simplex 2 virus (HSV), toxoplasmosis, hepatitis B and C, tuberculosis, and syphilis, they should be screened for these conditions as well. In high prevalence areas for perinatal HIV infection, tremendous increases in congenital syphilis have been observed. Although there is no information about the relative trans-mission rates of these infections to their newborn infants, there is theoretical concern that severely immunocompromised pregnant women may reactivate latent infections or transmit newly acquired organisms at a higer rate to their infants. Thus, it is important for the pediatrician to know the maternal stage of HIV disease and infection status for each opportunistic infection that may potentially infect the child.

Many HIV-infected women who are receiving various prophylactic and treatment modalities will become pregnant. Current recommendations are to consider treating HIV-infected women with zidovudine when CD4 counts drop below 500/mm³ and to give PCP prophylaxis with CD4 counts below 200/mm³ (85–87). For pregnant women who have CD4 counts that are between 200 and 500 cells/mm³ the risks and benefits of antiretroviral therapy should be discussed before therapy because of the effect on the fetus. Although the effect of trimethoprim-sulfamethoxazole (TMP/SMX) on the newborn infant is well known, there is less experience with zidovudine or other antiretrovirals (86). Preliminary studies in infants of mothers who received zidovudine indicate that there are no adverse effects on the infant. However, anemia and growth retardation noted in a few infants may have resulted from maternal zidovudine use (86). Medications for other maternal infections such as toxoplasmosis, *Mycobacterium avium-intracellulare*, *M. tuberculosis* (MTb), and CMV may have profound effects on the developing infant. The long-term impact of any or all of these on infected and uninfected infants is unknown. Nevertheless, when the mother's health requires these medications the indirect benefit to the fetus outweighs the risks. Thus the infant born to a woman who received antiretrovirals or other medications must be monitored closely for the first few years of life.

There is no consistent information to indicate that infant outcome is affected by mode of delivery. However, any invasive technique that could cause a break in the skin, such as scalp monitoring, fetal blood sampling, forceps, or suction may potentially increase the risk of transmission and should be avoided.

Immediate Care of Newborn Infant

Most HIV-infected infants are asymptomatic at birth, although infants born to drug using women may be jittery and irritable. However, there is a small group of infants that may present with HIV related symptoms and/or immunologic and hematologic abnormalities within the first few days of life. Rarely an infant may present with thrombocytopenia, anemia, and leukopenia. Some groups have noted an increased incidence of prematurity or low birth weight among infants born to HIV-infected women that may be related to drug use but can add the problems of prematurity to the infant's management (88, 89). Since premature rupture of membranes has been reported to occur frequently, infants may be at increased risk for sepsis in the newborn period (88). One group in the Bronx noted a four-fold increase in HIV seroprevalence among infants in the neonatal nursery when compared to the hospital in general (89). Although not found in all studies, this study found that infected infants were more likely to be small for gestational age and microcephalic (89). Additionally, there is increased incidence of twinning among infants born to HIV-infected women. It must be kept in mind that there may be discordant infection between twins, with twin A reported to be more frequently infected (16). All infants born to HIV-infected women should have a thorough physical examination looking for hepatosplenomegaly, diffuse adenopathy, microcephaly, petechiae and other skin infections. The clinician must remember the potential for other congenital and perinatal infections, and evaluation and treatment for these must be instituted if suspected. Other evaluations are outlined in Table 38.4. The minority of infants who are symptomatic in the neonatal period will most probably have a rapidly progressive course and must be monitored extremely closely.

Before discharge the mother should be given explicit instructions about breast feeding (13, 14, 17). In the United States breast feeding is not recommended due to the potential for infection from breast milk. However, in developing countries breast feeding is encouraged where water supply is suspect and availability of formula unreliable since the infant may otherwise die from infection or malnutrition.

The mother and infant should be seen within the first month of life for a thorough evaluation and to strengthen the relationship with the family. She should be given instructions as to signs and symptoms that should prompt her to call or bring the child for evaluation.

Care of Infant of Unknown HIV Status

Care of the infant born to an infected mother will generally require a consultation with a pediatric HIV specialist, but primary care can be given by the pediatrician. Once an infant is known to be HIV positive but not yet diagnosed to be infected (CDC classification P-O), he or she must be followed very closely in the first 6 months of life. Table 38.4 outlines suggested evaluations in the first 2 years of life. Access and availability of appropriate laboratories may limit the application of these suggestion at some sites and for some children. Because it is difficult to diagnose HIV infection in infants younger than 6 months and because of the potential for rapidly progressive disease, we suggest visits at least at birth and 1, 2, 3, and 6 months and then at 3 month intervals if asymptomatic. Specific diagnosis for HIV should be performed one time in the first month of life as close to birth as possible and then at least at 3 and 6 months of age. This could include HIV culture, PCR, or p24 antigen determinations depending on the availability to the clinician. HIV culture or PCR are the most sensitive and should be used for definitive diagnosis in the first 6 months of life. If not available p24 antigen determinations can be used in an infant older than 1 month. A combination of these will most quickly identify an infected child. In an asymptomatic or mildly symptomatic infant or child we suggest at least two positive results of culture/PCR/p24 antigen before considering a child infected and informing the parents or beginning antiretroviral therapy. A second confirmatory test should be obtained within 1 month of receiving the first positive result. If the child has definitive clinical and immunologic evidence of HIV infection as outlined by the

Table 38.4. Suggested Clinical and Laboratory Evaluation for Infant or Child Younger Than 2 Years Born to HIV-infected Women[a]

Evaluation	Birth	1–2 wk	1 mo	2 mo	3 mo	4 mo	5 mo	6 mo	7 mo	8 mo	9 mo	10 mo	11 mo	12 mo	15 mo	18 mo	21 mo	24 mo
History, PE	X	X	X	X	X	X	X	X	[b]		X			X	X	X	X	X
Developmental assessment	X	X	X	X		X		X			X			X	X	X	X	X
Height, Weight, HC	X	X	X	X		X		X			X			X	X	X	X	X
CBC platelets	X		X			X		X			X			X	X	X	X	X
Chemistry panel	X		X			X		X			X			X	X	X	X	X
Urinalysis	X		X			X		X			X			X	X	X	X	X
Immunoglobulins	X					X		X			X			X	X	X	X	X
ELISA/Western blot	X					X		X			X			X	X	X	X	X
Lymphocyte subsets	X		X			X		X			X			X	X	X	X	X
P24 antigen	X							X							X	X	X	X
HIV culture	X				X			X										
PCR	X				X			X										
CMV urine	X			X		X		X										
PPD control	Every 3–6 mo																	
Neurologic evaluation	CMV or toxoplasmosis																	
Ophthalmology evaluation	At 1–2 yr																	
Dental examination	Routinely at 2 yr or if indicated (i.e., speech delay or chronic otitis)																	
Audiology											X							
If mother positive or unknown																		
Hepatitis B serology	X																	
Syphilis serology	X[c]		X	X	X	X	X	X		X								
Toxoplasmosis (IgG, IgM)	X[b]		X	X	X	X	X	X				X		X	X			
For child infected or if clinically indicated																		
Chest X-ray	[d]																	
CT/MRI	[d]																	
Echo cardiogram	[d]																	
ECG	[d]																	

[a] PE, physical exam; HC, head circumference; CBC, complete blood count; CT, computed tomography; MRI, magnetic resource imaging; ECG, electrocardiogram.
[b] Every 3 mo after age 6 mo.
[c] If positive.
[d] Baseline, then if clinically indicated.

CDC, he or she can be considered presumptively infected with one culture or PCR or p24 antigen test. Appropriate HIV care including antiretroviral therapy can be instituted while awaiting confirmatory results. Since false-positive laboratory tests have been seen in the best of laboratories and mislabeling of specimens occurs, it is suggested that a repeat test be obtained. For the infant who has repeatedly negative results in the first 6 months of life he or she is most probably not infected. However, he or she should have a repeat Western blot at 12, 18, and 24 months of age before being definitively called a seroreverter.

Lymphocyte subsets should be obtained at 1, 2, and 6 months of age. Because some infected children can show a rapid drop in CD4 numbers in the first few months of life more frequent determinations may be necessary. If found to be stable they can be monitored every 3 months until age 2 years or until the child is found to be truly uninfected by culture, or PCR or has seroconverted to HIV antibody negative by ELISA. If an asymptomatic child seroconverts and has negative HIV specific diagnostic tests with normal immunologic workup and is older than 18 months he or she can be presumed to be uninfected. However, these children should be continued to be followed at 6-month intervals until 2 years of age and then at least yearly because of rare reports of infants found to be HIV infected after age 18 months despite repeated antibody testing or culture. This is important since the long term impact of maternal HIV infection on the uninfected infant is unknown. Additionally, infants of women who received antiretrovirals or other medications during pregnancy must be monitored for long term toxicity.

All HIV exposed infants should be evaluated for other infections. Since congenital toxoplasmosis has a grave prognosis in this population any child whose mother has antibody to toxoplasmosis should have an evaluation for congenital toxoplasmosis, especially if the mother has CD4 counts of <200 cells/mm³ (90). Because of the difficulty in the diagnosis of toxoplasmosis in the neonate, repeated serological evaluations for IgG and IgM antibodies are indicated. Similarly, if the mother has a history of ac-tive syphilis that was either untreated or inadequately treated, the infant must be evaluated and treated for possible congenital syphilis (91).

Presumptive PCP Prophylaxis

The CDC has outlined recommendations for PCP prophylaxis based on CD4 counts (see Chapter 21) (92). Any infant aged 1–11 months who has been found to have a CD4 count below 1500 cells/mm³, 12–23 months with CD4 count below 750/mm³, 24 months–5 years with CD4 count below 500/mm³, and >5 years with CD4 count below 200/mm³ should receive PCP prophylaxis. A repeat CD4 count should be obtained in 1 month and if still below the age appropriate cutpoint the child should remain on PCP prophylaxis until a definitive diagnosis of HIV infection is made. Since uninfected children rarely have CD4 counts this low, very few uninfected children will actually receive prophylaxis (79).

Immunization Schedule

Routine immunizations should be given to all HIV-positive children at the schedules outlined in Chapter 46 (93, 94). It is recommended that all children testing HIV positive receive inactivated polio vaccine and not live vaccine because of the theoretical possibility of vaccine associated polio both in the child and other HIV-infected persons. No household contacts should receive live oral polio vaccine. Because children born to HIV-infected women have been shown to develop early measles with severe symptoms it is important that all children receive their immunizations (95) (see Chapter 46). Children found to be infected should also be immunized with influenza vaccine at 1 year of age and then yearly thereafter. They should receive pneumococcal vaccine at 2 years of age (see Chapter 46). Any child who is unimmunized or thought to be unresponsive to immunization and is exposed to measles or varicella should receive immunoprophylaxis.

Care of Infant of Known HIV Status

Once children are known to be infected they must be monitored closely for their entire lives. Since HIV is a multisystem disease involving not only the immune system but every other system, the care and evaluation of an infected child should be performed by a physician with experience in HIV disease who has access to subspecialists. Table 38.5 outlines signs and symptoms and organ involvement and the most common AIDS indicator diseases that should prompt the involvement of a specialist in infants and children younger than 2 years. If a child is identified to be infected as a result of presenting clinical signs he or she should have all the baseline workup recommended for the child described earlier of unknown or of indeterminate status (Table 38.4). Also recommended is a baseline electrocardiogram, echocardiogram of the heart, and chest X-ray. These would then be repeated when clinically indicated.

Primary HIV-specific management includes antiretroviral therapy, specific antimicrobial prophylaxis for opportunistic infections, and aggressive supportive care. General supportive care includes case management with its components of psychosocial support, patient/family education and advocacy, as well as developmental intervention, nutritional supplementation, and pain management.

Prophylaxis of Opportunistic Infections

Prophylaxis of opportunistic and common infections in the HIV-infected infant is usually limited to those infectious agents to which a newborn or infant (younger than 2 years) is likely to be exposed. The treatment of specific complicating opportunistic infections is covered in Chapters 16, 17, 20–22. Since opportunistic infections in the HIV-infected infant are more likely to be a primary rather than a reactivated infection, as in adults, such infections have a graver prognosis. Thus, both primary and secondary prophylaxis becomes important. The following infectious agents merit consideration for prophylaxis in certain clinical situations.

The HIV-infected infant with depressed immune function and with severe recurrent bacterial and viral infections that would not be expected to occur in a child with normal humoral immunity should be considered for intravenous immunoglobulin prophylaxis (96–98). Infants may fail to make measles antibody after two immunizations. They should receive γ–globulin after a known exposure to measles, and if measles is endemic, they should be considered for monthly IVIG. A child exposed to measles should also receive immune serum globulin if the last dose of intravenous γ-globulin was given 2 weeks before the exposure. In addition, infants with thrombocytopenia (platelets <20,000) may benefit from intravenous γ-globulin in combination with antiretroviral therapy.

As previously discussed, PCP requires prophylaxis based on age adjusted CD4 counts and after treatment of PCP. TMP/SMX is recommended as first line therapy followed by dapsone. Although less optimal, prophylaxis with monthly infusions of intravenous pentamidine has been suggested as well (90). *M. tuberculosis* has become a major threat to infants from households with adult HIV-infected individuals who are at increasing risk of *M. tuberculosis*. All exposed infants should have an intermediate strength purified protein derivative and anergy panel skin testing. Infants younger than 2 years with a positive PPD with a negative chest X-ray should be given 9–12 months isoniazid (99). Some clinicians may initiate prophylactic therapy with a course of isoniazid even in those cases with a negative PPD. The treatment of multiply drug resistant tuberculosis is more complicated and is discussed in Chapter 16A. Children with CD4 counts below 100 cells/mm^3 are at risk for *M. avium intracellulare* infection (101) (see Chapter 16B). There is preliminary evidence that rifabutin may be an effective prophylaxis agent. The use of rifabutin in infants at risk of *M. avium* infection is currently being evaluated. Infants who have had *Candida* esophagitis or who have recurrent treatment resistant thrush may need long term prophylaxis with either oral imidazoles (3 times/week) or daily topical antifungal creams or suspensions. There have been a small number of HIV-infected children reported to have toxoplasmosis (90). In such circumstances the infant should be treated with pyrimethamine and sulfadiazine plus folinic acid. Some pediatric infectious dis-

Table 38.5.   Signs and Symptoms and Organ System Involvement in HIV-infected Infants and Children That May Need Further Evaluation and Subspeciality Involvement

General
  Night sweats
  Severe fatigue
  Recurrent fevers
  Weight loss
  Poor weight gain
  Poor growth
  Sepsis or bacteremia
  Diffuse or massive adenopathy
  Unusual abscesses
Central nervous system
  Developmental delay
  Hyperreflexia
  Hypertonicity
  Speech delay and learning disabilities
  Spasticity, spastic paresis
  Loss of milestones
  Progressive encephalopathy
  Seizures
  Meningitis
  Central nervous system neoplasm
  Central nervous system toxoplasmosis
  Congenital CMV
  Syphilis
Eye
  Retinitis
  Toxoplasmosis
  CMV
Dental
  Severe dental caries
  Delayed dentition
  Discoloration of teeth
Ears, nose, throat
  Recurrent herpes gingivostomatitis
  Recurrent and recalcitrant oral candidiasis
  Recurrent aphthous ulcers
  Continuous nasal discharge
  Chronic sinusitis
  Chronic otitis media
  Mastoiditis
  Parotid swelling, parotitis
Skin and nails
  Exzematoid rashes
  Chronic superficial fungal infections of
    skin and nails
  Severe cradle cap
  Unusual rashes
  Petechiae
  Severe molluscum contagiosum
  Severe warts
  Severe varicella

Severe and atypical measles rash
Severe and recurrent zoster
Clubbing
Gastrointestinal tract
  Hepatosplenomegaly
  Hepatitis: HIV, CMV, hepatitis B and C
  Colitis
  Recurrent diarrhea
  Severe and prolonged diarrhea: bacterial,
    protozoal, and viral (*Cryptosporidia, Isopora
    belli, Salmonella, Shigella, Giardia,*
    rotavirus, adenovirus, *C. difficile*)
Hematologic
  Anemia
  Thrombocytopenia
  Lymphopenia
  Thrombocytosis
  Neutropenia
Cardiac
  Tachycardia
  Congenital heart disease (?)
  Arrhythmias
  Pericarditis
  Myocarditis
  Endocarditis
Renal
  Proteinuria
  Hematuria
  Nephritis
  Frequent urinary tract infections
  Nephrotic syndrome
Pulmonary
  Persistent cough
  Tachypnea
  Hypoxia
  Wheezing
  Frequent pneumonias
  Atypical pneumonias
  Tuberculosis
  Chronic bronchitis
  Interstitial pneumonia
Most common AIDS indicator diseases in infants
  and children younger than 2 years
  PCP
  Frequent bacterial infections
  Lymphocytic interstitial pneumonitis
  Candida esophagitis
  Disseminated CMV infection
  Encephalopathy
  Candida of lung and bronchi

ease specialists have given a few HIV-infected infants with symptomatic recurrent mucocutaneous HSV or recurrent cutaneous disseminated varicella (after a treatment course with intravenous acyclovir) an oral prophylaxis regimen of acyclovir 3 to 5 times/week (100a,b). Children with CMV retinitis may need chronic suppressive therapy with gancyclovir or foscarnat. There does not appear to be any agent suitable for prophylaxis of *Cryptosporidium* or other parasitic gastrointestinal infections.

Nosocomial Infections in HIV-infected Infants

There are several other infectious agents that may be acquired in the community or as nosocomial infections from exposure in the hospital, outpatient clinic, or day care setting. They can have serious impact on the immunocompromised HIV-infected infant. These infections include respiratory syncytial virus *Parvovirus* B-19, hepatitis B, papilloma virus, rotavirus, and other viruses causing diarrhea. Bacterial pathogens causing diarrhea are *Salmonella/Shigella, Campylobacter, Clostridium difficile*. Skin infections can be caused by tinea. It is suggested that when possible CMV negative or filtered blood be used in all HIV-infected infants who receive transfusions. Infants who require placement of indwelling catheters for venous access, medication administration, and parenteral feeding also can develop hospital or community acquired infections with *Candida* and other fungal infections, as well as methicillin resistant *Staphylococcus aureus*, coagulase negative staphylococci and gram-negative bacteria (102, 103). Control of these nosocomial infections requires diligence to establish infection control procedures and a constant awareness by the medical team of the risks faced by the HIV-infected infant under their care.

Neurological Evaluation

The infant may have evidence of growth failure or progressive neurologic abnormalities before immune deficiency is severe. In the first 2 years of life infants may present with subtle signs of involvement of the central nervous system with hyperreflexia, developmental delays, or delay in speech (104–108). A subgroup may suddenly develop rapidly progressive signs of HIV-associated encephalopathy with spasticity, pseudobulbar palsy, and seizures. This is generally seen in children with significantly reduced CD4 counts. These abnormalities should prompt further investigations in consultation with a neurologist. A computed tomography or magnetic resonance imaging scan, a lumbar puncture, and an evaluation for central nervous system opportunistic infections should be instituted (see Chapters 24 and 35).

Antiretroviral Therapy

Currently it is advised that any child with symptomatic HIV infection or with significantly reduced CD4 counts for age should receive zidovudine (see Chapter 35). HIV-infected infants who have CD4 counts below 1750 cells/mm^3 at <12 months of age, below 1000 cells/mm^3 at 13–24 months, below 750 cell/mm^3 at 2–6 years, and below 500 cells/mm^3 in those older than 6 years have significantly reduced CD4 counts when compared with normal healthy children and with uninfected children born to infected women and should receive antiretroviral therapy or be considered for clinical treatment trials.

Only two antiretrovirals have been approved for use in children. Zidovudine is considered the treatment of choice for initial therapy of children infected with HIV. Dideoxyinosine has been approved for children who have experienced severe toxicities to zidovudine or have had progressive disease after zidovudine treatment. Children treated with zidovudine have shown a stabilization of CD4 counts, improved cognition and stabilization of neurologic disease, weight gain, and increased life span (109–112). Toxicities that require regular monitoring include anemia and neutropenia. Children who receive dideoxyinosine should be monitored for pancreatitis, peripheral neuropathy, and peripheral retinal pallor (113) (see Chapters 29 and 35).

Supportive Care

The supportive care provided to HIV-infected infants becomes more complicated as the primary HIV disease progresses. As the availability of antiretrovirals and new prophylactic regimes for opportunistic infection improves, the survival and longevity of even severely HIV-infected newborns and infants will improve. Thus, attention must be paid to supportive care that will have a significant impact on quality of life. Supportive medical services are best provided in the context of a case management team that has access to multiple subspecialistst and community resources. Several nonprimary HIV-specific interventions have been discussed including prophylaxis and neurodevelopmental assessment. We will conclude this chapter with a discussion of the importance of case management and psychosocial support services needed by families caring for the HIV-exposed newborn and the infant who becomes HIV infected. In this section we will address the important issues of nutritional assessment and intervention strategies as well as pain management.

Nutrition. During the first 6 months of life many HIV-infected children will have declining weight. This decline frequently precedes other HIV-associated clinical signs and is due to a decrease in muscle mass rather than body fat (114–116). HIV-infected children gain weight less well than uninfected children to seropositive mothers. Growth failure can be a marker for disease progression and can also serve as an indicator of therapeutic response (117, 118). HIV-infected infants have been shown to develop significant lactose intolerance compared with race matched uninfected infants. The documentation of malabsorption in HIV-infected infants by an abnormal D-xylose test usually indicates an enteric infection. In adults the time of death in AIDS patients has been directly related to loss of body cell mass and body weight. Indicators of malnutrition, body weight, and serum albumen closely correlate with time of death. Although such nutritional longitudinal data are just becoming available in children, it can be expected that malnutrition is important in the mortality and morbidity of perinatal HIV infection. Therefore, close nutritional evaluation including assessment of dietary intake, body composition, and laboratory markers of nutritional status should be part of routine care for HIV-infected infants. Aggressive nutritional intervention strategies must be implemented. In an infant that is not gaining weight despite receiving maximum calories, considerations should include the use of elemental diets, tube feeding, or parental alimentation if severe malabsorption is present. Those enteric infections known to be associated with HIV infection should be monitored by culture, smear, and, when necessary, biopsy. By introducing appropriate nutritional interventions early in the course of perinatal HIV infection, it may be possible to prevent malnutrition. The provision of adequate nutrition may help delay the progression of immunodeficiency and improve absorption of medication. The use of lactose-free and elemental diets in select HIV-infected infants may prove to be important therapeutic interventions that can modify the progression of HIV and improve quality of life.

Pain Management. The management of HIV infection and its complications results in considerable pain that is frequently undertreated. Such pain includes the acute and chronic pain related to the disease itself as well as pain from multiple diagnostic and therapeutic procedures and from toxicities to medications. If pain is suspected, the use of appropriate pain medications including aspirin, acetaminophen, codeine, morphine, and methadone should be initiated. All programs and physicians caring for HIV-infected infants should develop a pain assessment and management protocol. Nonpharmacological approachs to pain management (including relaxation, hypnosis, play therapy, visualization, and distraction) should be part of such protocols and applied especially for the pain related to procedures.

ADAPTATION OF RECOMMENDATION TO FOREIGN COUNTRIES

The suggestions for the medical management and care of the newborn and infant born to HIV-positive women as outlined in this chapter are not applicable to the developing world. As in the United States, most HIV-infected women and their children are poor with little access to prenatal and postnatal care. Although simple and relatively inexpensive, HIV serology is still not available in many areas of the world. HIV culture and PCR are unavailable in many parts of this country and will most likely not be available worldwide because of expense. The use of acid-dissociated P24 antigen may be more readily adapted and affordable for developing countries. CD4 count that is routinely available here is unavailable in many developing countries. Although dapsone and TMP/SMX are inexpensive and usually available, other antimicrobials useful in prophylaxis and antiretrovirals are generally not available.

CONCLUSION

Care of the child with HIV infection is complicated by the fact that it is most often a perinatal infectious disease. Health care providers must not only struggle with the diagnosis and medical management of this most complex of chronic diseases in the HIV-infected child but also respond to the overwhelming social problems that affect most of those families caring for these children, In general, families with HIV-infected children are extremely poor, with limited access and availability to health care and historically distrustful of our public health system. Frequently, the parents have had limited educational opportunities and difficulty in understanding the complexity of a disease that both they and their child have acquired. There are often cultural barriers to seeking and receiving health care by families with HIV who are multiracial and from varied ethnic backgrounds. The immediate problems of everyday life often are more consuming than the disease itself. In many cases, women are the single parent of an HIV-infected child, often without a job, sometimes homeless, and living with the psychosocial complications of drug use by themselves or their sexual partner. Families must deal with the uncertainty of the infection status of the newborn infant, and mothers must spend hours at the hospital seeing specialists for her child, while often neglecting her own medical needs. She must deal with issues of death and dying for both herself and her child often at an age when other young women are planning their futures. Thus, to successfully care for the infant born to infected women many services must be provided—legal advice, transportation, child care, respite care, hospice care, family counseling, and many other services (Figure 38.3). Many HIV-infected children require foster care, and providers must learn to deal with complicated confidentiality issues and guardianship. HIV is a multiorgan system disease, and it is essential for HIV are to be provided by a team of primary care providers, subspecialists, case managers, social workers, and psychologists. It is also essential to

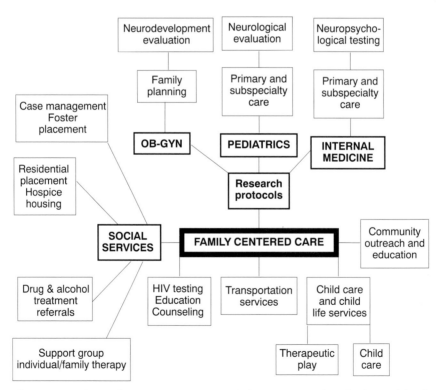

Figure 38.3.   Comprehensive services necessary for care. HIV-infected infant and family.

Table 38.6.   Team Members and Specialists Necessary for Care of HIV-infected Child

Team (to provide daily care)
   Infectious disease/immunology specialist
   Primary providers
   Social worker/case manager
   Nurses
Specialty to be consulted
   Neurology: every 3–6 mo and with developmental delays, microcephaly, and encephalopathy
   Neuropsychology/neurodevelopment: developmental delays
   Gastrointestinal tract nutrition: weight loss, chronic diarrhea, bloody stools, failure to thrive
   Ear, nose, throat: chronic otitis or sinusitis
   Ophthalmology: visual impairment
   Dental: severe dental caries
   Cardiology: cardiomyopathy
   Pulmonary: interstitial pneumonia, clubbing, recurrent pneumonia
   Renal: nephritis, nephrotic syndrome
   Dermatology: unusual skin rashes
   Physical therapy: encephalopathy
   Occupational therapy: encephalopathy
   Hearing and speech: speech delays

have strong ties to community organizations that can assist the families in providing services such as housing , food, clothing, and transportation. All of these are essential components in caring for a child born into a family with HIV infection.

FUTURE PERSPECTIVE

We have made great strides in the area of early diagnosis of HIV, but the availability of these tests must be established. To develop effective therapeutic strategies and vaccines, it is most important to have a better understanding of the timing of HIV infection. Current research is directed at determining the proportion of infants infected in utero compared with perinatally. Does the timing of infection explain why some children develop AIDS at 2 months and others are symptom free for 10 years? Should all infants be treated with antiretrovirals, or should only those who appear to have symptomatic progressive disease be treated? How many children are born with other congenital or perinatal infections, and how are such possible coinfections related to disease progression? Research should be directed at understanding the mechanism for the development and progression of central nervous system disease and the immunopathology of HIV infection in the neonate. Last, accurate markers for progression of disease are needed so that therapeutic modalities can be instituted before symptomatic disease.

References

1. Centers for Disease Control. Update: Acquired immunodeficiency syndrome—United States 1991. MMWR 1992;41:463–468.
2. Gwinn M, Pappaioanou M, George R, et al. Prevalence of HIV infection in childbearing women in the United States: Surveillance using newborn blood samples. JAMA 1991;265:1704–1708.
3. Novick LF, Berns D, Stricof R, et al. HIV seroprevalence in newborns in New York State. JAMA 1989;261:1745–1750.
4. Chu Sy, Buehler JW, Oxtoby MJ, et al. Impact of the HIV epidemic on mortality in children, United States. Pediatrics 1991; 87:806–810.
5. Chin J. Current and future dimensions of the HIV/AIDS pandemic in women and children. Lancet 1990;336:221–224.
6. Boylan L, Stein ZA. The epidemiology of HIV infection in children and their mothers-vertical transmission. Epidemiol Rev 1991;13:143–177.
7. Blanche S, Rouzioux C, Moscato MLG, et al. A prospective study of infants born to women seropositive for human immunodeficiency virus type 1. N Engl J Med 1989;320:1643–1648.
8. European Collaborative Study. Risk factors for mother-to-child transmission of HIV-1. Lancet 1992;339:1007–1012.
9. Ryder RW, Nsa W, Hassig SE, et al. Perinatal transmission of the human immunodeficiency virus type 1 to infants of seropositive women in Zaire. N Engl J Med 1989;320:1637–1642.
10. European Collaborative Study. Children born to women with HIV-1 infection: Natural history and risks of transmission. Lancet 1991;337:253–260.
11. Hutto C, Parks WP, Lai S, et al. A hospital-based prospective study of perinatal infection with

human immunodeficiency virus type 1. J Pediatr 1991;118:347–353.

12. Krivine A, Firtion G, Cao L, et al. HIV replication during the first weeks of life. Lancet 1992;339: 1187–1189.

13. Dunn DT, Newell ML, Ades AE, et al. Risk of HIV type 1 transmission through breastfeeding. Lancet 1992;340:585–588.

14. Ruff AJ, Halsey NA, Coberly J, et al. Breast-feeding and maternal-infant transmission of HIV type I. J Pediatr 1992;121:325–329.

15. Ehrnst A, Lindgren S, Dictor M, et al. HIV in pregnant women and their offspring: Evidence for late transmission. Lancet 1991;338:203–206.

16. Goedert JJ, Duliege AM, Amos C, et al. High risk of HIV-1 infection for first-born twins. Lancet 1991;338:1471–1457.

17. Van De Perre P, Simonon A, Msellati P, et al. Postnatal transmission of HIV type I from mother to infant: A prospective cohort study in Kigali, Rwanda. N Engl J Med 1991;325:593–598.

18. Lewis SH, Reynolds-Kohler C, Fox HE, Nelson JA. HIV-1 in trophoblastic and villous Hofbauer cells, and hematological precursors in eight-week fetuses. Lancet 1990;355:565–568.

19. Rossi P, Moschese V, Brodiden, PA et al. Presence of maternal antibodies to HIV-1 envelope glycoprotein gp-120 epitopes correlates with the uninfected status of children born to seropositive mothers. Proc Natl Acad Sci USA 1989;86:8055.

20. Goedert JJ, Mendez H, Drummond JE, et al. Mother-to-infant transmission of human immunodeficiency virus type 1: Association with prematurity or low anti-gp120. Lancet 1989;2:1351–1354.

21. Halsey NA, Markham R, Wahren D, et al. Lack of association between maternal antibodies to V3 loop peptide and maternal-infant HIV-1 transmission. J Acquir Immune Defic Syndr 1992;6: 153–157.

22. Parekh BS, Shaffer N, Pan CP, et al. Lack of correlation between maternal antibodies to V3 loop peptide of gp 120 and perinatal HIV-1 transmission. AIDS 1991;5:1179–1184.

23. Rogers MF, Thomas PA, Starcher ET, et al. AIDS in children: Report of the centers for disease control national surveillance, 1982 to 1985. Pediatrics 1987;79:1008–1014.

24. Scott GB, Hutto C, Makush RW, et al. Survival in children with perinatally acquired human immunodeficiency virus type 1 infection. N Engl J Med 1989;321:1791–1796.

25. Auger I, Thomas P, De Gruttola V, et al. Incubation periods for pediatrics AIDS patients. Nature 1988;336:575–577.

26. Blanche S, Tardieu M, Duliege AM, et al. Longitudinal study of 94 symptomatic infants with perinatally acquired human immunodeficiency virus infection. Am J Dis Child 1990; 144:1210–1215.

27. Tovo PA, De Martino M, Gabiano C, et al. Prognostic factors and survival in children with perinatal HIV-1 infection. Lancet 1992;339: 1249–1253.

28. Duliege AM, Messiah A, Blanche S, et al. National history of HIV type 1 infection in chil-

dren: Prognostic value of laboratory tests on the bimodal progression of the disease. Pediatr Infect Dis J 1992;11:630–635.

29. Krasinski K, Borkowsky W, Holzman RS. Prognosis of human immunodeficiency virus infection in children and adolescents. Pediatr Infect Dis J 1989;8:216–220.

30. Thomas P, Singh T, Williams R, et al. Trends in survival for children reported with maternally transmitted AIDS in New York City, 1982 to 1989. Pediatr Infect Dis J 1992;11:34–39.

31. Working Group on HIV Testing of Pregnant Women and Newborns. HIV infection, pregnant women, and newborns. JAMA 1990;264:2416–2417.

32. Lindsay ML, Peterson HB, Feng TI, et al. Routine antepartum human immunodeficiency virus infection screening in an inner-city population. Obstet Gynecol 1989;74:289–294.

33. Centers for Disease Control. Revision of the CDC surveillance case definition for acquired immunodeficiency syndrome. MMWR 1987:36:3S–9S.

34. Centers for Disease Control. Classification system for human immunodeficiency virus (HIV) infection in children under 13 years of age. MMWR 1987;36:225–253.

35. Rakusan TA, Parrott RH, Sever JL. Limitations in the laboratory diagnosis of vertically acquired HIV infection. J Acquir Immune Defic Syndr 1991;4:116–121.

36. Jackson JB, Ndugwa C, Mmiro F, et al. Non-isotopic polymerase chain reaction methods for the detection of HIV-1 in Ugandan mothers and infants. AIDS 1991;5:1463–1467.

37. Tudor-Williams G. Early diagnosis of vertically acquired HIV-1 infection. AIDS 1991;5:103–105.

38. Cassol SA, Lapointe N, Salas T, et al. Diagnosis of vertical HIV-1 transmission using the polymerase chain reaction and dried blood spot specimens. J Acquir Immune Defic Syndr 1992;5:113–119.

39. Comeau AM, Harris JA, McIntosh K, et al. Polymerase chain reaction in detecting HIV infection among seropositive infants: Relation to clinical status and age and to results of other assays. J Acquir Immune Defic Syndr 1992;5:271–277.

40. De Rossi A, Ades AE, Mammano F, et al. Antigen detection, virus culture, polymerase chain reaction and in vitro antibody production in the diagnosis of vertically transmitted HIV infection. AIDS 1991;5:15–20.

41. Petru A, Dunphy MG, Aximi P, et al. Reliability of polymerase chain reaction in the detection of human immunodeficiency virus infection in children. Pediatr Infect Dis J 1992;11:30–33.

42. Rogers MF, Ou CY, Rayfield M, et al. Use of polymerase chain reaction for early detection of the proviral sequences of human immunodeficiency virus in infants born to seropositive mothers. N Engl J Med 1989;320:1649–1654.

43. Krivin A, Yakudima A, Le May M, et al. A comparative study of virus isolation, polymerase chain reaction, and antigen detection in children of mothers infected with immunodeficiency virus. J Pediatr 1990;116:372–376.

44. Edwards JR, Ulrich PP, Weintrub PS, et al. Polymerase chain reaction compared with con-

current viral cultures for rapid identification of human immunodeficiency virus infection among high-risk infants and children. J Pediatr 1989;115:200–203.

45. Miles SA, Baldwin E, Magpantay L, et al. Early detection of HIV-1 infection in infants of seropositive mothers by acid dissociated HIV p24 antigen [Abstract TuB 0512]. Eighth International Conference on AIDS, Amsterdam, Jul 1992.

46. Burgard M, Rouzioux C, Blanche S, et al. 355 Viral cultures and antigenemia for the diagnosis of HIV infection in newborn: A three year experience [Abstract TuB 0511]. Eighth International Conference on AIDS, Amsterdam, Jul 1992.

47. Rakusan T, Sison A, Saxena E, et al. Detection and quantitation of HIV-I DNA in infants during the first two months of life [Abstract PoB 3661]. Eighth International Conference on AIDS, Amsterdam, Jul 1992.

48. Rich KC, Janda WM. Immune complex dissociated P24 antigen assay in infants and children of HIV infected women [Abstract PoB 3663]. Eighth International Conference on AIDS, Amsterdam, Jul 1992.

49. Kabagabo U, White C, Petru A, et al. Infants under 3 months of age produce detectable IgA specific antibody to HIV-I [Abstract PoA 2244]. Eighth International Conference on AIDS, Amsterdam, 1992.

50. Chandwani S, Moore T, Krasinski K, et al. Early diagnosis of HIV-I infected children by plasma P24 assay after immune complex dissociation [Abstract PoB 3633]. Eighth International Conference on AIDS, Amsterdam, Jul 1992.

51. Kovacs A, Xu J, Wong W, et al. Sensitivity of PCR by age in children [Abstract PoB 3700]. Eighth International Conference on AIDS, Amsterdam, Jul 1992.

52. Reuben JM, Bremer JW, Rosenblatt HM, et al. Diagnosis of HIV infection in early infancy: HIV culture, PCR, HIV+ specific IgA antibody [Abstract PoB 3648]. Eighth International Conference on AIDS, Amsterdam, Jul 1992.

53. Borkowsky W, Krasinski K, Polack H, et al. Early diagnosis of human immunodeficiency virus infection in children <6 months of age: Comparison of polymerase chain reaction, culture, and plasma antigen capture techniques. J Infect Dis 1992;166:616–619.

54. Andiman WA, Silva TJ, Shapiro ED, et al. Predictive value of the human immunodeficiency virus 1 antigen test in children born to infection mothers. Pediatr Infec Dis J 1992;11:436–440.

55. Palomba E, Gay V, Martio, MD, et al. Early diagnosis of human immunodeficiency virus infection in infants by detection of free and complexed p24 antigen. J Infect Dis 1992;165:394–395.

56. Comeau AM, Hsu HW, Schwerzler M, et al. Detection of HIV in specimens from newborn screening programs [Letter]. N Engl J Med 1992;326:1703.

57. Amadori A, De Rossi A, Chieco-Bianchi L, et al. Diagnosis of human immunodeficiency virus 1 infection in infants: In vitro production of virus-specific antibody in lymphocytes. Pediatr Infect Dis J 1990;9:26–30.

58. Quinn TC, Kline R, Halsey N, et al. Early diagnosis of perinatal HIV infection by detection of viral-specific IgA, antibodies. JAMA 1991;226:3439–3442.

59. Landesman S, Weibler B, Mendez H, et al. Clinical utility of HIV-IgA immunoblot assay in early diagnosis of perinatal HIV infection. JAMA 1991;266:3443–3446.

60. Weiblen BJ, Lee FK, Cooper ER, et al. Early diagnoses of HIV infection in infants by detection of IgA HIV antibodies. Lancet 1990;335:988–990.

61. Amadori A, Giaquinto C, Zacchello F, et al. In-vitro production of HIV-specific antibody in children at risk of AIDS. Lancet 1988;1:852–854.

62. Pahwa S, Chirmule N, Leombruno C, et al. In vitro synthesis of human immunodeficiency virus-specific antibodies in peripheral blood lymphocytes in infants. Proc Natl Acad Sci USA 1989;86:7532–7536.

63. Blanche S, Le Deist F, Fischer A, et al. Longitudinal study of 18 children with perinatal LAV/HTLV III infection: Attempt at prognostic evaluation. J Pediatr 1986;109:965–970.

64. Mayers MM, Davenny K, Schoenbaum EE, et al. A prospective study of infants of human immunodeficiency virus seropositive and seronegative women with a history of intravenous drug use or of intravenous drug using sex partners, in Bronx, New York City. Pediatrics 1991;88:1248–1256.

65. Johnson J, Nair P, Hines SE, et al. A natural history and serological diagnosis of infants born to human immunodeficiency virus-infected women. Am J Dis Child 1989;143:1147–1153.

66. Kamani N, Lightman H, Leiderman I, et al. Pediatric acquired immunodeficiency syndrome-related complex: Clinical and immunological features. Pediatr Infect Dis J 1988;7:383–388.

67. Mok JQ, De Rossi A, Ades AE, et al. Infants born to mothers seropositive for human immunodeficiency virus. Lancet 1987;1:1164–1168.

68. Borkowsky W, Paul D, Bebenroth D, et al. HIV infections in infants negative for anti-HIV by enzyme-linked immunoassay. Lancet 1987;1:1168–1171.

69. Nesheim S, Lee F, Sawyer M, et al. Diagnosis of human immunodeficiency virus infection by enzyme-linked immunospot assays in prospectively followed cohort of infants of human immunodeficiency virus-seropositive women. Pediatr Infect Dis J 1992;11:635–639.

70. Lee FK, Nahmias AJ, Lowery S, et al. Elispot: A new approach to studying the dynamics of virus-immunosystem intersection for diagnosis and monitoring of HIV infection. AIDS Res Hum Retroviruses 1989;5:517–523.

71. Ellaurie M, Burns ER, Bernstein LJ, et al. Thrombocytopenia and HIV in children. Pediatrics 1988;82:905–908.

72. Saulsbury FT, Boyle RJ, Wykoff RF, et al. Thrombocytopenia as the presenting manifestation of human T-lymphotropic virus type III infection in infants. J Pediatr 1986;109:30–34.

73. Kovacs A, Frederick T, Church J, et al. CD4 T-lymphocyte counts and *Pneumocystis carinii* pneumonia in pediatric HIV infection. JAMA 1991;265:1698–1703.

74. Denny T, Yogev R, Gelman R, et al. Lymphocyte subsets in healthy children during the first four years of life. JAMA 1992;267:1484–1488.

75. Monforte A, Novati R, Galli M, et al. T-cell subsets and serum immunoglobulin levels in infants born to HIV-seropositive mothers: A longitudinal evaluation. AIDS 1990;4:1141–1144.

76. McKinney RE, Wilfert CM. Lymphocyte subsets in children younger than 2 years old: Normal values in a population at risk for human immunodeficiency virus infection and diagnostic and prognostic application to infected children. Pediatr Infect Dis J 1992;11:639–643.

77. de Martino M, Tovo PA, Galli L, et al. Prognostic significance of immunologic changes in 675 infants perinatally exposed to HIV. J Pediatr 1991;119:702–709.

78. Wong WY, Pan L, Chan L, et al. Evaluation of current CDC recommendations for PCP prophylaxis in HIV positive children [Abstract PoB 3322]. Eighth International Conference on AIDS, Amsterdam, Jul 1992.

79. Frederick T, Kovacs A, Caldwell B, et al. CD4 counts and AIDS-defining conditions in infants and children with HIV infection [Abstracts PoC 4275]. Eighth International Conference on AIDS, Amsterdam, Jul 1992.

80. Butler KM, Husson RN, Lewis LL, et al. CD4 status and P24 antigenemia: Are they useful predictors of survival in HIV-infected children receiving antiretroviral therapy? Am J Dis Child 1992;146: 932–936.

81. Pahwa S, Lesser M, Paul M, et al. Correlation of T lymphocyte counts, lymphocyte function, viral load and survival in children with HIV infection [Abstract PoB 3860]. Eighth International Conference on AIDS, Jul 1992.

82. Rutherford GW, Oliva GE, Grossman M, et al. Guidelines for the control of perinatally transmitted HIV infection and care of infected mothers, infants and children. West J Med 1987;147:104–108.

83. MacDonald MG, Ginzburg HM, Bolan JC. HIV infection in pregnancy: Epidemiology and clinical management. J Acquir Immune Defic Syndr 1991;4:100–108.

84. Johnson JP, Vink PE, Hines SE, et al. Vertical transmission of HIV from seronegative or indeterminate mothers. Am J Dis Child 1991;145: 1239–1241.

85. Minkoff HL, DeHovitz JA. Care of women infected with HIV. JAMA 1991;2666:2253–2258.

86. Sperling RS, Stratton P, O'Sullivan MJ et al. A survey of zidovudine use in pregnant women with HIV infection. N Engl J Med 1992;326:857–861.

87. Heagarty MC, Abrams EJ. Caring for HIV-infected women and childern. N Engl J Med 1992;326: 887–888.

88. Minkoff H, Nanda D, Menez R, Fikrig S. Pregnancies resulting in infants with AIDS or AIDS-related complex. Obstet Gynecol 1987; 69:285–287.

89. Hand IL, Wiznia A, Checola RT, et al. HIV seropositivity in critically ill neonates in the South Bronx. Pediatr Infect Dis J 1992;11:39–42.

90. Mitchell CD, Erlich SS, Mastrucci MT, et al. Congenital toxoplasmosis occurring in infants perinatally infected with HIV-1. Pediatr Infect Dis J 1990;9:512–518.

91. Ikeda MK, Jenson HB. Evaluation and treatment of congenital syphilis. J Pediatr 1990;117:843–852.

92. Centers for Disease Control. Guidelines for prophylaxis against *Pneumocystis carinii* pneumonia for children infected with human immunodeficiency virus. MMWR 1991;40:1–13.

93. Immunization Practices Advisory Committee. Immunization of children infected with HIV-supplementary ACIP statement. MMWR 1988;37: 181–183.

94. Committe on Infectious Diseases, American Academy of Pediatrics. Report of the commitee on infectious diseases. 22nd ed. Elk Grove Village, IL: American Academy of Pediatrics, 1991:124–126.

95. Embree JE, Datta P, Stackiw W, et al. Increased risk of early measles in infants of HIV type I-seropositive mothers. J Infect Dis 1992;165: 262–267.

96. Pahwa S. Intravenous immune globulin in patients with AIDS. J Allergy Clin Immunol 1989; 84:625–631.

97. Ochs HD. Intravenous immunoglobulin in the treatment and prevention of acute infections in pediatric acquired immunodeficiency syndrome patients. Pediatr Infect Dis J 1987;6:509–511.

98. National Institute of Child Health and Human Development Intravenous Immunoglobulin Study Group. Intravenous immune globulin for the prevention of bacterial infections in children with symptomatic HIV infection. N Engl J Med 1991; 325:73–80.

99. Committee on Infectious Diseases, American Academy of Pediatrics. Chemotherapy for tuberculosis in infants and children. Pediatrics 1992;89:161–165.

100a. Jura E, Chadwick EG, Josephs SH, et al. Varicella-zoster virus infections in children infected with HIV. Pediatr Infect Dis J 1989;8:586–590.

100b. Lim W, Sadick N, Gupta A, et al. Skin diseases in children with HIV infection and their association with degree of immunosuppression. Int J Dermatol 1990;1:24–30.

101. Hoyt L. Oleske J, Holland B, Connor E. Nontuberculous mycobacteria in children with acquired immunodeficiency syndrome. Pediatr Infect Dis J 1992;11:354–360.

102. Leibovitz E, Riguad M, Chandwani S, et al. Disseminated fungal infections in children infected with HIV. Pediatr Infect Dis J 1991;10: 888–894.

103. Gleason-Morgan D,, Church JA, Bagnall-Reeb H, et al. Complications of central venous catheters in pediatric patients with acquired immunodeficiency syndrome. Pediatr Infect Dis J 1991; 10:11–14.

104. Aylward EH, Butz AM, Hutton N, et al. Cognitive and motor development in infants at risk for HIV. Am J Dis Child 1992;146:218–222.

105. Epstein LG, Sharer LR, Oleske JM, et al. Neurologic manifestations of human immunodeficiency virus infection in children. Pediatrics 1986;78:678–687.

106. Mintz M, Epstein LG. Neurologic manifestations of pediatric acquired immunodeficiency syn-

drome: Clinical features and therapeutic approaches. Semin Neurol 1992;12:51–56.

107. European Collaborative Study. Neurologic signs in young children with human immunodeficiency virus infection. Pediatr Infec Dis J 1990;9:402–406.

108. Belman AL, Diamon G, Dickson D, et al. Pediatric acquired immunodeficiency syndrome. Am J Dis Child 1988:142:29–33.

109. Pizzo PA, Eddy J, Falloon J, et al. Effect of continuous intravenous infusion of zidovudine (AZT) in children with symptomatic HIV infection. N Engl J Med 1988;319:889–896.

110. McKinney RE, Maha MA, Conner EM, et al. A multicenter trial of oral zidovudine in children with advanced human immunodeficiency virus disease. N Engl J Med 1991;324:1018–1025.

111. McKinney RE, Pizzo PA, Scott GB, et al. Safety and tolerance of intermittent intravenous and oral zidovudine therapy in human immunodeficiency virus-infected pediatric patients. J Pediatr 1990; 116:640–647.

112. DeCarli C, Fugate L, Fallon J, et al. Brain growth and cognititve improvement in children with human immunodeficiency virus-induced encephalopathy after 6 months of continuous zidovudine therapy. J Acquir Immune Defic Syndr 1991;4:585–592.

113. Butler KM, Husson RN, Balis FM, et al. Dideoxyinosine in children with symptomatic human immunodeficiency virus infection. N Engl J Med 1991;324:137–144.

114. McCorkindale C, Dybevik K, Coulston AM, Suchker KP. Nutritional status of HIV-infected patients during the early disease states. J Am Diet Assoc 1990;90:1236–1241.

115. Halsey NA, Boulos R, Holt E, et al, Transmission of HIV-I infections from mothers to infants in Haiti. JAMA 1990;264:2088–2092.

116. Kotler DP, Tierney AR, Wang J, Pierson Jr RN. Magnitude of body-cell-mass depletion and the timing of death from wasting in AIDS. Am J Clin Nutr 1989;50:444–447.

117. McKinney R, Katz SL, Wilfert CM, et al. Analysis of weight growth rates in children < 2 years old born to HIV infected mothers [Abstract 903]. 32nd Interscience Conference on Antimicrobial Agents and Chemotherapy, Anaheim, 1992.

39

Medical Management of Children and Adolescents with Hemophilia

Jonathan C. Goldsmith

CONGENITAL COAGULATION DEFECTS

Inherited bleeding disorders are a result of a deficiency or dysfunction of one of the glycoproteins known as clotting factors. Genetic aspects of hemophilia and the life-threatening nature of the abnormality were well described in ancient Hebrew writings (1). The disorders were first reported in modern times by Schönlein in the early 1800s. Several researchers confirmed the existence of two different forms of X-linked recessive inherited hemophilia in the 1950s. These disorders are known as hemophilia A or classical hemophilia (factor VIII or antihemophilic factor deficiency) and hemophilia B (factor IX deficiency or Christmas disease).

In the United States, there are between 15,000 and 20,000 individuals with hemophilia. For every five people with hemophilia A there is one with hemophilia B. Pathophysiologically, bleeding continues longer in hemophiliacs than in normals. The hallmark of hemophilia is bleeding into joint spaces. Over time this can lead to joint inflammation, deformity, diminished range of motion, and acute and chronic pain. In addition to joint and soft tissue bleeding, life-threatening bleeding can occur in the central nervous system. Substantial amounts of blood can also be lost from the gastrointestinal and genitourinary tracts without specific macroscopic lesions. Although the risk of intracranial bleeding related to birth trauma does not seem to be greater in hemophiliacs than full-term infants in general (2), postcircumcision bleeding is predictable. For one-third to one-half of those with hemophilia, there is no family history of the disorder. In those without an antecedent family history, bruising in toddlers can mistakenly raise suspicions of child abuse.

The clinical severity of hemophilia correlates with the plasma level of the deficient clotting factor. Approximately 60% of those with hemophilia have severe disease with <1% of the normal level of factor VIII or factor IX. They have "spontaneous" bleeding without recognized preceding injury and by adulthood may have advanced arthropathy affecting several joints. Some 15% of hemophiliacs have moderately severe disease with 1–5% of the normal amount of factor. These individuals have infrequent spontaneous bleeding-but predictable prolonged bleeding after trauma and surgery. By adulthood, those with moderately severe hemophilia may have one abnormal joint. The one-quarter of hemophiliacs with mild disease may not be recognized until adulthood after surgery or trauma, if they lead a somewhat restricted life in childhood. Family studies conducted after recognition of one individual with mild hemophilia often identify many similarly affected family members. Plasma factor levels must be determined by coagulation laboratories thoroughly familiar with clotting factor assays and their quality control. Techniques used in blood drawing in small

747

children can also affect results by improper anticoagulation. Specialized laboratories are also necessary adjuncts for the prudent management of hospitalized hemophiliacs undergoing diagnostic and therapeutic procedures.

HIV DISEASE IN HEMOPHILIACS

Hemophiliacs were inadvertently exposed to human immunodeficiency virus (HIV) in the late 1970s and early 1980s through their use of pooled clotting factor concentrates for the treatment of bleeding episodes. Factor concentrate lots used to treat hundreds of hemophiliacs for many months are prepared from plasma from more than 20,000 donors. Based on stored serum specimens subsequently analyzed for HIV antibody, half of all the hemophiliacs eventually infected with HIV were infected by January 1982 (3, 4). HIV antibody screening of plasma donors and heat or solvent/detergent inactivation of clotting factor concentrates has eliminated new HIV infections and reinfections. Boys with hemophilia treated in the United States since January 1, 1986, have no risk of HIV infection through the use of factor concentrates. Other blood components and those obtained outside the United States do not offer this high level of HIV safety.

The first AIDS case in a hemophiliac was reported in 1981 (5). Reports were then received in geometrically increasing proportions for 8 years. Since 1989 the case accrual rate has been constant: 8% of the hemophilic cases have occurred in children younger than 13 years; 37% have been reported in adolescents and young adults aged 13–29 years. In addition, it has been estimated that there are some 5000–7000 hemophiliacs with earlier stage HIV infection. In terms of the entire AIDS epidemic, 6% of pediatric cases have hemophilia as their HIV acquisition route, and ~30% of adolescent cases are individuals with hemophilia.

Differences in biochemical purification of the clotting factors provided important clues to the inactivation of HIV. Alcohol fractionation steps were employed in the purification of some factor IX complex concentrates in use in the early 1980s. These steps employing 20% ethanol were later

shown to inactivate HIV (6). Intravenous immunoglobulin G preparations used for passive immunotherapy are similarly purified from pooled human plasma and have been shown clinically to be free of HIV transmission risk.

Geographically, AIDS cases in hemophiliacs have been reported from all states and United States territories. The highest case rates/million population (≥12) have been reported from Mississippi, Missouri, and New Jersey. Early in the epidemic, the first AIDS cases in sparsely populated states were individuals with hemophilia. In many states, boys of school age with hemophilia and HIV infection pioneered approaches to school attendance.

In addition to the AIDS identifying opportunistic infections and cancers, other conditions associated with immunodeficiency are also fairly common in hemophiliacs. Pyarthroses were reported early in the HIV epidemic (7) and continue to be noted owing to *Staphylococcus aureus, Streptococcus pneumoniae,* and *Haemophilus influenzae* type b (8). Idiopathic thrombocytopenic purpura may affect up to 10% of hemophiliacs with HIV disease and can result in serious hemorrhagic complications (9). A few of these patients have been successfully subjected to splenectomy (10). Other therapies, such as intravenous immunoglobulin G, would also be appropriate. Risks of wound infection after splenectomy and other surgeries do not appear to be excessive in HIV-infected hemophiliacs (11).

There have been several aspects of the HIV epidemic that are unique to the hemophilic population. One of these is the occurrence of concurrent transfusion transmitted hepatotrophic viral infections. With first generation tests, between 70 and 90% of hemophiliacs have reactive hepatitis C serologies (12). As a result, elevated serum transaminases are very common. The use of potentially hepatotoxic nucleoside analogue agents required special evaluation in hemophiliacs before initiation of larger clinical trials. These preliminary studies did not demonstrate excessive toxicity or hypocoagulability of blood. As a result, liberalization of enrollment criteria with respect to liver function tests was made possible for hemophiliacs. In the face of immunodeficiency, hepatitis C infection has progressed more rapidly in some hemophiliacs, leading to death from hepatic failure or gastrointestinal hemorrhage caused by portal hypertension. In the mid-1980s, a few hemophiliacs with HIV disease underwent successful liver transplantation for hepatic failure with incidental cure of their coagulation defect (13). This major therapeutic intervention has more recently been restricted to individuals without known HIV infection. Interferon-α has been proposed as a treatment for hemophiliacs with histologically advanced liver disease. Preliminary results suggest that interferon can favorably affect chronic hepatitis infection (14). Trials of interferon in combination with nucleoside analogue agents for concurrent HIV infection are planned for the AIDS Clinical Trials Groups (ACTG) (protocol 203).

Cofactors for HIV progression have been postulated to explain more rapid deterioration in some individuals. Age at the time of HIV infection has been definitively shown to be a cofactor in large cohorts of hemophiliacs (15–17). The percentage of individuals with AIDS at 8 years of follow-up correlated with age (15). The approximate date of seroconversion in the cohorts was identified by analysis of stored serum samples. Results of one survey indicated that 13.5% of those ≤17 years old, 28.8% of those 18–34 years, and 43.7% of those 35–70 years progressed to AIDS by 8 years after seroconversion. The explanation for the favorable influence of youth on HIV progression is beginning to emerge. Analysis of lymphocyte subpopulations from children aged 0–5 years has confirmed the presence of higher numbers of CD4 cells, CD45RA cells, and activated B cells compared with adult hemophiliacs aged ≥25 years (18). The CD45RA subpopulation may suppress B cell responses by CD8 suppressor cell induction and activate cytotoxic T cells and natural killer cells by production of interleukin-2 and interferon-γ. Other clues to the pathogenesis of HIV disease in hemophiliacs can be derived from analysis of HIV antibody. Assessment of patient sera by indirect immunofluorescence in the mid–1980s indicated high titers of antibodies (19). These high titers might have been a result of the parenteral route of exposure and might have slowed the progression of HIV disease. This idea is being actively explored by passive immunotherapy with sera containing high titers of anti-HIV antibody and active immunization with whole virus and recombinant glycoproteins (20).

COMPREHENSIVE CARE

Patients and families with hemophilia have benefitted from a multidisciplinary comprehensive health care delivery system. In the mid-1970s the now Maternal and Child Health Bureau created predominantly university hospital based health professional teams focused on hemophilia care. Each team was headed by a hematologist with interest and ability in hemophilia care. A nurse-coordinator directed the daily operation of the hemophilia center. Part-time assistance was provided by medical social workers, physical therapists, dentists, orthopedic surgeons, specialized coagulation laboratories, psychologists, and blood banks as available at the various geographic sites. These individuals provided an integrated, prospective approach to a chronic disease marked by disability and premature death. Patients received at least annual assessment by the multidisciplinary team in addition to intercurrent care on a need basis. The annual evaluation consisted of visits with all members of the comprehensive team and formulation of a treatment plan that dealt with medical, social, school, nursing, physical therapy, and psychological issues.

The benefits of the comprehensive care system for individuals with hemophilia were substantial. Over the first ten years of Maternal and Child Health Bureau sponsored programs, the average age of hemophiliacs in the United States increased by ten years to more than 20. Despite the implementation of elective corrective orthopedic surgical procedures the average number of hospitalizations per patient per year declined from 1.9 to 0.3. Time lost from school fell dramatically from 14.5 to 4.3 days/year. Unemployment in adults fell from near 40% to <10% and in some regions to less than the overall unemployment rate. Costs of care also fell by nearly 75% per patient per year. The development and initiation of medically supervised home infusion therapy was a major factor in reducing the medical costs from $31,600 to $8,127 per year from 1975 to 1985. In addition to these tangible benefits, patients and families also developed autonomy and independence that permitted them to lead more fulfilling and productive lives (21).

The occurrence of HIV disease in hemophiliacs presented new challenges to the comprehensive care system. Children, adolescents, and adults with hemophilia and their families had to confront a new and life-threatening chronic disease. This situation of the superimposition of a second major illness on an antecedent one had not been previously addressed by health care teams. Families struggling for normalcy in the growth and development of their child with a bleeding disorder had to take on the additional challenges of a progressive virus disease with its societal judgments. Adults who had accommodated to their bleeding disorder through self-infusion therapy and sensible career choices found themselves at the beginning of a new maze with problems similar to those that they had surmounted years before. The confusion and in some cases despair confronting these individuals is self-evident. Families with hemophilia also have multigenerational issues that stem from the X-linked nature of inheritance of the disorder. Maternal guilt regarding the genetic transmission of the disorder was compounded by HIV infection in their children, brothers, and fathers in a few cases. These situations have some parallel features to nonhemophilic families where both parents and children are affected by HIV.

In addition to the problems faced by the consumers, the health care providers were also challenged. They had to address and resolve their feelings about the HIV epidemic that complicated the technological advances which they had promoted. Lyophilized clotting factor, which had facilitated many personal advances for individuals with hemophilia, turned out to be the vector for HIV infection in the same individuals. The health care team prescribed and administered many doses of clotting factor before risks were appreciated by the medical community.

Hemophilia treatment centers took several approaches to HIV disease. Some chose to learn on the job. Treatment center personnel made a concerted effort to learn about HIV disease, especially its evaluation and treatment, and offered these services through the long term personnel from the comprehensive care center. A slightly different approach consisted of incorporating infectious disease physician specialists into the comprehensive care team. A third approach involved referral of HIV-infected hemophiliacs to infectious disease specialists or HIV focused practitioners if available in the local community. Patients and families with long standing ties to a treatment team usually preferred the first model. However, this solution was not always practical nor preferred by the comprehensive care team.

A major initiative for treatment center teams in the HIV era was implementation of Risk Reduction Programs. Spouses and sexual partners of adult hemophiliacs and adolescents were taken as new clients of the treatment center. Teenagers were a special focus for these programs. The HIV-infected hemophiliac teenagers presented a unique opportunity to investigate strategies that could be applied to adolescents in general to reduce the sexual transmission of HIV. A cooperative agreement was created by the Centers for Disease Control, completed, and subsequently implemented in 1991 and 1992 by 11 hemophilia treatment centers at various locations in the United States. This Sentinel Evaluation Project seeks to assess knowledge, attitudes, beliefs, and behaviors in hemophilic teenagers with HIV disease. After individual interviews for recruitment, a mailed instrument was administered to 504 adolescent boys; 60% of those agreeing to participate returned the questionnaires. Knowledge bases about HIV infection and transmission were quite high in this select group of teenagers. Over 80% understood the importance of condoms in decreasing transmission of HIV and, in addition, two-thirds of the participants employed condoms every time they had sex. To try to generate and reinforce behavior change peer social activities will be conducted. Separate parental retreats will be scheduled to facilitate more intense interactions. These educational initiatives for decreasing HIV transmission are based on principles similar to those previously used in the hemophilic population to exchange hemophilia specific information. Successes in behavior modification in this highly medically sophisticated patient group are a necessary prerequisite for broader application of the techniques.

Although the HIV epidemic is centered in the more populous urban areas, people with hemophilia are more homogeneously dispersed throughout the United States. This feature created a significant problem for hemophiliacs in terms of access to new HIV therapeutics. A unique solution to this problem was developed by the National Hemophilia Foundation and medical leadership from the hemophilia treatment centers. An arrangement of regional coordinating centers in each of the ten federally designated geographic regions was created. The regional coordinating centers were responsible for data collection, protocol implementation, and technical assistance. Scores of hemophilia treatment centers made protocols available in diverse sites, monitored compliance, and collected data. The National Institute of Allergy and Infectious Diseases made resources available to staff the regional sites and to enroll patients in selected ACTG protocols. This AIDS Clinical Trials Unit "without walls" successfully completed ACTG 036, which demonstrated the benefits of zidovudine when compared with placebo in those with more advanced, but asymptomatic, HIV disease (22). Smaller numbers of patients also enrolled in dideoxycytosine and dideoxyinosine salvage protocols. Several hundred hemophiliacs with HIV infection are actively participating in ACTG 175 which evaluates nucleoside analog monotherapy combination therapy. This unique approach to clinical investigation of HIV therapies has served as an important demonstration project for enhancing access in future trials. Even in urban areas, creation of local neighborhood sites for clinical trials will be an important development to ensure patient access and accrual.

IMMUNOTHERAPY ASPECTS OF ANTIHEMOPHILIC FACTOR INFUSIONS

Since the advent of HIV disease, the immunologic status and treatment practices of hemophiliacs have been meticulously examined. The factor concentrates used to stop bleeding in hemophiliacs had very low specific activities until the late 1980s. As a result, patients were infused with large amounts of plasma proteins including fibrinogen and fibronectin. More recent studies have shown that clotting factor concentrates, but not purified factor VIII, impair in vitro lymphocyte responses (23–25). This suggested that hemophiliacs with HIV infection might have an additional immunological burden. A corollary question was whether changes in treatment practices could change the rate of progression of immunologic deterioration. A few studies have been conducted in matched cohorts of hemophiliacs receiving newer, purer clotting factors with specific activities of >1 and those being treated with less pure clotting factors. One study demonstrated no difference between the treatment groups in terms of decline in absolute CD4 lymphocyte counts (26). However, the two concentrates employed would qualify as higher purity, because both had specific activities of >1. In another study, the cohorts receiving the purer antihemophilic factor concentrates seemed to have more prolonged preservation of their CD4 lymphocyte counts (27). Presumably, preservation of this surrogate marker will correlate with delayed occurrence of AIDS identifying clinical events. Many clinicians have chosen to act on this data and treat all their patients with purer factor concentrates. This includes HIV-infected factor IX deficient patients now that purer coagulation factor IX concentrates are clinically available.

MANAGEMENT OF HEMOPHILIA: WHAT PRIMARY CARE PROVIDERS SHOULD KNOW

Bleeding complications in hemophilia are the result of prolonged hemorrhage after unnoticed or apparent trauma. Compared with normals, hemophiliacs bleed longer, although they bleed no more in a given time interval. Therefore, early clotting factor replacement infusion is the cornerstone of management.

The types of bleeding in children and adolescents with hemophilia are age dependent in most instances. Infants and toddlers have a pattern punctuated by oral and soft tissue hemorrhage. Eruption of deciduous teeth and frenulum tears can result in substantial blood loss if therapy is delayed. Intramuscular and soft tissue bleeding are the results of initial attempts to crawl and walk. Intra-articular bleeding, the hallmark of hemophilia, asserts itself as gait patterns become established. By age 8–10, many boys develop a "target" joint despite on-demand replacement therapy. These joints may account for 80% of the boy's bleeding episodes and set the stage for hemophilic arthropathy as an adolescent or adult. Without proper preparation, surgery, episodes of trauma, or invasive diagnostic tests can also result in life- or limb-threatening hemorrhage.

Clotting factor replacement therapy is determined by the nature of the bleeding episode and severity of the coagulation defect. Insertion of an intravenous needle or catheter rarely requires replacement therapy. However, an arterial stick for a blood gas determination requires treatment before and for 1–2 days after the procedure. A liver biopsy or appendectomy, respectively, would require coverage before and for 5–14 days after operation.

Hemophiliacs have benefitted by the first attempts to reduce the risk of transfusion transmitted viral illnesses. Before knowledge of HIV, it was appreciated that coagulation factor concentrates could transmit agents of hepatitis B and non-A, non-B hepatitis even if units of plasma with hepatitis B surface antigen were excluded from the donor pool. Methods of virus inactivation were investigated regarding their ability to render clotting factor concentrates noninfectious for hepatitis. A heat treatment process was licensed for antihemophilic factor in the United States in 1983. Concentrate was exposed to 60°C for 72 hours in the lyophilized state. Unfortunately, hepatitis transmission was not affected as assessed by serial transaminases. Also, in the early 1980s, others treated concentrates with tri-N-butyl phosphate (TNBP) cholate and demonstrated inactivation of lipid enveloped model viruses (28). With advancing knowledge, both types of processes were demonstrated to inactivate HIV (29). Concentrates are now treated with second generation

methods. Heating is generally performed as part of a pasteurization procedure (heating in the liquid state for 10 hr at 60°C), and the solvent detergent systems use TNBP with either polysorbate 80 or Triton X-100. HIV transmission has been eliminated by both methods, and hepatitis B and C transmission also appear to have been severely reduced (30). The demonstration that these types of procedures can successfully eliminate the risk of virus infection suggests that similar processes might be used to enhance the safety of single and multiple donor plasma products and holds the promise that virus inactivation of blood cell preparations can be performed.

Since 1983, the number and types of coagulation factor concentrates have increased rapidly. Dry heating processes (60–68°C for 30–60 hr) were demonstrated to inactivate HIV-1. Concentrates of this type typically had the symbol T or HT added to the established trade name. In late 1987 and early 1988, factor VIII products purified using murine monoclonal antibodies were introduced into clinical practice. Several logs of viral reduction were achieved by partitioning in the affinity process. One concentrate (Hemofil-M) used TNBP-Triton X-100 (a solvent detergent system) to achieve many additional logs of viral kill, whereas Monoclate used dry heat. Later the heating process was replaced by a pasteurization step (Monoclate-P) (see Table 39.1). These affinity purified clotting factor concentrates have specific activities of ≥2000 units/mg protein before the addition of albumin as a stabilizer in the final container. Conventionally purified factor VIII concentrates have specific activities from one (FVIII-SD, Humate-P) to ~10 (Profilate OSD, Koate-HP) to over 50 (Melate). Von Willebrand factor, a major impurity in Humate-P, makes it especially useful for the treatment of individuals with von Willebrand's disease who are unresponsive to Desmopressin. All viral inactivation techniques destroy potentially contaminating HIV-1 and -2. Heating in the liquid state (pasteurization), use of solvent detergent methods (TNBP + Triton X-100 or Polysorbate 80), and heating to 80°C additionally confer a high degree of hepatitis C inactivation.

Coagulation factor IX concentrates are preferred for replacement therapy of hemophilia B, because they do not contain other factors of the prothrombin complex (factors II, VII, and X) and as a result have a tremendously reduced risk of producing inappropriate thrombosis like the factor IX complex concentrates (see Table 39.2). Specific activities of the coagulation of factor IX concentrates range from ~75 (AlphaNine) to >150 (AlphaNine-SD and Mononine). Factor IX complex concentrates typically contain <5 units of factor IX/mg protein. Activated factor IX complex concentrates and porcine factor VIII (Hyate:C) are employed in the treatment of hemophilia A patients with acquired circulating anticoagulants (inhibitors).

Nonconcentrate based therapy is possible for individuals with mild hemophilia A and type I von Willebrand's disease. Desmopressin (Stimate) be given at a dose of 0.3 µg/kg IV in 20–50 ml normal saline over 20–30 min or 0.4 µg/kg SC. Factor VIII and von Willebrand factor levels will increase two- to five-fold over baseline. Laboratory monitoring is essential to evaluate the effectiveness of initial and subsequent (every 12–24 hr) doses.

Epsilon amino caproic acid (Amicar) and tranexamic acid (Cyklokapron) inhibit fibrinolysis. They are especially useful for oral bleeding after frenulum tears or dental eruption. An adjunctive infusion of clotting factor may be required. Amicar (50 mg/kg every 6 hr) or Cyklokapron (25 mg/kg every 8 hr) are given orally for 7–10 days. The liquid preparations are generally better tolerated.

Factor VIII produced by recombinant DNA technology has been in clinical trials

Table 39.1. Factor VIII Concentrates

Product and Manufacturer	Viral Inactivation Techniques	Clinical Use
Immunoaffinity purified		
Monoclate-P (Armour)	60°C × 10 hr, liquid state	Hemophilia A
Hemofil-M (Baxter-Hyland)	TNBP/Triton X-100, ≥25°C × ≥10 hr	Hemophilia A
Coagulation factor VIII (American Red Cross)	TNBP/Triton X-100, ≥25°C × ≥10 hr	Hemophilia A
Conventional purification		
Profilate OSD (Alpha)	TNBP/Polysorbate 80, 27°C × ≥6 hr	Hemophilia A
Humate-P (Behringwerke)	60°C × 10 hr, liquid state	von Willebrand's disease
Koate-HP (Miles-Cutter)	TNBP/Polysorbate 80, 27°C × 6 hr	Hemophilia A
Factor VIII-SD (New York Blood Center)	TNBP/cholate, ≥24°C × 6 hr	Hemophilia A
Melate (New York Blood Center)	TNBP/Polysorbate 80, ≥24°C × 6 hr	Hemophilia A
Hyate:C (Porton)	None (porcine)	Hemophilia A (inhibitor)

Table 39.2. Factor IX Concentrates

Product and Manufacturer	Viral Inactivation Techniques	Clinical Use
Coagulation factor IX		
AlphaNine (Alpha)	60°C × 20 hr, in *n*-heptane	Hemophilia B
AlphaNine-SD (Alpha)	TNBP/Polysorbate 80, 24–30°C × 6 hr	Hemophilia B
Mononine (Armour)	Sodium thiocyanate + ultrafiltration	Hemophilia B
Factor IX complex		
Profilnine HT (Alpha)	60°C × 20 hr, in *n*-heptane	Hemophilia B
Proplex T (Baxter-Hyland)	68°C × 144 hr, dry state	Hemophilia B
Konyne-80 (Miles-Cutter)	80°C × 72 hr, dry state	Hemophilia B
Bebulin (Immuno)	60°C × 10 hr at 1190 mbar + 80°C × 1 hr at 1375 mbar	Hemophilia B
Activated factor IX complex		
Autoplex (Baxter-Hyland)	68°C × 144 hr, dry state	Hemophilia A (inhibitor)
FEIBA (Immuno)	60°C × 10 hr at 1190 mbar + 80°C × 1 hr at 1375 mbar	Hemophilia A (inhibitor)

since 1987. The recent commercial availability of Recombinate (Baxter-Hyland) and Kogenate (Miles-Cutter) for the treatment of hemophilia A make "blood substitute" replacement therapy a reality.

Many minor bleeding episodes can be successfully treated with one infusion of factor concentrate, if administered in the first few hours after the onset of a spontaneous hemorrhage (see Table 39.3). However, many infusions may be required for successful performance of surgical procedures. Before major soft tissue surgery, 50 units/kg antihemophilic factor are infused. Then, half of the loading dose is given every 8 hr for 3–5 days, followed by the same dose every 12 hr for 3–5 days, followed by once daily infusions at the same dose for 3–5 days for a total of 10–14 days. Antihemophilic factor can also be administered by continuous intravenous infusion. The doses of coagulation factor IX are 35–40 units/kg for major surgery, with one-quarter of the loading dose given every 12 hr for 3–5 days, followed by the same dose at least once daily for a total of 10–14 days.

UNIQUE ASPECTS OF HIV DISEASE IN HEMOPHILIA

Management of HIV disease in hemophiliacs parallels that of others with HIV infection with some important differences. At the present time all hemophiliacs with HIV infection in the United States are older than 7 years. Although there are children of adult hemophiliacs with transplacental HIV infection, these younger children are unaffected by hemophilia. The female children are obligate carriers of the disorders, and the male children are unaffected, because hemophilia is an X-linked recessive disorder. Because the HIV-infected hemophilic

children are older than 7, their course more closely resembles that of adolescents and adults. Evaluation of these hemophiliacs presents some problems not encountered in other patient groups affected by HIV infection. Pulmonary presentations of opportunistic infections are common. However bronchoscopy and lavage and especially transbronchial biopsy could result in life-threatening bleeding in a hemophiliac. Before any procedure, persons with hemophilia must have their clotting defect corrected by the infusion of a sufficient amount of the deficient coagulation factor. For bronchoscopy and lavage, clotting factor should be administered for 3–5 days after the procedure. In general transbronchial biopsy should not be performed, even with adequate preoperative preparation. The risks of bleeding after the procedure in a vital, noncompressible area exceed those of the population in general. If an examination of lung tissue is mandatory, then a thoracotomy with careful attention to hemostasis under direct visualization is preferred. Clotting factor replacement may be required for 10–14 days after operation.

Central nervous system complications of HIV infection also require a different approach in the HIV-infected hemophiliac. Central nervous system bleeding is still a major complication of congenital bleeding disorders. Therefore, the HIV-infected hemophilic child or adolescent should first be infused with clotting factor, then evaluated with a computed tomography scan of the brain to determine if bleeding has occurred. In the face of persisting headache or focal neurologic findings, a magnetic resonance imaging scan is helpful to learn if there are white matter changes consistent with HIV infection, atrophy, or infectious/neoplastic processes. This two-step approach can be time consuming but is necessary in the HIV-infected hemophiliac.

HIV-infected hemophiliacs have an increased risk for the development of non-Hodgkin's lymphoma compared with the general population (31). Although no cases have been reported in those aged 0–9 years, the relative risk for age 10–19 years is 49. Prolonged survivals owing to therapeutic advances may increase this relative risk even further.

Table 39.3.   Initial Factor Concentrate Dosing[a]

Hemophilia A	
Minor bleeding	20–25 units/kg IV
Major bleeding	50 units/kg IV
Hemophilia B	
Minor bleeding	15–20 units/kg
Major bleeding	30–40 units/kg

[a]Minor bleeding, hemarthrosis, oral bleeding, hematuria, soft tissue bleeding; major bleeding, large joint hemarthrosis, preoperative, headache, or head trauma.

The impact of HIV disease on hemophilic boys' growth does not appear to be significant in the first few years after seroconversion (32). However, more recent analysis confirms impaired growth (33). To clarify the impact, nearly 350 hemophilic boys ages 6–19 were recruited in 1988 to participate in a Growth and Development Study at 14 Hemophilia Treatment Centers located throughout the United States. Subjects were enrolled from 4–7 years after being HIV infected through transfusion. One-third of the enrollees were HIV-negative boys with hemophilia. At baseline, the neuropsychological performance of the HIV infected and HIV negative groups was similar. Parents interviewed as part of the assessment reported more behavioral and emotional problems than would be expected in a group of similarly aged males. Overall performance of both groups was less than expected based on IQ scores (34). This might be related to the impact of hemophilia as a chronic disease and raises some interesting questions regarding the impact of a second chronic disease, HIV, on boys with hemophilia.

Hemophiliacs with HIV infection have been at the center of several societal controversies. Boys with hemophilia and HIV disease such as Ryan White from Indiana and the Ray family boys in Florida encountered discrimination when they attempted to attend publicly funded schools. These school aged children catalyzed public opinion. In some cases the results were quite negative with de facto expulsion. Ultimately many communities facing similar situations could allow HIV-infected hemophilic boys to attend public school and be treated with compassion. Evidence of the lack of HIV transmission in casual settings supported these decisions (35, 36). Work related discrimination has also been encountered by older hemophiliacs for many years because of their bleeding disorder, but in the last 10 years, HIV infection compounded the problem. The recently enacted Americans with Disabilities Act now provides legal redress for those encountering work or school related discrimination owing to HIV that has been defined as a disability.

Ten to 15 million Americans are transfused annually. The safety of the blood re-source is of special importance in the health care field. Screening of donated blood components for transfusion transmitted viral diseases has never been more thorough with testing for hepatitis B, hepatitis C, transaminases, and HIV-1 and -2 antibody. Hemophiliacs played a passive but critical role in identifying the transmission of these agents in blood components. The large plasma pools used to prepare clotting factor concentrates in effect amplified the risks for hemophiliacs. Hemophiliacs represent only 1% of those with AIDS; however because of their medical sophistication and national treatment center network, they have participated in and contributed to the rapidly advancing knowledge base about HIV disease far in excess of their relative numbers.

References

1. Ingram GIC. The history of hemophilia. J Clin Pathol 1976;29:469–472.
2. Goldsmith JC, Kletzel M. Risk of birth related intracranial hemorrhage in hemophilic newborns: Result of a North American survey. Blood 1990;76 (suppl):421A.
3. Evatt BL, Gomperts ED, McDougal JS, Ramsey RB. Coincidental appearance of LAV/HTLV-III antibodies in hemophiliacs and the onset of the AIDS epidemic. N Engl J Med 1985;312:483–486.
4. Eyster ME, Gail MH, Ballard JO, et al. Natural history of human immunodeficiency virus infections in hemophiliacs: Effects of T-cell subsets, platelet counts, and age. Ann Intern Med 1987;107:1–6.
5. Ehrenkranz NJ, Rubinin J, Gunn R, et al. *Pneumocystis carinii* pneumonia among persons with hemophilia A. MMWR 1982;31:365–367.
6. Wells MA, Wittek AE, Epstein JS, et al. Inactivation and partition of human T-cell lymphotropic virus, type III, during ethanol fractionation of plasma. Transfusion 1986;26:210–213.
7. Goldsmith JC, Silberstein PT, Fromm RE, Walker DY. Hemophilic arthropathy complicated by polyarticular septic arthritis. Acta Hematol 1984;71: 121–123.
8. Pappo AS, Buchanan GR, Johnson A. Septic arthritis in children with hemophilia. Am J Dis Child 1989;143:1226–1228.
9. Ragni MV, Bontempo FA, Myers DJ, Kiss JE, Oral A. Hemorrhagic sequelae of immune thrombocytopenic purpura in human immunodeficiency virus-infected hemophiliacs. Blood 1990;75:1267–1272.
10. Kim HC, Raska K Jr, Trooskin S, Saidi P. Immune thrombocytopenia in hemophiliacs infected with human immunodeficency virus and their response to splenectomy. Arch Intern Med 1989;149: 1685–1688.
11. Buehrer JL, Weber DJ, Meyer AA, et al. Wound infection rates after invasive procedures in HIV-1

seropositive versus HIV-1 seronegative hemophiliacs. Ann Surg 1990;211:492–498.

12. Brettler DB, Alter HJ, Dienstag JF, Forsberg AD, Levine PH. Prevalence of hepatitis C virus antibody in a cohort of hemophilia patients. Blood 1990;76:254–256.

13. Ragni MV, Bontempo FA, Lewis JH. Organ transplantation in HIV-positive patients with hemophilia. N Engl J Med 1990;322:1886–1887.

14. Makris M, Preston FE, Triger DR, et al. A randomized controlled trial of recombinant interferon-α in chronic hepatitis C in hemophiliacs. Blood 1991; 78:1672–1677.

15. Goedert JJ, Kessler CM, Aledort LM, et al. A prospective study of human immunodeficiency virus type 1 infection and the development of AIDS in subjects with hemophilia. N Engl J Med 1989;321:1141–1148.

16. Aledort LM, Hilgartner MW, Pike MC, et al. Variability in serial CD4 counts and relation to progression of HIV-1 infection to AIDS in haemophilic patients. Br Med J 1992;304:212–215.

17. Lee CA, Phillips AN, Elford J, et al. Progression of HIV disease in a haemophilic cohort followed for 11 years and the effect of treatment. Br Med J 1991;303:1093–1096.

18. Fletcher MA, Mosley JW, Hassett J. Effects of age on human immunodeficiency virus type 1-induced changes in lymphocyte populations among persons with congenital clotting disorders. Blood 1992;80:831–840.

19. Goldsmith JC, Dewhurst S, Hedenskog M, Casareale D, Volsky DJ. High prevalence and high titers of LAV/HTLV-III antibodies in healthy hemophiliacs in the midwestern United States. Am J Med 1986;81:579–583.

20. Redfield RR, Birx DL, Keeter N, et al. A phase I evaluation of the safety and immunogenicity of vaccination with recombinant gp160 in patients with early HIV infection. N Engl J Med 1991;324:1677–1684.

21. Pierce GF, Lusher JL, Brownstein AP, Goldsmith JC, Kessler CM. The use of purified clotting factor concentrates in hemophilia. Influence of viral safety, cost, and supply on therapy. JAMA 1989;261:3434–3438.

22. Merigan TC, Amato DA, Balsley J, et al. Placebo-controlled trial to evaluate zidovudine in treatment of human immunodeficiency virus infection in asymptomatic patients with hemophilia. NHF-ACTG 036 Study Group. Blood 1991;78:900–906.

23. Thorpe R, Dilger P, Dawson NJ, Barowcliffe TW. Inhibition of interleukin-2 secretion by factor VIII concentrates: A possible cause of immunosuppression in haemophiliacs. Br J Haematol 1989;71: 387–391.

24. Hay CRM, McEvoy P, Duggan-Keen M. Inhibition of lymphocyte IL-2 receptor expression by factor VIII concentrate: A possible cause of immunosuppression in haemophiliacs. Br J Haematol 1990;75:278–281.

25. Schulman S. Effects of factor VIII concentrates on the immune system in hemophilic patients. Ann Hematol 1991;63:145–151.

26. Mannucci PM, Gringeri A, de Biasi R, et al. Immune status of asymptomatic HIV-infected hemophiliacs: Randomized, prospective, two-year comparison of treatment with a high-purity or an intermediate-purity factor VIII concentrate. Thromb Haemost 1992;67:310–313.

27. de Biasi R, Rocino A, Miraglia E, et al. The impact of a very high purity factor VIII concentrate on the immune system human immunodeficiency virus-infected hemophiliacs: randomized, prospective, two-year comparison with an intermediate purity concentrate. Blood 1991;78:1919–1922.

28. Horowitz B, Wiebe ME, Lippin A, Stryker MH. Inactivation of viruses in labile blood derivatives. I. Disruption of lipid-enveloped viruses by tri(N-butyl) phosphate detergent combinations. Transfusion 1985;25:516–522.

29. McDougal JS, Martin LS, Cort SP, et al. Thermal inactivation of the acquired immunodeficiency syndrome virus, human T-lymphotropic virus-III/lymphadenopathy-associated virus, with special reference to antihemophilic factor. J Clin Invest 1985;76:875–877.

30. Mannucci PM, Schimpf K, Brettler DB, et al. Low risk for hepatitis C in hemophiliacs given high-purity, pasteurized factor VIII concentrate. Ann Intern Med 1990;113:27–32.

31. Rabkin CS, Hilgartner MW, Hedberg KW, et al. Incidence of lymphomas and other cancers in HIV-infected and HIV-uninfected patients with hemophilia. JAMA 1992;267:1090–1094.

32. Pasi KJ, Collins MA, Ewer AK, Hill FG. Growth in haemophilic boys after HIV infection. Arch Dis Child 1990;65:115–118.

33. Jason J, Gomperts E, Lawrence DN, et al. HIV and hemophilic children's growth. J Acquir Immune Defic Syndr 1989;2:277–282.

34. Loveland K, Stehbens J, Contant C, et al. The hemophilia growth and development study: Baseline neurodevelopmental findings. J Pediatr Psychol, in press.

35. Berthier A, Fauchet R, Genetet N, et al. Transmissibility of human immunodeficiency virus in haemophilic and nonhaemophilic children living in a private school in France. Lancet 1986;2: 598–601.

36. Lusher JM, Operskalski EA, Aledort LM, et al. Risk of human immunodeficiency virus type 1 infection among sexual and nonsexual household contact of persons with congenital clotting disorders. Pediatrics 1991;88:242–249.

40

Medical Management of Adolescents with HIV Infection

Donna Futterman and Karen Hein

Human immunodeficiency virus (HIV) infection and AIDS have had a profound social and medical impact on adolescents (1). By 1988, in the most recent national study, AIDS was the sixth leading cause of death among youth in the United States aged 15-24 years (2). Some 20% of the almost 250,000 AIDS cases in the United States as of 1992 are among young people age 20–29 years (3). Because there is an average 11-year period from HIV infection to the development of AIDS (4), most of these young adults were undoubtedly infected while teenagers.

HIV infection is a particular threat to adolescents because the behaviors that are associated with infection often begin during adolescence. Some key differences among HIV-infected adolescents, children, and adults are the proportion infected through sexual intercourse, disease progression, and access to medical care and prevention services (5). Adolescents may be given care in settings where young children or adults are cared for or in adolescent-specific sites. Regardless of the setting, age-specific elements of care should be addressed.

HIV TRANSMISSION AND RISK-RELATED ACTIVITIES

Perinatal transmission accounts for over 85% of AIDS cases among children younger than 13 years, with the remaining cases associated with the receipt of infected blood products. In contrast, ~65% of adolescents aged 13–19 years, and 90% of 20- to 24-year-

olds with AIDS, were infected through sexual exposure or intravenous drug use (3, 6).

It is during adolescence that most people consolidate their sexuality and first have sexual intercourse. Consequences of unprotected intercourse include sexually transmitted diseases (STD), unwanted pregnancy, drug addiction, and HIV infection. Late consequences of STDs include ectopic pregnancy, involuntary sterility, and cervical carcinoma. The three leading causes of death among United States adolescents are suicide, homicide, and accidents, which account for 75% of deaths in this age group. Along with AIDS, these three causes of death are often related to risk-taking activities by adolescents and are largely preventable. Yet responsibility for helping to create safer environments clearly lies with adults. Seat belts and helmets have helped lower rates of motor vehicle and bicycle fatalities. Similarly, condom use can lower rates of HIV, STDs, and pregnancy. Without adult involvement and support for expanding AIDS education, increasing condom availability in schools, and expanding access to health care, it is unlikely that teenagers will be able to implement prevention strategies by themselves.

Sexual Risk
Sexual Behaviors and Condom Use

HIV can be transmitted by all three forms of intercourse—vaginal, anal, oral—regardless of the sex of the partner (7). A recent

757

report from the national high school-based Youth Risk Behavior Survey (YRBS) showed that two-thirds of males and half the females had initiated sexual intercourse by age 17. One-quarter of the students reported four or more sexual partners by 12th grade (8). This study undoubtedly underestimates risk behavior among all adolescents, since out of school youth were not included. The average age of first intercourse in the United States is 16 years (8, 9). In some studies of urban adolescents the average age at first intercourse is as young as 12 years (10). Some 85% of pregnancies among adolescents are unintended, underscoring the extent of intercourse without effective contraception (11).

Condoms are the only form of protection against both pregnancy and STDs, including HIV. Widely varying rates of condom use have been reported in multiple studies. In the YRBS survey, among students who had sexual intercourse in the past 3 months, less than half used condoms during their last intercourse (8). In a national survey of adolescent males in 1988, 58% of those aged 17–19 years reported condom use at last intercourse, but these rates were significantly lower among males who had five or more sexual partners, had paid for sex, or used drugs intravenously (12). In another study conducted in the Midwest among females aged 12–19 years, only 50% reported that they had ever used condoms (13). In a survey of urban minority adolescent females, 26% reported engaging in anal intercourse, but condoms were used in only one-third of these encounters (14).

National health objectives for the year 2000 include the goal of increasing condom usage by sexually active adolescents aged 15–19 years. For females, the goal is to increase usage from the 1988 baseline of 26% up to 60%, and for males the goal is to increase usage from 57 to 75% (15). However, as of 1992, federally sponsored AIDS risk-reduction messages for teenagers do not encourage condom use, and network television does not carry condom advertisements.

Another major obstacle to risk reduction efforts is the lack of ongoing national research on adolescent sexuality. Two studies that sought to define new trends in adolescent and adult sexuality were canceled by the federal government in 1992 because of political opposition to explicit questions about sexual practices. These types of studies are crucial in designing prevention programs by providing details about the number and types of partners as well as frequency and type of intercourse and use of condoms (16).

Sexually Transmitted Diseases and Puberty

In the United States, the highest rates of STDs (i.e., gonorrhea, syphilis, and hospitalization for pelvic inflammatory disease) are seen among sexually active adolescents aged 13–19 (17). One in seven teens aged 15–19 get an STD each year (1). Worldwide, STDs are also concentrated among adolescents and young adults (18). Infection with other STDs (particularly genito-ulcerative infections, i.e., syphilis, herpes, and chancroid) facilitates transmission of HIV. Of note, the incidence of primary and secondary syphilis in the United States among all age groups increased 59% from 1986 to 1989 whereas gonorrhea rates decreased by 22% during that period (19). Acquisition of an STD also may serve as a marker for sexual behaviors that are associated with the spread of HIV (7, 20–22). In addition to increasing the risk of acquiring HIV, STDs have their own serious consequences. Infection with chlamydia or gonorrhea can cause infertility in females and males, and several strains of human papilloma virus have been linked to the development of cervical cancer.

The high rate of STDs among adolescents is due to an interaction of behavioral risks and physiologic susceptibility. HIV is a sexually transmitted pathogen, and its transmission dynamics reflect both host and viral factors (23). Host factors that facilitate the acquisition of HIV during adolescence include the development of the female genital tract during puberty. Menarche begins at an average age of 12 in the United States and is followed by a period of anovulatory cycles for months to years. The lack of progesterone that accompanies anovulatory cycles creates a more permeable cervical mucus that allows sperm and infectious agents in semen to more easily ascend into the upper genital tract. Early puberty is also characterized by ectopy (the extension of endocervical columnar cells onto the vaginal surface of the cervix). This single layer of columnar cells may be more susceptible to infection than the multilayer squamous epithelial cells that replace them as puberty proceeds (17).

Males Who Have Sex with Males and Lesbian Youth

There are subgroups of adolescents who are at higher risk of HIV infection than others. Male adolescents who have intercourse with other males are at particular risk for HIV given the high prevalence of HIV infection among gay and bisexual adult men. Between 17 and 35% of young males have had same sex experiences to orgasm (24), yet many of these adolescents do not identify themselves as gay or bisexual.

For those youth who are gay, societal and familial prejudices against homosexuality often interfere with their ability to build an integrated gay identity or "come out" to themselves and others. The prevention of open socialization with gay peers increases the pressure on gay adolescents to explore their sexuality in secretive and sometimes unsafe ways (25). Despite an abundance of safe sex messages aimed at the gay community, the gay adolescent who is in the process of "coming out" frequently does not have access to these safe sex messages or does not yet identify with the gay community and therefore ignores these messages. Gay male and lesbian adolescents may engage in heterosexual sex to hide their homosexuality from themselves and others (26), which can result in potential exposure to HIV infection. Lesbians can also become infected with HIV via their own or their partner's injection drug use (27).

Adolescent Females

Among females, adolescents are more likely than adults to become infected with HIV through sexual exposure than by injection drug use. A program that follows a large cohort of HIV-infected adolescents found that although 85% of females contracted HIV infection via heterosexual intercourse, very few were aware that their male partner had HIV infection at the time of

their exposure. Ongoing obstacles to safer sex included the need to convince male sexual partners to use condoms, fear that insistence on condom usage would disclose HIV status, desire to have a baby, and lack of availability of female-controlled safer sex method (28).

Runaway and Homeless Youth

Adolescents who engage in "survival sex" or the exchange of sex for money, drugs, food, or shelter are at particularly high risk for HIV infection. There are an estimated 900,000 teens who engage in some form of survival sex or "sex work," of whom two-thirds are female. Their average age is 15, and they engage in unprotected intercourse with many high-risk partners (29). There is some overlap between these teen sex workers and the estimated 1–2 million teenagers who run away each year. There are ~100,000-200,000 homeless teenagers (30). Many of these adolescents also survive on the streets by engaging in high-risk sexual behavior in exchange for food, shelter, protection, or companionship (31). Some adults may select adolescents as sexual partners because they think that they are less likely to have HIV or other STDs.

Sexual Abuse

Sexual abuse poses yet another risk for HIV transmission. Of reported sexual abuse cases, 17–30% of the victims are in the adolescent age group (32). In addition to direct risk from an HIV-infected abuser, sexual abuse puts adolescents at risk by increasing the likelihood of future high-risk behavior. Adolescents who have been sexually abused as children have a lower age of initiation both of intercourse and use of alcohol and illicit drugs (33). A study of adults examining risk behaviors for HIV reported a four-fold increase in prostitution (survival sex) among females and a eight-fold increase among males who had been sexually abused during childhood (34). Practitioners caring for sexually abused children and adolescents are recognizing the need to incorporate HIV counseling into evaluation protocols (35), and those caring for HIV-infected adolescents must also incorporate assessment of sexual abuse into their practice.

Substance Use

Drug use also puts adolescents at risk for HIV infection. The link among injection drug use, needle sharing, and AIDS was established within the first year of the reported epidemic. Injection drug use continues to be reported as the sole risk activity by 13% of 13–19-year-olds with AIDS in the United States (3). Various drugs can be injected including heroin, cocaine, amphetamines, estrogens (by youth seeking to be transsexuals), and anabolic steroids (by body builders and athletes). The percentage of adolescents who are administering these drugs intravenously and engaging in needle sharing practices is unknown, but the YRBS showed that 1.5% of high school students (2.3% of males and 0.7% of females) reported intravenous drug use. Risk behaviors tend to cluster, and among adolescents with four or more sexual partners, 5.1% reported intravenous drug use (8). In 1991, the Monitoring the Future longitudinal study released data showing a gradual decline in illegal drug use with; ~9% of high school seniors reporting that they ever used cocaine. Almost 4% reported using crack/cocaine, and 1.3% had used heroin. The peak age of initiation of cocaine use was 15–16 years. Illicit drug use was reported throughout the country. Almost half (48%) of high school seniors had tried an illicit drug, and 29% had tried an illicit drug other than marijuana (36). These studies did not include the estimated 15% of high school age youth who had dropped out of school and may be more heavily involved in substance abuse. Studies have shown adolescents to underreport substance use. In a study of pregnant teenagers, one-third of documented cocaine users consistently denied use (37).

Crack/cocaine use also appears to be highly associated with risk related sexual behaviors. Crack is a smokable form of cocaine that is inexpensive and rapidly addictive. Crack is also a sexual stimulant and disinhibitor that can increase sexual arousal while impairing judgment and self-control. Because it is so highly addictive, crack use has become associated with the exchange of sex for crack or money to purchase crack. (38). Crack use has recently been found to be associated with HIV infection among adolescents; nearly 40% of infected adolescents seen at an HIV clinic in New York City reported heavy crack use and denied intravenous drug use. Among youth using crack/cocaine, almost 80% reported survival sex (39). The Centers for Disease Control noted that cities reporting high levels of crack use are also reporting dramatic increases in other STDs, including syphilis and gonorrhea (40). In New York City, where cases of congenital syphilis rose precipitously from 60 per year in 1980–1986 to 1017 cases in 1989, a case control study reported a significant association with crack/cocaine use (41).

There are also a substantial number of adolescents who are using other substances (e.g., alcohol, marijuana, or "designer drugs") that can impair their judgment and increase the likelihood of engaging in risk related sexual and drug use behaviors. Use of these substances before or during intercourse can impair the adolescents' ability to practice safer sex.

Hemophilia and Blood Transfusions

Males with hemophilia who received HIV-infected clotting factors have a prevalence of HIV infection paralleling the severity of their clotting disorder. Among people with severe hemophilia, 75% are infected with HIV vs. 25% of those with mild hemophilia (42). Although hemophilia accounts for only 1% of adult cases of AIDS, among adolescent cases aged 13–19, 30% were caused by transfusion of infected blood products (3). Because all blood products have been tested for HIV since 1985, and clotting factors are now heat treated (providing additional protection against infection), transmission of HIV to people with hemophilia and other transfusion recipients has virtually ceased.

Adolescents infected via blood products (from one-time transfusions or because of chronic illnesses, such as sickle cell disease or cancer, which require multiple transfusions) may also engage in risky sexual behavior (i.e., intercourse without condoms). A study of adolescents with hemophilia demonstrated that, despite a good knowledge base about safe sex, only one of nine males who were having sexual intercourse consistently used condoms (43). Studies are underway to assess the types of interventions (including parent and peer involvement) that can successfully address risk behaviors in this population (44).

Congenitally Infected Adolescents

In the future, as more effective treatments are developed, more children who were congenitally infected with HIV will reach their adolescent years. Many cases of congenitally infected adolescents, aged 12 and older, have now been described (45, 46). An Italian multicenter study reported that 49% of surviving children had reached 9 years of age (47). Some issues facing these children include devastating multisystem illness, growth failure, delayed puberty, social isolation, and decisions regarding disclosure of HIV status.

HIV TESTING AND COUNSELING

As the benefits of early treatment of HIV infection have been demonstrated, the indications for HIV testing have increased. Although the presence of risk related activities can indicate which adolescents should be offered HIV counseling and testing, studies have shown that relying on risk assessments alone will miss a significant proportion of infected adolescents (48). Laws governing testing vary among states and have thus far focused on adults. Before the HIV epidemic, adolescents in all states had the right to consent for confidential diagnosis and treatment of STDs without parental notification or consent. However, many states have limited minors' access to contraceptive services and abortion through parental consent requirements. There are 22 states with regulations or laws specifically focused on adolescents and HIV testing, most give minors the right to HIV testing on their own consent. (49) Debates over the rights of minors to consent to confidential testing and mandatory testing programs in the Job Corps and military (50), the issue of parent and sexual partner notification, and persistence of discrimination against HIV-positive people highlight some complexities of counseling and testing adolescents for HIV.

Recommendations for counseling adolescents were developed in 1989 at a national consensus conference. Principles include 1) before and after test counseling must be offered and be developmentally and culturally appropriate; 2) adolescents capable of giving informed consent should be allowed to consent to HIV testing, preferably with a family member or other responsible adult who can provide emotional support during the testing process; 3) testing should be voluntary and not coercive or mandatory as a prerequisite for admission to programs; 4) confidentiality should be assured with special care taken in settings such as foster care, residential institutions, or detention facilities, 5) adolescents should be assured access to all appropriate research and treatment protocols (51).

Elements of HIV test counseling include: 1) an explanation of confidentiality and clarification of who will have access to test results; 2) assessment of the reasons for HIV testing and the adolescent's actual risk behaviors; 3) determination of the risks and benefits of HIV testing for the individual; 4) anticipation of reactions to a positive or negative test result. Written consent should be obtained, and positive or negative test results should always be given in person. Plans for partner and family notification should be developed according to local laws. Risk reduction information and strong linkages with medical and mental health referral resources should be available at all sites providing HIV testing for adolescents.

PROGRAM ISSUES

Comprehensive medical and psychosocial services require the services of a multidisciplinary team of providers trained in the specific developmental and physiological needs of adolescents. In addition to the medical services described below, the team must address issues such as crisis intervention, risk reduction, living wills and health care proxies and parent and partner notification. It is important to establish a mutual referral relationship with youth-serving, community based agencies and medical programs to facilitate referrals of at-risk and HIV-infected adolescents. An outreach strategy developed by one program in New York City initially targeted agencies serving runaway, homeless, and gay and lesbian youth. Later, relationships were forged with agencies with structured environments (such as drug treatment programs, foster care agencies, and court-related facilities) whose staff could facilitate referrals (39).

To attract and retain disenfranchised youth, programs must address three main barriers to care. 1) Payment: a sliding fee scale is needed to make services accessible to youth as is assistance in securing Medicaid and Social Security health benefits. 2) Accessibility: programs should assess their geographic accessibility and consider providing transportation subsidies for the patients; whenever possible, health professionals should be brought together at the clinic site rather than requiring multiple visits by patients. 3) Consent and confidentiality: policies must be established in accordance with local and institutional guidelines (39).

MEDICAL MANAGEMENT
Natural History and Staging Classifications

The natural history of HIV infection in all age groups has not yet been completely defined. The only longitudinal studies including adolescents were in people with hemophilia where adolescents had a slower rate of progression compared with young children or adults. Because most adolescents are infected when their immune system has already developed, the natural history of HIV in adolescents will most likely parallel that seen in adults.

Medical management of an HIV-infected adolescent begins with a staging evaluation to determine the risk of disease progression and the appropriate course of treatment. This assessment includes a characterization of the patient as asymptomatic, asymptomatic with persistent generalized lymphadenopathy, symptomatic with HIV-related symptoms, or having AIDS. The new surveillance definition for adolescent and adult cases of AIDS would add a CD4 count of $<200/mm^3$ and pulmonary tuberculosis, recurrent bacterial pneumonia, and invasive cervical cancer to the list of AIDS indicator diseases (52). Several classification systems have been in use including the Centers for Disease Control pediatric and adult classification of HIV/AIDS (53, 54) and the Walter Reed staging classification for Adults (55). The criteria used for these classification systems were not developed specifically for adolescents and thus might be modified as the natural history of HIV in adolescents is better understood.

Medical History

A medical history should assess prior illnesses or medical treatments that may be HIV related or affected by HIV disease progression (56). Evidence should be sought for the acute HIV seroconversion illness because this can help date HIV acquisition. Symptoms are frequently similar to a mononucleosis-like syndrome of fever, malaise, lymphadenopathy, and variable involvement of multiple organ systems (57). A medical history for late presenting, congenitally infected adolescents should include a history of their parents' drug use or risk behaviors.

Other elements of a medical history include 1) sexual and drug use history (see Tables 40.1 and 40.2); 2) prior illnesses, especially STDs, recurrent pneumonia, or tuberculosis which may reactive in the presence of HIV infection or during adolescence; 4) hospitalizations; 5) menstrual and pregnancy history; 6) use of condoms and contraception by males and females; 7) previous sources of medical care; 8) history of blood transfusions or receipt of blood products; 9) immunizations; 10) medications; 11) allergies, especially to medications; 12) family history (medical and psychiatric); 13) a nutrition and diet history. When working with adolescents, it is important to be both specific and concrete; for example an adolescent may not realize they had a sexually transmitted infection but might recall symptoms or taking medications.

A psychiatric history should include assessment of past and present functioning, depression, anxiety, psychosis, suicidal thoughts or attempts, medications, or hospitalizations. A social history should include current living situation (family, friends, alone, institution, homeless), history of foster care, arrest and jail history, literacy level,

Table 40.1.   Elements of a Sexual Risk History

1. At what age did you begin sexual intercourse (oral, vaginal, anal), and how old was your partner?
2. Do you have sex with men, women, or both?
3. Do you consider yourself heterosexual, homosexual, or bisexual?
4. Have you ever had the following sexual experiences; if so how often and with how many partners. Oral, vaginal, or anal intercourse? Receptive or insertive? What percentage of time were condoms used? Describe those experiences in the past month.
5. Describe the number of sexual partners you have had and their ages, and indicate if any of them had known risk factors for HIV infection.
6. Have you ever had an STD (name all of them, describe symptoms, ask for treatment history).
7. What forms of birth control have you used? Describe. Have you done anything to try and prevent STDs? What?
8. Have you ever been pregnant, had a baby, or had an abortion or miscarriage?
9. Have you used drugs or alcohol before or during sex?
10. Have you ever had sex in exchange for food, money, drugs, or a place to sleep or live?
11. Has anyone ever forced you to do something sexually that you did not want to do?
12. Do you have any questions or concerns about your current sexual experiences?
13. What are you doing to protect yourself and your sex partners from being infected with HIV?
14. What do you know about safe and safer sex? How do you feel about changing your sexual behaviors to prevent HIV infection? What sexual behaviors will you miss? How does your partner feel about safe sex?
15. Do you think condoms can prevent the spread of HIV and STDs? If so, what makes it hard for you to use condoms? Did you use a condom the last time you had intercourse? Why or why not?

Table 40.2.   Elements of a Drug Use History

1. Do you, your friends, or your sexual partners ever use any of the following: alcohol, marijuana, crack, cocaine, heroin, amphetamines, hallucinogens (LSD, PCP) barbiturates, sedatives, steroids. Are you using them in combinations? How?
2. For each drug describe: age of first use, frequency of use in past month, average daily use, and ways used (pills, snorted, smoked, injected).
3. In what settings do you use drugs: alone, with friends or lovers, at parties, where you buy the drugs (crack houses, shooting galleries)?
4. For those who have injected drugs, describe needle use: sharing frequency and with whom , use of works in shooting galleries, cleaning practices.
5. For those who smoke crack, describe frequency of use, percentage of use in crack houses, frequency of sex in crack houses and types of sex.
6. How do you get money to obtain drugs?
7. Have you ever had sex in exchange for drugs?
8. Have you ever had a medical problem (i.e. visited a doctor or hospital) or tried to hurt or kill yourself after drug use?
9. Have you ever been in trouble with the law, your family, school, or job, after drug use?
10. Do you think you are addicted to or have a problem with drugs?
11. Have you ever tried to "get off" drugs? What treatment programs have you tried? How else have you tried?

school and work status, and sources of financial and social supports, including who knows about HIV status.

Review of Systems

An HIV-oriented review of systems should include general assessment of weight loss or failure to gain weight during the growth spurt, fatigue, anorexia, nausea, prolonged or high fevers, night sweats, lymph node enlargement, or any skin lesions or rashes. The head, eyes, ears, nose, and throat (HEENT) review should note any visual or hearing changes, sinusitis, dysphagia, thrush, gum disease, tooth decay, or oral ulcers. Persistent cough or shortness of breath should be ascertained. Questions should be asked regarding diarrhea, abdominal pain or masses, and anal pain or discharge. Similarly, penile or vaginal pain, itching or discharge, herpes or other persistant infections should be noted along with any complaints of pelvic pain. A neuromuscular review should seek evidence of weakness, myalgia, or abnormal pain or sensations.

A neuropsychiatric review should ask for evidence of personality changes, dementia, depression, anxiety , thought disorders, or headaches. Of concern, is the evaluation of the adolescent for symptoms of post-traumatic stress disorder, a sequela of the often violent conditions in the lives of at-risk youth. For some of these complaints it may be difficult to distinguish those caused by HIV from those associated with less severe illnesses or with chronic use of illicit drugs.

Physical Examination

Because adolescence is characterized by dynamic changes in somatic growth and cognitive function, assessments should note the failure to progress as well as actual regression. A complete physical examination is performed with special attention to vital signs and growth assessment, including weight and height velocity. During puberty, weight is expected to double and height increase by 15–20%. Failure to gain weight or height at the expected rate during puberty may be significant. Normal ranges of pulse rate and blood pressure increase during adolescence (58). Nutritional status should be noted. Adolescence is a time when skin problems like acne can first present, but many other common dermatologic disorders are seen with HIV infection and may signal progression of disease.

The lymph nodes should be examined and lymphadenopathy fully described: location, number, size consistency, persistence. Adenopathy can be a sign of benign intercurrent illness or if confined to the inguinal area may be associated with sexually transmitted infections or with lower extremity trauma. Axillary adenopathy in the absence of upper extremity trauma is rarely seen in conditions other than HIV infection. Adolescence is a stage when lymphoid tissue normally begins to regress (58), but regression of adenopathy may also be seen in advanced AIDS.

An HEENT examination should include assessment of visual acuity, a fundoscopic examination and a thorough oral examination. Early oral *Candida* (thrush) can present as an erythematous, denuded patch on the mucous membrane rather than the more typical white plaques. Gum disease, or ulcers, and tooth decay are oftern seen in HIV-infected adolescents. The lungs and heart should be examined. An abdominal examination should note the presence of masses or hepatosplenomegaly.

The genitalia should be assessed including the sexual maturity staging of Tanner and Whitehouse describing the pubertal development of secondary sexual characteristics in pubic hair, female breasts, and male genitalia from stage 1 (prepubertal) through stage 5 (adult) (56). A yearly or twice yearly pelvic examination with appropriate laboratory tests and inspection for vaginal *Candida*, warts, or other lesions should be performed for females who have had sexual intercourse, have unexplained pelvic pain, or are over age 18. Presence of these lesions should be sought during the male genital examination. A rectal examination for herpes, warts, or other lesions is also needed for both females and males, including those who deny anal intercourse.

The neurologic examination should include a mental status assessment. It is not known how HIV infection will affect cognitive development in the adolescent. Assessment of the adolescent's ability to generalize or think abstractly is important in providing age apppropriate explanations to the patient. Neuropsychological testing should also be performed if neurologic involvement is suspected.

Laboratory Asessment

Laboratory assessment must consider adolescent-specific normal values where these are available and different from other age groups. Markers have been identified that are useful in assessing HIV disease state, predicting progression, and thereby guiding therapy; however, normal values during puberty have not been established. The most useful markers to date have been the lymphocyte cells, particularly the helper or CD4 lymphocyte, whose decline is associated with disease progression (60, 61). A CD4 count of <500/mm^3 is an indication of immune dysfunction and for the use of antiretrovirals. A report from a program seeing large numbers of HIV-infected adolescents indicated that almost 50% of the patients had CD4 of <500/mm^3 at presentation (39).

Simultaneous increases in β_2 microglobulin (a product of activated lymphocytes), neopterin (a product of activated macrophages) (60, 62), and HIV p24 antigen levels and a disappearance of antibodies to p24 (as measured by bands on the Western blot) are also viewed as markers of disease progression in adults (63, 64). Measurement of CD4 cell counts and percentages should be performed at baseline and at 3- to 6-month intervals (65, 66). It does not appear that adolescents have the same degree of hypergammaglobulinemia as has been seen in HIV-infected infants and children. It is highly recommended that the HIV antibody test be repeated for confirmation upon program entry (Table 40.3).

A complete blood count is necessary to assess the presence of anemia, lymphopenia, and neutropenia or decreased platelets. Normally during adolescence, hemoglobin increases in males 1–2 g/dl (58). A chemistry panel including evaluation of renal and liver function is advisable. HIV renal involvement may be accompanied by an increased blood-urea-nitrogen, creatinine, or potassium or decreased serum bicarbonate. Albumin will be decreased in the presence of chronic malnutrition or malabsorption. An elevated total protein will be present with an increased immunoglobulin fraction. Increased liver enzymes may denote liver involvement, but an elevated alkaline phosphatase can also be seen during the adolescent growth spurt (58) or with disseminated *Mycobacterium avium intracellulare*. An elevated lactate dehydrogenase may signal lymphoma or pulmonary disease, especially *Pneumocystis carinii* pneumonia.

All adolescents having intercourse should be screened for sexually transmitted pathogens because asymptomatic infections are possible. The work up of a patient for STDs includes serologic testing for syphilis and hepatitis, gonorrhea cultures (oral, genital, anal), a test for chlamydia (immunofluorescent slide test or culture), herpes culture, a Gram stain to detect inflammation or *Candida* in males and females or gonorrhea in males, KOH prep for *Candida*, and a "wet prep" for trichomonas or clue cells seen with bacterial vaginosis. HIV infection has been associated with a rapid progression of cervical neoplasia (67, 68), indicating the need for cervical cytology (Papanicolaou smear) every 6–12 months in HIV-infected, sexually experienced females (69–71). Preliminary evidence that colposcopic examinations may be abnormal in HIV-infected females with normal cervical cytology highlight the need for close follow-up. Further study is needed to determine the utility of anal cytology in males and females who engage in anal intercourse (72).

Table 40.3.   Intake and Suggested Intervals[a]

Laboratory Panel	
HIV antibody test	Repeat for confirmation, obtain informed consent
CD4+ T lymphocyte cells	Every 6 months when > 600/mm³
	Every 3 months when > 600/mm³
Complete blood count with differential	Every 6 months
Electrolytes, renal function, and liver enzyme panel	Every 6 months
Toxoplasmosis titer	Yearly
PPD with anergy panel	Every 6–12 months (with chest X-ray if anergic)
STD-gynecological, Genito-urinary Panel	
Hepatitis B serology	Before and after immunization (if needed)
Syphilis serology	Every 6 months
Gonorrhea culture (oral, genital, anal)	Every 6 months
Chlamydia (genital)	Every 6 months
Papanicolaou smear	Every 6–12 months (with colposcopy when needed)
Anal cytology[b]	
P24 antigen[b]	
β_2 microglobulin[b]	
Immunoglobulins[b]	

[a]Additional tests or modifications in schedules should be based on clinical status and sexual behavior.
[b]Optional, currently a research tool

A tuberculin skin test (PPD) with anergy panel (Merieux multitest or *Candida* and tetanus antigen) should be performed to assess the presence of tuberculosis infection and cell mediated immunity. Baseline chest X-ray should be obtained in those who are anergic to assess tuberculosis and to be used as comparison if respiratory symptoms develop. The chest X-ray is particularly valuable in patients with a history of pulmonary disease. Baseline titers for toxoplasmosis should be obtained because this infection can reactivate in HIV-positive adolescents. Serologic assessment of immunity to rubella should be performed in adolescent females.

Immunizations

Although there is sometimes a decreased antibody response to immunizations in immunocompromised patients, immunizations that are recommended for HIV adolescents include Pneumovax and a yearly influenza vaccine (73). Additionally, adolescents should receive vaccinations that are appropriate for their age such as diphtheria and tetanus and measles, mumps, and rubella (74, 75). Hepatitis B vaccine should be given to all adolescents who are not immune (76).

Treatments for HIV

Until 1989, virtually all the antiretroviral medications used in the treatment of HIV related illness were developed in clinical trials among children or adults. Although adolescents were included in clinical trials as of 1989, most were males with hemophilia. In 1992 seven clinical trial sites were funded to specifically focus on adolescents. In addition to issues of access and consent to participate in trials, care must be taken to include adolescent-specific normal laboratory test values when evaluating efficacy and toxicity of medications.

The dose, dose interval, toxicity, and effectiveness of various medications differ among the neonate, child, adolescent, adult, and elderly (77). During the adolescent years, there are gender-related changes in body composition. Proportional differences include greater increase in body fat among adolescent females and bone and muscle

mass among adolescent males (58). These differences in body habitus alter drug distribution and have a direct effect on drug dose. Changes in drug metabolism during adolescence affect drug half-life and therefore the dosing interval. Adolescents in Tanner stage 1 should receive pediatric dose schedules, and adolescents in Tanner stage 5 should receive adult dose schedules, regardless of their chronological age. Further studies are needed to determine appropriate dose schedules for adolescents in Tanner stages 2, 3, and 4.

Some of these age-related differences in response to medications have already been demonstrated. For example, prophylaxis against *Pneumocystis* pneumonia is recommended for HIV-infected patients with CD4 counts of $<200/mm^3$ (78). Young children have had fewer adverse reactions to trimethoprim-sulfamethoxazole than adults (79, 80). Similarly, children have had less hematologic toxicity than adults when taking high dose zidovudine (81, 82). Rates of adverse reactions in adolescents are unknown.

Extrapolating from adult data, adolescents should receive zidovudine when their CD4 cells are $<500/mm^3$ because of the demonstrated efficacy in delaying disease progression in asymptomatic persons (83, 84). Efficacy and minimal toxicity have been seen at doses of 200 mg every 8 hr. Toxicity is primarily related to anemia and neutropenia, emphasizing the need for close patient monitoring. Other licensed antiretrovirals include dideoxyinosine (125–200 mg every 12 hr) and dideoxycytidine (0.375–0.75 mg every 8 hr) in combination with zidovudine (85, 86). Because these medications can cause peripheral neuropathy and rarely pancreatitis, close monitoring is indicated. In the future, treatment options will increase as new medications are licensed by the Food and Drug Administration. Hopefully, with the expansion of clinical trials to include more adolescents, the recommended dosages will be based on scientific studies in this age group.

Adolescents should also be provided with prophylaxis against *Pneumocystis* pneumonia if they have had an episode of *Pneumocystis* pneumonia or if they have a CD4 count of $<200/mm^3$. The medication recommended for initial prophylaxis is trimethoprim/sufamethoxosole but if an allergic reaction develops, dapsone or aerosolized pentamidine should be employed (87, 88). Studies are underway to assess the efficacy of prophylaxis against such opportunistic infections as cytomegalovirus and *M. avium* complex.

A new initiative for adolescents has been launched through the AIDS Clinical Trials Group (ACTG). Protocol 220, a pre-enrollment protocol, has been approved for youth from 13 years up to their 21st birthday. This protocol will study variables affecting enrollment of adolescents into existing and future ACTG treatment protocols as well as adherence to quarterly standard of care follow-up (medical history, physical exam, laboratory assessments). A secondary objective of this study will be to describe the nature, stage, and progression of HIV infection in adolescents. This study opened for enrollment in the summer of 1993. Issues related to the ability of minor adolescents to consent to participate in clinical trials are being addressed by the Adolescent Working Group of the ACTG.

Compliance

Compliance with medical regimens is a challenge for all age groups. The unique issues for adolescents center on their developmental stage, life circumstances, and having nonjudgmental and knowledgable health care providers. For those who are HIV infected and asymptomatic but have an abnormal immune system, coming to medical providers and taking antiviral medications is an unwanted reminder of their potentially fatal disease. Concrete thought processes, "I feel and look good, how can I be sick?" may be combined with developmental self-perceptions of immortality and invincibility to intensify denial. These factors may decrease compliance with complicated medical regimens.

There is a documented decrease in compliance when using chronic therapies and complex regimens in all age groups (89). Adolescents should be assisted in developing plans to integrate medications into their daily life, and obstacles to this should be anticipated and discussed. Instruction should

be simple. Understanding by the patient should be elicited by asking for a repetition of the plan. Most adolescents will not respond to abstract notions of efficacy such as good health or longevity. Teenagers are more responsive to attempts to enhance their self-esteem by taking pride in reaching concrete goals that they have helped to set. Bolstering the patient's social supports (family, friends, agencies) is another strategy for encouraging compliance. Effective collaboration with youth serving, community-based agencies is also important in serving the many needs of HIV-infected adolescents.

For the subset of disenfranchised HIV-infected teens (homeless, prostitutes, drug addicted), compliance with medication schedules is often a much lower priotiy than securing food and a place to sleep. For these teens, money to purchase medications as well as literally having a place to keep their medicines loom large in the compliance equation.

Psychological Issues

Adolescents may have a wide range of psychological reactions to being informed they are infected with HIV. These reactions include fear, depression, and anxiety. These feelings are an appropriate response to their perceived losses including the loss of a healthy future and present health status. Many adolescents have difficulty understanding and believing the concept of disease latency and asymptomatic infection. This adds to the difficulty of motivating changes in risk related behaviors. For many, a positive test result represents a death sentence. However, a review of adolescents found no increase in suicide attempts and only a minimal increase in suicidal thoughts after finding out about positive HIV status (90). These findings of a lack of increase in suicidal behavior after testing HIV positive are similar to those reported in adults (91).

The issues of when and to whom one should disclose their HIV infection constantly confront the adolescent. Many appropriately fear the loss of support from family, friends, and present and future sexual partners. For many HIV-infected adolescents, particularly the girls, there is a great concern about their perceived inability to have children. Most feel ambivalent about wanting a child yet not wanting to pass on their infection. Some teens report a loss of interest in sexual intimacy, reflecting their "betrayal" at being infected through sexual intercourse. Others become empowered by strictly adhering to safe or safer sex guidelines or finding another HIV-infected partner with whom to have safer sex. Still others, in anger or denial of HIV infection, engage in uprotected intercourse. A nonjudgmental provider can help the adolescent voice their concerns and communicate honestly about their actual behaviors, which then serves as the basis for risk reduction strategies.

PREVENTION AND RISK REDUCTION

Prevention strategies are different for adolescents compared with adults. Cognitive styles of concrete thinking and perceptions of invulnerability may limit some adolescents' understanding of the future consequences of risky behavior. Adolescents therefore require very specific and practical information to help them understand their risk and how to change their behaviors. Principles of successful risk reduction strategies for adolescents include 1) helping the adolescent recognize their risk and feel that their actions can make a difference, 2) teaching and practicing risk reduction skills, 3) encouraging an environment and peer group that reinforces lower risk alternatives, and 4) repeating the messages that reinforce health promoting behaviors.

The further spread of HIV infection among adolescents can be curtailed only if prevention programs are widely disseminated and embraced (92, 93). Children and adolescents should be educated about HIV in their homes, schools, and communities before they begin to engage in risk related activities. Because family members may be reluctant to discuss sex and drug use, it is important to have resources available that can help families to begin a dialogue (94). There are excellent curricula available for school-based education programs; however, there have often been difficulties in implementing these curricula on a local level. In 1991, the New York City public school system began an innovative program to ex-

pand AIDS education and make condoms available in high schools serving ~250,000 students. However, there are continued struggles over whether the education message should be confined to a "moralistic" one urging sexual abstinence rather than a "realistic" one encouraging risk reduction (95). Many community organizations and youth serving agencies have combined their risk reduction messages with a broader health promotion message. They have also encouraged youth to become part of the compassionate response to AIDS by serving as peer educators and volunteers. Finally, the media and other cultural institutions have a major role in destigmatizing those at risk and promoting a more open discussion of specific AIDS prevention measures.

All adolescents, regardless of their risk, should be provided with information about HIV transmission and programs that will help them understand and modify risky behaviors. During adolescence, peer identification is a major factor in the young person's move from total dependence on family to independent functioning. This has provided the basis for many innovative HIV oriented peer education programs (96). Interventions for prevention and risk reduction should include three components: HIV/AIDS education, discussion of safe and safer sex including a condom demonstration, and exercises that will help adolescents develop decision making, assertiveness, and communication skills. For HIV-infected or high risk adolescents, the interventions should also be directed to the information obtained during an individualized risk assessment. Basic information about HIV infection, transmission, and prevention should be provided in a simple, straightforward manner (97). HIV/AIDS education should include a discussion about the differences between AIDS and HIV infection and between high and low risk behaviors.

Adolescents must learn that they can protect themselves by either 1) abstaining from or delaying sexual intercourse or 2) practicing safer sex by using condoms during sexual intercourse. The risks of unprotected vaginal, anal, and oral intercourse (without a condom) should be explained and these activities discouraged. Latex condoms with nonoxynol-9 spermicide, but not natural skin condoms, are effective at reducing one's risk for HIV transmission through sexual intercourse. Most adolescents have not had the opportunity to talk about condoms or learn how to properly use them. Adolescents are more likely to use condoms if they perceive them as enjoyable, and believe that they can effectively negotiate condom use with a sexual partner. Demonstrating their proper use and letting adolescents practice condom use on a penis model or their fingers can desensitize them and enable them to use condoms correctly. Role play exercises can also be used to help adolescents develop decision making, assertiveness, and communication skills for successfully negotiating risk reduction and condom use with a sexual partner and resisting peer pressure to use drugs and engage in unprotected intercourse (98).

For adolescents who are at a critical stage in the development of their sexual identity, sex should not be equated with possible death. The full range of options for expressing intimacy and sensuality should be presented. Differentiation between risk related intercourse and risk free "outercourse" may be useful. Outercourse can be defined as sensual touching on the outside of the body including kissing, massage, and masturbation. The challenge is to help adolescents learn how to explore their feelings and sexuality in ways that are safe and healthy. This is particularly important for gay and lesbian youth who face many obstacles in developing a positive identity.

FUTURE RESEARCH

HIV infection has clearly entered the adolescent population, although most infected youth are asymptomatic and unaware of their serostatus. The time for primary prevention alone has passed (99). Some questions that still must be answered follow. 1) Prevention and risk reduction. What are the most effective risk reduction programs for teenagers, and how can they be implemented in a timely manner? How can HIV-infected youth be helped to reduce or eliminate their ongoing risk related behaviors? 2) Progression of disease. What is the natural history of HIV infection in adolescents, and how does it compare with children and

adults? Are there factors related to adolescent physical development that accelerate or retard disease progression? How does the use of crack/cocaine or other illicit drugs affect the transmission and natural history of HIV infection? What are the important age- and sex-related differences in the use of therapeutics for HIV-related illnesses during adolescence? What strategies will work to enhance compliance with these regimens? 3) Health services. What are the most effective models of care to attract and retain high risk and HIV-positive youth over time? What are the costs of identifying and caring for HIV-infected adolescents? How will programs be funded to provide access for disenfranchised youth?

CONCLUSION

The number of reported adolescent AIDS cases has increased by 77% in the past 2 years (100). The extent of HIV infection among adolescents is unknown; many adolescents across the country are infected, and most adolescents in the country are at risk given the high rates of unprotected sexual intercourse and the increased presence of HIV. All primary care providers as well as adolescent medicine and other specialists caring for teenagers will play a vital role in helping to answer these critical questions as well as providing services to meet the needs of adolescents as this epidemic progresses.

References

1. DesJarlais D, Ehrhardt A, Fullilove, et al. AIDS and adolescents. In: Miller H, Turner C, Moses L, eds. AIDS: The second decade. Washington, DC: National Academy Press, 1990:147–252.
2. Novello A. Report of the secretary's work group on pediatric HIV infection and disease. Washington, DC: Department of Health and Human Services, Nov 1988.
3. Centers for Disease Control. HIV/AIDS Surveillance Report, 1992;Oct:1–18.
4. Brookmeyer R. Reconstruction and future trends of the AIDS epidemic in the United States. Science 1991;253:37–42.
5. Hein K. AIDS in adolescence: Exploring the challenge. J Adolesc Health Care 1989;10 (suppl): 10–35.
6. Vermund SV, Hein K, Gayle H, Cary J, Thomas P, Drucker E. AIDS among adolescents in NYC: Case surveillance profiles compared with the rest of the US. Am J Dis Child 1989;143:1220–1225.

7. Friedland GH, Klein RS. Transmission of the human immunodeficiency virus. N Engl J Med 1987;317:1125–1135.

8. Centers for Disease Control. Sexual behaviors among high school students—U.S. 1990. MMWR 1992;40:885–888.

9. Zelnik M, Shah FK. First intercourse among young Americans. Fam Plann Perspect 1983;15:64–70.

10. Hein K, Cohen MI, Marks A, et al. Age at first intercourse among homeless adolescent females. J Pediatr 1978;93:147–148.

11. National Research Council Panel on Adolescent Pregnancy and Child Bearing. In: Hayes CD, ed. Risking the future: Adolescent sexuality, pregnancy and child bearing. Washington, DC: National Academy Press, 1987:33–74, 95–121.

12. Sonenstein FL, Pleck JH, Ku LC. Sexual activity, condom use and AIDS awareness among adolescent males. Fam Plann Perspect 1989;21:152–158.

13. Orr D, Langefeld C, Katz B, et al. Factors associated with condom use among sexually active female adolescents. J Pediatr 1992;120:311–317.

14. Jaffe L, Seehaus M, Wagner C, Leadbeater B. Anal intercourse and knowledge of AIDS among minority-group adolescents. J Pediatr 1988;112:1005–1007.

15. Anonymous. Healthy children 2000: National health promotion and disease prevention objectives related to mothers, infants, children, adolescents and youth. Washington, DC: Department of Health and Human Services 1991:1–244.

16. Kost K, Darroch J. American women's sexual behavior and exposure to risk of sexually transmitted diseases. Fam Plann Perspect 1992;24:244–254.

17. Bell T, Hein K. The adolescent and sexuality transmitted diseases. In: Holmes K, ed. Sexually transmitted diseases. New York: McGraw-Hill, 1984:73–84.

18. Aral S, Holmes K. Sexually transmitted diseases in the AIDS era. Sci Am 1991:264:62–69.

19. Gershman K, Rolfs R. Diverging gonorrhea and syphilis trends in the 1980s: Are they real? Am J Public Health 1991;81:1263–1267.

20. Wasserheit J. Interrelationships between human immunodeficiency virus infection and other sexually transmitted diseases. Sex Transm Dis 1992;19:61–77.

21. Quinn TC. Evolution of the HIV epidemic among patients attending STD clinics. J Infect Dis 1992;165:541–544.

22. Hook EW. Syphilis and HIV infection. J Infect Dis 1989;160:530–534.

23. Holmberg SD, Horsburgh CR, Ward JW, Jaffe HW. Biological factors in the sexual transmission of human immunodeficiency virus. J Infect Dis 1989;160:116–125.

24. Remafedi G. Preventing the sexual transmission of AIDS during adolescence. J Adolesc Health Care 1988;9:136–143.

25. Martin AD. Learning to hide: The socialization of the gay adolescent. Ann Am Soc Adolesc Psychiatry 1982;10:52–65.

26. Paroski PA. Health care delivery and the concerns of gay and lesbian adolescents. J Adolesc Health Care 1987;8:188–192.

27. Chu S, Buehler J, Fleming P, Berkelman R. Epidemiology of reported cases of AIDS in lesbians, US 1980-89. Am J Public Health 1990;80:1380–1381.

28. Futterman D, Cohn J, Monte D, Shaffer N. HIV-infected adolescents: Risk behaviors and clinical status of a NYC cohort [Abstract Th 1560]. Eighth International Conference on AIDS, Amsterdam, 1992.

29. Sanders JM. Guidelines to health care providers of the sexually active adolescent. In: Schinazi RF, Nahmias AJ, eds. AIDS in children, adolescents and heterosexual adults. New York: Elsevier, 1988:350–351.

30. Sondheimer D. HIV infection and disease among homeless adolescents. In: DiClemente R, ed. Adolescents and AIDS: A generation in jeopardy. Newbury Park, CA: Sage, 1992:71–85.

31. Rotheram-Borus MJ, Koopman C, Haignere C, Davies M. Reducing HIV sexual risk behavior among runaway adolescents. JAMA 1991;266:1237–1241.

32. Hampton RL, Newberger EH. Child abuse incidence and reporting by hospitals: Significance of severity, class and race. Am J Public Health 1985;75:55–60.

33. Harrison PA, Hoffman NG, Edwall GE. Differential drug use patterns among sexually abused adolescent girls in treatment for chemical dependency. Int J Addict 1989;24:499–514.

34. Zierler S, Feingold L, Laufer D, Velentgas P, Kantrowitz-Gordon I, Mayer K. Adult survivors of childhood sexual abuse and subsequent risk of HIV infection. Am J Public Health 1991;81:572–575.

35. Yordan E, Yordan R. Sexually transmitted diseases and human immunodeficiency virus screening in a population of sexually abused girls. Adolesc Pediatr Gynecol 1992;5:187–191.

36. Johnston LD, O'Malley PM, Bachman JG. Drug use among American high school seniors, college students and young adults, 1975–1990. Rockville, MD: National Institute on Drug Abuse, 1991;1:1–199.

37. Zuckerman B, Amaro H, Cabral H. Validity of self-reporting of marijuana and cocaine use among pregnant adolescents. J Pediatr 1989;115:812–815.

38. Fullilove R, Fullilove M, Bowser B, Gross S. Risk of sexually transmitted disease among black adolescent crack users in Oakland and San Francisco, CA. JAMA 1990;263:851–855.

39. Futterman D, Hein K, Reuben N, Dell R, Shaffer N. HIV-infected adolescents: The first 50 patients in a NYC program. Pediatrics 1993;91:730–735.

40. Kerr P. Syphilis surge with crack use raises fear on spread of AIDS. NY Times Jun 29, 1988;B1,5.

41. Greenberg M, Singh T, Htoo M, Schultz S. The association between congenital syphilis and cocaine/crack use in NYC: A case-control study. Am J Public Health 1991;81:1316–1318.

42. Goedert JJ, Kessler CM. Aledort LM. A prospective study of human immunodeficiency virus type 1 infection and the development of AIDS in subjects with hemophilia. N Engl J Med 1989;321:1141–1148.

43. Overby KJ, Lo B, Litt IF. Knowledge and concerns about acquired immune-deficiency syndrome and their relationship to behavior among adolescents with hemophilia. Pediatrics 1989;83: 204–210.

44. Parsons J, Norman L, Maksoud J, et al. Attitudes toward interventions among adolescents with hemophilia and HIV and their parents. [Abstract]. J Adolesc Health 1993;14:53.

45. Lambert B. AIDS and children: Longer but troubled life. NY Times Nov 7, 1989; A1.

46. Grubman S, Oleske J. The maturation of an epidemic: Update on pediatric HIV Infection. AIDS in press.

47. Tovo P, DeMartion M, Gabiano C et al. Prognostic factors in survival in children with perinatal HIV infection. Lancet 1992:339:1249–1253.

48. D'Angelo LJ, Getson PR, Luban NLC, Gayle HD. Human immunodeficiency virus infection in urban adolescents: Can we predict who is at risk? Pediatrics 1991:88:982–985.

49. English A. Expanding access to HIV services for adolescents: Legal and ethical issues. In: DiClemente R, ed. Adolescents and AIDS: A generation in jeopardy. Newbury Park, CA: Sage, 1992;262:283.

50. Hein K. Mandatory HIV testing for youth: A lose-lose proposition. JAMA 1991;266:2430–2431.

51. English A, AIDS Testing and Epidemiology for Youth Work Group. AIDS testing and epidemiology for youth. J Adolesc Health Care 1989: 10 (suppl):52–57.

52. Centers for Disease Control. Addendum to the proposed expansion of the AIDS surveillance case definition. Washington, DC: Department of Health and Human Services, 1992:1–23.

53. Centers for Disease Control. Classification of HIV infection in children under 13 years of age. MMWR 1987;36:225–236.

54. Centers for Disease Control. Revision of the CDC surveillance case definition for acquired immune deficiency syndrome. MMWR 1987;36 (suppl)1–15.

55. Redfield RR, Wright DC, Tramont EC. The Walter Reed staging classification for HTLV-III/LAV infection. N Engl J Med 1986;314:131–132.

56. Futterman D, Hein K. Medical care of HIV-infected adolescents. AIDS Clin Care 1992;4: 95–98.

57. Tindall B, Cooper DA, Donovan B, Penny R. Primary HIV infection: Clinical and serological aspects. Infect Dis Clin North Am 1988;2:329–341.

58. Tanner JM. Growth at adolescence. 2nd ed. London: Blackwell Scientific, 1962.

59. Goodman Ds, Teplitz ED, Wishner A, et al. Prevalence of cutaneous disease in patients with AIDS or AIDS-related complex. J Am Acad Dermatol 1987;17:210–220.

60. Masur H, Ognibene FP, Yarchoan RY, et al. CD4 counts as predictors of opportunistic pneumonias in HIV infection. Ann Intern Med 1989;111:223–231.

61. Fahey JL, Taylor JMG, Detels R, et al. The prognostic value of cellular and serologic markers in infection with human immunodeficiency virus type 1. N Engl J Med 1990;322:166–172.

62. Lifson A, Hessel N, Buchbinder S, et al. Serum B_2-microglobulin and prediction of progression to AIDS in HIV infection. Lancet 1992;339:1436–1440.

63. Cooper EH, Lacey CJN. Laboratory indices of prognosis in HIV infection. Biomed Pharmacother 1988;42:539–546.

64. Eyster ME, Ballard JO, Gail MH, et al. Predictive markers for AIDS in hemophiliacs: Persistence of p24 antigen and low T4 count. Ann Intern Med 1989;110:963–969.

65. Hein K, Futterman D. Medical management in HIV-infected adolescents. In: Hauger S, Nicholas S, Caspe W, eds. Guidelines for the care of children and adolescents with HIV infection. J Pediatr 1991;119:S18–S20.

66. Centers for Disease Control. Guidelines for the performance of DC4+ T-cell determination in persons with HIV infection. MMWR 1992;41:1–17.

67. Maiman M, Fruchter R, Serur E, Boyce J. Prevalence of HIV in a colposcopy clinic. JAMA 1988;260:2214–2215.

68. Vermund S, Kelley K, Klein R, et al. High risk of human papillomavirus infection cervical squamous intraepithelial lesions among women with symptomatic HIV infection. Am J Obstet Gynecol 1991;165:392–400.

69. Centers for Disease Control. Risk for cervical disease in HIV-infected women-NYC. MMWR 1990;39:846–849.

70. Minkoff HL, DeHovitz JA. Care of women infected with the human immunodeficiency virus. JAMA 1991;88:2253–2258.

71. Hankins C, Hands M. HIV disease and AIDS in women: Current knowledge and research agenda. J Acquir immune Defic Syndr 1992;5:957–71.

72. Palefsky J, Gonzales J, Greenblatt R, et al. Anal intraepithelial neoplasia and anal papillomavirus infection among immunosuppressed homosexual males with group IV HIV disease. JAMA 1990; 263:2911–2916.

73. Centers for Disease Control. Recommendations of the immunization practices Advisory committee: Immunization of children with human immunodeficiency virus. MMWR 1988;37:181–183.

74. Peter G, ed. Immunization in special clinical circumstances: Adolescents and college populations. Report of committee on infectious diseases. 21st ed. Elk Grove Village, IL: American Academy of Pediatrics, 1988.

75. Centers for Disease Control. Measles prevention: Recommendations of the immunization practices advisory committee. MMWR 1989;38:1–18.

76. Collier AC, Corey L, Murphy VL, Handsfield HH. Antibody to the human immunodeficiency virus and suboptimal response to hepatitis B vaccine. Ann Intern Med 1988;109:101–105.

77. Hein K. The use of therapeutics in adolescence. J Adolesc Health Care 1987;8:8–35.

78. Centers for Disease Control. Guidelines for prophylaxis against PCP for persons infected with HIV. MMWR 1989;38 (suppl 5):1–9.

79. McSherry G, Wright M, Oleske J, Connor E. Frequency of severe adverse reactions to TMP-SMX and pentamidine among children with HIV infection[Abstract 1357]. 28th Interscience

Conference on Antimicrobial Agents and Chemotherapy, Los Angeles, 1988.

80. Gordon FM, Simon GL, Wofsy CB, et al. Adverse reactions to trimethoprim-sulfamethozaxole in patients with AIDS. Ann Intern Med 1989;100:495–499.

81. Pizzo PA, Eddy J, Falloon J, et al. Effect of continuous intravenous infusion of zidovudine (AZT) in children with symptomatic HIV infection. N Engl J Med 1988;319:889–896.

82. Fischl MA, Richmon DD, Causey DM, et al. Prolonged zidovudine therapy in patients with AIDS and advanced ARC. JAMA 1989;262:2405–2410.

83. National Institute of Allergy and Infectious Diseases. State of the art conference on AZT therapy for early HIV infection. JAMA 1990;363:1606–1609.

84. Volberding P, Lagakos S, Koch M, et al. Zidovudine in asymptomatic HIV infection: A controlled trial in persons with fewer than 500 CD4+ cells per cubic millimeter. N Engl J Med 1990;322:941–949.

85. Kahn J, Lagakos S, Richman D, et al. A controlled trial comparing zidovudine with didanosine in HIV infection. N Engl J Med 1992;327:581–7.

86. Meng T, Fischl M, Boota A, et al. Combination therapy with zidovudine and dideoxycytidine in patients with advanced HIV infection. Ann Intern Med 1992;116:13–20.

87. Centers for Disease Control. Guidelines for prophylaxis against PCP for persons infected with HIV. MMWR 1989;38 (suppl):1–7.

88. Soloway B, Hecht F. Changing approaches to prophylaxis for *Pneumocystis carinii* pneumonia. AIDS Clin Care 1992;4:61–65.

89 Litt IF, Cuskey WR. Compliance with medical regimens during adolescence. Pediatr Clin North Am 1980;27:3–15.

90. Futterman D, Hein K, Kipke M, HIV+ adolescents: HIV testing experiences and changes in risk-related sexual and drug use behaviors. [Abstract SC 663]. International Conference on AIDS, San Francisco, Jun 1990.

91. Perry S, Jacobsberg L, Fishman B. Suicidal ideation and HIV testing. JAMA 1990;263:679–682.

92. Hein K. Risky business: HIV in adolescents. Pediatrics 1991;88:1052–1054.

93. Rotheram-Borus MJ, Koopman C, Rosario M. Developmentally tailoring prevention programs: Matching strategies to adolescents' serostatus. In: DiClemente R ed. Adolescents and AIDS: A generation in jeopardy. Newbury Park, CA: Sage, 1992:212–229.

94. Hein K, DiGeronimo T. AIDS: Trading facts for fears: A guide for young people. New York: Consumer Reports Books, 1989.

95. National Research Council. AIDS and adolescents. In: Turner CF, Miller HG, Moses LE, eds. AIDS: Sexual behavior and intravenous drug use. Washington, DC: National Academy Press 1989:372–401.

96. Anonymous Peer education. Teens teaching teens about AIDS and HIV infection prevention. Washington, DC: Center for Population Options, 1989.

97. Kipke MD, Futterman DC, Hein K. HIV infection and AIDS during adolescence. Med Clin North Am 1990;74:1149-1167.

98. Kipke M, Boyer C, Hein K. An evaluation of an AIDS risk reduction and skills training program (ARREST). J Adol Health, in press.

99. Dubler N, Stern G. Illusions of immortality: The confrontation of adolescence and AIDS in America. Albany: New York State Department of Health, 1991:1–44

100. Select Committee on Children, Youth and Families. A decade of denial: Teens and AIDS in America. Washington, DC: House of Representatives, 102nd Congress, May 1992:1–394.

41

Obstetric Issues — Relevance to Women and Children

Howard L. Minkoff and Ann Duerr

The rate of new AIDS cases in the United States is rising more rapidly among women than it is among men, making AIDS the fifth leading cause of death of reproductive age women in this country. In some of the nation's cities it is already the leading cause of death among minority women of reproductive age. In addition to the litany of infectious complications that affect all human immunodeficiency virus (HIV)-infected individuals, women are subject to gender specific conditions such as a possibly more aggressive form of cervical neoplasia. Clearly perinatal transmission of HIV, although critically important, is not the only issue that encumbers seropositive woman. An appreciation of the social and clinical complexities that an infected women confronts will provide an appropriate context for discussions about interventions aimed primarily at pediatric prevention or palliation.

Providers of health care to women must now recognize the central role they play in this epidemic. Most women who see such providers, whether the clinicians be obstetrician/gynecologists, family practitioners or midwifes, see no other provider in a given year. Thus, if infected women are to be identified and given the opportunity to access new therapies, and if exposed neonates are to be identified in the neonatal period, these providers must recognize their responsibility to assure that all women have the opportunity to ascertain their serostatus for the sake of their children and themselves. Finally it must be recognized

that until the best interests of the mother and the child, vis à vis testing, converge, any program targeted solely to neonatal therapies or perinatal interventions will be destined to failure. This chapter is designed to serve as a primer for clinicians who are interested in the care of the mother as well as the child.

HIV TESTING OF WOMEN

Since testing for antibody to HIV became a practical clinical tool in 1985, various testing strategies have been proposed for women. Given the limited therapeutic armamentarium available for the care of women and children in the early 1980s, the driving force behind testing at the outset was to empower reproductive choice. Selwyn et al. (1) demonstrated early on, however, that at least among drug using women serostatus did not substantively alter the likelihood that they would elect to terminate pregnancy. Subsequently Sunderland and her colleagues (2) evaluated the reproductive choices of 98 drug and nondrug using seropositive women and 108 matched seronegative women. Although seropositive women were significantly more likely to abort an index pregnancy, only a small minority (18.8%) actually did so, and follow-up over the next year and a half showed a "catch up" with many seropositive women having one, two, or three subsequent pregnancies. Despite the fact that most evidence suggested, and recent data continue to suggest, that serostatus plays a marginal role at best in determining whether a woman will abort, it was still believed that each woman had the right to all information germane to her individual decision. The strategy that was most widely used at that time was selective offering of the test. Women who volunteered a history of risk behavior would have the advantages and disadvantages of the test discussed at their prenatal visit. Shortly thereafter, evidence of the failure of that approach began to be published. Several researchers compared HIV serosurveys with anonymously collected patient descriptors to which the surveys were linked and found that a large percentage of infected individuals had not acknowledged any risk behaviors (3). Results from a prospective study of 2724 pregnant women in Baltimore indicate that only 57% of seropositve women would have been detected if a targeted approach were used; the detection rate increased to 87% when all women were offered counseling and testing (4). At Bellevue, voluntary testing, based on active case finding and self identification, failed to detect 24 of 28 HIV-infected mothers (5). Since a history of intravenous drug use or sex with bisexual men is perceived to be a stigma to "main stream" society, many women, not surprisingly, did not choose to acknowledge these behaviors if the sole perceived advantage would be access to a test.

Informed by these reports, advocates of testing proposed strategies that reflected an understanding of the stigma attached to the acknowledgement of risk behavior. Many institutions, particularly those in high prevalence communities, moved in the direction of universally offering the test. As expected, it was then found that many women who at the time of pretest counseling acknowledged no risk, but whose test result confirmed an HIV infection, indeed knew their risk factor but chose not to discuss it until their serostatus had been established (6).

As interventions for both the mother and child were developed in the late 1980s many clinicians came to believe that merely "offering" the test was too passive a process. Given the medical advantage that accrued to the identified woman and her child it was felt that the imprimatur of the physician should be given to the test through the substitution of "recommending" for offering (7).

Currently many obstetrical services in high prevalence communities are recommending that all prenatal patients take an HIV test. There are clinicians who feel, however, that the time has come to go even further in testing. Some, who advocate either mandatory or "right of refusal" approaches to testing, do so based on the medical advantage for the child whose serostatus is known and the inability of the child to choose for itself. There is in fact debate between those who prioritize fetal/neonatal beneficence and those who believe that maternal autonomy should be paramount.

Pending a "cure" for the newborn or documentation in the peer reviewed literature of substantive improvement in the quality and quantity of life for the child based on available therapies, this debate will not be easily resolved. Current guidelines for obstetricians advocate testing but still strongly recommend that informed consent remain part of the pretest process.

The post-test counseling session for a seropositive woman should be planned before the woman arrives for her result. This planning includes a review of the woman's support network and the development of a follow-up plan for ongoing psychosocial support and medical evaluation. The clinician may find that the session proceeds more smoothly when it is conducted with two staff members present. An additional clinician familiar with counseling can act as a support person and can help assure that the patient understands the information being transmitted.

Women's reactions to learning they are HIV seropositive range from despair and anger to total denial and withdrawal (8). In general people react to learning this diagnosis in much the same way they have reacted to other stressful events in their lives. It is important to allow women sufficient time during the counseling session to work through some of these initial reactions. The experience of HIV counselors in Brooklyn is that the initial counseling session lasts between 45 and 75 min.

The content of the counseling that a woman receives if she is seropositive must be sufficient to assure an informed decision regarding reproductive choice. Information about the perinatal transmission of the virus, the consequence of pregnancy on the natural history of HIV disease, the natural history of pediatric HIV disease, and the therapeutic options for the woman should be described in lay language. If abortion is still an option, depending upon the woman's due date and the state's legal limit for abortion, the physician may choose to discuss it at this time. Liaison with psychosocial support services should be established and provided for the woman's decisions concerning pregnancy and other life issues.

INTERACTION OF HIV AND PREGNANCY

The biologic issues that most centrally form the content of counseling are the perinatal transmission rate of HIV and the consequence of pregnancy on the course of the mother's HIV infection. Perinatal transmission of HIV has been documented for almost a decade (9–14). The rate and determinants of that transmission, however, remain uncertain. Reported transmission rates have shown wide geographic variation ranging from 14 to over 50% (15). Biologic factors such as CD4 counts, viremia, recent seroconversion, and clinical illness may contribute to differing transmission rates (16–23). Additionally some work has focused on the role of maternal antibody on transmission although findings have not been uniform (24–30).

The timing of perinatal transmission also remains unclear with evidence to suggest both antepartum and intrapartum transmission (31–44). Although some evidence does point to intrapartum transmission there are no empiric data to support a protective effect to cesarean section, and, in fact, there are reports of infected babies who had been delivered abdominally. Clearly, the timing of perinatal transmission will have direct relevance to the design and ultimate success of trials designed to interrupt perinatal transmission (see below and Chapters 10C and 45).

Other pregnancy outcomes do not appear to be affected by serostatus, at least among asymptomatic patients. Birth weight and gestational age did not differ between HIV-infected drug using women and seronegative controls in reports from Britain (45) nor between seropositive and seronegative women from the United States regardless whether they had used drugs (46). Studies that included more symptomatic women, however, have reported higher prematurity rates and lower birth weights among seropositive women (47).

The possibility that pregnancy will modify the natural history of HIV disease is also still open. To understand the effect of pregnancy on the course of HIV disease it is essential for the clinician to understand both the normal immune response to foreign antigens and the effect of pregnancy on that response (48–50). The obstetric literature supports the hypothesis that a pregnant patient is more susceptible to various viral, bacterial, and fungal infections and is more likely to die from these infections than her nonpregnant counterpart. In an epidemic of Asian influenza, for example, 50% of women who died were pregnant, although pregnant women comprised only 7% of women in the reproductive age group (51). Similarly, infectious hepatitis reportedly carries a much higher mortality in pregnancy than in the nonpregnant state (52). Higher than normal isolation and infection rates have been reported among pregnant patients for other virus infections such as herpes, cytomegalovirus and poliomyelitis (53). Additionally, the severity of other infections such as malaria, toxoplasmosis, and listeriosis is greatly increased during pregnancy (53). Ascertainment bias, however, limits the reliability of much of these data.

Although a slight decrease in total immunoglobulins has been reported during pregnancy and somewhat reduced complement levels have been observed in the first trimester, these changes cannot account for the major decrease seen in immune response (54). Because the response to most infectious disorders noted above are cell mediated, it is thought that pregnancy may be associated with a decrease in cell-mediated immunity. The demonstrated ability of pregnant women to mount a satisfactory response to intradermal skin antigens, however, and their ability to reject skin grafts suggests that only certain selective functions of cell-mediated immunity are depressed during pregnancy (53). The main focus of interest has been on the role of lymphocytes in the depression of cell-mediated immunity.

It is not entirely clear in what manner T cell function is compromised in pregnancy. Sridama et al. (55) showed that there was a significant decrease in relative and absolute number of helper T lymphocytes (CD4) throughout pregnancy and the normalization of these cells occurred during the third and fifth month postpartum. No change in the ratio of other T cells was observed. Bailey et al. (56) also observed a decrease in T helper cells in pregnancy but thought patients had adequate T helper cell function as determined by in vitro immunoglobulin synthesis assay. They did not observe increased B suppressor activity and believed that a decrease in T helper cells was responsible for the immunodeficiency of pregnancy. A small but significant reduction in total circulating lymphocytes and the T helper subsets was reported by Vanderberken et al. (57), but no change in the T suppressor and cytotoxic cells (CD8) was found. In contrast, a progressive increase in the total number of T cells during the first two trimesters of pregnancy was reported by Fiddes et al. (58) and a decrease only noted in the third trimester. They also reported an increase in the T8 cells, which led to a significantly decreased T4 to T8 ratio. Glassman et al. (59) did not observe any significant alteration in the T cell subsets during pregnancy but reported significantly reduced B cells during the postpartum period.

Although the cited evidence is conflicting, most investigators agree that there is a decrease in cell-mediated immunity during pregnancy, a decrease probably mediated through an altered T helper cell-to-T suppressor cell ratio. Other factors contributing to the immunosuppression of pregnancy may be increased levels of total steroids and other pregnancy specific plasma proteins and hormones like human chorionic gonadotrophin, α-fetoprotein, and pregnancy-associated α$_2$-glycoprotein.

As noted, the multiple defects in the immune response seen in AIDS patients renders them susceptible to various opportunistic infections. Since pregnancy may also be associated with a significant depression of cell-mediated immunity, concern has been expressed that pregnancy could have an adverse effect on the natural history of HIV disease by enhancing the relative immunoincompetence. The initial reports of AIDS in pregnancy seemed to confirm this impression. The first five reported patients with cases of AIDS in pregnancy, all with opportunistic infection, died (60–62). As suggested by the authors, however, the poor outcome in pregnant women at that time may have represented reporting bias, delay in diagnosis and treatment, or an actual worsening of the infection in pregnancy. In one report on the follow-up of 34 HIV-positive mothers for a mean of 27.8±21.6 months, it was found that 15 of the women had developed AIDS or AIDS-related complex (63). This was higher than the expected progression of the disease in nonpregnant patients and suggested that perhaps pregnancy was responsible for the acceleration of their illness. A definite conclusion could not be drawn from that report since the mothers were identified through the birth of a child who developed AIDS and thus may be representative of a cohort with advanced immunocompromise. Several controlled studies have been reported in which HIV-positive mothers have been prospectively followed. Schaefer et al. (64) followed 32 HIV-positive women and 40 HIV-negative women during pregnancy and 6 months after delivery and did not observe any clinical progression of illness during pregnancy among seropositive women. Nine percent of patients developed signs of clinical worsening during postpartum observation. The authors believed that pregnancy had only a minor effect on the course of HIV disease. Bigger et al. (65) showed that the direction of immunologic changes seen in HIV-positive mothers was the same as that in HIV-negative control pregnancies except that drops in CD4 counts were 10-20% greater among seropositive women.

Other investigators have failed to show any evidence of disease progression during pregnancy. In a follow-up of 88 postpartum patients, MacCallum et al. (66) were unable to demonstrate any adverse effect of pregnancy on the course of HIV disease.

Similarly, Berrebi et al. (67) followed 23 pregnant patients and their matched seropositive nonpregnant controls for 2 years after delivery and could not find any statistical difference in the number of opportunistic infections between the two groups.

At present, a significant influence of pregnancy on the course of HIV disease has not been documented. The available evidence suggests that pregnancy may exert only a minor influence on the progression of disease. More prospective, long-term studies are needed before the impact of pregnancy will be clearly delineated.

CARE OF HIV-INFECTED PREGNANT WOMEN

The guiding principal in the care of pregnant women with any medical complication is to provide the ideal standard of care in an unmodified fashion unless there is compelling evidence that the standard presents an unacceptable risk to the fetus. In the latter circumstance the counsel of the mother is sought to best balance the benefits and burdens to the mother and child of utilizing an alternative approach. That same principal should stand for HIV-infected women, and there are very few examples of therapies that need to be modified because of pregnancy. Thus at the outset the clinician should assure that the usual interventions are in place. Pneumovax vaccine, influenza vaccine, and hepatitis vaccine should be administered if necessary (7). Testing should be performed to detect any sexually transmitted diseases such as syphilis, gonorrhea, and chlamydia. The woman should be evaluated for tuberculosis and toxoplasmosis.

During the antepartum period clinicians should be wary of nonspecific symptoms that may, in other circumstances, be attributed to pregnancy per se. Fatigue and weight loss are common in early pregnancy but may be harbingers of HIV symptomatology. Upper respiratory tract symptoms (e.g., fever and tachypnea) particularly warrant aggressive investigation. Patients should be encouraged to report all symptoms immediately. Nutritional counseling should be instituted if difficulty is encountered in maintaining appropriate weight gain. Although no cofactors have proved to adversely affect the rate of disease progression, it seems prudent to advise patients to avoid factors shown to alter T4-to-T8 ratios (sleep deprivation, stress) or enhance viral replication in vitro (e.g., antigenic stimulus, infections). Alcohol and illicit drugs should be discouraged.

The timing of the institution of many HIV therapeutic agents are currently related to CD4 counts. These counts should therefore be followed closely during pregnancy. Several authors reported that pregnancy per se will lead to changes in the CD4 count so a more frequent approach to monitoring may be warranted (7, 48, 68). Although some component of the decline of CD4 counts among seropositive women during pregnancy may be attributable to pregnancy, the prognostic significance of a low count cannot be assumed to be less reliable than in nonpregnant populations. In at least one small study the incidence of serious infectious morbidity among HIV-infected pregnant women with low counts was remarkably high (69). Among 16 patients whose CD4 count dropped below 300 mm^3, three developed opportunistic infections, one developed pneumonia and one had an intra-abdominal abscess. No serious infectious morbidity was seen among 40 seropositive women whose counts remained above 300 mm^3 throughout the pregnancy.

The standard approach to the utilization of prophylaxis against *Pneumocystis carinii* pneumonia can therefore, be maintained during pregnancy because the risk of *P. carinii* pneumonia in the mother far outweighs the risk to the fetus from therapy. Women whose CD4 counts drop below 200 mm^3 should be given either pentamidine or trimethoprim-sulfamethoxazole prophylaxis. Aerosolized pentamidine has the advantage of less frequent side effects and extremely low blood levels; but access to the aerosol form may not be readily available to all women, and its use has been associated with breakthrough of *P. carinii* (70, 71). Trimethoprim-sulfamethoxazole is readily available and highly effective. Although adverse maternal reactions are common (most commonly rash), neonatal consequences have not been serious, and kernicterus has not been reported in settings in which sulfa derivatives were not also used during the neonatal period. Although trimethoprim-sulfamethoxazole appears to provide more effective prophylaxis (70, 71) the specific drug that is used is probably less important than the fact that some therapy is prescribed during gestation.

Antiretrovirals have been recommended for nonpregnant individuals whose CD4 counts drop below 500 mm^3 (72). The degree of advantage to starting therapy at that level, as opposed to lower levels has recently been brought into question (73). Certain unique considerations have a bearing when deciding whether to use antiretrovirals during pregnancy. Although concerns about adverse fetal effects have to be addressed, the potential beneficial effects on vertical transmission must also be considered. Pharmacokinetics studies to date have shown that the drug will cross the placenta and achieve relatively high concentrations in the fetus and placenta within several hours of maternal dosing (74). Although animal data are, on the whole, reassuring in regard to teratogencity, one study has caused concern. Among rats exposed to zidovidine (ZDV) throughout their lives, 10% of the females were found to have nonmetastasizing vaginal tumors at the time of their deaths. Several factors make the relevance of these findings to humans highly tenuous. First, rats excrete ZDV and its metabolites in their urine, whereas humans do not, second, rats soil the vaginal vault with urine. It is questionable therefore whether in utero exposure to ZDV in humans will have the same potential for adverse sequelae as that seen in the rat model. The reported experience among humans exposed to ZDV during pregnancy although, small has not been worrisome. Sperling et al. (75) reported 43 women who took varying doses of ZDV for varying periods of time during gestation. No teratogenic effects were noted. The most common adverse sequela was anemia in the newborn, which often took place in a setting in which anemia might have been anticipated in any event (e.g., prematurity). Given the small sample size and short follow-up, however, the possibility of teratogenicity must still be entertained. Conversely, since ZDV acts to prevent reverse transcription of RNA the possibility also exists that its use in pregnancy could lower the perinatal viral transmission rate. This consideration is the basis for an ongoing placebo controlled trial that is discussed in "Prevention of Perinatal Transmission."

The intrapartum management of the HIV-infected mother is minimally affected by serostatus, although to some extend the care of all mothers and neonates in the labor and delivery suite has been altered by the HIV epidemic. The introduction of universal precautions into the labor and delivery area has changed some standards in that setting. Delee suctioning, for example, is no longer performed with suction generated by a clinician. The mucous trap is now attached to wall suction. With this new approach caution must be exercised lest excessive pressure be utilized that could theoretically damage the neonate's intestinal tract. It has been recommended that less than 140 mm/Hg be used (7).

Concerns about fetal scalp electrodes and scalp clips continue to be voiced. These concerns are based on the documented presence of virus in the vaginal secretions and the prolonged contact, that the fetus might have in the hours before birth, after the membranes have ruptured, with those virus particles. Some component of the fetus' protection at that point could be intact skin. Thus, piercing that skin to obtain a scalp blood sample or placing an electrode into the skin which could then act as a "wick" pose a theoretical risk of inoculating the fetus with virus. Very scant empiric data exist which address this concern. Although some investigators have reported that infants who underwent the types of invasive procedures described above were no more likely to become infected than infants not so exposed, the size of the cohorts was too small to have the requisite statistical power to eliminate the level of risk generally associated with needle stick injuries. Thus clinicians must continue to balance the theoretical risk of these procedures with the clinical benefit to be derived from their performance, and "routine" use should be avoided.

Data available on the relation of the mode of delivery to infant's serostatus do not support modification of current obstetrical guidelines. Many HIV-infected children have been delivered by cesarean section. Note, however, that few of the reports on infection and mode of delivery have commented on the status of membranes or the duration of labor, and none had sufficient sample size to eliminate the possibility of some ameliorating effect of operative delivery. Given the reported effect of birth order on neonatal infection among twins, with first born twins being at increased risk (42), and the presence of virus in vaginal secretions, the possibility that cesarean section could be beneficial cannot be eliminated. It is also possible that some form of vaginal antisepsis could also be of benefit. Pending the documentation of benefit from these approaches, the continued utilization of obstetrical indications for cesarean section seems warranted.

The clinician's responsibilities in the postpartum period include a continuation of universal precautions that should be extended to the neonate, a proscription of breast feeding (in developed countries), and appropriate referral of mother and child to physicians with expertise in the management of HIV disease. As soon as the child is born universal precautions should be exercised by its care providers. Gloves should be worn until all secretions have been removed from the skin.

The mother should be advised of the risks related to breast feeding. Sporadic, anecdotal reports have appeared in the literature for years that document transmission of HIV through breast milk (76–79). Most of the initial reports described mothers who had received blood transfusions in the early postpartum period. The assumption in these cases was that the mother was seronegative before the transfusion, although as a rule, serostatus had not been documented before the transfusion. In the succeeding months the children in these reports were found to be HIV infected. Subsequent cohort studies have, in general, verified the potential of HIV-infected mothers to transmit virus in the neonatal period through breast milk. Van de Perre et al. (80) followed 16 mothers who seroconverted during a mean follow-up of 16.6 months postpartum. Postnatal seroconversion occurred in four of the five infants born to mothers who seroconverted during

the first 3 months postpartum and in four of the ten who seroconverted between months 4 and 21 (one infant was excluded because of a positive polymerase chain reaction at birth). In all cases the infant seroconverted during the same 3-month period as the mother. Again, it appears that seroconversion in the mother denotes a particularly risky period from the point of view of virus transmission (80), in keeping with the known viremia associated with primary infection and seroconversion (81). Bulterys et al. (82), using the polymerase chain reaction to detect HIV in colostrum and breast milk, reported a 20% positivity rate overall, with somewhat higher rates in colostrum than in postneonatal milk samples. A prospective study of HIV-seropositive women and their infants also found evidence of HIV-infected cells in breast milk (83). Approximately half of breast milk samples taken 15 days postpartum and 20% of breast milk samples taken 6 months postpartum were positive for HIV-1 by polymerase chain reaction. Although all women were HIV seropositive during pregnancy and in utero transmission could not be differentiated from transmission occurring during or after delivery, it is noteworthy that the of HIV-infected cells in early breast milk was associated with HIV infection in the child, even after correcting for maternal immune status. The follow-up studies reported to date have not generally demonstrated a large difference in seroprevalence between breast fed and non breast fed cohorts. Recommendations to avoid breast feeding in the setting of HIV infection would seem prudent for developed parts of the world where safe alternatives to breast milk are readily available. Conversely, benefit/burden analyses clearly demonstrate the inappropriateness of the same approach in parts of the world where bottle feeding is not a practical alternative and where the consequences of proscribing breast milk would be far more detrimental to the health of HIV-exposed children than would be the risk of acquiring the virus (84).

NOSOCOMIAL RISK

An important concern of clinicians who care for HIV-infected parturients is the risk of nosocomial acquisition of HIV. The concern of obstetricians is heightened by the fact that theirs is a surgical subspecialty and by evidence of nosocomial risks in their field. Rates of hepatitis B, before hepatitis vaccine programs, for example, were high among obstetricians, and cluster outbreaks of hepatitis among patients of obstetrician/gynecologists have been reported. These facts reinforce the need for rigorous implementation of universal precautions by clinicians caring for parturient women (85).

Universal precautions require appropriate equipment and garb to prevent contact between skin and secretions and rapid cleansing to remove any secretions that contact skin. Therefore, during the delivery process clinicians should don water impermeable gowns and wear gloves (85). Splatter can occur, potentially contaminating the conjunctivae, so that goggles should also be worn (85). Since many injuries occur when needles are resheathed, needles should be immediately disposed of, unsheathed, in impenetrable disposal boxes (85). To avoid the need to carry unsheathed needles through wards, these boxes should be placed in all areas where needles might be used.

The operating suite poses particular risks to obstetricians during cesarean sections (86). Holes are found in gloves in as many as 15% of cases. Some studies have shown that these tears occur most often on the subordinate index finger, suggesting that the surgeon has been feeling for the placement of the needle (87). Although that technique may occasionally be unavoidable deep in the pelvis, this is rarely true during closure. Surgeons must reacquaint themselves with appropriate instruments for retraction and grasping to decrease reliance on their fingers. An additional safeguard is the use of "double gloving." Only one-third of tears in an outer glove will be accompanied by tears in an inner glove. The inner glove is generally a half size larger than standard while the outer glove is the surgeon's usual size. Finally a kidney basin can be used as a "way station" for sharp instruments during the procedure. The nurse then places requested sharps into the basin from which the surgeon retrieves them and vice versa. This technique avoids "blind" passes between operating room personnel.

PREVENTION OF PERINATAL TRANSMISSION

Despite dramatic improvements in the therapies available for the care of infected children, their prognosis remains grim. The need remains, thus, for continued attention to mechanisms to prevent the vertical transmission of HIV from the infected mother. Many theoretic underpinnings of a well designed assault on transmission however, still need to be addressed. The rates, timing, and determinants of transmission all must be known to optimize the design of intervention studies.

Unless the background rates of transmission are known it is difficult to obtain the appropriate power for a study and determine the sample size needed to demonstrate the protective effect of a pharmacologic intervention. Knowledge of the timing of transmission will inform the decision about timing of intervention, and the determinants of transmission must be known to assure that study groups start with similar background risks. As has been noted previously, knowledge in all these areas is accumulating.

Despite the array of scientific questions that remain open, trials are already underway to measure the efficacy of several interventions, and other protocols are under active development. The first large scale trial to be instituted was the AIDS Clinical Trials Group study 076, a trial of ZDV in late pregnancy, intrapartum, and the early neonatal period. Approximately 700 women will have to be enrolled in either the active (drug) or placebo arms of this study before the success of this approach can be gauged. This trial was preceded by pharmacokinetic studies of ZDV in pregnancy that demonstrated the passage of the agent and its metabolites into the fetal compartment. Experiments in animal models also suggested that the agent may be of benefit if given before challenge with the virus. At the time of this writing well over half the needed number of participants have been recruited, and efficacy cannot be commented upon. A preliminary analysis is being conducted in the fall of 1993.

The next agent scheduled to enter large scale trials will be HIV immunoglobulin (HIVIG). HIVIG is an immunoglobulin obtained from HIV-infected, asymptomatic volunteers. It has no p24 antigen and has high titers of antibody against p24 and components of the viral envelope. Initial studies suggested that HIV immune plasma can neutalize circulating infectious HIV (88, 89). More recent studies in nonpregnant individuals have documented some beneficial effects on the rates of change of CD4 counts with the administration of HIVIG. The perinatal trials of HIVIG will focus on women who are already on ZDV for maternal indications. The cohort under study will be more immunocompromised than that involved in 076 because those women must not have an indication for ZDV lest they be excluded. It is reasonable to hypothesize therefore that the HIVIG cohort's background transmission rate may be somewhat higher. In the HIVIG trial women will be randomized to receive either HIVIG and ZDV or intravenens immunoglobulin and ZDV. One concern about the use of HIVIG is a shift toward baseline levels that has been seen in the CD4 counts of nonpregnant individuals after their course of therapy has been completed.

Soluble CD4 is a molecule that is similar to the antigen found on the surface of cells to which HIV binds. This molecule has been bound to IgG to prolong its half-life and to facilitate transport across the placenta. In theory it will act as a "false receptor" for HIV so that the virus will not be free to bind to fetal cells. There are some data from animal work to support that theory. Phase I trials (safety and pharmacokinetics) of soluble CD4, however, have not provided encouraging results, and the pharmaceutical manufacturer has withdrawn the agent from trial.

Other areas of "intervention" research are ongoing. These include vaccines and monoclonal antibodies. It is hoped that these modalities will result in fetal protection via either passive or active immunity against key components of the virus. It is unclear at the moment which, if any, portion of the virus must be blocked if fetal infection is to be prevented.

WOMEN'S ISSUES

It is becoming increasingly clear that gender specific conditions will affect the course of HIV disease for women. What is also clear is that gender has important consequences of a nonbiologic nature that may also adversely affect the course of disease in women. Gender and/or childbearing capacity have had an impact on the ability of women to obtain the resources needed to negotiate their lives as infected individuals in this society. Access to resources as diverse as drug rehabilitation, standard therapeutic agents, and experimental protocols have all been limited for women.

A significant percentage of HIV-infected women acquire their infection through the use of intravenous drugs (90), and many of them are identified as seropositive through contacts with perinatal HIV testing programs. The chance that they will receive adequate care and follow-up for themselves, and hence be able to provide a reasonable environment for their children, is contingent on the provision of addiction services. It is therefore quite disconcerting to note that pregnancy often creates a significant barrier to many treatment programs in certain areas of the country.

Pregnancy also has been a barrier to access to standard therapeutic agents for HIV-infected women. Initial guidelines recommended that consideration of pentamidine be deferred, for example, until the completion of pregnancy (91). Thus a women whose CD4 count was <200 mm^3 early in pregnancy faced an approximate risk of 10% of acquiring a potentially lethal, often preventable pneumonia before the end of her gestation. Adhering to that recommendation would have placed obstetricians in the position of treating their patients' welfare as a secondary consideration and of supplanting the mother's rightful primacy as fetal advocate. Beyond these first principles, note that no particular risk has been associated with pentamidine to justify that recommendation and that serious pneumonia during pregnancy, even if not lethal, has been associated with preterm births and cannot be considered in the best interests of the fetus. Although current guidelines no longer recommend deferment of *P. carinii* prophylaxis during pregnancy (92), these "reflex" exclusions are emblematic of the difficulties confronting the seropositive women who conceives.

The difficulty these women have in obtaining drugs extends beyond difficulties in acquiring agents used as part of standard care of HIV-infected individuals. If anything, access to treatment trials is even more circumscribed. Indeed, until very recently national trials often expressly excluded not only pregnant and lactating women, but also women of childbearing capacity. Many institutional review boards and pharmaceutical industry protocols still contain similar exclusionary language. Thus for the individual who has failed standard therapy and for whom treatment trials are the sole remaining hope, gender can be a powerful obstacle. Recent Supreme Court rulings may have relevance in this regard. In the Johnsons Control case it was held that the possibility of exposure to teratogens was not sufficient justification to exclude women from a work place. The individual woman was allowed to strike the balance between the potential adverse consequences of exposure and loss of employment opportunities. The opportunity to participate in trials in which the benefit/burden considerations are equivocal would allow the same opportunity in research that the court allowed in employment.

References

1. Selwyn PA, Carter RJ, Schoenbaum EE, Robertson VJ, Klein RS. Rogers MF. Knowledge of HIV antibody status and decisions to continue or terminate pregnancy among intravenous drug users. JAMA 1989;261:3567–3571.
2. Sunderland A, Minkoff HL, Handte J, Moroso G, Landesman S. The impact of human immunodeficiency virus serostatus on reproductive decision of women. Obstet Gynecol 1992;7916:1027–1031.
3. Barbacci M, Repke J, Chaisson R: Routine prenatal screening for HIV infection. Lancet 1991;337:709–711.
4. Landesman S, Minkoff HL, Holman S, McCalla S, Sijin O. Sero Survey of Human Immunodeficiency Virus infection in Parturient. JAMA 1987;258:2701–2703.
5. Krasinski K, Borkowski W, Bebenroth D, Moore T. Failure of voluntary testing for human immunodeficiency virus to identify infected parturient women in a high-risk population [Letter]. N Engl J Med 1988; 318:185.
6. Minkoff HL, Landesman SH, Delke I, et al. Routinely offered prenatal HIV testing. N Engl J Med [Letter] 1988;319:1018.
7. Anonymous. Human immunodeficiency virus infections. College Obstet Gynecol Technical Bull (Revised) 1992;169:1–11.
8. Holman S, Sunderland A, Brethard M. Counselling of the HIV infected pregnant woman. Clin Obstet Gynecol 1989;32:486–491.
9. Centers for Disease Control. Unexplained immunodeficiency and opportunistic infections in infants, New York, New Jersey and California. MMWR 1982;31:665–667.
10. Joncas JH, Delage G, Chad Z, Lapointe N. Acquired or congenital immune deficiency syndrome in infants born to Haitian mothers [Editorial]. N Engl J Med 1983;308:842.
11. Rubenstein A, Sicklic M, Gupta A, et al. AIDS with reversed T4 to T8 ratios in infants born to promiscuous and drug addicted mothers. JAMA 1983; 249:2350–2356.
12. Oleske J, Minnefor A, Cooper R, et al. Immune deficiency syndrome in children. JAMA 1983;249:2345–2349.
13. Cowen MJ, Hellmar G, Chudwin D, Wara DW, Chang RS, Ammann A. Maternal transmission of acquired immune deficiency syndrome. Pediatrics 1984;73:382–386.
14. Thomas P, Jaffe H, Spira TJ, et al. Unexplained immune deficiency in children: a surveillance report. JAMA 1984;252:639–644.
15. European Collaborative Study. Risk factors for mother to child transmission of HIV-1. Lancet 1992;339:1007–1112
16. D'Arminio MA, Ravizza M, Muggiasca ML, et al. HIV-infected pregnant women: Possible predictors of vertical transmission [Abstract WC 49]. Seventh International Conference on AIDS, Florence, Jun 1991.
17. Hague RA, Mok JYQ, MacCallum L, et al. Do maternal factors influence the risk of HIV? [Abstract WC 3237] Seventh International Conference on AIDS, Florence, Jun 1991.
18. Van de Perre P, Simmon A, Msellanli P, et al. Mother-to-infant postnatal transmission of HIV-1: A cohort study [Abstract WC 33]. Seventh International Conference on AIDS, Florence, Jun 1991.
19. Kreiss J, Datta P, Willerford D, et al. Vertical transmission of HIV in Nairobi: Correlation with maternal viral burden [Abstract WC 3062]. Seventh International Conference on AIDS, Florence, Jun 1991.
20. Boue F, Pons JC, Keros L, et al. Risk for HIV-1 perinatal transmission vary with the mother's stage of HIV infection [Abstract Thc 44]. Sixth International Conference on AIDS, San Francisco, Jun 1990.
21. St. Louis ME, Kabagabo U, Brown C, et al. Maternal factors associated with perinatal HIV transmission [Abstract WC 3207]. Seventh International Conference on AIDS, Florence, Jun 1991.
22. Burns D, Muenz L, Walsh J, et al. Correlation of perinatal transmission of HIV-1 with mother's lowest prepartum CD4 level [Abstract 463]. 31st International Conference on Antimicrobial Agents and Chemotherapy, Chicago, Oct 1991.
23. Tibaldi C, Palomba E, Ziarati N, et al. Maternal factors influencing vertical HIV transmission [Abstract WC 3277]. Seventh International Conference on AIDS, Florence, Jun 1991.
24. Rossi P, Moschese V, Broliden PA, et al. Presence of maternal antibodies to human immunodeficiency virus 1 envelope glycoprotein gp120 epi-

topes correlates with the noninfective status of children born to seropositive mothers. Proc Natl Acad Sci USA 1989;86:8055–8058.

25. Broliden PA, Moschese V, Ljungren K, et al. Diagnostic implications of specific immunoglobulin G patterns born to HIV infected women. AIDS 1989;3:577–582.

26. Goedert J, Mendez H, Drummond JE, et al. Maternal infant transmission of HIV Type 1: Association with prematurity or low anti-qp120. Lancet 1989;2:1351–1353.

27. Devash Y, Calvelli T, Wood DG, et al. Vertical transmission of HIV is correlated with absence of high affinity/avidity maternal antibodies to the gp120 principal neutralizing domain. Proc Natl Acad Sci USA 1990;87:345–349.

28. Shaefer N, Parekh BS, Pau CP, et al. Maternal antibodies to V3 loop peptides of gp120 are *not* associated with lack of HIV-1 perinatal transmission [Abstract WC 49]. Seventh International Conference on AIDS, Florence, Jun l991.

29. Allain JP, Matthew T, Coombs R, et al. Antibody to V3 loop does not predict vertical transmission of HIV [Abstract WC 2263]. Seventh International Conference on AIDS, Florence, Jun 1991.

30. Ugen KE, Goedat JJ, Boyer J, et al. Vertical transmission of HIV infection. Reactivity of maternal sera with glycoprotein 120 and 41 peptides from HIV type 1. J Clin Invest 1992;89:1923–1930.

31. Lapointe N, Michaud J, Pekovic D, Chausseau, Dupuy JP. Transplacental transmission of HTLV-III virus [Letter]. N Engl J Med 985;312:1325.

32. Marion RW, Wiznia AA, Hutcheon G, et al. Human T cell lymphotrophic virus type embryopathy. A new dysmorphia syndrome. Am J Dis Child 1986;140:638–640.

33. Nicolas S. Is there an HIV associated facial dysmorphism? Pediatr Ann 1988;17:353.

34. Qazi QH, Sheikh TM, Fikrig S. Lack of evidence for craniofacial dysmorphism in perinatal HIV infection. J Pediatr 1988;112:7–11.

35. Courgnaud V, Laure F, Barin F, et al. In utero HIV-1 transmission identified through PCR [Abstract MBP-1]. Fifth International Conference on AIDS, Montreal, Jun 1989.

36. Soeiro R, Rashbaun WF, Rubenstein A, Lyman WD. The incidence of human fetal HIV-1 infection as determined by the presence of HIV-1 DNA in abortus tissues [Abstract WC 3250]. Seventh International Conference on AIDS, Florence, Jun 1991.

37. Courpotin C, Israel G, Dubeaux D, et al. Predictive value of HIV replication in cell culture in babies born to seropositive mothers. Lancet 1988;2:1074–1074.

38. Fleury HJA, Delord B, Douard D, Interet de la mise enculture systematique du VIH chez les enfants nes de mieres infectees [Abstract TBP245]. Fifth International Conference on AIDS, Montreal, Jun 1989.

39. Borkowski W, Krazinski K, Paul D, et al. Human immunodeficiency virus type 1 antigenemia in children. J Pediatr 1989;114:940–945.

40. Ehrnst A, Lindgren S, Dictor, et al. HIV in pregnant women and their offspring: Evidence for late transmission. Lancet 1991;338:203–207.

41. Hanson CG, Shearer WT. Pediatric AIDS: Diagnosis of HIV infection in infants and children.

In: Feigin RD, Cherry JD, eds. Textbook of pediatric infectious diseases, 3rd ed. Philadelphia: WB Saunders 1992.

42. Goedert JJ, Duliege AM, Amos CI, Felton S, Biggar RJ. High risk of HIV-1 infection for first born twins. Lancet 1991;338:1471–1475.

43. Landesman S, Weiblem B, Mendez H, et al. Clinical utility of HIV-IgA assay in the early diagnosis of perinatal HIV infection. JAMA 1991;266:3443–3446.

44. Quinn TC, Kline RL, Halsey N, et al. Early diagnosis of perinatal HIV infection by detection of viral specific IgA antibodies. JAMA 1991;266:3439–3442

45. Johnstone FD, MacCullum L, Brettle R, Inglis JM, Peutherer JF. Does infection with HIV affect the outcome of pregnancy?' Br Med J 1988;296:467.

46. Minkoff HL, Henderson C, Mendez H, et al. Pregnancy outcomes among women infected with HIV and matched controls. Am J Obstet Gynecol 1990;163:1598–1603.

47. Ryder RW, Nsa W, Hassig SE, et al. Perinatal transmission of the human immunodeficiency virus type 1 to infants of seropositive women in Zaire. N Engl J Med 1989;320:1637–1642.

48. Nanda D, Minkoff HL. HIV in pregnancy-transmission and immune effects. Clin Obstet Gynecol 1989;32:456–466.

49. Claman HN. The biology of the immune response. JAMA 1987;258:2834.

50. Nosal Gustave JV. The basic components of the immune system. N Engl J Med 1987;316:1320.

51. Bowen DL, Lane HC, Fauci AS. Immunopathogenesis of the acquired immunodeficiency syndrome. Ann Intern Med 1985;103:704.

52. Freeman DW, Barno A. Deaths from influenza epidemic associated with pregnancy. Am J Obstet Gynecol 1969;78:1172.

53. Weinberg ED. Pregnancy associated depression of cell mediated immunity. Review of infectious diseases. 1984;6:814.

54. Gall S. Maternal immune system during human gestation. Semin Perinatol 1977;1:119.

55. Sridama V, Pacini F, Yang SL, et al. Decreased level of helper T cells: A possible cause of immunodeficiency in pregnancy. N Engl J Med 1982;307:352.

56. Baily K, Herrod HG, Younger R, Shaver D. Functional aspects of T-lymphocyte subsets in pregnancy. Obstet Gynecol 1985;66:211.

57. Vanderberken Y, Vheghe MP, Velespesse G, et al. Clin Exp Immunol 1982;48:1118.

58. Fiddes TM, O'Reilly DB, Cetrulo CL, et al. Phenotypic and functional evaluation of suppressor cells in normal pregnancy and in chronic aborters. Cell Immunol 1986;97:407–418.

59. Glassman AB, Bennet CE, Christopher JB, Self S. Immunity during pregnancy: Lymphocyte subpopulations and mitogen responsiveness. Ann Clin Lab Sci 1985;15:357–362.

60. Minkoff HL, DeRegt RH, Landesman S, Schwarz R. *Pneumocystis carinii* pneumonia associated with acquired immunodeficiency syndrome in pregnancy: a report of three maternal deaths. Obstet Gynecol 1986;67:284–287.

61. Wetli CV, Roldan EO, Fujaco RM. Listeriosis as a cause of maternal death: An obstetric complication

of the acquired immunodeficiency syndrome
(AIDS). Am J Obstet Gynecol 1983;147:7–9.

62. Jensen LP, O'Sullivan MJ, Gomez-del-Rio M, et al.
Acquired immune deficiency syndrome in pregnancy. Am J Obstet Gynecol 1984;148:1145–1146.

63. Minkoff H, Nanda D, Menez R, Fikrig S.
Pregnancies resulting in infants with acquired immunodeficiency syndrome or AIDS related complex. Obstet Gynecol 1987;69:285

64. Schaefer A, Grosch-Woerner I, Friedman W,
Kunzer R, Mielke M, Jimenez E. The effect of pregnancy on the natural course of HIV disease
[Abstract 4039]. Fourth International Conference
on AIDS, Stockholm, Jun 1988.

65. Bigger RJ, Pahwa S, Landesman S, Goedert JJ.
Helper and suppressor lymphocyte changes in
HIV-infected mothers and their infants [Abstract
4031]. Fourth International Conference on AIDS,
Stockholm, Jun 1988.

66. MacCallum LR, France AJ, Jones ME, et al. The effects of pregnancy on the progression of HIV disease [Abstract 4032]. Fourth International
Conference on AIDS, Stockholm, Jun 1988.

67. Berrebi A, Kobuch WE, Puel J, et al. Influence of
pregnancy on human immunodeficiency virus disease. Eur J Obstet Gynecol 1990;37:211–217

68. Biggar RJ, Pahava S, Minkoff HL, et al. Immunosuppression in pregnant women infected with
human immunodeficiency virus. Am J Obstet
Gynecol 1989;161:1239–1244.

69. Minkoff HL, Willoughby A, Mendez H, et al. Serious
infections among women with advanced HIV infection. Am J Obstet Gynecol 1990;162:30–34

70. Schneider M, Hoepelman A, Schattenkerk J, et al.
A controlled trial of aerosolized pentamidine or
trimethoprim-sulfamethoxazole as primary prophylaxis against *Pneumocystis carinii* pneumonia in
patients with human immunodeficiency virus infection. N Engl J Med 1992; 327:1836–1842.

71. Hardy D, Feinberg J, Finkelstein D, et al. A controlled trial of trimethoprim-sulfamethoxazole or
aerosolized pentamidine for secondary prophylaxis of *Pneumocystis carinii* pneumonia in patients with the acquired immunodeficiency syndrome. N Engl J Med 1992;327:1842–1848.

72. Volberding P, Lagakos S, Koch M, et al.
Zidovudine in asymptomatic human immunodeficiency virus infection. A controlled trial in persons
with fewer than 500 CD4-positive cell per cubic
millimeter. N Engl J Med 1990;322:941–949.

73. Editorial. Zidovudine for symptomless HIV infection. Lancet 1990:335:821–822.

74. Little BB, Bawdon RE, Christmas JT, Sobhi S,
Gilstrap LC. Pharmacokinetics of azidothymidine
during late pregnancy in Long-Evans rats. Am J
Obstet Gynecol 1989;161:732–734.

75. Sperling RS, Stratton P, OB/GYN Working Group of
ACTG. Treatment options for HIV virus infected pregnant women. Obstet Gynecol 1992;79:443–447.

76. Zeigler JB, Cooper DA, Johnson RO, et al. Postnatal
transmission of AIDS associated retrovirus from
mother to infant. Lancet 1984;1:896–898.

77. Lepage P, Van de Perre P, Caraël M, et al.
Postnatal transmission of HIV mother to child
[Letter]. Lancet 1987;2: 400.

78. Weinbreck P, Loustaud V, Denis F, et al. Postnatal
transmission of HIV infection [Letter]. Lancet
1988;1:482.

79. Colebunders R, Kapita B, Nekwei W, et al.
Breastfeeding and transmission of HIV [Abstract
5103]. Fourth International Conference on AIDS
Stockholm, Jun 1988.

80. Van de Perre P, Simonon A, Msellati P, et al.
Postnatal transmission of human immunodefi-
ciency virus type 1 from mother to infant. N Engl J
Med 1991;325:593–598

81. Daar E, Moudgil T, Meyer R, Ho D. Transient high
levels of viremia in patients with primary human
immunodeficiency virus type 1 infection. N Engl J
Med 1991;324:961–964.

82. Bulterys M, Chao A, Farzadegan H, et al. Detection
of HIV-1 in breast milk, multiple sexual partners
and mother-to-child transmission of HIV-1: A cohort study [Abstract ThC 1524]. Eighth International
Conference on AIDS, Amsterdam, Jul 1992.

83. Van de Perre P, Simonon A, Hitimana D, et al.
Infective and anti-infective properties of breastmilk
from HIV-1-infected women. Lancet 1993;341:
914–918.

84. Hu D, Heyward W, Byers R, et al. HIV transmission from breastfeeding: policy implications
through a decision analysis model. AIDS 1992;
6:1505–1514.

85. Centers for Disease Control. Recommendations for
prevention of HIV transmission in health-care settings. MMWR 1987;36;2S–18S.

86. Panlilio A, Welsh B, Bell D, et al. Blood and amniotic fluid contact sustained by obstetric personnel
during deliveries. Am J Obstet Gynecol 1992;
167:703–708.

87. Tokars J, Bell D, Culver D, et al. Percutaneous injuries during surgical procedures. JAMA 1992;167:
2899–2904.

88. Jackson G, Rubenic M, Knigge M, et al. Passive
immunoneutralization of HIV patients with advanced AIDS. Lancet 1989;2:647–651.

89. Karpas A, Hill F, Youle M, et al. Effects of passive
immunization in patients with AIDS-related complex and AIDS. Proc Natl Acad Sci USA 1988;85:
9234–9237.

90. Ellerbrock T, Bush T, Chamberland M, Oxtoby M,
Epidemiology of women with AIDS in the United
States, 1981 through 1990. A comparison with
heterosexual men with AIDS. JAMA 1991;265:
2971–2975.

91. Centers for Disease Control. Guideline for prophylaxis against *Pneumocystis carinii* pneumonia for
persons infected with human immunodeficiency
virus. MMWR 1989;38:1–9.

92. Centers for Disease Control. Recommendations for
prophylaxis against *Pneumocystis carinii* pneumonia for adults and adolescents injected with human
immunodeficiency virus. MMWR 1982;41(RR-
4):1–11.

42

Nursing Roles in Care of Child and Family

Mary G. Boland and Sheila J. Santacroce

Human immunodeficiency virus (HIV) infection in children is a worldwide problem and not confined to selected communities, cities, or countries. Knowledge regarding the diagnosis, management, and treatment of children with HIV infection continues to increase, requiring that nursing practice keep pace. The progressive nature of the disease and psychosocial issues complicate nursing care of the child with HIV infection. It is critical that management and treatment begin early; if the signs and symptoms are recognized, the effects of the illness can be minimized through supportive and antiretroviral therapies. This chapter will discuss the care of the infant and child with perinatally transmitted HIV infection utilizing a comprehensive and family centered approach, recognizing that nurses provide care in various settings and circumstances in both the developing and developed world. The authors recognize that nurses assume responsibility for much of the management of care, particularly in secondary and tertiary care settings in the developed world. Our intent is to provide a framework that integrates current scientific information with existing nursing practice.

PRINCIPLES OF CARE

HIV infection meets the definition of chronic illness as "a condition with a protracted course which can be progressive and fatal, or associated with a normal life span despite impaired physical and mental functioning" (1). Because children with chronic illnesses constitute an increasing percentage of patients there has been substantial

interest in the impact on the children, their families, and the health care system. As we improve our interventions for HIV infection, we are making steady progress toward improving the life span of infected children and adults. Commonalities with other childhood illness are evident as are the differences in both the issues faced by children and families and the demands placed on nurses and other providers.

When an illness is chronic and of extended duration, the family is impacted as well as the child. Although both parents are responsible for the care, mothers and fathers play different roles with the mother assuming responsibility for maintenance of the family as a unit while also serving as the physical caretaker of the ill child in most families. The mothers of HIV-infected children are themselves infected and can suffer from feelings of guilt, low self-esteem, and worthlessness. Some families are fragile because of difficulties that predated the diagnosis of HIV infection, such as drug and alcohol abuse. Some children may not know their biological parents as a result of placement with relatives or foster or adoptive parents early in life. Regardless of the form of the family or the emotional, social, or financial difficulties it faces, it is the substance of the relationships that are sustaining to the child. The family unit, with its various configurations, struggles to respond to the diagnosis of HIV. Families face the loss of the chronically ill child and adult throughout their lives, resulting in feelings of chronic sorrow. Often, family members experience physical fatigue and health problems combined with serious ongoing social and financial stressors. Even when there is adequate health insurance, other expenses such as transportation to clinics and time lost from work can stress a family's budget. Financial problems are intensified when there is inadequate or no health insurance. As HIV-infected parents become ill, their ability to care adequately for the infected child may decrease. The family requires more support to meet the needs of each member and to maintain the family system.

Some HIV-infected children have been receiving care for as long as 9 years and have yet to develop AIDS. Their long-term survival may be attributed to continuous care as well as the unique characteristics of their particular infection. In many families, the demands of the child are part of a larger quilt of multiple needs that exist within the family unit. Service providers have recognized that caring for children within such complicated and complex family situations requires the development of new approaches and models for service delivery.

When provided with the opportunity, families speak clearly about their needs and wants in relation to care. At an invitational family meeting on pediatric AIDS, families identified easy access and constant availability of a single identified person (either physician, nurse, or social worker) as the one factor that enabled them to care effectively for their child. Additionally, family to family support and a belief in hope that is shared by health care, education, and social service personnel were identified as helping biological, extended, and foster families. The families described as least helpful services provided in a piecemeal fashion, with the family responsible for locating and coordinating services. Even when the quality of actual health care is excellent, the family members reported feeling angry, stressed, and overwhelmed when forced to find and coordinate ancillary services (2).

Although families can describe their needs and the number of children with chronic illness is increasing, the delivery of health care in the United States continues to be oriented toward treatment of acute episodic illness. The variation in expectations between chronically ill consumers and acute care providers can lead to conflict and a struggle for control. In one study, families felt this struggle was second only to the uncertainty surrounding the child's survival (3). Yet, the parent and provider must come to some resolution if care is to adapt to the realities of their child's complex and ongoing health status. Over time, an ongoing involvement with one provider, can develop into a trusting relationship. However, this process is not easy. It requires the ability to assess the family's adaptation to the child's condition and also a willingness to share what has traditionally been the territory of professional care providers. Initially, a formal assessment of the family structure (household members, pattern of drug and alcohol use, sources of support, and previous stressors) is helpful in identifying needs and resources available to help care for the family. Such an assess must be ongoing because changes occur frequently in disorganized families.

Because of the multiple and varying needs of the HIV-infected child, parents will develop relationships with providers that evolve over time. As parents become increasingly knowledgeable about health care delivery they see an ongoing need to negotiate the health care system. Nurses must be willing to invest in the development of a nurse patient/parent relationship where both acknowledge the limitations of existing knowledge and service delivery but negotiate an alliance that acknowledges and respects the experiences of both the child/parent and nurse.

A complex interaction occurs among chronic illness, the family's response, and the child's developmental status. Changes in all three occur simultaneously: the child develops, the chronic condition changes as it follows its course, and the family changes through its life cycle and its adaptation to the child's unfolding condition (4). Care for most HIV-infected children requires lifelong treatment involving multiple drug regimens with oral and intravenous treatments and complex medical interventions (5). As care proceeds, nurses must be sensitive to changes in the child, the child's medical condition, and the family situation.

The dynamic of the ongoing care needs of multiple family members and the inability to separate the health and social service needs of families has served as a catalyst for the development of new approaches to the care of HIV-infected children. Typically, such programs attempt to provide comprehensive services throughout the continuum of wellness and illness incorporating concrete social services with health care. The organization and structure of such programs varies with each community, but it is clear that such cooperative efforts are having an impact on the delivery of services (6). The multiple providers involved with a family must develop mechanisms that assure coordination and collaboration (7). A failure to do so can result in fragmentation, duplication of services, manipulation of service providers, and staff or agency splitting.

Planning Nursing Care

Nurses have played a central role in building and staffing networks for HIV-infected infants, children, and families. The range of services needed may include hospital and ambulatory based care, counseling, child development services, home care, hospice care, transportation, housing, food, and financial and legal assistance. Longer survival creates a demand for health services over an extended period and in multiple settings, including long-term care facilities, day care centers, and schools. Nurses will continue to be a key source of support in providing critical health care. Hospital and community based nurses contribute to successful patient outcomes when they function as case managers who link children and their families with the services they need. They can become the link between the family and the child's medical team, deliver high-tech care, reinforce teaching, and provide emotional support. Many community nursing agencies provide other home based services such as home health aides, therapists, nutritionists, nutritionists, and social workers. Although case management has various definitions and can be provided by several providers in many settings, case management delivered by nurses is generally linked to the delivery of health care services either at the primary or tertiary level. Most definitions of case management incorporated client intake and assessment, service planning, referral and system linkage, monitoring of service, and advocacy on behalf of clients. At times, the case management may be informal and consist of coordination of services. At other times, the role may be formalized and the process specifically defined and evaluated (8).

When planning nursing care for an individual with HIV infection the complete spectrum of disease must be considered. HIV-infected children will continue to require multiple services in various settings. During their treatment, a child and family can expect to encounter many nurses performing multiple roles. Because, for many nurses, their practice is dictated by the requirements of the setting or position, there is a temptation to narrow the nursing focus to the immediate needs of the child in a particular setting. However, the scope of nursing need for the child is broad and will change with symptoms, treatment, and disease progression. The nurse who combines excellent clinical and interpersonal skills with sensitivity and respect for children and a willingness to educate and support the child and caretakers can make a tremendous difference in the quality of life for that child and family (Table 42.1). It is well accepted that nursing care of children is a family centered subspecialty, but pernatally transmitted HIV infection is forcing the evolution of a new dimension to family centered care. The nurse can no longer define her patient as the ill child when both adults and children are infected and require care. To provide the continuous care dictated by the chronicity of the disease the caretaker must be engaged and the needs addressed as defined by the families. Nurses must understand that many disorganized families are action oriented, moving from one crisis to the next with little energy or interest for dealing with needs that appear not to be acute. Health care services that are perceived as "doing nothing" (i.e., no prescription, procedure, treatment, or improvement in condition) may be viewed as valueless. Denial is the most commonly used defense and breaks down, sometimes only temporarily, when faced with dramatic signs of illness. Therefore, there is potential for a clash between the values of highly trained professionals focused on health needs and families fighting to survive.

Scope of Nursing Practice

As the care of HIV infection increases in complexity, nurses will serve in expanded

Table 42.1.   Concepts Essential for Nurses Caring for Children with HIV

A basic understanding of
  Immunology and nursing implications
  Etiology of HIV infection
  Epidemiology of HIV infection in children
  Centers for Disease Control classification for HIV in children
  Methods of diagnosis
  Prognosis and course of illness

An ability to
  Perform a nursing assessment of symptoms, including development evaluation
  Perform an ongoing family assessment, including caretakers' need for support
  Develop a plan for nursing and family management of symptoms
  Conduct developmentally appropriate child and family education

An awareness of
  Treatments available for combating HIV infection in children
  Common therapies for treating specific viral and bacterial infections
  High risk for child abuse and neglect in children with HIV, hallmarks of abuse, and responsibility
    to report
  Community resources and mechanisms for referral
  Availability of medical research protocols and mechanisms for referral
  Issues facing families of children with a chronic fatal illness
  Professional responsibility to provide care and maintain confidentiality
  Obligation to use universal precautions

roles as direct providers of care and treatment, including prescription of medication and performance of invasive procedures. Certified Pediatric Nurse Practitioners, by virtue of their training and certification, can function in all care settings performing physical examinations, triaging sick children, prescribing medications, and performing procedures under the guidelines of individual state nurse practice acts. Laws governing nursing practice have been revised in several states to include this authority and to provide direct third party reimbursement for nurses who meet the licensing and certification standards for advanced practice. Guided by clinical practice protocols the care of persons with HIV and AIDS already has become the responsibility of nurses in secondary and tertiary care center (9). In academic research settings nurses are responsible for implementation and management of protocols related to clinical research and investigational drug therapies.

CLINICAL ISSUES

Identification of Infected Infants

Advances in routine prophylaxis of HIV-associated infections and antiretroviral therapy minimizes and delays the onset of symptoms and prolongs the lives of children with HIV infection. Therefore, infants at risk must be identified at birth and ideally, prenatally through voluntary, confidential testing or newborn screening programs (10, 11). Nurses practicing in the area of women's health should become skilled in counseling women. Testing should be offered to all women of childbearing age, regardless of pregnancy status and not based solely on self-identified risk factors, allowing for informed reproductive decisions before pregnancy and more complete identification of infected women (12). Pediatric nurses should have a high index of suspicion and raise the issue of testing for HIV infection for infants born to mothers at risk or those who exhibit symptoms suspicious of immunodeficiency (11) (see Chapter 1, 12, and 38).

Screening and Diagnosis

When testing for HIV is offered, it is always accompanied by culturally sensitive counseling. Before testing, the nurse informs the woman being tested or the parent/guardian of the child that the test being offered is for HIV, why HIV is suspected, and why testing is desirable and discusses HIV test interpretation and the implication for adults and children, available treatments for HIV/AIDS, as well as HIV transmission risks and prevention. Written informed consent is obtained.

Test results are only given in person to the individual tested (in the case of children, the parent or guardian). The nurse counsels the woman concerning the meaning and implication of results as well as HIV infection risk reduction strategies before giving the results. Test result disclosure usually causes an emotional response that limits the usefulness of discussing health-related issues later (13). She is offered referrals for clinical care and psychosocial support. The nurse should discuss appropriate person with whom the woman should discuss her diagnosis, emphasizing sexual partners, assisting the woman in developing a plan for such discussions, and anticipating possible reactions. Prevention of HIV transmission, including safer sex, and risks to infants born to infected women are included in the counseling session.

Because infants born to infected women retain maternal HIV antibodies for as long as 15 months after birth, the enzyme-linked immunosorbent assay and Western blot reveals the mother's status-possibly the first confirmation of her infection (14). The nurse must be prepared to support the mother's emotional response to the personal implications of her child's test.

When a child is found to be HIV infected (or seropostive and younger than 18 months), the parent is informed that the child is at risk for AIDS. The course of the illness is again described, including the fatal outcome. Emphasis is placed on treatment opportunities for prolongation of life and minimized disability. Caretakers are taught by the nurse that certain conditions must be evaluated immediately by a physician: fever, because of increased risk of serious bacterial infection; rapid breathing, because of the subtle onset of *Pneumocystis carinii* pneumonia and its seriousness for infants; and changes in mental status, because of implications as evidence of meningitis. The caretakers is also strongly advised that all medical care providers should be informed of the child's HIV status to ensure appropriate and rapid evaluation of the child with an impaired immune system. The nurse validates that the caretaker can use and read a ther-

mometer through direct observation. One is provided if there is none available at home. *P. carinii* pneumonia prophylaxis is initiated for the child older than 1 month until adequacy of immune function can be determined (see Chapter 21). The nurse informs the caretaker of the importance of the medication, dose, schedule, and potential side effects. A referral is made immediately to a center with expertise in caring for children with HIV infection for further evaluation and initiation of therapy when indicated. When the diagnosis is made at a referral center, local care providers are informed with the parents' consent, and a public health nurse referral is strongly recommended for ongoing evaluation and parent support.

When HIV infection is diagnosed in an older child, the issues of revealing the diagnosis to the child must be raised with caretakers. Parents often express concern about the child's potential reaction to the diagnosis and the reaction of others if the child shares the information with friends or teachers. Parents often initially refuse, but eventually agree, to informing children, particularly when the child becomes symptomatic and treatment is initiated or changed. When consent is given, developmentally appropriate information is presented to the child. Parents often appreciate the support of the medical team in explaining the diagnosis to children through preparation for the discussion, their presence during the discussion by the parents, or by their presentation of the information to the child in the parents' presence. Validation that child heard the information correctly is essential. A difficult area for parents to discuss is the mode of acquisition, especially when congenital infection is related to the parent's sexual activity or drug use. Children handle the diagnosis well, and many state they knew or had strong suspicions but felt unable to ask the parents for confirmation (15) (see Chapters 43, 50, and 51).

Treatment

As it has become apparent that therapy prolongs life and improves symptoms, treatment has become recommended for children before the onset of profound clinical symptomatology and immune devastation. Current research efforts focus on evaluation of new agents as well as maximizing the effect of known agents through testing of combination therapies (see Chapter 35). Strategies to delay the onset of serious symptoms in children with HIV infection include efforts to block replication of HIV, to prevent and specific infectious agents, and to strengthen the immune system (Table 42.2).

Prevention of Complications

Major responsibilities of the professional nurse in caring for the child with HIV infection include protecting health, promoting growth and development, minimizing disability related to HIV, and maximizing the quality of life.

Infection

Infection in the child with HIV is a major cause of morbidity, disability, and death. Nursing efforts are focused on the prevention of infection. Hygiene measures are initiated in the home and in the hospital with an emphasis on hand washing before and after patient contact and handling of secretions, such as with changing diapers. Homes should be assessed for the availability of a clean water supply and ability to provide appropriate storage for foods and medications. Personal hygiene measures including oral cavity and skin care should be reviewed with caretakers to prevent infection and minimize discomfort.

Immunization is critical in the prevention of communicable diseases (see Chapter 46) (16). Also all health care personnel working with HIV infected children must meet recommendations for measles vaccination and should receive influenza virus vaccine when offered to prevent transmission of these illnesses to their patients (17). Immunization status of the child should be evaluated at each medical visit and outstanding doses given then to improve compliance and ensure protection. Children with HIV infection should be routinely assessed for exposure to *Mycobacterium tuberculosis*. Nurses should instruct caretakers in the procedure for reporting results. Public health nurses are available to visit homes, evaluate responses, and report findings to the HIV team.

Children with HIV infection often cannot produce functional antibody. Immune serum immunoglobulin infusions may be initiated in select children to decrease the incidence of serious bacterial and viral infections.

Parents are taught to monitor and assess their children for signs of infection, including fever, rapid or shallow breathing, change in level of consciousness, diarrhea for more than one day, or onset of rash. Of particular significance is *P. carinii* pneumonia. Efforts are made to identify children at risk and attempt prevention through the prophylactic use of selected chemotherapeutic drugs such as trimethoprim-sulfamethoxazole (Bactrim). Any child who presents with symptoms of infection should be seen immediately for a medical assessment and *Pneumocystis* considered, even if the child is receiving prophylaxis. All health care personnel evaluating a child should be informed of the HIV status so an appropriate work up is undertaken.

Varicella presents a problem to the child with HIV infection. Parents should request that their child's teacher, school nurse, and parents of playmates inform them if classmates or playmates develop chicken pox. Varicella zoster immunoglobulin is administered within 96 hrs of a significant exposure to varicella zoster. Children who visit clinics or are hospitalized are placed in isolation for 10–21 days after exposure (17). If varicella develops, acyclovir is administered intravenously. Strict isolation is enforced until all lesions have crusted. Nursing measures include skin care, maintenance of hydration, management of fever, provision of comfort measures, and assessment for dissemination of disease. HIV infected parents or contacts of a child with varicella are at minimal risk if they have had chicken pox before acquiring HIV. Health care workers who are susceptible to varicella zoster should not be assigned to children with active illness (18).

Many infants and children with HIV have chronic problems with oral thrush, *candida* diaper dermatitis, and esopageal candidiasis. Nursing measures include instructing parents in assessment of the infection, administering antifungal medications for maximum effectiveness, providing adequate hydration, nutrition, and skin care, and managing pain. Whenever a child with HIV infection and fever presents to medical care, the nurse should asses the caretakers' ability for follow-up and adherence to prescribed care measures, understanding and skills, and likelihood of returning for reevaluation if the child worsens. Although some nonserious causes of fever may be managed at home, not all caretakers can do so. Follow-up by telephone or visit is established before discharge, and means of contacting the health care team are identified (19).

Children with HIV infection experience neutropenia related to their illness as well as to its treatment. Recombinant growth factors have the potential for ameliorating or eliminating myelosuppression and its associated risks (20). Children who are neutropenic and have fever should be evaluated immediately: obtain and assess a history and obtain cultures of urine, stool, blood, posterior pharynx, and any obvious lesions or wounds. If the child has an indwelling central venous access device, blood cultures are obtained from the port of each lumen an appropriately labeled. A chest X-ray is obtained, and oxygen saturation is measured using pulse oximetry; the need for other diagnostic tests is considered and therapy initiated without delay.

Bleeding

Anemia and thrombocytopenia are common findings in the child with HIV infection (see Chapter 32). Children will often undergo complete assessments to determine the causes of these problems. Others will improve with the initiation of antiretroviral therapy. Some children will require replacement through transfusion, infusion of intravenous immunoglobulin or steroids for management of an autoimmune process. Erythropoietin has been helpful in the management of anemia in children with renal disease and may be indicated in HIV infection. Nursing management of symptoms related to anemia include cardiovascular and respiratory assessment and initiation of measures to conserve energy. Caretakers of children with thrombocytopenia are instructed in prevention of injury, inspection of body secretions for fresh or old blood and safe application of pressure to injury or needle puncture sites. Universal precau-

tions are utilized whenever the potential for contact with bloody secretions exists.

Impairment in Respiratory Function

Lung disease is responsible for most morbidity and mortality associated with pediatric HIV infection. Problems include lymphoid intersitial pneumonitis complex, *P. carinii* pneumonia, bacterial pneumonia, and viral infections and malignancies (see Chapter 13, 16, 19, 21, 25, and 33). Nurses should instruct caretakers in the respiratory assessment of the child (awareness of baseline status and changes in respiratory rate, cough, color, nasal flaring, distress with feeds, change in energy level, and breathing difficulty and reporting of significant findings. Instruction is also given in positions for children that may ease respiration and provision of adequate rest. Home oxygen may be prescribed, and caretakers will need instruction in its safe use. Method of home heating should be explored; oxygen should not be used in a room with open flame kerosene heaters. Many caretakers will be aware that the acute pulmonary problems associated with HIV are life threatening and need increased support during the diagnostic and acute phases.

Neurodevelopmental Disorders

Neurodevelopmental impairment is the most devastating effect of HIV infection in children. Many children additionally suffer the sequelae of maternal drug use during pregnancy. Central nervous system impairment can also be a symptom or result of other infections that occur in HIV infected children. All children at risk for or known to have HIV infection should have baseline and routine neurodevelopmental evaluations by an expert (see Chapter 23). Caretakers should be aware of the potential for impairment and their child's status and be vigilant for signs of failure to progress or loss of milestones. Children with delays, even minimal, should be referred for physical, occupational, and developmental intervention to maximize potential and minimize disability. Ideally, such intervention should be in the local community or at home with the primary caretakers' partici-

Table 42.2.   Medications Commonly Prescribed for Children with HIV[a]

Medication	Indication	Dose	Side Effects/Toxicities/Comments	Nursing Interventions
Therapy aimed at combating HIV				
Azidothymidine (zidovudine)	Proven HIV infection with CD4+ count inadequate for age; HIV encephalopathy or other symptoms of disease	PO: <13 yr 180 mg/m² q 6hr; >13 yr 100 mg 5 times daily; IV: 480 mg/m² daily continuously or 120 mg/m² infused over 1 hr q 6 hr when drug cannot be delivered by mouth or in children with progressive encephalopathy not responsive to oral drug	Neutropenia, anemia; Increased mean corpuscular volume; Myopathy, particularly in lower extremities (uncommon); Hyperactivity; Short serum half-life	Carefully follow CBC with differential; Helps as monitor of compliance; Monitor serum levels of muscle enzymes; observe gait; monitor for signs of muscle weakness, tenderness, wasting; Elicit history of sleep difficulties, distractibility, change in school performance; may need further evaluation and referral. Families must be educated concerning need for drug administration q 6 hr and assisted with identifying a schedule allowing ease of compliance, especially during school day and night sleep
Videx	Same, but less beneficial for central nervous system disease	90–150 mg/m² BID given PO	Drug is acid labile; Variable absorption of drug even when taken under optimal circumstances, especially in children with gastrointestinal symptomatology; Drug is suspended in magnesia and alumina; Peripheral neuropathy correlated with administration in adults; Pancreatitis associated with high doses (540 mg/m²/day) or concurrent use of pentamidine; Peripheral retinal depigmentation observed with high doses	Instruct family to administer drug to child 30 min before or 1 hr after meals; Careful monitoring of clinical response by history taking, physical examination, neurodevelopmental assessment, and laboratory evaluation; Participation in therapeutic drug monitoring; Suspension may cause diarrhea and require taking alumina hydroxide before each dose; Discuss potential with family; observe child for signs of pain, changes in gait, complaints of numbness, pain or tingling in hands or feet, or signs of constipation. Monitor serum amylase, lipase, and triglycerides before initiation of drug and routinely throughout therapy; Teach family to immediately report abdominal pain, nausea, or vomiting; avoid caffeine, carbonated drinks, and chocolate, all of which can cause GI symptoms; Careful monitoring for vision complaints

Table 42.2.—*continued*

Medication	Indication	Dose	Side Effects/Toxicities/Comments	Nursing Interventions
Zalcitabine (ddC)	Same, but less beneficial for central nervous system disease	Dose and schedule not yet established for children. Recommended for use only in alternating or combination schedules with AZT to alleviate toxicity and limit the emergence of drug-resistant strains.	Ulcers in oral cavity and on tongue and lips

Erythematous maculopapular rash on trunk and extremities, including palms

Reports of peripheral neuropathy in adults | Inform family of potential
Inspection of oral cavity
Teaching concerning oral hygiene to prevent infection
Monitor oral intake/hydration status
Monitor for signs and symptoms of pain
Inform family of potential
Inspect skin for occurrence of rash

Inform family of potential
Observe for symptoms, inlcuding change in gait, refusal to walk, jaw pain, complaints of numbness, pain, tingling, and complaints of constipation |

Prevention and treatment of concurrent infections

Medication	Indication	Dose	Side Effects/Toxicities/Comments	Nursing Interventions
Trimethoprim-sulfamethoxazole (Septra, Bactrim)	Treatment of PCP	5 mg/kg q 6 hr IV or PO trimethoprim	Anemia, neutropenia, thrombocytopenia, rash, fever, Stevens-Johnson syndrome	Monitor CBC and differential
Educate caretakers concerning potential for side effects; impress need for visit to medical care provider if fever/rash occur for assessment
Inform caretakers of devasting impact on infants and discourage discontinuation of prophylaxis without consulting an HIV specialist
Monitor renal function
	Prophylaxis of PCP in child with inadequate CD4+ counts, in any child with a history of previous PCP infection, or in seropositive infant <1 yr with presence of HIV related symptoms	75 mg/m^2 BID on Mon, Tue, and Wed only or daily	Interstitial nephritis	

Table 42.2.—*continued*

Medication	Indication	Dose	Side Effects/Toxicities/Comments	Nursing Interventions
Pentamidine (Pentam 300, Lomidine)	Treatment of PCP; Prophylaxis of PCP (when child hypersensitive to TMP-SMX or bone marrow suppression interfering with antiretroviral therapy)	4 mg/kg IV q 24 hr; 4 mg/kg IV q month; 300 mg via aerosol q month in children old enough to follow directions	Hypotension related to rate of infusion; Hypoglycemia with chronic use; Bronchospasm related to aerosol administration; Necessitates cooperation of child for effective delivery of medication via aerosol; Burning in back of throat, metallic taste in mouth during inhalation; No data concerning efficacy of aerosol or intravenous pentamidine in children as prophylaxis	Administer over 60–90 min with monitoring of blood pressure throughout infusion; Dextrostick 45 min into and after infusion; Monitor for effects especially when used with other drugs (ddI, ddC) with pancreatic toxicity; Assess for history of prior bronchospasm during therapy; Administered by a respiratory therapist using a Respirgard II jet nebulizer; frequent pulmonary assessment; medication and equipment available for treatment of acute respiratory distress; premedication may be necessary; Room used for administration must be ventilated according to OSHA standards; Careful assessment of child's development and emotional ability to cooperate with a long and somewhat unpleasant procedure; Allow careful use of hard candies and flavored drinks during treament.
Intravenous immunoglobulin	Prevention of serious bacterial infections in children and hypogammaglobulinemia; treatment for thrombocytopenia	400 mg/kg IV q month	Potential for adverse events including pyrogenic reactions, systemic reactions, cardiovascular manifestations, or hypersensitivity; Interferes with immunogenicity of measles, mumps, rubella vaccine; Consider home administration in appropriate families under constant supervision of a Registered Nurse	Inform parents; emphasize need to report fever, shortness of breath, rapid respirations, cough immediately to a health professional aware of child's HIV status; Epinephrine immediately available; Administer using an escalating rate regimen with monitoring of patient throughout and vital sign assessment before rate escalation; May require premedication with hydrocortisone; Plan measles, mumps, rubella administration 3 months after last dose; readminister vaccine if immunoglobulin administered within 14 days after immunization

Table 42.2.—*continued*

Medication	Indication	Dose	Side Effects/Toxicities/Comments	Nursing Interventions
Nystatin (Mycostatin)	Mild mucocutaneous candidiasis	1–6 ml PO each cheek 4–5 times daily after feeding for oral lesions	Prolonged use safe but may cause problems with dentition in older children related to sugar content of suspension	Instruct family in oral hygiene measures
	Candida diaper dermatitis	Apply creme in thin film to diaper area after thorough cleansing 4–5 times daily for diaper dermatitis	Frequency of administration difficult to comply with, and families often cease therapy when plaques not visible; *Candida* diaper dermatitis frequently occurs coincidently with oral disease	Instruct family of need to continue therapy beyond resolution of visible lesions; Assist family in identifying a schedule to optimize compliance; Assess diaper area; Anticipate occurrence of diaper area lesions and provide therapy
Ketoconazole	Severe or recalcitrant mucocutaneous esophageal candidiasis	3.3–6.6 mg/kg in one daily dose PO for mucocutaneous	Potential hepatotoxicity	Evaluate liver function before and during therapy
	Candida diaper dermatitis	Apply creme in thin film to diaper area once daily after thorough cleansing	Should *not* be taken with antacids; best absorbed when taken after a fatty meal or with milk products; Potential for rash, pruritus	Assist families in determining optimum dosing schedule, especially those whose children also receive ddl
Amphotericin	Invasive or disseminated candidiasis; Cryptococcal disease	Assess febrile/hemodynamic response with test dose 0.1 mg/kg/day; after 1 week of therapy, may give double daily dose on alternate days; duration of therapy depends on type and extent of infection	Fever with shaking chills; Abnormal renal function (hypokalemia, elevated serum creatinine, and BUN hypomagnesemia); Consider outpatient and home infusion for appropriate children and families when acute illness resolved	Inform family, monitor child, prevent skin injury; Premedication with Tylenol and hydrocortisone may reduce systemic reactions; Demerol IV for shaking chills; monitor platelet count; Monitor and replace electrolytes; Monitor renal function; Referral to experienced home health agency for teaching and at home supervision as well as laboratory evaluation

Table 42.2.—*continued*

Medication	Indication	Dose	Side Effects/Toxicities/Comments	Nursing Interventions
Drugs used to mediate toxic effects of therapy				
Granulocyte colony-stimulating factor Neupogen, Filgrastin)	Neutropenia related to antiretroviral therapy or HIV infection itself	1–20 μg/kg daily and titrated to maintain absolute neutrophil count between 2 and 6000 cell/mm^3	Mild fever, althralgia, myalgia, headache, nausea, rash and swelling at injection site Medication is administered SC	Assess child for symptoms, teaching regarding symptom management Assess family for ability and willingness to administer injections to their child Educate family and back-up concerning home injection therapy Make appropriate home health referrals for monitoring of injection administration, support and potential administration of drug Arrange for home/community laboratory evaluation and reporting to prescribing physician
			Doses are titrated in response to blood work values	
Erythropoeitin (Eprex)	Chronic, transfusion dependent anemia related to drug therapy or HIV related autoimmune phenomena	50–100 IU/kg IV or sq 3 times q wk; dose reduced when hemoglobin level reaches 10–11.5 g/dl	May cause hypertension in children with renal disease related to increased blood viscosity Adequate iron stores; ferritin necessary for optimum response Drug given IV or SC	Monitor blood pressure Obtain laboratory evaluation before initiation of therapy; initiate iron therapy if needed Assess family for ability and willingness to administer injections to their child Educate family and back-up in medication administration Appropriate home health referrals for monitoring, support, medication administration Arrange for home/community laboratory evaluation and reporting to prescribing physician Inform family
			Doses are titrated in response to blood work values	
			Mild skin rash may occur	

^{a}CBC, complete blood count; GI, gastrointestinal; AZT, azidothymidine; PCP, *P. carinii* pneumonia; ddI, dideoxyinonsine; ddC, dideoxycytodine; TMP-SMX, trimethoprim-sulfamethoxazole; OHSA, Occupational Health and Safety Administration; BUN, bloodurea-nitrogen.

pation. Children with HIV are eligible for special services, including Early Intervention Programs, because of risk for delay and potential learning problems. Nurses should become familiar with resources in their state and make appropriate referrals (21, 22). Hospitalized children benefit from developmentally appropriate infant stimulation, play programs, and participation in the hospital school program.

Alterations in Fluid Balance

Children with HIV infection are at risk for fluid and electrolyte imbalance related to the impact of the virus on the gastrointestinal tract, kidneys, and other vital organs and the impact of other infectious diseases (see Chapter 20, 27, and 29). Imbalances may become severe and life threatening. The nurse should be cognizant of these imbalances, their causes, signs, and symptoms, nursing interventions, and potential medical management. Nurses assess fluid intake and output, body weight, and tissue turgor. Blood and urine laboratory values are obtained and evaluated for indications of imbalance.

Children with HIV infection can suffer from diarrhea and breakdown of diaper area skin. Stools should be routinely sent for culture, even when recently evaluated. Caretakers should inspect stool for occult and fresh blood. A skin care plan is established. Instruction is given in maintaining hydration, and necessary diet changes are made. Intravenous fluid and electrolyte therapy may be warranted to correct imbalances.

Alterations in Nutrition

Children with HIV infection often experience marked failure to thrive and multiple nutritional deficiencies related to problems that increase caloric needs, interfere with food intake, and reduce nutrient absorption. Nurses should routinely obtain information concerning feeding history, occurrence of fever, vomiting, diarrhea, or other problems. Height, weight, and head circumference measures are made and plotted on growth charts. Prevention of weight loss should be a goal (23, 24). Dietary referrals are made for assistance in the establishment of nutritional intervention. Children may

enjoy and accept nutritional supplements given with meals and for snacks. If adequate oral consumption fails, total enteral nutrition is an alternative. These are always supplemented with oral feeds to maintain oral motor capabilities. Families and caretakers should be instructed in feeding tube placement, insertion site care, potential complications associated with tube feedings, signs and symptoms of distress, and interventions.

Children with HIV infection may have abnormal gastrointestinal motility and malabsorption. Intravenous nutrition is an option for the child with functional impairment of the gastrointestinal tract or inability to tolerate enteral feeds. The decision to initiate parenteral feedings must be made in conjunction with the child's guardian and in consideration of impact on the family's life. Careful assessment must be made of the caretakers' ability to manage the care, the availability, skill, and willingness of respite caretakers, the presence of supportive home health services, and the appropriateness of the home environment (25). Total parenteral nutrition (TPN) is infused through a central venous access device. Partially implanted devices (single or multiple lumen Broviac or Hickman catheters) are generally chosen for infusions of several hours duration, particularly in mobile, curious children. Totally implanted devices (Port-A-Cath, Infus-A-Port, Mediport) are useful for infusions of short duration administered under close supervision, such as in a hospital or clinic setting (26). Both allow delivery of highly concentrated, complex formulas containing nutrients essential to the promotion of weight gain, wound healing, and growth. TPN is always initiated slowly and gradually advanced. Infusion patterns are chosen to stimulate normal eating and to allow for family and child freedom. Infusion pumps are used to maintain constant infusion rates as well as tapering with the initiation and completion of each infusion to prevent hyperglycemia and hypoglycemia. Infusions of TPN are not interrupted, increased to maintain schedule, or discontinued abruptly. When formulas prescribed are not immediately available, 10% dextrose may be used temporarily.

Children who receive TPN are carefully monitored for complications related to the infusion such as glucose intolerance electrolyte imbalances, hepatic or pancreatic dysfunction and cardiac or respiratory distress(27). Meticulous care of the central venous access device and handling of all tubing and connections is essential to prevention of infection and catheter related sepsis. Good hand washing precedes all manipulations. Catheter insertion sites and tunnels are assessed at least daily. Skin is cleansed with povidine-iodine, and all tubings, ports, and lines are cleansed with alcohol. Site dressings should be maintained in a clean, dry, and occlusive state. Dressings are changed and catheters flushed according to established institution and agency protocols. Procedures assessments are documented in the medical record, and any findings of concern are immediately communicated to the physician.

Home infusion therapy of TPN or other medications is an option for children who are medically stable but in need of continued support. Normal life is supported, and costs are markedly reduced. However, home intravenous therapy is complex with little room for error. Families and responsible individuals are identified before discharge planning along with experienced home health agencies skilled or at least willing to care for children with human immunodeficiency virus infection on a long-term basis. Opportunities for teaching, demonstration, and performance are offered until the caretaker and at least one other committed adult exhibits competence in initiating and discontinuing TPN, providing catheter care, and identifying catheter, pump, and TPN-related problems (infection, obstruction, dislocation, air in line, disconnection, or breaks) and appropriate interventions. Written materials are provided, including telephone numbers for emergency contacts. All families will require at least daily visits by the home health nurse for about the first week of home therapy with long-term support and assessment as needed (28). Revision of the home plan and increased assistance will be needed if the caretaker develops physical disability or dementia.

Facilitating Coping with Spectrum of Illness

From the anticipation of the diagnosis and beyond the death of a child from AIDS, families of children with HIV infection are challenged by the crises and stresses of a chronic and fatal illness. Although the illness trajectory is unique for each child with HIV, every child will eventually develop symptoms of infection and begin antiretroviral therapy. Currently, once treatment is initiated, some therapeutic intervention will be necessary for the duration of the child's life. Adherence to lifelong administration of medication to a child at multiple times during the day and at night is a challenge for any caretaker. When treatment is initiated, relevant laboratory evaluations and physical symptoms should be carefully reviewed and demonstrated to the caretakers as well as anticipated effects of treatment. Parents may express reluctance to initiate therapy because of their experiences with side effects related to particular antiretrovirals. Many parents benefit from talking with other experienced parents about children's reactions. Information is provided about dose and schedule. A nurse can assist the parent in identifying a schedule that optimizes the therapeutic effect of the drug and fits into the family's and child's schedule. Oral syringes, individually marked for dosing amount, can be dispensed and assist parents in administration of correct amounts of medication, particularly those who may not be able to see small numbers or lines on a syringe. Medication timers and reminders can be offered and are of great assistance to families with many responsibilities. A social worker should be involved in assessing the family's ability to pay for treatment and in obtaining financial assistance when needed. Some families are reluctant to obtain antiretrovirals in their home community, fearing the pharmacist will immediately know the diagnosis, and would prefer purchasing the medication at the medical center or need a referral to another pharmacy. That pharmacy should be contacted before the referral to assess the availability of the drug in a pediatric formulation. We have found it helpful to request a home visit by a public health nurse within days after initiation of therapy to verify that drug was obtained and is properly stored and administered. For some families, we recommend drawing up each day's dose in syringes at one time. A nurse should estimate the family's compliance with medication administration at each visit by asking the parent for information concerning dose schedule, missed doses, and any difficulties encountered with problem doses such as those late at night or during the school day. Zidovudine usually causes a rise in red blood cell mean corpuscular volume, and watching the pattern of that parameter may offer an estimate of compliance. Reviewing laboratory findings and physical symptoms as well as any changes in weight, well-being, energy level, and appetite are helpful in demonstrating to parents the impact and progress of therapy. Engaging parents in following the progress of the child on therapy by teaching them signs of improvement and symptoms of progress reinforces the importance of their role. Information concerning compliance is also obtained from children themselves. School-age children and those older can be encouraged to work with their caretakers to remember medication doses. Any treatment is most effective when given as recommended because with the currently limited number of therapies for HIV, each must be maximized. Information concerning compliance must be sought in objective and nonjudgmental ways, acknowledging the difficulties of administering medication long term to children but emphasizing treatment to prolong life and minimize symptoms.

Terminal Care

There comes a time in the course of a child's struggle with AIDS that treatment options for HIV and its associated problems have been exhausted. When the family and the health care team agree that this point has been reached, interventions are focused on reducing pain and suffering, encouraging communication, and supporting the adaptive coping strategies of the child and family. The discussion of a *Do Not Resuscitate* order with the family defines the child's status and clarifies the focus for nursing interventions. The family has an opportunity to discuss their wishes concerning heroic measures. Many express guilt at not "doing everthing," and others have long accepted the inevitability of death for this child. All caretakers, family and professional, are given time to come to closure with the child, to anticipate their loss, and to prepare for death.

The dying child has the same developmental needs as other children of the same age. Consistency in the providers of nursing care promotes security in the child. Providing good physical care for the child assists the nurse in establishing a trusting relationship with the family. Care focuses on prevention of infection, maintenance of adequate fluid balance, prevention of constipation, maintenance of hygiene support of self care, promotion of effective breathing patterns, provision of diversion, provision of adequate sleep and rest, assistance with mobility, and adequate relief from pain. Children with HIV may have family members with current or past difficulties with drug use. The potential for abuse of the child's pain medications must be considered in the development of an appropriate pain management plan for the child. Hospice programs in the hospital or at home are available to families of children with HIV (see chapter 44). For many reasons, home care is not for everyone. The nurse must assess the family structure, functioning, and resources as well as its ability to assume the physical and emotional responsibilities of caring for a dying child at home. Families may live in crime ridden areas or distant rural communities inaccessible to nursing supports. Hospice services should be offered to families well in advance of a terminal event to maximize utilization of services and allow the development of relationships. When a referral is made to a hospice agency, the nurse should assess the agency's experience in caring for children and for people with HIV before demographic data are given. Whether home care or hospitalization is chosen, families are assured the they will not be abandoned and that plans might be changed; home or rehospitalization remains an option. Every effort is made to guide the family in making choices that they can live with after the child's death.

ADMINISTRATIVE ISSUES
Confidentiality

Nurses have access to a great deal of confidential information as a condition of their work. With this ready access comes the responsibility to protect and maintain the confidentiality of the patient. The nursing profession has addressed this in the American Nurses' Association code of ethics that states "The nurse safeguards the client's right to privacy by judiciously protecting information of a confidential nature" (29). Further, health care facilities have adopted policies specifically stating the responsibility of providers to protect information related to all patients receiving care.

The advent of HIV and AIDS brought the issues of confidentiality and privacy to the forefront as the public health and advocacy systems struggled with the need for reasonable and rational policies that balanced patient confidentiality and protection of the public. Information on HIV serostatus reported to state health agencies and the federal Centers for Disease Control is protected under state and federal confidentiality regulations. Many states have passed legislation to define the limits of confidentiality to protect the infected person from the sequelae of disclosure that have included stigmatization and loss of employment, housing, and health insurance. Some infected children have been unable to go to school, and uninfected children of an infected parent or sibling have also been kept out of school. Sharing information indiscriminately with other staff members could cause harm. As a result, institutions have developed policies and procedures to assure compliance with state legislation. Administrators should review their policies to assure they are adequate to protect children and families. Nurses should look to the policies and procedures of their facilities for guidance regarding confidentiality in their individual work setting. To assist programs and agencies in formulating their own confidentiality policies, the American Bar Association has developed model AIDS/HIV policy and procedures. With a focus on HIV-infected persons with developmental disabilities, it provides direction on disclosure of information within and outside agencies as well as notification of sexual or needle sharing partners. The American Bar Association reminds us that the duty to maintain confidentiality derives from an individual's right to privacy. The right to privacy is established by federal and state constitutions and their respective regulations. Once a professional relationship begins, a duty or obligation is placed upon the service provider to protect the individual's rights (30) (see Chapter 49).

Access to information regarding HIV status is necessary for a nurse to provide care to the whole person and to serve as an advocate for the client (31). For providers aware of the HIV diagnosis, accidental rather than intentional disclosure of diagnosis related information is more likely to occur. Typically, a casual discussion of a patient condition in the elevator or a patient clipboard left in a conference room used by parents results in disclosure of diagnosis to a visitor, staff member, or another parent. In both inner city and rural communities, patients and staff live in the same communities and may be related through ties of church, school, sports, or employment. Nurses must exercise discretion in everyday conversations held with other professionals and at nurse stations to be sure that confidentiality of the patient is protected within their unit and agency. HIV status is disclosed to colleagues on a need to know basis. There is no need to inform other parents on the unit about the diagnosis.

Family to family networking is a source of strength to many parents who meet and become acquainted through their contacts in the hospital or treatment programs. The informality created through these networks often extends to nurse and other care providers who may develop relationships over a period of years with groups of families. Nurses must remember that information related to diagnosis and management of an individual child should never be shared between families. This can be difficult because family members may compare and contrast the treatment of children, but the nurse must adhere to strict limits regarding such disclosures.

Prevention of Occupational Transmission

Although HIV is not easily spread, the potential for occupational transmission from an infected patient to a nurse exists. When providing patient care, all patients must be considered to be potentially infected and their blood and body fluids treated accordingly. The Centers for Disease Control and Occupational Safety & Health Administration have provided guidelines, and agencies have developed policies over the past several years to protect staff and patients. Needle stick injuries pose the greatest threat to nurses and are more likely to occur when units are understaffed or nurses are inexperienced. The intravenous tubing-needle assemblies, "piggyback" or "intermittent," have a higher risk of needle stick injury than any other devices. Exposed needles dangling from unintentionally disconnected secondary medication sets and needles that protrude from disposable containers also result in needlesticks. In response to this risk, the medical products industry has begin to develop new and safer systems for nurses and other providers whose work places them at risk for exposure to infected blood and body fluids, and the Food and Drug Administration recommends that needleless systems or recessed needle systems replace hypodermic needles for accessing intravenous lines (32). Convenient placement of needle disposal containers, monitoring and communication of needle stick injuries, and education have been shown to decrease needle stick injuries in health care workers (33). Even more important than observing universal precautions is understanding why the precautions have been established and how they halt transmission. The greatest potential for occupational transmission comes from incorrect or incomplete implementation of procedures. Conversely, familiarity can lead to a casual approach to infection control. As nurses get to know a particular patient or work extensively with HIV-infected patients they can minimize risk and become lax in adhering to procedures that protect them from exposure to infected blood and body fluids.

All children find invasive procedures difficult and can respond with physical aggression to the perceived threat. Such situations are not only traumatic for the child but place physicians and nurses at risk for potential exposure when confronted with an angry child. The use of developmentally appropriate techniques to prepare children can be helpful. At the Children's Hospital AIDS program (Newark, NJ), simple behavioral interventions such as distraction, visualization, and self-hypnosis are used for venipuncture, spinal tap, and other invasive procedures. These are simple to teach to staff and children and have proven to be effective with children of all ages. Similar techniques are used for children with other chronic illnesses, such as cancer, and have been found to be effective. Institutionalization of such behavioral approaches into nursing practice guarantees that they will be used consistently. The benefits include minimizing acute and chronic trauma to children, decreased anxiety for parents as clinic visits become less threatening to child, decreased anxiety around invasive procedures for patient and nurse, and decreased risk of occupational transmission to staff.

Supervisors can validate the importance of infection control through orientation with new staff, dissemination of new information at staff meetings, assuring adequate supplies and staffing, and formal monitoring of compliance.

Staff Support

Staff nurses report a strong sense of satisfaction from working with children with HIV/AIDS. They have been able to help patients live longer and to have a positive influence on the quality of their lives. Many providers find a sense of accomplishment and challenge in working exclusively with HIV-infected children.

Yet the work is not easy or without stress. Psychosocial stressors on nurses and other health care workers include fear of contagion and transmission, discomfort with homosexuality and drug use, intensive complicated care, repetitive grief, facing one's own mortality, and conflict over goals of treatment (34). Suggested interventions include education, informal peer support, support groups, and administrative support (35). Despite the recognition that caretaking can be stressful and can lead to burnout, there has been little research focusing on identifying stressors and developing of interventions to support the retention of professional caretakers of persons with HIV. Because the direct caretakers witness, on a daily basis, suffering and death they are constantly challenged to maintain their competence and sense of control in situations that threaten their self-esteem and professional competence. Personal values, cultural background, and religious ideals are challenged. Stresses also result from the uncertainty and discomfort nurses feel in relating to parents who may continue to abuse drugs and alcohol and retain legal custody while unable to assume caretaking responsibility for their children. The intense physical care needs of hospitalized and dying children can result in emotional and physical fatigue. For some children, the hospital nurses become "family" and suffer the pain and loss that occurs as the disease progresses. While dedicated to prolonging life and providing an acceptable quality of that life, nurses are expected to implement treatments that can lead to debilitating and painful side effects. Such situations lead to concerns regarding the benefit to the child an erupt into conflicts among staff and between physicians and nurses. Death of the child becomes a personal loss, and multiple deaths can leave a staff drained as they struggle to deal with grief and bereavement that frequently cannot be acknowledged to each other or within the institution.

Agencies must recognize the stressors faced by direct care providers and accept that HIV/AIDS care is different. A proactive approach that recognizes the potential for stress and uses multiple strategies to deal with the manifestations of stress is necessary. The needs of nurses working on inpatient units differ from those of nurses working in ambulatory based HIV specific care and research programs. Inpatient nurses see the most severe spectrum of disease without the opportunity to care for the asymptomatic HIV-infected child or the child who is receiving TPN at home and doing well. Demands of inpatient care are such that these nurses are the least likely to receive ongoing support or have access to planned stress management interventions. Hospitals that care for large numbers of children will need to consider how to provide access to interventions including clear consistent policies and procedures for care, regular updates of HIV care, continuous communication between nurses and staff of the HIV care program, support groups, and access to mental health consultants.

Nurses in HIV care programs develop relationships with children and families that are continuous throughout the illness. The caretaking style of nurses includes needing to be needed, increased susceptibility to overinvolvement, and investing more emo-

tional energy than is helpful to either the nurse or family (36). Assistance may be needed to identify reasonable boundaries for involvement and preserve the nurse's role as a professional. As the condition of the child worsens, nurses struggle with feelings of powerlessness and incompetency as all their treatments and experience cannot change the outcome. Their grief and loss is intensely personal and must be recognized. The ability to attend funerals and maintain contact with the family is important to the nurse as well as the parent. Healing and memorial ceremonies designated specifically for staff to acknowledge the loss at a personal level can be helpful. The death of the parent to AIDS contributes to the stress of staff as they must put their own feelings aside to assist the child and surviving family members or work with a child welfare agency to place the child or children. Then they must begin the process of education and teaching with the new caretakers. Sadly, for some children members of the medical team are the most consistent figures in their life.

AIDS organizations are beginning to recognize and accept grief as an organizational and a personal issue. Agencies that have begun formal programs report that liberal leave and vacation policies, employee support groups, and management training are effective antidotes to stress. Explicit in these programs is the willingness to provide staff with opportunities to deal with their feelings of grief in a constructive manner that also benefits the organization through decreased sick time and increased staff retention (37).

Organizational structure and management style are closely related to employee satisfaction. Programs with a structure and culture that supports an interactional rather than a command and control style of management are more likely to be successful in serving people with HIV, retaining staff, and acomplishing their goals. Because our group at the Children's Hospital AIDS Program is diverse in age, gender, cultural and ethnic background, professional discipline, and job responsibilities we have discovered through trial and error that we need various options that can be used by some or all of the group. These range from the purely recreational to the therapeutic and are done both at work and outside of work. The pace at work makes it difficult to bring everyone together, so we have found off-site retreats to be effective for team building as well as program evaluation. Since much of the stress comes from the demands of medical care and research, it has been crucial to have physician participation. The impetus and planning of our program came from the nurses and social workers and the administrative staff. At the core of any intervention is the creation of an organizational climate the supports and nurtures its staff, enabling them to care competently and effectively for their patients.

RESEARCH ISSUES

Participation in biomedical research is the standard of care for the child with HIV infection. Nurses are critical to the care of children with HIV infection, particularly as members of the medical research team. Nurses are in an ideal position to educate families about clinical trials as part of care, and identify children and families eligible and able to participate in medical research. They are family advocates in ensuring informed consent for those who may feel uncomfortable questioning physicians or who feel there is no other choice than participating in research owing lack of insurance or fears of abandonment by the health care team. Nurses assess and refer families to support services needed to facilitate participation in research such as transportation and home health care. Nurses communicate with local caretakers concerning the protocol and their role in the child's care. They educate the family, local caretakers, and hospital staff concerning the treatment plan, new pharmacologic agents, and the child's response to therapy. Nurses collect, report, organize, and analyze data concering the child's compliance, response to therapy, and possible related side effects and toxicities. Nurses work with families to manage symptoms related to HIV and its treatment.

For nurses to further influence the health of children with HIV infection, these children must become a focus of concern for clinical nursing research. A particular priority area is the development of innovative programs for prevention and education among vulnerable groups such as sexually active adolescents, injection drug users, alcohol abusers, pregnant women and their newborns, homeless youth, and youth belonging to racial and ethnic minorities (38). Additional areas of high priority for nursing research include 1) management of pain and other symptoms related to HIV infection, 2) supportive care needs of children with HIV and their caretakers, 3) methods for case management in the tertiary care center, at home, and in the community, 4) methods for maintaining adequate nutrition in children with HIV, 5) models for providing hospice care to families with HIV, and 6) models for accessing natural social systems as part of the continuum of care given the dire predictions for congential HIV infection (39, 40). Investigation in these priority areas will assist in the theory development for pediatric HIV infection nursing practice and improve the care offered to the children and families affected by HIV.

SPECIAL ISSUES
Urban Challenges

Until recently, HIV infection among children had been a disease of large metropolitan areas. New York City, northern New Jersey, and Miami were the first communities to report HIV in children, and they continue to report significant numbers of AIDS cases. They have been joined by many other metropolitan areas and rural areas (especiatly in the southern United States) reporting increasing rates of HIV seroprevalence in women and infants. A nurse working in communities with such high seroprevalence must be prepared to deal with HIV infection regardless of her work setting, but, more important, she or he must be aware of the burden faced by individuals and the community at large.

Urban areas face problems that lack easy definition and make placing of blame difficult. Loss of jobs, aging housing, flight of the middle class to the suburbs, failing public schools, and aging health care institutions all existed before the emergence of HIV. Although inner cities have been the focus of much public policy debate, the enthusiasm and efforts of the 1960s and 1970s to reverse the decline of urban areas have been dampened by fear, complexity, and cynicism (41). Nurses working in inner cities do not need to read policy reports to understand the difficulties facing the cities. They see, on a daily basis, individuals struggling with hopelessness, fighting poverty, and lacking any alternatives to the drugs and violence that control their lives. These same problems exist and are less appreciated in smaller metropolitan and rural communities. Primary health care is not readily available, leading to misuse of emergency rooms and inpatient hospitalization. Home health services, increasingly available in suburban communities, either cannot be provided because the physical safety of nurses cannot be guaranteed, or third party providers, including Medicaid, will not reimburse services at a rate that allows agencies to remain financially viable. The lack of a service infrastructure and the misuse of existing services seriously compromises the delivery of comprehensive care to families. Although care of medically complex children might challenge the most stable families, the special problems of chronically ill children who come from poor families are particulary difficult. The very children who need the most have the least available (44).

Current seroprevalence rates indicate that although HIV has spread throughout the United States, urban areas will continue to have the largest numbers of infected persons. However, heterosexually acquired HIV has spread most rapidly in the southern United States, particularly in rural populations. Pediatric HIV/AIDS is overwhelmingly a disease of African-Americans, Haitians, and Latinos. Minority populations in this country suffer poorer health, evidenced by more illnesses and a higher incidence of disease, and they die in larger numbers than the nation as a whole (43). HIV has worsened the problems by increasing the demand for services in communities that have been unable to provide adequate care for poor minority populations.

Geography is involved because the ethnic population served varies among urban areas. While recognizing the ethnic communities are not monolithic, it is helpful to be aware of the particular cultural beliefs and experiences of the community, particularly related to health care and the small and large institutions that provide such services. Client heterogeneity and use of multiple services can complicate the provision of care.

Family participation must be sought when developing a plan of care to assure that is realistic based on the circumstances of the individual family. An idealistic, aggressive plan may not be feasible given various factors such as lack of telephone, no refrigeration, no transportation, and so forth. The list of potential problems is long. Typically, a family member will be reluctant to share such information, particularly if living in conditions they feel reflect poorly on the family. At other times services may be refused because the family wishes to protect their privacy, worries about disclosure of the diagnosis, or is concerned about immigration status. Nurses and physicians are forced to move from the ideal to the real and to accept compromise. This is difficult given our use of advanced technology and desire to provide the latest and best treatments.

Chemical dependency involving alcohol and/or drugs (prescription, nonprescription, and injection) is a problem for many families. Commonly, more than one drug will be abused, and many parents will use drugs and alcohol. Such substance abuse has a behavioral and emotional effect on the ability to parent. The drug use brings its own problems and may prevent the parent from caring in a responsible manner for the child. Addicted parents may not see that they could choose to seek treatment. They may not believe options are available or that treatment could be successful. This sense of hopelessness contributes to a feeling of being trapped by both the illness and the substance abuse. Finally, substance abuse can impair the ability to accept responsibility for the care of a sick child. Understanding the behavioral components of substance disorders will alleviate anxiety associated with confronting substance abuse and will help the nurse to regard the addicted adults as persons caught in an illness from which they cannot escape without assistance. Nurses dealing with addicted parents need to recognize and learn to deal with the behavioral manifestations of addiction. Such parents may use flattery, intimidation, manipulation, and/or anger in their attempts to get their own way with staff members. These parents are adept at turning one staff member against another, thus creating dissension between and among providers and agencies. Specific in service education on dealing with substance abuse may be necessary to provide nurses with the skills to deal comfortably with such parents.

Families with a history of problems are usually involved with multiple agencies either by choice or because of referrals from agencies identifying needs. The nurse should not expect the family to volunteer such information unless asked directly. Even then, the parent may deny involvement of agencies such as child welfare and drug treatment programs. If a trusting relationship develops, this information may be disclosed at a later time.

Case management may be provided by several agencies and may be designated for one individual or the family unit. This service is mandated for several federal and state programs such as Early Intervention, Medicaid (in some states), mental health services, and drug treatment programs. The service is also offered through community based AIDS service organizations, community health agencies, foster care agencies, and AIDS health care programs. Families under the supervision of child welfare agencies receive case management mandated either by state law or the courts. Confiden-tiality laws in individual states may prohibit agencies from sharing information or working collaboratively. Therefore, the concept of a single designated case manager is not realistic and must be modified based on the needs of families, legal mandates, and services existing within communities. Yet these multiple managers should have as a goal assuring access to services and enhancing the quality of life for the child and family. Not infrequently, agencies work independently without knowledge of the other services. Multiagency case management may be needed but requires a willingness to communicate between agencies. In some instances, meetings of the case managers are useful in assuring that all parties are working with the same information base and that services are appropriate to the needs of the child and family. Unfortunately, none of these case managers can obtain nonexistent but needed services and are sometimes as powerless as their clients when faced with service gaps.

Rural Settings

HIV infection is the most significant public health problem facing Americans today. Many associate HIV and its related problems of poverty and drug abuse with the inner cities. In fact, rural residents themselves have denied the possibility of AIDS in their communities. HIV has reached the rural areas of the nation. In North Carolina, a largely rural state with several moderate-sized cities, the HIV seroprevalence among women giving birth in 1992 statewide was 2.23/1000. Among black women, the rate was 5.98 statewide (North Carolina HIV/STD Control Branch, July 1993). HIV seropositive mothers are equally distributed between rural and urban settings. Plotting the counties of residence for HIV seropositive children known to the Duke University center demonstrates an initial clustering of cases along the interstate highways. Initially mothers reported migration from rural areas to the northeast United States and back after the birth of a child or diagnosis with HIV for the support of their extended families. Currently most women who have acquired HIV in North Carolina had done so through heterosexual transmission. Grandmothers bring their grandchildren to rural areas where their foster care stipends afford a higher standard of living than in cities and to escape the hardships of city life. Accessing services is not easier in rural areas. Children seropositive for HIV require specialized health care services, generally available in academic tertiary care centers. Such facilities in rural areas may serve children with HIV in entire states or regions. Average length of travel time for children to care in North Carolina is 3 hr with transportation generally provided by social service or volunteer agencies transporting several children and guardians. Social Service transportation is accessible to only mother and child. Extended family members cannot come to clinic for information about HIV. It is more difficult to assess the family and their interactions and to identify who in the family is willing and able to care for the child. Generally, grandmothers or other extended family members assume care if the mother becomes ill or disabled. Rural elderly, however, have higher rates of poverty and more chronic illness than the national average (45). When a child is hospitalized, mothers most frequently return to their homes to care for other children. Discharge teaching can be difficult to achieve and hospitalizations unnecessarily prolonged. Informed, willing, and experienced local community health care providers are difficult to identify in some counties. Fragile rural health care systems have almost no tolerance for new patients with HIV who will eventually need complex and expensive care (45). When referrals are made, families are reluctant to disclose the diagnosis of HIV to local caretakers because of concerns about anonymity and confidentiality in small, rural communities where residents are often well-known or related to one another. Children with HIV participate in research protocols and may become candidates for high-tech home care with indwelling central catheter and infusions of medication or nutrition. Home care plans can be challenging to implement with large distances to emergency care for equipment repair and for visits from home health nurses for supervision, support, quality assurance, and delivery of supplies. Local care providers sometimes have only theoretical knowledge of the use of high tech devices. Safety issues must be considered and extensive initial training with ongoing support offered to physicians and nurses. Adaptations in the physical structure of the home may be required to use biotechnology in a rural environment. Local providers are an invaluable resource, and many children would be denied access to the state-of-the-art care they deserve were it not for their interest and efforts. These providers should be involved, informed, and consulted at all stages of the illness for the best outcome for the child and family.

Respite and psychosocial support services are critical to the survival of families caring for children with HIV. Anonymity and confidentiality are often issues. Often families will accept support and more willingly disclose sensitive information to helpers from outside their culture or community when informal networks are least likely to overlap and privacy is protected. Cultural sensitivity on the helpers' part is essential.

Priorities for rural areas are education concerning HIV infection and the reality of the infection in rural populations with an emphasis on prevention, screening, identification, and referral. Formal health care systems must anticipate increased demands on their services and develop plans for response. Academic centers must work in collaboration with community agencies to provide care for families. Care must be centralized given long travel times, and ideally, pediatric/primary HIV, adult HIV, as well as obstetric/gynecologic care can be offered at one institution. Physicians and nurses in university settings must conduct formal and informal educational programs concerning HIV. Finally, informal support systems in rural care areas must be improved to allow more effective use of formal services by rural families (46).

Developing Countries

Although much attention has been paid to HIV infection in the United States and western Europe, the impact will be the greatest on developing nations (see Chapter 3). For many of these nations, the inability to screen blood will result in transfusion related cases in children. Certain countries are reporting sexually transmitted infection in children and young adolescents who have been working, usually involuntarily, in the sex industry. Seroprevalence rates in women have been high in Africa, but countries in Asia, Latin America, and eastern Europe are now reporting cases of infection in children transmitted perinatally. Heterosexual transmission, rather than intravenous drug use, is responsible for infection in women in their childbearing years.

Although nursing education and practice varies between countries, the International Council for Nurses has defined a Code for Nurses. This Code states "The nurse's responsibility is to those people who require nursing care" and that the nurse " . . . in providing care, promotes an environment in which the values, customs and spiritual beliefs of the individual are respected . . . " and " . . . Holds in confidence personal information and uses judgement in sharing information" (47). International Council for Nurses has reaffirmed this Code in response to HIV infection and recognizes that a broad range of nursing skills are necessary to provide optimal care in whatever setting it is needed (48). The term "nurse" can be used to indicate multiple roles and services provided by individuals with variable educational preparation and clinical responsibility. Specialty nursing practice is not well developed. Nurses in developing nations may lack the status and power necessary to assure that they are provided with the necessary education to deal with the HIV epidemic. The International Council of Nurses, working with the Global Program on AIDS of the World Health Organization, has been providing nursing education in several countries and publishes an HIV/AIDS newsletter that is distributed through their member organizations. In addition, several publications specific to nursing practice in the developing world have been developed. HIV specific education and clinical training is available for nurses through government and privately funded training programs.

Limited clinical resources for diagnosis and treatment are the greatest obstacle and force nurses to improvise to provide care. In many communities, nurses have taken the responsibility of caring and are involved in prevention and education as well as care of the sick and dying. Much of the work takes place in hospitals and at the community level. Constrained by limited availability of medications and other treatments, the care offered is supportive and nursing intensive. Much information presented in this chapter can be adapted for use in the developing world.

Beause children and their parents may be unable to utilize health services because of cost of care and medicines and/or lack of transportation, they will be cared for in their homes during the chronic and terminal phases of disease. A lack of medications or inability to purchase them forces caretakers to rely on traditional healing practices and palliative therapies. Nurses are in a position to educate family members and train volunteer community members to provide home visits and supportive care. Such programs are especially necessary in high incidence countries where infected persons may live in rural villages and lack access to ongoing professional nursing care.

Third world countries with their large populations of infected women and children may be approached by pharmaceutical companies interested in conducting clinical research trials of new drugs. Such trials can offer early access to new drugs, access to new technology, and economic benefit to the community (49). Nurses will need to participate in the development or local procedures to review the ethical and clinical justifications for the studies and assure that local values and culture are considered.

SUMMARY

When dealing with HIV infection nurses are asked to broaden their concept of family centered care to incorporate ill family members and sometimes to work with successive families in caring for an individual child. The chronicity of the disease requires that a child receive a range of nursing services in various settings. Nurses must be prepared to offer high quality technologically advanced care combined with basic interventions to meet needs for comfort and support. As the member of the health team with a holistic approach and the ability to bridge the hospital, home, and community nurses will continue to be critical in the care of children with HIV infection.

References

1. Mattsson A. Long-term illness in childhood: A challenge to psychosocial adaptation. Pediatrics 1972;50:801–809.
2. McGonigel M. Family meeting on pediatric AIDS. Washington, DC: Association for Children's Health, 1988.
3. Thomas R. The stuggle for control between families and health care providers when a child has complex health care needs. Zero Three 1988:15–18.
4. Jessop DJ, Stein REK. Meeting the needs of individuals and families. In: Stein R, ed. Caring for children with chronic illness. New York: Springer, 1989:63–74.
5. Abrams EJ, Nicholas SW. Pediatric HIV infection. Pediatr Ann 1990;19:482–487.
6. Conviser R. Caring for families with HIV: Case studies of pediatric HIV/AIDS demonstration projects. Newark: National Pediatric HIV Resource Center, 1991.
7. Novella AC. A guide: family-centered comprehensive care for children with HIV infection. Washington, DC: Department of Health and Human Services, 1991.
8. Boland M. Supporting families caring for children with HIV infection. In: Anderson G, ed. Courage to care responding to the crisis of children with AIDS. New York: Child Welfare League of America, 1990: 65–76.
9. Flaskerud J. Overview: HIV disease and nursing. In: Flaskerud J. Ungvarski P, eds. HIV/AIDS A

Guide to Nursing Care. Philadelphia: WB Saunders 1991:1–29.

10. Task Force on Pediatric AIDS. Perinatal human immunodeficiency (HIV) testing. Pediatr AIDS HIV Infect Fetus Adolesc 1991–1992;3:95–98.

11. Nair P. Early identification of HIV infection in children. Pediatric AIDS HIV Infect Fetus Adolesc 1992, 3:40–44.

12. Partridege JC, Sokal KB, Song DF, et al. Maternal history does not predict perinatal HIV exposure [Abstract]. Pediatr Res 1990;27:1492

13. Witt RC, Silvestre AJ, Rinaldo CR, et al. Guidelines for disclosing HIV antibody test results to clients. Nur Pract 1992:17:55–63.

14. Husson RW, Cornean AM, Hoff, R. Diagnosis of human immunodeficiency virus infection in infants and children. Pediatrics 1990;86:1–10.

15. Tasker, M. How can I tell you? Secrecy and disclosure with children when a family member has AIDS. 1st ed. Bethesda, MD: Association for the Care of Children's Health, 1992.

16. Committee on Infections Diseases, American Academy of Pediatries. Report of committtee on infectious diseases, 22nd ed. Elk Grove Village, IL: American Academy of Pediatrics, 1991.

17. Markowiz LE, Orenstein NA. Measles vaccine. Pediatr Clin North Am 1990;37:603–625.

18. Josephson A, Karantil L, Gombert M. Strategies for management of varicella-susceptible health care workers after a known exposure. Infect Control Hosp Epidemiol 1990;11:309–313.

19. Rostad ME. Curent strategies for managing myelosuppresion in patients with cancer. Oncol Nursing Forum 1991;18(suppl):7–15.

20. Nicholas S. Management of the HIV positive child with fever. J Pediatr 1991;119:521–524.

21. Butler C, Hittelman J, Hanger S. Approach to neurodevelopmental and neurologic complication in pediatric HIV infection. J Pediatr 1991;119:2:541–546.

22. Task Force on Pediatric AIDS. Education of children with immunodeficiency virus infection. Pediatric AIDS HIV Infect Fetus Adolesc 1990–1991;3:99–102.

23. Prestidge LL, Klish WJ. Pediatric HIV infection and wasting. Semin Pediatr Infect Dis 1990;1:73–76.

24. Nicholas SW, Leung J, Fennow I. Guidelines for nutritional support of HIV infected children. J Pediat 1991;119:559–562.

25. Boland MG. The child with HIV infection. In: Durham JD, Cohen FL, eds. The person with AIDS: Nursing perspectives. 2nd ed. New York: Springer, 1991:332–333.

26. Marcoux C, Fishers S, Wong D. Central venous access devices in children. Pediatr Nurs 1990;16:123–133.

27. Worthington PA, Wagner BA. Total parenteral nutrition. Nurs Clin North Am 1989;24:355–369.

28. Rivard WA. Parent instruction manual for home parenteral nurtition. Oncol Nurs Forum 1990;17:435–436.

29. Anonymous. Code for nurses with interpretive statements. Kansas City, MO: Amercian Nurses' Association, 1985.

30. Rennert S. AIDS/HIV and confidentiality: Model policy and procedures. Washington, DC: American Bar Association, 1991.

31. Grady C. Ethical aspects. In: Flaskerud JH, Ungvarski PJ, eds. HIV/AIDS. A guide to nursing care. 2nd ed. Philadelphia: WB Saunders, 1991:4–439.

32. Food and Drug Administration. FDA safety alert: Needlestick and other risks from hypodermic needles on secondary I.V. administration sets-piggyback and intermittent I.V. Rockville, MD: Department of Health and Human Services. Apr 1992.

33. Haiduven DJ, DeMaio TM, Stevens DA. A five year study of needlestick injuries; significant reduction associated with communication, education, and convenient placement of sharps containers. Infect Control Hosp Epidemiol 1992:13:265–271.

34. Flaskerud J. Psychosocial aspects. In: Flaskerud JH, Ungvarski PJ, eds. HIV/AIDS. A guide to nursing care. 2nd ed. Philadelphia: WB Saunders, 1991:267–274.

35. Bolle J. Supporting the deliverers of care: Strategies to support nurses and prevent burnout. Holistic Nurs Pract 1989:3:63–71.

36. Barnsteiner J, Gillis-Donovan J. Being related and separate: A standard for therapeutic relationships. Am Maternal Child Nurs 1990;15:223–228.

37. Soos J. Caring for the AIDS caregiver: An evaluation of staff burnout at Shanti Project and a benefit-cost analysis of the "staff care plan" [Dissertation]. Berkeley: University of California, 1991.

38. Larson E, Ropka ME. An update on nursing research and HIV infection. Image: J Nurs Scholarship 1991;21:4–12.

39. Benedict S. Nursing research priorities related to HIV/AIDS. Oncol Nurs Forum 1990;17:571–573.

40. Busby A. Rural nursing research priorities. J Nurs Adm 1992;22:50–56.

41. Edelman P, Radin B. Serving children and families effectively: How the past can help the future. Washington, DC: Education and Human Services Consortium, 1991.

42. Kohrman A. Medical technology: Implications for health and social service providers. In: Hochstadt N, Yost D, eds. The medically complex child. The transition to home care. Chur, Switzerland: Harwood Academic, 1991:3–14.

43. Payne KW, Ugarte CA. The office of minority health resource center: Impacting on health related disparities among minority populations. Health Educ 1989;20(5):6–8.

44. Gwinn M, Pappaioanou M, Geroge JR, et al. Prevalence of HIV infection in child bearing women in the United States. JAMA 1991;265:1704–1708.

45. National Rural Health Association. Rural Health Care News. 1990; Jul-Aug:1–2.

46. Busby A. Rural nursing research priorities. J Nurs Admin 1992;22:50–56.

47. Anonymous. Code for nurses. Geneva: International Council of Nurses, 1973.

48. Anonymous. Guidelines for nursing management of people infected with human immunodeficiency virus (HIV). Geneva: World Health Organization, 1988.

49. Barry M. Ethcial dilemmas with economic studies in less-developed countries: AIDS research trials. IRB 1991;13:8–9.

Psychosocial Support for Child and Family

Lori Wiener and Anita Septimus

Within the second decade of the AIDS epidemic, profound and devastating psychosocial problems confronting human immunodeficiency virus (HIV)-infected children and their families continues (1). The unique social issues and challenges that HIV presents to families have been well documented. These include the difficulty in sharing their child's diagnosis with relatives, friends, neighbors, and employers as well as isolation, social stigma, depression, grief, disorientation, inability to sustain normal routine, and threat to family integrity (2).

A child with AIDS usually identifies a whole family at risk of infection. AIDS disrupts the family equilibrium by placing a dark and frightening cloud over their future. Drug use was initially associated with over 70% of the families of children with AIDS, and many of these families had problems that antedated infection with HIV. Moreover, over 80% of these families are from minority backgrounds, many of whom are already burdened by poverty, discrimination, and weak support systems (3) (see also Chapter 52). Because of their severe socioeconomic vulnerability, most of these families may already be known to multiple social service agencies when confronted with the diagnosis of an HIV infection in one or more family members. The additional burden of HIV infection can overwhelm already weak coping capacities, pushing vulnerable families into disorganization and crisis.

Although many issues related to chronic and acute childhood illness are appreciated by pediatric health professionals, the special

constellation and intensity of the problems facing families affected by HIV are unparalleled in modern health care (4). A major debilitating factor, unique to this disease, is that AIDS may cause acute and probably fatal illness in more than one family member over time. Frequently, these families are without savings, employment, income, insurance, legal counsel, and medical or social support, which increases the vulnerability to depression (5). Accordingly, the aim of care must be child centered and family focused (6) and necessitates comprehensive and coordinated medical and psychosocial care by a specialized multidisciplinary health care team.

This chapter addresses the impact of HIV on the family. Stresses of the disease and common emotional reactions faced by children, parents, and siblings are identified. Special attention is given to families, emphasizing the needs of women and minorities and the problems created by poverty and drug abuse. Interventions and strategies are aimed at building on family strengths through early intervention, providing support, handling interagency linkages, and serving as advocates.

STAGES OF DISEASE

Diagnosis: A Time of Initial Crisis

Similar to the diagnosis of other life-threatening illness, the family's response to the diagnosis of AIDS in a child can include shock, fear, guilt, disbelief, anger, and sadness. Because of the implications of the diagnosis and a wish to reverse the outcome, it is not unusual for parents to request repetition of diagnostic tests. Once the HIV status is accepted, families often describe a feeling of disorganization and of being overpowered. They also experience some anticipatory grief reactions as they begin to mourn the loss of the hopes and dreams of the family's future together (7). Of parents who are infected themselves, many describe overwhelming sadness at the realization that they might not be able to have more children or that they might die before their child. Recognition that they might not be able to provide their child with care, comfort, and love is often described as being too painful to bear. Parents may also feel helpless and angry.

When the diagnosis is made, parents tend to worry about caretaking issues (especially if one or both parents are ill), available support systems, and how best to keep the child's diagnosis confidential. Almost all affected families are immediately concerned about potential societal discrimination and ostracism as well as isolation from their family, extended family members, and friends. In light of the AIDS climate these concerns have proved to be realistic. Maladaptive responses by parents at the time of diagnosis (or at other times throughout the child's illness) can include denial of the diagnosis, the need for therapeutic intervention, and depression, renewed or continued substance abuse, self blame, or the blaming of others.

Clinical Syndromes

Neurologic consequences of HIV infection are among the most difficult manifestations of the disease for parents to cope with. Parents struggle with feelings of helplessness, sadness, anger, and anticipatory mourning when the infant does not develop normally, has behavioral disorganization, or shows overt evidence of dementia. As the child becomes increasingly dependent, parents grieve for the child's losses and are faced with making new and difficult adjustments. Sometimes, it is only when the child develops visible and profound impair-

ments that the full implications of the disease becomes an emotional reality.

Terminal Illness

One of the most challenging clinical tasks throughout the child's illness is helping families plan realistically for the future. Because of the unpredictable nature of HIV, it is not always possible to plan for the child's final days or weeks. When the child becomes terminally ill, parents need assistance with decisions regarding how aggressively to pursue further medical interventions. For example, do they want the child to be resuscitated and possibly placed on mechanical ventilation? They may also need assistance deciding whether they want their child to die in the hospital or at home. Dignified care for the child must be advocated regardless of their choice for terminal care. However, in many geographic areas, home care and hospice programs may be limited owing to lack of insurance or resources available for persons with AIDS. In such cases, the social worker needs to be creative in obtaining quality care for the child at home.

COMMON EMOTIONAL REACTIONS FACED BY CHILDREN AND FAMILIES
Children
Birth through Preschool

Identification of a seropositive infant can raise significant problems for the family, especially the biological mother, who may be just learning of her own infection at the same time she discovers that she has infected her child. Comprehensive family support and follow-up is needed to help parents get through this crisis, and reduce their anxiety and feelings of helplessness. If abandoned by professionals and friends they may decompensate (2, 8). This may result in leaving the child in the hospital or in continual or renewed substance abuse by the parents.

Children younger than 2 years cannot grasp the concept of illness and death. The psychological trauma of the diagnosis falls primarily on their caretakers (9). Infants and toddlers are most concerned with immediate events (physical trauma) and separation from their parents. Parents struggle with having their child hospitalized and the anticipated permanent separation from their child after death. Depending on the age and developmental stage of the child, comprehension of hospitalization and adaptation to frequent separations from the parents may be difficult. Parental emotional distress will be defined largely by their ability to help the child deal with repeated hospitalizations and medical procedures (9).

Young children are most worried about medical tests and procedures. Children as young as 4 or 5 begin to conceptualize death as a process involving physical harm. An honest approach to hospitalization and medical procedures is imperative. Telling the child that he or she is going to the hospital or that a needle stick will hurt briefly and that it is okay to cry lets him or her know that their feelings are validated. Preparing for medical procedures through medical play or coloring books that illustrate the procedure has also been beneficial for many children.

School-age Children

Some children who have acquired HIV from contaminated blood products may also be burdened by a preexisting condition (such as hemophilia or cancer) (10). Caring for a child with a chronic or acute illness has a lasting impact on the family. Parents have had to relinquish control and depend on a medical system for answers. For many of these families, the uncertainty of the prognosis for the primary medical condition is compounded by the uncertainty of the progression of HIV infection to full-blown AIDS (10). The majority have acquired their disease perinatally and may only begin to develop symptoms of AIDS later in childhood.

The diagnosis of a serious illness often prompts a barrage of questions (11). Many parents remain ambivalent about whether to inform their child about their infection. This decision is often based on several realistic concerns, including fear of abandonment by family and friends, the effect that disclosure might have on siblings, concerns about the loss of employment or housing, and worries that the child will be unable to keep this information to himself or herself (12). Parents may also withhold the diagnosis to protect their child from painful realities (such as how they became infected and/or discussions about death) and wish to preserve their child's happy childhood without burdening them with the knowledge of their life-threatening disease for as long as possible (13). However, children, seeing their parents upset and hearing a lot of medical talk often suspect that they are more seriously ill than they are being told. Families find themselves further burdened by a lack of candor within the home where they might benefit from being able to talk openly about the situation. Both the child and the family can be caught in a conspiracy of silence. Family decisions about the diagnosis must take several factors into consideration, including the psychological effects on the child and family, coping abilities, and environmental and social support systems they might mobilize. Despite legitimate reasons to keep the HIV diagnosis a closely guarded secret, many parents yearn to leave the world of concealment and lies, which is in conflict with their own moral values (13). When families do decide to reveal the diagnosis, they often need help doing so in a style appropriate to the child's motor and cognitive development.

It has been demonstrated that by the age of 10 or 11, children who have been diagnosed with cancer understand death as permanent and universal with a total cessation of all bodily sensation (14). Some begin developing philosophical views of life and death. Answering a child's question about whether he or she will die from their disease is extremely difficult for most parents. The child's worst fears are often associated with abandonment, not death. They worry about how their parents will cope and the pain and suffering their parents might experience. These issues should be openly and honestly discussed. When a parent cannot face these questions alone, engaging the help of the social worker or other mental health professional can be most beneficial.

Parents have concerns about whether they need to inform the school of their child's diagnosis. School-age children with HIV infection have become the focus of teachers, parents, other students, and neighbors (3) (see

Chapters 48 and 49). For some students, fear of ostracism and rejection have resulted in low self-esteem and anxiety regarding returning to the classroom. This issue needs to be dealt with openly and honestly by the child, teachers, and principal. Other children have returned to the classroom to find their teachers to be compassionate and sensitive to their individual learning needs. This process occurs when adequate education of school staff takes place.

The child must be reassured that he or she did not cause the illness. This can be particularly difficult for a parent when one parent is struggling with his or her own feelings of guilt. Simple explanations about the virus and medical procedures are important so that medical interventions are not perceived as punishment.

Adolescents

The particular developmental task of adolescence lends a special poignancy to the problem of the diagnosis of an HIV infection (10) (see also Chapter 39). Characteristically, adolescents are narcissistic and optimistic, have a strong sense of invulnerability and immortality, are prone to peer pressure, and have a limited ability to conceive of long-term consequences of current behavior. In adolescence the personality components established during childhood are examined, reworked, and reaffirmed, and a struggle between balancing a sense of omnipotence and a sense of impotence is common. The diagnosis of HIV infection during this time often produces denial, fear, or withdrawal. Denial—a belief that the outcome will be reversed—and fear that others will find out are the most common initial reactions among adolescents. The fear of being rejected by one's peers is often greater than the fear of dying from the disease.

AIDS affects all spheres of an adolescent's life. The infection is most frequently acquired through heterosexual and homosexual behavior as well as drug use. Adolescents are more likely to have experienced disruption in their lives before becoming ill (15). Adolescents with hemophilia or another pre-existing medical condition often describe tremendous resentment of being struck with a double diagnosis and life filled

with restriction. The most damaging result of HIV infection on the adolescent is its effect on the formation of relationships outside the family. Critical issues to be addressed include the difficulty of informing sexual partners, the use of "safer sex" practices and alternative sexual expression, fear of the conclusions that peers may reach about how the virus was acquired, and feeling defiled, guilty, or sexually abnormal. The enforced dependency on family and the medical community is exceedingly difficult for adolescents (10) and an approach that focuses on the value of the individual and his need and right to care for himself is essential. The cruicial question, "Will I ever be able to marry and have children," will demand open and honest discussion (16). These anxieties can lead to poor school performance, depression, isolation and resentment (10), and acting-out behavior.

Parents and Guardians

Guilt

Regardless of the mode of acquisition, all parents experience some degree of guilt pertaining to their child's diagnosis of AIDS. Parents whose history includes intravenous drug use or sexual promiscuity bear the additional guilt of having placed their children at risk. Partners of individuals involved in the high-risk behavior experience additional emotional reactions. If they had not been aware of their partner's life-style, feelings of resentment, anger, betrayal, and inadequacy are common (17). Parents who sanctioned a blood transfusion or infusion of coagulation factors may experience guilt at having done so, especially if the procedure occurred subsequent to the identification of the AIDS virus but before the availability of blood screening tests. Mothers of hemophiliacs often express guilt about passing on hemophilia, and now another life-threatening condition has resulted from the treatment. Parents of hemophiliacs may also feel an enormous sense of responsibility for actually being the ones to infuse their child with the contaminated blood. Those who requested and were not permitted to donate their own blood often harbor resentment toward the medical community and additional guilt for not pursuing the issue further. Health care providers need to listen and be supportive. When focusing on guilt, it is important to help parents differentiate between cause and intent. That is, it may have been their behavior or actions that cause their child harm (7).

Anger

Anger is a prominent emotion for some families. Parents may be angry at the child's health care providers for not addressing the risks associated with transfusions or clotting agents. Some of this anger can also be directed against homosexuals and drug users who voluntarily donated the "contaminated" blood. This may even result in parents refusing to use existing support services primarily established by the gay community. Anger that is directed at specific individuals is often short-lived but may resurface at different points during the child's illness. The degree of anger toward the medical system and medical personnel also depends on how compassionately the information regarding their or their child's infection was given and how their health care providers have responded to them since the diagnosis. Parents draw strength when a forum is provided to express their emotional reactions and anger. Families seem to move past this phase when reassured of ongoing comprehensive medical and psychosocial family care.

Task Overload

Caring for a child with an HIV infection is generally time-consuming, burdensome, and unpredictable. This is especially true for single parents and families already faced with poverty and multiple daily demands. Struggling to work, maintain a home, sustain a family life, care for other children, and comply with frequent medical appointments can be virtually impossible. Owing to new fears of overt discrimination, many families have the additional burden of keeping the truth to themselves.

Isolation

Most families report that they are unwilling to share their child's diagnosis with friends and relatives. The loss of social support results in isolation, which contributes to depression and to difficulty in accomplishing family tasks. Sometimes it is only when the parents become ill and the family is at the height of vulnerability that rejection is risked through the disclosure of the diagnosis. Interventions should be designed to help family members anticipate the reactions of their community and of individuals with whom they are considering sharing the diagnosis (9). Each family's wishes regarding the confidentiality of their child's infection must be viewed as their inviolable right, because it is often their only measure of control over their situation (9).

Depression

A reactive depression may result from facing HIV infection of the family, and parents may also have a chronic depressive state that is a result of the coexistence of multiple problems. These problems include the stress of single parenthood, substance abuse, socioeconomic problems, rejection of family and friends, emotional isolation, loss of employment, and illness.

Studies of depression in women show that the main precipitating cause is not grief itself but the hopelessness that precedes the grief (18). This is particularly germane for poverty stricken single mothers who may be barely coping with existing problems. Their perception of hoplessness precedes the acquisition of HIV and is compounded by the suffering and fatality of infection. Inpatient psychiatric referrals may be indicated when suicide risk is high, as illustrated in the following vignette.

A woman found out that she was HIV positive when her 9-month baby was diagnosed with AIDS. At age 26 she had known little happiness or stability. She could remember only years of trauma, losses, poverty, drug addiction, violence, abuse, and now AIDS. She was accustomed to the idea that she would die young and possibly violently. She did not feel that she deserved to live longer than her mother, who had died at age 28 and left four daughters orphaned. Yet the idea of dying a painful, slow death was unacceptable and she said obsessively that she would smother her baby and then put a gun to her head. Out of rage, despair, and guilt she refused to care for her baby. A 2-week emergency psychiatric hospitalization and follow-up therapy sessions proved beneficial; she was able to care for her child until the child's death at age 2. She still receives counseling (8).

Fears of Multiple Losses

After the initial shock, anger, and blame, parents begin to mourn for multiple losses. These include the potential loss of their child, the loss of their dreams for the family's future together, the loss of bearing or fathering more children, the loss of pleasurable activities that may have led to infection, the loss of trust either in a medical system or in women or men who may have infected them, the loss of self-esteem, loss of sexuality, and the loss of a sense of invulnerability.

Tragic loss often leaves deep wounds that heal with time. As pediatric AIDS families struggle through the possible loss of multiple members, we must recognize that every loss represents a challenge to each family's integrity. Families need psychological support in grieving each loss as it occurs. Only then can they gather the strength and courage to go on living one day at a time.

SPECIAL CONSIDERATIONS
Extended Family Caretakers

The tragic loss of multiple members within families puts a crushing burden on the most fragile and vulnerable group of women. Grandmothers and great-grandmothers are increasingly called upon to care for HIV-infected infants and children besides caring for their own children who are dying of AIDS.

These crises are particularly traumatic for such elderly women who have already experienced an unusual amount of death and tragedy within their lifetime owing to violent crimes, drug use, and a life filled with poverty and oppression. Through a sensitive, caring response, individual and group support, respite care, and the availability of in-home support, these women can continue to carry on their difficult responsibilities while working through the painful consequences of AIDS and multiple deaths.

Siblings

Siblings of chronically or acutely ill children are severely emotionally affected. The burden and grief borne by the parents of a terminally ill child are so great that the ensuing problems of siblings may fade in comparison. As a result, the pain, fear, and confusion felt by siblings can be easily ignored. Family life is strengthened when individuals can share information and feelings and can communicate openly a sense of hope and trust in the future. Families who choose not share the HIV diagnosis with a child's siblings may block healthy expression of feelings needed in a time of crisis. So much energy is expended to keep the secret of AIDS that family members lose a sense of the other's feelings.

In many cases, both the infected child and siblings know or suspect the presence of HIV or AIDS but are also painfully aware of the absolute need in the family to keep the secret. A 6-year girl illustrated this point when she and her 11-year sister were watching an AIDS program on television. The 6-year-old responded by saying: "This is exactly what I have, I have AIDS. I know it, but please don't tell Mommy; it would just kill her." When open communications between siblings and between parents are blocked, it is detrimental to the family.

Envy and rivalry between children exist in every family. In HIV-infected families, uninfected siblings tend to feel resentment of the special medical care and parental attention given to the sick child. They are burdened with jealously and, subsequently, experience guilt for escaping the affliction. In many families in which more than one sibling is infected, siblings worry that they too will become ill and die. They often describe themselves as looking into a mirror—fearing the pain and suffering they may have to face in the future and the effect it will have on their families. Children whose parents are infected fear abandonment and worry about who will care for them if their parents die. They frequently express a desire to be part of that decision-making process. Family support and counseling are therefore vital in helping families renegotiate the siblings' roles in terms of age, maturity, and competence. Older siblings are encouraged to become more active in helping, caring, and nurturing the HIV-infected child without assuming the adult role. In general, siblings feel loneliness and loss while the child is hospitalized and fear becoming ill or dying themselves; expression and resolution of these feelings is crucial.

Support groups for siblings of HIV-infected children are potentially very helpful, but they cannot be established as long as parents feel the need to keep the diagnosis a secret. Support groups for siblings at the Albert Einstein Medical Center with a selected group of teens who had been told of their family's HIV illness demonstrated the positive and therapeutic impact of sharing knowledge of AIDS. Their parents reported that the group improved their child's school performance, decreased anger toward the HIV-infected parent, lowered anxiety as well as reduced negative and envious behavior toward the ill child. The group therapists noted that the siblings in the group demonstrated heightened sensitivity, empathy, sense of self worth, and responsibility within both the family and society. In fact, with their increased awareness about the disease, many siblings began to channel their energy toward improving knowledge about AIDS in their communities. Parents also reported that the group improved relationships with their children, and as a result a stronger and more intimate bond between them was created.

Another example of support are the summer camps for HIV-infected children and their families that have operated in the summers of 1989, 1990, 1991, and 1993 (see Table 43.1). Having the whole family participate in the camp experience has allowed siblings the opportunity to be a part of the family drama. It opened their eyes and hearts to the situation of their ill brother or sister, removed misconceptions and fantasies about the illness, and created deeper love and understanding while paving the way for more open communication once the family returned home. Support groups and more camp initiatives are needed to counteract the loneliness and isolation experienced by siblings of HIV-infected children.

Women and Minorities

AIDS is moving across the nations of the world and is taking young women in its path. Women of minorities, primarily blacks and Hispanics, have been most affected. According to the Centers for Disease Control, the incidence of AIDS among Hispanic women is over 11 times that of white women. In New York City, AIDS has already become the primary cause of death for all women 25–34 years old.

Both in black and Hispanic communities, sexual practices reflect the established sex roles in which women are dominated by men and have fewer privileges. Women report that protection is used infrequently despite its necessity because they may fear violence or rejection from their partners. The fear of AIDS is not sufficient to fight these inhibitions and often increases the anxiety of women. More minority women are becoming knowledgeable about HIV owing to forceful outreach and education, but their lack of economic and personal freedom prevents them from integrating their knowledge into preventive behavior. They often feel disempowered, alienated from traditional sources of help and support, and, as a result, stigmatized. Historically, these women have been tangled in a web of poverty, illness, and oppression; by the dictates of racism and poverty, they are disempowered and disenfranchised (19). In general, these women lack a community of support such as that shared by gay men.

However, HIV-infected women come from all walks of life, and the social issues transcend socioeconomic class, race, and cultural boundaries. Important issues include isolation and lack of support because the infection is often kept secret; grief over the loss of body image, sexuality, and childbearing potential; need for medical care, child care, and related services; need for counseling and support to make decisions about conception and pregnancy; lack of an organized advocacy network; loss of self-esteem; sense of responsibility after watching a child deteriorate and die; and the stigma that "women with AIDS are all drug users or prostitutes who infect their children" (20). All women need emotional, financial, medical, and legal support in minimizing their isolation while maximizing empowerment and self-respect.

Poverty, Drug Abuse, and AIDS

HIV is infecting our most disadvantaged people. Infected children are predomi-

Table 43.1. Summer Camps

Camp Sunburst: serves children with HIV/AIDS and their families.
    National AIDS Project
    148 Wilson Hill Rd.
    Petaluma CA 94952
    707-769-0169
Summer Program of Herbert G. Birch: serves children with HIV/AIDS and their families.
    Herbert G. Birch Services Summer Camp Program
    145-02 Farmers Blvd.
    Springfield Gardens NY 11434
    718-528-5754
Camp Chrysalis: serves children and their families who are affected by HIV/AIDS in Maine.
    Camp Chrysalis
    Waldo-Knox AIDS Coalition
    PO Box 990
    Belfast ME 04915
    207-338-1427
St. Claire's Summer Camp: serves children with HIV/AIDS and their families.
    AIDS Resource Foundation for Children
    182 Roseville Ave.
    Newark NJ 07107
    201-483-4250
Camp Dream Street: serves children with cancer, blood disorders, and other life-threatening illnesses.
    Dream Street Foundation
    9536 Wilshire Blvd. Suite 310
    Beverly Hills CA 90212
    310-274-7227
Camp Heartland: serves children infected and affected by HIV/AIDS.
    Camp Heartland Project
    4565 N Green Bay Ave.
    Milwaukee WI 53209
    414-264-6161 or 414-242-6487
The Hole In The Wall Gang Camp: serves children with cancer and other serious blood conditions who, because of their disease, its treatment, or its complications, cannot attend an ordinary summer camp.
    The Hole In The Wall Gang Camp
    565 Ashford Center Rd., PO Box 156
    Ashford CT 06278
    203-429-3444
Several Hemophilia Camps accept children with hemophilia and HIV into their summer programs; ask for a camp directory.
    National Hemophilia Foundation
    1-800-42-HANDI

nantly in single-parent families (natural, foster, or adoptive mother). The recent and alarming increase of crack use adds another dimension. Traditional social welfare methods are less effective with addicted mothers. The ethical dilemma of providing financial help that may be diverted to more drugs is an everyday occurrence.

Impoverished people with AIDS, especially intravenous drug users and their children, have special health problems and may require longer hospitalizations because they have no place to go (21). Efforts aimed at AIDS prevention must address the elimina-

tion of poverty. Innovative ways of raising self worth and providing opportunities for education and employment are essential for the control of HIV infection. Traditional and nontraditional culturally sensitive and ethnically specific services for women are desperately needed, especially in urban and minority communities (22).

INTERVENTIONS

Early Intervention

The initial visit to the health care center is a critical but often neglected point for psychosocial intervention. After the initiation of a psychosocial assessment and assurance of ongoing support services by the social worker, infusing hope in the context of AIDS is a most effective way of imparting coping skills. Family members often refer to this as a positive attitude. A pattern of mutual trust, strength, and hope is established in the professional relationship that in turn generates more positive attitudes and nurturance. Imparting hope should begin at the initial visit and permeate all services. Parents are often confused about AIDS, having gained conflicting information from friends and the media. Through compassionate and accurate education about the infection and its treatment and information regarding treatment options, much anxiety and despair can be alleviated. Therefore, at the end of the initial evaluation, the health care team, including the physicians, primary nurse, nurse practitioner, and social worker, should meet with each family. Usually within a month of diagnosis, when intensive early supportive intervention is provided, parents can move from the panic of the initial diagnosis to acceptance and realistic expectations (8).

Clinical support services are essential for medical care and to assure children equal access to therapeutic trials (23). The authors have found that clinical support services are utilized best when the provider can establish an ongoing, stable, nurturing, and nonthreatening relationship with parents either before the initial clinical or hospital visit through telephone contact or immediately after entering a medical system.

Psychosocial Assessment

Through collaborative and multidisciplinary efforts, a health care team can provide comprehensive care that supports the entire family throughout the illness (24, 25). An essential component of this approach is a psychosocial assessment that identifies each family's strengths and vulnerabilities (Table 43.2). With such an assessment, the team can then best anticipate the psychological adjustment of families and plan appropriate interventions. The assessment should be obtained as soon after the family presents to the medical center as possible but may need to be obtained over a course of visits. An assessment of family functioning is assisted by using genograms, which indicate family transmitted diseases such as AIDS as well as dysfunctional patterns such as alcohol and substance abuse (Table 43.2). A genogram may answer such basic questions as the number of family losses or who may be available to the children in case the parent becomes too ill to provide care (Fig. 43.1). Once the psychosocial assessment and genogram are complete, clinical interventions and community interagency linkages can be initiated to assist families in coping with the enormous tasks at hand.

Mental Health Services

AIDS is clearly a family disease and no family member remains unaffected or unchanged by the experience. An initial assessment determines the family's ability to cope with problems and evaluates their specific needs and resources. Important issues include providing emergency food or housing, facilitating proper medical care, and helping mothers place their children in day care, educational settings, or respite care. A needs assessment has also identified that parents are interested in information pertaining to HIV infection, available treatment, and assistance dealing with the disclosure of the diagnosis (26). With treatment and supportive care options now available, children may live longer, and the disease has become a more chronic illness creating a cumulative psychological burden requiring various modalities of intervention (27).

Crisis Intervention

Crisis intervention has emerged as the predominant psychotherapeutic modality used in assisting families throughout the illness. With targeted and timely interventions—such as psychiatric referral for suicidal patients, emergency shelter for families who have lost their housing, and grief counseling for parents who have lost a child—parents are provided with immediate assistance and are allowed to express their despair, their often unbearable isolation, and their multiple fears. A range of individ-

Table 43.2.   Psychosocial Assessment of Anticipated Family Adaptation

Family constellation
   Biological as well as adoptive/foster/extended family members
History of illness
   Route of transmission, history of symptoms
Child's personality profile
   Preillness
      Relationship with parents, siblings, peers
      Functioning in school and play
      Coping abilities
      Existing standardized test information
      Prior losses
   Current
      Knowledge and reaction to diagnosis
      Words used to describe infection
      Beliefs, attitudes, expectations
      Coping abilities
      Ability to deal with separation
      Energy level, mood
      Behavioral changes at home, school, play
      Revelation to any friends
      School's understanding of child's situation
Family History
   Family beliefs, attitudes, expectations regarding illness, treatment, death
   Who in the family is aware of diagnosis?
   Reactions of family members/friends/neighbors
   Quality of relationships with extended family members
   Coping abilities during previous crises
   History of depression and/or nonprescribed drug and alcohol use
   History of previous losses
   Nature and stability of residential/occupational arrangements
   Sources of emotional and financial support; availability of medical insurance
   Cultural/religious beliefs
   Health status of all family members
Community Support
   Involved community agencies
   Social work involvement

ual therapy interventions can also be of assistance. To the extent that these young, dying adults who are losing their young children can express their emotions, they can be helped through their ordeal (8).

Individual Counseling

Play therapy is a powerful tool for the young children in creating a structure in which he or she can express and work through feelings and fears of isolation, separation, and abandonment. Play therapy provides a safe atmosphere where the child learns new skills in coping with invasive medical procedures while reenacting previous traumas (28). Play and verbal techniques help the older child share, relive, reenact, and resolve traumatic life events.

For children who suffer from encephalopathy or are nonverbal, what cannot be "told" can possibly be played out or depicted in drawings or paintings. Common themes include fear of others finding out their diagnosis and being rejected, guilt related to their illness and how it has affected the whole family, concerns over their parents' health status, and inability to talk openly with their parents about dying.

Several difficult and delicate subjects will arise when working with parents and family members around their various AIDS-related problems. Supportive and insight oriented therapy can enhance family coping skills and assist in complex decisions and dilemmas such as planning future pregnancies, making educated decisions concerning sexual intimacy, and helping parents express

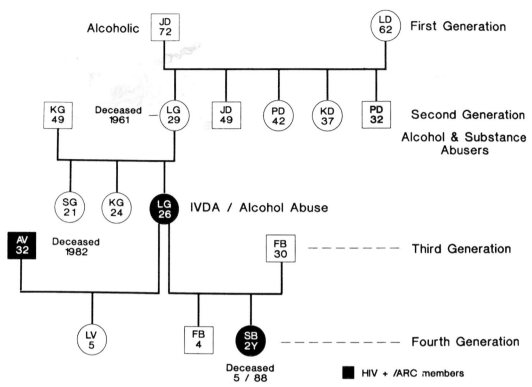

Figure 43.1. Four generation genogram of an HIV/AIDS family. *ARC*, AIDS-related complex.

their denial, fear of death, and anger. It allows them to prepare for death by setting conditions, discussing burial, and arranging for eventual care for their children. Careful discussion of these topics may trigger deep emotions but can lead to a sense of liberation and increased hopefulness. Most issues can also be successfully addressed in couple, family, or group settings. If hospital resources do not include counseling services, local AIDS organizations often have listings of local psychotherapists who accept Medicaid reimbursement or see clients on a sliding-fee basis.

Couple and Family Counseling

Many families experience serious conflict in marital or significant relationships because of unresolved blame, guilt, anger, lack of support, and fears of contagion, loss, and death. Other couples need informed and educated reassurance in continuing intimate relationships, since they often react to HIV infection by either completely withdrawing from each other or by refusing to alter their sexual behavior at all. Consequently, couple and family counseling are treatment modalities of great assistance to many families. The goals typically focus on promoting adaptive functioning, problem solving, and changing overt behavior, as well as modifying systemic family processes, including communication and interpersonal relationship difficulties (29). The child cannot be treated in isolation (30). Family interventions, involving as many family members as possible, must aim at restructuring the family in a realistic way that respects the kinship system, sibling system, and a three- to four-generation hierarchy. This does not necessarily follow traditional family restructuring, but these systems can be effectively reorganized with realistic expectations while families are strengthened at a most crucial point in life.

There may be an immediate indication for couple, family, or group therapy. These may include history of serious injury to the child inflicted by parents; explosive, sociopathic, or severe parental psychosis; and active parental substance abuse. In such situations referrals by the social worker, physician, or nurse need to be made to protective psychiatric care or drug treatment services. A family plagued by poverty and drug abuse for protracted periods may be overwhelmed by the tasks of parenting and family life (31). Establishing a sense of trust and stability and some balance in the family system is essential to first engage family members in the health care system and then in individual or family treatment (29).

Group Support

No matter what the circumstances, most individuals both need and have the capacity to relate to others. Most parents of HIV-infected children have a strong need to talk to others faced with the same situation and to help new families learning of their child's infection. The benefits of support groups for parents and guardians of HIV-infected children are two-fold. First, a support group can provide a safe atmosphere and a comfortable environment for open discussion of issues. In such a setting, new attitudes and coping styles can be developed. Second, support groups provide an opportunity to ventilate and share the experiences of feeling alienated as a result of this disease (32). The isolation parents feel upon diagnosis and the resulting helplessness is eased by seeing and talking to others in the same situation. As parents confide, share, and discuss forbidden areas (such as the kinds of behavior that led to infection or thinking about their child's funeral) they feel less singled out, their problems become less unique and less unusual, and they often feel less overwhelmed and frightened by them (33). In fact, the bond between group members is often so immediate and strong that the group becomes perceived as the surrogate family much needed in time of crisis and isolation. Parents often share telephone numbers and addresses and become available to each other on a regular basis. Several themes continue to emerge in support groups for parents or guardians of HIV-infected children: feelings of guilt and responsibility; anger and disbelief about the diagnosis; the need to lie to others; the loss of life as it once was; disclosure of the diagnosis to the child; impact of the disease on relationships with significant others, marriage partners, or other family members; comfort in religion or spiritual beliefs; the pain of watching their children lose ground; and the fear of either having to go on with life without their child or the fear of their child having to through life without them by their side (1). Practical advice regarding benefits, child care, school, becoming actively involved in the child's medical treatment, and talking to their children, other family members, friends, neighbors, and dates is also common. The most intense and intimate interchanges occur around the loss of a child's developmental milestones, the loss of a child's eyesight, and the anticipation of a child's death and the meetings after a death.

For parents who are emotionally vulnerable, the group can offer a wide range of role models with whom they can interact. Most groups for parents of HIV-infected children have been hospital based and open-ended, with no time limits set for length of involvement. They are most frequently run by social workers or other mental health professionals specifically trained in group treatment. Groups consisting of approximately six to ten members are ideal, because this allows both for interactions to occur and for individual needs to be met. The groups do not need to be separated by modes of acquisition of HIV. In fact, by hearing the pain and suffering others experience, members have developed increased empathy for others and new values and attitudes regarding their own situation. The most difficult parents to engage in group support on any regular basis are those who remain drug dependent.

For those who are either uncomfortable sharing their feelings face-to-face, who fear loss of confidentiality, or who have limited time or access to support groups in their community, a telephone support group may be very helpful. Through the Pediatric Branch of the National Cancer Institute telephone support groups for HIV-infected girls, siblings of infected children, infected and noninfected mothers, infected and noninfected fathers, foster and adoptive mothers, and grandmothers and grandfathers who are primary caretakers have been offered. Initially this intervention was offered as part of a study examining the usefulness of telephone support groups as a therapeutic support modality. The posttest questionnaires supported the impression that the groups were helpful, with 85% of the members reporting that they felt better about themselves since starting the group; 83% of the members also felt better about their ability to cope, and 80% felt better ability to handle their child's illness. Six months after the completion of the group, the participants were asked again how they felt about the group experience. Eighty-five percent felt better about their ability to cope since starting the group, 74% felt better about their ability to handle their child's problems, and 85% continued to feel better about themselves since the group began (34). Telephone group support has now been incorporated into our ongoing psychosocial support program.

The preventive and healing qualities of group support have far-reaching implications. However, group support is not for everyone. Members must be willing to confront what the future may bring in the words, the faces, and the physical conditions of the other group members (35).

ADVOCACY AND INTERAGENCY LINKAGES

Flexibility and creativity in using one's self requires the social worker or mental health professional to let go of certain fixed roles in dealing with parents in favor of others that may be uncomfortable, unfamiliar, and of less professional status (36). Children with AIDS and their families experience a multitude of simultaneous needs that require networking with complex systems and agencies. Many parents are already accustomed to contact with multiple agencies and workers within any given day. The workers in these agencies are often perceived as judgmental and even as obstacles to the services they need. Persistent efforts toward engaging parents are needed. Outreach is a key component of engaging and assisting parents of HIV-infected children, and a case management model has been most effective. Entering the parent's world through action, such as providing respite care and negotiating frustrating

public assistance agencies, is often viewed more favorably than offering mental health support services (36). The following are the most common areas where advocacy services are needed.

School Advocacy

Parents who have informed the school of their child's diagnosis and advocated for their child to remain in the classroom have been involved in unpredictable school battles (see Chapters 48 and 49). Some parents have utilized legal interventions to assist in this process. Unfortunately, some of these school cases have become highly publicized incidents of discrimination, some with accompanying acts of violence. This has led many parents to remain anonymous and to keep the diagnosis from the school for as long as possible. Fortunately, the number of situations where legal intervention is needed is being drastically reduced as school districts are beginning to develop their own HIV policies, and certain states have adopted "no-disclosure" laws (see Chapter 49). Nevertheless, the anxiety associated with informing school personnel about their child's diagnosis and fear of disclosure is tremendous. The health care team can assist families with the school process in several ways. These include 1) informing parents of a child's right to an education; 2) meeting with school officials and school personnel to educate them about HIV infection as well as apprise them of the individual needs of a specific child; 3) accompanying parents to school board meetings when they feel this would be of support; 4) providing consultation to teachers and principals in talking to the other classmates about HIV and AIDS; and 5) providing up-to-date information to the school pertaining to the child's progress once the child has reentered the classroom. The degree of involvement between the health care team and a particular child's entrance in the school will vary. Some parents require enormous support getting through the process. Other school districts have established policies, and little assistance is needed. In some cases, staff members have been subpoenaed to testify that a child should be in school.

Pediatricians and social workers can be essential during litigation, serving as expert witnesses in court or as respected sources of information for the school board and the public in general (37). Families have been deeply grateful for the time devoted by health care team members in their efforts toward coordinating their child's attendance in school. The publication entitled *Someone at School Has AIDS: A Guide to Developing Policies for Student and School Staff Members Who Are Infected with HIV* is available by the National Association of State Boards of Education. This can be especially helpful to school districts working toward establishing their own policy guidelines. Each state may have separate laws, and the health care team should be apprised of the law.

Legal Interventions

Legal intervention has become a critical component in caring for children and families with AIDS (see Chapter 49). Legal intervention may be needed to prospectively plan for the child's health care and custody arrangements (38). Early discussions of the future are indicated when the parents are HIV positive, especially when their symptomatology includes signs of neuropsychiatric sequelae. Assisting parents in identifying future care providers for their children, ensuring a durable power of attorney, and arranging legal custody is best done as early as possible. This can prevent a crisis when the parents become unable to provide care for the child, participate in decisions regarding their child's care, or die. It reaffirms parents' control over their family situation and it reassures their children about who will raise them. If family members or others are not identified, foster care may be needed.

Substance Abuse Programs

HIV infection in young children has been inextricably linked to drug use in adults (1). Substance using women are a primary concern because 80% of HIV infected women are of childbearing age (39). The pervasive destructive effects of drug addiction on an individual's capacity to function in daily life are well appreciated (40). These women rarely seek AIDS counseling before having children. Many crack-addicted women are so absorbed in their addiction that they do not receive prenatal care or consider the implications to their unborn or newborn babies. Persons who are drug addicted are being turned away from drug programs or being put on long waiting lists. They need these programs to wean themselves from drugs: innovative, accessible, and available drug treatment programs and residential settings equipped to care for HIV-infected women and children are desperately lacking. Recovering substance abusers are at risk for renewed abuse and require extensive support services, especially when their child dies. Outreach to substance abusers, with sensitivity to their existential struggle and premorbid history, is crucial. Meanwhile, infants and children of drug addicted parents are being referred to protective services and need foster care placement until their parents can provide safe homes for them. Protective service referrals and out of home placements (often involving frequent moves and a series of primary caretakers for the infants or child) are often routine interventions (40).

Protective Services

The question of whether to refer a family to protective services is influenced by many factors. These include the professional's previous experience with protective services and the current health status of child and parents. One's outrage at neglect or abuse directed against children and a wish to protect them may clash with one's sensitivity to the rights of parents to raise their children without interference in ways that are consistent with their cultural and personal belief systems (36). The need to act in the best interest of the child must remain the health care provider's first priority. Complicating factors include the parents' own health status and the limited number of available foster families to care for HIV-infected children at the time they are taken out of their home. Identifying extended family members who are willing, invested, and able to provide proper and loving care for the HIV-infected child is the first alternative, followed by the lengthy search for a foster home placement.

Foster Care

Child welfare traditionally has emphasized family cohesion (reunification), but in extreme cases equal consideration should be given to placing the child in a more nurturing environment. Foster placement can be an extremely rewarding experience for both the child and family. Foster parents, who have made a commitment to care for HIV-infected children, have for the most part been courageous and excellent care providers. They have formed particularly strong emotional attachments to the children. In fact, many foster parents have explored ways to adopt their foster children. Currently, the adoption process takes approximately 18 months to 4 years. Adoption of these children can be a complicated process that often leaves parents feeling abused by the system rather than appreciated for their ultimate expression of love and devotion.

Ideally, foster parents should be given authority through prompt legal guardianship to make decisions regarding medical procedures and treatments as well as education and recreational options for their foster children. This would necessitate new approaches to care within the child welfare field where the child's rights are the focus instead of those of the biological parents.

Foster home placements also present additional psychosocial challenges. For the older child placed in foster care after the loss of his or her parents there are several significant losses: loss of relationships within the family; loss of neighborhood friends and teachers; loss of the self as a member of a nuclear family; and, most importantly, fear of the loss of one's own life. It is not unusual for the child to panic when he or she develops any of the symptoms suffered by the deceased parent. Loss has also been observed as a key issue for foster parents. The following comments are frequently heard: "I was not supposed to get this attached." "I never thought it possible that I could love this child as much as I love my own," I never planned on becoming a parent. Now I can't imagine not being one." Like all biological parents, foster parents may need help in coping with feelings of loss and impending separation.

Case Management

Children with AIDS and their families typically require intensive social and financial support, concrete services such as shelter, food, clothing, and transportation to health services, legal guidance, specialized home care or day care programs, mental health services, and substance abuse assistance. Children experience a wide range of illnesses demanding different levels of care. At the acute stages, they require inpatient hospital care. When stabilized, they can be cared for at home with adequate medical and social services. Whenever possible, health care services should be delivered at home to provide a stimulating and nurturing environment (see Fig. 43.1, 43.2). In response to the complex needs of HIV-infected families, medical facilities in large epicenters established comprehensive family AIDS centers as far back as 1983. These centers provide a full range of medical AIDS-related services utilizing the case management model. State and federal agencies are now utilizing a task force of skilled social workers to test different case management models, most particularly family case management models. Such HIV/AIDS case management models could promote earlier and better prevention and service delivery, increase medical compliance while reducing duplication of services and reduced use of entitlement through empowerment and higher functioning. Whether case management is hospital based or community provided, close linkage is needed to maximize a continuum of quality care for each child and family (see also Chapters 42 and 44).

Terminal Illness

When there is consensus between the staff and family that the terminal phase is near, the family should be encouraged to decide where the child's final days will be spent. The health care team must support their decision and accept a possible change of mind should circumstances change (41). It is usually when the child is medically stable that parents find it least frightening to talk about terminal care and to begin thinking about future care needs for the child and family (42). Families welcome help in making connections with community re-

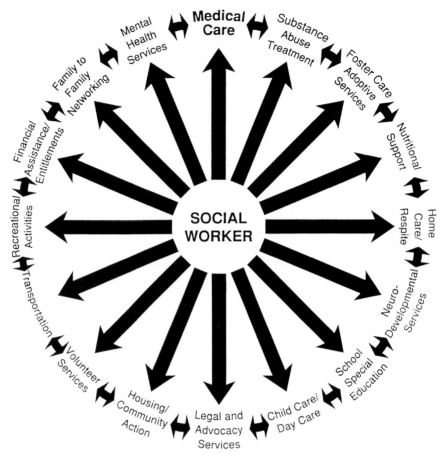

Figure 43.2.   HIV-infected children and families: case management approach to care and interagency linkages toward comprehensive family-based care.

sources and clergy as well as assessing local supports for the period after death. Children often obtain great satisfaction by being able to make a wish of their own through organizations such as the Make-A-Wish Foundation or Starlight Express.

Owing to an inability to care for their child, a minority of parents decide to relinquish their children before their death. However, in most cases, the child stays with the parent until the time of death. Many community AIDS organizations offer free legal services, and parents should be encouraged to make a will. A videotape made by the parent and left for the child has also been extremely therapeutic and beneficial to many (43). It provides a parent with an opportunity to say good-bye to his or her child and to share many thoughts that either the child would be too young to understand at the time of the parent's death or that the

parent had been reluctant to express face to face. For children old enough to appreciate such a tape, it has provided them with the strength to face their own disease and a sense of security in knowing the intensity of their parent's love. The timing of such tapes is important. The parent should be in relatively good physical health, because children want to remember their parents as "looking good." Parents should also be psychologically prepared to undertake such an emotionally difficult process. In our experience, these tapes are best made with a social worker or mental health professional with whom the parent has worked closely.

For those parents who are not able to or comfortable with making a videotape, other ways to create a feeling of remembrance are needed. For example, creating a memory book (an album of photographs and stories), leaving special jewelry or clothing, or writing poems or letters have also been extremely useful memories for children.

If possible, children should be allowed to have as much interaction as possible during the terminal phase of their parent's illness. If the dying parent or sibling cannot have visitors, ways to maintain the closeness between them are important. Telephone contact, handmade cards and presents, and other concrete items help the child feel connected and assist in processing the death and his or her loss (44). If the child is terminally ill and the parent(s) cannot visit, the same interventions have proved very useful.

Spirituality

Inevitably AIDS touches the painful issues of death and dying that are most powerfully denied in our society. Belief in God and spirituality is a great source of strength for us to respect and to tap. The time comes in each patient's life when he or she must face death. This transition from life should be as peaceful and loving as possible.

Many children have left this world with such beautiful acceptance and expressions of peace and love that they have become our teachers in this domaine. Such as 10-year Shari who fought her illness valiantly for 2 years. But during her last struggle she turned to her mother and all the medical people around her and clearly said, "There is nothing more for me here, I want to return to God." Six-year Jessica looked at her mother in the Emergency Room and said "Mommy, I love you but I want to return to God's house." Eight-year Billy quietly asked his grandmother if he could go be with Jesus. These examples have powerfully taught us about the importance of spiritual belief and faith.

Clearly, when we can support children and their parents in their spiritual quest with respect, love, and empathy, we are fortunate to help ease their transition from this world with peace. Helping families make the connection with someone who shares their spiritual faith is an important service that should not be ignored.

Bereavement

Parents express profound grief as they face their child's death. Regardless of the extent to which they believed themselves to be prepared, the actual death of the child initiates an extended period of grieving that is both intense and slow to resolve (41). In fact, the impact of the child's illness and death on the family continues long after the child has died. Parents describe still lying to friends and neighbors years later about the cause of death. Because of such isolation and unresolved mourning, pathologic grief reactions are common. Aborted or pathologic mourning may have long-term effects. Parents who are infected themselves often express suicidal ideation, feeling as if they have nothing to live for except waiting to become symptomatic themselves and join their child in death.

Follow-up calls after the child's death, assessing bereavement, making referrals for ongoing mental health services, helping parents reconnect with others, and, in turn, providing them with a sense of purpose by helping others in a similar situation are essential interventions (1). Many parents received tremendous support at the hospital from other parents, support groups, and staff members. When the child dies, this routine is aborted, and parents experience this as another loss. Inviting all families that have lost a child back to the hospital together on a yearly basis may provide them with a sense of continuity, support, and usefulness to others. Bereavement groups specifically for parents who have lost a child to AIDS can also have enormous psychological benefit. The goal of mourning is to lessen the pain of loss and the allowance of enriched memories. This can be accomplished by providing parents with the opportunity to reflect on and review the illness-dying experience until acceptance occurs (45). Ongoing availability and interest in the health of these families after a child's death should become an integral component of psychosocial support programs.

MULTIDISCIPLINARY APPROACH

The complexity of caring for children with AIDS and their families requires multifaceted assistance from a highly specialized multidisciplinary team. The needs of these families exceed the resources of any single discipline. Multidisciplinary staff members should include physicians, nurses, social workers, psychologists, psychiatrists, physical therapists, occupational therapists, speech therapists, nutritionists, pharmacists, recreational therapists or child life specialists, educators, and chaplains. The team approach provides comprehensive medical and psychosocial care to the entire family in the medical setting while coordinating the child and family care with community resources. Meetings scheduled on a regular basis and attendance by the entire team are essential.

PSYCHOSOCIAL STRESS ON STAFF

Parents often view the medical center as the only safe place where they feel free to vent their fears, frustrations, anger, grief, and overwhelming social and economic problems (4). This places a great sense of responsibility on the health care team. The poor prognosis for the infant coupled with the likely infection and potential for illness and death in the parents creates enormous stress for the providers of care. As the number of children with HIV infection increases, staff members do not have the time to absorb the pain and recuperate from multiple losses (46). Fear of contagion, stigma associated with the work, professional isolation, lack of support from family and friends, and decreased job satisfaction are other factors that contribute to stress among caretakers (47).

The emotional drain is the most likely cause of staff burnout. The hopelessness of the family with HIV infection can evoke a sense of helplessness in the worker attempt-

ing to serve the family. Health professionals my feel overwhelmed by the need, emotional deprivation, deteriorating health, and dependency of the families (36). Staff members may wish to rescue families. Others may have difficulty empathizing with the parents' circumstances and life-styles that may be so different from their own. Conversely, some staff members find that the parents' experiences of intense loneliness, depletion, and hopelessness stir up similar feelings in themselves (36). Many providers find themselves feeling angry and helpless when parents continue to engage in high-risk behavior, place others at risk, or fail to return for follow-up appointments or administer the child's medications. At the same time these parents can also be tender, courageous, and appreciative (21). As a result, practitioners may withdraw from, reject, or over-invest in a family's life to overcome feelings of frustration, anger, helplessness, and hopelessness in the face of enormous unfulfilled needs (36). Clearly, a high level of dedication and skill and a supportive work milieu are vital to all practitioners in this field to counteract burnout while providing families with sensitive and human care (Table 43.3).

CONCLUSION—-CHALLENGES AND FUTURE DIRECTIONS

Caring for children with AIDS and their families requires compassionate, multifaceted assistance to the entire family. Parents need support. Professionals must mobilize family support in the care of the children.

The complexities associated with HIV infection transcend the medical aspects of the

Table 43.3.   Reducing Stress in Work Place

Goals	Interventions
Maintain level of positive involvement in work	Find ways of releasing tension and "refueling" (32), such as staff retreats
Avoid miscommunication about patient care and staff responsibilities	Frequent multidisciplinary staff meetings
Enhance professional growth and self-esteem	Opportunities for writing, presenting one's work, ongoing education; professional reward system
Stay in touch with one's feelings; review personal doubts	Availability of staff support group and informal peer support
Balance issues of living with those of dying	Balance between direct clinical work and other responsibilities; see children enjoying life outside of clinic such as at camp

disease. The disease will always test a family's emotional stability. Marshaling social and community support is invaluable for most families. Some families will choose to network with other families and receive support from their community. Most families, however, utilize support well and benefit from the assistance available to them through a comprehensive multidisciplinary care team approach. Therefore, all psychosocial models must coordinate care between the hospital, home, and community while incorporating ongoing clinical assessments of a family's changing needs. They must also focus on each family's strengths and resources and not be blinded by their often overwhelming vulnerabilities.

The challenges facing professionals caring for HIV-infected children are formidable. Enabling families to find meaning in life, praising their survival skills, and tapping new sources of psychic strength, courage, and resiliency are the essence of this demanding yet rewarding work.

References

1. Wiener LS, Moss H, Davidson R, Fair C. Pediatrics: The emerging psychosocial challenges of the AIDS epidemic. Child Adolesc Social Work J 1992;9:381–407.
2. Septimus A. Psycho-social aspects of caring for families of infants infected with human immunodeficiency virus. Semin Perinatol 1989;13:49–54.
3. Rogers MP, Thomas PA, Starcher ET, Noa MC, Bush TJ, Jaffe HW. Acquired immunodeficiency syndrome in children: Report of the Centers for Disease Control National Surveillance, 1982 to 1985. Pediatrics 1987;79:1008–1014.
4. Cooper ER, Pelton SI, LeMay M. Acquired immunodeficiency syndrome: A new population of children at risk. Pediatr Clin North Am 1988;35:1365–1387.
5. DesJarlais DC, Friedman SR, Strug D. AIDS and needle sharing within the IV-drug use subculture. In: Feldman D, Johnson T, eds. The social dimension of AIDS. New York: Praeger, 1986:121–126.
6. Boland MG. Management of the child with HIV infection: Implications for service delivery. In: Report of the Surgeon General's workshop on children with HIV infection and their families. Rockville, MD: Dept. of Health and Human Services, 1987:42.
7. Boland M, Tasker M, Evans P, Keresztes J. Helping children with AIDS. The role of the child welfare worker. Public Welfare 1987;45:23–29.
8. Septimus A. Caring for HIV-infected children and their families: Psychosocial ramifications. In: Anderson G, ed. Carriage to care. Washington, DC: Child Welfare League of America, 1990.
9. Lewert G. Children and AIDS. Soc Casework 1988;69:348–354.
10. Waters BGH, Ziegler JB, Hampson R, McPherson AH. The psychosocial consequences of childhood infection with human immunodeficiency virus. Med J Aust 1988;149:198–202
11. Lansky S, List MA, Ritter-Sterr C. Psychiatric and psychological support of the child and adolescent with cancer. In: Pizzo PA, Poplack DG, eds. Principles and practice of pediatric oncology. Philadelphia: JB Lippincott, 1989:885–896.
12. Olson RA, Huszti HC, Mason PJ, Seibert JM Pediatric AIDS/HIV infection: An emerging challenge to pediatric psychology. J Pediatr Psychol 1989;14:1–21.
13. Tasker M. How Can I Tell You? Association of the Care of Children's Health, 1992.
14. Easson WM. The dying child: The management of the child or adolescent who is dying. 2nd ed. Springfield, IL: Charles C Thomas, 1981.
15. Schonberg SK. Adolescents and AIDS. J Adolesc Health Care 1989;10:4s.
16. Miller R, Goldman E, Bor R, Kernoff P. AIDS and children: Some of the issues in haemophilia care and how to address them. AIDS Care 1989;1:59–65.
17. Jue S. Identifying and meeting the needs of minority clients with AIDS. In: Leukefeld CG, Fimbres M, eds. Responding to AIDS: Psychosocial initiatives. Silver Spring, MD: National Association of Social Workers, 1987:65–79.
18. Brown G, Harris T. Social origins of depression: A study of psychiatric disorder in women. New York: Free Press, 1978.
19. Zuckerman C, Gordon L. Meeting the psychosocial and legal needs of women with AIDS and their families. NY State Med 1988;88:619–620.
20. Wofsy CB. Intravenous drug abuse and women's issues. In: Report of the Surgeon General's workshop on children with HIV infection and their families. Rockville, MD: Dept. of Health and Human Services, 1987:32.
21. Heagarty MC. AIDS: A view from the trenches. Issues Sci Technolo 1987;Winter:112–117.
22. Wiener LS. Women and human immunodeficiency virus: A historical and personal psychosocial perspective. Social Work 1991;36:375–378.
23. Howard J, Beckwith L, Rodning C, Kropenske V. The development of young children of substance-abusing parents: Insights from seven years of intervention and research. Zero Three. 1989;9:8–12.
24. Hersh SP, Wiener LS, Psychosocial support for the family of the child with cancer. In: Pizzo PA, Poplack DG, eds. Principles and practice of pediatric oncology. Philadephia: JB Lippincott, 1989:897–913.
25. Christ GH, Wiener LS, Psychosocial issues in AIDS. In: DeVita VT, Hellman S, Rosenberg SA, eds. AIDS: Etiology, diagnosis, and prevention. Philadelphia: JB Lippincott, 1985:275–297.
26. Falloon J, Eddy J, Wiener L, Pizzo PA. Human immunodeficiency virus infection in children. J Pediatr 1989;114:1–30.
27. Balfer ML, Krener PK, Black Miller F. AIDS in children and adolescents. J Am Acad Child Adolesc Psychiatry 1988;27:147–151.
28. Greenacre P. Play in relation to creative imagination. Psychoanal Study Child 1959;14:61–81.

29. Klavins Simring S, Mishne JM. Family treatment. In: Ehrenkranz SM, Goldstein EG, Goodman L, Seinfeld J, eds. Clinical social work with maltreated children and their families. New York: New York University Press, 1989;62–78.

30. Mishne JM. Individual treatment. In: Ehrenkranz SM, Goldstein EG, Goodman L, Seinfeld J, eds. Clinical social work with maltreated children and their families. New York: New York University Press, 1989:38–61.

31. Weitzman J. Engaging the severely dysfunctional family in treatment: Basic considerations. Fam Process 1985;15:473–485.

32. Grant D. Support groups for youth with the AIDS virus. Int J Group Psychother 1988;38:237–250.

33. Gitterman A, Shulman L. Mutual aid groups and the life cycle. Itasca, IL: FE Peacock, 1986.

34. Wiener LS, DuPont E, Davidson R, Fair C. National telephone support groups: A new avenue toward psychosocial support for HIV-infected children and their families. Social Work Groups, in press.

35. Morin SF, Charles KA, Malyon AK. The psychological impact of AIDS on gay men. Am Psychol 1984;39:1288–1293.

36. Goldstein EG, Gonzales-Ramos G. Toward an integrated clinical practice perspective. In: Ehrenkranz SM, Goldstein EG, Goodman L, Seinfeld J, eds. Clinical social work with maltreated children and their families. New York: New York University Press, 1989:21–37.

37. Blackman JA, Appel BR. Epidemiologic and legal considerations in the exclusion of children with AIDS, cytomegalovirus or herpes simplex virus infection from group care. Pediatric Infect Dis 1987;11:1011–1015.

38. Chachkes E. Women and children with AIDS. In: Leukefeld CG, Fimbres M, eds. Responding to AIDs: Psychosocial initiatives. Silver Spring, MD: National Association of Social Workers, 1987:51–64.

39. Centers for Disease Control. Human immunodeficiency virus infection in the United States. A review of current knowledge. MMWR 1987:36:56.

40. Weston DR, Ivins B, Zuckerman B, Jones C, Lopez R. Drug exposed babies: Research and clinical issues. Zero to Three. 1989;9:1–7.

41. Howell DA, Martinson JM. Management of the terminally ill child. In: Pizzo PA, Poplack DG, eds. Principles and practice of pediatric oncology. Philadelphia: JB Lippincott, 1989:991–1002.

42. Wiener LS, Fair C, Pizzo PA. Care for the child with HIV infection and AIDS. In: Goltzer S, Armstrong-Dailey A, eds. Hospice care for children. New York: Oxford University Press, in press.

43. Taylor-Brown S, Wiener L. Making videotapes of HIV-infected women for their children. Families Soc 1993;74:468–480.

44. Dubik-Unruh S. Children of chaos: Planning for the emotional survival of dying children of dying families. Palliat Care 1989;5:10–15.

45. Koch CB, Herman J, Donaldson MG. Supportive care of the child with cancer. Semin Oncol 1974;1:81–86.

46. Bolle JL. Supporting the deliverers of care: Strategies to support nurses and prevent burnout. Nurs Clin North Am 1988;23:843–850.

47. Wiener LS, Seigel K. Social workers' comfort in providing services to AIDS patients. Social Work 1990;35:18–25.

44

Respite and Terminal Care for Children with HIV Infection and Their Families

Ann Armstrong-Dailey and Cindy Fair

Children are not supposed to die. The death of a child violates society's norms and is not what parents and health care providers expect and desire for that child. But children do die.

According to former Surgeon General C. Everett Koop in 1986, "approximately 100,000 children in the United States die annually. Many more will be diagnosed with life-threatening illness. Most parents of dying children want involvement and some control over their children's care" (1). The United States General Accounting Office notes that "nationally, between 10 and 15 percent of all children have a chronic health condition, ... and about 10 percent of them—or 1 million children—have a severe form of it" (2).

The Pediatric AIDS Coalition's 1991 Legislative Agenda states that "the incidence of HIV infection among infants, children, adolescents and women continues to rise unabated" (3). Current Centers for Disease Control and Prevention statistics show that through June 1993 6013 cases of AIDS had been reported in children aged 0–19 years.

Children with life-threatening or terminal conditions and their families are often a forgotten population within our health care delivery system. Many of these children die alone and afraid. In addition, the emotional strain and grief faced by the families of these children is overwhelming. There is a great need for improved care of these children and families worldwide. As the AIDS virus continues spreading to newborn in-

fants, this need for comprehensive children's hospice care will only increase.

Kathy, a 15-year-old from the Pacific Northwest, provides an example of the extraordinary complications faced by children with AIDS. When Kathy was 7 years old, she was hit by a car while riding her bike. In receiving a transfusion in the hospital, she contracted the human immunodeficiency virus (HIV) virus. Living in a rural community she and her family have lived the past 8 years with Kathy's illness a secret. Even other family members do not know that Kathy has AIDS.

In addition to the normal stresses felt by families when a child is dying, this family was facing it alone. Deep feelings of isolation developed. Kathy's older brother, unable to express his feelings, attempted suicide. Kathy's father and mother both work, making it very difficult to care for Kathy when she is too sick to go to school. Even transportation to the urban hospital where Kathy receives treatment is a challenge, especially on work days. The hospital staff, recognizing these stresses, recommended psychosocial support for the family from the outset.

Over the past 8 years, Kathy's condition has deteriorated. She is often home from school in a lot of pain. Unfortunately, since her parents both have to work, they cannot be with her. Realizing the situation, Kathy's social worker recommended hospice and respite care. It took months of effort on the social worker's part to convince Kathy's physician and nurses that hospice care would be appropriate—they felt it would be a sign of giving up.

This family, however, was barely hanging together. They were told about the option of hospice care and wanted to receive it. They have now been receiving hospice care for over a year, and, with this increased level of support, the entire family can cope much better and is growing together during this tough time, rather than breaking apart.

The hospice program coordinates emotional and psychological support for Kathy's brother who is now in college and respite and home care so that Kathy can still be at home and receive the care she needs and so that her parents can work without the burden of guilt. This hospice program even collected money this past spring to buy Kathy a party dress for her first dance. Kathy and her family, while still facing the stresses of a terminal illness, at least have appropriate support to enable them to accept the reality that her time is limited and to live life to its fullest for as long as they have together.

The partnership of hospice programs and hospitals, and among health care professionals of all disciplines, is essential to achieve appropriate support. Children's hospice is a concept of care for children and adolescents facing a life-threatening condition. Hospice care can take place in the patient's home, inpatient hospice, hospital, or other appropriate location. In hospice care, the term "patient" refers to the patient as well as the patient's immediate support system, be it family or significant others.

Children's hospice care equally addresses the individual needs of the patient and family including the developmental, psychological, spiritual, and physical aspects of care. Support of anticipatory grief begins at the time of referral. Bereavement support is provided to the family for at least 1 year after the death of the child. Services must include, but are not limited to, those of medical, psychosocial, spiritual, bereavement, and any additional services necessary for appropriate care of the patient and family. Registered nurse consultation must be made available 24 hr/day as needed by the patient and family.

Children's hospice care facilitates the participation of parents in the role of primary caretaker and supports the inclusion of the patient and family in the decision making process to the best of their capabilities and desires. The hospice team is designed to support the patient and family, and this team receives support from many areas including extensive education and training programs.

Children with AIDS have special needs that require modifications to the provision of traditional hospice care services. The unpredictable prognosis of the AIDS patient and, typically, their family's inaccessibility to health services present special challenges to the provision of appropriate care.

NEEDS PARTICULAR TO HIV-INFECTED CHILDREN
Initiation of Care

Traditionally accepted admission criteria for the provision of hospice care are set at the 6-month prognosis. Importantly, the child with AIDS typically has a life expectancy of more than 6 months and often needs many of the multidisciplinary services provided by hospice programs before the final 6 months of life.

Since professional staff may be reluctant to state a specific prognosis because of the variation and uncertainty about the clinical course of each child with AIDS, the difficulty of estimating life expectancy for AIDS patients is further complicated. A child with AIDS will go through various degrees of illness and may face life-threatening illnesses several times. Paul Brenner, Executive Director of Montgomery Hospice Society in Rockville, MD, notes that AIDS does not necessarily progress along a predictable path (P. Brenner, personal communication, 1992). Each time that child takes on a new infection, the child and family face the possibility of death and need the specialized support provided through hospice care. There are also times, such as when the family cannot appropriately care for their child at home—when the child is dependent on a respirator or cannot take food—that admission to the hospice program could be necessary. When it comes to children with AIDS, the decision regarding when to admit a child to a specific program of care must be on a case by case basis.

Children often require active treatment during the terminal phase of their illness. Health care providers and families alike support aggressive noninfectious treatment of complications. Children with AIDS can develop a variety of both infectious and noninfectious complications, many of which are treatable or respond to supportive care. Accordingly, the decision to abandon active interventions must balance the prospect for benefit, even if only transient, against the child's comfort and sense of well-being. The distinction between active and palliative treatment can be very unclear for a child with AIDS. Thus, traditional approaches are becoming more flexible, providing the blend of aggressive and palliative care that these children frequently need.

Families must be made aware of all care options available from the time of diagnosis so that comprehensive multidisciplinary support can be provided when they need it. Each plan of care should be individualized and flexible, with the emphasis of treatment on caring in addition to "curing." Plans of care must consider that many interventions are appropriate and that curative treatment and hospice care are not mutually exclusive.

Accessibility of Care

A disproportionate number of mothers of HIV-infected children "are black and Hispanic, live in poverty and lack access to health and social services. . . . In addition, a large and growing proportion of mothers of infants with AIDS suffer from serious substance abuse problems and are unable to care for their infants once discharged from the hospital" (3). The family may not have access to transportation to and from a clinic. Insurance is normally exhausted or nonexistent. Housing may be substandard, food and medicine in short supply, and employment unobtainable.

A Government Accounting Office survey showed that parents of ill children encounter difficulties in "paying for services, because of insurance coverage limitations, copayments, and deductibles; parents have large out-of-pocket expenses. . . . they ex-

pend considerable time and effort before they can locate providers and get the services needed. Parents lack a focal point to contact when they need help" (2).

Caretaker

Children and families with AIDS require comprehensive multidisciplinary care. For infants, children, and youth with HIV and AIDS, basic health care is essential, as are specialized medical services, educational services, and mental health and developmental services. For HIV-infected youth, and parents, drug treatment may also be needed. With these multidisciplinary needs, active service coordination is essential.

Children and families coping with AIDS at home need home health nurses who are experienced in pediatric home care and home health assistants to provide support to the family. Specific complications may require physical, speech, respiratory, and intravenous therapy. The responsibilities of the primary caretakers who may themselves have HIV infection lead quickly to burnout and make it essential for the providers to receive appropriate support themselves.

According to Glenn Ann Martin RN, MN, MS, "a good staff support group serves four important functions: 1) Allows an outlet to express feelings in a safe, accepting atmosphere without fear of reprisal; 2) Provides an opportunity for caregivers to ask for help and to affirm themselves as competent caregivers; 3) Gives the careperson the chance to hear others express similar feelings and conflicts, and a chance to affirm others; and 4) Provides a forum for problem analysis and resolution" (4).

Aspects of Care

Care for children and families with AIDS includes the full array of health care disciplines: physicians, nurses, psychologists, social workers, therapists, teachers, clergy, et al. The psychosocial aspects of this illness require particular attention in AIDS cases because of the stigma attached to the disease and because of the fact that entire families are often infected. "Parents may experience social isolation, stress from financial burdens such as costs and/or loss of income, a sense of loss of control, guilt, a lack of confidence in their parenting abilities, anxiety about the child's medical condition, current problems with drug addiction, and/or grief about their child's and possibly their own or a spouse's impending death" (5). Uninfected siblings and teens with AIDS often require additional supportive services and counseling.

We must all remember that "children with AIDS can be touched, hugged and loved. It is the responsibility of all care providers involved to assure that their lives are of the best quality possible" (5).

ALTERNATIVES FOR AVAILABLE CARE

Children with AIDS are cared for in various settings. Hospital care or inpatient hospice care are options used when extensive physical treatment or supervision is needed or when the child's family cannot care for the child at home. In some cases when children are abandoned in an inpatient setting, or when the child's immediate family is deceased, foster care can provide a home for the child with AIDS. As with many chronic illnesses, home care is the most popular alternative. Commonly parents will want to provide as much care to their children themselves as possible.

Each community has its own unique resources available to children with life-threatening conditions and their families. Some have already developed comprehensive multidisciplinary programs of care, whereas others may have a home care program only. However, every community has the potential, and probably many existing pieces, of children's hospice care. Through local churches, children's hospitals, support groups, community organizations, home care programs, respite programs, and so forth, the community can work together to coordinate existing services to meet the needs of these children and families.

As the AIDS patient population continues to dramatically increase, so does the need for such basic support services. In providing such support to children with AIDS, the primary caretakers may need a break in the provision of care or support with some daily routines and activities. To provide such relief, a growing number of programs are offering opportunities for respite care. Respite care is a key component of support that can truly benefit the family unit and the health care providers throughout the illness.

RESPITE CARE
What Is Respite Care?

Respite care is one of many social supports that can uphold and facilitate the adaptive coping of children and families living with HIV. Respite care is a community service for families to provide periods of short-term care for individuals with disabilities (6). Historically, respite services have been organized for caretakers of patients with Alzheimer's disease and families of children with developmental disabilities such as autism and mental retardation. Within the field of developmental disability, respite care has been cited by parents and professionals as both a crucial preventative and emergency service (7). Typically, respite care is utilized by parents or primary caretakers to attend to the needs of other family members, keep appointments, or simply relax.

Respite care differs from other services in that it is not necessarily treatment oriented; rather it enables caretakers to tend to other needs. The principal focus of respite services is the family, not simply the patient. The goal of respite care is to support the family unit and reduce family stress.

There are two primary models of service delivery designed to meet the goals of respite care: in home services and out of home services (6). In home services include homemaker services, sitter/companion programs, and parent trainer services. Homemaker services are provided by a trained homemaker. Services are usually available 7 days/week in 4- to 8-hr shifts. Sitter/companion programs provide short-term respite in the family's home; the family is paired with one sitter/companion who provides respite services on a regular basis. The parent trainer model is similar to the sitter/companion services in that respite care is provided by the same person. However, this model also utilizes individuals from the family's informal support network; relatives, friends, and neighbors are recruited and trained to provide respite.

Out of home services include family care services, respite providers' homes, and respite residences. Family care services and services given in the respite provider's home are similar. The distinguishing factor is that family care providers are state licensed and may care for more than one child at a time. Respite residences are free standing centers that provide residential services to individuals with disabilities.

Children with AIDS and their families are similar to those who have traditionally received respite services. However, there are significant differences. Families living with HIV face the pressures of caring for a child who is seriously ill as well as dealing with the economic concerns and social stigma that accompany AIDS. Communities that traditionally rally to support families in times of illness may not be willing or equipped to respond to those with HIV infection. The advent of AIDS challenges the existing respite care programs to accommodate the many needs of families with HIV-infected children.

Why Is Respite Needed?

The demands placed on all caretakers of an HIV-infected child are great. Even when a child is relatively healthy, a parent must manage the administration of medicine and attend frequent clinic appointments. As the disease progresses there may be an increased need for actual physical care. A child who is cognitively and/or motorically impaired because of neurological effects of the virus will require vigilant supervision. Increasingly complex medical regimes also add to the burden of caring for an infected child. Numerous hospitalizations and eventually the need for terminal care combine to create immeasurable stress for the caretaker and family.

Families living with HIV are also often plagued with other difficulties such as poverty, drug abuse, and violence (8). Social problems coupled with a chronic and ultimately fatal disease can leave a family struggling to meet the needs of a sick child. Respite care can support the family so that the needs of the child and family are met.

Who Needs Respite?

Each family living with AIDS is unique and possesses a unique set of strengths and vulnerabilities. Respite care can foster the strengths and offset a family's vulnerabilities by providing services that are tailored to meet the specific needs of an individual family.

Special consideration must be given to the infected parent/child unit. Most children with HIV acquired their disease vertically from an infected mother. As a result, care providers must consider that not only is a parent coping with the demanding tasks of caring for a chronically ill child, they are also dealing with their own illness and possibly that of their partner. In the absence of support from an extended family, physical and emotional exhaustion may take a mounting toll on the HIV-infected parent's ability to care for themselves and their family (9). Respite care can ultimately play a crucial role in supporting family integrity and stability by providing time for parents to tend to other pressing needs. For example, respite care can provide the opportunity for parents to tend to their own health needs.

Grandparents often become involved as a primary caretaker for an HIV-infected grandchild as a result of the illness or death of the child's parents. They may have the duty of caring for both their infected adult child and grandchild.

Task overload and emotional/physical sequelae is a distinct danger for grandparents. Grandparents also have their own health needs that can be overlooked in the face of a child's illness. Respite services can ameliorate the effects of such stressors by providing homemaker services and encouraging grandparents to attend to their own health concerns.

Another group of primary caretakers who can profit from the same reprieve from their duties are foster parents. Often, they have all the emotional responses as well as the responsibilities of the biological parents. They may also be dealing with negative reactions from family and friends surrounding the purposeful addition of an infected child to the community. Foster parents often have their own or other foster children who need and deserve attention. Respite care can enable foster parents to attend to their own needs as well as those of other family members.

A group often neglected by health related services are uninfected siblings. In families with a chronically ill child, older brothers and sisters are often recruited to provide care for their sibling (10). Older children with infected parent(s) may also have the double responsibility of caring for their parent(s). As one eloquent 10-year girl stated, "The hardest thing about having a Mommy with AIDS is having to take care of her when Daddy is not home." Respite services can support healthy siblings in two manners. First, respite providers can care for the infected children, thus allowing the primary caretaker to spend time with other children in the family. Second, respite providers can spend individual time with healthy children. Many healthy children receive less attention than their sick sibling. Extra attention from nurturing adults is welcome.

The infected child can also directly benefit from respite services. Respite services for the infected child must be determined by the status of his or her health. A child who is relatively healthy may enjoy activities outside the home or hospital, whereas a more impaired child may prefer to play a game or read a book.

When Is Respite Needed?

Child and family specific respite services can appreciably improve a child's quality of life and support the entire family throughout the disease. Optimally, respite services should be provided as a component of comprehensive services made available to the family upon diagnosis. If presented in this manner, respite care is more likely to be utilized on regularly rather than only when a crisis occurs. Clearly respite care should be utilized during crisis periods such as illness of parent or child. However, if the family is already familiar with the concept of respite care it will prove more helpful and less stressful.

Respite care is especially useful when a child is hospitalized. Parents often do not want to leave their child unattended in the hospital. Respite workers can assist by relieving parents at the hospital so they can attend to other needs or catch up on much needed sleep. Longer term respite care is appropriate if a parent is hospitalized or is in need of

drug rehabilitation. In situations such as this a child (and siblings) would most likely need out of home services.

During the terminal phase of AIDS, respite workers work directly with hospice organizations. The role of respite workers is often indistinguishable from that of hospice workers. Respite for family members during this time is critical since the family will be experiencing physical and emotional exhaustion.

Where Is Respite Available?

There are several options to consider when seeking respite care services. Respite care is an integral component of most hospice programs. Often, state funded organizations that provide various services to people with AIDS also provide respite care. Private or nonprofit AIDS organizations usually have respite care as a component of assistance. Foster care agencies often have respite care built into existing programs to provide support to foster parents caring for medically fragile children. In some communities, religious institutions have joined forces to respond to the respite needs of those infected with HIV (11).

Respite care services can usually be accessed by the caretaker alone. It is not necessary to receive a referral from a particular agency to secure services. There are no national guidelines that determine how care is accessed, how care will be delivered, or who is eligible. These policies will vary among communities.

The costs of respite services also vary. Many programs use volunteers to provide respite care services, whereas others use paid staff. There is no federal ruling mandating that respite services be provided to families with HIV. It is possible that respite care would be provided if the child qualified for services under Public Law 99-147, which extends special education services to handicapped children from birth to age 3 years; however, the level of implementation of this act varies among states. Determining the availability of respite services in a given community can be challenging, but the fruits of such labor are very meaningful. Table 44.1 lists some available respite care resources.

CARE CENTERS AND FACILITIES

Care locations available to AIDS patients are often different from those available to children with other illnesses or conditions. HIV-infected or AIDS children often receive treatment in specialized tertiary care hospitals. These centers employ staff specially trained for the unique complications experienced in children with AIDS. They also have the latest diagnostic capabilities, treatment regimens, and technological advances.

When their child is not receiving inpatient treatment, families usually want to bring the child home for care. Because of the complicated care required for HIV-infected or AIDS children, specially trained home care professionals can enable this to occur. When chronically ill children and their parents look for services after the child's discharge, they turn to the health care and support service providers in their area. Home care programs and hospice programs can be of significant importance to these families in locating and arranging for care for their child at home.

Children's Hospice International's 1989 survey showed that 52% of children's hospice related services are being provided through community based organizations, whereas 25% are hospital based. Over half serve urban and rural areas combined. A growing number of programs, such as Grandma's House in Washington DC, are being developed specifically to care for children with AIDS.

Table 44.1.   Respite Care Resources

A Guide for the Implemention of a Respite Care Program School of Hope 819 South Laurel Hope AR 71801 501-777-4501	**Respite Care Manual** Temporary Care Services Inc. PO Box 542 Cambridge MA 02238 617-492-4630
Respite Care Archdiocese of Denver Respite Care Program 1050 S. Birch St. Denver CO 80222 303-759-5150	**Giving Families a Break: Strategies for Respite Care** Meyer Children's Rehabilitation Institute 444 South 44th St. Omaha NE 68131 402-559-7467
For This Respite, Much Thanks (program development) United Cerebral Palsy Association, Inc. 1522 K St. NW Suite 1112 Washington DC 20005	**Alta Mira Specialized Family Services** 1221 Isleta Blvd SW Albuquerque NM 87105 505-873-0600
Respite Companion Program Model Publication Division, NCA 600 Maryland Ave. SW West Wing, 100 Washington DC 20024 202-479-1200	**How to Begin a Respite Progam in a Rural Area: Provider Training Manual** Las Cumbres Learning Services PO Box 740 Los Alamos NM 87544 505-672-1791
How To Manual for Providing Respite Care for Family Caregivers Project Share Box 2309 Rockville, MD 20852 301-231-9539	**Zia Respite Service** 900 First St. Alamagordo NM 88310 505-437-3040
Providing Respite Care: Training Program for Respite Care Providers and Home Health Aides Social Policy Research Group 210 Commercial St. 3rd Floor Boston MA 02109 617-723-7030	**Care Break** 7110 Penn Av. Pittsburgh PA 15208 412-371-8903 **Texas Respite Resource Network** Santa Rosa Health Care Corporation PO Box 7330 San Antonio TX 78207-3198 512-228-2794

RESOURCES

Hospice programs, hospitals, foster parent agencies, and special support groups worldwide are developing to meet the rapidly increasing needs of children with life-threatening conditions and their families. Children with HIV and AIDS are of particular concern as their numbers are the most dramatically increasing.

Although the numbers of children and women who are HIV infected continue to multiply, the impact of pediatric AIDS and HIV infection on the health care delivery system is far greater than even the numbers suggest. Late in their illness, children with AIDS may have frequent admissions to hospitals. Costs for specialized treatments for AIDS children tend to be higher, yet these families tend to fall into the lower income brackets and are thus heavily dependent on public support and insurance.

To meet these needs, hospices and home care programs nationwide are doing what they can to provide appropriate support within the care system and to provide the much-needed resources and professional assistance. Table 44.2 lists some valuable resources for children and families with AIDS. Table 44.3 lists pediatric and AIDS hotlines.

Table 44.2.   AIDS Resources for Children and Families

Newsletters and Information	Educational Materials
AIDS Information Sourcebook Oryx Press 4041 North Central Ave. Suite 700 Phoenix AZ 85004 800-279-6799	**America Red Cross** HIV/AIDS Education National Capital Chapter 2025 E. St. NW Washington DC 20006
Children with AIDS Newsletter of The Foundation for Children with AIDS Inc. 77B Warren St. Brighton MA 02135 617-783-7300	**Criteria for Evaluating and AIDS Curriculum** National Coalition of Advocates for Students 100 Boylston St. Suite 737 Boston MA 02116 617-357-8507
Children with HIV/AIDS: A Sourcebook for Caring NACHRI 401 Wythe St. Alexandria VA 22314 703-684-1355	**Materials Catalog America Responds to AIDS** Department of Heatlth and Human Services Public Health Service Centers for Disease Control National AIDS Information and Education Program Atlanta GA 30333
Pediatric AIDS Coalition 1331 Pennsylvania Ave. NW Suite 721 North Washington DC 20004 800-336-5475	**PBS AIDS Video Series** PBS Video News Special Editions 1320 Braddock Pl. Alexandria VA 22314 1-800-424-7963
Child Welfare and AIDS Project 1950 Addison St. Suite 104 Berkeley CA 94204 415-643-7020	**Health Link: The Nation's Education for Health** News Magazine National Center for Health Education 30 East 29th St. New York NY 10016
Child Welfare League of America 440 First St. NW Suite 310 Washington DC 20001 202-638-2952	
Dept. of Health and Human Services Public Health Service, National AIDS Clearinghouse PO Box 6003, Rockville, MD 20850 800-458-5231	

Table 44.3.   AIDS Hotlines

Children's Hospice International
   Provides resources and referrals to children
   with life-threatening conditions, their families
   and health care professionals
	1-800-2-4-CHILD

Mothers of AIDS Patients (MAP)	619-234-3432

National AIDS Hotline
   24-hr service 7 days/week to respond to any
   questions that adult or young person may
   have about HIV infection and AIDS
	1-800-342-AIDS

Spanish	1-800-344-SIDA
Hearing impaired	1-800-AIDS-TTY
National Institute of Health Pediatric Branch	301-402-0696/0697
National Pediatric HIV Resource Center	1-800-362-0071
Pediatric AIDS Coalition	1-800-336-5475

CONCLUSION

Children's hospice provides support and care for children who are seriously ill so that their lives can be as full as possible. Hospice care neither hastens nor postpones death. Hospice care focuses on patient and family needs to the extent possible. This requires considerable flexibility on the part of hospice workers and other caretakers involved with the hospice programs, since every patient and every family present different needs, hopes, values, religious beliefs, and prior experiences with death.

It is these aspects of children's hospice care that make it especially suited for the care of HIV-infected children and their families throughout the illness. Hospice denotes a philosophically "old-fashioned" approach to medical care and services, which focuses on helping people with expected relatively short life spans to live their remaining lives to the fullest without pain, with choices and dignity, and with family support.

Former Secretary of Health and Human Services, Otis R. Bowen, noted "children's hospice care facilitates the participation of parents in assuming the role of primary caregiver. It supports the inclusion of the patient and the family in the decision-making process to the best of the family's capability and commensurate with their desires. . . . Hospice is a concept of care which can take place in a hospital, at home or in a residential care setting" (12).

Application of the hospice concept can significantly enhance the lives of dying children, their families, and their health care providers. Without hospice oriented support and practical assistance to pediatricians, nurses, other health care professionals, and family members, too many of these children face death with unnecessary physical pain, loneliness, and isolation. Children with life-threatening conditions, their families, and caretakers must deal with the pain, grief, fear, frustration, and profound sense of guilt and failure that inevitably accompany the prospect of a child's death.

According to Milton Glatt, MD, a child psychiatrist, "whenever incurability is confused with untreatability, an attitude (either expressed or tacit) of "there is nothing more I can do" often results. However, much can be done to aid the child with the life-threatening condition and his family in coping with the stress and fears involved in dealing with the likely death. Children's hospice care can turn this potentially devastating experience into one of growth for a child and his support system" (M. Glatt, personal communication, 1989).

Children with HIV or AIDS and their families face a multitude of special challenges. There are many avenues of support available to help them cope. Respite care, as one aspect of a comprehensive children's hospice care regimen, can bring great relief to a family needing support. These multidisciplinary aspects of care can ensure that the child and family can truly live each remaining day in as much comfort as possible. Children's hospice care affirms life and living.

References

1. Koop C. Enriching the circle of care: Children's Hospice International Pediatric Hospice Conference. Alexandria, VA: Children's Hospice International, 1986:1.
2. General Accounting Office. Health care. Home care experiences of families with chronically ill children. Washington, DC: Government Printing Office, 1989:1,19.
3. Anonymous. 1991 Legislative Agenda. Washington DC: Pediatric AIDS Coalition, 1991:1.
4. Martin GA. 1985 Pediatric Hospice Conference Report. Alexandria, VA: Children's Hospice International, 1985:59.
5. Berry RK. Home care of the child with AIDS. Pediatric Nursing, 1988;14:341–342.
6. Powell T, Ogle P. Brothers and sisters: Addressing unique needs through respite care services. In: Respite care. Baltimore: Paul H. Brooks, 1986.
7. Levy J, Levy P. Issues and models in the delivery of respite services. In: Respite care. Baltimore: Paul H. Brooks, 1986.
8. Septimus A. Psycho-social aspects of caring for families of infants infected with human immunodeficiency virus. Semin Perinatol 1989;13:349.
9. Meyers A, Weitzman M. Pediatric HIV disease: The newest chronic illness of childhood. Pediatr Clin North Am 1991;38:169–194.
10. Travis G. Chronic illness: Its impact on child and family. Stanford: Stanford University Press, 1976.
11. Shelp E, DuBose E, Sunderland R. The infrastructure of religious communities: A neglected resource for care of people with AIDS. Am J Public Health 1990;80:970–972.
12. Bowen OR. Children's hospice international opening ceremonies. Alexandria, VA: Children's Hospice International, 1986.

SECTION VI

Prevention, Education, and Public Policy Issues

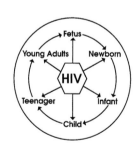

Passive Immunization Strategies for HIV-infected Children

Lynne M. Mofenson and Stephen A. Spector

Immunoglobulin preparations, particularly intravenous immunoglobulin (IVIG), have been used successfully as antibody replacement for the prevention (pre-exposure prophylaxis) of recurrent infections seen in congenital or acquired immunodeficiency disorders, as postexposure prophylaxis or treatment for certain defined infectious exposures (e.g., immunoprophylaxis for neonates born to hepatitis B-infected mothers), and as an immunomodulatory substance (e.g., treatment of idiopathic thrombocytopenic purpura).

Pre-exposure prophylaxis might be expected to be most effective for prevention of infections with common pathogens, since IVIG contains a wide spectrum of antibodies against commonly encountered organisms, based on the immunologic experience of the donor population. The success of such an approach is dependent on the concentration of desired antibody in the IVIG preparation, adequate dosing to maintain protective antibody levels between IVIG infusions, and the presence of at least partially functioning nonspecific defense mechanisms (such as phagocytic cells and complement). IVIG has been most successful when used as replacement therapy for the prevention of common infections in patients with a defined singular defect in an otherwise intact immune system. Pooled IVIG has had less success when used in more complex combined immunodeficiency states or as prophylaxis for infections with less common pathogens.

A different situation is encountered in patients with established infections. In these patients, high concentration of specific antiviral or antibacterial antibody may be required to achieve a therapeutic effect. Hyperimmune preparations may be necessary to achieve and maintain antibody levels that are adequate to eradicate or modify an established infection. In some situations, particularly in certain viral infections, antibody alone may be insufficient.

IVIG has also been used as an immunomodulatory agent in the treatment of diseases with inflammatory or autoimmune manifestations. Understanding the complex process of immunoregulation and the role of antibody in such regulation has undergone marked advances in the past decade. The antigen-binding region of an immunoglobulin molecule, the idiotype, can itself be recognized by the immune system as an antigen, with the formation of antiidiotypic antibody. These antibodies can further generate their own antiidiotype response with the formation of anti-antiidiotypic antibody, and so on; the resulting idiotypic network has been proposed as the major mechanism for immune system self-regulation (1). Theoretically, IVIG preparations might be expected to contain a diverse number of antibodies with differing antiidiotype specificity because of the normal presence of antiidiotype antibodies in an individual (2, 3). Immunomodulatory effects of IVIG could occur via several mechanisms: neutralization of autoantibody

841

by complexing with antiidiotypic antibody, preventing reaction of the autoantibody with self-antigen; enhancement of T cell suppressor function through binding of antiidiotypic antibody to certain T cell receptors, activating production of specific suppressive lymphokines; downregulation of B cell function through binding of antiidiotypic antibody to the B cell receptor for antigen, decreasing autoantibody production; binding of antiidiotypic antibody to active C3 fragments, causing inhibition of complement-mediated tissue damage; or saturation of Fc receptors on reticuloendothelial system cells, thereby reducing interaction with and clearance of autoantibody-antigen complexes (3).

In pediatric human immunodeficiency virus (HIV) infection, IVIG has been used for its antigen-specific and immunomodulatory functions. After a general discussion of currently available IVIG preparations, this chapter will focus on the use of immunoglobulin in pediatric HIV infection for preexposure prophylaxis of bacterial and viral infections; postexposure prophylaxis or treatment of established infections such as hepatitis B, measles, cytomegalovirus, and parvovirus B19 infections; and use as an immunomodulator for HIV-associated thrombocytopenia. We will also discuss the potential use of hyperimmune HIV intravenous immunoglobulin (HIVIG) for prevention of vertical HIV transmission.

PASSIVE IMMUNOPROPHYLAXIS PREPARATIONS

IVIG

In the mid 1940s, Cohn and colleagues (4) developed a method for fractionating human plasma with cold ethanol that enabled the production of concentrated and relatively pure γ-globulin preparations. Cohn Fraction II has as its main protein component IgG immunoglobulin, present as monomers, dimers, and aggregates (the latter two components are artifacts generated during the fractionation process). When given intravenously, IgG aggregates can cause spontaneous activation of the complement cascade through binding of the Fc portion of the aggregated immunoglobulin to Fc receptors on comple-

ment, producing significant vasomotor symptoms and anaphylaxis. Therefore, dosage of standard immunoglobulin is limited by the necessity of intramuscular injection, allowing maximum doses of only 100-150 mg/kg. Moreover, because of slow absorption from the muscle depot, peak serum levels are not achieved for several days.

During the late 1970s, various techniques were developed to prevent IgG aggregation and render human-derived IgG safe for intravenous infusion. These techniques include enzymatic cleavage with pepsin or plasmin; chemical modification by reduction and alkylation, sulfonation, or β-propirolactone treatment; incubation at low pH; or physical removal of aggregates by isolation with polyethylene glycol, the use of anion exchangers such as diethylaminoethyl (DEAE)-Sephadex, or diafiltration and ultracentrifugation (5). Amino acids (glycine), albumin, and/or sugars are added to purified preparations as stabilizers to prevent reaggregation and protect IgG during lyophilization. This has enabled the development of several (IVI) products that allow patients to receive rapid and repeated administration of physiologic or supraphysiologic doses of IgG with little discomfort or risk.

All products currently available in the United States are prepared by the Cohn-Oncley procedure (or a modification thereof) and differ primarily in the procedures utilized to prevent IgG aggregation. Enzymatically treated IVIG has a shorter biologic half-life and a disturbed IgG subclass distribution; chemically treated IVIG lacks the IgG_3 subclass, and some of the Fc-related function is altered; anion exchange preparations are poor in the IgG_4 subclass but have the lowest IgA content (6). Although these preparations may vary in their concentration of specific antibody and IgG subclasses, most preparations retain the physiologic properties of native IgG, and for most patients the products are equally efficacious (2). Table 45.1 compares the seven licensed IVIG preparations available in the United States (2, 6-13). Except one product available only in a liquid formulation, all products are lyophilized and require reconstitution just before use.

All products have minimal anticomplementary activity. Plasma products in the United States are screened for hepatitis B surface antigen, HIV antibody, and elevated (above twice upper normal limits) alanine aminotransferase levels. Screening for antibody to hepatitis C is also performed by some manufacturers and will be implemented soon by others, as will screening for hepatitis B core antigen (2). Since IVIG is a biologic material prepared from pooling plasma from 3000 to 6000 donors, the preparations will contain at least some antibodies against virtually all common human pathogens. However, there may be variation among lots in the antibody titer against specific pathogens (10, 14).

Although IVIG allows the delivery of large volumes of immunoglobulin without the pain of intramuscular injection, the use of IVIG is expensive. Substantial amounts of plasma are required, because 1 unit whole blood provides only 2–3 ml IgG (5). Product costs are generally five to ten times those for standard immunoglobulin, to which must be added the costs of intravenous administration and monitoring during infusion. Costs may vary in different locales; the average wholesale price of products available in the United States range from $35 to $65 per gram, before adding administrative costs for infusion (i.e., equipment, clinic space, nursing time) (2). The annual wholesale cost to provide 400 mg/kg IVIG monthly to an infant weighing 10 kg ranges from $1680 to $3120, with administrative fees approximately doubling the annual wholesale figures. Recent studies have demonstrated that IVIG infusions can be administered safely at home, with substantial cost savings for children and adults with primary immunodeficiency (15–17). Subcutaneous rapid infusion of IVIG (34–40 ml/hr) administered at home with a small portable pump, has also been successful in a small number of children with primary immunodeficiency (18). Subcutaneous infusion appears to yield serum IgG concentrations similar to those obtained after intravenous infusion, and may provide an efficient, less expensive, and less invasive method of administration.

Administration of IVIG usually requires 1–3 hr. The infusion is begun at a slow rate (e.g., 0.01–0.02 ml/kg/min). If this is tolerated, the infusion can be increased as tolerated to a maximum rate of 0.04 ml/kg/min, although rates up to 0.08 ml/kg/min have been tolerated safely. If a reaction is anticipated, premedication with aspirin or diphenhydramine can be given 1 hr before infusion.

IgG levels increase in a dose-dependent fashion immediately after infusion. In general, for each 100 mg/kg IgG infused, peak serum IgG level rises ~200 mg/dl (19). IgG levels drop off rapidly for 1–3 days immediately after the infusion owing to equilibration in the body compartments. Levels then fall exponentially with a half-life of ~20 days; however, there is individual variation in half-life, with a range of 11–44 days (13, 19). IgG half-life may be reduced with hypercatabolic states or in patients with hypergammaglobulinemia (20). In patients with hypogammaglobulinemia, serial trough IgG determinations are recommended to optimize dose and infusion interval, targeting a trough IgG level of 500 mg/dl or more (21).

Recommendations for IVIG use in HIV-infected children have been empiric and based on regimens similar to those used for patients with primary immunodeficiency; in National Institutes of Health (NIH) sponsored clinical trials, IVIG was administered in a dose of 400 mg/kg every 28 days. However, in HIV-infected children, most of whom have hypergammaglobulinemia, it is possible that higher or more frequent dosing may be needed because reduced IgG half-life in hypergammaglobulinemic patients. Pharmacokinetic studies of IVIG in HIV-infected patients have not been published. However, recent data from the National Institute of Child Health and Human Development (NICHD) IVIG Clinical Trial indicate that the optimal dose and frequency of IVIG in HIV-infected children may be yet to be determined (22, 23). Among patients with entry CD4+ lymphocyte counts of ≥200/mm³ (those in whom efficacy was observed), 161 IVIG patients received 3,148 infusions and 152 placebo recipients received 2,885 infusions, with an average infusion interval of 30 days in both arms. Infections were categorized by type and by days elapsed since previous infusion (1-10, 11–20 or 21–35 days), and rate per

Table 45.1. Chararacteristics of Immunoglobulin Preparations for Intravenous Use Licensed in the United States[a]

Trade Name and Date Licensed	Preparation and Formulation	Manufacturer	Comments
Gamimune-N, 2/28/86	Isolated from effluent III by diafiltration and ultrafiltration at acid pH pH 4.25, 5% IgG solution stabilized with 10% maltose Liquid	Miles Inc, Cutter Biological, 400 Morgan Ln, West Haven, CT 06516	Does not require reconstitution Normal IgG subclass distribution Approximate IgA content 270 µg/ml Contraindicated in selective IgA deficiency
Gammagard, 2/18/86	Isolation with polyethylene glycol, ultrafiltration, DEAE-Sephadex adsorbed pH 6.8, stabilized with 2% glucose Other additives: 0.2% polyethylene glycol, 0.3% albumin, 0.3 M glycine, 0.15 M NaCl	Baxter Healthcare Corp, Hyland Division, 550 N Brand Blvd, Glendale, CA 91203	Requires reconstitution with sterile water for injection USP to 5% solution Normal IgG subclass distribution on average; some reports indicate that preparation is IgG_4 depleted Low IgA preparation: approximate IgA content 0.4–1.9 µg/ml Not contraindicated in IgA deficiency
Gammar-IV (formerly Perimmun), 12/14/89	Lyophilized Isolation with polyethylene glycol, low-ionic strength ethanol pH 6.8, stabilized with 5% sucrose Other additives: 3% albumin, 0.5% NaCl Lyophilized	Armour Pharmaceutical, Suite 200, 920A Harvest Dr, Blue Bell, PA 19422	Requires reconstitution with sterile water for injection USP to 5% solution Normal IgG subclass distribution Approximate IgA content 20 µg/ml Contraindicated in selective IgA deficiency May be given to diabetics (sucrose)
Iveegam, 4/8/88	Immobilized trypsin treatment followed by polyethylene glycol/hydroxyethyl starch fractionation pH 6.8, stabilized by 5% glucose	Immuno-US Inc, 1200 Parkdale Rd, Rochester, MI 48307-1744	Requires reconstitution with sterile water for injection USP to 5% solution Low IgG_3 subclass Moderately low IgA; approximate IgA content >5 µg/ml

Table 45.1.—*continued*

Trade Name and Date Licensed	Preparation and Formulation	Manufacturer	Comments
PolyGam	Other additives: 0.5% polyethylene glycol, 0.3% NaCl. Lyophilized. Isolated by polyethylene glycol, diafiltration, ultrafiltration, DEAE-Sephadex ion exchange chromatography. pH 6.8, stabilized with 2% glucose	Baxter Healthcare Corp, Hyland Division, 550 N Brand Blvd, Glendale, CA 91203	Contraindicated in selective IgA deficiency. Requires reconstitution with sterile water for injection USP to 5% solution. Normal IgG subclass distribution. IgA depleted; approximate IgA content <10 µg/ml
	Other additives: 0.3% albumin, 0.2% polyethylene glycol, 0.3 M glycine, 0.15 M NaCl. Lyophilized	Distributed by American Red Cross Blood Services, Washington, DC 20006	Not contraindicated in IgA deficiency
Sandoglobulin, 6/7/84	Isolated by incubation of IgG at acid pH 4 with trace pepsin. pH 6.6, stabilized with 10% sucrose. Lyophilized	Swiss Red Cross Central Laboratory Transfusion Service, Wankdorfstrasse 10, 3000 Berne 22, Switzerland. Distributed by Sandoz Pharmaceuticals Corp, Route 110, East Hanover, NJ 07936	Requires reconstitution with normal saline to 3 or 6% solution. Has been given as 12% solution at up to 0.25 ml/kg/min. Approximate IgA content 720 µg/ml. Contraindicated in selective IgA deficiency
Venoglobulin-I, 10/13/88	Isolated by polyethylene glycol fractionation and DEAE-Sephadex treatment. pH 6.8, stabilized with 2% mannitol. Other additives: 1% albumin, <0.6% polyethylene glycol, 0.5% NaCl. Lyophilized	Alpha Therapeutic Corp, 555 Valley Blvd, Los Angeles, CA 90032	Requires reconstitution with sterile water for injection USP to 5% solution (incompatible with D5W). Normal IgG subclass distribution. Approximate IgA content 24 µg/ml. Contraindicated in selective IgA deficiency

[a]Data from manufacturer's product inserts and Buckley and Schiff (2), Fischer (10), Greenbaum (11), and Tankerdsley (12). USP, United States Pharmacopeial.

100 patient-years were calculated. The greatest reduction in serious and minor bacterial and virus infections occurred early in the interval after infusion, with attenuation of benefit later in the interval, and further diminishing benefit after 21 days postinfusion. To maintain IgG levels capable of preventing bacterial and virus infections in HIV-infected children during the interval between infusions, an increased dose or frequency of infusion may be needed in some patients. However, because this would dramatically increase the cost of IVIG, further study, including pharmacokinetic evaluation, is required.

Adverse Reactions to IVIG Therapy

Adverse reactions to IVIG administration can be local or systemic. Local reactions are due to administration technique, e.g., phlebitis and tissue extravasation.

The incidence of systemic side effects ranges from 3 to 12% and does not appear to be dose related (20). Systemic vasomotor reactions are rarely severe enough to warrant discontinuation of therapy. Most adverse effects are minor and include nausea, vomiting, abdominal pain, chills, flushing of the face, sweating, chest tightness, shortness of breath, headache, dizziness, backache, muscle cramps, and joint pains. More severe reactions, such as hypotension, loss of consciousness, or anaphylaxis, are rare, and may be more common in agammaglobulinemic or hypogammaglobulinemic patients (19).

Systemic reactions can be caused by several mechanisms: antigen-antibody interactions; activation of the complement system, possibly by residual IgG aggregates; true hypersensitivity reactions; and reactions to stabilizers, preservatives, or contaminants in the IVIG preparation.

Antibody-antigen reactions are most often seen in a- or hypogamma-globulinemic patients treated with IVIG for the first time or in patients retreated after a therapy-free interval of several weeks to months (19). Repeated infections in such immunodeficient patients may lead to antigenic overload and may predispose to sudden formation of antigen-antibody complexes with rapid intravenous infusion of corresponding antibodies, causing activation of the complement system and provoking a systemic reaction. These reactions can be avoided by starting the infusion very slowly.

As many as 42% of patients with solitary IgA deficiency syndromes may have anti-IgA antibodies, which can predispose to rare, more severe reactions if the IVIG preparation used contains even low levels of IgA (13). Such patients should receive IVIG containing little or no detectable IgA (19) (Table 45.1); screening for anti-IgA antibody is not necessary.

Reactions tend to occur early in the IVIG infusion and may be related to the rate of infusion. Most of these effects can be prevented or aborted by stopping or decreasing the rate of infusion for 15–30 minutes.

As with other blood products, the possibility of transmission of blood-borne infectious agents is of concern. Virus partitioning and inactivation by the cold ethanol fractionation and incubation steps of the manufacturing process result in substantial reduction (log kill of over 10^6 viral units/ml) or elimination of hepatitis B virus and infectious retroviruses, including HIV (23, 24). All donor plasma used in the manufacture of commercial products currently available in the United States is screened for hepatitis and HIV, and potentially infectious units are excluded. There has been no documented transmission of HIV infection or hepatitis by any preparation currently available. The risk of infection secondary to infectious contamination of currently available IVIG preparations is felt to be minimal (2), but because of the theoretical risk, IVIG should only be used in children for clinical disease for which there is demonstrated efficacy.

IVIG FOR PRE-EXPOSURE PROPHYLAXIS OF INFECTIONS IN HIV-INFECTED CHILDREN
Rationale

Although B and T cell dysfunction are seen in HIV-infected adults and children, the consequences of B cell dysfunction may be more pronounced in children, particularly those with vertically acquired infection. In adults, even if response to new antigens is diminished, pre-existing memory cells provide some measure of immunity from infection with common pathogens. However, if defective B-cell function occurs early in life, before the development of specific memory cells, severe and recurrent infection with otherwise common organisms may result.

In children with HIV infection, recurrent infection with common bacterial and viral organisms is a frequent and early manifestation of HIV disease. Although AIDS in adults is associated with the development of infections with opportunistic organisms, development of recurrent systemic infection with common encapsulated bacteria is so common in HIV-infected children that the federal Centers for Disease Control (CDC) modified the pediatric AIDS case definition in 1987 to include recurrent serious bacterial infection as an AIDS indicator disease (25).

Significantly increased frequency of invasive pneumococcal disease has been reported in several studies (26–28). In one population-based cohort, the annualized rate of pneumococcal bacteremia, 6.7 episodes/100 patient-years (29), was twice that observed in children younger than 6 years with sickle cell anemia (3.2/100 patient-years) (30) and seven times that reported in adults with AIDS (31). Recurrent episodes of pneumonia, often without an identified origin, also cause significant morbidity (32, 33). In addition, recurrent minor bacterial infections such as otitis media are common in HIV-infected children (34). Serious infection with common viruses has also been reported, including death secondary to measles (35–42).

The clinical similarity between the types of bacterial and viral infections observed in HIV-infected children and those observed in children with congenital humoral immunodeficiencies formed the rationale for the evaluation of IVIG for infection prophylaxis in pediatric HIV-infected patients. In the latter half of the 1980s, several investigators published reports indicating potential benefit of IVIG for the prevention of infections in HIV-infected children. There have been six published case reports, involving a total of 61 patients, and three comparative reports, involving a total of 51 treated patients, on the use of IVIG as pre-exposure prophylaxis for infections (43–51).

Except for one small comparative study in an adolescent hemophiliac population that did not show benefit of IVIG for infection prophylaxis (51), the other studies reported various benefits from IVIG therapy including decreased infections and hospitalizations, improvements in growth and survival, decline in p24 antigen, and improvement in immunologic abnormalities. Reported immunologic benefits included declines in elevated lactate dehydrogenase levels, improved suppressor cell function, enhanced mitogen response, and improvement in CD4+ lymphocyte count.

However, interpretation of these reports was difficult because of the lack of controls in most of the studies, the small number of children studied, the retrospective nature of some of the studies, and the lack of standardized patient evaluation and follow-up. Moreover, the investigators used widely varying regimens of IVIG. Further, in some instances the product used was produced before HIV antibody screening of blood products was initiated in 1985 and may have contained antibody to HIV.

Therefore, the NIH has sponsored two randomized, placebo-controlled, double-blind clinical trials to evaluate the efficacy of IVIG for infection prophylaxis in HIV-infected children. The trials were designed to evaluate two dissimilar populations. The patients enrolled in the NICHD IVIG Clinical Trial generally had mild to moderate HIV disease, and although zidovudine (ZDV) therapy was permitted after study entry, it was not designed to evaluate combination therapy in this patient population. In contrast, the patients in the AIDS Clinical Trial Group (ACTG) Protocol 051 had moderate to severe HIV disease (AIDS or AIDS-related complex), and for this group the trial was designed to evaluate the efficacy of IVIG in combination with ZDV.

NICHD IVIG Clinical Trial

The NICHD IVIG Clinical Trial was a randomized, double-blind, placebo-controlled multicenter trial conducted between March 1988 and January 1991. Subjects included 376 asymptomatic but immunologically abnormal or clinically symptomatic HIV-infected nonhemophiliac children younger than 13 years; mean follow-up was 17 months. The children were categorized into two groups according to CD4+ lymphocyte count (<200 or >200/mm^3) at entry into the study and by history of AIDS-defining opportunistic or recurrent serious bacterial infections (CDC Pediatric Class P-2-D-1 or P-2-D-2). Most children (83%, 313 of 376) had an entry CD4+ count of 200/mm^3 or above. Although all enrolled children had some clinical or laboratory abnormalities caused by HIV infection, 53% had only mild HIV disease; 13% were clinically asymptomatic with laboratory abnormalities only (CDC Pediatric Class P-1-B), and 40% had only mild, nonspecific symptoms of HIV disease with CD4+ lymphocyte counts of >500/mm^3, such as enlarged lymph nodes or parotitis (CDC Pediatric Class P-2-A) or mild lymphoid interstitial pneumonitis (CDC Pediatric Class P-2-C); 22% had a history of AIDS-defining infections.

Children were seen monthly for examination and infusion, and information regarding all intercurrent infections, medications, and hospitalizations was routinely collected. Serious bacterial infections were classified as either lab proven or clinically diagnosed. Lab proven serious bacterial infections were defined as bacteriologically confirmed episodes of meningitis, bacteremia, osteomyelitis, septic arthritis, acute mastoiditis, abscess of internal organ, acute pneumonia, or acute sinusitis. Clinically diagnosed serious infections were defined as episodes of acute pneumonia or sinusitis without defined microbiologic etiology that met predetermined clinical and radiologic criteria (52). Minor bacterial, serious and minor viral, and opportunistic infections were classified as lab proven if an organism was isolated by culture, detected by antigen or histology findings, or diagnosed by specific antibody testing. If the evaluating physician reported a clinical syndrome consistent with a bacterial (e.g., otitis media), viral (e.g., exanthem illness), or opportunistic etiology (e.g., oral thrush), the episode was classified as clinically diagnosed.

Prophylaxis against *Pneumocystis carinii* pneumonia (PCP) with trimethoprim-sulfamethoxazole (TMP-SMX) on a 3 consecutive days/week regimen and use of antiretroviral therapy at any time after study therapy were permitted according to the prevailing standard of care as determined by the patient's physician with consent of the parent or guardian.

Initial results, based on data collected through October 1990, have been published (53). IVIG was found to significantly increase the time free of serious bacterial infections (particularly invasive disease caused by *Streptococcus pneumonae* and episodes of acute pneumonia, most of which were clinically-diagnosed) in HIV-infected children with entry CD4+ counts of ≥200/mm^3 (relative risk 0.58, 95% confidence interval 0.39–0.86, $P = 0.009$) but not in children with entry CD4+ lymphocyte counts <200/mm^3. Additionally, there was a significant decrease in the number of acute care hospitalizations per 100 patient-years in IVIG-treated children with entry CD4+ counts of >200/mm^3 (relative risk 0.65, 95% confidence interval 0.38–0.91, $P = 0.03$)

A further analysis evaluated the efficacy of IVIG for prevention of a broader spectrum of infection types in patients over a longer follow-up, through the date of actual study termination, January 1991 (54). Analysis was focused on the study group in whom efficacy was observed previously, i.e., children with entry CD4+ counts of >200/mm^3. Minor bacterial infections and serious and minor virus infections together occurred five times more frequently than serious bacterial infections, the primary end point of the study. Lab proven serious bacterial infections accounted for only 27% of reported serious bacterial infections. Opportunistic infections were relatively rare in this population, occurring at a rate similar to lab proven serious bacterial infections. In IVIG-treated children with CD4+ lymphocyte counts of >200/mm^3, a significant decrease was observed in the rates of serious and minor virus infections, minor bacterial infections, as well as serious bacterial infections (Table 45.2). However, there was no apparent difference between treatment arms in the rate of opportunistic fungal and protozoan infections, including PCP, regardless of entry CD4+ lymphocyte count.

Detailed analyses were performed to evaluate the effect of PCP prophylaxis and ZDV therapy on the observed efficacy of IVIG in reducing bacterial and viral infections

Table 45.2.   Number and Rate of Selected Infections by Infection Type in Study Patients with Entry CD4+ Count of ≥200/mm³ According to Treatment Arm

Type of Infection	Immunoglobulin (n = 161 patients; total follow up = 250.2 patient-yr)		Placebo (n = 152; total follow up = 226.1 patient-yr)	
	No. of episodes	Rate/100 patient-yr	No. of episodes	Rate/100 patient-yr
Serious bacterial	66	26.4[b]	109	48.2
Lab proven	15	6.0	33	14.6
Clinical diagnosis	51	20.4	76	33.6
Minor bacterial	288	115.1[c]	361	159.7
Lab proven	27	10.8	45	19.9
Clinical diagnosis	261	104.3	316	139.8
Serious and minor viral	90	36.0[d]	122	54.0
Lab proven	11	4.4	20	8.8
Clinical diagnosis	79	31.6	102	45.1
Opportunistic	25	10.0	30	13.3
Lab proven	4	1.6	7	3.1
Clinical diagnosis	21	8.4	23	10.2

[a]Data from NICHD IVIG Clinical Trial, March 1988–January 1991.
[b]$P = 0.002$, comparing rate/100 patient-years, immunoglobulin vs. placebo.
[c]$P = 0.02$, comparing rate/100 patient-years, immunoglobulin vs. placebo.
[d]$P = 0.01$, comparing rate/100 patient-years, immunoglobulin vs. placebo.

(55, 56). Fifty percent of patients with entry CD4+ counts of >200/mm³ had received TMP-SMX for PCP prophylaxis (50% of placebo and 49% of IVIG patients) and 45% had received ZDV (47% of placebo and 44% of IVIG patients). Time to initiation of therapy was similar in each group. In addition, proportional hazards modeling indicated that neither PCP prophylaxis or ZDV independently accounted for the benefit observed with IVIG.

In patients with entry CD4+ count below 200/mm³, no significant difference was observed in the rate of serious and minor bacterial, viral, and opportunistic infections between IVIG and placebo arms.

There was no overall difference in mortality rates between IVIG and placebo recipients. However, recent analysis of cause of death indicates that most patients who died had CD4+ lymphocyte count below 200/mm³ before death. In addition, half the children with serious infection present at death had an opportunistic infection, for which IVIG did not demonstrate prophylactic efficacy (57).

Earlier reports had suggested that IVIG prophylaxis might be associated with beneficial effects on CD4+ cell count (44, 49). Recent analysis of serial CD4+ lymphocyte monitoring during the NICHD IVIG Clinical Trial indicates that IVIG was associated with a statistically significant slowing of age-adjusted CD4+ cell decline in children with entry CD4+ counts of >200/mm³ (age adjusted CD4+ cell loss of 3.5 cells/mm³/month in IVIG patients compared with 17.0 cells/mm³/month in placebo patients, $P = 0.01$) (58). Whether this benefit was due to a direct immunomodulatory effect of IVIG or an indirect consequence of the antigen-specific function of IVIG (i.e., by decreasing intercurrent bacterial and viral infections that might activate HIV replication and subsequent CD4 cell destruction) is subject to further study.

Beneficial effects of IVIG for infection prophylaxis and slowing CD4+ lymphocyte decline were confined to those children with entry CD4+ counts of >200/mm³. However, because of the small number of children with entry CD4+ counts below 200/mm³ (50 patients), the ability of the study to detect clinically relevant differences in IVIG efficacy in this population was very limited.

It is possible that adjunctive therapy with IVIG is most effective in those children with mild to moderate immunologic dysfunction who have some remaining T helper cell function. Qualitative defects in T helper cell function occurring in a distinct and progressive pattern, before CD4+ cell decline, have been described in HIV-infected children and adults, with progressive loss of

T helper response to recall antigen followed by alloantigen and finally mitogen stimulation (59–62). Progressive functional loss has been correlated with CD4+ cell decline over time. In HIV-infected children, a CD4+ count below $200/mm^3$ has been significantly associated with loss of response to all antigenic stimuli. However, loss of T helper response could occur even when the CD4 count was above $200/mm^3$ (62). In addition, in HIV-infected children, the stage of T helper deficit correlated with risk of infection; the earliest dysfunction observed with HIV infection, loss of recall antigen T helper cell response, was associated with an increased risk of bacterial infections, whereas more progressive dysfunction observed later in HIV disease, was associated with decline in CD4+ lymphocyte count and with increased risk of opportunistic infection. Therapies, such as IVIG, that may be successful at one level of immune dysfunction may not be sufficient with increasing levels of dysfunction.

In some studies, ZDV has been demonstrated to improve T helper and other immune cell function (63–65). It is possible that ZDV, by delaying immunologic deterioration, could prolong an infection "risk-free" period, during which adjunctive immunotherapy may not be necessary. Alternatively, it is possible that in children with more advanced disease (such as those who did not benefit from IVIG in the NICHD IVIG Clinical Trial), the combination of enhanced immune function with ZDV administered with IVIG may provide benefit. Although ZDV therapy did not affect the results of the NICHD IVIG Clinical Trial, the trial was not designed to evaluate the efficacy of IVIG in children receiving ZDV.

AIDS Clinical Trial Group Protocol 051

The second NIH trial, ACTG Protocol 051, was a double-blind, randomized, placebo-controlled multicenter trial to evaluate IVIG in HIV-infected children with AIDS or AIDS-related complex who were receiving ZDV. This trial, which began in October 1988 and ended in August 1992, enrolled 262 HIV-infected children (including hemophiliacs) between 3 months and 12 years of age; mean age at entry was 3.7 years, similar to that of the NICHD IVIG Clinical Trial (3.3 years). A total of 255 patients were evaluable for analysis; mean follow-up time was 25.5 months.

All patients in the study had moderate to severe HIV disease, either CDC defined AIDS (children with lymphoid interstitial pneumonitis alone (CDC Pediatric Class P-2-C) were excluded unless they required supplemental oxygen and steroids) at study entry or AIDS-related complex (defined as 1) two or more of the following major criteria: failure to thrive, persistent or recurrent oral thrush, and/or entry CD4+ count behavior below $500/mm^3$; or 2) one major criteria in combination with minor symptoms such as chronic diarrhea, lymphadenopathy, organomegaly, cardiomyopathy, nephropathy, thrombocytopenia or recurrent herpes simplex or zoster infection). Twenty-nine percent (74 of 255) of subjects had entry CD4+ counts of $<200/mm^3$ compared with 13% (50 of 376) in the NICHD IVIG Clinical Trial.

Children were stratified at study entry by history of recurrent serious bacterial infections, prior ZDV therapy, and PCP prophylaxis with TMP-SMX. Thirty-three percent (83 of 255) of subjects were receiving PCP prophylaxis with TMP-SMX at study entry, 29% (36 of 126) of placebo patients, and 36% (47 of 129) of IVIG patients. Fewer patients, 14% (53 of 376), in the NICHD IVIG Clinical Trial received TMP-SMX prophylaxis at study entry (15% of placebo and 13% of IVIG patients).

Preliminary analysis of the study has been completed, focusing on the time to the first lab proven serious bacterial infection and survival. A total of 53 patients had one lab confirmed serious bacterial infection, 31 in placebo and 22 in the IVIG group. The estimated relative risk of lab confirmed serious bacterial infection for IVIG recipients was 0.63 (95% confidence interval 0.36–1.08, $P = 0.09$ univariate log-rank analysis).

Dissimilar to the NICHD IVIG Clinical Trial, in a subgroup analysis by entry CD4 lymphocyte count below or above $200/mm^3$, there was not evidence of a differential IVIG effect. The relative risk of serious lab proven bacterial infection in IVIG recipients compared with placebo recipients was 0.51 (95% confidence interval 0.21–1.25, $P = 0.13$) for the 74 patients with entry CD4+ counts of <200/mm^3. The relative risk was 0.67 (95% confidence interval 0.33–1.33, $P = 0.25$) for the 181 patients with entry CD4+ counts of ≥200/mm^3. Therefore, in children with AIDS or advanced AIDS-related complex receiving ZDV, the entry CD4 count did not define a population responding to IVIG.

Subgroup analysis by TMP-SMX prophylaxis at entry indicated that the effect of IVIG appeared to be different for patients receiving TMP-SMX prophylaxis at the time of study entry. A significant effect of IVIG was observed only for the 171 patients not receiving TMP-SMX prophylaxis from study entry. In this subpopulation, the relative risk of serious lab proven bacterial infection for IVIG recipients was 0.42 (95% confidence interval 0.21–0.86, $P = 0.015$). There was no apparent benefit from IVIG for the 83 patients receiving TMP-SMX prophylaxis from study entry. The two-year event rate for first serious lab confirmed bacterial infection was 24.5% in IVIG compared with 17.6% in placebo patients (relative risk of 1.34, 95% confidence interval 0.50–3.64, $P = 0.56$).

During the initial year of enrollment PCP prophylaxis was not permitted except in patients with a history of lab confirmed PCP, whereas during the second year primary prophylaxis at entry was allowed if CD4+ count was <500/mm^3. TMP-SMX prophylaxis appeared to provide some protection from development of lab proven serious bacterial infection in children regardless if they entered the study during the first or second year of accrual. Although the NICHD IVIG Clinical Trial did not observe an influence of TMP-SMX prophylaxis on the beneficial effect of IVIG in their patient population, the patient population was healthier and the number of patients receiving TMP-SMX from study entry fewer. Although neither ACTG 051 nor the NICHD trial was designed to compare the effectiveness of TMP-SMX compared IVIG for infection prophylaxis, it is possible that TMP-SMX used for PCP prophylaxis could also provide effective prophylaxis against bacterial infections. In the initial study by Hughes and colleagues (66), of daily TMP-SMX for PCP prophylaxis in cancer pa-

tients, a decrease in bacterial infections as well as PCP was observed.

No difference in overall survival was observed between IVIG and placebo patients in either study, nor was or by receipt of a difference in survival if patient received TMP-SMX prophylaxis from study entry.

Further analyses are planned, including the impact of IVIG on clinically, diagnosed serious bacterial infections, minor bacterial infections, serious and minor virus infections, and CD4+ cell decline. Analysis of ACTG 051 in conjunction with the NICHD IVIG Clinical Trial will be needed before definitive recommendations concerning the use of IVIG in HIV-infected children can be made.

IVIG FOR POSTEXPOSURE PROPHYLAXIS OR TREATMENT OF ESTABLISHED INFECTION

Once an HIV-infected child has a defined infectious exposure, the use of passive immunization as postexposure prophylaxis to prevent infection or ameliorate the severity of disease is recommended for certain diseases, such as measles, varicella zoster, and hepatitis B. Measles exposure is treated with administration of standard intramuscular immunoglobulin. Prevention of varicella zoster is most reliably accomplished by administration of a high titered, hyperimmunoglobulin preparation. HIV-infected children who are receiving IVIG who have a known measles or varicella exposure should also receive appropriate prophylaxis with intramuscular immunoglobulin or varicella zoster immunoglobulin if it is more than 2 weeks since their last dose of IVIG.

The Public Health Service has recommended that all infants receive hepatitis B immunization, regardless of maternal hepatitis B infection status (67). In addition, infants born to hepatitis B surface antigen carrier mothers should also receive passive immunization with high-titered hyperimmunoglobulin within 12 hr of birth.

The use of immunoglobulin preparations to treat an established infection is more controversial. There have been only anecdotal reports of the use of IVIG in the treatment of certain viral or opportunistic infections.

CMVIG for Treatment of Cytomegalovirus Infection

IVIG and hyperimmune cytomegalovirus immunoglobulin (CMVIG) have been used alone and in combination with ganciclovir for the treatment of cytomegalovirus pneumonia in immunosuppressed patients after allogenic bone marrow transplantation, with somewhat conflicting results (68–72). A lack of therapeutic efficacy has been demonstrated in established cytomegalovirus disease when CMVIG is used alone for treatment of bone marrow recipients with cytomegalovirus pneumonia (68). However, the combination of IVIG or CMVIG with ganciclovir has been more promising in some small preliminary reports. In one study from New York City using historical controls, patients receiving combination therapy had improved survival (7 of 10 survived) over patients receiving only single agent therapy (none of 11 patients survived) (69). In another small study from Seattle that compared combination therapy with antiviral therapy alone, improved survival was also noted with combination therapy (52% compared with 15%) (70). However, the European Bone Marrow Transplant Group recently reported a retrospective study on 49 allogeneic bone marrow transplant recipients who developed cytomegalovirus interstitial pneumonia, all of whom received ganciclovir and high dose IVIG (although regimen and type of immunoglobulins varied between sites) (71). Response to treatment was observed in 35%, and survival for 30 days after cytomegalovirus diagnosis was only 31%, substantially less than previously reported. Additionally, the authors did not find any difference between the use of standard IVIG and hyperimmune CMVIG nor did they find that the immunoglobulin dose influenced survival, leading to the conclusion that immunomodulatory rather than cytomegalovirus-specific effects of IVIG may be most important in treatment. At present, recommendations regarding the use of immunoglobulin preparations for treatment of established cytomegalovirus infection in organ transplant patients is controversial, but most centers treat cytomegalovirus pneumonia with both ganciclovir and IVIG.

The success of ganciclovir for the prevention of cytomegalovirus disease in bone marrow transplant recipients will, hopefully, decrease the need for acute treatment of disease in most patients (72).

There are no published data regarding IVIG treatment or prophylaxis of cytomegalovirus in HIV-infected patients, nor are there current data to suggest that IVIG has benefit in treating cytomegalovirus syndromes.

IVIG for Treatment of Parvovirus B19-associated Anemia

Recently, human parvovirus B19, the causative agent of the common childhood illness erythema infectiosum (or fifth disease), has been implicated as a cause of severe chronic anemia in patients with congenital or acquired immunodeficiencies, including both adults and children infected with HIV (73–75). In an uncontrolled study involving six HIV-infected adults with red cell aplasia caused parvovirus, administration of IVIG, 400 mg/kg/day for 5–10 days, resulted in prompt reticulocytosis and a rise in hemoglobin level; relapse occurred in two patients who were successfully retreated (73). In patients with relapse 6 months after initial therapy, empiric maintenance treatment with 400 mg/kg IVIG monthly may be beneficial. Nevertheless, treatment failures with IVIG have also been described (76).

IMMUNOMODULATORY USE OF IVIG IN HIV-INFECTED CHILDREN: THROMBOCYTOPENIA

Thrombocytopenia is a well-known complication of HIV infection, thought to be a result of the polyclonal stimulation of B cells and hypergammaglobulinemia with the production of platelet-associated antibodies (77). The incidence of HIV-related thrombocytopenia in symptomatic HIV-infected children is said to be 13% (78), and may be the presenting manifestation of HIV. The immune mechanism in HIV-associated thrombocytopenia has some similarities to and differences from classic immune thrombocytopenic purpura. The differences concern primarily the specificity of the platelet-associated antibodies. Anti-HIV antibodies form a principal component of platelet bound IgG and IgM in the HIV-infected patient, but other antibodies seen in classic immune thrombocytopenic purpura are also found. Decreased platelet survival and splenic sequestration appear common to both types of thrombocytopenia.

Based upon the successful use of IVIG for childhood immune thrombocytopenic purpura, IVIG has been given with some success to children with HIV-associated thrombocytopenia, although the benefit is transient in some cases (78–84). The mechanisms for IVIG efficacy in childhood or HIV-associated immune thrombocytopenic purpura are not fully understood. An important mechanism of action may be blockade of Fc receptors, resulting in a decrease in immune clearance of antibody-coated platelets. Other potential mechanisms include antiidiotypic antibody complexing to autoantibody, thereby preventing binding to platelet membrane; immunoregulation via antiidiotype antibody, resulting in diminished autoantibody production; and alteration in Fc receptor expression.

As an alternative form of γ-globulin therapy for thrombocytopenia, anti-Rh (anti-D) antibodies have been utilized in Rh-positive patients (85, 86). Advantages of this form of treatment are that a much lower dose of γ-globulin is possible, infusion time is significantly reduced to <10 min (compared with 2-4 hr with IVIG), and there are fewer side effects. This form of therapy does not work for Rh negative patients and splenectomized patients (86) and has not been studied in HIV-infected patients with thrombocytopenia.

Antiretroviral therapy with either ZDV or dideoxyinosine has also been associated with increased platelet count in some children. The combined use of ZDV and IVIG appears to have been beneficial for pediatric patients in a few reported cases (84). HIV-associated thrombocytopenia and treatments are discussed in detail elsewhere.

POTENTIAL FUTURE THERAPY AND PROPHYLAXIS: HYPERIMMUNE HIV IMMUNOGLOBULIN

The prolonged latency between infection with HIV and the onset of AIDS suggests that the host immune response against the virus may be involved in mitigating HIV infection (87). The humoral and cellular immune factors associated with protection against infection or development of disease, once infected, are incompletely understood and are an active area of research. As discussed earlier in Chapter 10C, there have been conflicting reports regarding the potential protective effect of maternal neutralizing antibody on vertical transmission of HIV, particularly antibodies to the V3 loop of gp120 envelope protein. Although specific virus epitopes associated with protective antibody have not been completely defined, there is increasing evidence that maternal immune status has an association with transmission risk to the infant. Additionally, there is evidence for genetic variation of HIV in an infected individual over time. Virus mutations may be associated with changes in biological properties of the virus, such as virulence or cell tropism (88). Within the host, there may be immune selection for HIV variants that can escape neutralization; such variants could have altered biologic properties associated with disease progression and possibly vertical transmission (89, 90). Active immunotherapy (discussed in Chapter 47) and passive administration of HIV-specific antibodies to boost the host immuneresponse against HIV are being evaluated for treatment of HIV-infected individuals as well as for prevention of vertical transmission.

Passive immunization with HIV hyperimmunoglobulin (HIVIG) could prevent or modify HIV infection directly by neutralization of free virus or by prevention of virus binding or fusion with target cells or indirectly by eliminating infected cells via antibody-dependent cell-mediated cytotoxicity or antibody-mediated complement fixation. A broad spectrum of HIV neutralizing antibodies can be obtained from healthy HIV-seropositive donors to produce a purified virus-inactivated HIVIG preparation. Monoclonal antibody preparations may offer the advantage of mass production of a specific antibody against a specific antigenic target without the potential risk, albeit small, of adventitious infection from human-derived blood products.

One major difficulty in the development of HIVIG preparations and monoclonal antibody "cocktails" is defining which antibodies, if any, confer protection in vivo. Neutralizing antibodies can be found in the serum of HIV-infected patients, and there is some evidence that the presence of such antibodies may correlate with disease stability. Several investigators have reported an association of neutralizing antibody with a more favorable clinical course in HIV-infected children (91, 92). If distinct virus epitopes can be identified that are associated with development of antibodies with broad, group-specific neutralizing capacity, a preparation of one or more human monoclonal antibodies could provide optimal treatment. However, if neutralizing antibody proves to be strain specific or if neutralization escape variants are important in vertical transmission and/or disease progression, a polyvalent HIVIG preparation will probably be necessary.

It is possible that HIV antibody could enhance rather than reduce target cell infection. This could occur through the development of antibody-virus complexes that would permit uptake of virions in the form of immune complexes by Fc receptors on macrophages or complement-antibody-virus complex uptake via the complement receptors found on macrophages, monocytes, and dendritic cells (93). Antibody-mediated enhancement of viral entry into macrophages has been well described in the case of flaviviruses such as dengue and yellow fever viruses (94) and also with animal retroviruses. However, in these cases, enhancing antibodies were distinct from the neutralizing antibodies that block virus infection. There is some in vitro evidence that antibody may facilitate HIV infection by both Fc as well as complement-mediated pathways in conditions of low antibody concentration in human cell lines and blood mononuclear cells (95). However, this effect was not demonstrated on freshly isolated normal human peritoneal macrophages and blood monocytes (96).

Although possible enhancement of virus infection, mediated by immune-complexed virus and Fc or complement receptors, is of concern, in vivo animal trials of HIV or simiar immunodeficiency virus vaccine or passive immunoprophylaxis have not shown evidence of enhancement of infection upon subsequent challenge with virus.

Initial studies of passive immunization to prevent viral infections in animal models, using low dose HIVIG and high titer virus challenge, did not demonstrate protection; however, with a lower virus challenge dose and the higher dose of HIVIG (10 ml/kg), protection was observed in a chimpanzee challenged with virus 1 day after receiving antibody (97). Additional animal studies had promising results. In a cynomologous monkey model, using both HIV-2 and simian immunodeficiency virus (SIV_{sm}) hyperimmune serum and live virus intravenous challenge, passive immunization successfully prevented infection of immunized animals when compared with control, unimmunized animals (98). In chimpanzees, high dose HIVIG (10 ml/kg, producing a p24 antibody titer in the animal of 1:640 at the time of challenge) protected against an intravenous challenge of live virus (99). A passive immunization preparation consisting of mouse-human chimeric IgG_1 monoclonal antibody specific for the principal neutralizing domain of the V3 loop of gp120 HIV-1 IIIb was successful in preventing HIV infection in a chimpanzee model (100). Such data suggest a potential in vivo protective effect of anti-V3 loop antibody.

The safety and toxicity of several HIVIG preparations have been evaluated in several small phase I studies of HIV-infected individuals (101–105). In one study, a highly purified human immunoglobulin containing high titers of antibody to HIV structural proteins with considerable functional activity in virus neutralization and antibody-dependent cellular cytotoxicity assays was prepared from plasma of asymptomatic HIV-seropositive subjects with CD4+ counts of ≥400/mm³. HIVIG was found to be safe and well-tolerated when used at doses of 50 and 200 mg/kg. No evidence of enhancement of HIV infection was observed. After infusion, there was disappearance of circulating p24 antigen in antigen-positive patients, a prolongation in the time to plasma virus culture positivity, and an increase in HIV neutralizing antibody. Reported clinical improvements such as increased Karnofsky rating and weight gain were noted in some patients, although the data were anecdotal in nature.

Analogous results were reported by Karpas and colleagues (103), using a similar preparation, with reductions in HIV viremia by polymerase chain reaction sustained clearance of p24 antigen, and stabilization of CD4+ counts in patients with AIDS-related complex but not AIDS. Vittecoq and colleagues (106), using heat-treated plasma from healthy HIV seropositive donors, also reported decreased antigenemia and clinical stabilization during treatment in nine patients compared with nine controls receiving HIV antibody-negative plasma 6. However, the investigators noted a possible "rebound" effect with increased p24 antigenemia and clinical deterioration in some treated patients when transfusions were stopped.

Thus, preliminary data in humans demonstrate that HIVIG is safe and well tolerated in HIV-infected persons, produces demonstrable neutralizing capacity in vitro, and appears to have pharmacokinetics similar to IVIG. The data from animal studies, and the preliminary epidemiologic data regarding vertical HIV transmission in humans, indicate that HIV antibody may provide some protection against infection. On the basis of this preliminary information, two phase II/III clinical trials to evaluate the efficacy of HIVIG for the prevention of vertical transmission of HIV are under development, sponsored by the NIH. One proposed study is a multicenter, randomized, controlled trial to evaluate the efficacy, safety, and tolerance of the combination of HIVIG (in a dose of 200 mg/kg administered monthly during pregnancy and to the newborn within 12 hr of birth) and ZDV (administered during pregnancy, intrapartum, and to the newborn for 6 weeks after birth) for the reduction of vertical HIV transmission in HIV-infected pregnant women receiving ZDV for medical indications during pregnancy. Comparison will be made with IVIG and ZDV administered similarly. This trial, which will enroll 400 HIV-infected pregnant women, began during the fall of 1993.

REFERENCES

1. Burdette S, Schwartz RS: Idiotypes and idiotypic networks. N Engl J Med 1987;317:219–224.
2. Buckley RH, Schiff RI: The use of intravenous immune globulin in immunodeficiency diseases. N Engl J Med 1991;325:110–117.
3. Dwyer JM: Manipulating the immune system with immune globulin. N Engl J Med 1992:326:107–116.
4. Cohn EJ, Strong LE, Hughes WL, et al: Preparation and properties of serum and plasm proteins. I. A system for the separation into fractions of the protein and lipoprotein components of biological tissues and fluids. J Am Chem Soc 1946;68:459–475.
5. Sandberg ET: Intravenous immunoglobulin preparations. Semin Pediatr Infect Dis 1992;3:144–146.
6. Skvaril F, Gardi A. Differences among available immunoglobulin preparations for intravenous use. Pediatr Infect Dis J 1988;7:S34–S48.
7. Colomb MG, Drouet C, Law DTW, Painter RH. Structural and biological properties of three intravenous immunoglobulin preparations. In: Morell A, Nydegger UE, eds. Clinical use of intravenous immunoglobulins. London: Academic 1986: 27–36.
8. Herrera AM, Saunders NB, Baker JR. Immunoglobulin composition of three commercially available intravenous immunoglobulin preparations. J Allergy Clin Immunol 1989;84:556–561.
9. Lundblad JL, Londeree N. The effect of processing methods on intravenous immmunoglobulin preparations. J Hosp Infect 1988;12:D3–D15.
10. Fischer GW. Uses of intravenous immune globulin to prevent or treat infections. Adv Pediatr Infect Dis 1992;7:85–108.
11. Greenbaum BH. Differences in immunoglobulin preparations for intravenous use—a comparison of six products. Am J Pediatr Hematol Oncol 1990;12:490–496.
12. Tankersley DL. Intravenous immunoglobulins—past, present and future. Consensus development conference on intravenous immunoglobulin: Prevention and treatment of disease, Bethesda, MD: National Institutes of Health, 1990:21–24.
13. Berkman SA, Lee ML, Gale RP. Clinical uses of intravenous immunoglobulins. Ann Intern Med 1990;112:278–292.
14. Fischer GW, Hemming VG, Hunter KW, et al. Intravenous immunoglobulin in the treatment of neonatal sepsis: Therapeutic strategies and laboratory studies. Pediatr Infect Dis J 1986;5:S171–S175.
15. Ochs HD, Lee ML, Fischer SH, Delson ES, Chang BS, Wedgwood RJ. Self-infusion of intravenous immunoglobulin by immunodeficient patients at home. J Infect Dis 1987;156:652–654.
16. Ryan A, Thomson BJ, Webster ADB. Home intravenous immunoglobulin therapy for patients with primary hypogammaglobulinemia [Letter]. Lancet 1988;2:793.
17. Kobayashi RH, Kobayashi AD, Lee N, Fischer S, Ochs HD. Home self-administration of intravenous immunoglobulin therapy in children. Pediatrics 1990;85:705–709.
18. Gardulf A, Hammarstrom L, Smith CIE. Home treatment of hypogammaglobulinaemia with subcutaneous gammaglobulin by rapid infusion. Lancet 1991;338:162–166.

19. Pirofsky B. Intravenous immune globulin therapy in hypogammaglobulinemia. Am J Med 1984;76: 53–60.
20. Ochs HD, Fischer SH, Wedgewood RJ, et al. Comparison of high-dose and low-dose intravenous immunoglobulin therapy in patients with primary immunodeficiency diseases. Am J Med 1984;76:78–82.
21. Rosenblatt HM. Primary immunodeficiency disorders and the rational use of intravenous immunoglobulin. Semin Pediatr Infect Dis 1992;3: 150–156.
22. Mofenson LM, Moye J, Lischner H, et al. Occurrence of infections and time from infusion in HIV-infected children in a clinical trial of immunoglobulin [Abstract 2]. Seventh Annual Conference on Clinical Immunology, Philadelphia, Nov 1992.
23. Mitra G, Wong MF, Mozen MM, McDougal JS, Levy JA. Elimination of infectious retroviruses during preparation of immunoglobulins. Transfusion 1986;26:394–397.
24. Centers for Disease Control. Safety of therapeutic immune globulin preparations with respect to transmission of human T-lymphotropic virus type III/lymphadenopathy-associated virus infection. MMWR 1986;35:231–233.
25. Centers for Disease Control. Revision of the CDC surveillance case definition for acquired immunodeficiency syndrome. MMWR 1987;36(suppl 1S).
26. Krasinski K, Borkowsky W, Bonk S, et al. Bacterial infections in human immunodeficiency virus-infected children. Pediatr Infect Dis J 1988;7:323–328.
27. Bernstein LJ, Krieger BZ, Novick B, et al. Bacterial infection in the acquired immunodeficiency syndrome of children. Pediatr Infect Dis J 1985;4: 472–475.
28. Roilides E, Marshall D, Venzon D, Butler K, Husson R, Pizzo PA. Bacterial infections in human immunodeficiency virus type 1-infected children: The impact of central venous catheters and antiretroviral agents. Pediatr Infect Dis J 1991;10:813–819.
29. Hsu H, Moye J, Ng P, et al. Pneumococcal bacteremia in children with HIV infection [Abstract WB 2062]. Seventh International Conference on AIDS, Florence, Jun 1991.
30. Zarkowsky HS, Gallagher D, Gill FM, et al. Bacteremia in sickle hemoglobinopathies. J Pediatr 1986;109:579–585.
31. Redd SC, Rutherford GW, Sande MA, et al. The role of human immunodeficiency virus infection in pneumococcal bacteremia in San Francisco residents. J Infect Dis 1990;162:1012–1017.
32. Marolda J, Pace B, Bonforte RJ, Kotin NM, Rabinowitz J, Kattan M. Pulmonary manifestations of HIV infection in children. Pediatr Pulmonol 1991;10:231–235.
33. Principi N, Marchisio P, Tornaghi R, et al. Occurrence of infections in children infected with human immunodeficiency virus. Pediatr Infect Dis J 1991;10:190–193.
34. Principi N, Marchisio P, Tornaghi R, et al. Acute otitis media in human immunodeficiency virus-infected children. Pediatrics 1991;88:566–571.

35. Chandwani S, Borkowsky W, Krasinski K, Lawrence R, Welliver R. Respiratory syncytial virus infection in human immunodeficiency virus-infected children. J Pediatr 1990;117:251–254.
36. Janner D, Petru AM, Belchis D, Azimi PH. Fatal adenovirus infection in a child with acquired immunodeficiency syndrome. Pediatr Infect Dis J 1990;9:434–436.
37. Hughes WT, Parham DM. Molluscum contagiosum in children with cancer or acquired immunodeficiency syndrome. Pediatr Infect Dis J 1991; 10:152–156.
38. Jura E, Chadwick EG, Josephs SH, et al. Varicella-zoster virus infections in children infected with human immunodeficiency virus. Pediatr Infect Dis J 1989;8:586–590.
39. Markowitz LE, Chandler FW, Roldan EO, et al. Fatal measles pneumonia without rash in a child with AIDS. J Infect Dis 1988;158:480–483.
40. Nadel S, McGann K, Hodinka RL, Rutstein R, Chatten J. Measles giant cell pneumonia in a child with human immunodeficiency virus infection. Pediatr Infect Dis J 1991;10:542–544.
41. Centers for Disease Control. Measles in HIV-infected children. MMWR 1988;37:183-186.
42. Krasinski K, Borkowsky W. Measles and measles immunity in childern infected with human immunodeficiency virus. JAMA 1989;261:2512–2516.
43. Silverman BA, Rubinstein A. Serum lactate dehydrogenase levels in adults and children with AIDS: Possible indicator of B cell lymphoproliferative and disease activity; effect of IVIG on enzyme levels. Am J Med 1985;78:728–736.
44. Gupta A, Novick BE, Rubinstein A. Restoration of suppressor T-cell functions in children with AIDS following intravenous gamma globulin treatment. Am J Dis Child 1986;140:143–146.
45. Wood CC, McNamara JG, Schwarz DF, et al. Prevention of pneumococcal bacteremia in a child with ARC. Pediatr Infect Dis J 1987;6:564–566.
46. Schaad UB, Gianella-Borradori A, Perret B, et al. Intravenous immune globulin in symptomatic paediatric human immunodeficiency virus infection. Eur J Pediatr 1988;147:300–303.
47. Williams PE, Hague RA, Yap PL, et al. Treatment of human immunodeficiency virus antibody children with intravenous immunoglobulin. J Hosp Infect 1988;12(suppl D):67–73.
48. Hague RA, Yap PL, Mok JYQ, et al. Intravenous immunoglobulin in HIV infection: Evidence for efficacy of treatment. Arch Dis Child 1989;64: 1146–1150.
49. Calvelli TA, Rubenstein A. Intravenous gamma globulin in infant-acquired immunodeficiency syndrome. Pediatr Infect Dis J 1986;5;S207–S210.
50. Siegal FP, Oleske JM. Management of the acquired immunodeficiency syndrome: Is there a role for immune globulins? In: Morell A, Hydeggar AE, eds. Clinical use of intravenous immunoglobulins. London: Academic, 1986:373–384.
51. Wagner N, Bialek R, Radinger H, et al. Intravenous immunoglobulins in HIV-infected hemophiliac children and adolescents: A randomized controlled trial over 24 months [Abstract WB 2067]. Seventh International Conference on AIDS, Florence, Jun 1991.

52. Mofenson L, Riqau-Perez JG, Nugent R, Cadden C, IVIG Clinical Trial Study Group. Pneumonia diagonsis in human immunodeficiency virus-infected children in a clinical trial of intravenous immunogloblin [Abstract 495]. 30th Interscience Conference on Antimicrobial Agents and Chemotherapy, Atlanta, Oct 1990.

53. NICHD IVIG Clinical Trial Study Group. Efficacy of intravenous immunoglobulin for the prophylaxis of serious bacterial infections in symptomatic HIV-infected children. N Engl J Med 1991; 325:73–80.

54. Mofenson LM, Moye J, Bethel J, et al. Prophylactic intravenous immunoglobulin in HIV-infected children with CD4+ counts of 0.20×10^9/L or more: Effect on viral, opportunistic and bacterial infections. JAMA 1992;268:483–488.

55. Mofenson LM, Bethel J, Moye J, et al. Effect of intravenous immunoglobulin, PCP prophylaxis and AZT on prevention of infections in HIV-infected children [Abstract 1008]. American Pediatric Society & Society for Pediatric Research, Baltimore, May 1992.

56. Mofenson LM, Shearer WT, Moye J, et al. Manipulating the immune system with immune globulin [Letter]. N Engl J Med 1992;326;1636–1637.

57. Mofenson LM, Moye J, Nugent R, et al. Serious infection and mortality in HIV-infected children in a clinical trial of intravenous immunoglobulin [Abstract 908]. 32nd Interscience Conference on Antimicrobial Agents and Chemotherapy, Anaheim, Oct 1992.

58. Mofenson LM, Moye J, Bethel J, et al. Effect of intravenous immunoglobulin (IVIG) on CD4+ cell decline in HIV-infected children in a clinical trial of IVIG prophylaxis [Abstract PoB 3449]. Eighth International Conference on AIDS, Amsterdam, Jul 1992.

59. Shearer GM, Clerici M. Early T-helper cell defects in HIV infection. AIDS 1991;5:245–253.

60. Clerici M, Stocks NI, Zajac RA, et al. Detection of three distinct patterns of T helper cell dysfunction in asymptomatic, human immunodeficiency virus-seropositive patients. J Clin Invest 1989;84: 1892–1899.

61. Lucey DR, Melcher GP, Hendrix CW, et al. Human immunodeficiency virus infection in the US Air Force: Seroconversions, clinical staging and assessment of a T helper functional assay to predict change in CD4+ T cell counts. J Infect Dis 1991;164:631–637.

62. Roilides E, Clerici M, DePalma L, Rubin M, Pizzo PA, Shearer GM. Helper T-cell responses in children infected with human immunodeficiency virus type-1. J Pediatr 1991;118:724–730.

63. Rinaldo C, Huang XL, Piazza P, et al. Augmentation of cellular immune function during the early phase of zidovudine treatment of AIDS patients. J Infect Dis 1991;164:638–645.

64. Roilides E, Venzon D, Pizzo PA, Rubin M. Effects of antiretroviral dideoxynucleosides on polymorphonuclear leukocyte function. Antimicrob Agents Chemother 1990;34:1672–1677.

65. Clerici M, Landy AL, Kessler HA, et al. Reconstitution of long-term helper cell function after zidovudine therapy in human immunodeficiency virus-infected patients. J Infect Dis 1992; 166:723–730.

66. Hughes WT, Kuhn S, Chaudhary S, et al. Successful chemoprophylaxis for *Pneumocystis carinii* pneumonitis. N Engl J Med 1977;297: 1419–1426.

67. Centers for Disease Control. Hepatitis B Virus: A comprehensive strategy for eliminating transmission in the United States through universal childhood vaccinations—recommendations of the Immunization Practices Advisory Committee (ACIP). MMWR 1992;40:RR13.

68. Reed EC, Bowden RA, Dandliker PS, Gleaves CA, Myers JD. Efficacy of cytomegalovirus immunoglobulin in marrow transplant recipients with cytomegalovirus pneumonia. J Infect Dis 1987;156:641–645.

69. Reed EC, Bowden RA, Dandliker PS, et al. Treatment of cytomegalovirus pneumonia with ganciclovir and intravenous cytomegalovirus immunoglobulin in patients with bone marrow transplants. Ann Intern Med 1988;109:783–788.

70. Emanuel D, Cunningham I, Jules-Elysee K, et al. Cytomegalovirus pneumonia after bone marrow transplantation successfully treated with the combination of ganciclovir and high-dose intravenous immune globulin. Ann Intern Med 1988; 109:777–782.

71. Ljungman P, Engelhard D, Link H, et al. Treatment of interstitial pneumonitis due to cytomegalovirus with ganciclovir and intravenous immune globulin: Experience of European Bone Marrow Transplant Group. Clin Infect Dis 1992;14:831–835.

72. Bowden RA, Meyers JD. Prophylaxis of cytomegalovirus infection. Semin Hematol 1990;27:17–21.

73. Frickhofen N, Abkowita JL, Safford M, et al. Persistent B19 parvovirus infection in patients infected with human immunodeficiency virus type 1: A treatable cause of anemia in AIDS. Ann Intern Med 1990;113:926–933.

74. Griffin TC, Squires JE, Timmons CF, et al. Chronic human parvovirus B19-induced erythroid hypoplasia as the initial manifestation of human immunodeficiency virus infection. J Pediatr 1991;118:899–901.

75. Nigro G, Gattinara GC, Mattia S, Caniglia M, Fridell E. Parvovirus-B19-related pancytopenia in children with HIV infection [Letter]. Lancet 1992;340:115.

76. Bowman CA, Cohen BJ, Norfolk DR, et al. Red cell aplasia associated with human parvovirus B19 and HIV infection: Failure to respond clinically to intravenous immunoglobulin. AIDS 1990;4:1038–1039.

77. Oksenhendler E, Seligmann M. HIV-related thrombocytopenia. Immunodeficiency Rev 1990;2:221–231.

78. Ellaurie M, Burns ER, Bernstein LJ, et al. Thrombocytopenia and human immunodeficiency virus in children. Pediatrics 1988;82:905–908.

79. Saulsburg FT, Boyle RJ, Wykoff RF, et al. Thrombocytopenia as the presenting manifesta-

tion of human T-lymphotrophic virus type III infection in infants. J Pediatr 1986;109:30–34.

80. Weinblatt ME, Scimeca PG, James-Herry AG, et al. Thrombocytopenia in an infant with AIDS [Letter]. Am J Dis Child 1987;141:15.

81. Boppana SB, Frenkel LD. Thrombocytopenia in an HIV-seropositive infant. Ann Allergy 1988;61: 12,57–59.

82. Kurtzberg J, Friedman HS, Kinney TR, et al. Management of human immunodeficiency virus-associated thrombocytopenia with intravenous gammaglobulin. Am J Pediatr Hematol Oncol 1987;9:299–301.

83. Leipnitz G, Kohler M, Pindur G, et al. AIDS-related thrombocytopenia. Experience of a medium-term treatment with intravenous IgG in haemophilia B patients. Vox Sang 1989;56:57–58.

84. Pahwa S. Intravenous immune globulin in patients with acquired immune deficiency syndrome. J Allergy Clin Immunol 1989;84:625–631.

85. Oksenhandler E, Bierling P, Brossard Y, et al. Anti-Rh immunoglobulin therapy for human immunodeficiency virus-related thrombocytopenic purpura. Blood 1988;71:1499–1502.

86. Bussel JB, Graziano JN, Kimberly R, et al. Intravenous anti-D treatment of immune thrombocytopenic purpura: Analysis of efficacy, toxicity, and mechanism of effect. Blood 1991;77:1884–1893.

87. Fauci AS, Gallo RL, Koenig S, et al. Development and evaluation of a vaccine for human immunodeficiency virus infection. Ann Intern Med 1989;110:373–385.

88. Johnson MA, Cann AJ. Molecular determination of cell tropism of human immunodeficiency virus. Clin Infect Dis 1992;14:747–755.

89. Wolinsky SM, Wike CM, Korber BT, et al. Selective transmission of human immunodeficiency virus type-1 variants from mothers to infants. Science 1992;255:1134–1136.

90. Tremblay M, Wainberg MA. Neutralization of multiple HIV-1 isolates from a single subject by autologous sequential sera. J Infect Dis 1990;162: 735–737.

91. Robert-Guroff M, Oleske JM, Connor EM, Epstein LG, Minnefor AB, Gallo RC. Relationship between HTLV-III neutralizing antibody and clinical status of pediatric AIDS and ARC cases. Pediatr Res 1987;21:547–550.

92. Ljunggren K, Moschese V, Broliden PA, et al. Antibodies mediating cellular cytotoxicity and neutralization correlate with a better clinical stage in children born to human immunodeficiency virus-infected mothers. J Infect Dis 1990;161:198–202.

93. Bologenesi DP. Do antibodies enhance the infection of cells by HIV? Nature 1989;340:431–432.

94. Halstead SB. Pathogenesis of dengue: Challenges to molecular biology. Science 1988;239:476–481.

95. Takeda A, Tuazon CU, Ennis FA. Antibody-enhanced infection by HIV-1 via Fc receptor-mediated entry. Science 1988;242:580–583.

96. Bakker LJ, Nottet HSLM, de Vos M, et al. Antibodies and complement enhance binding and uptake of HIV-1 by human monocytes. AIDS 1992;6:35–41.

97. Shadduck PP, Weinberg JB, Haney AF, et al. Lack of enhancing effect of human anti-human immunodeficiency virus type 1 (HIV-1) antibody on HIV-1 infection of human blood monocytes and peritoneal macrophages. J Virol 1991;65:4309–4316.

98. Prince AM, Reesink H, Pascual D, et al. Prevention of HIV infection by passive immunization with HIV immunoglobulin. AIDS Res Hum Retroviruses 1991;7:971–973.

99. Putkonen P, Thorstensson R, Ghayamizadeh L, et al. Prevention of HIV-2 and SIVsm infection by passive immunization in cynomolgus monkeys. Nature 1991;352:436–438.

100. Eichberg JW: Experience with seventeen HIV vaccine efficacy trials in chimpanzees [Abstract FA 2]. Seventh International Conference on AIDS, Florence, Jun 1991.

101. Emini EA, Scheif WA, Murthy K, et al. Passive immunization with a monoclonal antibody directed to the HIV-1 gp120 principal neutralizing domain confers protection against HIV-1 challenge in chimpanzees [Abstract ThA 64]. Seventh International Conference on AIDS, Florence, Jun 1991.

102. Jackson GG, Perkins JT, Rubenis M, et al. Passive immunoneutralization of human immunodeficiency virus in patients with advanced AIDS. Lancet 1988;2:647–652.

103. Karpas A, Hill F, Youle M, et al. Effects of passive immunization in patients with acquired immunodeficiency syndrome-related complex and acquired immunodeficiency syndrome. Proc Natl Acad Sci USA 1988;85:9234–9237.

104. Karpas A, Hill F, Gazzard B, et al. Passive immunization in ARC and AIDS patients: Persistent neutralization of HIV-1 as monitored by polymerase chain reaction [Abstract ThB 85]. Seventh International Conference on AIDS, Florence, 1991.

105. Cummins LM, Weinholt KJ, Matthews TJ, et al. Preparation and characterization of an intravenous solution of IgG from human immunodeficiency virus-seropositive donors. Blood 1991;77: 1111–1117.

106. Vittecoq D, Mattlinger B, Barre-Sinoussi F, et al. Passive immunotherapy in AIDS: A randomized trial of serial human immunodeficiency virus-positive transfusions of plasma rich in p24 antibodies versus transfusions of seronegative plasma. J Infect Dis 1992;165:364–368.

46
Immunizations for HIV-infected Children

Samuel L. Katz

Throughout the world immunization has become the essential cornerstone of ideal child health supervision and where appropriately practiced has resulted in striking reductions of vaccine preventable diseases. In the United States for example, the numbers of reported cases of diphtheria, tetanus, pertussis, paralytic polio, measles and congenital rubella have been reduced by greater than 97–99% when 1992 data are compared with those of the years of peak incidence (Table 46.1). These records of achievement have been eroded, however, when access to health care has been restricted for some deprived populations and have resulted in outbreaks such as the measles experience of 1989–1991 (1) in this country. From a global perspective, the World Health Organization's Expanded Program on Immunization (EPI) has striven since 1977 to provide requisite vaccines to infants throughout the world with increasing coverage of the target populations each year. Although the EPI goals have not yet been fully achieved, the decreased numbers of deaths from measles, pertussis, neonatal tetanus, and tuberculosis are encouraging and provide impetus to the full extension of the program to all infants in all nations (2). The basic EPI schedule (Table 46.2) has been developed to provide protection as early in life as possible against those diseases with the highest morbidity and mortality among children at risk. With the availability of new vaccines and the assessment of their potential benefits, the program has been augmented in some areas to include these immunogens (e.g., hepatitis B). Figure 46.1 illustrates the numbers of cases occurring and those prevented in developing countries in 1990 for four selected infectious diseases. Goals of the pro-

Table 46.1. Maximum and Current Morbidity of Vaccine Preventable Diseases in the United States[a]

	Peak Year	1992
Diphtheria	206,939 (1921)	4
Tetanus	1,560 (1923)	42
Pertussis	265,269 (1934)	3,359
Paralytic polio	21,269 (1952)	4 (suspected, under review)
Measles	894,134 (1941)	2,200
Rubella	57,686 (1969)	148
Congenital rubella	20,000 (1964–1965)	9
Mumps	152,209 (1968)	2,460

[a]Data from Centers for Disease Control.

gram include the eradication of paralytic polio by the year 2000 and a 95% reduction in measles deaths plus a 90% reduction in measles cases by 1995.

Because the incidence of pediatric human immunodeficiency virus (HIV) infection is highest in some nations where EPI's efforts are most focused, the questions of successful immunization of children with immunocompromise and the duration of protection provided by standard vaccines become crucial in determining whether the progress to date will continue or will be altered by failure of vaccination among HIV-infected children whose immune systems are compromised. To date, data do not indicate a loss of effectiveness of the programs, but this is a dynamic situation where expanded coverage is reaching larger numbers of children overall so that vaccine failures or breakthroughs among HIV-infected youngsters might not yet have become apparent in overall statistics. It has become increasingly important to obtain information on vaccine efficacy and safety among individual HIV-infected children for their own well-being and to predict trends among large populations of such children.

Table 46.2.   EPI Vaccine Schedule[a]

Age	Vaccines
Newborn	BCG, TOPV, (HB)[b]
6–8 weeks	DTP, TOPV 2, (HB 2)
10–12 weeks	DTP 2, TOPV 3
14–16 weeks	DTP 3, TOPV 4
9 months	Measles (HB 3)

[a] TOPV, trivalent oral poliovirus vaccine; HB, hepatitis B; DTP, diphtheria, tetanus, pertussis.
[b] Currently recommended only in selected regions with high rates of endemic hepatitis B infections.

GENERAL CONSIDERATIONS

The problem of vaccine safety and efficacy for HIV-infected children is multifactorial. In addition to the expected ontogeny of the infant immune system, there are the superimposed perturbations induced by HIV infection (see Chapter 9). Immune responsiveness to vaccine antigens will vary with the degree of deficiency present at the time of any immunization. Because the infant vaccine recipient will in nearly all instances be seeing these antigens for the first

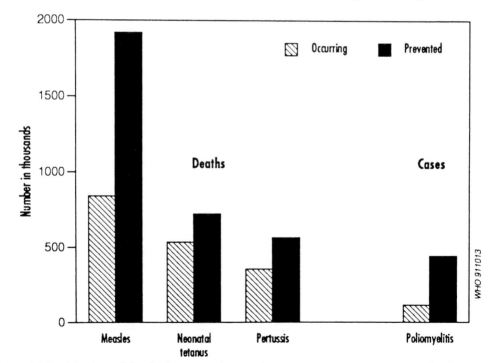

Figure 46.1.   Number of deaths from measles, neonatal tetanus, and pertussis and number of cases of paralytic poliomyelitis occurring and prevented by immunization (EPI) in 1990 in developing countries. From World Health Organization. EPI for the 1990's. Geneva: WHO, Mar 1992.

time, it is not a matter of recall so much as primary response that therefore invokes multiple T and B cell functions and interactions modulated by lymphokines. Over 90% of infected infants will have acquired their HIV infection vertically so that its effects may already be operational in the early weeks and months of life when vaccines are first administered. Because of technical ease of assessment, serum antibodies are most frequently checked as a surrogate of immunity, but increasingly laboratories are also assessing cellular and mucosal responses. With inactivated antigens, most often administered parenterally, the principal response is a humoral immune one, and there is no unusual risk to the immunocompromised recipient. At worst, the individual would fail to respond. At best, a satisfactory antibody rise would result with varying duration of persistence. With live replicating vaccines, there may well be a variety of immune responses including humoral antibody, secretory antibody, and cellular immunity. An example would be measles virus vaccine where secretory IgA, lymphocyte proliferative responses, and humoral antibodies have been demonstrated after successful vaccination (3). However, in the immunocompromised host, these vaccines carry the potential liability of unchecked replication with an agent attenuated for the normal host, producing serious disease in the immunocompromised recipient. Again, measles vaccine provides an example with an often cited pair of leukemic children who developed giant cell pneumonia after receipt of an earlier measles vaccine in the late 1950s (4). In areas where the naturally acquired infection (tuberculosis, measles, polio) poses a serious threat, the hypothetical risk of vaccine induced illness may be justifiable. As noted below, with polio there is the alternative of enhanced inactivated poliovirus vaccine (EIPV), rendering the question moot. With tuberculosis and measles there is no alternate choice.

Likelihood of exposure to vaccine preventable diseases varies greatly in different settings, and even within one country there may be enormous variance in transmission. Infants and children in urban day care centers are exposed to a great variety of viral, and some bacterial, pathogens in contrast to children dwelling in rural and suburban homes. An example is hepatitis A for which an experimental vaccine is under test in this country and already licensed in several European nations (5). Occult infection has been documented in day care settings without any morbidity among the children themselves but with transmission and resultant overt hepatitis among adult caretakers and parents. There are no reports of exaggerated disease among HIV-infected infants who acquire the same virus. Although tuberculosis has become a significant problem, especially with multiply drug resistant strains, among HIV-infected adults in some major cities (6), it has not yet become a major pediatric problem. The exposure of infants and children to tuberculous relatives or other infected adults poses a significant threat. In developing nations the EPI relies heavily on BCG administered in the newborn period to protect against widespread tuberculosis. Its use in the United States has been minimal, but a reevaluation of policies is underway.

These examples serve only to illustrate the variability that exists in assessing the benefits and risks of immunization procedures among HIV-infected children in different settings. Another variable relates to the age at which the diagnosis of HIV infection can be established in perinatally exposed infants. Several vaccines are recommended in the first 2 months of life, before definite HIV infection may have been proven in some infants. Because ~70% of them will prove to be uninfected, the uncertainties focus on those 30% who are incubating infection but may not yet be detected or proven.

A final concern that has been raised is whether the introduction of new antigens by stimulating macrophages and lymphocytes that may harbor quiescent HIV might activate virus replication and thereby accelerate the progress of the underlying infection. It is difficult to acquire precise data with which to confirm or reject that hypothesis, but to date it has not been found to be of other than hypothetical concern. One study has reported a peak rise in quantitative HIV viremia shortly after administration to adults of influenza virus vaccine, but this was brief and unaccompanied by any detectable clinical deterioration (7).

Infants and children of HIV antibody positive mothers should be immunized according to the recommendations of the Committee on Infectious Diseases of the American Academy of Pediatrics (8) and the Advisory Committee on Immunization Practices of the United States Public Health Service (9). Both groups have promulgated special recommendations for these children in contrast to "normal" ones. These recommendations are reviewed and revised on a regular basis to provide timely and appropriate policy based on the constantly accumulating information regarding experience with vaccines and with the naturally occurring infections in HIV children at risk. The Committee on Infectious Diseases of the American Academy of Pediatrics publishes a compendium of its recommendations every 2 or 3 years in its official report (The Red Book). Updated Academy recommendations may also be found in issues of the monthly journal *Pediatrics*. Advisory Committee on Immunization Practices publishes its recommendations frequently throughout the year in the Morbidity and Mortality Weekly Reports or its supplements.

SCHEDULES

Because HIV-indeterminate or -infected infants will be seen regularly for both primary care and evaluation of their status, a schedule can be devised to provide them all the recommended immunizations but with no more than two injections at any one visit. (In most instances they will also undergo phlebotomy for samples to detect virus, P24 antigen, CD4 counts, and immunoglobulins and/or other tests.) For humane reasons keeping the number of needle sticks to an irreducible minimum is warranted, and a suggested schedule (Table 46.3) incorporates all recommended vaccines but never with more than two injections per visit. Hopefully the multivalent combined antigens that are undergoing tests will soon become available (On 30 March 1993 the Food and Drug Administration approved for licensure a combined DTP-Hib conjugate vaccine for use in this country for children aged 2 months to 5 years.) so that the requisite numbers will be even further reduced (e.g., diphtheria, tetanus, pertussis and *Haemophilus influenzae* type B conjugate

combined in one injection). With HIV cultures and/or polymerase chain reaction at least 90% of vertically infected infants can be identified by age 6 months. This will assign them to that group of children for whom such a rigorous schedule of immunization is recommended. At present it is not yet agreed that children who are culture and polymerase chain reaction negative on two occasions after the first months of life can be declared uninfected with certainty until they have seroreverted by both enzyme-linked immunosorbent assay and Western blot, varying from ages 9 to 18 months. Therefore a significant number of youngsters who eventually turn out to be noninfected may follow this schedule through the first year of life. Other than the substitution of EIPV for oral poliovirus vaccine (OPV) and the recommendation of influenza virus vaccine, this departs minimally from the recommended schedule for normal infants and children. Justification for an aggressive immunization program for children suspected to be HIV infected is substantiated by the severity and prolongation of clinical manifestations that they may undergo with naturally acquired infections

Table 46.3. Suggested Schedule for Immunization of P-0 and HIV-infected Infants

Age	Vaccines[a]
Newborn	HB 1
1 month	HB 2
2 months	DTP 1, HIB 1
3 months	EIPV 1
4 months	DTP 2, HIB 2
5 months	EIPV 2
6 months	DTP 3, (HIB 3 or HB 3)[b]
7 months	(HB 3), Flu 1
8 months	Flu 2
12 months	HIB 3 or 4[c], EIPV 3
15 months	MMR 1, (DTaP 4)[d]
18 months	(DTaP 4)[d]
24 months	Pneumo 1

[a]HB, hepatitis B; DTP, diphtheria and tetanus toxoids with pertussis whole cell; EIPV, enhanced inactivated poliovirus vaccine; HIB, *H. influenzae* type B conjugate; flu, influenza virus vaccine; MMR, measles, mumps, rubella; DTaP, diphtheria and tetanus toxoids with acellular pertussis; pneumo, 23 valent pneumococcal polysaccharide.
[b]If primary series for HIB requires three doses, HB 3 may be postponed until next visit; if only two HIB doses are required, HB 3 may be given at 6-month visit.
[c]Third or fourth dose of HIB dependent on which vaccine had been used previously.
[d]DTaP can be administered at either a 15- or 18-month visit.

(see Chapters 13, 16, and 19). In some instances knowledge of acute exposure to an infection may permit administration of an immunoglobulin that may modify or abort the infection (see Chapter 45). It is important to appreciate that if the child is maintained on monthly intravenous immunoglobulin, the response to live virus vaccines measles-mumps-rubella (MMR) will be prevented by neutralization of the infecting attenuated viruses. To assure an uninterrupted immunization process, it may be necessary to postpone intravenous immunoglobulin for as long as 3 months (10) and then to delay the resumption of globulin for at least another 4–6 weeks.

MEASLES

Of all the vaccine preventable diseases, measles is the one that has been most frequently cited for its aggravated severity and complications in immunocompromised patients, including HIV-infected children. In a review of the literature, the case fatality rate for measles in HIV-infected individuals was 40% (11). Data such as these have raised concern about how best to protect children from this infection. The safety of live attenuated measles virus vaccine has not as yet been challenged in infected youngsters, but its efficacy is variable and to a great extent unpredictable. Both the major advisory committees recommend its use in both P-0 as well as HIV-infected infants at the usual age (12, 13) whether symptomatic or asymptomatic. Because of the uncertainty of initial response to vaccine and the duration of protection conferred, symptomatic HIV-infected children exposed to measles should also receive immunoglobulin prophylaxis (0.5 ml/kg with a maximum of 15 ml) regardless of when they received their vaccine. If the patient is on an intravenous immunoglobulin regimen, and has received intravenous immunoglobulin within the past 2–3 weeks, additional globulin is unnecessary.

One study has suggested that infants of HIV-infected mothers are susceptible to measles with an increased risk at an earlier age, regardless of whether they are infected (14). Apparently the transplacental transfer of maternal specific antibody to measles is diminished in those infants (presumably because of lower maternal titers). As a result,

their risk of acquiring measles before the recommended age of vaccination (9 months, see Table 46.2) was nearly four times greater than that of control infants born to HIV-seronegative mothers. An early study in this country showed only two of eight symptomatic HIV-infected children responsive to measles vaccine and only three of 24 children studied retrospectively to possess protective antibodies. Subsequent studies (15, 16) have tried to look prospectively at this question. Of 39 measles antibody negative children who were appropriately vaccinated, 19 remained antibody negative, 13 (33%) became antibody positive, and two were equivocal. With an aggressive measles intervention program, of their total cohort of 127 HIV-infected children, 34% remained antibody negative despite vaccine. There seemed to be a significant correlation with CD4 counts at the time of immunization. Those with mean CD4 counts of 1334 ± 681 cells/ml responded, whereas those with 463 ± 349 were the nonresponders. Cooper and colleagues (17) studied a group of 17 children who were either P-1 or P-2 and found that only nine responded with protective levels of antibody after a single dose of MMR. Of interest was their observation that a greater number of HIV-infected children responded to the rubella component of MMR (17).

More difficult to quantitate has been the decay in antibody observed among HIV-infected children after an initially positive response to vaccine. Using both an indirect enzyme immunoassay method as well as microneutralization, Walter and his colleagues (18) demonstrated that a significant portion of 28 infected children responded to measles vaccine and retained detectable antibody for 12 months after immunization (79%). However, when they were tested again 36 months after immunization, only 58% retained antibody. On every determination, the titers obtained were significantly lower than those of uninfected infants.

BCG

The other live vaccines that have been used in HIV-infected infants are BCG and OPV. Embree (19) described 120 infants of HIV-positive mothers who were given BCG without any untoward effects; 70%, however, failed later to respond to purified protein derivative testing. BCG vaccine has been safe when given to HIV-infected infants in the newborn period, as recommended by EPI, but conversion to a positive tuberculin test has been less frequent (33%) when contrasted to uninfected infants where an 83% skin test conversion has been observed (20). Concern persists regarding complications or dissemination of BCG in HIV-infected recipients. Five children (Haiti, Canada, Zaire) are reported to have undergone probable BCG dissemination before their death from AIDS in the first year of life (21). A recent description of an increasing incidence of BCG lymphadenitis and abscesses among infant recipients in Haiti (22) did not reveal any correlation to the prevalence of HIV among this population.

The most complete prospective studies reported to date enrolled 422 newborns in Kigali, Rwanda, immunized with BCG during the first week of life and included a 6-month follow-up at which time 377 infants were examined for the presence of a BCG scar and their response to skin testing with 10 IU tuberculin (23). HIV infection had been confirmed in 204 of their mothers. Of 33 infants known to be HIV infected, three had no detectable BCG scar. Sixteen of the 33 were nonreactive to the tuberculin skin test (49% in contrast to 9% of the infants of HIV-negative mothers). The absence of adverse effects of BCG supports its continued use in newborns living in areas of high tuberculosis endemicity but with an awareness that successful immunization may be achieved less frequently than in noninfected infants. The theoretical, but unproven, asset has been proposed that BCG might also provide some degree of cross-protection against the atypical mycobacteria to which HIV-infected children are highly susceptible.

POLIO

Because a nonreplicating poliovirus vaccine is available, safe, and immunogenic, it is recommended for infants of HIV-positive mothers instead of OPV in those countries and situations where it is economically and logistically feasible. For the EPI, OPV is still

used (Table 46.2) because it is most inexpensive and far more adaptable to the circumstances in developing nations. Despite the widespread use of hundreds of millions of doses of OPV in such settings, no cases of paralytic sequelae have been reported in either the recipients or their contacts. Nevertheless, in the United States and other western nations, EIPV has been routinely recommended for immunization of the infants of HIV-infected mothers. This adds three more injections to the schedule for the first 2 years of life, but these can be integrated as shown in Table 46.3. HIV-infected adults who were immunized early in life with poliovirus vaccines have been shown to respond appropriately to EIPV boosters (24). Barbi and colleagues (25) studied 43 children of HIV-seropositive mothers who at age 8 months were given two doses of EIPV. Neutralizing antibody responses to all three poliovirus serotypes developed in 88% of the children, whereas 100% had antibodies to at least two types. There were no statistically significant differences noted in either the rate of response or the titers of antibody between those children who proved to be HIV infected and those who seroreverted. One year later 16 of the children received a booster dose of EIPV with similar responses again in both infected and noninfected individuals. This favorable response with multiple doses of these inactivated antigens seems more favorable than that observed after single doses of live vaccines (e.g., measles and BCG).

DTP

In contrast to EIPV, the results with diphtheria, tetanus, pertussis immunization of HIV-infected children have sometimes been disappointing. Poor antibody responses to both diphtheria and tetanus toxoid have been recorded in symptomatic HIV-infected children (26). Those infants who have been immunized early at 6, 10, and 14 weeks, however, have demonstrated more adequate antibody responses to the two toxoids (27). Because there is still uncertainty about which antigens of bordetella pertussis are responsible for the development of protective immunity, antibody responses to whole cell or acellular pertussis antigens have not been helpful as yet. In various studies, from 40 to 100% of HIV-infected children have developed protective levels of tetanus antitoxin. For diphtheria, the range is from 18 to 72% (28).

HEPATITIS B

Because many of the same risk factors associated with maternal to fetal transmission of HIV infection may also be present for hepatitis B, immunization with the recombinant vaccine has been encouraged, even before the current recommendations for universal neonatal vaccination. A study by Zuin and colleagues in Milan (29) demonstrated an impaired response among HIV-infected children. Fifty-one infants of seropositive mothers were followed after vaccination with the standard three-dose schedule (at 0, 1, and 6 months). Of 18 infants who proved to be HIV infected, 14 responded with protective antibody levels. In contrast, 32 of 33 uninfected infants delivered to HIV-positive mothers responded with appropriate titers. In a 24-month follow-up, 93% of the seroreverters maintained protective levels, whereas only 25% of the HIV-infected children demonstrated antibodies to hepatitis B surface antigen titers greater than 10 mIU/ml. These results contrast with those noted above for EIPV and demonstrate once again the necessity to study each vaccine separately rather than to generalize from the results with one or another inactivated or live product.

PNEUMOCOCCAL

The results in HIV-infected children given pneumococcal vaccines of multivalent type have been variable. In general, however, responses have been poorer than in control uninfected children of similar age. In one study only one of 11 HIV-infected children responded to three of four serotypes (types 3, 7F, 9N 14) when tested 4 weeks after a single dose. Eight of nine uninfected control children responded adequately to three or four serotypes. The vaccine used was the 23-valent product (30). Similar studies in adults have shown poor response among those with CD4 counts of <500 so that administration has been recommended as early as possible in the course of infection. However, these results in children aged 2–9 years offer no significant encouragement. One adult study (31) suggested that response to pneumococcal vaccine improved significantly after the first 4 weeks of zidovudine therapy.

INFLUENZA VIRUS

Influenza virus vaccine has been variably recommended by both advisory committees for symptomatic children but not for those without symptoms. This may be logical from one perspective but appears self defeating since, in general, one would anticipate that in earlier HIV infection before cellular functions had diminished, the likelihood of an appropriate response would be enhanced. Studying both single and two dose regimens for influenza virus vaccine administration to HIV-infected children, Chadwick et al. (32) found that either schedule resulted in lower hemagglutination inhibition antibody titers among the infected children than among uninfected age-matched controls.

HAEMOPHILUS INFUENZA TYPE B CONJUGATE

Because several invasive *H. influenza* B infections have been reported in HIV-infected men (33), studies of their response to *H. influenza* B conjugate vaccines have been undertaken (34). These indicated that initial anti-polyribosyl-ribitol-phosphate antibody titers were lower than in seronegative individuals but that immunization with conjugate vaccine early in the course of HIV infection was likely to produce a protective level of antibody. As discussed previously, this undoubtedly reflects a recall phenomenon rather than a primary response to the antigen. Surprisingly, there is a scarcity of data regarding similar studies in HIV-infected infants and children, although the vaccine is recommended and routinely administered to infants of HIV-infected mothers. Indacochea and colleagues (35) demonstrated a satisfactory response to HbOC vaccine at 2, 4, and 6 months in five HIV-infected infants, four of whom achieved titers of >1 μg/ml. Using another *H. influenza* b conjugate, Walter et al. (36) immunized nine HIV-infected infants and found that their geometric mean titers (GMT) of anti-polyribosyl-ribitol-phosphate antibodies after two doses were significantly lower (GMT 0.46) than those assayed in uninfected controls (GMT 4.06). Two of nine infected children achieved titers greater than 1 μg/ml, whereas seven of 12 uninfected subjects exceeded that titer. Expanded studies of this nature are needed accompanied by long-term follow-up to assess the persistence of antibody and its efficacy in preventing infection and illness.

NEW VACCINES

Over the coming years several new vaccines are anticipated to be introduced for infant and childhood immunization. One that has remained imminent for nearly a decade in the United States is varicella-zoster virus. This is a live attenuated vaccine that will therefore carry the same concerns as all actively replicating agents in immuno-compromised children. One report of 11 HIV-infected children who received live attenuated OKA-Merck vaccine without any adverse effects found that only three of 11 susceptibles developed demonstrable antibodies that disappeared rapidly over the next 3–12 months (37). Further studies will be required to determine the immunogenicity, safety, and efficacy of this vaccine in HIV-infected children. One reassuring precedent is the extensive series of trials conducted by Gershon and her collaborators (38) in children with leukemia. These studies confirm that a two-dose schedule of vaccine was highly effective in inducing antibody and preventing chickenpox among the recipients. When breakthrough infections did occur, they were generally of a very mild nature. Additionally, the recipients over a period of 5–10 years had a significantly lower rate of zoster than that recorded among leukemic children who underwent natural chickenpox (39).

Other anticipated vaccines may include respiratory syncytial virus, conjugated pneumococcal and meningococcal antigens, group B streptococcal, various herpesviruses (cytomegalovirus, herpes 1 and 2,

Epstein-Barr), and hepatitis A among others. In each instance, it will be necessary to conduct careful studies to determine the initial immune response, the occurrence of possible adverse events, the persistence of antibody, and the degree of protection provided HIV-infected children by these products. The incentive to protect these highly susceptible individuals against vaccine-preventable infections should provide ample stimulus for the organization and conduct of such studies.

CONCLUSIONS

HIV-infected infants and children require careful and continuing investigations of their responses to vaccines. In each instance, the individual vaccine must be evaluated, because generalizations cannot be drawn from one to another. Also, it will be equally important to assess their safety, immunogenicity, and efficacy at varying stages of the HIV infection. From initial data, and from theoretical expectation, children earlier in their infection should be more responsive and more likely to maintain immunity than those children who are later in the course of their HIV-induced immunodeficiency and eventually AIDS. To employ vaccines in the most beneficial fashion for this ever increasing population of patients in need, governmental agencies, academic investigators, and pharmaceutical firms will need to collaborate in developing the data base on which to formulate appropriate recommendations. Until there is a successful preventive (or even therapeutic) vaccine for HIV, one of the least expensive and most effective ways of preventing some of the viral and bacterial infections to which these children are highly susceptible will be the judicious use of available vaccines.

References

1. Katz SL. Measles in the United States: 1989 and 1990. Adv Pediatr Infect Dis 1991;6:79–90.
2. World Health Organization. EPI for the 1990s. Geneva: WHO, Mar 1992.
3. Preblud SR, Katz SL. Measles vaccine, In: Plotkin SA, Mortimer EA Jr, eds. Vaccines. Philadelphia: Saunders, 1988;182–222.
4. Mitus A, Holloway A, Evans AE, Enders JF. Attenuated measles vaccine in children with acute leukemia. Am J Dis Child 1962;103:413–418.

5. Bancroft WH. Hepatitis A vaccine. N Engl J Med 1992;327:488–490.

6. Beck-Sague C, Dooley SW, Hutton MD, et al. Hospital outbreak of multidrug-resistant *Mycobacterium tuberculosis* infections. JAMA 1992;268: 1280–1286.

7. Ho DD. HIV-I viraemia and influenza {Letter}. Lancet 1992;339:1549.

8. Report of Committee on Infectious Diseases. 22nd ed. Elk Grove Village, IL: American Academy of Pediatrics, 1991.

9. Advisory Committee on Immunization Practices. Use of vaccines and immune globulins in persons with altered immunocompetence. MMWR 1993; 42(RR-4):1–18.

10. Siber GR, Werner BG, Halsey NA, et al. Interference of immune globulin with measles and rubella immunization. J Pediatr 1993;122:204–211.

11. Kaplan LJ, Daum RS, Smaron M, McCarthy CA. Severe measles in immunocompromised patients. JAMA 1992;267:1237–1241.

12. Advisory Committee on Immunization Practices. Immunization of children infected with human immunodeficiency virus: Supplementary statement MMWR 1988;37:181–183.

13. Committee on Infectious Diseases. Measles: Reassessment of the current immunization policy. Pediatrics 1989;84: 1110–1113.

14. Embree J, Datta P, Stackiw W, et al. Increased risk of early measles in infants of human immunodeficiency virus 1-seropositive mothers. J Infect Dis 1992;165:262–267.

15. Krasinski K, Borkowsky W. Measles immunity in children infected with human immunodeficiency virus. JAMA 1989;261:2512–2516.

16. Palumbo P, Hoyt L, Demasio K, et al. Population-based study of measles and measles immunization in human immunodeficiency virus-infected children. Pediatr Infect Dis J 1992;11:1008–1014.

17. Cooper ER, Pelton SI, Brena A. Response to measles and rubella vaccine in children with HIV infection [Abstract PoB 3678]. Eighth International Conference on AIDS, Amsterdam, Jul 1992.

18. Walter EB, Katz SL, Bellini WJ. Measles immunity in HIV-infected and HIV-infected control children [Abstract]. Pediatr Res 1993;33:186A.

19. Embree J. Safety and efficacy of immunizations with live vaccines [Abstract MGO 23]. Fifth International Conference on AIDS, Montreal, Jun 1989.

20. Lallemant-Lecoeur S, Lallemant M, Cheynier D, et al. BCG immunization in infants born to HIV-1 seropositive mothers. AIDS 1991;5:195–199.

21. Ninanae J, Grymonprez A, Burtonboy G, et al. Disseminated BCG in HIV infection. Arch Dis Child 1988;63:1268–1269.

22. Bonnlander H, Rossignol AM. Complications of BCG vaccinations in rural Haiti. Am J Public Health 1993;83:583–585.

23. World Health Organization. BCG immunization and paediatric HIV infection. Wkly Epidemiol Rec 1992;18:129–132.

24. Vardinon N, Handsher R, Burke M, et al. Poliovirus vaccination responses in HIV-infected patients: Correlation with T4 cell counts. J Infect Dis 1990;162:238–241.

25. Barbi M, Bardare M, Luraschi C. Antibody response to inactivated polio vaccine (E-IPV) in children born to HIV positive mothers. Eur J Epidemiol 1992;8:211–216.

26. Borkowsky W, Steele CJ, Grubman S, et al. Antibody response to bacterial toxoids in children infected with human immunodefiency virus. J Pediatr 1987;110:563–566.

27. Ryder RW, Oxtoby MJ, Mvula M, et al. Safety and immunogenicity of BCG, DTP, and OPV in newborn children in Zaire infected with HIV-1. J Pediatr 1993;122:697–702.

28. Onorato IM, Markowitz LE, Oxtoby MJ. Childhood immunization, vaccine-preventable diseases and infection with human immunodeficiency virus. Pediatr Infect Dis J 1988;6:588–595.

29. Zuin G, Principi N, Tornaghi R, Paccagnini S. Impaired response to hepatitis B vaccine in HIV infected children. Vaccine 1992;10:857–860.

30. Mulligan MJ, Sperduto AR, Peter JB, et al. Decreased response to pneumococcal vaccine in children with HIV infection [Abstract]. Pediatr Res 1993;33:176A.

31. Glaser JB, Volpe S, Aguirre A, et al. Zidovudine improves response to pneumococcal vaccine among persons with AIDS and AIDS-related complex. J Infect Dis 1991;164:761–764.

32. Chadwick EG, Decker MD, Yogev R, et al. Serologic response to a two-dose regimen of inactivated influenza vaccine in HIV-infected children [Abstract]. Pediatr Res 1993;33:164A.

33. Steinhart R, Reingold AL, Taylor F, et al. Invasive *Haemophilus influenzae* infections in men with HIV infection. JAMA 1992;268:3350–3352.

34. Steinhoff MC, Auerbach BS, Nelson KE, et al. Antibody responses to *Haemophilus influenzae* type B vaccines in men with human immunodeficiency virus infection. N Engl J Med 1991;325: 1837–1842.

35. Indacochea FJ, Insel RA, Hamiton BL. Immunogenicity of *H. influenzae* type B (Hib) CRM 197 conjugate vaccine (HbOC) in young HIV-infected (HIV+) infants [Abstract]. Pediatr Res 1992;31: 165A.

36. Walter EB, Rosenfeld E, Edwards KM, et al. Immunogenicity of *Haemophilus influenzae* type B (HIB) polysaccharide-neisseria meningitidis outer membrane protein (PRP-OMP) conjugate vaccine in children with HIV infection [Abstract 977]. 32nd Interscience Conference on Antimicrobial Agents and Chemotherapy, Anaheim, 1992.

37. Garcia M, Villota J, Cilleruelo MJ, et al. Evaluation of varicella-zoster virus (VZV) infection and immunity after VZV vaccination in HIV-infected children [Abstract PoB 3852]. Eighth International Conference on AIDS, Amsterdam, Jul 1992.

38. Gershon AA, Steinberg SP. Varicella Vaccine Collaborative Study Group. Persistence of immunity to varicella in children with leukemia immunized with live attenuated varicella vaccine. N Engl J Med 1989;320:892–897.

39. Hardy I, Gershon AA, Steinberg SP, et al. The incidence of zoster after immunization with live attenuated varicella vaccine—a study in children with leukemia. N Engl J Med 1991;325:1545–1550.

Current Status of Vaccines for HIV

M. Juliana McElrath and Lawrence Corey

INTRODUCTION

Importance of Developing an HIV Vaccine

Human immunodeficiency virus (HIV) infection has continued to spread rapidly throughout the globe and imposes a serious threat to the health and economic welfare of most regions of the world. There are several biological, epidemiological, and behavioral characteristics of HIV that make the development of an effective vaccine one of the most important global research projects of our time. Control of the spread of HIV is a formidable goal. Infection is invariably subclinical, or mildly symptomatic (1), making prompt diagnosis of new cases unlikely even in the most sophisticated of medical settings. Once infected, HIV can be detected in genitorurinary secretions and blood within 2–4 weeks (2, 3) and persists to death, in most cases a period of more than 10 years (4). This prolonged period of consistent infectivity is nearly unprecedented for such a severe infectious disease. Current therapies do not decrease viral infectivity from genitourinary secretions (5). In addition, persistent excretion of virus in the genitourinary tract means that any epidemiological and behavioral control must be vigilant for extended periods. As with most other sexually transmitted diseases, the vast majority of infection occurs when the source contact is in the subclinical or asymptomatic period. As such, there is an ever increasing reservoir of persons capable of transmitting this infection, leading to the extension of the epidemic. Perhaps most disconcerting is that control of the behav-

ioral aspects of spread such as modifying sexual activity and injection drug use involves complex social, political, and economic issues that are often outside the purview and control of health care providers. Even the most well funded HIV control program is lacking in the fundamental resources to effectively and permanently solve the behavioral and economic problems that are key to the control of this infection. The most successful model for reducing the actual worldwide incidence and prevalence of infection of a pathogen has been the development and implementation of a vaccine, an immunogen that can stimulate host immunity. reduce infection or the excretion of virus from potentially infected sites upon subsequent exposure to the agent (6).

Goals of an HIV Vaccine

The last decade has brought forth knowledge illustrating both the difficulty in and the potential for developing an effective HIV vaccine. The ultimate goal of HIV vaccine development is to produce an immunogen that, when administered to healthy HIV-seronegative persons, would protect them from acquisition of infection by the virus, what some have termed "sterilizing immunity" (7). Ultimately one would like the exposed immunized individual to have no evidence of infection with HIV or if infected to have no evidence of infectious virus at mucosal surfaces, in blood or other organs that may promote further spread. Several daunting issues about developing an HIV vaccine are the extended time (birth through the sexually active years) that infection may be acquired, the multiple means by which infection is spread, (blood and sexual activity), and the recognition that both cell associated and cell free virus can induce infection (8). Thus, the length of time an immunization is required to maintain host immunity at "protective" levels must be prolonged. There are, however, circumstances in which protection is needed in the short term, such as in the HIV-exposed infant, the HIV-exposed health care worker, and an individual involved in a new high-risk encounter. An immunogen that could be selectively administered as prophylaxis after exposure to HIV, for example during the perinatal period or after needle stick injury or high risk sexual exposure, may also prove to be of great benefit. Unfortunately, recent studies suggest that the incubation of HIV, i.e., from exposure to the first demonstration of HIV in peripheral blood mononuclear cells, is often < 2 weeks (2, 3), making active immunization in the unprimed seronegative individuals difficult. Traditionally, the instillation of passive immunoprophylaxis (discussed below) has been more effective in such a situation.

Although sterilizing immunity is the ultimate goal, an HIV vaccine that markedly limits infection in the host, especially one that markedly decreases or even prevents detectable levels of HIV in genital secretions or blood as well as delays progression of symptomatic HIV infection would also be of utility. Although there are logistic problems inherent in the use and testing of such a product, many successful vaccines have produced such an effect and led to successful control of disease. Recent studies have also indicated that HIV antigens can induce novel immune responses to the virus already infected with the virus (9). As such, use of these immunogens to delay the progression of HIV disease has been under intense investigation. Whether such an immunotherapeutic vaccine will be clinically useful remains to be determined.

Measures of Vaccine Activity

Perhaps the most basic and formidable problem in developing an HIV vaccine is our lack of understanding of what immune responses are necessary to preventing and containing HIV-1 infection (10). Studies of the natural history of HIV-1 have provided important insights into the role of many aspects of the humoral and cellular immune responses containing infection, but proof of a serological or cell-mediated immune marker associated with reduction in virus spread or resolution of infection has been elusive. In fact, some authorities feel, that in humans there is no "protective immune response" to HIV (11). We will analyze current information on humoral, cellular, and local immune responses, recognizing that a wide range of host immune responses operate in concert and synergistically and it is likely that the best immunogens will elicit a broad spectrum of host immune responses to heterogeneous HIV-1 antigens.

Antibodies

In many virus infections, especially those in which transmission is mainly through extracellular cell-free virus, the presence of antibodies in blood and on mucosal surfaces, which are the initial site of infection, constitute the most important aspect of host protection (12). Antibodies that bind to virus and prevent cellular attachment and/or mediate cytolytic responses decreasing the quantity of the virus below detectable levels have in many situations been the mainstay of successful vaccines, e.g, poliomyelitis (13). As such, antibodies that inactivate virus in vitro either through neutralization or antibody-dependent cellular cytotoxicity have had the greatest correlation with protection against infection or resolution of infection (14). The role of neutralizing an antibody-dependent cellular cytotoxicity antibodies in HIV-1 infection is unclear. Some studies have shown that persons with higher levels of neutralizing antibodies, especially to the strain of virus with which they are infected (autologous), have a slower rate of progression than those who possess lower levels of neutralizing antibodies (15,16). However, such analyses are fraught with difficulty in that changes in virus phenotype and genotype (antigenic drift) occur over time. Additionally, autologous strains may differ significantly from the prototype strains used in the virus neutralization assay. In addition, even when autologous strains are cultured in vitro, this selects one "quasi-species" from the many viruses currently replicating in the patient (17). This may not be the predominant pathogenic strain of virus.

The principal neutralizing domain of HIV-1 is the hypervariable region on the envelope called V3 loop (18). Over the course of infection, most persons develop point mutations in this region`that reduce the ability of antibody to neutralize virus. Thus envelope virus "escape" variants emerge (19). Recently, studies of acute HIV-1 infection have shown that clearance of virus from plasma appears to occur before the development of detectable levels of V3 loop and neutralizing antibodies to the autologous isolate, suggesting other factors contribute to clearing virus from plasma (20).

On the positive side, perhaps the strongest evidence for the importance of neutralizing antibodies occurs from animal model studies. In the chimpanzee model, passive administration of high titered HIV-1 antibodies can prevent infection (21). High titered monoclonal antibodies that neutralize virus can prevent infection against homologous but not heterologous viruses (22). In the simian immunodeficiency (SIV) model, immunogens that induce neutralizing antibodies have been shown to protect animals against subsequent challenge with homologous isolates; lower levels of protection are associated with heterologous isolate challenge. However, the duration and titer of neutralizing antibodies in these macaque studies are transient, and the correlation between neutralization and protection with various vaccine products has been incomplete at best (23).

One area in which neutralizing antibodies have been less demonstrably important has been in prevention of maternal to fetal transmission. In many perinatally transmitted infections, high titers of neutralizing antibodies can prevent maternal-to-infant transmission, (e.g., neonatal herpes simplex virus infection) (24). In other infections, such as human cytomegalovirus infection, which is associated with transmission of virus infected cells, neutralizing antibodies at the onset of delivery do not appear to prevent infection in the infant but are associated with a marked reduction in subsequent disease (25). Some studies have suggested that high levels of neutralizing antibodies may be correlated with a reduction in perinatal transmission (26, 27); others have shown little or no correlation (28, 29). The problem is confounded because transplacental as well as intrapartum exposure to virus are modes of infection for the infant. Overall, most authorities believe that because HIV is found in plasma and cell free genital secretions, neutralizing antibodies are a necessary but not a sufficient correlate of protection. It is apparent from the passive immunization experiments that to be effective, neutralizing antibodies must be present at high titer, persistent and broadly reactive against a wide variety of circulating strains.

Mucosal Immune Responses

Because most HIV infections are acquired through sexual transmission, the presence of HIV-specific mucosal antibodies is assumed to be of importance. Unfortunately, little is known about the role of mucosal antibodies play reducing the acquisition of any sexually transmitted pathogens, let alone HIV (30). Among HIV-infected persons, antibodies to HIV are detected in saliva and genitourinary secretions (31–33). These antibodies are predominantly IgG, and their presence in secretions may be the result of transudation from serum. In selected instances, locally produced anti-HIV secretory IgA has been detected. However, little is known about the association between secretory IgA antibodies and virus excretion in genitourinary secretions and whether mucosal antibody responses influence acquisition in the neonate or sexual partner. In the SIV model an inactivated vaccine that was able to induce mucosal antibody responses detected by Western blotting and enzyme immunoassay subsequently protected against mucosal challenge to the homologous virus strain (34). As such, there is increasing interest in the ability of immunogens to induce mucosal immunity. At present information of currently tested vaccines to elicit and maintain mucosal antibodies to HIV is unavailable.

T Cell Responses

Several lines of evidence suggest that an effective HIV immunogen must induce long lasting T cell responses to HIV. In vitro CD8+ T cells will reduce the spread of infection in tissue culture and can eradicate HIV from chronically infected cell lines (35, 36). In addition, patients early in the disease have greater cytotoxic T lymphocyte responses to HIV than those later in the disease (37). Whether this relates to CD4+ helper dysfunction or an altered depletion of CD8+ cytotoxic T lymphocyte (CTL) precursors or both remains to be determined. One of the great mysteries of HIV infection is the high frequency of HIV specific cytotoxic T lymphocytes that are found in the peripheral blood of HIV-infected persons. It is the first disease in which the frequency of HIV T lymphocytes has allowed the direct cloning of antigen specific T cells from peripheral blood without prior amplication of precursor (38). Cytotoxic T lymphocyte responses have been directed to various HIV epitopes including the structural (env (39–41), gag, and pol) (42, 44 gene products, and the nef and rev regulatory gene products (42, 43). Immunogens that induce CD8+ CTL activity may have a broader range of effectiveness in reducing or eliminating virus infected cells early in infection. As such, there has been a quest to develop immunogens that induce CD8+ CTLs or to use immunogens in concert with adjuvants that will enhance CTL activity to HIV antigens.

T cell helper responses, determined by lymphoproliferation to various HIV-1 antigens and mitogens, have been examined at various stages of HIV disease (45, 46). Persons with higher levels of intact T cell responses appear to have a more prolonged asymptomatic clinical course than those who do not. As described earlier, the clearance of virus from plasma in those with acute symptomatic HIV infection has not been correlated with the development of neutralizing antibody (20). The role of cell-mediated immune responses (CD4 helper and CD8+ killing) in this process is being explored. However, the exact nature of the cell-mediated immune response that is most closely related to controlling HIV replication and maintaining immunologic function in the host is unclear. Similarly, the type and degree of T cell responses necessary to achieve protection against challenge in animal models is undefined. Adoptive transfer experiments or experiments in which protection from challenge in animal models is lost after depletion of antigen specific cells have not been performed. As such, current data do not provide sufficient information to determine the T cell responses to HIV-1 envelope proteins that correlate with protection.

Additional measurements of T cell function such as in vitro lymphokine production to antigens (interferon-2, interferon-α, interferon-4, interferon-6) and delayed hypersensitivity testing to skin test antigens have also been assessed in HIV-seropositive individuals and many HIV-uninfected recipients of HIV vaccines (47–49). The role of these assays in predicting disease progression and protection is unclear. All these assays have advocates; many are technically difficult, and quantitation of the responses adds another degree of difficulty. Few of these assays have as yet been employed in vaccine trials in animal models, and their role in predicting activity of an immunogen in vivo is unclear. It is clear that this is one of the areas of greatest scientific need and discovery in the field of HIV vaccines.

ANIMAL VACCINE STUDIES
Models

The development of animal models is important in understanding HIV pathogenesis and for designing strategies for prevention and treatment of HIV infection. Unfortunately, the inadequacies of existing models have contributed to a large obstacle toward progress in HIV vaccine research (see Chapter 10B). There is no relatively inexpensive and readily available animal model that can be experimentally infected with HIV-1 which will lead to an AIDS-like illness similar to that found in human disease. However, the identification of a new nonhuman primate model and the development of a monkey-human immunodeficiency virus hybrid are recent achievements that offer promise in improving the pace of vaccine studies. The features of the existing and new experimental models are described in Table 47.1 and discussed in detail below.

SIV infection in macaques, particularly *Macaca mulatta* (rhesus) and *M. fascicularis* (cynomolgus), is one established model for identification of candidate vaccines for testing in humans. This model has the advantage of eliciting immune abnormalities and an AIDS-like disease in its host within months to years, depending on the infecting SIV strain (49). Disadvantages of the system include the use of SIV, a close relative of HIV-1 but with known differences in immunodominant envelope regions (50). Unlike HIV-1, HIV-2 can infect rhesus and cynomolgus macaques, but the development of immunodeficiency is rare (51–53).

Two new macaque models await further study to determine their overall utility in HIV-1 vaccine research. A recent report by Agy and associates (54) describes the ability to infect pigtail macaques (*M. nemestrina*) with either cell associated or cell free suspensions of HIV-1. Although a portion of the animals have developed rash and lymphadenopathy characteristic of HIV-1 illness, it is not yet known if the persistent infection will lead to an AIDS-like illness in the infected animals. Another promising strategy in the developmental stage is the construction of a hybrid virus called SHIV, which contains HIV-1 *env*, *tat*, and *rev* genes with the remaining full complement of SIV genes (55). The chimeric virus can infect and produce viremia in cynomolgus macaques (*M. fascicularis*), and experiments are in progress to determine whether infected animals develop immunodeficiency disease similar to AIDS.

Numerous studies of HIV-1 infection have been performed in the chimpanzee, and to a lesser extent in the gibbon (56–58). Although the animals develop virus infection of peripheral blood lymphocytes and virus-specific antibody responses after inoculation, they show no evidence of an AIDS-like disease. The scarcity and expense of using chimps, combined with their failure to develop immunodeficiency, limit the use of the chimp/HIV-1 model in large-scale comparative vaccine trials.

Severe combined immunodeficient mice reconstituted with human peripheral blood leukocytes (hu-PBL-SCID) can be infected with various HIV-1 strains at low doses (59). This model provides an easily accessible, relatively inexpensive model for studying candidate HIV vaccines through adoptive transfer experiments. A potential drawback

Table 47.1.   Animal Models for Vaccine Studies

Animal	Virus	Disease	Comments
Rhesus, cynomolgus, and pigtail macaques	SIV_{mac} SIV_{sm}	Acute illness, AIDS-like illness, and death	Good animal availability; less relevant to HIV disease
Pigtail macaque	HIV-1	Acute illness, AIDS-like illness unknown	Good animal availability; needs further study
Rhesus, cynomolgus, and pigtail macaques	HIV-2	AIDS-like illness rare	HIV-2 genetically more related to SIV than HIV-1
Cynomolgus macaque	SHIV	Unknown	Chimeric virus lacking HIV-1 structural proteins; needs further study
Chimpanzee, gibbon	HIV-1	No AIDS-like illness	Endangered animal species, expensive
hu-PBL-SCID mouse	HIV-1	Fall in CD4 cells, altered immune function	Persistence of infection and CD8 cells unclear

with this model is that functional CD8+ T cells do not persist in the reconstituted animals and that HIV-1 infection appears to spread rapidly and ablate T cells rather than create a chronic persistent infection.

One advantage of the HIV-1 animal models is that they provide a consistent model to challenge the primate with prototype and/or clinical HIV isolates. They have utility in determining whether a particular immunogen or immuization regimen will produce sterilizing immunity. Therefore these models have been extensively utilized in exploratory studies of candidate HIV-1 vaccines.

Vaccine Trials in Animal Models

SIV Protective Vaccines

Optimism toward the development of a vaccine that can protect against HIV-1 infection stems from the recent vaccine protection studies that have been reported in the macaque/SIV, chimp/HIV, and hu-PBL-SCID/HIV-1 models. These findings are summarized in Table 47.2 and presented below.

At least 19 experiments (reviewed in Ref. 23) have shown partial to complete protection of macaques against intravenous or intramuscular homologous SIV challenge after 3 to 6 immunizations with whole inactivated SIV formulated with various adjuvants (60, 61). The antibody responses in the protected animals typically decline after boosting, and no anamnestic response is detected with challenge. Cross protection against intravenous challenge with low dose heterologous SIV strains has been reported, although the duration of protection appears to be shorter (<3 months) than with homologous virus challenge (>8 months). Significant protection against intravenous challenge with cell associated SIV has not been shown. Recently, however, Cranage and colleagues (34) were able to demonstrate protection of 4 rhesus macaques, previously immunized and resistant to intravenous SIV challenge, against intrarectal SIV challenge after vaccination and boosting with inactivated SIV. This is the first report of protection against a mucosal challenge mediated by vaccination in the

Table 47.2.   Protection Induced by Vaccination in Animal Models[a]

Vaccine	Animal	Challenge	Protection	Comments
Whole inactivated SIV	Macaque	SIV	Partial or complete	Extends to heterologous strains
Live attenuated SIV	Macaque	SIV	Partial or complete	Duration of protection long-lived
SIV vac/env + gp160	Macaque	SIV	Complete	Needs confirmation: no human cellular products
SIV envelope peptide	Macaque	SIV	Partial or complete	Abortive infection
HIV-1 rgp120	Chimp	HIV-1	Complete	Correlate of protection: anti-V3 binding antibodies
Hyperimmune IgG, anti-V3 monoclonal antibody	Chimp	HIV-1	Complete	V3 loop region important correlate for protection
CD4 immunoadhesin	Chimp	HIV-1	Complete	Pre- and postexposure protection
Adoptive transfer: PBL from vaccinees	hu-PBL-SCID	HIV-1	Partial to complete	Waning immunity after rgp160 boost

[a]V3, V3 region of HIV-1 envelope; PBL, peripheral blood lymphocytes.

macaque/SIV model. Thus far, none of the SIV vaccines administered parenterally have provided protection against cell free SIV vaginal transmission, although evidence for local IgG and IgA production in the vagina and genital lymph nodes has been found in macaques immunized with SIV *gag* particles conjugated with cholera toxin subunit (62).

Protection of macaques against SIV infection has been extended with the use of killed SIV-infected human T cells as immunogens (63). Unfortunately, recent experiments in the same laboratory have shown that two of four macaques vaccinated with uninfected human T cells were also protected against SIV challenge (64). The investigators and others have discovered that the best immune correlate of protection was anticellular rather than anti-SIV antibodies (65). These findings, a potential setback in the macaque/SIV vaccine studies, have emphasized the necessity of designing vaccine trials in which the challenge virus stock is grown in mononuclear cells compatible with the host species. However, the addition of "anticellular" immune responses to those specific for HIV-1 antigens may be one way to enhance protective immunity.

One of the recent advances in SIV vaccine studies has been the first evidence that recombinant envelope vaccines can protect against SIV challenge. Four *M. fascicularis*, immunized with recombinant vaccinia virus expressing SIVmne gp160 and boosted with gp160 derived from baculovirus-infected cells, were protected for 1 year against subsequent low-dose intravenous challenge with the homologous virus (66). Other vaccinia recombinant SIV *env* and multiple gene products trials from several laboratories using different strains for immunization and challenge have thus far been unsuccessful, despite the development of strong antibody titers against the immunogen (reviewed in Ref. 60). Although the results using vaccinia recombinants appear mixed, this approach appears to offer promise and awaits confirmation by other investigators.

Two vaccine strategies have induced immune responses that suppress but do not eliminate SIV infection upon challenge. These include immunization with recombinant SIV envelope peptides (67) and attenuated SIV live vaccine (69). In a recent study by the Desrosiers laboratory (68), rhesus monkeys vaccinated with live SIV deleted in *nef* were completely protected against intravenous challenge with fully pathogenic SIV. This live attenuated vaccine has provided the greatest success in achieving protection in the SIV model than any approach to date. It is conceivable that the initial transient infection may stimulate a stronger, more durable immune response. However, it is improbable that a live attenuated HIV vaccine would be used in humans in the near future because of concerns that the virus may revert to a virulent strain.

Pre- and Postexposure Prophylaxis in Macaques

Passive immunization with SIV$_{sm}$ or HIV-2 pooled high dose immune sera has induced protection in cynomolgus monkeys intravenously challenged 6 hr later with cell free homologous SIV or HIV-2, respectively (69). Although the design of these studies was optimized to test the hypothesis of protection with pre-exposure prophylaxis, and is unlikely to be mimicked in human clinical settings, the findings support the potential utility of passive immunization with high titer anti-HIV human antibodies to protect against accidental percutaneous exposures or vertical transmission during labor and delivery.

Several laboratories have shown that the course of infection with SIV was markedly altered for those animals that were not protected by pre-exposure administration of inactivated or modified whole virus vaccination (60, 70, 71). The animals appeared partially protected from SIV disease and survived longer than the unimmunized animals. However, studies employing similar vaccines in animals already infected with SIV have failed to demonstrate any improvement in SIV immune response or disease course (63, 72).

Chimp/HIV Vaccine Trials

The first successful HIV-1 immunization and protection study in chimpanzees was reported by Berman and associates in 1990 (73), who immunized animals with either mammalian-derived recombinant envelope glycoprotein gp120 or its precursor gp160. After HIV-1 challenge, only the gp120 immunized animals were protected, despite the presence of neutralizing antibodies in both groups when tested in vitro. The investigators found that the only humoral component that correlated with protection which was present in the gp120 but not gp160 immunized animals was antibody directed to the third hypervariable or V3 domain of the envelope. Additional evidence of the importance of the V3 domain in protection was reported by Girard et al. (74) who found two of three chimps immunized with various HIV immunogens and boosted with synthetic V3 immunogens were protected against HIV-1 challenge.

The protective role of antibodies against V3 loop gained additional support from recent passive immunization studies in chimpanzees by Emini et al. (22). One chimpanzee received anti-V3 domain-specific neutralizing monoclonal antibody 24 hr before intravenous virus challenge, and the second animal received the same immunogen 6 hr after virus challenge. Both animals were protected against HIV-1 infection. In a subsequent report, Prince et al. (21) were able to protect a chimpanzee with a low challenge dose of HIV-1 using high titer HIV-1 immunoglobulin from the pooled plasma of healthy HIV-infected persons with high titer neutralizing antibody.

Another important gp120 domain for neutralization of virus is the CD4 binding domain. Ward et al. (75) treated two chimpanzees with a hybrid CD4 immunoadhesin molecule 8 and 1 hr before HIV-1 exposure and found that the immunogen mediated protection against infection. The gp120 CD4-binding domain is a conformational epitope that exhibits broad neutralizing activity against diverse variants of HIV-1 and, like the V3 domain, appears to be of potential usefulness in achieving protection against HIV-1 through vaccination.

Significant progress in vaccine research was demonstrated by the ability to achieve protection for extended periods in three chimpanzees against challenge with HIV-infected cells by using a mixture of immunogens and boosting with V3 loop peptides (76). This work provides encouragement

that it may be possible to elicit long lasting protective immunity against cell associated HIV-1, which may be the more common mode of HIV-1 transmisson.

Hu-PBL-SCID Mice Protection Studies

Transfer of peripheral blood lymphocytes from human volunteers immunized with vac-env and boosted with rgp160 into hu-PBL-SCID mice resulted in protection in those animals receiving cells from three of four donors (77). As the interval between boosting of the vaccine and challenge increased, the ability of the reconstituted mice to resist HIV challenge was lost. In other studies, the transfer of human cytotoxic T lymphocytes specific for Nef peptides conferred partial protection against HIV-1 (78).

Correlates of Immunity for Protection against SIV and HIV

As discussed earlier, the mechanisms of vaccine protection in the macaque/SIV models remain unclear. Neutralization titers elicited with whole inactivated SIV vaccines in the protected animals were generally much lower than those demonstrated with natural SIV infection, and relative levels did not correlate with protection upon SIV challenge (23). The SIV envelope region equivalent to the HIV-1 V3 loop is much more conserved (50), and the correlation between neutralizing antibodies directed to this region and protection against SIV infection is not strong. In the SIV model, neutralizing sites other than V3 may be of greater importance for protective immunity. The recent report by Stott et al. (64) confirmed by other laboratories (65), demonstrating that protection against SIV infection using inactivated SIV vaccines appears to correlate with antibodies directed against cells in which virus was grown rather than virus antigens, complicates the interpretations of previous vaccine studies with inactivated SIV.

Both neutralizing antibody activity and T cell responses against SIV envelope were elicited in macaques protected with the vac-env vaccine followed by gp160 boosting (66). However, similar immunologic responses have been demonstrated with other vaccinia recombinant SIV envelope vaccine trials in animals that were not protected upon challenge (23). The collective results of vaccine studies in the chimp/HIV model support the protective nature of the anti-V3 loop domain (79). In addition, antibody directed against the gp120 domain responsible for binding to the CD4 receptor elicits broadly reactive neutralizing activity that can mediate protection upon challenge. As such, immunizing agents that can induce antibody reactivity to both the V3 loop and the CD4-binding domain have been investigated most intensively.

STATUS OF HIV-1 VACCINE TRIALS

The last 5 years have brought a considerable increase in testing of candidate HIV vaccine products, especially subunit envelope proteins. As described earlier, much work in this field has been directed at envelope based vaccines because of the role neutralizing antibodies and antibody-dependent cellular cytotoxicity are likely to play in preventing acquisition of infection.

The approaches reflecting the diversity of scientific thought on likely vaccine candidates are shown in Tables 47.3 and 47.4

which list the types of vaccines that are under development and that have entered clinical trials. One overriding concern in developing HIV vaccines is that of safety. This is reflected in 1) concern whether vaccination can subsequently enhance HIV-1 infection upon exposure to the agent; 2) the importance of distinguishing vaccination from natural infection and the fact that an effective immunogen may produce a positive HIV serologic test, which may complicate such diverse issues as military service, medical coverage, and travel; 3) the importance of counseling participants enrolled in trials on the experimental nature of the products and their unproven role in protection against subsequent contact with HIV-1.

Manufacturers have largely restricted HIV vaccine research to subunit vaccines, an approach that more likely guarantees safety and allows the easy differentiation between vaccination and natural infection through the use of available technology. In contrast, HIV vaccine research in animal modes has largely utilized inactivated or altered live virus vaccines. However, there are myriad logistic differences in the manufacture of a whole inactivated vaccine. Safety to laboratory workers involved in the manufacture of a vaccine that requires growth of

Table 47.3. Types of HIV Vaccines and Their Current Clinical Status[a]

Type of Vaccine	Testing Status
Live attenuated	None
Inactivated whole virus	None
Recombinant subunit proteins (HIV envelope proteins)	
gp160: baculovirus vector/alum	Phase II trials complete
gp160 vaccinia infected Vero cells	Phase I
gp120 CHO cells (IIIB and MN strains)	
Alum adjuvant	Phase II
QS 21 adjuvant	Phase I
gp120: CHO cells, SF-2 strain in MF-59 adjuvant	Phase II
gp120 yeast, SF-2 strain: MF-59 anf MF-59 MTP adjuvant	Phase II
Fusogenic envelope peptides	Phase I
gp120-cocktails	Phase I
p24-T4 particles	Phase I
Envelope stripped particles, incomplete Freund's adjuvant	(Seropositive phase II)
Modified live virus vectors	
Vaccinia/gp160 recombinant	Phase II
Vaccinia (vac/gag/pol) construct	Phase I
Avipox (gp160)	Phase I
Combination	
vac-env gp160 followed by recombinant gp160 or gp120	Phase I

[a]CHO, Chinese hamster ovary.

Table 47.4.   Vectors under Investigation for Use as Modified Live Virus Vaccines

Vaccinia
Avipox
Adenovirus
Rhinovirus
BCG
Salmonella
Hepatitis B
Adeno-associated virus

large quantities of infectious HIV-1 and the adequacy of inactivation procedures are of concern. This is especially pertinent as current assays to detect HIV are relatively insensitive. There is also a concern about inoculating even inativated HIV-1 nucleic acids. As such, no pharmaceutical manufacturer to date has utilized the inactivated whole virus HIV vaccine approach in clinical trials. One group has utilized HIV-1 particles that are stripped of gp120 and then inactivated, essentially an inactivated core protein vaccine, but only in HIV-infected volunteers (47). More recently, recombinant technology has been utilized to manufacture uninfectious "particles" by transfecting mammalian cells with recombinant viruses containing HIV-1 core and envelope proteins. This approach may thus achieve the advantages of a whole inactivated vaccine, i.e., a particle or conformation of both envelope and core immunogens. Similarly, the assurance of safety from an attenuated live virus mutant is also years away.

HIV Recombinant Proteins

Several HIV-1 recombinant proteins have entered phase I testing in humans. Most have been envelope based products. Two products have used the entire HIV-1 envelope, gp160, one purified from the recombinant protein made in baculovirus-infected insect cells and one purified from a vaccinia gp160 recombinant that expresses gp160 in Vero cells. Others have omitted the transmembrane portion of the HIV-1 envelope. These gp120 products are made in Chinese hamster ovary (mammalian) cell cultures. In addition, nonglycosylated 55,000-molecular weight envelope protein made in yeast has also been under development. Many of

these vaccine products were initially derived from the prototype HIV-LAI, which is an uncommon isolate from American and European HIV-infected patients. Because of the necessity of trying to develop strains in which neutralizing antibodies are more closely related to strains prevalent in the community, many of these vaccine approaches are being modified to incorporate an HIV-1$_{mn}$-like strain. Much of the phase I testing of HIV-1 vaccines in the United States is conducted through the five AIDS Vaccine Evaluation Units sponsored by the National Institutes of Health. To date, over 15 separate studies have been performed with candidate HIV-1 vaccines, and over 800 persons have been enrolled in clinical trials of these products. No serious adverse reactions have been noted, and side effects have been related to local immune responses that have varied with vaccine product and adjuvant. Dropouts from clinical trials have been infrequent, and as described below, almost all these vaccines have proven to be in some way immunogenic.

gp160 PROTEINS

A series of trials utilizing doses from 40 to 160 mg of a recombinant baculovirus-derived product, HIV-LAI gp160, have been conducted by several investigative teams. The rgp160 is clearly immunogenic; increasing doses are associated with increasing antibody titers to the immunogen and to denatured HIV proteins and EIA antibodies to gp160 (80). Unfortunately, however, antibody responses to the immunogen tend to be transient and rapidly fall, even with multiple boosts. A vaccination regimen of four 320-μg doses administered at 0, 1, 6, 12, and 18 months produces antibody responses that are detectible for 6–9 months after immunization by Western blot and EIA assays. However, neutralizing antibodies are seen in only about 30% of vaccines, are of low titer, and are of short duration (3 months) and directed only to the homologous HIV-1 (81). Development of this gp160 baculovirus-derived protein for use in HIV-1 seropositives (see below) is proceeding (9), but in noncomparative studies the gp120 products in Chinese hamster ovary cells have elicited higher levels of neutralizing antibodies to HIV-1. The gp160 protein purified from gp160-infected Vero cells has been studied less extensively and at lower doses than gp160 baculovirus-derived protein, also appears to be immunogenic, and has shown somewhat higher reactogenicity with respect to local reactions compared with the baculovirus-derived gp160 (82). It is of interest to examine preliminary data that compared with studies using gp120 proteins. The two gp160 products appear to elicit poorer neutralizing antibodies, suggesting that there may be "immunosuppressive" elements on gp41 that may influence the humoral immune responses to these proteins.

gp120 PROTEINS

The gp120 vaccines made in Chinese hamster ovary cells have provided the most optimism concerning the use of a recombinant envelope protein for an immunoprophylactic vaccine. Two separate vaccines have been evaluated by the National Institute of Allergy and Infectious Diseases AIDS Vaccine Evaluation Group (AVEG), one an HIV-1 IIIB rgp120 protein in an alum adjuvant and its counterpart derived from the HIV/MN strain and the other an rgp120 protein derived from the HIV-1 SF-2 strain, an isolate from an HIV-infected patient in San Francisco. The rgp120 (HIV-1 SF-2 strain) is mixed with an adjuvant called MF-59, which is an oil emulsion that enhances immunogenicity. By using vaccine regimens of 0, 1, 6, or 8 months, both mammalian-derived rgp120 vaccines have elicited neutralizing antibody titers to the homologous HIV strain in 70–90% of recipients when measured 2–4 weeks after the third dose (83, 84). The duration of neutralizing antibody titer is under study. The neutralization titers appear about 20-fold lower than those seen in asymptomatic seropositives infected with HIV. But other aspects of immunogenicity such as binding titers to the immunogen itself, gp120, appear similar to those seen in asymptomatic seropositives. Both vaccines elicit antibodies to the CD4 binding site of HIV-1, and both vaccines have been well tolerated. Further phase II testing of these vaccines is underway, and the goal is to evaluate the immunogenicity of these proteins in a more general population, including sexual partners of HIV seropositives and persons attending sexually transmitted diseases clinics who are thus at higher risk for acquiring HIV infection.

Another envelope-based product made in a yeast protein of 55,000 molecular weight has also entered into clinical trials and has also been well tolerated (85). It has been made from the SF-2 strain of HIV-1 and also includes the MF-59 adjuvant described above. Of interest, neutralizing antibody titers have been seen in 50–70% of recipients at almost similar titers to those of the fully glycosylated mammalian-derived gp120 product. This is of interest in that it suggests that neutralizing epitopes of the SF-2 strain of HIV-1 are directed at many non-V3 nonglycosylated sites.

Are these recombinant envelope proteins sufficiently immunogenic to warrant continued evaluation? The utility of the recombinant soluble proteins is primarily directed toward the development of humoral antibodies. At present, neutralizing antibodies have been active against the homologous virus type and appear to be of somewhat lower magnitude than those seen in HIV-1 seropositive individuals. However, testing of sera from HIV-1-uninfected volunteers immunized with these regimens against a battery of recent isolates in the United States and Europe is underway. In addition, cocktails of gp120 antigens from vaccine strains are being prepared to evaluate multivalent vaccines that may elicit a broader immune response. None of the recombinant soluble proteins have elicited detectable CD8+ CTL activity. As discussed above, further work on correlates of protection will need to be developed to determine the extent to which these vaccines are appropriate for movement into large scale efficacy trials.

Modified Live Virus Vaccines

Because infection with cell associated HIV has been well demonstrated, vaccine regimens that will elicit cytotoxic T cell responses are under development. Traditionally, live attenuated vaccines have been the model used to enhance cell mediated immune responses and long lasting protective immunity. As discussed earlier, this appears to be a remote possibility for use as an HIV vaccine in humans because of safety considerations. To combine the advantages of live virus and subunit approaches, investigators have inserted HIV-1 genes into live virus vectors. Administration of the vector elicits immune responses to both the vector and the desired HIV gene product. Several such approaches have been described (Table 47.4) that include viral, mycobacterial, and bacterial delivery systems.

The modified subunit vaccine that has received the most testing in the HIV area has been a vaccinia recombinant in which the HIV-1 gp160 gene has been inserted (vac-env) (86). A vaccinia recombinant that includes *env* and other genes (*gag* and part of *pol*) has also been developed (87). The vac-env vaccine has entered phase I studies. It has been shown to be genetically stable and to induce both humoral and cellular immune responses to HIV envelope (88, 89). One major limitation with the use of a vaccinia recombinant has been that those who have had previous vaccinia immunization, even if distant in time, mount a strong anamnestic response to vaccinia such that the immune response to HIV gp160 is often inferior and obscured. Vaccinia naive subjects respond much better immunologically. The cellular immune responses to gp160 in vaccinia naive subjects are stronger and of longer duration than those of recombinant proteins, consistent with the paradigm that these live virus vectors elicit better cellular responses than recombinant proteins. However, recombinant soluble proteins appear to induce antibodies of grater magnitude and frequency.

As a means of augmenting the advantages of both responses, investigators have begun to develop HIV vaccines that can be used in combination regimens. The regimen that has been investigated more closely has been the combination of vaccinia recombinant "priming" followed by recombinant subunit protein boosting. This appears to offer some advantages of both types of vaccine approaches. Immunization with vac/env elicits the T cell priming such that subsequent recombinant protein boosting results in more marked neutralizing antibodies than either vaccine alone (90, 91). The combination vaccine regimen has, to date, been the only one that has been associated with the induction of major histocompatibility complex class I restriced CD8+ CTL responses to HIV envelope (90, 92). Further studies of combination approaches in which the subunit gp120 proteins are used as the boosting vectors are underway.

Nonetheless, vaccinia as a vector offers several concerns. One advantage of vaccinia is that recombinant protein inoculated in a localized area can be contained by a bandage, and hence under carefully controlled conditions spread to immunosuppressed patients can be minimized if not eliminated. However, under field conditions in developing countries, containment may be more difficult to achieve, so a safer vector is desired. Approaches taken to circumvent this limitation have been to construct an attenuated recombinant vaccinia or to use relatively less infectious pox viruses. One candidate under development is a canary pox vector. This virus can infect avian fibroblasts but induces one round of replication in the human host (93). Because it causes an abortive infection, the risk of transmission to immunocompromised patients is minimized. Recombinant avipox has been used to immunize against rabies glycoproteins (94) and an avipox gp160 recombinant is about to enter human clinical trials in the United States. Another approach is to insert HIV-1 into BCG vaccine (95). This vector appears to offer similar advantages to vaccinia with the potential benefit that if necessary antimycobacterial therapy could be utilized to contain the recombinant. Other approaches include the use of recombinant adenovirus and *Salmonella* vectors. These vectors offer the attractiveness of oral administration, prolonged replication, and perhaps induction of enhanced mucosal immunity. However, the issues of inapparent immunization through fecal-oral spread of live vaccine strains will have to be handled both from an investigation and liability point of view.

Although there are several lines of evidence, as discussed above, to show that envelope proteins are essential in the pathogenesis and potential protection against HIV, there are also data to suggest that other virus structural proteins may be important in protection and should be considered in the development of candidate immunogens to HIV. Perhaps the best evidence for this relates to the HIV Gag protein. In HIV-seropositive patients the predominant CD8+ CTL responses are directed against the nonenvelope gene products including Gag and reverse transcriptase proteins (38). Similarly, anti-p24 antibodies decrease over time as HIV p24 antigen increases over time in HIV disease, which suggests that immune responses to epitopes of the Gag protein may be important in pathogenesis. The inclusion of HIV Gag proteins in HIV immunogens has been approached in a manner similar to HIV envelope (96). A Gag particle vaccine has been developed in which whole HIV virions are treated with a detergent, which removes the envelope protein, and then inactivating it with Formalin. Similarly, a recombinant approach has been utilized in which *gag* gene products are made in a yeast vector. In addition, a peptide vaccine containing the p18 product has been synthesized and utilized in clinical trials. Work on these vaccines is still in its infancy.

Vaccines that include both *env* and *gag* gene products offer theoretical advantages of both approaches. Again, work in this area is just being initiated. A vaccinia recombinant that includes HIV envelope with a truncated *gag-pol* gene is entering clinical trials (87), and noninfectious particles containing the same structural genes have been snythesized by several groups.

ROLE OF HIV VACCINES IN PREGNANCY AND INFANTS

Immune Responses

Prevention of vertical transmission of HIV infection is a high priority in the design of vaccine trials in both HIV-uninfected and -infected individuals. The long-term goals of developing vaccines in the maternal-infant setting are to delay progression of HIV-1 infection in the HIV-infected mother and to prevent transmission of HIV-1 infection in the fetus or neonate. The mechanisms of transmission of HIV infection from mother to fetus or neonate are under study and bear relevance to the design and implementation of any intervention intended to prevent this process. However, the urgent need to halt the spread of neonatal infection precludes further delays of perinatal vaccine trials, and it is hoped that as the trials proceed, information regarding transmission and pathogenesis can be obtained simultaneously.

Strategies to modify HIV-1 infection in pregnant women by immunization have had to await safety information from nonpregnant seronegative and seropositive vaccine trials (see Table 47.1). Certainly, immune responses may be altered as a result of pregnancy alone, which may contribute to increased host susceptibility to various pathogens, including HIV-1 infection. In a prospective study of immunologic changes during and after pregnancy in women from high risk groups, the loss of CD4+ cells in HIV-infected pregnant women was more rapid than in the postpartum period (97). A higher rate of disease progression has been reported in those mothers who transmit HIV-1 to the infant than in those who bear uninfected infants (98), but this may relate to more advanced disease at the onset of pregnancy. However, there is no evidence that AIDS progresses at an accelerated rate in pregnancy. Undoubtedly, the pregnant HIV-1-infected woman may benefit as much if not more from any intervention that demonstrates promise in the nonpregnant infected individual.

Evidence from various case reports indicates that vertical transmission of HIV-1 infection may occur during the intrauterine, peripartum, or postpartum period. Risk factors in HIV+ mothers reported to be associated with vertical transmission include CD4 counts of <400 cells/μl, advanced HIV-1 disease, p24 antigenemia, and previous delivery of HIV+ offspring (99). Prematurity may correlate with an increased incidence of HIV-1 infection in the newborn. Although the data are conflicting, some studies have indicated that HIV+ pregnant mothers with high HIV-1 anti-gp120 antibody titers, specifically to the V3 loop region, are less likely to transmit HIV infection to their offspring (26, 27). Cessation of breast feeding could reduce the incidence of postpartum vertical transmission of HIV-1 from the infected mother to child (100), but the magnitude of this reduction is undefined.

It is believed that most HIV-1 infection of the fetus occurs during the perinatal period, a time when immunization is more likely to be successful in the prevention of peripartum transmission. If the fetus is infected in utero before identification of the mother as pregnant and HIV infected, obviously vaccination is unlikely to reverse this event. Second, the maximum transfer of maternal IgG through the placenta to the fetus occurs toward the later stages of pregnancy (101), which is thereby more likely to be of benefit in preventing perinatal transmission rather than earlier intrauterine transmission.

There are two theoretical concerns for the fetus with active maternal immunization: antigenic tolerance and enhancement of infection. Ideally, the immune system should respond to foreign antigen but ignore self antigens. Immunological tolerance in humans is believed to evolve during the perinatal period with the exposure of self antigens to immature lymphocytes. Several mechanisms have been proposed for the induction of tolerance in B and T lymphocytes, including clonal deletion, clonal anergy, and suppression (102, 103). Among the relevant HIV and SIV animal models, vertical transmission has not been demonstrated. There is no evidence to support the possibility that the fetus will develop tolerance or active immunity with active HIV-1 vaccination of the mother. But because the induction of T cell tolerance during the fetal period is believed to terminate before birth, and optimal transfer of maternal IgG antibody to the fetus is reportedly within the last month of gestation, active immunization of the mother is a potentially important strategy to investigate.

Alternatively, there is the possibility that induction of immune responses in the pregnant HIV+ woman may lead to antibody-mediated enhancement in the mother and/or the fetus. Enhancing antibodies, distinct from neutralizing antibodies, facilitate uptake of virus by binding of the virus-antibody complex to the Fc and/or complement receptor of the host cell (104, 105). This phenomenon has been described in several in vitro virus infection systems, and there is some evidence to suggest that the effect may exacerbate disease in vivo owing to dengue, West Nile, and yellow fever viruses.

Antibody-mediated enhancement has been reported in vitro with HIV-1 infection through both the Fc and complement-mediated mechanisms, but there is no evidence that antibody-mediated enhancement has a significant impact on clinical HIV-1 disease, nor has such an effect been relevant in HIV-1 or SIV vaccine trials with subsequent viral challenge in animal models (106).

Immune based intervention in the maternal-infant setting is likely to involve both active and passive immunization. In the long term, the most reasonable approach would include active immunization of the mother as early as the second trimester of pregnancy, followed by active and passive immunization of the newborn analogous to that used to prevent hepatitis B transmission in neonates from mothers who are carriers. To carefully assess the safety and immunogenicity induced by immunization, the active and passive strategies must initially be examined in separate trials. The relevant approaches under study or planned is outlined in Table 47.5 and described below.

Phase I Trials

Two phase I placebo-controlled trials (AVEG 102 and 104) in HIV-1-infected pregnant women using recombinant envelope products are scheduled to begin in 1993 under the sponsorship of the National Institutes of Health Vaccine Research and Development Branch. The objective of these studies is to evaluate the safety and immunogenicity of the candidate vaccine in asymptomatic HIV+ mothers and the passive acquisition of vaccine-specific antibody in the infant. Each volunteer will receive up to five immunizations during pregnancy, with an option for additional boosts postpartum. Should these studies conclude that the immunogens are safe for the mother and fetus, and induce or boost responses to HIV-1 specific epitopes in the mother, expanded phase II and efficacy trials will likely be considered. It is reasoned that stimulation of maternal HIV-specific immune responses through active immunization may reduce the quantity of cell free and/or cell associated HIV-1 in the mother, as well as induce antibody that upon migration through the placenta to the fetus may neu-

Table 47.5.   HIV Vaccine Studies Relevant to Maternal to Infant HIV-1 Transmission

Trial	Vaccine	HIV-1 Strain	Vaccine Developer	Target Population	Comments
AVEG 007B	rgp120	SF-2	BIOCINE	HIV uninfected	Five 1-month injections; similar schedule in pregnancy trials
AVEG 003	rgp160	LAI	MicroGene Sys	HIV uninfected	Same product to be tested in AVEG 102; safety in seronegatives
AVEG 009	rgp120	MN	Genentech	HIV uninfected	Same product to be tested in AVEG 104; safety in seronegatives
Army	rgp160	LAI	MicroGene Sys	HIV uninfected	Same product to be tested in AVEG 102; safety in seropositives
AVEG 103	rgp120	SF-2	BIOCINE	HIV infected	Safety data regarding immunization in seropositives
AVEG 102	rgp160	LAI	MicroGene Sys	HIV infected pregnant women	Up to five immunizations; placebo control; 18-month follow-up, option of booster postpartum
AVEG 104	rgp120	MN	Genentech	HIV infected pregnant women	Up to five immunizations; placebo control, 18-month follow-up; option of booster postpartum
ACTG 185	Hyper HIV IgG	Pooled HIV + plasma	Unknown	HIV infected pregnant women	Combined trial with zidovudine HIVIG to be given monthly to women and within 12 hr of delivery to newborn

tralize potential HIV-1 in the fetus. It will be important to assess any measurable effects on the maternal virus burden before the initiation of larger trials.

HIV hyperimmune globulin (HIVIG), containing concentrates of high antibody titers to HIV-1 structural proteins derived from pooled plasma of asymptomatic HIV+ persons, has been evaluated in a few small phase I human studies (107). These studies have demonstrated that the product is safe and well tolerated at 50–200 mg/kg and that no enhancement of HIV-1 infection occurs. A phase II/III study (AIDS Clinical Trials Group 185) began in September 1993 to investigate the potential for HIVIG in combination with zidovudine to prevent vertical HIV-1 transmission. The large multicenter study has

been delayed because of liability concerns by the manufacturer of the HIVIG (108).

Potential obstacles remain before moving forward with the investigation of immunization in the maternal-infant setting. One major limitation in proceeding with perinatal intervention trials is the relatively large number of HIV+ mother-infant pairs needed to determine clinical efficacy. Competing chemotherapeutic studies reduce the availability of volunteers eligible to enroll in future vaccine studies. Understanding and compliance with the protocols may be difficult for those women who belong to high risk behavior groups, particularly because the theoretical risk associated with vaccination must be carefully explained and understood. Legal issues concerning liability and indemnification must be seriously addressed by the national governmental agencies. Expansion of trials outside the United States should be considered, but the infrastructure to conduct these trials must be in place.

Despite these barriers, the momentum to intervene in HIV-1 perinatal transmission is now apparent, and it is anticipated that future studies will be designed so that the findings from each can be assessed in parallel. Furthermore, the vaccine trials will hopefully provide new information on the natural history of HIV-1 infection during pregnancy and infancy and will expand our knowledge about the correlates of immunity to prevent HIV-1 infection that will be useful in development of preventive HIV-1 vaccines.

SUMMARY

In conclusion, the area of HIV vaccine development has proceeded at a steady pace in the last 4–5 years. Several candidate immunogens and approaches have been identified that have given promising leads, especially with respect to eliciting neutralizing antibodies to HIV-1. The vaccines have shown excellent safety, indicating the feasibility of developing a safe HIV vaccine that will be well tolerated and that is immunogenic. The issues facing vaccine developers are whether characteristics of correlative immunity can be defined and the type of immune response that will provide long lasting protection against a wide variety of strains and protect from sexual and parenteral exposure to virus be produced. The magnitude of the HIV problem suggests that there will be enormous benefits if we can set realistic expectations for an HIV vaccine. Most authorities do not feel that a first generation vaccine will achieve the 95% protective efficacy seen with polio and measles. However, a vaccine that will reduce the incidence of infection and transmissibility by 60–70% would still have an enormous impact upon slowing the incredible spread of this fatal disease and offer enormous potential economic and humanitarian benefit to developed and underdeveloped countries. As such, the rapid development and testing of an HIV vaccine seems to be the highest priority research in the field of HIV, if not all infectious diseases.

References

1. Fauci AJ. Immuno pathogenic mechanisms in human immunodeficiency virus (HIV) infection. Ann Intern Med 1991;114:678–693.
2. Daar ES, Moudgil T, Meyer RD, Ho DD. Transient high levels of viremia in patients with primary human immunodeficiency virus type 1 infection. N Engl J Med 1991;324:961–964.
3. Clark SJ, Saag MS, Decker WD, et al. High titered cytopathic virus in plasma of patients with symptomatic primary HIV-1 infection. N Engl J Med 1991;324:954–960.
4. Pantaleo G, Grazios C, Fauci AJ. The immunopathogenesis of human immunodeficiency virus infection. N Engl J Med 1993;328:327–335.
5. Herrin Y, Mandelbrot L, Henrion R, Pradinaud R, Coulaud JP, Montagnier L. Virus excretion in the cervicovaginal secretions of pregnant and nonpregnant HIV-infected women. J Acquir Immune Defic Syndr 1993;6:72–75.
6. Fauci AS, Gallo RC, Koenig S, Salk J, Purcell RH. Development and evaluation of a vaccine for human immunodeficiency virus (HIV) infection. Ann Intern Med 1989;110:373–385.
7. Bolognesi DP. AIDS vaccines: Progress and current challenges. Ann Intern Med 1991;114:161–162.
8. Bolognesi DP. HIV immunization. Fresh pathways to follow. Nature 1990;344:818–819.
9. Redfield RR, Birx DL, Ketter N, et al. A phase I evaluation of the safety and immunogenicity of vaccination with recombinant gp160 in patients with early human immunodeficiency virus infection. N Engl J Med 1991;324:1677–1684.
10. Ada G, Koff W, Petricciani J. The next steps in HIV vaccine development. AIDS Res Hum Retroviruses 1992;8:1317–1319.
11. Sabin AB. Improbability of effective vaccination against human immunodeficiency virus because of its intracellular transmission and rectal portal of entry. Proc Natl Acad Sci USA 1992;89:8852–8855.
12. Bolognesi DP. Prospects for prevention of and early intervention against HIV. JAMA 1989;261:3007–3013.
13. Fox JP. Modes of action of poliovirus vaccines and relation to resulting immunity. Rev Infect Dis 1984;6:5352–5355.
14. Weinhold KJ, Lyerly HK, Matthews TJ, et al. Cellular anti-gp120 cytolytic reactivities in HIV-1 seropositive individuals. Lancet 1988;1:902–905.
15. Albert J, Abrahamsson B, Nagy K, et al. Rapid development of isolate-specific neutralizing antibodies after primary HIV-1 infection and consequent emergence of virus variants which resist neutralization by autologous sera. AIDS 1990;4:107–112.
16. Arendrup M, Nielsen C, Hansen JES, Pederson C, Mathiesen L, Nielsen JO. Autologous HIV-1 neutralizing antibodies: Emergence of neutralization-resistant escape virus and subsequent development of escape virus neutralizing antibodies. J Acquir Immune Defic Synd 1992:5:303–307.

17. Meyerhans A, Cheynier R, Albert J, et al. Temporal fluctuations in HIV quasispecies in vivo are not reflected by sequential HIV isolations. Cell 1989;58:901–910.
18. LaRosa GJ, Davide YP, Weinhold K, et al. Conserved sequence and structural elements in the HIV-1 principal neutralizing determinant. Science 1990;249:932–935.
19. Simmonds P, Zhang LQ, McOmish F, Balfe P, Ludlam CA, Leigh Brown AJ. Discontinuous sequence change of human immunodeficiency virus (HIV) type 1 *env* sequences in plasma viral and lymphocyte-associated proviral populations in vivo: Implications for models of HIV pathogenesis. J Virol 1991;65:6266–6276.
20. Ariyoshi K, Harwood E, Chiengsong-Popov R, Weber J. Is clearance of HIV-1 viremia at seroconversion mediated by neutralising antibodies? Lancet 1992;340:1257–1258.
21. Prince AM, Ressink H, Pascual D, et al. Prevention of HIV infection by passive immunization with HIV immunoglobulin. AIDS Res Hum Retroviruses 1991;7:971–973.
22. Emini EA, Schlief WA, Nunberg JH, et al. Prevention of HIV-1 infection in chimpanzees by gp120 V_3 domain-specific monoclonal antibody. Nature 1992;355:728–730.
23. Gardner MB, Hu S-L. SIV vaccines, 1991—a year in review. AIDS 1991;5:S115–S127.
24. Brown ZA, Benedetti J, Ashley R, et al. Neonatal herpes simplex virus infection in relation to asymptomatic maternal infection at the time of labor. N Engl J Med 1991;324:1247–1252.
25. Medearis DN Jr. CMV immunity: Imperfect but protective. N Engl J Med 1982;306:985–986.
26. Goedert JJ, Mendez H, Drummond JE, et al. Mother-to-infant transmission of human immunodeficiency virus type 1: Association with prematurity and low anti-gp120. Lancet 1989;2: 1351–1354.
27. Rossi P, Moschese V, Broliden PA, et al. Presence of maternal antibodies to human immunodeficiency virus 1 envelope glycoprotein gp120 epitopes correlates with the uninfected status of children born to seropositive mothers. Proc Natl Acad Sci USA 1989;86;8055–8058.
28. Parekh BS, Shaffer N, Parr CP, et al. Lack of correlation between maternal antibodies to V_3 loop peptides of gp120 and perinatal HIV-1 transmission. AIDS 1991;5:1179–1184.
29. Halsey NA, Markham R, Wahren B, Bonloc R, Rossi P, Wigzell H. Lack of association between maternal antibodies to V_3 loop peptides and maternal-infant HIV-1 transmission. J Acquir Immune Defic Syndr 1992;5:153–157.
30. Forrest BD. Mucosal approaches to HIV vaccine development. AIDS Res Hum Retroviruses 1992; 8:1523–1526.
31. Behets FM, Edidi B, Quinn TC, et al. Detection of salivary HIV-1 specific IgG antibodies in high-risk populations in Zaire. J Acquir Immune Defic Syndr 1991;4:183–187.
32. Shoeman RL, Pottathid R, Metroka C. Antibodies to HIV in saliva. N Engl J Med 1989;320:1145–1146.
33. Archibald DW, Witt DJ, Craven DE, Vogt MW, Hirsch MS, Essex M. Antibodies to human immunodeficiency virus in cervical secretions from women at risk for AIDS. J Infect Dis 1987;156: 240–241.
34. Cranage MP, Baskerville A, Ashworth LAE, et al. Intrarectal challenge of macaques vaccinated with formalin-inactivated simian immunodeficiency virus. Lancet 1992;339:273–274.
35. Walker CM, Moody DJ, Stites DP, Levy JA. CD8+ lymphocytes can control HIV infection in vitro by suppressing virus replication. Science 1986;234:1563–1566.
36. Tsubota H, Lord CI, Watkins DI, Morimoto C, Letvin NL. A cytotoxic T-lymphocyte inhibits AIDS virus replication in peripheral blood lymphocytes. J Exp Med 1989;169:1421–1434.
37. Hoffenbach A, Langlade-Demoyen P, Dadaglio G, et al. Unusually high frequencies of HIV-specific cytotoxic T lymphocytes in humans. J Immunol 1989;142:452–462.
38. Walker BD, Plata F. Editorial review: Cytotoxic T lymphocytes against HIV. AIDS 1990;4:177–184.
39. Plata F, Autran B, Pedroza-Martins L, et al. AIDS virus-specific cytotoxic T-lymphocytes in lung disorders. Nature 1987;328:348–351.
40. Walker BD, Chakrabarti S, Moss B, et al. HIV-specific cytotoxic T-lymphocytes in seropositive individuals. Nature 1987;328:345–348.
41. Koenig S, Earl P, Powell D, et al. Group-specific, MHC class-I restricted cytotoxic responses to HIV-1 envelope proteins by cloned peripheral blood T-cells from an HIV-1-infected individual. Proc Natl Acad Sci USA 1988;85:8638–8642.
42. Riviere Y, Tanneau-Salvadori F, Regnault A, et al. Human immunodeficiency virus-specific cytotoxic responses of seropositive individuals: Distinct types of effector cells mediate killing of targets expressing gag and env proteins. Virology 1989;63:2270–2277.
43. Nixon DF, Townsend ARM, Elvin JG, Rizza CR, Gallwey J, McMichael AJ. HIV-1 gag-specific cytotoxic T-lymphocytes defined with recombinant vaccinia virus and synthetic peptides. Nature 1988;336:484–487.
44. Walker BD, Flexner C, Paradis TJ, et al. HIV-1 reverse transcriptase is a target for cytotoxic T-lymphocytes in infected individuals. Science 1988;240:64–66.
45. Lange HC, Depper JM, Greene WC, Whalen G, Waldmann TA, Fauci AS. Quantitative analysis of immune function in patients with the acquired immunodeficiency syndrome. Evidence for a selective defect insoluble antigen recognition. N Engl J Med 1985;313:79–84.
46. Miedema F, Petit AJC, Terpstra FG, et al. Immunological abnormalities in human immunodeficiency virus (HIV)-infected asymptomatic homosexual men. J Clin Invest 1988;82:1908–1914.
47. Slade H, Turner J, Abrams C, Coulo D, Salle J. Immunotherapy of HIV-seropositive patients; preliminary report on a dose-ranging study. AIDS Res Hum Retroviruses 1992;8:1329–1331.
48. Clerici M, Stocks Ni, Zajac RA, et al. Detection of three distinct patterns of T helper cell dysfunction in asymptomatic, human immunodeficiency virus-seropositive patients. J Clin Invest 1989;84: 1892–1899.

49. Letvin NL, Daniel MD, Sehgal PK, et al. Induction of AIDS-like disease in macaque monkeys in T-cell tropic STLV-III. Science 1985;230:71–73.

50. Putney S. The principal neutralization determinant of SIV is different from HIV-1 [Abstract THA 14]. Seventh International Conference on AIDS, Florence, Jun 1991.

51. Dormont D, Livartowski J, Charmaret, et al. HIV-2 in rhesus monkeys: Serological, virological and clinical results. Intervirology 1989;30(suppl 30):59–65.

52. Putkonen P, Bottiger B, Warsedt K, Thorstensson R, Albert J, Biberfeld G. Experimental infection of cynomolgus monkeys (*Macaca fascicularis*) with HIV-2. J Acquir Immune Defic Syndr 1989;2: 366–373.

53. Nicol I, Flammino-Zola G, Dubouch P, et al. Persistent HIV-2 infection of rhesus macaques, baboons and mangabeys. Intervirology 1989;30: 258–667.

54. Agy MB, Frumkin LR, Corey L, et al. Infection of *Macaca nemestrina* by human immunodeficiency virus type-1. Science 1992;257:103–106.

55. Li J, Lord CI, Haseltine W, Letvin NL, Sodroski J. Infection cynomologus monkeys with a chimeric HIV-1/SIV$_{mac}$ virus that expresses the HIV-1 envelope glycoproteins. J Acquir Immun Defic Syndr 1992;5:639–646.

56. Alter HJ, Eichberg JW, Masur H, et al. Transmission of HTLV-III infection from human plasma to chimpanzees: An animal model for AIDS. Science 1984;226:549–552.

57. Fultz PN, McClure HM, Swenson RB, et al. Persistent infection of chimpanzees with human T-lymphotropic virus type III/lymphadenopathy associated virus: A potential model for acquired immunodeficiency syndrome. J Virol 1986;58: 116–124.

58. Goudsmit JC, Debouck C, Meloen RH, et al. Human immunodeficiency virus type 1 neutralization epitope with conserved architecture elicits early type-specific antibodies in experimentally infected chimpanzees. Proc Natl Acad Sci USA 1988;85:4478–4482.

59. Mosier DE, Gulizia RJ, Baird SM, Wilson DB, Spector DH, Spector SA. Human immunodeficiency virus infection of human PBL-SCID mice. Science 1991;251:791–794.

60. Desrosiers R, Wyand M, Kodana T, et al. Vaccine protection against simian immunodeficiency virus infection. Proc Natl Acad Sci USA 1989;86: 6353–6357.

61. Murphey-Corb M, Martin LN, Davison-Fairburn B, et al. A formalin-inactivated whole SIV vaccine confers protection in macaques. Science 1989; 246:1293–1297.

62. Lehner T, Bergmeier LA, Panagiotidi C, et al. induction of mucosal and systemic immunity to a recombinant simian immunodeficiency viral protein. Science 1992;258:1365–1368.

63. Stott EJ, Chan WL, Mills K. Preliminary report: Protection of cynomolgus macaques against simian immunodeficiency virus by fixed infected-cell vaccine. Lancet 1990;336:1538–1541.

64. Stott EJ, Kitchin PA, Page M, et al. Anticell antibody in macaques. Nature 1991;253:393.

65. Langlois AJ, Weinhold KJ, Matthews TJ, Greenberg ML, Bolognesi DP. The ability of certain SIV vaccines to provoke reactions against normal cells. Science 1992;255:292–293.

66. Hu S-L, Abrams K, Barker GN, et al. Protection of macaques against SIV infection by subunit vaccines of SIV envelope glycoprotein gp160. Science 1991;255:456–459.

67. Shafferman A, Jahrling PB, Benveniste RE, et al. Protection of macaques with a simian immunodeficiency virus envelope peptide vaccine based on conserved human immunodeficiency virus type 1 sequences. Proc Natl Acad Sci USA 1991;88: 7126–7130.

68. Daniel MD, Kirchloff F, Czajak SC, Sehgal PK, Desrosiers RC. Protective effects of a live attenuated SIV vaccine with a deletion in the *nef* gene. Science 1992;258:1938–1941.

69. Putkonen P, Thorstensson R, Ghavarnzadeh L, et al. Prevention of HIV-1 and SIV^{sm} infection by passive immunization in cynomolgus monkeys. Nature 1991;352:436–438.

70. Sutjipto S, Pedersen N, Miller CJ, et al. Inactivated whole simian immunodeficiency virus vaccine fails to protect rhesus macaques from intravenous or genital mucosal infection but delays the subseqent disease course of intravenously exposed animals. J Virol 1990;64:2290–2294.

71. Marthas ML, Sutjipto S, Higgins J, et al. Immunization with a live, attenuated simian immunodeficiency virus (SIV) prevents early disease but not infection in rhesus macaques challenged with pathogenic SIV. J Virol 1990;64:3694–3700.

72. Gardner JB, Jennings M, Carlson JR, et al. Post-exposure immunotherapy of simian immunodeficiency virus (SIV)-infected rhesus with an SIV immunogen. J Med Primatol 1989;18:321–328.

73. Berman PW, Gregory TJ, Riddle L, et al. Protection of chimpanzees from infection by HIV-1 after vaccination with recombinant glycoprotein gp120 but not gp160. Nature 1990;345: 662–625.

74. Girard M, Kieny M-P, Pinter A, et al. Immunization of chimpanzees confers protection against challenge with human immunodeficiency virus. Proc Natl Acad Sci USA 1991;88:542–546.

75. Ward RHR, Capon DJ, Jeh CM, et al. Prevention of HIV-1 IIIB infection in chimpanzees by CD4 immunoadhesin. Nature 1991;352:434–436.

76. Fultz PN, Nara P, Barre-Sinoussi F, et al. Vaccine protection of chimpanzees against challenge with HIV-1-infected peripheral blood mononuclear cells. Science 1992;256:1687–1690.

77. Mosier DE, Gulizia RJ, MacIsaac PD, et al. Resistance to HIV infection of SCID mice reconstituted with periperal blood leukocytes from donors vaccinated with vaccinia-gp160 and recombinant gp160. Proc Natl Acad Sci USA 1993; 90:2243–2247.

78. Groopman JE. Of mice, monkeys and men. Nature 1991;349:568-569.

79. Biberfield G, Emini EA. Progress with HIV vaccines. AIDS 1991;5(suppl 2):5129–5133.

80. Dolin R, Graham B, Greenberg S, et al. The safety and immunogenicity of a human immunodeficiency virus type 1 (HIV-1) recombinant gp160

candidate vaccine in humans. Ann Intern Med 1991;114:119–127.

81. Keefer M, Belshe R, Clements ML, et al. Safety and immunogenicity of a baculovirus-derived HIV-1 IIIB recombinant gp160 vaccine (VaxSyn[(R)]) [Abstract PoA 2228]. Eighth International Conference on AIDS, Amsterdam, Jul 1992.

82. Belshe R, Clements ML, Dolin R. Safety and immunogenicity of fully glycosylated rgp160 IIIB vaccine in low risk volunteers [Abstract PoA 2432]. Eighth International Conference on AIDS, Amsterdam, Jul 1992.

83. Clements ML, Belshe R, Duliege AM, et al. Safety and immunogenicity of IIIB rgp120/HIV-1 vaccine in seronegative volunteers [Abstract MoA 0026]. Eighth International Conference on AIDS, Amsterdam, Jul 1992.

84. Chernoff D, Kahn J, Sinangil F, et al. Phase I dose escalation MTP-PE study of an HIV-1 gp120 vaccine in seronegative adults [Abstract MoA 0025]. Eighth International Conference on AIDS, Amsterdam, Jul 1992.

85. Dolin R, Corey L, Graham B, et al. Safety and immunogenicity of an HIV vaccine candidate, Env 2,3 in combination with MTP-PE/MF59 [Abstract PoA 2226]. Eighth International Conference on AIDS, Amsterdam, Jul 1992.

86. Hu SL, Kosowski SG, Dalyrmple JM. Expression of AIDS virus envelope in recombinant vaccinia viruses. Nature 1986;320:537–539.

87. Panacali DL, Mazzara G, Sullivan JL, et al. Use of lentivirus-like particles alone and in combination with live vaccinia-virus-based vaccines [Abstract]. AIDS Res Human Retroviruses 1992; 8:1449.

88. Cooney EL, Collier AC, Greenberg PD, et al. Safety of and immunological response to a recombinant vaccinia virus vaccine expressing hIV envelope glycoprotein. Lancet 1991;337:567–572.

89. Graham BS, Belshe RB, Clements ML. Vaccination of vaccinia-naive adults with HIV-1 gp160 recombinant vaccinia (HIVAC-le) in a blinded, controlled, randomized clinical trial. J Infect Dis 1992;116:244–252.

90. Cooney EL, McElrath MJ, Corey L. Enhanced immunity to HIV envelope elicited by a combined vaccine regimen consisting of priming with a vaccinia recombinant expressing HIV envelope and boosting with gp160 protein. Proc Natl Acad Sci USA 1993;90:1882–1886.

91. Graham BS, Matthews TJ, Belshe RB, et al. Augmentation of human immunodeficiency virus type 1 neutralizing antibody by priming with gp160 recombinant vaccinia and boosting with rgp160 in vaccinia-naive adults. J Infect Dis 1993;167:533–537.

92. Siliciano RF, Bollinger RC, Callahan KM. Clonal analysis of T-cell response to the HIV-1 envelope proteins in AIDS vaccine recipients. AIDS Res Hum Retroviruses 1992;8:1349–1352.

93. Taylor J, Paoletti E. Fowlpox virus as a vector in non-avian species. Vaccine 1988;6:466–468.

94. Cadoz M. Immunization with canarypox virus expressing rabies glycoprotein. Lancet 1992;339: 1429–1432.

95. Aldovini A, Young RA. Humoral and cell-mediated immune responses to live recombinant BCG-HIV vaccines. Nature 1991;351:479–482.

96. Kahn JO, Stites DP, Scillian J, et al. A phase I study of HGP-30, a 30 amino acid subunit of the human immunodeficiency virus (HIV) p17 synthetic peptide analogue subunit vaccine in seronegative subjects. AIDS Res Hum Retroviruses 1992;8:1321–1325.

97. Biggar RJ, Pahwa S, Minkoff H, et al. Immunosuppression in pregnant women infected with human immunodeficiency virus. Am J Obstet Gynecol 1989;161:1239–1244.

98. Minkoff H, Nanda D, Menez R, Filerig S. Pregnancies resulting in infants with acquired immunodeficiency syndrome or AIDS-related complex: Followup of mothers, children, and subsequently born siblings. Obstet Gynecol 1987;69: 286–291.

99. Ukwa HN, Graham BS, Lambert JS, Wright PF. Perinatal transmission of human immunodeficiency virus-1 infection and maternal immunization strategies for prevention. J Obstet Gynecol 1992;80:458–468.

100. Van de Peare P, Lepage P, Homsy J, Dabis F. Mother-to-infant transmission of human immunodeficiency virus by breast milk; presumed innocent or presumed guilty? Clin Infect Dis 1992; 15:502–507.

101. Sidiropoulos D, Herrmann U, Morell A, von Muralt G, Barandum S. Transplacental passage of intravenous immunoglobulin in the last trimester of pregnancy. J Pediatr 1986;109:305–308.

102. Schwartz RH. Acquisition of immunologic self-tolerance. Cell 1989;57:1073–1081.

103. Wraith DC, McDevitt HO, Steinman L, Acha-Onbea H. T cell recognition as the target for immune intervention in autoimmune disease. Cell 1989;57:709–715.

104. Homsy J, Meyer M, Tateno M, Clarkson S, Levy JA. The Fc and not CD4 receptor mediates antibody enhancement of HIV infection in human cells. Science 1989;244:1357–1360.

105. Robinson WE Jr, Montefiori DC, Gillespie DH, Mitchell WN. Complement-mediated, antibody-dependent enhancement of HIV-1 infection in vitro is characterized by increased protein and RNA synthesis and infectious virus release. J Acquir Immune Defic Syndr 1989;2:33–42.

106. Bolognesi DP. Do antibodies enhance the infection of cells by HIV? Nature 1989;340:431–432.

107. Mofenson LM, Wright PF, Fast PE. Summary of the working group on perinatal intervention. AIDS Res Hum Retroviruses 1992;8:1435–1438.

108. Cohen J. Did liability block AIDS trial? Science 1992;257:316–317.

48

Medical Issues Related to Provision of Care for HIV-infected Children in Hospital, Home, Day Care, School, and Community

Stephen Chanock and R. J. Simonds

Like all children, children with human immunodeficiency virus (HIV) infection live, play, learn, and are cared for in many settings. To protect HIV-infected children and their caretakers, family, and playmates from acquiring transmissible infections, those responsible for the care of children should exercise safe infection control practices that include 1) using recommended procedures to reduce the risk of disease transmission, 2) educating children and their care providers regarding transmission of HIV and other infectious agents in a way that neither minimizes nor exaggerates risk, and 3) promoting understanding, confidentiality, and compassion for children with HIV infection. To provide guidance for implementing such practices, this chapter reviews how HIV is transmitted, including the presence of HIV in various body fluids and the risk of transmission after various exposures, and provides specific guidelines for preventing the transmission of HIV and other infections in the particular settings where children are cared for. For specific details of the management of other infections, the reader is directed to Chapters 13–22.

HIV TRANSMISSION

The serious nature of HIV infection, the presence of HIV in various body fluids, and the close contact that children often enjoy with their playmates and caretakers have combined to generate considerable concern about HIV transmission in homes, schools, health care facilities, day care centers, and playgrounds. Unfortunately, the lack of understanding of how HIV is transmitted has sometimes led to fear and ostracism of children with HIV infection in situations that present no discernible risk to others. However, the understanding of HIV transmission that has accumulated over the past decade has promoted a rational approach to prevention and in most cases allayed unwarranted fears.

Presence of HIV in Body Fluids

The replication cycle of HIV occurs exclusively within infected cells, although HIV may also be found extracellularly when new progeny viruses are released from the cell by budding. HIV preferentially infects and replicates in cells expressing the CD4 antigen, the ligand for viral attachment and subsequent cell entry (1, 2). These cells include a subset of helper T lymphocytes, monocytes, and macrophages. Using an in situ polymerase chain reaction technique, researchers have estimated that 0.1–13% of peripheral blood mononuclear cells from an HIV-infected person may contain HIV, depending on the stage of infection (3). Free HIV, not associated with cells, has also been isolated from plasma, cerebrospinal fluid, and other body fluids (4–6).

In view of the wide distribution of lymphocytes and monocytes in the body, it is not surprising that HIV has been isolated from many body fluids, although HIV transmission is most commonly associated with exposure to body fluids, such as blood or semen, that are especially rich in lymphocytes and monocytes. The efficiency of recovery of virus from various fluids appears to be proportional to the density of lymphocytes and monocytes in the fluid. HIV has been isolated from blood (7), semen (7), vaginal and cervical secretions (8), amniotic fluid (9), breast milk (5), alveolar fluid (10), saliva (11–13), tears (14), throat swabs (15), and cerebrospinal fluid (6). HIV nucleic acid sequences have been detected in urine by polymerase chain reaction (16). HIV has not been isolated from stool or vomitus; however, these fluids theoretically may contain HIV if contaminated with blood.

The presence of HIV in saliva and tears is particularly relevant to questions regarding the possibility of HIV transmission to and from children. HIV was detected in saliva from 1 of 73 adults with HIV infection in one study (11), in 3 of 55 in a second (12), and in 8 of 20 in another (13). Nine of 19 throat swabs from HIV-infected children in one study contained HIV (15). Although such swabbing is likely to result in contamination with lymphocytes from the tonsils or pharynx, the authors noted that the virus was also found in cell free supernatants. HIV was isolated from tears from one of seven infected persons (14). Despite these findings, no case of transmission attributed to exposure to saliva or tears has been reported.

Mechanism of HIV Transmission

Conditions for transmission of HIV require sufficient quantity of the virus and a portal of entry that permits establishment of infection of host cells. HIV transmission occurs primarily in three types of settings: 1) from a mother with HIV infection to her newborn during pregnancy, delivery, or breast feeding; 2) by direct inoculation of infected blood or blood-containing tissues through transfusion of blood or blood products, transplantation of organs or certain tissues, reuse of contaminated needles or other injection equipment, or penetrating injuries with needles or other sharp objects contaminated with blood; 3) between sex partners through contact of infected semen, vaginal or cervical secretions, or blood with anal or genital mucosa (17). HIV transmission after contact of blood with mucous membranes or nonintact skin has also been reported rarely in health care settings. HIV transmission has not been reported through inhalation of aerosols, bites from bloodsucking insects, or ingestion of food prepared or served by an infected person.

Risk of HIV Transmission

Several factors may contribute to the efficiency of HIV transmission, including the volume of blood or other inoculum, the titer of HIV in the inoculum (which may be related to the stage of infection), antiretroviral therapy received by the source person, the route of exposure (e.g., intravenous infusion vs. contact with a mucous membrane), and possibly factors particular to the strain of HIV. Considerable data have been collected to address the risk of HIV transmission following different routes of exposure. The risk of HIV being transmitted to a recipient of a transfusion of HIV-infected blood is at least 95%, and the risk of transmission to the newborn of an infected mother is between 13 and 40% (see Chapter 10C). HIV transmission during vaginal or anal intercourse or through sharing needles for injection has been responsible for most AIDS cases in the United States, but the risk for transmission after single or multiple exposures by these routes is more difficult to quantify.

Percutaneous or Mucocutaneous Blood Contact

Prospective studies have estimated the risk of HIV transmission after a single percutaneous exposure to HIV-infected blood to be 0.3% (95% confidence interval 0.13–0.70%) (18–20). In addition to those factors affecting transmission discussed previously, factors that may increase the risk of transmission after percutaneous exposure include injury with a hollow-bore rather than solid-bore needle, increased depth of needle penetration, and penetration through bare rather than gloved skin (21). HIV transmission after cutaneous or mucous membrane exposure to HIV-infected blood has been reported (22, 23). However, because HIV transmission has not been reported among health care workers prospectively monitored after more than 1000 cutaneous or mucous membrane exposures (18–20), the risk of transmission after such exposures cannot be determined but is probably much less than that after percutaneous exposure. In these studies, the upper bounds of the 95% confidence intervals for the risk of HIV transmission after mucous membrane or skin contact with infected blood are 0.3 and 0.04%, respectively. All reported cases of transmission after mucocutaneous exposure have involved blood contact with mucous membranes or with skin that was apparently not intact because of eczema or other lesions.

"Casual" Contact

The risk of HIV transmission from the type of ordinary contact that is common among children in households, schools, day care centers, and other out of home child care settings, if it exists, is extremely small. Several sources of data support this conclusion. First, various studies addressing HIV infection among adult and child household members of infected persons have shown that, among more than 1000 household contacts studied, the only persons infected with HIV were those with other risks for infection (24–40, Table 48.1). Second, no cases of HIV transmission caused by such contact have ever been substantiated. Finally, none of the more than 200,000 cases of AIDS reported to Centers for Disease Control (CDC) have been attributed to such contact.

Several household studies documented no HIV transmission despite the presence of household activities that might be expected to involve contact with blood or other body fluids (Table 48.2). Because HIV has been isolated from saliva (11–13), biting and kissing have been considered as exposures of particular concern. Biting is common among young children (41), al-

Table 48.1.   Summary of Published Studies of HIV Seroprevalence among Persons Having Only Household Contact with HIV-infected Persons in the United States and Europe

Reference	No. Index Persons		No. Persons with Contact[b]		No. HIV Positive	No. Persons yr of Contact	Time	Location
	Total	Children[a]	Total	Children[a]				
Redfield et al. (24)	2	0	3	3	0	N/A	1983–1984	United States
Kaplan et al. (25)	4	4	4	0	0	12	1983–1984	Newark
Jason et al. (26)	34		62		0		1983–1984	United States
Berthier et al. (27)	24	24	70	70	0	146	1983–1985	France
Fischl et al. (28)	45	0	29	0	0	58	1983–1985	Miami
Melbye et al. (29)	14		26		0		1984	Denmark
Lawrence et al. (30)	29	24	39	13	0	65	1984	St. Louis
Brettler et al. (31)			51		0	95	1984–1987	Massachusetts
Friedland et al. (32)	90	0	206	155	0	320	1984–1987	New York City
Biberfeld et al. (33)	29	20	56	20	0	111	1985	Sweden
Romano et al. (34)	43		69	14	0		1985	Italy
Lusher et al. (35)	183		304	≥22	0	605	1985–1989	United States
Muntean et al. (36)	18	18	45		0		1986[c]	Austria
Madhok et al. (37)	10		23		0		1986[c]	Scotland
Peterman et al. (38)	88	0	63	19	0	142	1988[c]	United States
Berntorp et al. (39)	19		21		0	42	1988	Sweden
Rogers et al. (40)	25	25	89	10	0	115	1990[c]	United States
Total	657	115	1167	326	0[d]	1711		

[a]Children generally defined as ≤18 years old; age cut-off different or not specific in some studies. Information not always available.
[b]Excludes persons with other risks for HIV infection (e.g., sex partners of index persons, children born to mothers with HIV infection, injection drug users).
[c]Year of publication of report.
[d]Rate of infection in persons with only household contact = 0/1711 person-year of contact (95% confidence interval = 0–0.18/100 person-years of contact).

Table 48.2.   Number of HIV-seronegative Persons Reporting Various Interactions with HIV-infected Household Contacts in Three Studies

Household Interaction	No. in Study with Interaction			
	Rogers et al. (40)	Friedland et al. (32)	Lawrence et al. (30)	Total
Slept together	27	78		105
Bathed together	25	21		46
Kissed on lips	52	36		88
Shared comb	49	134		183
Shared toilet	19	192		211
Shared toothbrush	14	27		41
Shared eating utensil	39	80		119
Gave injections	4		25	29

though bites that result in blood contact are rare. Biting has been suggested, although not proven, as a possible mode of HIV transmission in two brief case reports (42, 45). In the first report, the sibling of a child infected with HIV by a transfusion was found to be infected, and the only exposure that was described was a bite that did not break the skin. In the second case, a woman who possibly had other risk factors for HIV infection became infected around the time that she was bitten by her HIV-infected sister, who had blood in her mouth at the time of the bite. In contrast, four studies of a total of 22 persons who were bitten by HIV-infected persons found that none of the bitten persons became infected (40, 44–46). In one of these studies (46), 30 staff members were bitten, scratched, or spat upon by an institutionalized person with HIV infection and aggressive behavior; none had seroconverted after 4–6 months of follow-up. In addition, Rogers et al. (40) documented lack of HIV infection in seven persons who bit HIV-infected children. Although data addressing the risk of HIV transmission from biting are limited, such transmission appears unlikely unless blood is inoculated percutaneously by the bite.

One study suggested that blood contamination of saliva as a result of tooth brushing or passionate kissing might create a risk of HIV transmission during passionate kissing or kissing after brushing teeth (47). However, kissing has not been proven to be a mode of HIV transmission.

These data indicate that HIV is rarely, if ever, transmitted among children and adults in circumstances relevant to children's care, education, and play activities.

Because of this, the presence of HIV infection per se should not restrict children from participating in athletics, day care, and school in most cases; appropriate precautions should routinely be followed.

PREVENTION OF HIV TRANSMISSION

Knowledge of the risk of transmission of HIV and other blood-borne pathogens led to the development of universal precautions to prevent percutaneous, mucous membrane, and skin exposures to blood-borne pathogens, including HIV, in health care settings (48–50). The principles of universal precautions include the use of safe practices and appropriate barrier precautions when contact with blood or certain body fluids of any patient is anticipated. Under universal precautions, all patients are considered to be potentially infected with a blood-borne pathogen because the patient's infection status is often unknown. Universal precautions apply only to body fluids that may transmit blood-borne pathogens (Table 48.3). The most likely of these to be present in child care settings are blood and body fluids containing blood.

Detailed recommendations regarding universal precautions have been published (48–50). Additionally, employers of health care workers and others should be aware of regulations issued by the Occupational Safety and Health Administration to reduce occupational exposure to blood-borne pathogens (51). The principles underlying universal precautions are also applicable outside of health care settings, such as in schools, day care centers, playing fields, and the home.

Table 48.3.   Universal Precautions to Prevent Transmission of Blood-borne Pathogens

HAND WASHING IS NECESSARY AFTER PHYSICAL CONTACT WITH ALL PATIENTS
Body fluids to which universal precautions apply
    Blood
    Any body fluid containing visible blood
    Semen and vaginal secretions
    Body tissues
    Cerebrospinal, synovial, pleural, peritoneal, pericardial, amniotic fluid
Examples of procedures for which gloves are recommended (masks, gowns, and eye protection if
    splattering is likely)
    Intubation
    Endoscopy
    Dental procedures
    Wound irrigation
    Phlebotomy
    Finger and heel sticks
    Arterial puncture
    Vascular catheter placement
    Tracheostomy suctioning
    Rinsing of used instruments
    Lumbar puncture
    Amniocentesis
    Puncture of other cavities (e.g., pleural, pericardial, peritoneal, and synovial)
    Cleaning newborns
Body fluids and procedures for which hand washing is sufficient for preventing blood-borne
    pathogens (unless fluid contains blood)[a]
    Urine
    Stool
    Vomitus
    Tears
    Nasal secretions
    Oral secretions
    Diaper changing
Special precautions for other body fluids (see text)
    Breast milk
    Saliva

[a]Gloves may be required to prevent transmission of other pathogens.

To prevent percutaneous exposures to blood-borne pathogens, including HIV, injuries with needles or other sharp items contaminated with blood must be avoided. Strategies to avoid such injuries include handling needles and other sharp instruments safely (e.g., not recapping, bending, or breaking needles; disposing of sharp items in puncture-resistant containers), using self-sheathing needles or other mechanical devices shown to reduce the risk of injury to health care workers, and limiting unnecessary use of needles. To prevent skin and mucous membrane exposures, appropriate barrier precautions should be used when contact with blood or other body fluids is anticipated. Gloves should be used for touching blood, body fluids requiring universal precautions, mucous membranes, and nonintact skin of all patients and for handling items soiled with blood or body fluids requiring universal precautions (Table 48.3). Masks, protective eyewear, and gowns should be used when splashes to the face or body may be expected. Hands should be washed immediately after contact with blood and after removal of gloves. Nondisposable instruments or devices that enter sterile tissue or through which blood flows should be sterilized after use; under no circumstances should needles, syringes, or other such equipment be used for more than one person without sterilization. Finally, blood and blood-containing fluids spilled on environmental surfaces should be promptly removed and contaminated surfaces cleaned with bleach (diluted 1:10 to 1:100, depending on the amount of organic material present) or other Environmental Protection Agency-approved disinfectant; gloves should be worn always during cleaning and decontaminating procedures.

Although universal precautions do not apply to human breast milk or saliva, some precautions against exposure to these fluids may be necessary. Because breast feeding has been implicated in the transmission of HIV infection from mother to infant, it may be prudent to wear gloves in situations where exposure to human breast milk is possible. Gloves should also be worn for contact with oral mucosa, for endotracheal suctioning, and for other oropharyngeal procedures that involve exposure to blood-contaminated saliva. Gloves need not be worn when feeding a child or cleaning oral secretions that do not contain visible blood. However, gloves should be worn when changing diapers that contain bloody stools and when handling other body fluids with visible blood.

Health Care Settings

Providing health care routinely involves using needles and other sharp objects, being potentially exposed to blood, and caring for persons who may be infected with blood-borne pathogens. For these reasons, appropriate infection control practices must be emphasized wherever health care is provided, including hospitals, outpatient facilities, and homes. Regardless of the setting, an effective infection control program has several important components. All persons providing medical or nursing care should receive training in infection control practices and be capable of carrying them out. Hand washing facilities and adequate supplies of necessary items, such as gloves, sterile needles and syringes, and puncture-resistant containers must be readily available and conveniently located. Sterilization facilities must be available when nondisposable instruments are used. Bleach (diluted 1:10 to 1:100, depending on the amount of organic material present) or other approved disinfectant should be available for wiping surfaces after spilled blood has been properly cleaned and contaminated materi-

als appropriately disposed (48). Sharps disposal containers should be placed out of the reach of children, and special care must be taken to exclude young children from settings where exposure to someone else's blood or to sharp objects used for another person is possible. Finally, a program for continuing education regarding infection control and ongoing monitoring of compliance with infection control policies can help ensure that recommendations are followed.

Hospitals

Additional considerations are needed for delivery rooms, emergency rooms, and operating rooms, places where the potential for exposure to blood is increased and where the prevalence of HIV infection among patients may be high. In various CDC studies, cutaneous, mucous membrane, or percutaneous blood contact was reported during 30% of vaginal deliveries, 43% of cesarean deliveries, 4% of emergency room procedures, and 30% of operating room procedures (52–54). In another CDC study, percutaneous injuries were observed in 7% of operative procedures (55). The prevalence of HIV infection among women delivering children in the United States is 0.15% overall but is over 4% in some hospitals (56, 57). The prevalence of HIV infection among adults is as high as 6–9% in some urban emergency rooms (52, 58) and 14% in some hospitals (59).

In the delivery room, appropriate barrier precautions should be used, including wearing gloves and gown when touching the placenta and when handling the newborn until blood and amniotic fluid have been removed from the infant's skin. Mechanical suction should be used when suctioning the newborn. In the nursery, gloves should be worn for umbilical cord care. In the absence of other indications, infants born to mothers with HIV infection need not be isolated from other patients. Donor breast milk (from someone other than the natural mother) should not be given unless the donor is HIV seronegative (60).

In the emergency room and intensive care unit, gloves, gowns, other barriers, and puncture-resistant containers must be easily accessible for emergency situations. Although HIV transmission has not been reported by mouth to mouth resuscitation, to minimize the need for this procedure, mouthpieces, resuscitation bags, or other ventilation devices should be available for use in areas in which the need for resuscitation is predictable. To prevent percutaneous injuries during suturing, instruments rather than fingers should be used whenever possible to manipulate tissue being sutured.

In diagnostic centers, special care is necessary to minimize inadvertent injection of blood from one patient to another during procedures such as nuclear medicine scans that involve withdrawal and reinjection of blood (61).

Other Health Care Settings

Infection control practices should be no less vigilant in other health care settings such as clinics, offices, or homes. Common play areas on pediatric wards, in clinics, and in offices should be closely supervised by staff trained to recognize and manage situations such as bleeding episodes that may pose a risk of disease transmission. However, children with HIV infection need not be excluded or separated from other children. Toys may be shared among all children, but they should be cleaned and disinfected before being used by another child if they are contaminated by blood.

Four reports have suggested the possibility of HIV transmission during the provision of health care at home (62–65). With increasing use of home parenteral therapy for HIV infection and other conditions, ensuring appropriate infection control practices in all homes in which such therapy is provided is essential (66, 67).

Schools

The well publicized instances of discrimination against children with HIV infection at school are particularly unfortunate because they cause unnecessary pain and anguish for children and their families while propagating the unfounded notion that HIV is likely to be transmitted in schools. No cases of HIV transmission in school have

been reported, and current epidemiologic data do not justify excluding children with HIV infection from school or isolating them in school to protect others. Children with HIV infection should be able to participate in all school activities with the same considerations as other children, to the extent that their health permits. Guidelines for the education of children with HIV infection (68, 69) and for the development of school policies (70) have been published.

Like other children with special health needs, children with HIV infection benefit from educational programs that provide needed medical services, such as management of emergencies and administration of medications. Moreover, a sound educational program can help create a more accepting environment for children with HIV infection. Evaluating each child's medical and educational needs on a case by case basis, with ongoing communication among the family, health care providers, and school health staff, can optimize benefits to the child (71). All educational institutions should have a policy regarding students and staff who have HIV infection.

Until children with HIV infection are no longer stigmatized and discriminated against, confidentiality will remain an important issue. The right to privacy must always be protected; a child's HIV status should be disclosed only with the informed consent of the parents or other legal guardians and, when age appropriate, assent of the child.

The persons aware of the child's HIV infection can be limited to those who need such knowledge to care for the child. In most cases, such persons include the school medical advisor, school nurse, and teacher. Because administration of HIV-related medications in school may compromise confidentiality, when possible the infected child should be encouraged to self-administer medications, with the approval of the school nurse or medical advisor. Children can use nearly all services for children with special needs without revealing their HIV status. Blood exposures from fights, unintentional injuries, nosebleeds, shed teeth, menstruation, and other causes may occur at school. All schools should be capable of handling blood and blood-containing body fluids using principles of universal precautions: readily available supplies (e.g., gloves, disposable towels, and disinfectants) should be provided, and all staff, including teachers, athletic coaches, cafeteria workers, and maintenance workers, should be educated in proper infection control.

Athletics

Many children and adolescents enjoy sports; one-third of girls and one-half of boys in United States high schools participated on varsity or junior varsity teams in 1990 (72). Participation in some contact sports may increase a child's risk of exposure to blood: forceful contact with hard surfaces, equipment, or other players may result in laceration or abrasion, and close player to player contact may lead to direct exposure to another person's blood. Nonetheless, the risk of HIV transmission during sports is extremely low. Despite the large number of persons participating in contact sports, only one case of HIV transmission attributed to sports has been reported worldwide (73). In this case, transmission was reported to have resulted from a collision that produced lacerations with copious bleeding and exchange of blood during a soccer match, but other modes of transmission were not satisfactorily excluded in the young man who became infected. Hepatitis B virus transmission during sports has been reported once, among high school sumo wrestlers (74).

The American Academy of Pediatrics (AAP), the National Collegiate Athletic Association, the National Football League, and the World Health Organization have published guidelines addressing HIV infection and sports (75–78). Athletes with HIV infection should be permitted to participate in competitive sports at all levels. However, because of the potential risk to the athlete's own health and the theoretical risk of HIV transmission to others during contact sports, athletes with HIV infection interested in participating in contact sports such as wrestling, boxing, or football should be evaluated on a case by case basis. This evaluation should consider such factors as the likelihood of blood contact (e.g., intramural touch football vs. varsity tackle football), the athlete's propensity to bleed (e.g., thrombocytopenia), and the presence of skin lesions that cannot be covered during active sport. The AAP recommends that an HIV-infected athlete considering a sport such as football or wrestling should be informed of the theoretical risk of transmission to others and be encouraged to consider another sport (75). The athlete's physician should be directly involved in the decision regarding participation. Last, organized athletic programs should develop policies regarding blood exposure.

The right to privacy should be protected; an athlete's HIV status need not be revealed to other players. On the playing field, contact by trainers and first aid providers with blood should be minimized by following appropriate infection control, including promptly cleaning blood from skin with soap and water and from surfaces such as wrestling mats with a 1:100 bleach solution; immediately controlling bleeding by covering abrasions, lacerations, or other lesions; using gloves or other barriers when attending to wounds; and avoiding reuse of sponges, water, or other first aid items to care for injuries involving blood. Finally, the leadership role enjoyed by many coaches may provide them the opportunity to educate athletes and others about the risk of HIV transmission through unprotected sex and through the sharing of needles or syringes for injection of anabolic steroids or other drugs (79, 80).

Day Care Centers

No cases of HIV transmission in out of home child care settings have been reported. Furthermore, the lack of HIV transmission following household exposure to persons, including children, with HIV infection argues against a significant risk of HIV transmission through the types of contact that occur routinely in child care settings. Therefore, CDC, AAP, and the American Public Health Association have recommended that children with HIV infection be allowed to attend child care in most cases (69, 81, 82). Several considerations should be weighed when deciding about enrollment, including the child's propensity for aggressive biting, the child's likelihood of having uncontrollable bleeding episodes, the presence of oozing skin lesions that cannot be covered, and the child's immune function. The child's physician should be directly involved with the decision about whether to enroll a child in day care. Day care center staff with HIV infection who adhere to infection control precautions may care for children unless they have conditions that would place them at increased risk of transmitting infection, such as open skin lesions that cannot be covered, diarrhea from infectious agents (such as cryptosporidiosis), or pulmonary tuberculosis (82).

The confidentiality of children attending child care must be protected to the greatest extent possible. A child's HIV status should be disclosed only with the informed consent of the parents or other legal guardians and then only to those who need such knowledge to care properly for the child. In general, at least one staff member should be aware of the child's immunodeficiency so that potential exposures to blood-borne or other infections can be managed appropriately.

Because child care settings may contain children who are unknowingly infected with HIV or other blood-borne infections, staff members should adopt routine procedures for handling blood and other body fluids of all children (see above). They also should be diligent in recognizing and managing exposures of all children to common childhood infections. The staff should notify the local health department and parents of all children of any exposures to tuberculosis, varicella, measles, or other communicable disease. Children who are immunosuppressed because of HIV infection or other reasons may be particularly susceptible to infection with such gastrointestinal pathogens as *Cryptosporidium*. Staff should be alert to exposures to these types of infections and notify parents if such an exposure occurs. Parents also should be notified of outbreaks caused by respiratory syncytial virus or *Salmonella* because immunodeficient children may develop serious illness if infected.

In some communities, day care centers designed to meet the special medical, developmental, and other needs of children with HIV infection may be available. These centers may afford a supportive environment for children with HIV infection but are not intended to be used for the purpose of excluding these children from other day care centers.

Adoption

Children with HIV infection deserve the same access to foster care and adoption as other children (83). Because caring for a child with HIV infection entails heavy responsibility, prospective foster or adoptive parents should know both the diagnosis and prognosis of the child. When possible, children at risk for HIV infection should be tested before placement. If the child is at risk for maternally acquired HIV infection, the biologic mother should be asked to consent to testing. If timely consent is not possible, most states have developed other methods, including the use of court orders, to evaluate the need and arrange for testing if indicated. In addition, in some areas HIV testing is encouraged to promote the timely placement of children. Because most HIV-seropositive children are born to mothers with HIV infection, great care is required to protect the biologic mother's right to confidentiality when testing the child.

Adoptive or foster parents of HIV-seropositive children must understand and practice infection control precautions. However, at the same time, they should be reassured of the negligible risk of HIV transmission by routine household contact. To prepare for possible medical emergencies, the parents should understand the importance of prompt attention to such signs as fever or respiratory distress.

Adoptive or foster parents of children who are HIV seropositive but whose diagnosis has not been confirmed by definitive testing (e.g., culture, polymerase chain reaction, or antibody test after age 18 months) should be informed of the risk of the child's being infected and encouraged to have the child further evaluated with more definitive tests or follow-up antibody testing. Assistance in using appropriate medical, psychological, and community resources also should be provided.

Management of Occupational Exposure to HIV

The potential for occupational exposure to HIV in the medical work place has led many medical centers to formulate protocols for rapidly evaluating exposures and, on the basis of determined risk, consider the need for immediate initiation of antiretroviral therapy. The United States Public Health Service has published detailed recommendations for management of occupational exposures to blood and body fluids that may contain HIV (84) (see Table 48.3). This document defines an exposure that may place a person at risk for HIV infection as

> . . . a percutaneous injury (e.g., a needlestick or cut with a sharp object), contact of mucous membranes, or contact of skin (especially when the exposed skin is chapped, abraded, or afflicted with dermatitis or the contact is prolonged or involving an extensive area) with blood, tissues, or other body fluids to which universal precautions apply . . . (84).

Recommended management includes reporting exposures promptly, evaluating the nature of the exposure, counseling the exposed person regarding management, and testing the source person (with consent) for hepatitis B surface antigen and HIV antibody. Evaluation should include determining the likelihood that the exposing fluid contains HIV, the concentration of HIV in the fluid, the volume of fluid, and the route of exposure. If the source person is known to be infected with HIV or refuses testing, the exposed person should be evaluated for HIV infection as soon as possible, and if seronegative, be retested periodically for at least 6 months. During the follow-up, the exposed person should seek medical evaluation for any acute illness, refrain from blood, semen, and organ donation, and take measures to prevent sexual transmission of HIV.

The United States Public Health Service reviewed the existing literature on the use of azidothymidine (AZT) for postexposure prophylaxis and determined that data are inadequate to establish its efficacy or safety (84). None of the nearly 300 health care workers who have been prospectively monitored after receiving AZT following exposure to HIV have seroconverted (85). However, because the risk of HIV transmission from a needlestick injury is only ~0.3%, a prohibitively large number of exposures would need to be evaluated to demonstrate efficacy. Several case reports documenting the failure of AZT to prevent infection have been published (86). In some of these cases, a large inoculum of HIV was injected accidentally, but in others, the health care worker sustained only a needlestick injury. Nevertheless, in the absence of conclusive data, many medical centers have adopted a protocol for offering AZT chemoprophylaxis as one alternative after occupational exposures. Most infectious disease consultants recommend that, when given to adults, AZT prophylaxis should begin as soon as possible (preferably within several hours) after exposure at a dose of 200 mg every 4 hr for 4–6 weeks. No data have been published on the use of zidovudine prophylaxis for children who have been exposed to HIV, and the Public Health Service did not consider children in its recommendations. The decision to begin AZT therapy should be made in consultation with trained personnel, and AZT, if given, should be administered under the care of a physician who will monitor for possible drug-related toxicities. In instances in which the source person is at risk for HIV infection but has an unknown HIV infection status, the decision about beginning chemoprophylaxis will need to be made without knowledge of the source person's HIV status. Many programs offer chemoprophylaxis conditionally for several days while the source person is being evaluated.

Because blood or body fluid exposures also may occur in the home or elsewhere (e.g., needlestick injury by family member providing home medical care), access to information regarding postexposure management should be available to persons outside medical centers. Some circumstances may be difficult to evaluate, such as that of a child who is found playing in the street with a needle of unknown source and who has evidence of a scratch. In these situations, personal physicians or other medical advisors could evaluate the exposure and advise regarding prophylaxis in consultation with infection control experts.

ISOLATION FOR OTHER INFECTIONS

The immunosuppression resulting from HIV infection leaves many HIV-infected children susceptible to other infectious diseases, including opportunistic infections and more severe cases of infection with common childhood bacterial, viral, and parasitic pathogens. Furthermore, these infections may be transmitted to other children, including those without HIV infection. During the past decade, experience in managing infectious complications of immunodeficiency in children has increased rapidly. This section reviews current knowledge about the prevention of transmission of other infections in settings where HIV-infected children are cared for.

General Considerations

Although protecting a child from all infections is impossible, health care and family providers should strive to minimize the risk of acquiring other infections by HIV-infected children in their care. The most important practice to emphasize is appropriate hand washing in all settings, particularly when children with HIV infection may be present.

Table 48.4 lists many infections to which children with immunodeficiency may be es-

Table 48.4. Specific Precautions for Common Childhood Infections[a]

Organism	Special Precautions — Hospital[b]	School?	Day Care?	Comments
Candida	None	No	No	Ubiquitous
Cytomegalovirus	None	No	No	Ubiquitous
Coccidioidomycosis	None	No	No	No person to person transmission
Cryptococcus	None	No	No	No person to person transmission
Cryptosporidia	Enteric	No	Yes	Exclude child with diarrhea
Epstein-Barr virus	None	No	No	Ubiquitous
H. influenza	Respiratory	No	No	Prophylaxis of contacts[e]
Hepatitis B	None	No	Yes	Avoid biting and blood contact[e]
Histoplasmosis	None	No	No	No person to person transmission
Herpes simplex	Contact	No	Yes	Exclude child with mouth sores and drooling
Influenza	Contact	No	No	Common in winter
Isospora hominis	Enteric	No	Yes	Pathogenicity negligible in immunocompetent children
M. avium-intracellulare	None	No	No	No person to person transmission
Measles	Respiratory	Yes	Yes	Exclude child until resolved[e]
Pertussis	Respiratory	Yes[c]	Yes[c]	Exclude child until treated[e]
Pneumococcus	None	No	No	Ubiquitous in normal children
Pneumocystis carinii	None[d]	No	No	Ubiquitous
Respiratory syncytial virus	Contact	No	No	Common in winter and spring
Rotavirus	Enteric	No	Yes	Exclude child with diarrhea
Salmonella	Enteric	No	Yes	Exclude infected child until three stools negative
Staphylococcus	Contact	Yes[c]	Yes[c]	Exclude child until resolved
Streptococcus	Contact	Yes[c]	Yes[c]	High rate of carriage among children
Syphilis	Drainage/secretion[c]	No	No	Should have been treated in infancy
Toxoplasma	None	No	No	No person to person transmission
Tuberculosis	Acid-fast bacilli	Yes	Yes	Until treated (see text)
Varicella zoster	Respiratory	Yes	Yes	Exclude child until lesions scabbed

[a]Adapted from Ref. 103 and edition 1. Universal precautions are applicable in all circumstances. In addition, these are general guidelines; other infection control considerations may apply in certain situations.
[b]Recommendations from Ref. 87.
[c]Precautions can be discontinued once the patient has been on therapy for at least 24 hr.
[d]Respiratory isolation has been recommended by some (104).
[e]Immunization recommended for all children.

pecially susceptible and indicates which precautions are necessary to prevent hospitalized children from transmitting the infection to children with HIV infection and others (87). Recommendations concerning attendance in school or day care for children with these infections are also offered. The principles behind these precautions also may be applicable in other settings, such as family gatherings or recreational programs.

Most opportunistic infections cannot be prevented by protecting against person to person exposure, since they are associated more with immunosuppression than with exposure. For instance, potentially pathogenic organisms such as *Candida* and *Mycobacterium avium-intracellulare* are ubiquitous, and many children may be colonized during the first years of life but generally do not develop symptomatic infection unless they become immunodeficient.

Many pathogens that infect children with HIV infection are prevalent among all children. For example, many immunocompetent children are colonized with *Haemophilus influenzae* or *Streptococcus pneumoniae* in the respiratory tract without illness, whereas children with HIV infection and immunodeficiency are more likely to have invasive and recurrent infections with these organisms. In most cases, because these organisms are ubiquitous and because school, day care, and other social activities provide important advantages, children with HIV infection would not greatly benefit by exclusion to avoid these exposures.

Children with HIV infection and other immunodeficiencies frequently require hospitalization and may account for a significant proportion of the patient population in some hospital wards. Therefore, special precautions are necessary to prevent nosocomial transmission of certain organisms (see Table 48.4) that may infect immunocompetent as well as immunodeficient hospitalized children.

Certain infections can be prevented by active or passive immunization. The schedule of active immunizations recommended by CDC, AAP, and the Immunization Practices Advisory Committee of the Public Health Service for HIV-infected children is similar to that for other children in most situations (see Chapter 46) (88, 89). Because children with HIV infection are susceptible to severe and sometimes fatal complications of vaccine preventable diseases, all children must receive all recommended immunizations on schedule. In addition, if an exposure to certain infections occurs, prophylaxis can be given by administration of specific immunoglobulins (e.g., hepatitis B, varicella) or of nonspecific immunoglobulin (e.g., hepatitis A, measles).

Specific Conditions

Gastrointestinal and Respiratory Infections

Acute diarrheal illnesses, which are common and often highly contagious in children, may be especially severe in children with HIV infection (see Chapter 20). Because most pathogens that cause infectious diarrhea are readily transmissible, especially among children in diapers, and because children may be particularly contagious during the initial phase of diarrhea, children with and without HIV infection who have acute diarrhea should be excluded from group day care until the diarrhea has abated. During an outbreak of diarrheal illness in a day care center or school, meticulous hand washing should be stressed to prevent further spread of the pathogen, particularly among young children.

Children are commonly infected with respiratory virus infections, particularly with respiratory syncytial virus, parainfluenza, influenza, or rhinovirus (see Chapter 19). These infections are rarely serious in HIV-infected children unless the child has an underlying cardiac or pulmonary disease (e.g., cardiomyopathy or lymphoid interstitial pneumonitis) or unless a bacterial superinfection follows. However, since children with HIV infection and cardiopulmonary compromise or extreme immunodeficiency may be more prone to the severe consequences of respiratory virus infection, these children should be carefully evaluated before being recommended for attendance in settings such as day care where frequent exposure to respiratory pathogens is likely.

Measles is highly contagious and appears to result in considerably higher morbidity and mortality in children with HIV infection (90) (see Chapter 19). All children with documented or presumed measles should be excluded from school or day care, and children with HIV infection who are susceptible to measles should not attend during an outbreak of measles among school or day care contacts.

In some cases, children with HIV infection who are infected with certain gastrointestinal or respiratory pathogens (e.g., *Cryptosporidium* or respiratory syncytial virus) may pose a more prolonged risk of transmitting the infection to others because immunosuppressed persons may continue to shed the organism for a longer duration than others. This prolonged infectivity should be considered when applying appropriate infection control precautions to children with these infections in hospitals, day care centers, and schools.

Varicella-Zoster Virus Infection

Varicella is highly contagious, and nearly all children become infected during childhood (see also Chapter 18). Because children with depressed immune function may have more severe infections (91) or may suffer chronic or recurrent infections, all children with varicella should be excluded from school or day care until all vesicles are crusted over. Hospitalized children with documented or suspected varicella or with a bona fide exposure to varicella should be placed immediately in strict isolation until no longer potentially contagious. Susceptible children exposed to varicella should receive varicella-zoster immunoglobulin within 96 hr to prevent or minimize the severity of infection (92).

Tuberculosis

Disease caused by *M. tuberculosis*, unlike diseases caused by other mycobacteria, presents a considerable risk of being transmitted to others (93) (see Chapter 16A). Specific infection control guidelines have not been established for tuberculosis (TB) in children with HIV infection, although such guidelines for TB in adults with and without HIV infection have been published (94).

TB is most often acquired through inhalation of aerosolized organism-bearing droplet nuclei. TB in normal children is not usually contagious for several reasons: 1) children usually carry a small bacillary burden; 2) extrapulmonary TB, which is more common in children than in adults, is not contagious except in unusual circumstances (e.g., aerosolization during debridement procedures or direct inoculation of infected tissue into a host); 3) cavitary tuberculous lung disease, which is associated with contagion, is uncommon in children; and 4) a child's cough may be less able to generate an aerosol adequate to transmit organisms.

Several important factors may affect the control of TB transmission among children with HIV infection. First, the ability of skin testing to diagnose recent acquisition of TB may be hampered by anergy to cutaneous skin test antigens such as tuberculin (PPD). Second, HIV infection may modify the spectrum of disease caused by *M. tuberculosis*, resulting in unusual clinical presentations that may delay diagnosis. Third, clinical experience with children infected with both HIV and TB is limited, and the extent to which a depressed host response may result in a higher bacillary burden and increased contagiousness is unknown.

Acid-fast bacilli precautions are indicated if pulmonary TB is suspected (87). Pulmonary TB should be suspected if a child is at risk for TB and has a cough or respiratory distress. The presence of pulmonary disease can usually, but not always, be confirmed by a chest radiograph that shows an infiltrate, cavitation, effusion, or adenopathy. Suspicion of contagious pulmonary TB is greatly increased by the presence of acid-fast bacilli in a sputum smear, although adequate sputum samples may be difficult to obtain from children. In some cases, acid-fast bacilli may be isolated from gastric or bronchoalveolar washings. If any of these smears are positive for acid-fast bacilli, the child should remain on acid-fast bacilli precautions until treatment has begun, cough has abated, and, when possible, a decrease in the number of acid-fast bacilli on smear has been demonstrated. Because of the possible increasing prevalence of multidrug-resistant isolates (95), culturing the organism and doing susceptibility testing are also important.

Children with recently diagnosed tuberculosis should not attend social programs until therapy has been initiated and the child is no longer considered infectious. Because new cases of TB in children are a result of exposure in the home or community, diagnosis of TB in a child should stimulate investigation of contacts who may have been the source of infection; these include family members, other caretakers, and other persons with close contact with the child. Therefore, a new diagnosis of tuberculosis in an adult should prompt a thorough investigation of all contacts, particularly when the adult provides or cares for children with HIV infection. If a contact is found to have contagious TB, other children and adults who may have been exposed to this contact should also be evaluated for TB. During contact evaluation, negative tuberculin skin test results should be interpreted in light of the immune status of the contact, since low CD4 counts may be associated with skin test anergy (96). In addition, contacts who have symptoms suggestive of TB should receive a full medical evaluation regardless of skin test results.

Health care providers of children at risk for TB, such as those sharing households with persons with HIV infection, should inquire routinely about the presence of TB among the child's contacts so that the child can be evaluated for TB as soon as possible after a potential exposure.

The reader is strongly encouraged to remain aware of recommendations by the CDC, the American Thoracic Society, the AAP, and other organizations. Chapter 16A also should be consulted for a more in-depth discussion of tuberculosis control measures.

Hepatitis B Virus Infection

Because hepatitis B virus is transmitted in ways similar to HIV, children born to mothers with HIV infection may also be exposed to hepatitis B virus, either perinatally or, to a lesser extent, in the home. All newborns should receive a complete hepatitis B vaccination series (97). Any child who shares a household with a hepatitis B surface antigen carrier should be vaccinated against hepatitis B (98). Children with HIV infection who receive hepatitis B vaccine should be serologically evaluated for immunity after vaccination (87).

PREVENTION OF TRANSMISSION OF INFECTION FROM HEALTH CARE WORKERS TO CHILDREN
Blood-borne Infections

Hepatitis B virus has been transmitted to patients from health care workers infected with hepatitis B virus who test positive for hepatitis Be antigen. In all cases, transmission occurred in association with a major break in standard infection control practices or from unintentional injury to the infected health care worker during invasive procedures (99). One case of HIV transmission from an infected health care worker to patients was reported recently (100), specifically from a dentist to five patients who had invasive procedures. This case is the only reported instance of HIV transmission from a health care worker to patients, and available data indicate that the risk of such transmission is very small (101).

Factors that may increase the risk of transmission of blood-borne infections in health care settings include major breaks in standard infection control practices (e.g., not wearing gloves during invasive procedures) and unintentional injury to the infected health care worker during invasive procedures (e.g., incurring needle stick while suturing in areas where visibility is impaired). The likelihood of a patient being exposed to a health care worker's blood is greater for those procedures that involve digital palpation of a needle tip in a body cavity or the simultaneous presence of the health care worker's fingers and a needle or other sharp object in a poorly visualized or highly confined anatomic site. In addition to the type of procedure, the technique, skill, and medical status of the individual health care worker may influence the potential for exposure to the worker's blood. The risk of blood exposure for both patients and health care workers can be minimized by the use of safer instruments and techniques and appropriate barrier precautions. Health care workers who might be exposed to blood should receive hepatitis B vaccine, preferably before any occupational exposures can occur. Health care workers who have exudative lesions or weeping dermatitis should refrain from all direct patient care until the condition resolves. If the health care worker must remain on duty, lesions or wounds should be covered with gloves or other barrier protection. Health care workers with HIV infection who adhere to universal precautions and who do not perform invasive procedures pose no risk for transmitting HIV to children. Recommendations for preventing HIV and hepatitis B virus transmission to patients have been published (99).

Other Infections

To prevent the transmission of other infections from health care or child care workers to children, meticulous hand washing before contact is extremely important. Moreover, work restrictions may be necessary for workers who have certain infections (102). Health care or child care workers with active pulmonary or laryngeal tuberculosis should be excluded from patient or child care until adequate treatment is instituted, cough is resolved, and three consecutive sputum smears are free of bacilli. Asymptomatic workers receiving preventive therapy for tuberculosis should be allowed to continue working. Workers with acute symptoms of diarrheal illness should not provide direct patient or child care, and those found to be infected with *Salmonella* should continue to be excluded until two consecutive stool specimens taken at least 24 hr apart are free of *Salmonella*. Workers with herpetic whitlow or other open or draining lesions should refrain from direct patient or other child contact until all lesions have healed or have been covered adequately. Any health care or child care worker with active measles, mumps, rubella, or varicella and any susceptible worker who has been exposed to these infections should not have direct contact with children while they are potentially contagious. Workers with herpes zoster should not have direct contact with patients or children who are immunosuppressed until all lesions have crusted, unless the lesions can be covered and there is no chance for exposing patients to vesicle fluid. To protect HIV-infected children from respiratory viral infections, caretakers and providers should be vaccinated against influenza, and in particular, if possible, those known to be infected with respiratory syncytial virus or influenza should not have direct contact with children with HIV infection.

Principles underlying infection control guidelines for health care workers (102) and day care center workers (82) may also be applicable for other adults caring for children (e.g., coaches, teachers, and parents). For example, an adult caretaker with diarrhea caused by *Cryptosporidium* or *Salmonella* should take appropriate precautions.

CONCLUSION

Children with HIV infection deserve the same rights to health care, privacy, education, and social interactions that other children enjoy. If appropriate guidelines are followed, these rights can be respected without additional risk to the health or safety of the child or others. Educated and caring health care professionals can both provide appropriate health care to these children as well as help the community to better understand HIV infection and the needs of infected children.

Because recommendations may change, care providers should regularly consult medical literature and specifically follow updated recommendations of the AAP, the CDC, and other organizations.

References

1. Fauci AS, Schnittman SM, Poli G, Koenig S, Pantaleo G. Immunopathologic mechanisms in human immunodeficiency virus (HIV) infection. Ann Intern Med 1991;114:678–693.
2. Levy JA, Kaminsky LS, Morrow WJW, et al. Infection by the retrovirus associated with the acquired immunodeficiency syndrome. Ann Intern Med 1985;103:694–699.
3. Bagasra O, Hauptman SP, Lischner HW, Sachs M, Pomerantz RJ. Detection of human immunodeficiency virus type 1 provirus in mononuclear cells by in situ polymerase chain reaction. N Engl J Med 1992;326:1385–1391.
4. Michaelis BA, Levy JA. Recovery of human immunodeficiency virus from serum [Letter]. JAMA 1987;257:1327.
5. Thiry L, Sprecher-Goldberger S, Jonckheer T, et al. Isolation of AIDS virus from cell-free breast milk of three healthy virus carriers. Lancet 1985;2:891–892.

6. Ho DD, Rota TR, Schooley RT, et al. Isolation of HTLV-III from cerebrospinal fluid and neural tissues of patients with neurologic syndromes related to the acquired immunodeficiency syndrome. N Engl J Med 1985;313:1493–1497.

7. Ho DD, Schooley RE, Rota TR, et al. HTLV-III in the semen and blood of a healthy homosexual man. Science 1984;226:451–453.

8. Vogt MW, Witt DJ, Craven DZ, et al. Isolation patterns of the human immunodeficiency virus from cervical secretions during the menstrual cycles of women at risk for the acquired immunodeficiency syndrome. Ann Intern Med 1987;106: 380–382.

9. Mundy DC, Schinazi RF, Gerber AR, Nahmias AJ, Randall HW Jr. Human immunodeficiency virus isolated from amniotic fluid. Lancet 1987;2:459–460.

10. Ziza J-M, Brun-Vezinet F, Venet A, et al. Lymphadenopathy-associated virus isolated from bronchoalveolar lavage fluid in AIDS-related complex with lymphoid interstitial pneumonitis [Letter]. N Engl J Med 1985;313:183.

11. Ho DD, Byington RE, Schooley RT, Flynn T, Rota TR, Hirsch MS. Infrequency of isolation of HTLV-III virus from saliva in AIDS [Letter]. N Engl J Med 1985;313:1606.

12. Levy JA, Greenspan D. HIV in saliva [Letter]. Lancet 1988;2:1248.

13. Groopman JE, Salahuddin SZ, Sarngadharan MG, et al. HTLV-III in saliva of people with AIDS-related complex and healthy homosexual men at risk for AIDS. Science 1984;226:447–449.

14. Fujikawa LS, Palestine AG, Nussenblatt RB, Salahuddin SZ, Masur H, Gallo RC. Isolation of human T-lymphotropic virus type III from the tears of a patient with the acquired immunodeficiency syndrome. Lancet 1985;2:529–530.

15. Kawashima H, Bandyopadhyay S, Rutstein R, Plotkin SA. Excretion of human immunodeficiency virus type 1 in the throat but not in urine by infected children. J Pediatr 1991;118:80–82.

16. Li JJ, Huang YQ, Poiesz BJ, Zaumetzger-Abbot L, Friedman-Kien AE. Detection of human immunodeficiency virus type 1 (HIV-1) in urine cell pellets from HIV-1-seropositive individuals. J Clin Microbiol 1992;30:1051–1055.

17. Curran JW, Jaffe HW, Hardy AM, et al. Epidemiology of HIV infection and AIDS in the United States. Science 1988;239:610–616.

18. Gerberding JL, Bryant-LeBlanc CE, Nelson K, et al. Risk of transmitting the human immunodeficiency virus, cytomegalovirus, and hepatitis B virus to health care workers exposed to patients with AIDS and AIDS-related conditions. J Infect Dis 1987;156:1–8.

19. Henderson DK, Fahey BJ, Willy M, et al. Risk for occupational transmission of human immunodeficiency virus type 1 (HIV-1) associated with clinical exposures. Ann Intern Med 1990;113:740–746.

20. Marcus R, CDC Cooperative Needlestick Study Group. Surveillance of health-care workers exposed to blood from patients infected with the human immunodeficiency virus. N Engl J Med 1988;319:1118–1123.

21. Mast ST, Gerberding JL. Factors predicting infectivity following needlestick exposure to HIV: An in vitro model [Abstract]. Clin Res 1991;39:58A.

22. Centers for Disease Control. Update: Acquired immunodeficiency syndrome and human immunodeficiency virus infection among health-care workers. MMWR 1988;37:229–234, 239.

23. Gioannini P, Lucchini A, Sinicco A, Paggi G, Cariti G, Giachino O. HIV infection acquired by a nurse. Eur J Epidemiol 1988;4:119–120.

24. Redfield RR, Markham PD, Salahuddin SZ, et al. Frequent transmission of HTLV-III among spouses of patients with AIDS-related complex and AIDS. JAMA 1985;253:1571–1573.

25. Kaplan JE, Oleske JM, Getchell JP, et al. Evidence against transmission of human T-lymphotropic virus/lymphadenopathy-associated virus (HTLV-III/LAV) in families of children with the acquired immunodeficiency syndrome. Pediatr Infect Dis J 1985;4:468–471.

26. Jason JM, McDougal JS, Dixon G, et al. HTLV-III/LAV antibody and immune status of household contacts and sexual partners of persons with hemophilia. JAMA 1986;255:212–215.

27. Berthier A, Fauchet R, Genetet N, et al. Transmissibility of human immunodeficiency virus in haemophilic and nonhaemophilic children living in a private school in France. Lancet 1986;2:598–601.

28. Fischl MA, Dickinson GM, Scott GB, Klimas N, Fletcher MA, Parks W. Evaluation of heterosexual partners, children, and household contacts of adults with AIDS. JAMA 1987;257:640–644.

29. Melbye M, Ingerslev J, Biggar RJ, et al. Anal intercourse as a possible factor in heterosexual transmission of HTLV-III to spouses of hemophiliacs [Letter]. N Engl J Med 1985;312:857.

30. Lawrence DN, Jason JM, Bouhasin JD, et al. HTLV-III/LAV antibody status of spouses and household contacts assisting in home infusion of hemophilia patients. Blood 1985;66:703–705.

31. Brettler DB, Forsberg AD, Levine PH, Andrews CA, Baker S, Sullivan JL. Human immunodeficiency virus isolation studies and antibody testing. Arch Intern Med 1988;148:1299–1301.

32. Friedland G, Kahl P, Saltzman B, et al. Additional evidence for lack of transmission of HIV infection by close interpersonal (casual) contact. AIDS 1990;4:639–644.

33. Biberfeld G, Bottiger B, Berntorp E, et al. Transmission of HIV infection to heterosexual partners but not to household contacts of seropositive haemophiliacs. Scand J Infect Dis 1986;18:497–500.

34. Romano N, De Crescenzo L, Lupo G, et al. Twin routes of transmission of human immunodeficiency virus (HIV) infection in a family setting in Palermo, Italy. Am J Epidemiol 1988;128:254–260.

35. Lusher JM, Operskalski EA, Aledort LM, et al. Risk of human immunodeficiency virus type infection among sexual and nonsexual household contacts of persons with congenital clotting disorders. Pediatrics 1991;88:242–249.

36. Muntean W, Zenz W, Zaunschirm W, Teubl I, Heinz FX. HTLV-III antibody status in household

contacts of seropositive hemophiliacs. Blood 1986;67:1780–1781.

37. Madhok R, Gracie JA, Lowe GDO, Forbes CD. Lack of HIV transmission by casual contact [Letter]. Lancet 1986;2:863.

38. Peterman TA, Stoneburner RL, Allen JR, Jaffe HW, Curran JW. Risk of human immunodeficiency virus transmission from heterosexual adults with transfusion-associated infections. JAMA 1988;259:55–58.

39. Berntorp E, Christensen P, Lindvall K. Lack of transmission of HIV to sexual and non-sexual contacts to HIV seropositive haemophiliacs following preventive information. Scand J Infect Dis 1990;22:279–282.

40. Rogers MF, White CR, Sanders R, et al. Lack of transmission of human immunodeficiency virus from infected children to their household contacts. Pediatrics 1990;85:210–214.

41. Garrard J, Leland N, Smith DK. Epidemiology of human bites to children in a day-care center. Am J Dis Child 1988;142:643–650.

42. Wahn V, Kramer HH, Voit T, Bruster HT, Scrampical B, Scheid A. Horizontal transmission of HIV infection between two siblings [Letter]. Lancet 1986;1:694.

43. Anonymous. Transmission of HIV by human bite [Letter]. Lancet 1987;2:522.

44. Drummond JA. Seronegative 18 months after being bitten by a patient with AIDS. JAMA 1986; 256:2342–2343.

45. Shirley LR, Ross SA. Risk of transmission of human immunodeficiency virus by bite of an infected toddler. J Pediatr 1989;114:425–427.

46. Tsoukas CM, Hadjis T, Shuster J, Theberge L, Feorino P, O'Shaughnessy M. Lack of transmission of HIV through human bites and scratches. J Acquir Immune Defic Syndr 1988;1:505–507.

47. Piazza M, Chirianni A, Picciotto L, Guadagnino V, Orlando R, Cataldo PT. Passionate kissing and microlesions of the oral mucosa: Possible role in AIDS transmission. JAMA 1989;261:244–245.

48. Centers for Disease Control. Recommendations for prevention of HIV transmission in health-care settings. MMWR 1987;36(suppl 2S):1S–18S.

49. Centers for Disease Control. Update: Universal precautions for prevention of transmission of human immunodeficiency virus, hepatitis B virus, and other bloodborne pathogens in health-care settings. MMWR 1988;37:377–382, 387–388.

50. National Commission on AIDS. Preventing HIV transmission in health care settings. Washington, DC: Government Printing Office, 1992.

51. Occupational Safety and Health Administration. Occupational exposure to bloodborne pathogens. Fed Register 1991;56:64175–64182.

52. Marcus R, Culver D, Bell D, et al. Risk of human immunodeficiency virus infection among emergency department workers. Am J Med 1993;94: 363–370.

53. Panlilio AL, Foy DR, Edwards JR, et al. Blood contacts during surgical procedures. JAMA 1991;265:1533–1537.

54. Panlilio A, Welch B, Bell D, et al. Blood and amniotic fluid contact sustained by obstetric personnel during deliveries. Am J Obstet Gynecol 1992; 167:703–708.

55. Tokars JI, Bell DM, Culver DH, et al. Percutaneous injuries during surgical procedures. JAMA 1992;267:2899–2904.

56. Gwinn M, Pappaioanou M, George JR, et al. Prevalence of HIV infection in childbearing women in the United States. JAMA 1991;265:1704–1708.

57. Novick LF, Berns D, Stricof R, Stevens R, Pass K, Wethers J. HIV seroprevalence in newborns in New York state. JAMA 1989;261:1745–1750.

58. Kelen GD, DiGiovanna T, Bisson L, Kalainov D, Sivertson KT, Quinn TC. Human immunodeficiency virus infection in emergency department patients. JAMA 1989;262:516–522.

59. Janssen RS, St Louis ME, Satten GA, et al. HIV infection among patients in U.S. acute care hospitals. N Engl J Med 1992;327:445–452.

60. Arnold LDW, Tully MR, eds. Guidelines for the establishment and operation of a human milk bank. West Hartford, CT: Human Milk Banking Association of North America, 1992.

61. Centers for Disease Control. Patient exposures to HIV during nuclear medicine procedures. MMWR 1992;41:575–578.

62. Centers for Disease Control. Apparent transmission of human T-lymphotrophic virus type III/lymphadenopathy-associated virus from a child to a mother providing health care. MMWR 1986;35: 76–79.

63. Centers for Disease Control. HIV infection in two brothers receiving intravenous therapy for hemophilia. MMWR 1992;41:228–231.

64. Grint P, McEvoy M. Two associated cases of the acquired immunodeficiency syndrome (AIDS). Communicable Dis Rep 1985;42:4.

65. Koenig RE, Gautier T, Levy JA. Unusual intrafamilial transmission of human immunodeficiency virus [Letter]. Lancet 1986;2:627.

66. Simmons B, Trusler M, Roccaforte J, Smoth P, Scott R. Infection control for home health. Infect Control Hosp Epidemiol 1990;11:362–370.

67. Anonymous. Caring for someone with AIDS. Atlanta: Centers for Disease Control, 1991.

68. American Academy of Pediatrics Task Force on Pediatric AIDS. Education of children with human immunodeficiency virus infection. Pediatrics 1991;88:645–648.

69. Centers for Disease Control. Education and foster care of children infected with human T-lymphotrophic virus type III/lymphadenopathy-associated virus. MMWR 1985;34:517–521.

70. Fraser K. Someone at school has AIDS. Alexandria, VA: National Association of State Boards of Education, 1989:1–35.

71. Santelli JS, Birn AE, Linde J. School placement for human immunodeficiency virus-infected children: The Baltimore city experience. Pediatrics 1992;89:843–848.

72. Centers for Disease Control. Vigorous physical activity among high school students—United States, 1990. MMWR 1992;41:33–35.

73. Torre D, Sampietro C, Ferraro G, Zeroli C, Speranza F. Transmission of HIV-1 infection via sports injury [Letter]. Lancet 1990;335:1105.

74. Kashiwagi S, Hayashi J, Ikematsu H. An outbreak of hepatitis B in members of a high school sumo wrestling club. JAMA 1982;248:213–214.

75. American Academy of Pediatrics, Committee on Sports Medicine and Fitness. Human immunodeficiency virus [acquired immunodeficiency syndrome (AIDS) virus] in the athletic setting. Pediatrics 1991;88:640–641.

76. Anonymous. AIDS and intercollegiate athletics. In: NCAA sports medicine handbook. Overland Park, KS: National Collegiate Athletic Association, 1992.

77. National Football League. HIV/AIDS-related policies. New York: National Football League, Aug 1992.

78. Anonymous. Global programme on AIDS. Consensus statement from consultation on AIDS and sports. Geneva: World Health Organization, 16 Jan 1989.

79. Scott MJ, Scott MJ Jr. HIV infection associated with injections of anabolic steroids. JAMA 1989;262:207–208.

80. Sklarek HM, Mantovani RP, Erens E, Heisler D, Niederman MS, Fein AM. AIDS in a bodybuilder using anabolic steroids [Letter]. N Engl J Med 1984;311:1701.

81. American Academy of Pediatrics Committee on Infectious Diseases. Health guidelines for the attendance in day-care and foster care settings of children infected with human immunodeficiency virus. Pediatrics 1987;79:466–471.

82. Anonymous. Caring for our children. Washington, DC: American Public Health Association and Elk Grove Village, IL: American Academy of Pediatrics, 1989:231–236.

83. American Academy of Pediatrics Task Force on Pediatric AIDS. Guidelines for human immunodeficiency virus (HIV)-infected children and their foster families. Pediatrics 1992;89:681–683.

84. Centers for Disease Control. Public Health Service statement on management of occupational exposure to human immunodeficiency virus, including considerations regarding zidovudine use. MMWR 1990;39(RR-1):1–14.

85. Henderson DK. Post-exposure chemoprophylaxis for occupational exposure to HIV-1 [Abstract]. Am J Med 1991(suppl 3B):312S.

86. Bell DM, Curran JW. Human immunodeficiency virus infection. In: Bennett JV, Brachman PS, eds. Hospital infections. Boston: Little, Brown, 1992:823–848.

87. Report of Committee on Infectious Diseases. 22nd ed. Elk Grove Village, IL: American Academy of Pediatrics, 1991.

88. Onorato IM, Markowitz LE, Oxtoby MJ. Childhood immunization, vaccine preventable diseases and infection with human immunodeficiency virus. Pediatr Infect Dis J 1988;6:588–595.

89. Centers for Disease Control. Recommendations of the Immunization Practices Advisory Committee (ACIP) on immunizations of children infected with human T-lymphotrophic virus type III/lymphadenopathy virus. MMWR 1986;35:595–598, 603–606.

90. Krasinski K, Borkowsky W. Measles and measles immunity in children infected with human immunodeficiency virus. JAMA 1989;261:2512–2316.

91. Shepp DH, Dandliker PS, Myers JD. Treatment of varicella-zoster virus infection in severely immunocompromised patients. N Engl J Med 1986;314:208–212.

92. Recommendations of Immunization Practices Advisory Committee: Varicella-zoster immune globulin for the prevention of chicken pox. Ann Intern Med 1984;100:859–865.

93. Bloom BR, Murray CJL. Tuberculosis: Commentary on a reemergent killer. Science 1992;257:1055–1064.

94. Centers for Disease Control. Guidelines for preventing the transmission of tuberculosis in healthcare settings, with special focus on HIV-related issues. MMWR 1990;39(RR-17):1–29.

95. Beck-Sague C, Dooley SW, Hutton MD, et al. Hospital outbreak of multidrug-resistant *Mycobacterium* tuberculosis infections. JAMA 1992;268:1280–1286.

96. Centers for Disease Control. Purified protein derivative (PPD)-tuberculin anergy and HIV infection: Guidelines for anergy testing and management of anergic persons at risk of tuberculosis. MMWR 1991;40(RR-5):27–33.

97. Centers for Disease Control. Hepatitis B virus: A comprehensive strategy for eliminating transmission in the United States through universal childhood vaccination. MMWR 1991;40(RR-13):1–25.

98. Centers for Disease Control. Protection against viral hepatitis: Recommendations of the Immunization Practices Advisory Committee (ACIP). MMWR 1990;39(RR-2):1–22.

99. Centers for Disease Control. Recommendations for preventing transmission of human immunodeficiency virus and hepatitis B virus to patients during exposure-prone invasive procedures. MMWR 1991;40(RR-8):1–8.

100. Ciesielski C, Marianos D, Ou CY, et al. Transmission of human immunodeficiency virus in a dental practice. Ann Intern Med 1992;116:798–805.

101. Chamberland ME, Bell DM. HIV transmission from health care worker to patient: What is the risk? Ann Intern Med 1992;116:871–873.

102. Polder JA, Tablan OC, Williams WW. Personnel health services. In: Bennett JV, Brachman PS, eds. Hospital infections. Boston: Little, Brown, 1992:31–61.

103. Garner JS, Simmons BP. Centers for Disease Control guideline for isolation precautions in hospitals. Infect Control 1983;4(suppl):245–325.

104. Walzer PD. *Pneumocystis carinii*—new clinical spectrum. N Engl J Med 1991;324:263–265.

49

Legal Issues Relevant to HIV-infected Children in Home, Day Care, School, and Community

David L. Katz

In 11 years, human immunodeficiency virus (HIV) has generated more litigation than any disease in history. The care of children with HIV infection raises myriad legal issues including protection of confidentiality, prevention against discrimination of access to public education in the regular classroom, prevention of access to community services such as day care and medical care. Additionally, the legal issues include assessing child capacity as applied to informed consent and the refusal or withdrawal of treatment, as well as determining who, in a foster care situation, may consent to medical care. Two major areas—protecting confidentiality and preventing discrimination in the education system—encompass the legal difficulties encountered most frequently by the HIV-infected child and his or her care providers. Hence, these two areas receive the greatest attention in this chapter.

This chapter focuses on legal issues specific to community services; however, health care professionals should be aware of the many additional legal issues that may become relevant, if not critical, during the course of caring for an HIV-infected child. Further, from the outset it is emphasized that effective advocacy for the child with HIV infection only begins with a basic comprehension of the relevant federal and state statutes, regulations, and case law. This is a general guideline to help the nonlegal reader understand some of the legal issues relevant to HIV-infected children. To this end, constitutional law, federal legislation, state policies, and local practices are simplified and presented in a nonlegal vernacular. Legal cases are discussed in a summary format, either where the United States Supreme Court decided a case of particular relevance or where a lower court case illustrates how a pertinent policy or issue not yet decided by the Supreme Court was addressed and decided by our judicial system.

Once generally familiar with the technicalities of the laws and the cases, it is important that affected groups such as parents of HIV-infected children, medical and legal care providers, and HIV-infected children themselves become social and political advocates. This is true for three reasons. First, laws are often enacted but not enforced effectively (e.g., civil rights legislation passed in the 1960s was widely ignored in practice for decades). Second, as originally enacted, laws frequently contain significant deficiencies (i.e., the laws are inapplicable to particular populations, individuals, or institutions). Third, laws and the rights and/or entitlements recognized therein are fluid. Through community and judicial interpretation, and through legislative amendments, laws continuously evolve. For a minority population (e.g., children infected with HIV), group support, organization, and activity are particularly important vehicles through which social and political strength may be obtained. Active lobbying by minority groups may create a political voice through which they may successfully effect changes in enforcement patterns and/or in the substantive law (see Chapter 54 for a more detailed discussion of advocacy). Thus, an appreciation of the current cases and laws relevant to children with HIV infection is a necessary but not sufficient prerequisite to effective legal care for these children.

CONFIDENTIALITY

In addition to the protections offered by antidiscrimination laws, HIV-infected persons may have independent legal protections against unauthorized disclosure of their medical diagnosis and related information. Generally, where one reasonably expects information communicated to another to be protected against unwanted disclosure to a third party, a duty of confidentiality may be said to arise. A breach of this duty occurs when an individual under such a duty either intentionally discloses the protected information without consent or fails to reasonably ensure that the information is protected (1).

Beyond any basic harm suffered from the breach itself, other more specific interests may be affected. Madison Powers identifies three categories of threats to interests that might be harmed by the unwanted disclosure of HIV status: 1) interference with the HIV-infected person's ability to make medical decisions; 2) damages to the person's reputation, social standing, and social relationships; and 3) discrimination in the availability of a wide variety of social services and opportunities (1). The last two categories are most germane to the child with HIV infection. Social relationships in and out of the school environment may be irreparably harmed by untimely and/or insensitive disclosures. Further, discrimination in the form of attempted exclusion from the classroom or day care may result. The antidiscrimination statutes discussed in this chapter provide the child with some protection, but it should be clear that, as a preventive measure, increased confidentiality de-

creases discriminatory behavior directly because fewer persons possess knowledge that a given child has HIV infection.

Protection against disclosure of medical information may be analyzed legally as a right contained within the more broad "right to privacy." Although the United States Supreme Court has never found the Constitution to contain express language defining such a right, the Court has held privacy to be a "fundamental right" derived indirectly from the Constitution (2). In theory, this line of cases provides informational privacy protection. However, the Supreme Court has significantly narrowed the scope of protection on this basis. Examining a case of state-sanctioned information disclosure (New York maintained a prescription drug registry that identified patients who were receiving certain narcotic medications), the Supreme Court upheld the state system even while acknowledging that patient stigmatization might result and could adversely affect a patient's decision whether to seek or to continue treatment (3). In dicta, the Supreme Court granted that, in certain circumstances, unwanted disclosures of personal information would constitute an unconstitutional invasion of privacy. Unfortunately, the limitations set forth in that and subsequent cases significantly narrowed constitutional protection with the result that where informational privacy protections exist, generally they are found in statutes or judicially developed common law (1).

For example, several states have passed legislation recently that specifically targets HIV information for protection against unauthorized disclosure (4–7). However, even strong HIV confidentiality statutes contain exceptions including permissible disclosure to protect third parties at risk of HIV transmission (1, 5). Although HIV information has not received similar attention through enacted federal legislation, the Privacy Act of 1974 prohibits, with numerous exceptions, a federal agency that holds information (including medical history) from disclosing that information to the public or to other federal agencies (8).

Two major holders of personal information present the greatest confidentiality concerns to the HIV-infected child: 1) the physician and extended medical community and 2) those within the educational system. The widely diverse circumstances in the clinical, research, and related health settings and the vast educational system present inherent practical difficulties in successfully providing full security for such highly personal information. However, the enactment of state statutes containing penalty provisions for breaches of confidentiality has advanced the goal of achieving increased privacy protection for these children and their families.

Physicians and Other Medical Staff

Frank, honest communication between patient and physician is critical in establishing the basis for accurate diagnosis and treatment. Further, trust between doctor and patient is enhanced by the expectation of privacy or nondisclosure. Information obtained and exchanged within the physician-patient relationship is considered by most lay persons and physicians alike to be confidential. Many cite the Hippocratic Oath as one important code setting forth such a principle:

> Whatever, in connection with my profession, or not in connection with it, I may see of the men which ought not be spoken abroad I will not divulge as reckoning that all should be kept secret (9).

Although the Hippocratic Oath and other codes (e.g., the American Medical Association's Code of Ethics) appear to carry substantial weight in judicial and legislative decision-making, significant legal impediments exist in any attempt to rely on such sources for legal authority. While the majority of states recognize through statute some form of a physician-patient "privilege," its application is restricted to judicial proceedings. Further, no federal law expressly recognizes this privilege. Entirely separate in coverage and purpose is the more general duty of nondisclosure. Although this latter right of confidentiality may be recognized by statute, the current health care system (which involves clinicians, researchers, laboratory technicians, blood bank personnel, insurance company and other third party payors) conspicuously obscures the boundaries within which reasonable expectations may be said to lie regarding physician behavior (i.e., the steps a physician would be expected to take to ensure protection against disclosure).

Additionally, the scope of the privilege or right recognized by each law is limited by three variables: 1) the context in which the privilege or right attaches (i.e., disclosure during judicial proceedings vs. more general settings); 2) the persons to whom such a privilege or right attaches (i.e., solely the physician vs. others in the health care system); and 3) the legally recognized exceptions to the privilege or the right to confidentiality. In interpreting state statutes, the courts have identified but not fully resolved these issues.

Physician-patient privilege statutes vary from state to state but generally are laws prohibiting in specific circumstances physicians from disclosing information that 1) was acquired in the physician's professional capacity *and* 2) was necessary for the diagnosis and treatment of the patient. A critical limitation inheres in all privilege statutes; i.e., the protection of information conveyed in the course of the professional relationship applies only to unwanted disclosure in judicial proceedings (1). Thus, the many nonjudicial contexts such as day care, discussion and transfer of insurance information, and communications within the education system are not covered by the narrow scope of the privilege.

As a result of this severe limitation, many jurisdictions have moved to expand protection by enacting more general nondisclosure legislation. Physicians should be aware that the modern trend is to hold the physician liable for unauthorized disclosures of medical information even in the nonjudicial setting (1). Depending on the jurisdiction, a cause of action seeking monetary damages may be available to the private litigant. The claim may be permitted based on a theory of tort liability for injuries that resulted from unauthorized disclosures. In other words, a tort classified as a "breach of the duty of confidentiality" or as an "invasion of privacy" provides the legal basis for a claim. Other courts have found that a duty of confidentiality arises from an implied condition in the doctor-patient contract, and a breach of this condition forms a legal basis for recovery (1).

The health care delivery system of the 1990s contains realities that result in many persons other than the primary treating physician having access to a patient's record. Such persons include researchers, nurses, technicians, administrative staff, and third party payor personnel. At least one commentator has argued that the modern system has left confidentiality (as traditionally understood and practiced in medicine) a decrepit concept (10). Further, most—but not all—judges have been unwilling to hold nonphysician health care professionals to the same duty of confidentiality applied to physicians. This reluctance stems, in part, from the courts' view that the special contractual relationship between physician and patient is not found with other personnel (1). Thus, a jurisdiction that holds a duty of confidentiality to attach to the physician on behalf of the patient may not extend the duty to others in the health care delivery system. In such jurisdictions, the patient who suffers unwanted disclosure by a nonphysician in a judicial or nonjudicial proceeding may be without a legal cause of action. Certainly judicial and/or legislative extensions of the right to confidentiality vary greatly from state to state.

Even in jurisdictions that have enacted statutory recognition of the patient right to confidentiality, the right is weakened by numerous legal exceptions. For example, within the judicial context, the court may compel disclosure in a wide range of circumstances such as where the health status of the plaintiff or the medical records are material issues in the litigation, where the court seeks to "protect individual or societal interests," or where the court determines it is in the "interest of justice" (1). Within the context of the federal government, the Federal Bureau of Investigation and the Internal Revenue Service possess authority broad enough to obtain patient identifiable information.

Finally, in varied form, all states have enacted some sort of mandatory reporting of HIV status. The required information may or may not include patient identifiable data. Where public health reports or other disclosure by a physician is statutorily required or permitted, immunization from liability generally may be assumed, but the issue should be researched. Notably, even the most stringent HIV confidentiality statutes contain exceptions including permissible (not mandatory) disclosure by the physician for the protection of third parties substantially at risk of infection (1). Thus, while the protection against nondisclosure of highly personal medical information has strong historical, professional, and moral underpinnings, it is recognized in a widely variable fashion among the states and, when recognized, is subject to severe limitations.

New developments in tort law have created an additional wrinkle in the problem of confidentiality for the HIV-infected person in the medical setting. As a result of recent so-called "duty to warn" cases, health professionals treating HIV-infected persons will occasionally be forced to confront the issue of whether to break confidentiality out of a legal duty to protect a third party. Some courts have found that professionals (e.g., psychologists and physicians) who are in a "special" relationship with a patient have a duty to warn and protect known potential victims from the patient's threatened actions (1, 11).

In the celebrated Tarasoff case in California, the court held that a psychologist was liable to a patient's former girlfriend when the psychologist heard during a therapy session the patient's threats to kill his ex-girlfriend and the patient later committed the murder (12). This duty to protect third persons appears to have most applicability to nonmedical situations involving adult patients. However, because of the severe physical harm suffered by most persons with HIV infection scenarios involving an HIV-infected minor (or, of course, an HIV-infected adult) may be envisioned in which physicians may find themselves wondering about liability stemming from a possible duty to warn.

For example, an adolescent with HIV infection who reports an intent to engage in unsafe sexual behavior with an identified partner or to share hypodermic needles with identifiable others places the physician in a difficult ethical and legal position. The physician may feel he or she is under an affirmative legal obligation to breach the duty of confidentiality. Although this author knows of no cases where a court has held a physician liable for damages for failure to warn a third party of the danger of HIV exposure or transmission, a related and particularly unsettling case was decided in 1991 against a hospital. In Johnson v. West Virginia University Hospitals, Inc., a policeman was called to an emergency room to help subdue a patient. During a struggle, the patient bit the officer, puncturing the skin, and the officer later learned the patient had AIDS. The emergency room staff, who knew the patient's diagnosis, had not notified the policeman. The policeman contended he would have handled the situation differently had he been informed. The policeman developed severe anxiety and a fear of contracting AIDS. He sued the hospital for emotional distress and was awarded $1.9 million for his "reasonable fear" (13, 14).

Among the many disturbing aspects of this case was 1) the court's unwillingness to instruct the jury to link reasonable fear to the statistical likelihood of developing AIDS or to the lack of scientific evidence supporting HIV transmission through biting or saliva and 2) that the officer was found to have maintained a reasonable fear of developing AIDS to the time of trial despite the fact that it was now 3 years after the incident and he had not seroconverted (13, 14). Unfortunately, the legal system all too often appears to deliver unreasonable and uneducated decisions. Hope must be held that such court decisions will be few and far between with the more educated opinions becoming the precedents upon which future cases will rely. Recommendations from the scientific community (e.g., National Institutes of Health consensus statements, Centers of Disease Control (CDC) guidelines) play an increasingly important role in judicial thinking. Indeed, the United States Supreme Court has advised that "courts normally should defer to the reasonable medical judgments of public health officials" (15).

Generally, the crux of these cases for a court, and the major question for any physician confronting a situation involving mandatory or permissive disclosure, will be whether a third party truly is at substantial risk of HIV transmission. This determination must be medically reasonable based on the facts at hand. A physician concerned with liability may best resolve a dilemma by 1) checking the regulations in his or her jurisdiction; 2) reviewing the most current guidelines and recommendations published by groups such as the American Academy of Pediatrics (AAP) and the CDC regarding reduction of the risk of HIV transmission; and 3) discussing the situation with a knowledgeable attorney in the jurisdiction (16–19).

Public Educators and Staff

Much of the previous analysis applies where the educational institution is simply the recipient of confidential information. A separate situation arises however where the school or school system holds medical information on a student and chooses to disclose this information. A minority of states have enacted required notification statutes under which the department of public health must notify designated school officials (see Table 49.1). We believe such statutes are harmful, unnecessary, and should be repealed. Justification for required notification usually is based on claims that the informaton will help decrease the risk of HIV transmission in the classroom. It appears clear that if school personnel are trained and required to use CDC-recommended universal precautions in all situations involving blood and other body fluids, the HIV transmission risk will be reduced to the greatest extent possible.

Most often, the school will possess HIV status information on a child because the parents have volunteered the information to selected school officials. A parent may elect to share such information for a variety of reasons including to enable the child to receive medications at school, to help safeguard against transmission of opportunistic infections from others to the HIV-infected child and of secondary infections from the HIV-infected child to other students, to help plan in advance for anticipated absences, and to attempt through selective disclosure to increase HIV awareness in a fashion likely to benefit the child.

Table 49.1.   Required Notification Statutes[a]

State	Statute	Year Enacted	Requirement
Arizona	HB 2126	1988	Director of the Department of Health must notify local school district that a pupil is HIV positive
Illinois	HB 2044	1987	Department of Health must notify principal of HIV-infected child's school of child's identity; principal may as necessary disclose child's identity to the school nurse and the child's teachers
	HB 4005	1988	If an HIV-infected child is enrolled in a public school, the principal must disclose child's identity to the superintendent of the school district where the child resides
Nevada	SB 49, Ch. 450	1991	Health authority and the principal must notify the superintendent of the school district of the presence of HIV within a school in the district
South Carolina	HB 2807	1988	Superintendent of the school district, nurse, or health professionals assigned to a public school attended by a child with HIV infection must be notified

[a]Compiled from data provided by AIDS Policy Center, Intergovernmental Health Policy Project, The George Washington University, 1992.

Here, in contrast to the medical setting, relevant federal legislation exists that provides informational privacy protection to students and their families. The final regulations, entitled Family Educational Rights and Privacy, were revised and issued by the Department of Education in 1988 (20). These regulations implement the Family Education Rights and Privacy Act of 1974, as amended, which was enacted as section 438 of the General Education Provisions Act (21). With a few specific exceptions, the regulations apply to all educational institutions or agencies to which funds have been made available by the Department of Education. Additionally, former students are covered under the statute's definition of student and are entitled to the same protections as students in attendance.

Included are institutions where funds are provided to students attending the agency or institution for educational purposes (e.g., under the Pell Grant Program and the Guaranteed Student Loan Program) (20). Notably, the protections against unauthorized disclosure do not apply to records of a student who is 18 years or older or who is attending an institution of postsecondary education that are 1) made or maintained by a physician or other recognized professional or paraprofessional acting in his or her professional capacity or assisting in a paraprofessional capacity; 2) made, main-

tained, or used only in connection with the student's treatment; and 3) disclosed only to individuals providing the treatment (20).

The regulations provide for confidentiality of personally identifiable information held by an educational agency or institution through a general rule that states that, prior to disclosure, a signed and dated written consent must be obtained from an eligible student (18 years old or attending an institution of postsecondary education) or from the student's parent. Unfortunately, this rule, which appears to provide clear and strong privacy protection, is weakened by numerous exceptions. The most relevant exception to the HIV-infected student is the situation where unconsented disclosure is permitted in connection with a "health or safety emergency."

The regulations state that prior consent is not required in an emergency if knowledge of the information is necessary to protect the health or safety of the student or others (20). Prior regulations required the disclosing entity to include four specific criteria in determining whether such information could be disclosed. The new, revised regulations removed these criteria, thereby permitting the educational institution or agency to make a determination absent federal regulation. Thus, an obvious potential weakness in the regulations was created—the method by which a particular school makes such a determination is not subject to a federal standard.

Conversely, a state or local community may always provide greater protection than that stemming from federal law, and some have moved in that direction. For example, the Department of Education in Michigan drafted and released the Education Model Communicable Disease Policy, which follows the federal regulations but contains additional protections (22). Questions and concerns regarding the federal confidentiality requirements may be addressed to personnel either in the Office of Special Education and Rehabilitative Services, Department of Education: 202-205-5465, or in the office of Family Policy and Regulatory Staff, Department of Education: 202-401-2057.

ANTIDISCRIMINATION LAWS

The HIV-infected child and family may suffer discrimination in innumerable settings ranging from denial of community and medical services to denial of housing opportunities to social isolation. It is beyond the scope of this chapter to analyze substantively all relevant antidiscrimination legislation. Thus, one area, education, has been selected for detailed examination. While federal legislation will be emphasized because it sets forth the mandatory minimum protections to be provided children (i.e., a state or local community may choose to enact greater protections), examples of state and local policy will be discussed.

Education is a fitting choice for three reasons. 1) Pediatric patients spend the majority of their time outside the home in educational institutions, hence discrimination in this setting is extremely problematic for the child and family. 2) The factors leading to discrimination in the education setting (e.g., irrational fears of HIV transmission, the wide variation of state and local practices) mirror those found in other settings. 3) Federal statutes exist and serve as models for future legislation. Although education is the focus here, those caring for the child with HIV infection should be aware that additional antidiscrimination statutes exist and often are useful to the child and family in noneducation settings. For example, families of children with HIV infection receive antidiscrimination protection in buying or renting housing through the Fair Housing Amendments Act of 1988 (23).

Federal Legislation

In considering discrimination problems within the education system for children with HIV infection, two major pieces of federal antidiscrimination legislation apply: Section 504 of the Rehabilitation Act of 1973 (§ 504) (24) and the Americans with Disabilities Act (ADA) (25). A third piece of legislation, the Education for All Handicapped Children Act (EHA) (26), subsequently renamed the Individuals with Disabilities Act (IDEA) (27) potentially could provide additional benefits to HIV-infected children but thus far has not proved useful in this context (Table 49.2). Older legislation and cases use the outdated term "handicapped," while newer statutes and cases employ the term "disability," which is preferred by members of the disability community and their advocates (28). Intermittent use here of the term handicapped results solely from the fact that most case law cited was generated under the older statute.

Further, § 504 and the ADA overlap significantly in the protections provided to the HIV-infected child. Additionally, concerning this specific application, the two statutes appear to operate in a virtually identical fashion (29). Thus, for the general educational purposes of this chapter, these two statutes will often be discussed together. Future litigation based on HIV discrimination may well use the ADA preferentially because it is the more recent statute, it provides greater coverage in some areas, and it has an accompanying legislative history that includes specific references to disability and discrimination based on infection with HIV.

In order to receive protection under § 504 and/or the ADA, a child must be handicapped/disabled. The ADA defines a person with a disability as one who

1. Has a physical or mental impairment which substantially limits that person in one or more major life activities; or
2. Has a record of such a physical or mental impairment; or

Table 49.2.   Education of HIV-infected Children: Federal Legislation

Statute	Administering Agency and Department	Relevant Coverage
Section 504 of the Rehabilitation Act of 1973	Department of Education, Office of Civil Rights	Public schools and those private schools that receive federal funds are prohibited from discriminating against children with HIV infection
Americans with Disabilities Act (Titles II and III)	Department of Justice, Civil Rights Division	Public and private schools regardless of whether they receive federal funds may not discriminate against children with HIV infection
Individuals with Disabilities Education Act	Department of Education, Office of Special Education and Rehabilitative Services	Children with specific impairments resulting in a need for a specially designed education and related services are guaranteed the right to such education and services (not yet applied successfully to children with HIV infection)

3. Is regarded as having such a physical or mental impairment (25).

The Rehabilitation Act of 1973 employs the same wording to define a handicapped individual. Early legal arguments that HIV-infected persons met the first prong of the definition by virtue of a physiologic impairments (e.g., hematologic, lymphatic, neurologic, respiratory) substantially limiting a major life activity (e.g., caring for one's self, breathing, walking, seeing, working) were persuasive. At least one court held specifically that learning is a major life activity (30), and the Department of Education adopted this view in its regulations (31). However, the asymptomatic individual presented problems for the courts, and the issue of contagiousness created additional difficulties for plaintiffs.

In Arline, the United States argued that contagious diseases (tuberculosis in that case) were not handicaps under § 504. The Supreme Court (giving great weight to an amicus brief filed by the American Medical Association) disagreed and held that the teacher with tuberculosis was handicapped (the extent of her respiratory illness was more than sufficient to establish substantial limitation of a major life activity) (15, 32). The next problem for the Court's determination was whether Arline was "otherwise qualified" because § 504 provides that no "otherwise qualified" handicapped individual shall, solely because of his or her handi-

cap, be excluded from an applicable program. In finding that Arline was otherwise qualified, the Supreme Court held that contagiousness did not preclude an individual from being handicapped and, if handicapped, from being otherwise qualified.

In a footnote, the Court stated its test for permissible exclusion: an individual posing a significant risk of communicating an infectious disease to others would not be otherwise qualified if reasonable accommodation would not eliminate the risk (15). Finally, the Supreme Court concluded that Arline had been fired not because of her impairment but due to fears of her contagiousness. The Court stressed that discrimination on this basis was impermissible.

This decision led to a number of positive legal developments. First, some courts extended the Arline holdings and suggestions to cases involving persons with HIV infection holding, for example, exclusion of an HIV-infected individual would be lawful *only* if there was a significant risk of HIV transmission (32, 33). Second, courts began to look to the scientific community for guidance on the issue of significant risk.

The CDC guidelines from 1985 include the following recommendations:

1. For most infected school-aged children, the benefits of an unrestricted setting would outweigh the risks of their acquiring potentially harmful infections in the setting and the apparent nonexistent

risk of transmission of HIV. These children should be allowed to attend school and after-school day care and to be placed in a foster home in an unrestricted setting; and

2. For the infected preschool-aged child and for some neurologically handicapped children who lack control of their body secretions or who display behavior, such as biting, and those children who have uncoverable, oozing lesions, a more restricted environment is advisable until more is known about transmission in these settings. Children infected with HIV should be cared for and educated in settings that minimize exposure of other children to blood or body fluids (17).

As more data become available, successive consensus reports and policy recommendations even less restrictive in nature were published by other organizations (16, 44). The CDC itself gave informal endorsement to the more permissive guidelines set forth by the National Association of State Boards of Education in 1989 (19, 34).

The judicial practice of granting substantial deference to guidelines and recommendations published by the scientific community is particularly important to the HIV-infected child. In this area of rapidly expanding knowledge, published medical consensus is a critical vehicle through which the court keeps educated. The medical and scientific community should not underestimate the vital nature of updating these reports. For example, the CDC official guidelines are now more than 7 years old and should be revised.

Fortunately, in a relatively short time, a vast amount of scientific information became readily available. Armed with these data, the courts routinely began to find that children with HIV infection presented no significant risk of transmitting HIV in the classroom and, therefore, could not be excluded. These decisions included HIV cases where a student was hemophilic, had a cold sore, and had oral thrush (35), where a 6-year mentally disabled child lacked control of her bodily fluids (36), and where a child had previously bitten another student (37). In fact, to our knowledge, every such case

litigated under § 504 eventually resulted in a victory for the child. Today it is apparent that concerns for the classroom (i.e., HIV or secondary infection transmission to other children) and concerns for the HIV-infected child (i.e., acquisition of infections from other children) in almost all cases can and must be handled through a nondiscriminatory means that avoids exclusion of the child.

Finally, while debated in and out of the courts for some years, there is now widespread agreement that a child with asymptomatic HIV infection meets the first prong of the definition (28, 29). The United States as part of its argument in Arline maintained that asymptomatic persons with HIV infection were not handicapped for purposes of § 504. Significantly, the United States subsequently reversed its position (29). In a memorandum to Arthur B. Culvahouse, Jr., counsel to President Reagan, the Department of Justice's Office of Legal Counsel set forth its legal opinion, which concluded that individuals with asymptomatic HIV infection did meet the first prong of the definition and, therefore, were covered under § 504 (29, 38). This is in accord with the numerous judicial decisions holding HIV infection alone to be a handicap covered by § 504 (37, 39, 40).

In addition, an asymptomatic child is covered under the third prong if perceived or regarded as having a physical or mental impairment substantially limiting a major life activity of the child. The memorandum from the United States Department of Justice supports this view, noting that in addition to coverage under the first prong, an individual with asymptomatic HIV infection may be protected under the third prong because a covered entity may regard such a person as being substantially limited in a major life activity (38). Moreover, whereas questions pertaining to coverage under § 504 for HIV-infected persons were not resolved for many years, the ADA clearly grants the symptomatic and asymptomatic child protection under the first prong and likely provides coverage under the third prong as well (28). Thus, although the legal reasoning at times appears obscure, inconsistent, and confusing, a clear and widespread consensus had developed: the antidiscrimination provisions of § 504 and the ADA apply to symptomatic and asymptomatic children with HIV infection.

As a final matter, one cannot end the analysis at this juncture. A concluding two-part query must be answered: 1) is the child "otherwise qualified" to participate in the contested activity; this question is critical because discrimination against a child with HIV infection does not violate the statute unless the child is "otherwise qualified"; and 2) even if the child is not otherwise qualified, is the school or institution able to compensate for the lack of qualification by making a "reasonable accommodation"; this is required by the regulations and was approved by the Supreme Court in Arline (29). For example, a child seriously ill with HIV infection might become impaired to the point of being incapable of fully performing certain physical activities (e.g., sports, activities involving lifting, exercises) (29). In such circumstances, exclusion from the particular activity though discriminatory is not prohibited by the statute.

However, a child who requires a slower pace of walking secondary to a decreased respiratory capacity should not be excluded from a field trip to a museum because reasonable accommodation is possible.

Questions concerning the responsibilities of schools and the rights of HIV-infected school children under § 504 may be directed to the regional Offices of Civil Rights established by the Department of Education (Table 49.3). Questions concerning coverage under the ADA may be addressed to the Department of Justice, Civil Rights Division: 202-514-0301; TDD: 202-514-0716.

The third statute, the EHA, provides for specially designed education programs and services for children whose handicap necessitates such programs. Under the EHA, a child is handicapped if he or she is mentally disabled, hearing impaired or deaf, speech or vision impaired, suffers a serious emotional disturbance, is orthopaedically impaired, suffers a specific learning disability, or suffers "other health impairment," such

Table 49.3.   § 504 Questions—Offices of Civil Rights, Department of Education

Region	States	Telephone Number
I	Connecticut, Maine, Massachusetts, New Hampshire, Rhode Island, Vermont	617-223-9662 TDD 617-223-9695
II	New Jersey, New York, Puerto Rico, Virgin Islands	212-264-4633 TDD 212-264-9464
III	Delaware, District of Columbia, Maryland, Pennsylvania, Virginia, West Virginia	215-596-6772 TDD 215-596-6794
IV	Alabama, Florida, Georgia, North Carolina, South Carolina, Tennessee	404-331-2954 TDD 404-331-7816
V	Illinois, Indiana, Minnesota, Michigan, Ohio, Wisconsin	312-886-3456 TDD 312-353-2541
VI	Arkansas, Louisiana, Mississippi, Oklahoma, Texas	214-767-3959 TDD 214-767-3639
VII	Iowa, Kansas, Kentucky, Missouri, Nebraska	816-891-8026 TDD 816-374-6461
VIII	Arizona, Colorado, Montana, New Mexico, North Dakota, South Dakota, Utah, Wyoming	303-844-5695 TDD 303-844-3417
IX	California	415-556-7000 TDD 415-556-6806
X	Alaska, Hawaii, Idaho, Nevada, Oregon, Washington, American Samoa, Guam, Trust Territory of the Pacific Islands	206-553-6811 TDD 206-553-4542

that special education and related services are required (26). A child with symptomatic HIV infection might come within any one of the categories listed while an asymptomatic child could be considered impaired under the "other health impaired" or possibly the "serious emotional disturbance" (awareness of HIV status by the child might lead to emotional stress) categories (29). Definitionally, EHA's "other health impaired" and § 504's "physical or mental impairment" are comparable; the regulations defining the two sets of terms include substantial overlap (29).

Thus, under the EHA, a child with HIV infection whose impairment(s) require specially designed education should be guaranteed this education as part of the right to a free appropriate education. Unfortunately, in the few decisions addressing HIV-infected children under the EHA, the courts have held such children were not within the EHA's definition of handicapped while they were handicapped under § 504 (29, 41, 42). However, no court foreclosed successful application of the EHA to HIV-infected children in a future case. Each court simply found the child at issue not to be handicapped based on the facts of the case.

Interestingly, in two of these cases (42, 43) the party arguing for EHA coverage was the school, which after excluding a child with AIDS was the defendant in a § 504 suit brought by the child. In each instance, the school unsuccessfully defended its actions by arguing that the child was obligated to exhaust EHA remedies (29). This raises the possibility that a school may attempt to use the EHA (IDEA) to effect a discrimination against a child with HIV infection. In other words, a school may claim that an HIV-infected child "requires" placement in a special education program as a means to separate the child from the regular classroom.

As a general policy, children with chronic illnesses, including HIV, should not be separated from their classmates. These children should be afforded the access and benefits of the regular classroom and activities. While individualized attention and care to special health needs is of critical importance, placement in special education programs and classrooms should be avoided if possible.

In its 1990 policy statement on children with health impairments in schools (43), the AAP stated that although educational planning should take into account the limitations placed on children with chronic illness, they "deserve access to basic educational services and the broader range of school activities such as clubs, student government, and athletics." A 1991 AAP policy statement specifically addressing the education of HIV-infected children elaborated, stating that such children in most cases do not need their health protected by exclusion from the school. The statement asserted that these children "should not be excluded from school for the protection of other children or personnel, nor should they be isolated within the school setting. Participation in school provides a sense of normality for the HIV-infected child and offers opportunities for socialization that are important" (44).

Thus, while the EHA (IDEA) is not currently of major use to HIV-infected children, hopefully future amending regulations, the ADA, and/or litigation under any of these statutes will more clearly establish the right under necessary circumstances to a special education and related services for children with HIV infection.

State Regulations and Local Policies

Although federal laws technically set the legal standards to which all states must adhere, the story only begins with the enactment of such legislation. First, statutory language is always subject to varied interpretation. In this vein, states and local communities may be openly hostile to what they see as federal intrusion into local affairs. Such communities typically will go to great lengths to "read" their practices and policies as consistent with federal law. Even absent malicious or provincialistic intent, a community policy inconsistent with federal mandates may take years to be recognized and altered.

Second, where state or local practices operate arguably in violation of federal law, enforcement of the federal standard becomes an issue with corrective action often delayed until a successful lawsuit forces the change. Third, a state or community may choose to offer broader rights or protections to its residents than those provided through the federal statutes. Therefore, in order to fully evaluate the legal conditions in a given school district, one must look beyond the federal laws to the state and the local policies.

States traditionally are accorded a fair amount of autonomy in running their educational programs. States, in turn, set forth general standards yet commonly grant a large measure of independence to the local school districts. There are approximately 15,000 school districts in the United States. Whereas school district policies are chiefly documents of communication and must reflect the legal standards and guidelines (45), it is apparent that throughout the country discrete policies on children with HIV infection will deviate greatly from one another.

The National Association of State Boards of Education (NASBE) recognizes the diversity among the many school districts. Without authority to promulgate regulations, NASBE addresses issues important to the districts and occasionally drafts model policies as guidance. Its guidance policies on children with HIV infection at school, published in 1989 (34), proved to be considerably influential. Though significantly more permissive than the official CDC guidelines (i.e., directing that HIV-infected children with biting behavior or lacking toilet training remain in the classroom, directing against a prohibition of contact sports), the CDC commended and informally endorsed the NASBE model policies.

A number of school districts subsequently drafted policies for HIV-infected students that, by incorporating the NASBE models, provided protections to HIV-infected children beyond those required under federal legislation. Unfortunately, many other school districts retain outdated and/or incomplete policies. For example, in a national survey of school districts it became evident that only a small minority of school districts had policies that appropriately required formal consent by the HIV-infected child or the parent prior to disclosure of HIV status to others (45).

Additionally, the health care provider and advocate must not forget something all too clear to children with HIV infection and their families: irrational fears and prejudices are not necessarily quieted or altered by judicial or legislative fiat. While legal directives may be relatively clear, individuals nevertheless possess the means and the power to frustrate functional operation of such mandates. Often the laws on paper bear no resemblance to the living reality. Newspapers continue to document harassment of HIV-infected children and their families so severe that, in effect, they are denied the protection of the antidiscrimination laws.

For example, in August of 1992 when a 7-year child with HIV infection indicated that she wished to attend the public elementary school in Lakeland, Florida, her family received death threats, and a large community meeting was held where many spoke out against permitting the child to attend the school (47). Thus, although federal legislation and judicial decisions are beginning to make headway in the fight against discrimination, local school districts and communities often lag far behind in implementing antidiscrimination measures and working successfully to alter attitudes.

LESS COMMON LEGAL ISSUES
Contact Sports

Contact sports including wrestling, football, rugby, and soccer have a high frequency of minor traumatic injuries resulting in bleeding (nosebleeds, abrasions). Because of this exposure to blood, a theoretical risk of HIV transmission exists. There are no documented cases of HIV transmission in any athletic setting; however, one undocumented case from Italy of possible HIV transmission during a collision between two soccer players was reported in 1990 (46).

In 1988, one court ordered a school to admit a 12-year child with HIV infection and also directed that the child could not participate in contact sports (35); however, the issue of the HIV-infected child who wishes to engage in contact sports has not been addressed subsequently by the courts or legislatures. In its 1989 model policies, NASBE recommended against prohibiting the HIV-infected student from participation in contact sports. NASBE noted that if CDC universal precautions were followed with any injuries involving blood, there would be no cause for concern of HIV transmission (34). The AAP addressed this issue in a 1991 report by its Committee on Sports Medicine and Fitness (48). The AAP recommendations include

1. Athletes infected with HIV should be allowed to participate in all competitive sports. This advice must be reconsidered if transmission of HIV is found to occur in the sports setting.
2. A physician counseling a known HIV-infected athlete in a sport involving blood exposure, such as wrestling or football, should inform him or her of the theoretical risk of contagion to others and strongly advise the student to consider another sport.
3. The physician should respect a HIV-infected athlete's right to confidentiality. This includes not disclosing the patient's status of infection to the participants or the staff of athletic programs.
4. All athletes should be made aware that the athletic program is operating under the policies in Recommendations 1 and 3.
5. Routine testing of athletes for HIV infection is not indicated (48).

The AAP recommendations reflect the prevailing medical knowledge of HIV transmission and should serve as guidelines for schools and children with HIV infection. If after receiving advice a child with HIV infection chooses to participate in a contact sport, litigation might ensue. Consistent with their analyses in cases where HIV-infected children seek admission to the regular classroom, courts probably would employ a "significant risk test" in resolving a dispute over whether a child with HIV infection may participate in a contact sport. At present, the scientific data convincingly support prohibiting any comprehensive restriction from contact sports.

Foster Care

Because of the complex relationships among HIV infection, drug use, prostitution, poverty, and child abuse and neglect, an increasing number of children with HIV

infection are entering the foster care system. Under nonfoster care circumstances, the parent(s) generally hold a right to make medical decisions on behalf of the child. This includes the ability to consent to HIV testing and to medical treatments whether routine or investigational. In foster care situations, the issue is complicated by the increased number of potentially involved parties (the biological parents, the foster parents, and the state) (49).

Laws governing the responsibilities of parents and foster parents vary among states, but the traditional rule is that parents retain the right to consent or to withhold consent for medical care. At first impression, this appears logical and just. Most parental rights are not terminated by foster care placement. Unlike adoptive parents, foster parents are intended as temporary custodians. In fact, federal law directs child welfare agencies to make reasonable efforts to place foster children back in their original home (49, 50). Yet, there are many situations where the foster parents are the more "involved" and available party. In such circumstances, it might be appropriate for the foster parents to possess a right of consent (perhaps nonexclusive). However, clearly the potential for confusion and conflict increases proportionally to the number of involved parties, and the law prefers clarity where possible. Perhaps in part because of feared disputes, state laws currently preserve the traditional rule.

However, where a court places a child in the care of a protective agency, the agency is given a right to consent. In these situations, the agency's relationship to the foster child is viewed legally as one of *in loco parentis* (i.e., being a legal replacement for the parent and thus charged with the parental rights, duties, and responsibilities). Thus, although foster parents are not given the right to consent, the agency may consent to medical care and treatment.

Plainly, the parents and the agency may disagree in a particular situation about whether medical care is desirable. Jurisdictions differ in their approaches to resolving differences between the parties. Many adopt policies similar to that of New York City where, under the rationale that legal custody lies with the commissioner of the child welfare agency, the commissioner is endowed with the ultimate responsibility for the foster care child's medical care. The policy directs that routine medical care decisions require only the commissioner's consent, whereas parental consent should be sought for nonroutine and emergency medical care (49).

Clearly, under this type of policy medical care including HIV testing and various treatment protocols must be categorized by the jurisdiction. Equally as plain is the potential for litigation where parties disagree about the necessity and/or the desire for medical care. Among the many issues raised by HIV infection are those of stigma and discrimination. A parent may seek to avoid any medical intervention, particularly HIV testing, which through problems in maintaining confidentiality could lead to these problems. Interestingly, at present, only two states (Illinois and Louisiana) expressly grant the agency authority to consent (without parental concurrence) to HIV testing of a child taken into temporary custody (51). In sum, increasing numbers of HIV-infected children and children at risk for HIV infection are being placed in foster care. The set-

ting of foster care raises numerous legal and ethical issues concerning appropriate care for these children. A concerned health care provider must critique the pertinent regulations in the jurisdiction.

CONCLUSIONS

The numbers of children with HIV infection continue to rise. Our medical and legal systems confront new challenges in resolving serious problems faced by these children and their families. The legal issues relevant to HIV-infected children are numerous. Federal and state legislation has begun to address the more easily identified and defined concerns of confidentiality and discrimination, but even there, coverage varies and enforcement is onerous. Advocates must familiarize themselves with the existing law and then seek to extend and expand rights and protections. Throughout this chapter, representative legal decisions have been cited. These judicial opinions are examples of the emerging case law addressing relevant legal issues for HIV-infected children and their care providers. Table 49.4 lists some of the significant cases and

Table 49.4.   Significant Legal Decisions

Case	Relevant Holding
Doe v. Centinela Hospital (1988)	Learning is a "major life activity" for purposes of meeting the statutory definition of handicapped or disabled
School Board of Nassau County, FL v. Arline (1987)	A person with a contagious disease (tuberculosis in this case) may be considered handicapped if a "major life activity" is substantially limited; further, contagion alone does not preclude the individual from being "otherwise qualified" for purposes of statutory protection and discrimination on that basis is impermissible
Chalk v. United States District Court, Central District of Cal. (1988)	Exclusion of an HIV-infected person is lawful only if a significant risk of HIV transmission exists
Doe v. Dalton Elementary School District No. 148 (1988)	Child with HIV infection, hemophilia, a cold sore, and oral thrush did not present a significant risk of HIV transmission in the classroom
Martinez v. School Board of Hillsborough County, FL (1988)	Mentally disabled child with HIV infection who lacked control of her bodily fluids did not present a significant risk of HIV transmission in the classroom
Thomas v. Atascadero (1987)	Child with HIV infection who had bitten another student did not, without more, present a significant risk of HIV transmission in the classroom; further, asymptomatic HIV infection meets the statutory definition of handicapped for purposes of coverage under § 504
Local 1812, American Federation of Government Employees v. Dept of State (1987)	Asymptomatic HIV infection meets the statutory definition of handicapped for purposes of coverage under § 504

Table 49.5. Organizations with Legal Expertise Concerning HIV Infection

Organization	Telephone Number
AIDS Project of the ACLU	212-994-9800 (extension 545)
National Lawyers Guild AIDS Network	415-824-8884
National Center for Youth Law	415-543-3307
National Association of Protection and Advocacy Systems	202-408-9514
Washington Lawyers Committee for Civil Rights, Disability Rights Council	202-682-5900
Local bar association	Listed under state bar association

includes a capsule summary of the legal holding.

As new knowledge in science and medicine becomes available, courts must be informed and educated. Although the emotional, financial, and time costs are enormous, the legal system, when used appropriately, can provide significant assistance to children, their families, and society. Although legal directives do not immediately result in attitudinal alteration, enforced compliance of the law over time will help reduce or eliminate some of the most profound fears and prejudice. Many public and private organizations have legal expertise in dealing with issues related to HIV infection. Any one of these groups may be able to provide legal assistance with a particular child or situation. An extremely abbreviated list of such organizations is presented in Table 49.5.

References

1. Powers M. Legal protections of confidential medical information and the need for antidiscrimination laws. In: Faden R, Geller F, Powers M, eds. AIDS, women, and the next generation: Towards a morally acceptable public policy for HIV testing of pregnant women and newborns. New York: Oxford University Press, 1991:221–255.
2. Griswold v. Connecticut, 381 U.S. 479, 484 (1965).
3. Whalen v. Roe, 429 U.S. 589 (1977).
4. Rothenberg K. AIDS: Creating a public health policy. 48 Maryland Law Review 1989:170–176.
5. California Health and Safety Code, sec. 199.21 West 1988 and subsequent amendments contained in Ch. 1216 (1988 Sessions Laws).
6. Massachusetts General Laws Annotated ch. 111, § 70F West 1988.
7. Hawaii Revised Statutes, sec. 325–101 1988.
8. 5 U.S.C. 552 (1982).
9. Quoted in Britton A. Rights to privacy in medical records. J Legal Med Jul-Aug 1975;3:30.
10. Seigler M. Confidentiality in medicine—a decrepit concept. N Engl J Med 1982;307:1518–1521.
11. Ginzburg H. Legal issues in the medical care of HIV-infected children. In: Pizzo PA, Wilfert CM, eds. Pediatric AIDS: The challenge of HIV infection in infants, children, and adolescents. Baltimore: William & Wilkins, 1991:756–764.
12. Tarasoff v. Regents of the University of California, 17 Cal. 3d 425, 441, 131 Cal. Rptr. 14, 27, 551 P.2d 334, 347 (1976).
13. Johnson v. West Virginia Hospitals, Inc., No. 19678, slip op. (W.Va., Nov 21, 1991) (rehearing denied, Feb 13, 1992).
14. Goldberg S. AIDS phobia: Reasonable fears or unreasonable lawsuits? ABA J Jun 1992;78:88.
15. School Board of Nassau County, Fla v. Arline 480 U.S. 273 (1987).
16. American Academy of Pediatrics Task Force on Pediatric AIDS: Pediatric guidelines for infection control of human immunodeficiency virus (acquired immunodeficiency virus) in hospitals, medical offices, schools and other settings. Pediatrics 1988;82:941–944.
17. Centers for Disease Control. Education and foster care of children infected with human T-lymphotropic virus type III/lymphadenopathy-associated virus. MMWR 1985;34:517–521.
18. Centers for Disease Control. Update: Universal precautions for prevention of transmission of human immunodeficiency virus, hepatitis B virus, and other bloodborne pathogens in health-care settings. MMWR 1988;37:377–387.
19. Centers for Disease Control. Guidelines for prevention of transmission of human immunodeficiency virus and hepatitis B virus for health-care and public-safety workers. MMWR 1989;38(suppl 6):1–37.
20. 53 Federal Register No. 69, Apr 11, 1988:11942–11958.
21. 20 U.S.C. 1232g (1988).
22. Michigan Department of Education Model Communicable Disease Policy. Lansing, MI: Michigan Department of Education, 1991.
23. 42 U.S.C. §§3601–3619 (1989 Supp.).
24. 29 U.S.C. §794 (1988).
25. 42 U.S.C.A. §§12101–12213 (West Supp. 1991) and 47 U.S.C.A. §§225, 611 (West 1991).
26. 20 U.S.C. §§1401, 1411–1420 (1988).
27. 20 U.S.C. §§1400–1485 (Supp. II 1990).
28. Feldblum CR. The Americans with Disabilities Act: Definition of disability. Labor Lawyer 1991;7:11.
29. Buss WG. Educating children with human immunodeficiency virus. In: Wiley Law Publications, eds. AIDS and the law. 2nd ed. New York: Wiley & Sons, 1992:105–150.
30. Doe v. Centinela Hospital, No. CV 87–2514 PAR (PX), 1988 U.S. Dist. Lexis 8401 (C.D. Cal 1988).

31. 34. C.F.R. §104.3(j)(2)(ii)(1990).
32. Hanlon SF. School and day care issues: The legal perspective. In: Pizzo PA, Wilfert CM, eds. Pediatric AIDS: The challenge of HIV infection in infants, children, and adolescents. Baltimore: Williams & Wilkins, 1991:693–703.
33. Chalk v. United States District Court, Central District of Cal., 840 F.2d 710 (9th Cir. 1988).
34. Fraser K. Someone at school has AIDS. Alexandria, VA: National Association of State Boards of Education, 1989.
35. Doe v. Dalton Elementary School District No. 148, 694 F. Supp. 440 (N.D. Ill 1988).
36. Martinez v. School Board of Hillsborough County, Fla., 692 F. Supp. 1293 (M.D. Fla. 1988) vacated and remanded, 861 F. Supp. (11th Cir. 1988).
37. Thomas v. Atascadero, 662 F.2d 376 (C.D. Cal. 1987).
38. Douglas W. Kmiec, Acting Asst Atty Gen, Office of Legal Counsel, Dept of Justice [Memorandum], Sep 27, 1988.
39. Local 1812, American Federation of Government Employees v. Dept of State, 662 F. Supp. 50 (D.D.C. 1987).
40. Ray v. School District of DeSoto County, 666 F. Supp. 1524 (M.D. Fla. 1987).
41. Robertson v. Granite City Community Unified School District No. 9, 684 F. Supp. 1001 (S.D. Ill. 1988).
42. Doe v. Belleville Public School, 672 F. Supp. 342 (S.D. Ill. 1987).
43. American Academy of Pediatrics. Policy statement on children with health impairments in schools. Am Acad Pediatr News 6(7); Jul 1990:17.
44. American Academy of Pediatrics. Policy statement on education of children with HIV infection. Am Acad Pediatr News 7(6) Jun 1991:20–21.
45. Anonymous. HIV/AIDS policy review, draft copy. Alexandria, VA: National School Boards Association, 1992.
46. Torre C, Sampietro C, Ferraro G, Zeroli C, Speranza F. Transmission of HIV-I via sports injury. Lancet 1990;335:1105.
47. Booth W. Quayle taunted on AIDS during Florida bus trip. Washington Post, Aug 24, 1992:A8.
48. Nelson MA, Goldberg B, Harris SS, Landry GL, Orenstein DM, Risser WL. Committee on sports medicine and fitness. Human immunodeficiency virus [acquired immunodeficiency syndrome (AIDS) virus] in the athletic setting. Pediatrics 1991;88:640–641.
49. Palacio C, Weedy C. Treatment issues regarding children in foster care. In: Pizzo PA, Wilfert CM eds. Pediatric AIDS: The challenge of HIV infection in infants, children, and adolescents. Baltimore: Williams & Wilkins, 1991:569–576.
50. Adoption Assistance and Child Welfare Act of 1980,42 U.S.C. 670.
51. States with HIV/AIDS Foster Care Legislation. AIDS Policy Center, Intergovernmental Health Policy Project, The George Washington University, Aug 1992.

50
Speaking with Children and Families about HIV Infections

Carolyn Keith Burr and L. Jean Emery

Children, even young children, are increasingly aware of human immunodeficiency virus (HIV) and AIDS through the media, through school, and at home. Their concerns and questions need to be addressed in an informed and compassionate way. How can health and social service professionals help children understand HIV/AIDS and assist families in responding to their questions and concerns? This chapter offers some guidance on these issues by focusing on the knowledge and skills that adults, both parents and professionals, need when speaking with individual children about HIV and AIDS. Principles of children's cognitive development regarding illness—central to appropriately speaking with children about AIDS—will be presented. The chapter also addresses the special issues of talking with children who are themselves infected with HIV or are personally affected because of a family member or friend who is infected with HIV.

In addition to helping children understand both AIDS as an illness and the prevention of HIV transmission, professionals and parents speaking with children want to teach empathy and compassion toward those affected by HIV/AIDS. Both the attitudes of trusted adults and the content of teaching materials can help children separate the illness from the persons affected by HIV and foster positive attitudes toward affected individuals.

Speaking with children about HIV/AIDS is challenging for professionals and families because it raises the difficult topics of sexuality, illness, and death and the values and feelings associated with them. By providing a framework for discussion and resources to enhance the discussion, the authors hope to provide professionals with a starting point for an ongoing response to children's concerns about HIV/AIDS.

CHILDREN AND HIV IN COMMUNITY CONTEXT: FAMILY, SCHOOLS, AND THE MEDIA
Family's Role

Much of what children learn about HIV/AIDS will be from their family. Families, in their daily life, provide children with a range of information, beliefs, and attitudes about health and illness. Some families place a high value on healthy behaviors and teach children about diet, hygiene, and safety at an early age. Other families simply model the behaviors they wish their children to follow and discuss health concerns only when someone is ill or when a child raises a question.

The family's own attitudes and knowledge about illness will influence their approach to explaining HIV/AIDS to the child. Adults may have only a limited understanding of illness causation. They may know that illness is caused by bacteria or viruses but have little knowledge of how disease occurs on a cellular or organ system level. Parents still explain that an ear infection is caused by "not wearing a hat" or that colds are caused by "getting your feet wet." Families' knowledge of HIV may be limited to what they have gleaned from the lay press. Professionals must assess the parents' knowledge level and provide information and written resources that will increase their understanding of HIV (Table 50.1). Community or workplace based AIDS edu-

cation, such as that available through the American Red Cross and others, is important in increasing adults' knowledge of HIV.

Families hold values and beliefs that will influence what they say to their children. Some families may have negative attitudes toward homosexuals or intravenous drug users and may believe that "AIDS is punish-

Table 50.1.   Resources for Parents and Families

Author and Title	Publisher and Date	Description
What Should You Tell Your Infected Child about AIDS?	*Common Sense about AIDS:* Supplement to *AIDS Alert.* American Health Consultants, Nov 1992	Brief article gives practical advice from professionals
Quackenbush M, Villarreal S. *Does AIDS Hurt? Educating Young Children about AIDS*	Network Publications, a division of ETR Associates, Santa Cruz, CA, 1988	Suggestions for teachers and other care providers of children younger than 10
Aunt Rita's Patient: A Story about AIDS, Teacher's Guide	American Red Cross, St. Paul, MN; available from local American Red Cross chapters 1989	Teacher's guide to a book for older school-age children teaching AIDS awareness, prevention, and compassion for person with HIV
Dumas LS. Why did Uncle Tommy die? Talking with your child about AIDS. In: *Talking with Your Child about a Troubled World*	Ballantine Books, New York, 1992	Chapter outlines techniques for telling children about AIDS and helping them face the death of a loved one to AIDS
What Shall I Tell My Child? Parent Information Booklet	Children's Hospital AIDS Program, 15 S. 9th St., Newark, NJ 07107, 1990	Suggestions on HIV disclosure to families of infected children; English and Spanish versions
Hausherr R. *Children and the AIDS Virus: A Book for Children, Parents, and Teachers*	Clarion Books, New York, 1989	Simple explanation of immune system, how HIV attacks it, and what can be done to prevent it; pictures and main text for young readers and informational subtext for adults
Berger L, Lithwick D, and Seven Campers. *I Will Sing Life: Voices from the Hole in the Wall Gang Camp*	Little, Brown, Boston, 1992	Chapter written by a young teenager with perinatally acquired HIV; describes own experience with disclosure and coping with HIV; suitable for preadolescent and adolescents
Steinhart B. *Living with HIV: Talking with Your Child*	National Hemophilia Foundation, New York, 1990	Pamphlet provides guidance to parents for talking with their child who has hemophilia and HIV
Tiffany J, Tobias D, Raqib A, et al. *Talking with Kids about AIDS: A Program for Parents and Other Adults Who Care*	Cornell University, Department of Human Service Studies, Van Rensselaer Hall 184, Ithaca, NY 14853, 1991	Manual suggests ways to talk with children in specific age groups

ment for misdeeds." Professionals are not likely to change strongly held beliefs completely, but they can provide information about HIV transmission that can allay fears about casual transmission in the school or community.

Families may have concerns about discussing HIV/AIDS with their children because of the issues of sexuality, drug use, and death that will inevitably arise. Parents must be offered guidance to address these issues in a developmentally appropriate manner. Professionals should consider the following questions as they work with families. How has the family answered other questions about sexuality and death when the child has raised these topics? Have they laid a groundwork of openness by answering questions from the child? Can parents determine the meaning behind the child's questions about AIDS?

Quackenbush and Villarreal (1), in their guide to educating children younger than 10 years about AIDS, suggest that children may ask questions for many reasons including general information-seeking and curiosity, concern about their own welfare, concern about the welfare of family members or friends, or simply seeing the reaction from adults. They suggest that parents look for opportunities to bring up the topic of AIDS in the context of discussions about health, sexuality, or "things that frighten people" and use these discussions to reinforce the family's values about compassion, death, and substance abuse, for example. They remind parents that they need not know all the answers and that parents may need to take a short time to think about responses before answering their child's questions. Parents, they note, may make mistakes in fielding questions, but, by establishing an ongoing dialogue with their children, they will have the opportunity to approach answers more completely in the future.

Using metaphors and examples is helpful to children as they begin to come to terms with some of the more difficult issues raised by HIV/AIDS. Children who understand that sexual behavior and needle sharing can put a person at risk for HIV may wonder why a person engages in those behaviors. An adult can explain that sometimes people do not know the full extent of the risk they are taking; e.g., they used drugs before it was known that AIDS was transmitted by needles or that everyone take some risks that can have serious consequences without always thinking things through. An example from a child's life can be helpful: "Sometimes when you are playing soccer in the yard, the ball gets kicked into the street and you run out to get it. You know that you should stop and look for cars before you go into the street, but sometimes in the excitement of the game you forget, and run into the street. Usually nothing happens except that you get yelled at by a grown-up, but you could have been hit by a car. You didn't mean to be careless, but you were. Sometimes the same kind of thing happens with adult behaviors and some of those behaviors result in exposure to HIV."

HIV/AIDS and Schools

HIV and AIDS have become a concern for schools for two reasons—1) the integration of HIV prevention education into health education and other areas of curriculum and 2) the issues surrounding admitting children with HIV into school settings because of transmission fears. A discussion of school based HIV prevention is beyond the scope of this chapter, but many materials have been developed and can be accessed through the Centers for Disease Control National AIDS Clearinghouse's School Health Education Database.

As children with HIV infection and AIDS are living longer healthier lives, their need for participation in all of the usual growth and socialization experiences of young children—day care, play groups, and school—has become more apparent. The perceived need for prevention education, however, has not always translated into acceptance of HIV-affected children and families into schools and communities.

At first, the "innocent victims" aspect of the disease was used by some as a way to differentiate among those infected by HIV. But schools and communities soon realized that fear of transmission of the virus had to be addressed to prevent that fear from crowding out consideration and compassion for the children and families affected by the virus. The ignorance, fear, near hysteria, and discrimination that was the country's initial response to AIDS in the adult population infuenced the response of communities to the issues of serving children with AIDS. In some communities, all the negative dynamics prevalent in responses to adults with AIDS spilled over into similar reactions to children. Thus, families have been cautious in sharing information about children's HIV status beyond their care providers and the family.

The reactions of persons living in small towns all over America was sensitively detailed. The volatile issue of children with HIV infection living in communities and attending schools was documented by Kirp and Epstein (2). Both positive and compassionate and negative, crass, and dangerous reactions to these situations were carefully provided. A home of children with AIDS was burned; death threats were made against households of young persons with HIV, and families affected by the disease were shunned—leading to isolation, often self-imposed, for families affected by AIDS. In other communities, families' disclosure of HIV led to support and assistance from the community.

Education of School Administrators, Staff, and Parents

The unpredictability of community response has led to a reticence among parents of children with HIV to share personal medical information beyond the family. One explanation is that misunderstandings about the disease are due to lack of education about the HIV virus and how it is transmitted. A carefully structured, ongoing education and training program about HIV/AIDS for the schools is an important beginning to a more measured response to AIDS in the school. By educating school administrators, teachers, parents, and the community about HIV, the school can create an environment that accepts HIV-affected persons and allows for HIV education, including prevention education, to occur. One such approach is suggested in the Child Welfare League of America guide for child day care providers (3). In their

model, a specific school staff member is assigned to become the "AIDS expert" and to develop an educational/training course that includes information about basic medical facts, issues of transmission of infectious diseases, progression of HIV after exposure, HIV testing, psychosocial issues for children with HIV/AIDS and their families, and age-appropriate education on HIV/AIDS for the children themselves.

The National Association of State Boards of Education has published a comprehensive guide to policy and procedure development for schools that examines issues of confidentiality policies, approaches to dispelling myths about transmission, and techniques for infection control (4). The Pediatric AIDS Foundation has produced a book and video set that is designed to assist communities to accept HIV-positive children in school (5). The guide outlines an approach to a community meeting and provides a video for use at that meeting as well as a video to help adults talk with children about HIV. A video and discussion guide about school-age children and HIV infection from the Child Welfare League of America (6) offers information for parents and care providers about the basics dynamics of children with HIV entering school.

Disclosure of a child's HIV diagnosis to selected professionals in the school setting can have positive benefits to the child's health and educational program as well as providing a source of support to families. No documented account of transmission of HIV has been traced to casual contact, such as is encountered in daily activity in a school setting. A child may be on medication or a special diet. In addition, children with HIV infection may be particularly vulnerable should there be an outbreak of chickenpox in the school. Depending on the age and emotional status of the child, she or he may also need and welcome emotional support from appropriate school staff members.

School settings clearly provide a place where children can learn HIV prevention. In addition they can provide all children with the learning experience that children with HIV, like children with other chronic illnesses, are more similar than different from them. By working proactively with school staff, health and social service professionals have an opportunity to reach children with accurate compassionate information about HIV, its prevention, and the persons who are living with it.

Children and Media

As with many issues in our society, the media is important in providing children with information about HIV/AIDS and in shaping their attitudes toward it. Television, especially, has been identified by children as a primary source of their knowledge about HIV/AIDS (7, 8). That information comes from TV in various ways—public service announcements, educational programs, news items on scientific breakthroughs or well-known people with AIDS, and HIV/AIDS in the stories of evening programs. TV movies, and daytime dramas. When current and accurate, information about HIV can add to the knowledge of older children. For younger children, TV information may cause them concern or fear. Unfortunately, public misconceptions, fear of contagion, and moral judgments may predominate in the news and do not help provide objective information. Professionals and parents must be ready to talk with children and to respond to their questions and concerns in a developmentally appropriate way.

CHILDREN'S UNDERSTANDING OF ILLNESS

To speak appropriately with children about HIV, professionals and families need an awareness of how children think about illness. Children's understanding about illness causality is different from that of adults, not simply because children lack knowledge about illness but because as their cognitive processes develop so does their ability to understand illness. The work of Piaget (9) describes the logic of children's understanding of space, time, causality, and number that follows a predictable sequence and is developmentally based. Bibace and Walsh (10) have applied those concepts in studying children's understanding of illness. They describe six stages of children's concepts of illness—their understanding of illness, its cause, and its cure. The most significant factor in the progress through these stages is the child's differentiation between self and other (11). They have also examined children's understanding of AIDS in a study of 60 children in three age groups (5–7 years, 8–10 years, and 11–13 years) representing the three major phases of cognitive development (12). They found that children's causal thinking about AIDS follows the same developmental sequence as that for other illnesses. Adapting the Concepts of Illness Protocol (10) to AIDS, they interviewed children using specific questions about the definition, cause, treatment, and prevention of AIDS. The responses were scored using the Developmental Conceptions of Illness Category System, which organizes the data according to the three major developmental levels or ways in which people think about illness. The results of this study provide the most systematic developmental analysis of children's understanding of AIDS.

Several authorities have recommended utilizing developmentally based approach to AIDS education for children (13, 14). Little specific guidance has been offered, however, on how to apply developmental concepts to speaking with children about AIDS concretely. The work of Bibace and Walsh (11, 12, 15) provides a foundation of children's developmental understanding of illness that, when combined with the work of others, can give specific guidance to professionals and parents speaking with children about HIV/AIDS.

Researchers have struggled with how to determine which children are in which developmental level of understanding of illness. The developmental sequence of illness understanding, as that of other cognitive areas such as time and conservation, follows a logical sequence over time but does not exactly correlate with age from child to child. However, chronological age has been chosen by most researchers as the index of cognitive development, since in normal children, age is highly correlated with cognitive stage (12). Children with developmental delay may be at a less advanced cognitive stage, however. Familiarity with the cognitive developmental stages enables the professional to tailor information to the needs of the child and family.

Prelogical Thinking

Children aged 2 to 7 years utilize what Piaget characterized as prelogical thinking. They cannot distance themselves from the environment and are egocentric; thus they cannot distinguish between their perspective and that of others. They focus on events that are external and observed and have little understanding of events that are internal or unseen. They do not distinguish between cause and effect or they link them through magical thinking (15). Older children in this stage can describe a cause for illness, which they can differentiate from the symptoms or effects, but they cannot link the cause to the effect.

Young children need their questions and concerns about HIV/AIDS addressed. These questions may arise in discussions about health and illness in general or in response to hearing about HIV/AIDS in the community or media. Since they cannot differentiate cause and effect and do not have concepts of the inner workings of the body, details of HIV prevention education ("Use condoms when having sex." "Don't share dirty needles.") are inappropriate for children at this age. However, simple hygienic measure, such as not touching someone else's blood and washing one's hands, can provide a basis for more specific HIV education later.

Magical thinking, however, may cause young children to have irrational fears about disease and illness, so professionals and families answering questions about AIDS should focus on managing fears. Children should be encouraged to talk about their worries. Gentle questioning about what a child knows or has heard can often uncover the worry and can help the adult assess the level of the child's knowledge and interest. Reassurance from an authority figure—a parent, teacher, or health professional—usually allays the child's concern (15). When there is media coverage of a well-known person with AIDS, children may worry that they can catch it or that someone they love may become ill. Reassurance that "AIDS is a bad illness, but it is hard to catch" and responses to specific concerns ("You can't catch it from hugging or kissing") should satisfy the child. More detailed explanations of sexual transmission or needle sharing behaviors require an understanding of cause and effect that the young child does not have. Parents should be encouraged to develop an ongoing dialogue with children about sensitive issues such as sexuality and death, and providers should offer guidance to parents in approaching these topics (Tables 50.1 and 50.2).

Concrete Logical Thinking

In the next developmental stage—concrete logical thinking—seen in children approximately ages 7–10 years, children differentiate more between self and other, can begin to differentiate between internal and external body events, can begin to understand inner bodily functions, can link cause and effect, and are more relativistic in their thinking (15). Children define illness and AIDS in terms of specific symptoms experienced by the body. Early in this stage, illness is described as affecting only the surface of the body, whereas older children can describe effects on internal body systems.

Since children in this cognitive stage have better understanding of cause and effect, HIV/AIDS education can include concrete examples of causes of AIDS (e.g., sharing dirty needles when using drugs) as well as concrete examples of ways in which HIV is not transmitted (e.g., kissing people, mosquitos, sharing a comb) (15). Children in this stage can also better understand the cause of HIV and its impact on body systems.

One study of 5th graders found that while their knowledge level was high (>90%) regarding needle sharing and sexual contact as transmission routes, 30–50% thought HIV could be transmitted through other activities—kissing, mosquito bites, sharing a comb (7). This finding may indicate that although media messages regarding transmission are being heard, children also need specific information about concrete ways in which AIDS is not transmitted to alleviate their fears.

Another study of 147 children aged 6–12 years found that their awareness and accurate knowledge regarding AIDS increased steadily through the school years (8). Television was identified as their source of HIV information by over half the 4th–6th graders, with parents seen as the source by another 20–30%, and school and friends identified as the major source by only ~10%. Knowledge also seemed to influence attitudes, with 60% of 4th graders believing that children with AIDS should not be allowed to attend school with other children, whereas only 9% of 5th and 6th graders held that belief. Table 50.2 contains several resources appropriate for children in this age group.

Formal Logical Thinking

The cognitive developmental level of children approximately age 11 and older—formal logical thinking—enables them to see themselves as distinct from but related to others. They can explain cause and effect in a more complex way and describe multiple factors that can influence events. These children can understand, for example, that persons with HIV can stay healthier through medications, by the quality of their care, and because of their attitude. Illness is viewed as a malfunction of internal processes that may result in internal and external symptoms (15). Because of their more sophisticated cognitive processes, children in this stage can understand the mechanisms of prevention and that they can avoid AIDS through their actions (Table 50.2).

SPECIAL SITUATIONS IN SPEAKING WITH CHILDREN ABOUT HIV

Affected Child

Children who personally know someone who is HIV infected—a friend, family member, teacher, or classmate—have special needs when the topic of HIV/AIDS is discussed. Their sense of vulnerability regarding HIV is likely to be increased. Uninfected children in families where perinatal transmission of HIV has occurred may have multiple family members infected with HIV—mother, father, siblings. In some families, members from multiple generations

may be infected, including grandparents, aunts, or uncles.

Affected children may wonder how the person contracted HIV and if they are also at risk. They should be reassured that casual transmission does not occur but should also be taught the basics of universal precautions in the home. If the adult with HIV is the child's parent, the child should be told that she or he is not at risk ("You were born before Mom was infected with the virus") or that the child's HIV status is known ("We had you tested for HIV and you don't have it"). Disclosure of diagnosis to a child can be painful for the parent with HIV infection. The parent may be experiencing guilt over the risk behaviors that caused the HIV and fears the anger or rejection of the child. In clinical practice, parents can be reminded that they never intended to cause harm and that they did not intentionally place themselves or their child at risk for HIV. This approach can help them cope with the guilt and pain.

Whether the person with HIV infection is a family member or an acquaintance, these situations also provide the opportunity to discuss the needs for compassion, acceptance, support, and friendship of all persons with HIV. The family may need to discuss the fact that persons with HIV are sometimes discriminated against or shunned because of their illness but that such attitudes reflect prejudice and fear. The love and support of friends and the community are important for persons with HIV.

Children need factual information not only about transmission but also about the course of illness. The media often gives the impression that once someone is HIV positive, they have AIDS, and AIDS is fatal. Children in the concrete logical stage of illness causation may believe that because HIV can cause death, it does so immediately. Children must be told that adults can live many years before HIV makes them sick and that even when they begin to have symptoms, there are medicines that can help them.

The media and, in some cases materials developed for children, often portray pediatric HIV as an illness with which children die within 1 or 2 years of diagnosis. In fact, children with HIV are living longer health-

Table 50.2.   Resources for All Children

Author and Title	Publisher and Date	Description	Age Group
Aiello B, Shulman J. *Friends for Life*	Kids on the Block Series, Twenty-First Century Books, 38 S. Market St., Frederick, MD (301-698-0210), 1988	Fifth graders learn about HIV when they discover an adult friend is infected with HIV	10 and over
Aunt Rita's Patient: A Story about AIDS	American Red Cross, St. Paul, MN; available from many local American Red Cross chapters, 1989	Two children learn about HIV prevention, AIDS, and empathy for persons with AIDS	9–12 (grades 4–6)
Fassler D, McQueen K. *What's a Virus Anyway? The Kids' Book about AIDS*	Waterfront Books, 98 Brookes Ave, Burlington, VT 05401, 1990	Discussion of viruses and how they make you sick, the AIDS virus, and how it is and is not transmitted; illustrated with pictures drawn by children; stresses that persons with HIV "are just like everybody else"; English and Spanish versions	6–11
Hausherr R. *Children and the AIDS Virus: A Book for Children, Parents, and Teachers*	Clarion Books (Houghton Mifflin imprint), 52 Vanderbilt Ave., New York, NY 10017, 1989	Simple explanation of immune system, how HIV attacks it, and what can be done to prevent it; pictures and main text for young readers and informational subtext for adults	7 and over
Koch J. *AIDS: A Primer for Children*	Barrent Publications, 1025 Northern Blvd., Roslyn, NY 11576 (516-365-4040), 1989	Simple explanation of how germs cause illness including HIV; explains that AIDS is not transmitted through casual contact; encourages children to ask questions; English and Spanish versions	7–10
Merrifield M. *Come Sit With Me*	Women's Press, 517 College St., Suite 233, Toronto, Canada M6G 4A7 (416-921-2425), 1990	Story of Nicholas, a child with AIDS, who is initially rejected at nursery school; a classmate's mother, a physician, provides AIDS education to other parents in school to overcome fear; provides reassurance from mother/physician authority figure that HIV is not spread through casual contact and utilizes egocentric perspective of young child	4–7

Table 50.2.—*continued*

Author and Title	Publisher and Date	Description	Age Group
Sanford D. *David Has AIDS*	Multnomah Press, 10209 SE Division St., Portland, OR 97266 (800-547-5890), 1989	Story of boy with hemophilia and AIDS who is befriended by another boy; religious beliefs of child and family help them prepare for his death	7–10
Shilling S, Mossburg M. *My Friend . . . and AIDS: A story of friendship in a world with AIDS*	A Way With Words Publishers, P.O. Box 934, Parker CO, 80134, 1988	Photo book describes friendship between two boys, one of whom has hemophilia and HIV	7 and older
Starkman N. *Z's Gift*	Comprehensive Health Education Foundation, 22323 Pacific Hwy. S., Seattle, WA 98198 (206-824-2907), 1988	Story of Z who learns his teacher has AIDS. Family physician speaks to parents about HIV and its transmission; describes Z's compassion and caring toward the teacher and how he copes with her death	7 and older
Swain J, Schilling S. *"My Name is Jonathan (and I have AIDS)"*	Prickly Pair Publishing, 9628 W. Oregon Pl, Denver, CO 80226 (303-986-3503), 1989	Picture book of the daily life of a 6-year-old with transfusion-acquired HIV including HIV transmission, medical procedures, and interactions with friends	7 and older
Tasker M. *Jimmy and His Family*	Association for the Care of Children's Health, 7910 Woodmont Ave., Suite 300, Bethesda, MD 20814 (301-654-6549), 1992	Illustrated book provides first person account of a boy living with AIDS, the love and support of his family, and safety of living with someone with HIV; English and Spanish versions	7 and older

ier lives because of new medications and better management. Discussions with children about the course of illness should include both honesty and hope.

Disclosure of someone's diagnosis of HIV to a child can be complicated not only by the child's developmental understanding but also by considerations of the need for confidentiality about the diagnosis. Because of fear that a child may tell others, a family may not feel it can tell a child about the HIV diagnosis of a family member or friend. Persons with HIV and their families fear discrimination, stigmatization, and reprisals if their HIV status is known. Families must consider how and when to tell a child. They can consider whether this is a child who can understand that "some things can be talked about within the family but not with everyone." Disclosure of diagnosis is a process that is ongoing. Children may need to ask questions that the family may have already answered; their understanding and need for information will change as they develop.

Child with HIV Infection

The disclosure to a child of his or her own diagnosis of HIV infection can be difficult and complicated. The family must consider whether they are ready for the child to know and what they will do if the child inadvertently learns. Knowing the child's cognitive level and having some idea of his or her understanding of illness causation can help the family decide what they want to tell the child. Because of the developmental delays that can be caused by HIV, a child's chronological age may be a less useful guide for determining the child's understanding of illness. The family may benefit from the assessment of the child's developmental level by a psychologist as they consider what to say and when. Table 50.3 provided suggested resources for talking with children with HIV infection.

HIV-affected families are coping with many issues in addition to HIV. They may be dealing with poverty, poor housing, lack of access to health and social services, and drug use. Families of children with transfusion-acquired HIV may be dealing with another chronic illness—hemophilia or heart disease, for example—in addition to HIV. These other issues often complicate the process of disclosure and may undermine the family's ability to support the child during the disclosure process. Professionals' support for families can be a critical ingredient during this process.

Families of children with HIV utilize coping strategies similar to those of families with other chronically ill children. They assign meaning to the illness through a religious philosophy ("God doesn't give us more than we can handle") or by seeking scientific and medical explanations (16). They may cope by seeking to share the burden of the illness within the family and community (17). Although many families have drawn on the strength of their extended family for emotional support and assistance with concrete tasks, the illness of multiple family members or the family dysfunction that preceded the illness may limit the family's ability to do so. Families may be unwilling to seek community support because of the stigma of AIDS. Health and social service providers caring for the child and family may be called upon to provide that emotional support.

Disclosure may occur regardless of whether the family is ready. Children have learned their HIV diagnosis from overhearing conversations among medical professionals or from taunts on the street. When one child confronted her aunt with "Do I have AIDS?" the aunt was honest and reassuring. "You are one of God's special angels," she told her and assured her of the family's love and care. Some children may react angrily, become withdrawn, or seem not to react at all.

Disclosure of HIV diagnosis is a process that unfolds over time. Information that is helpful and satisfactory to a child at one point may need expansion and clarification later. The experience of therapists leading a group of school-age children who know their diagnosis of HIV seems to suggest that children must work through their fears of what will happen when they die: (will they be alone when they die? will they have a blanket in the casket?) before they can more on to other issues (S. Lewis, personal communication, 1992). Once the child knows his or her HIV diagnosis, the family and professionals

Table 50.3.   Resources for HIV-infected Children[a]

Author and Title	Publisher and Date	Description	Age Group
Baker LS. *You and HIV: A Day at a Time*	WB Saunders, Curtis Center, Independence Square W, Philadelphia, PA 19106, 1991	Well written, detailed book describes workings of body, immune system, viruses, and HIV replication; chapters discuss opportunistic infections, antiretroviral therapy, and other aspects of treatment; best utilized in small sections with guidance from a family member or professional	10–adult
Lebien S. *Our Immune System*	Immune Deficiency Foundation, P.O. Box 586, Columbia, MD 21045 (410-461-3127), 1990	Brochure explains how immune system works, roles of immunoglobulins, T cells, and B cells and how infections make you sick and how they are treated	7–10 and older
Saidi P, Lerner A, Clemow L. *Defending the Castle*	Univ. of Medicine and Dentistry of NJ, Robert Wood Johnson Medical School, NJ Regional Hemophilia Program, 378C, 1 Robert Wood Johnson Pl., New Brunswick, NJ 08903, 1989	Analogy of a castle is used to describe body and immune system, with HIV as attacker; includes information on risky behavior and relationship of HIV and hemophilia	11 and older
Tasker M. *Jimmy and the Eggs Virus*	Children's Hospital AIDS Program, 15 S. 9th St., Newark, NJ 07107 (800-362-0071), 1988	Jimmy learns that he has AIDS, not "eggs," virus and handles his fears; introduces health professionals and children he meets and describes how talking about HIV can help it be less frightening; useful in disclosing HIV diagnosis to children	7 and older

[a]General resources for children are also appropriate for HIV-infected children when shared with them by an adult.

should look for opportunities to clarify and validate the child's understanding.

Mary Tasker's (18) provides an indepth exploration of issues of disclosure to children of their diagnosis. Using the experience of parents and families, Tasker provides a framework for understanding the complex issues surrounding disclosure while leaving it to families to decide if, how, and when disclosure should occur.

Support groups for HIV-affected families by agencies such as the Family Place in Newark, New Jersey (19) can be helpful in the disclosure process. Interaction within these groups helps families continue to absorb the meaning of this disease to their children and to themselves. The group setting offers a forum for sharing information and feelings and dealing with the issues of grief and loss. The resultant discovery of a universality of experience often helps participants combat the isolation encountered as a result of HIV infection in the family. Decision making about whether or when to disclose HIV to persons in the school or community is facilitated. Members of the group learn together and strengthen both their spirit and their ability to educate others.

RESOURCES FOR CHILDREN, FAMILIES, AND PROFESSIONALS

The resources listed in Tables 50.1–50.3 include selected materials for children, families, and professionals that can be helpful in speaking with children about HIV. Many other materials are available for children regarding HIV prevention programs in the school and community. New materials for talking with HIV-affected and -infected children are being developed. The Centers for Disease Control National AIDS Clearinghouse (1-800-458-5231) provides access to databases for educational materials for children including books, videos, comic books, and coloring books. The National Pediatric HIV Resource Center (1-800-372-0071) serves as a resource for professionals as a part of their training, technical assistance, and resource development activities.

CONCLUSION

An adult who speaks with a child about HIV and AIDS needs to be knowledgeable and have an assessment of the child's level of cognitive development and understanding of illness. Often, parents or professionals are confronted with the need to respond to a child's question or concern without being prepared for it. By taking a moment to reflect and to clarify with the child the meaning of the question, the adult can respond in a sensitive and developmentally appropriate way. By being open to a child's questions and promoting an atmosphere where questioning is encouraged, the adult lays the groundwork for continuing discussions about HIV and AIDS. Such discussions prepare children to learn more about their bodies, about illness and illness prevention, and about empathy and compassion for persons affected by HIV.

Families of children infected with HIV or closely affected by it face difficult issues in sharing the HIV diagnosis with a child. Disclosure of diagnosis is a dynamic process that can be assisted by sensitivity to the child's readiness for receiving information, understanding of his or her cognitive developmental level, and support for the child and family during the process.

Professionals caring for children in the community and for children infected and affected by HIV must be committed to maintaining an informed, sensitive, and compassionate approach to speaking with children about HIV both in their formal provider roles and in their roles in the backyards and playgrounds of the community.

References

1. Quackenbush M, Villarreal S. Does AIDS hurt? Educating young children about AIDS. Santa Cruz: Network Publications, 1988.
2. Kirp DL, Epstein S. Learning by heart: AIDS and schoolchildren in America's communities. New Brunswick: Rutgers University Press, 1989.
3. Child Welfare League of America. Serving children with HIV infection in child day care: A guide for center-based and family day care providers. Washington, DC: Child Welfare League of America, 1991.
4. Anonymous. Someone in school has AIDS: A guide to developing policies for students and school staff members who are infected with HIV. Alexandria, VA: National Association of State Boards of Education, 1989.
5. Sega Charitable Trust & Pediatric AIDS Foundation. A guide for communities—video and discussion guide. Santa Monica: Pediatric AIDS Foundation, 1992.

6. Child Welfare League of America. Caring for school-age children with HIV infection—video and discussion guide. Washington, DC: Child Welfare League of America, 1991.

7. Brown LK, Nassau JH, Barone VJ. Differences in AIDS knowledge and attitudes by grade level. J School Health 1990;60:270–275.

8. Fassler D, McQueen K, Duncan P, Copeland L. Children's perceptions of AIDS. J Am Acad Child Adolesc Psychiatry 1990;29:459–462.

9. Piaget J. The origins of intelligence in children. New York: International Universities Press, 1952.

10. Bibace R, Walsh ME. Developmental stages in children's conceptions of illness. In: Stone GC, Cohen F, Adler N, eds. Health psychology. San Francisco: Jossey-Bass, 1979:285–301.

11. Bibace R, Walsh ME. Development of children's concepts of illness. Pediatrics 1980;66:912–917.

12. Walsh ME, Bibace R. Children's conceptions of AIDS: A developmental analysis. J Pediatr Psychol 1991;16:273–285.

13. Centers for Disease Control. Guidelines for effective school health education to prevent the spread of AIDS. MMWR 1988;37(S-2):1–14.

14. Helgerson S, Petersen L, AIDS Education Study Group. Acquired immunodeficiency syndrome and secondary school students: Their knowledge is limited and they want to learn more. Pediatrics 1988;81:350–355.

15. Walsh ME, Bibace R. Developmentally-based AIDS/HIV education. J School Health 1990;60:256–261.

16. Holladay B. Challenges of rearing a chronically ill child. Nurs Clin North Am 1984;19:361–368.

17. Venters M. Familial coping with chronic and severe childhood illness: The case of cystic fibrosis. Soc Sci Med 1981;15A:289–297.

18. Tasker M. How can I tell you? Bethesda: Association for the Care of Children's Health, 1992.

19. Child Welfare League of America. Living with loss: Children and HIV—video and discussion guide. Washington, DC: Child Welfare League of America, 1991.

51

Children Speaking with Children and Families about HIV Infection

Lori Wiener, Aprille Best, and Alexandra Halpern

The occurrence of a life-threatening illness during childhood has a profound effect on the psychological, social, and spiritual integrity of the family unit. When the life-threatening illness is human immunodeficiency virus (HIV), families are faced with additional challenges. Multiple family members are often infected, ill, or dying. The diagnosis of HIV also carries a stigma that results in the diagnosis frequently being kept secret. Children are often the last to whom the diagnosis is revealed. Even when children are aware of the diagnosis, there is a great attempt to withhold information about the severity of their illness, and the impact the disease is having on their family's ability to survive emotionally and financially. Children, however, sense stress and often know how sick they are and whether they are going to die before they, or their parents, have been told. In fact, it is not unusual for the child to withhold such information from their parents in an attempt to protect them from further worry, hurt, guilt, or pain. Indeed, the child often senses more accurately what the parent can tolerate than the parent senses how much the child can assimilate, and the child acts accordingly (1).

The medical and social consequences of HIV/AIDS are well documented now in both the medical literature and the popular media. Yet one aspect of the pediatric AIDS epidemic is largely unreported, i.e., the experiences and perspectives of children themselves. As a defensive means to protect children from the painful realities of illness and death, there is a tendency to try and help them escape from the potential consequences of their situation. John Allen (1988) and other Jungian counselors have described ways to restore the authenticity of the child's own visionary activity, so that problems can be expressed, traumas enacted, pain felt, and eventually reparation and healing can occur (2). It has been our experience that when HIV-infected children are provided a safe, nonthreatening, and protected space with someone they trust, the "inscapes" into their inner world are not only revealed, but enormous healing is facilitated. The challenge to therapists is to recognize and not abdicate their personal responsibility in this.

This chapter consists of a collection of thoughts, feelings, fears, anxieties, and images revealed by 24 HIV-infected children and eight noninfected siblings during clinical interviews. Methods and intervention strategies will be described. Different stages in the disease cycle as perceived by children will be shown. Specific developmental considerations and recurrent emotional themes will be reviewed with emphasis on example stories and drawings. The authors want to give special thanks to the children who shared their inner world with us and their parents for allowing us to now share them with you.

METHODS AND INTERVENTIONS

The material that is presented in this chapter was obtained through two clinical interventions: incomplete stories and drawings. (A more comprehensive sample of drawings and writings by HIV-infected children and their siblings will be presented in a book entitled *Be a Friend: Children Who Live with HIV Speak*, to be published by Albert Whitman in 1994.) Both these interventions allow children the opportunity to express themselves and reveal their inner life through a medium they enjoy, such as telling or writing stories and using materials with which they are familiar: computer, markers, crayons, pencils, and/or paint.

Children become verbally defended at a very early age and adept at covering their feelings. By drawing on the inherent fantasy nature of children we can cut through barriers and defenses much more quickly than is usually possible in verbal therapy with this age population. The result is concrete. The more we understand about what the child is feeling the more interventions or models of support we can offer the entire family. It is important to remember that a natural part of working with children is working through resistance. They may enjoy drawing and writing stories but may still resist intervention, fearing that they will reveal some content with which they will be unable to come to terms. It is for this reason that the relationship between the child and the therapist is the most important ingredient that allows the process of healing to occur.

Therapeutic Relationship

The therapeutic relationship and alliance is essential and begins as soon as the child begins drawing or writing his or her own story. Although beginners are advised to seek supervision in the use of play and interpretation as a therapeutic tool (3), imaginative expression in the presence of a therapist with no interpretation helps children release some of the power of symbols and their emotions at a critical moment in their lives (4–7). The main task is to nurture the child and the child's images (2). Simply being with the child and talking about the content of the picture in the third person ("I notice you've drawn a monster that is bigger than you; I wondered what the monster is thinking . . . feeling . . . and planning to do next") can help alleviate some of the loneliness and isolation that seriously ill children often feel (2). Children can also move through the psy-

chological process of initial loss, pain, and hopelessness to self-control, flexible mastery, and acceptance in this way. With each new awareness achieved through drawings and writings, the child becomes more comfortable, expansive, and secure. As this process occurs, more profound and previously unrevealed issues can be addressed (8). Indeed, the art of children experiencing physical illness and uncertain futures offers an opportunity for unconscious acceptance and conscious resolution. Children tend to hold onto any adult who they feel may somehow be able to help them grow through frightening situations, and therefore the therapist has the tremendous responsibility to honor the effort and truly respect the work of each child (9).

Incomplete Stories

Questions such as "tell me what you are feeling" will most often result in a one word answer. Incomplete sentences such as "I often wonder . . ." or "If only . . ." allows a child to express the thoughts they both wonder about and wish for in a nonthreatening style. The interviewer then has the opportunity to comment on the child's responses and encourage elaboration on selected topics. After the children have become comfortable writing their own stories, they frequently choose their own story titles. The titles clearly reflect either where they are in their disease course or issues of utmost importance to them at that time. Examples of such titles and stories are "What I Want My Mommy to Know," "Me and My Friends," "The Pro's and Con's of Telling Others," and "How HIV Really Is." If the content is, or becomes, too difficult, drawings are another vehicle for children to express what they cannot, or will not, say in words. Verbally adept children can cover masterfully, and art penetrates that defense and reveals what words shield.

Drawings

Art is another vehicle for expression of feelings and a way to reveal inner thoughts, fears, and turmoil. Children experience a sense of mastery when they complete drawings, and their finished works, especially when accompanied by a story, also help bolster self-esteem and self-efficacy (10). Drawings are a symbolic portrayal of the children's feelings, perceptions, and reactions to their situation.

Both stories and drawings represent a form of communication that reveals the inner world of the child and provides children with the opportunity to psychologically master the situations in their life that feels insurmountable. In addition, being able to express through play, writing, or drawing many of the issues not being openly discussed at home can provide a means for relieving tension and building rapport with someone outside the family. During every hospital visit, each child is offered the opportunity to work with their social worker. This includes giving form to their feelings through the use of play with dolls, puppets, and storytelling. Others choose to write their "own book," which helps validate their experiences and give their life a sense of importance. The book is left in the social worker's office, and upon each return clinic visit, the child is offered the opportunity to write a new "chapter." Each chapter in the book represents the unfolding of their journey of living with HIV. It is this journey that will now be described.

EMOTIONAL RESPONSES TO DISEASE
Learning of the Diagnosis

Diagnosis is clearly a crisis point for children, although the child's initial response may be more related to the emotional state of their parent when disclosing this information. When offered the opportunity, children find it helpful to talk and/or write about what they remember about learning of their diagnosis. The following story and Figure 51.1 illustrate how vivid these memories may be for children.

How HIV Really Is

When I first found out about my HIV infection I was driving in the car with my mother.

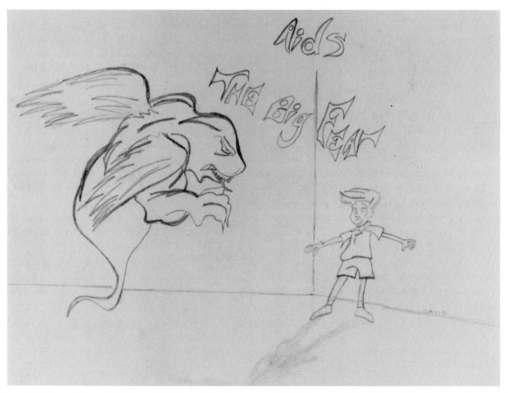

Figure 51.1. Although Figure 51.1 speaks eloquently to this 14-year boy's fear, an outcome of its production is in the encouragement of the young artist's talents—a boost to self-esteem and, as a talent recognized and encouraged, a vehicle for acceptance among peers.—David, age 14.

She told me that I only have 6 months to live. That is what the doctors told her. She also told me that I would be sick from now on out and that I would start losing friends if I told anybody about it. I started crying and so did she. She pulled the car over and hugged me but we almost had an accident doing so. That was six years ago.

I did not get to go to school no more because the school did not want me to attend. They got me a home tutor instead. Then in 1988 I started coming to NIH. The first time was really hard. I stayed there for three months because I was real sick and too sick to start a protocol. When I got better I started treatment and then began coming to NIH every month. All the people that I have met are real friendly and made me feel happy, accepted and that I have a life to look forward to. I am doing real well and I am even in school. I feel hopeful about the future and would love to be a truck driver when I grow up.

It is real hard to get stuck with needles alot and to know that you may not live long. I get scared going to bed sometimes worrying that I will not wake up.

For those of you who are HIV positive remember to keep God in your heart and to pray everynight. Pray for HIV to go away and for everything to be alright for all of us. Pray for people to be more accepting and so we can all be much happier.

—Damen, age 15

Recognition of Clinical Symptoms

Most children express very little about how they feel toward living with HIV. As clinical symptoms of HIV develop, it is often unclear to parents or health care providers just what children perceive the virus is doing to their bodies. Figures 51.2–51.7 are a response to the question: "If HIV had a face, what would the face look like?" The virus is often a "monster" that is significantly larger than the child. It is common for children to fantasize about becoming friends with the virus and in essence fighting "a war" together. Others, like Figures 51.6 and 51.7, use intellectual defenses to gain a sense of mastery.

Drawings also allow children to communicate with their health care providers about their individual symptoms. In this re-gard an illuminating open-ended question "What does HIV look like inside your body?" has been both revealing and useful in terms of understanding the child's concerns and diagnosing medical problems (see Figs. 51.8–51.10).

Feeling Different: Feeling Sick

HIV-infected children struggle with the many ways they perceive themselves as different from their peers. Other children are most often well and do not have to spend time in a clinic, take medication, or require hospitalizations for specific illnesses or infections. HIV-infected children frequently find themselves behind in school work because of repeated absences. Another factor that adds to their sense of being different is the real disparity in their physical appearance. These children often grow up smaller and weaker than their peers and siblings. Being different, looking different, and feeling different are common themes that the following stories reflect.

When You Have AIDS

Hi. My name is Tanya. I have AIDS and everyone is different than I am. It feels terrible to have AIDS because my tummy hurts alot and because, if my friends find out, they wouldn't want to play with me. When I told the kids at school I had AIDS they made fun of me. I told them by accident. Now I want to run away from school. I wish I were not an AIDS patient. I wish I did not have to take medicine.

When you have AIDS you feel bad alot, even when you don't have a high fever. I am different from everyone. AIDS patients hurt alot. It is going to take a long time to get rid of (my) AIDS and by the time I do I will be too old to live a long while. I'll only live a little while. In the meantime, my friends only understand I have a catheter. They don't understand my AIDS. I wish they would understand. I wish they would know the truth. I wish they would be my friends forever. But now I am learning to live with my AIDS. If you have AIDS, be proud of who you are. We have to stick together.

—Tanya, age 6

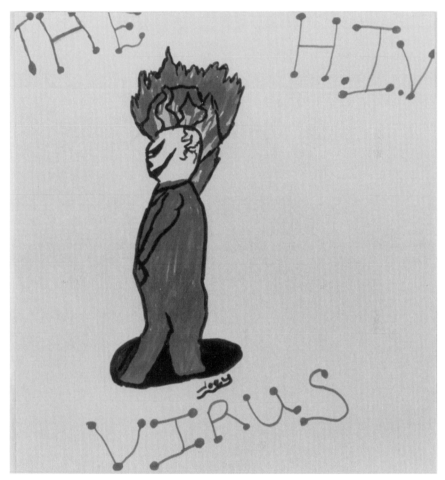

Figure 51.2.—Joey, age 12.

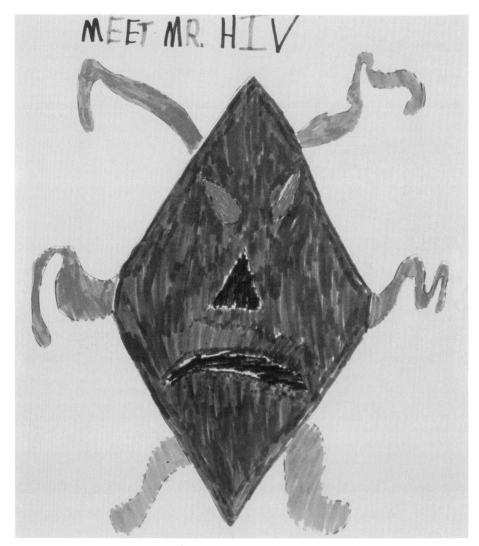

Figure 51.3.—Brett, age 11.

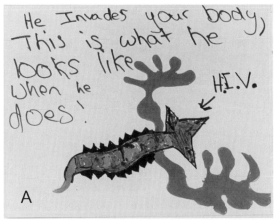

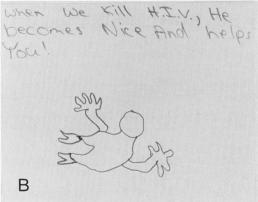

Figure 51.4.—Dawn, age 10.

The issues of feeling different also transcend to their siblings as the following stories and Figure 51.11 demonstrate.

What It Is Like Having HIV

Sometimes you feel sad and you wish your brother and your sister had it. You don't think it is fair that you've got something they don't. You think "Why do I have to have it?" but I, BJ have it. I wish there was a cure for us that have HIV because we would be well again. I wouldn't have the trouble of carrying this medicine that is going to my heart. Don't you wish that too?

Some people treat you like you can't do this or you can't do that and ALL I want is to do things anybody else can do. Like climb monkey bars or big toys. I want to be normal. Don't you?

—*BJ, age 10*

What It Is Like When You Have HIV and Your Brother or Sister Doesn't

Sometimes it doesn't feel fair that your sister or brother doesn't have AIDS because they don't have to take any medication or worry about anything. If your brother or sister doesn't have AIDS they don't have to worry so much about what other people know about them or what they will think about them if they found out. Sometimes you wish that your brother or sister would have the same thing that you do, so that they would know what it is like. But you also don't want them to be sick. It is difficult when your younger brother or sister grows faster than you do and you end up wearing their hand me down clothes instead of it being the other way around. Sometimes it is nice to get all the attention but your brother or sister may not like that and want some of the attention themselves.

—*Becky, age 8*

Terminal Illness

Am I going to die? Almost every child asks this question at some point during his

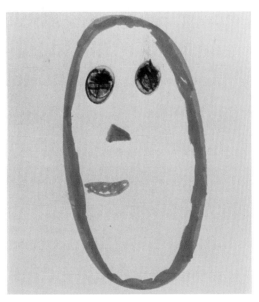

Figure 51.5.   You are about to make me suffacate. . . . I hate you because you do bad things to my body. . . . All you ever do is kill my cells. . . . I wish you weren't so mean. . . . You are stupid. . . . Go pick on someone your own size. . . . If you keep killing all of my cells you are going to die and so am I. . . . Get out of here. . . . Leave me alone. . . . Don't be such a red monster. . . . Let's be friends!—Sara, age 10; Jonathan, age 9.

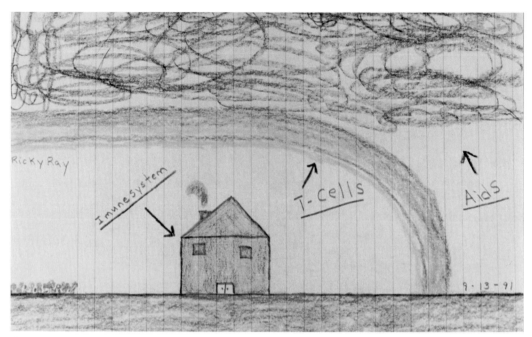

Figure 51.6. Houses appear frequently in the spontaneous drawings of children. In drawing them, children are unaware that they are telling more about themselves then they have drawn. This is eloquently demonstrated in Figure 51.6. While seeming to address the issues of what the AIDS virus looks like, this 14-year boy symbolically addresses his need for values usually associated with home and family: security, affection, a place to grow and be. Note that this boy's parents were anticipating a physical change of homes, and this child was seeking to solidify an important personal relationship at the time of this drawing.—Ricky, age 14.

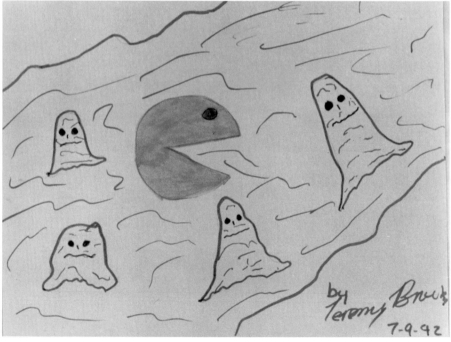

Figure 51.7. This is what the HIV virus looks like. It is like lots of Pac Mans (T cells) which the ghost kills in a stream of blood. The ghost is HIV. The ghosts outway the T cells. My T cell is scared. Because I only have one T cell.—Jeremy, age 12.

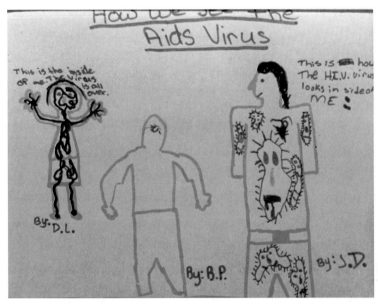

Figure 51.8.   The external shape of the bodies are all drawn in yellow. This choice of color as an outline vs. the rich colors and much more detailed drawing used in depicting the AIDS virus shows how visible these children feel the AIDS virus is and how exposed (transparancy of color of their bodies) they feel. Lack of detail to their physical bodies contrasted to the detail given to the virus-shows the feelings of helplessness these children live with facing something over which they have no control.— DL, age 10; BP, age 10; JD, age 12.

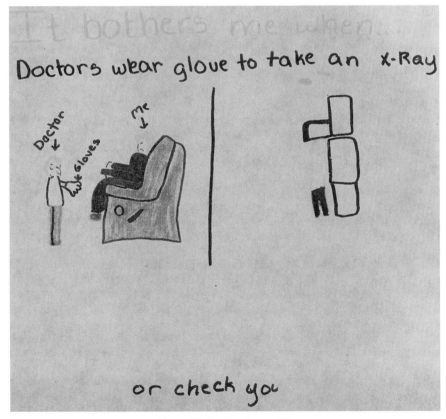

Figure 51.9.—Jamie, age 13.

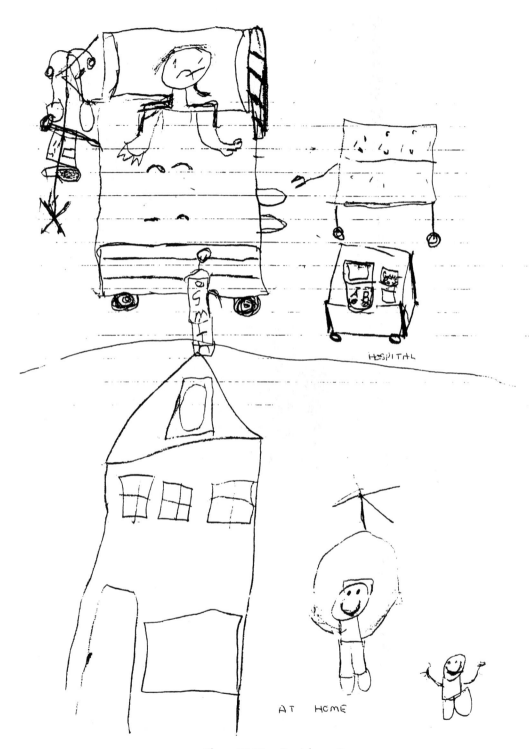

HOSPITAL

AT HOME

Figure 51.10.—Daniel, age 9.

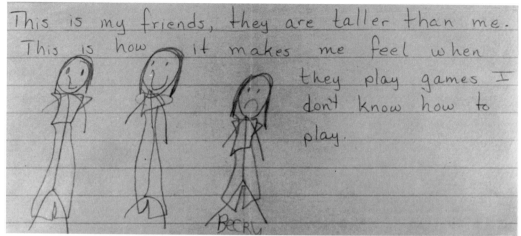

This is my friends, they are taller than me. This is how it makes me feel when they play games I don't know how to play.

BECKY

Figure 51.11. Drawings help assess the developmental and cognitive functioning of the child. Although the figure drawings appear to reflect an intelligent child who is cognitively functioning at an appropriate level for her age, the few lines to depict the bodies and the "see through" figures depict the depth, impotency, and low self-esteem she feels. In understanding this, the therapist is then empowered by the child to offer assistance that the child cannot find within herself. In effect, the child has given the therapist a mandate. Notice that this young artist has omitted hands and feet—pretty important parts of the body for "game playing"—which more eloquently than her words shows how deeply being "left out" affects her.—Becky, age 8.

or her illness. For some, it comes around the time they learn of their diagnosis. It may first be asked when a friend or parent dies but could easily come "out of the blue" while driving in a car, while eating dinner, or in the middle of the night. It may be approached during a fight such as "Why can't I do this, I am going to die soon anyway!" For others, the issue of dying is first approached when the child becomes terminally ill (Fig. 51.12). Unfortunately, for others, it is never asked, mostly because the child fears the answer or is worried that talking about dying will be too disturbing to their parent who is working so hard to do everything they can to keep them alive. All children want to be remembered and they appreciate being able to talk about how they want to be remembered. They also benefit from being able to express their thoughts and worries for their family's future after they are gone. The following stories illustrate this point. Figure 51.13 depicts a lack of investment in life and ambivalence that many terminally ill children experience.

You could die from AIDS. When you do your mommy and daddy will be very sad be-cause they wouldn't have a child anymore. But you will always be remembered. My mommy and daddy would always think of me and they will keep all my stuff in my room like my toys and pictures and my books. I always want them to remember me saying "I love you." They will always remember me sucking my thumb and wanting me to "STOP!"

—Hydeia, age 6

I Often Wonder . . .

I wonder why they can't find a cure for HIV. If they can't find a cure then I can get real sick and get AIDS. I wonder what that would be like. I think that would be hard. I might get real, real sick and die. That would be scary. The hardest part about dying would be missing my family. But I would see them in heaven one day and I know they would love me forever.

I wonder what heaven is like. But when I get to heaven I won't have to worry about anything. Doctors or medicine or pain. I think heaven is happy, pretty, and friendly. Lots of yellow, pink, and purple.

I hope they find a cure so I won't still have to worry about HIV while I am in heaven.

—Rachael, age 8

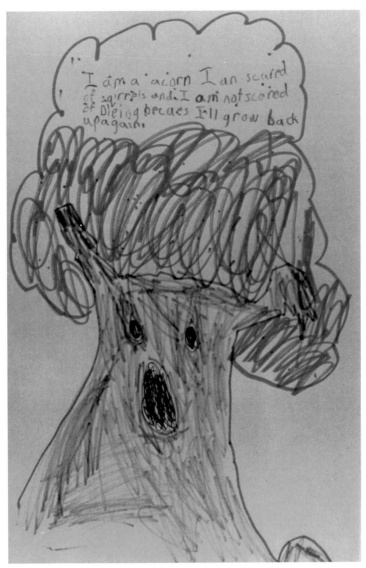

Figure 51.12. *I am an acorn. I am scared of sqirrels and I am not scared of dieing becues I'll grow back up again.* Feelings about death are clearly il-

lustrated, yet this drawing also demonstrates functioning on developmentally appropriate level.—BJ, age 9.

I Often Wonder . . .

I often wonder how often I'm going to get sick and what will happen to me during those times. I worry about how much energy I could lose and if the day would come that I wouldn't be able to play sports or to play with my friends.

I often wonder how much longer in life I have. Sometimes I think I only have months to live; other times I'm more hopeful and I think I'll live at least a couple more years.

The thought of not living long scares me. Especially dying. I worry most about what my

dying will do to my family. I want them to be able to go on with their lives and not be depressed all the time. In fact, if I was in Heaven and looking down on my family I would want to see them getting along with each other, and remembering me having a lot of fun with my friends always being over.

—Kevin, age 13

Clearly, the range of reactions to death is great. Some children exhibit depression with outbursts of anger and anxiety, whereas

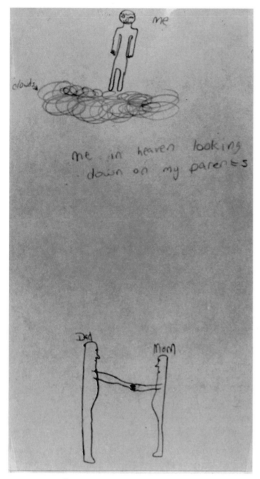

Figure 51.13.—Kevin, age 13.

others are astoundingly courageous and steadfast in the face of death (1). Each child is an individual, and all that has gone on in her or his life and illness will be a contributing factor to the child's behavioral and emotional reactions.

What Is Heaven Like?

Clearly, children think a lot about heaven. They spontaneously make references to life after death and express curiosity about the nature of existence (11). Most children are not very frightened of the dying process. Their fears surround being alone, the physical sensations surrounding the time of death, and the actual separation from their loved ones. Discussions about death and an afterlife are most common after the loss of a friend(s) from AIDS. Each death of someone they knew well is very difficult for HIV-infected children to cope with as they often wonder when their turn will come and if their experience will be the same as the person who has just died. Children benefit when provided the opportunity to remember as much as they can about each person they had known and lost. Figures 51.14–51.16 illustrate the images several children have about the friends that they have lost and about what heaven will be like.

DEVELOPMENTAL CONSIDERATIONS

Understanding the developmental stages of each child furthers the therapist's ability to be accepting and present at the precise level of the child. This is crucially important when one is trying to comprehend the complexity and dichotomy separating cognition and affect. How can we continue to view the child as a whole if we separate all the parts? This challenge remains the central issue of therapy. In a sense we are asking the final question: How can we help children find resolution in their internal conflicts and feel whole?

Spontaneous art expression can be counted on to fulfill at least two objectives. According to Naumberg (12) the art may show the steps by which the child's unconscious was gradually released through the symbolic expression of the art. Second, the art may suggest the possibilities inherent in such a procedure for the therapist to obtain valuable material bearing on both diagnostics and therapy. The child trusts that we can and will understand this. However, to understand, we must consider not only the disease state but the age and developmental level from which each child operates.

Birth through Latency

The very young child is mostly concerned with the separation and withdrawal that occur when hospitalized and the discomforts of the illness. The amount of emotional and symbolic material a child shares is often dependent on the sensitivity and skill of the adult (2). Nevertheless, the young child should be given the opportunity on different occasions to express his or her concerns through play with toys, dolls,

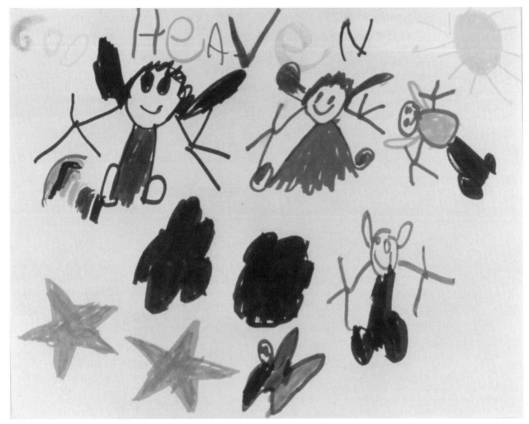

Figure 51.14.   I often wonder what Heaven is like. I think there is angels all over, baby angels and grown up angels. I also think my friends are there and are happy. When I die I will see them there. I think I too will be happy in Heaven.—Hydeia, age 6.

and/or sand art and through spontaneous storytelling and drawings (1). Young children do not express ideas in their drawings; rather they express *what* they feel and *how* they feel. These drawings can be an important method in understanding the young child's feelings and providing helpful clues to personality and personal problems and concerns (13).

School Age Children

Whether to disclose the diagnosis to others and concern over how others, especially friends, will respond to the diagnosis are often the most crucial issues with which school age children (as well as adults) struggle. Role playing possible scenerios is often helpful. School age children frequently enjoy writing their own books, especially when the diagnosis is not shared with their friends. In deciding whether to share the diagnosis with others, children benefit from being able to weigh the "pros and cons" of disclosing their diagnosis as the following story illustrates.

The Pros and Cons of Telling Other People My Diagnosis

Sometimes I want to tell people about my virus, but then I think about the Pro's and Con's. Some Pro's that I think about are that I wouldn't have to hide anything or lie anymore. I feel bad about lying, but then again, I can't tell anyone. I like coming to NIH because I can say it without having to worry about the way that people take it.

But then there's always the Con's. People could just forget about the facts and just get away from me. They could tell their parents, but then the parents would maybe want to get me out of the school, but from my point of view, they have nothing to worry about. Another Con could be that the people that I tell

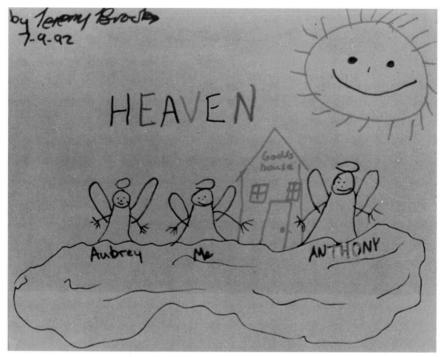

Figure 51.15. Heaven is a very special place. It is special because nothing bad happens to you there. No illness. You get to see loved ones who have passed on. I will get to see lots of people in Heaven. Like a lot of kids I knew. And a lot of adults too. That will be really neat. The hardest part about going to Heaven will be missing people who are here on Earth. Like my mom. The best part is that mom and I will be together again one day, forever.—Jeremy, age 12.

and that I trust to keep it a secret could tell someone else and then they would tell everyone else so then everyone would get away from me. Even if I tell them and they know the facts, they just wouldn't understand. Then there are always the people who won't believe me or the facts.

—Jamie, age 10

Being asked questions and having to answer questions is a source of enormous stress for most HIV-infected children. Some children do not want others to find out about their infection to avoid having to respond to other peoples' questions. The following story reflects this sentiment.

What It Is Like When Friends Find Out about Your HIV Infection

When friends find out they ask you all kinds of questions. Like "How did you get AIDS?" and "What is it like to have AIDS?" and "Do you have to take lots of medicines?" and "Is it scary to have AIDS?" I like when people ask

"When are you going to get well" and "I hope you get well soon." The questions that I hate when people ask are "You'll never get well" and "Can I catch your illness." I would like everyone to know that please do not be scared of us, we have feelings too, it is not so easy to live with AIDS, be nice and treat us like everyone else. The worst thing about having AIDS is not knowing if people will be your friends. So please be our friends. We need you to be our friends.

—Becky, age 8

A minority of children have decided to go "public." That is, they have been open with their friends, neighbors, teachers, and, for some, the media such as television and newspaper reporters. This is an important decision that must be carefully weighed in light of the family needs, resources, as well as the emotional climate of their community toward AIDS. The following story describes the decision of a 15-year boy to "go public" and the effect it has had on his ability to cope.

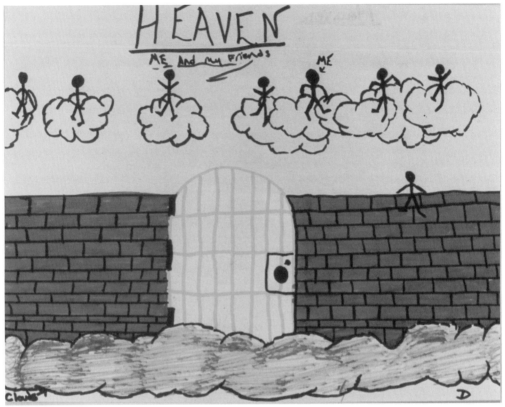

Figure 51.16. In this 10-year boy's illustration of heaven, use of intellectualization as a defense is most prominent. His investment in the art is centered on the wall which is solid and literally blocks his acceptance of reality. The opening into emptiness suggests an emptiness "beyond the door" and could be an acknowledgement that this defense is beginning to weaken.—Joey, age 10.

What It Feels Like Going Public

I had known about my HIV infection for five years before I decided to go public. During those five years it was really scary. I walked around knowing but not telling anyone that I had the disease. I was always worried that someone was going to figure it out and about what would happen if they did. The worst situation that I thought of was everybody would call me names, no-one would play with me or even be near me. I also imagined getting cut at school and having to tell everyone right then and there. I worried about this most of the time. Finally it got to the point where I couldn't hold back anymore and I had to tell someone. I was really nervous about what their response was going to be but I felt whatever it was it had to be better than lying all of the time. I wondered if people would come to my house to play once they found out, if people would throw rocks at my house or smash the windows. But let me tell you what happened.

I told my best friend first. We were playing Nintendo and I said "Matt, you know I have AIDS don't you?" and he said "Ya, but that's O.K. I'll still be your friend." I didn't know for sure that Matt had known but I thought he might since my mom had just told his mom about it. Boy, did I feel alot better. It even gave me the courage to tell someone else. And then someone else until I went completely public.

I am so glad that I did go public because now I am not scared all the time anymore about losing my friends if/when they found out my diagnosis. I don't worry anymore that when I go into the hospital or if I got real sick they would figure it out. So if you go public it makes you feel a lot better. Living with HIV is hard enough. Lying on top of it and always fearing rejection makes it that much harder.

—Kevin, age 15

Me and My Friends

It is very hard to make friends and to lose them. This is what I remember most about each one of the kids I have gotten to know and love. Jeff loved rude dog. He was always nice. Michelle was a cute baby and she always kept Ernie on her leg. Cory was funny, real nice and smiled alot. Ezra was also cute, he had a beautiful face. Aubrey always knew what she wanted and was funny too.

All of these friends had AIDS. They fought hard to live. Now when I think of them I feel sad because they had a chance to live but they died and I knew them all real well. I think they are all in heaven together now, having a party or something. It makes me feel better to think of them all together because that makes it all seem less scary.

—Joey, age 11

A turning point for many HIV-infected school age children is being able to reach out to other infected children and share what living with HIV is like for them from day to day. When fears associated with confidentiality prevent this in a face to face meeting, becoming a pen pal can be therapeutic for both children. For those children who are not comfortable communicating with others, asking them what they would like the world to know about HIV/AIDS often produces previously unrevealed content. When provided the opportunity, HIV-infected children have a wonderful way of teaching children and adults about what they feel should be known about this disease as the following story illustrates.

What I Want the World to Know

Having AIDS is not fun. It sometimes makes you not feel very good and not want to do very much. If some people tease you it is not funny because you might get sick and one day people may tease you. I like when people treat me nice and I don't like it when people tease me. It is not funny.

—Hydeia, age 7

Other school age children use writing as a means of reflecting upon what their life is like and would have been like without AIDS.

I Often Wonder . . .

I often wonder what my life would be like if I didn't have AIDS. I think my life may not have been much different.

But if I didn't have AIDS I would eat more and not be so skinny. I would not have to get needle sticks or take medicine that tastes sick. I would not have to get up at 11 pm or at 7 am to take medicine and I would be able to eat whenever I wanted.

If I didn't have AIDS I would not have to worry about dying from it. My parents would probably be the same though whether or not I had AIDS. But if I didn't have AIDS they would not have to worry so much about me. It's hard for me to see my parents worry.

I often wonder how other children without AIDS learn to appreciate life. That's the best part about having AIDS.

—Brett, age 11

Concerns about the impact of the disease on the family is a theme that is evident throughout most sessions with HIV-infected children. Figure 51.17 illustrates how children often feel torn and pulled in different directions. The two leashes demonstrate the tug children feel to be well and to keep things on an even keel. Children tend to worry about the impact of their illness on their siblings, the family's financial situation and their parents' marriage. It is helpful when they are allowed to express these concerns. The first story was written by a 9-year boy during a lengthy hospitalization and the second by a 14-year boy after a serious infection.

I Often Wonder . . .

I often wonder how I could become a millionaire.

I also wonder if they can make a cure to make me better!

I often wonder what my life would be like if I didn't have AIDS. I think I would be a normal human being and we would be a normal family.

—Daniel, age 9

How HIV Has Affected My Family

HIV has affected my family a lot. Let's start with my mom. She is always worried

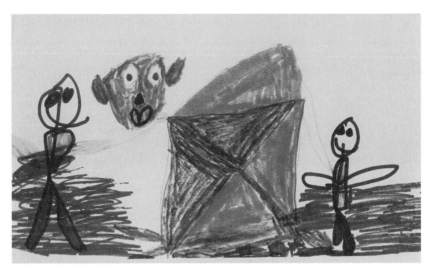

Figure 51.17. This drawing by a 9-year boy indicates developmental arrest, which can also assist physicians in their recommended interventions. The most positive aspect of this picture is the solid sense of self of this child who is able to "hold on" in the face of tremendous upheaval.—John, age 9.

about how I am doing. She is always checking my temperature, feeling my head to see if it is warm, and she frequently asks me "How are you doing?" My dad on the other hand I know is worried but he doesn't talk to me about it. He works less since I have been diagnosed so that he can do more stuff with me and my family together. I like that alot! In fact he feels like a whole different person since I was diagnosed with HIV. My sister is 16 years old. I don't think she has changed very much. We still fight but I know that she loves me and if I got real sick she would be right there for me.

If I didn't have HIV my family would be different. They would be happier because they wouldn't have to worry all the time about me having a life-threatening disease and if or when I would get real sick. I also think HIV has made my family closer. Family togetherness means more to them now. Like we take long vacations together and talk more to each other. That's the best part about all of this.
—Kevin, age 14

Adolescence

Because of multiple developmental considerations, coping with HIV is both complex and challenging for adolescents (Fig. 51.18). The diagnosis of HIV infection often produces denial, fear, anger, and withdrawal, and owing to the need for peer ac-

ceptance, the fear of being rejected by one's friends is often greater than the fear of dying from the disease. Consequently, HIV-infected adolescents frequently live in emotional isolation and are at high risk for depression, acting-out behaviors, and suicide. Adolescents' creative activity can be utilized to help the therapist with the initial establishment of a relationship. A therapeutic alliance is essential, and when this is established individual sessions are extremely useful. Because of fear, anxieties, and frequent early resistance, it is important to accept all early attempts of self-expression (14). Within the hospital setting, activities that can be performed in a group are sometimes met with less resistance than individual sessions. Drawings, writings, and group activities reduce isolation and allow HIV-infected adolescents the opportunity of knowing that their fears, concerns, and worries are acceptable, and they learn to understand themselves better. Figure 51.19 was done in the clinic by five HIV-infected adolescent boys. It is important to allow the adolescents to take most of the initiative for the theme and development of each group project.

A PARENT WITH AIDS

When a child's parent is also HIV infected, the parent's concerns about the stability of home and family are magnified.

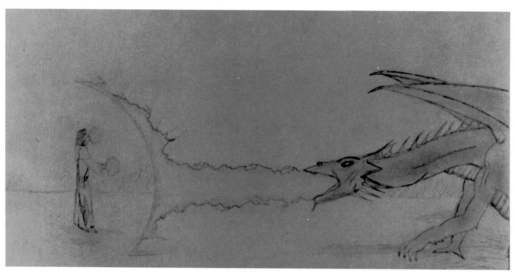

Figure 51.18. Encouragement of this young artist to continue to draw his "creatures" as a way to externalize his demons is an important step in helping him come to terms with his diagnosis. The powerful dragon's fire cannot destroy the supreme being in his protected place. However, one wonders how long this small figure can hold out against the seeming relentless pursuit of the monster.—Wayne, age 17.

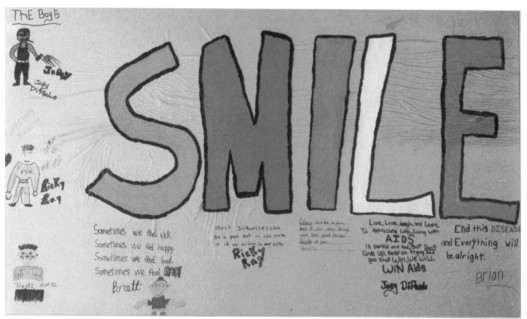

Figure 51.19.—**S,** *Sometimes we feel sick. Sometimes we feel happy. Sometimes we feel bad. Sometimes we feel RAD!*—Brett, age 12. **M,** *Most sicknesses can be a pain but we can make it if we believe in our selfs.*—Ricky, age 14. **I,** *Illness can be a pain, but it can also bring out the good things* *Inside of you.*—Travis, age 10. **L,** *Live, love, laugh, and learn to Appreciate Life. Living with AIDS is painful and sad, But Don't Give Up. Keep on trying And you shall Win. We will Win AIDS.*—Joey, age 12. **E,** *End this DISEASE, and Everything will be alright.*—Brian, age 16.

Their parent may be hospitalized at the same time that they are. They may be at very different points in their disease. Parents tend to sacrifice their own health by putting their child's health care needs before their own. As a result, children worry about their parent(s) and feel guilty, angry, and sometimes resentful when they have to take medicine and their parent(s) do not. Children are very sensitive to upsets and changes in the family. The following piece and Fig. 51.20 by an 11-year girl illustrate these concerns precisely.

If Only . . .

. . . If only my mother and I didn't have HIV then my whole family wouldn't have to go through what they have to go through.

. . . If only my dad would be able to talk to us about us being sick.

. . . If only we didn't have to worry so much about money.

. . . If only my mom would stop being so stubborn and start taking some medicine so that she would not get sick.

. . . If only the world would be a more understanding place.

—Dawn, age 11

Other children are realistically concerned about losing both parents. When one parent dies, the other parent grieves along with the child. However, frequently, the surviving parent finds it too difficult and "close to home" to talk about the deceased parent at any

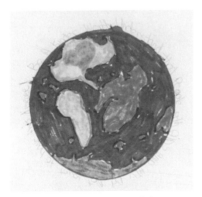

Figure 51.20.—Words encircling globe: *Be A Kinder World. Understand that People with AIDS and HIV Did Not want to have this disease!*—Dawn, age 11.

length. Children worry about what will happen to them if the other parent dies. They benefit greatly by being able to share their thoughts and concerns. Parents benefit from learning how to communicate with their child openly and honestly about their own health status and future plans for their child in the case that they can no longer care for their child. The first story was written by an 11-year boy whose sister was in the intensive care unit with severe pancreatitis. The content, anticipated multiple deaths including one's own death, is not uncommon among HIV-infected children.

It's Hard Losing Someone You Love

Have you ever lost anybody you loved? Do you know how it feels? Do you know what to do? Do you know what to say? What do you do? What do you say except you love them.

My dad died when I was 7. I didn't know what to say at first when my mom told me that my dad died. I will never forget those words: "Ricky, Dad died." I didn't know what to feel. I just started to cry. And cry. Now that I am 11, I remember lots of bits and pieces about my dad. I wish I could remember more but I guess what I remember mostly is how much he loved me and how much I loved him.

My dad is in Heaven. So are a lot of other people who I have known. So will I be, and my mother, and my sister one day. I hope that day will not be too soon.

—Ricky, age 11

This second story was written by a 4-year-old 6 months after her mother's death. Until this time, there had been no dialogue with her father about where she would go if he died. A plan was able to be instituted shortly after this story was written.

My mommy lives in heaven. Her eyelashes go down instead of up because she is dead. My mommy is happy in heaven but I miss her. If I could tell my mommy something I would tell her that I miss her and that I wish that she didn't die. She knows how much I love her. I told her that before she died and that I did not want her to die until I died. I think I am going to die too in a little while when I grow up. Like in 90 days or so. That's a long time. GOD is in heaven too. He lives in heaven. GOD always has people around him and he swims in the sky. He has pink whiskers, red hair and two feet. My mommy is with GOD right now. She can hear him but she can't talk to him because she is dead. She can only hear me if I speak into a loud speakerphone. One day I went to a memory place and said into a loud speakerphone and said Memory of my Mama. I was holding a candle in my hand carefully. The memory was that I loved my mommy. My father misses my mommy too. I don't remember when she died. It was a long time ago. Sometimes I worry that my daddy will die too. Then I would be alone. He would be in heaven with my mommy.

—Marilyn, age 4

LOSING A PARENT

Although HIV-infected children worry about the health of their infected parent(s) they are most concerned about their parents' death. This is a common theme expressed in the therapeutic situation. The following letter and drawing (Fig. 51.21) was written by a 10-year girl during her clinic visit while her own mother was hospitalized in another state. Both the letter and her drawing express her anticipatory fears and grief.

Dear Mom,

I miss you. Sometimes I get scared when you get sick. I worry that you will not come home. I want you to take care of yourself. If you ever got real sick will you tell us? I worry too much. I worry most about you because you might get sick, not tell me and die. If you died I would be really upset and sad and cry a whole lot. I cried last night because I missed you so much. Sometimes I worry about me getting sick too and what you would do if I got real sick. Like would you cry or would you come see me in the hospital? If you were in the hospital I want to come see you.

Sometimes I even think about heaven. It is quiet and peaceful there and I know that you and I will be there together one day.

Mommy I love you and know you love me.

—Sara, age 10

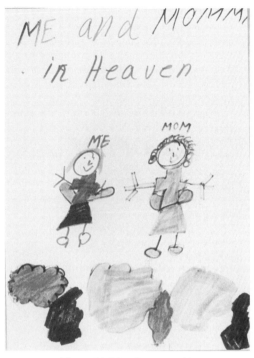

Figure 51.21.—Sara, age 10.

The child who has lost a parent is a child at risk for psychiatric difficulties. The factors associated with an increased risk of psychological morbidity for children after the death of a parent or sibling are described elsewhere (8, 15). Several interventions, however, including letters and drawings have been a highly effective technique for children whose parents have died. It allows them to feel connected to their deceased parent and to visualize where they are. Often, with proper support, children feel comfortable writing letters to or about their parent for the first year after their parent's death. After that time, they are frequently able to talk openly about their experiences and memories. Helping children make "a memory book" of photographs or a collage of their most precious memories of their parent ("monuments") can also assist children in dealing with their grief. Figure 51.22 was made 1 month after the death of this 5-year girl's mother, and the following letter was written 5 months after the mother's death during a routine clinic visit.

Mommy I want you to know everything. Like how tall I am today, that I did really good with my shot, that I am going home from the hospital today and that I am starting Kindergarten next week. I am going to wear my dress which has flowers on it and is black to my first day of school.

Most of all Mommy I want you to know that I miss you and that I think about you all the time. I miss you the most when I am crying. I wish I could fly up there to the sky to be with you. I know that you're not sick anymore and I hope that you are happy.

—*Cassie, age 5*

SIBLINGS

Comprehensive medical and psychosocial management includes how the illness affects the child's siblings. All siblings of an HIV-infected child, regardless of whether they are HIV-infected themselves, are emotionally affected by its destructive impact on the family. The stress of having to lie about the true nature of the illness is tremendous, and the impact of lying requires special attention. The following story demonstrates the often silent thoughts, fears, and confusion non-HIV–infected siblings experience. Figures 51.23–51.28 further illustrate several siblings' attempts to cope with the impending loss of a brother or sister and in one case (Fig. 51.27) the loss of three brothers.

The Hardest Thing about All of This

The hardest thing about all of this is my brother. My brother is HIV and he bugs me.

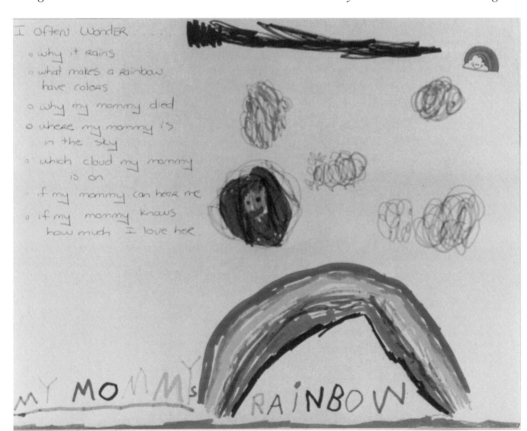

Figure 51.22. *I Often Wonder/why it rains/what makes a rainbow have colors/why my mommy died/where my mommy is in the sky/which cloud my mommy is on/if my mommy can hear me/if my mommy knows how much I love her.* Once again an eloquent example of the inner world as expressed in the symbols for life and rebirth—being rendered in painful disarray. Healing for this child has already begun as expressed in her beautiful letter. Internally the impact of her mother's death still weighs as heavily (as the rainbow is drawn), but this child shows appropriate expressions of grief, loss, and the healing process.—Cassie, age 5.

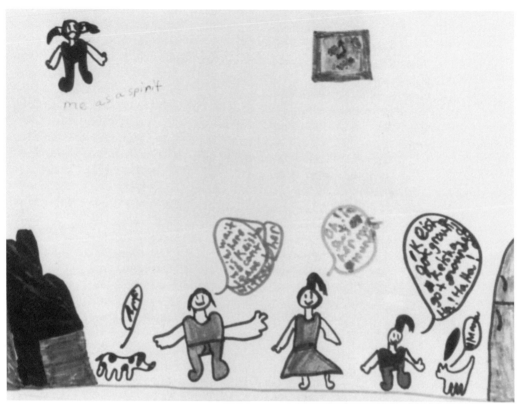

Figure 51.23. *Me as a spirit.   Arf.   Wait. Where is Keisha we can't leave without her. Oh!! She is in her room grounded.   Keisha got grounded. Keisha got grounded. Ha! Ha! Ha! Meow.*—Keisha, age 10.

He gets alot of attention especially when he almost died. Sometimes when he gets alot of attention I feel left out. When he gets new toys and Nintendo tapes I often get nothing. That makes me feel sad. Sometimes I feel angry when my mother is busy and can't help me with my homework. She is busy with all kinds of activities related to my brother and HIV. I also get angry when I don't have anyone to play with and my brother gets to bring his friends over. I also get scared. AIDS scares me because I am afraid that my brother will die. I always had a brother and I don't know how it would feel not to. Sometimes he wants me to sleep in his bed with him maybe because he is scared too. He doesn't talk to me about what it is like to have HIV. But I haven't asked him either. I told my best friend. She told me she would not tell her family but she did tell them. It worked out O.K. and she is still my best friend. If I could change anything in the whole wide world it would be to get rid of AIDS and that no kids would be sick. I really want my brother to know that I love him even if I don't always show it. There are just some times that I have to hit him back.

—Lauren D, age 10

There are a growing number of children in this country who are at risk of losing not only a brother or sister but perhaps one or both parents as well. The following story is just one example of the many concerns with which these children must live a daily basis.

I Often Wonder . . .

. . . I often wonder what will happen to my family because of AIDS. I wish my sister would be alright but I know she may not be. I wish my mother would start relaxing and not jump to conclusions about my sister so quickly. I also wish my mother will continue to feel well. . . . I also wish I could not lie about my sisters and mothers health. Lying is hard to keep

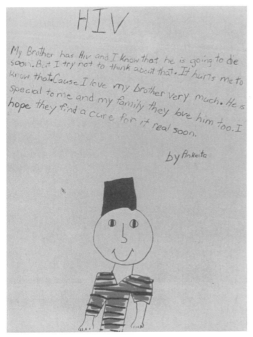

Figure 51.24.   *My Brother has HIV and I know that he is going to die soon. But I try not to think about that. It hurts me to know that. Cause I love my brother very much. He is special to me and my family they love him too. I hope they find a cure for it real soon.*—Ankeita, age 11.

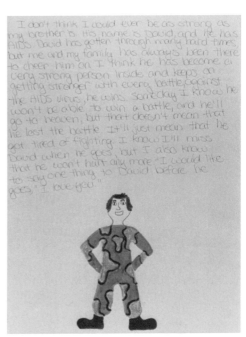

Figure 51.25.   *I don't think I could ever be as strong as my brother is. His name is David, and he has AIDS. David has gotten through many hard times, but me and my family has always been there to cheer him on. I think he has become a very strong person inside and keeps on getting stronger with every battle, against the AIDS virus, he wins. Someday I know he won't be able to win a battle, and he'll go to heaven, but that doesn't mean that he lost the battle. It'll just mean that he got tired of fighting. I know I'll miss David when he goes, but I also know that he won't hurt any more. I would like to say one thing to David before he goes, "I love you."*—Diane, age 13.

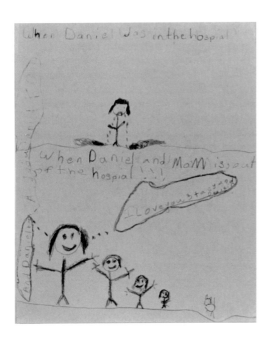

Figure 51.26.   Top, *When Daniel was in the hospial!* Bottom, *When Daniel and Mom is out of the hospial!!!*—Stacy, age 7.

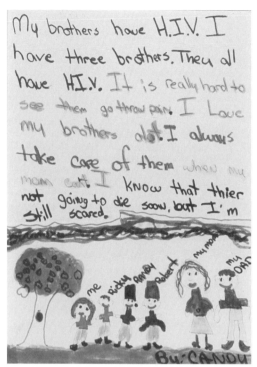

Figure 51.27. *My brothers have H.I.V. I have three brothers. They all have H.I.V. It is really hard to see them go throw pain. I Love my brothers alot. I always take care of them when my mom can't. I know that thier not going to die soon, but I'm still scared.—Candy, age 11.*

straight and I feel like I could just tell the truth and get the monkey off my back.
—Melissa, age 13

CONCLUSION

Throughout this chapter, the children's words and pictures speak about what it is like to face HIV and go through the struggle of trying to understand illness, relationships, and people. Children have no problem talking about important matters. However, distilling their many thoughts, passionate pleas, doubts, worries, hopes, dreams, and stories into one chapter is difficult. Hopefully, not too much has been sacrificed in what they have said (16). Like adults, each child whose work is reflected in this chapter responded differently to his or her illness. Each had unique struggles to overcome. Each has had a different experience in terms of others accepting them and their disease, yet all of them, without exception, had the courage to face their own

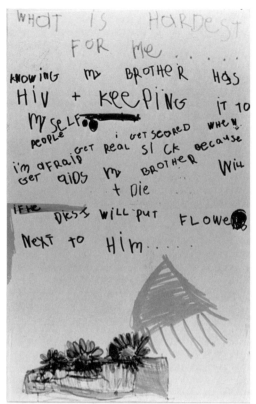

Figure 51.28. *What is hardest for me . . . . . knowing my brother has HIV and keeping it to myself. I get scared when people get real sick because I'm afraid my brother will get AIDS and die. If he dies I will put flowers next to him. . . . . —Lauren W, age 7.*

fears and express themselves symbolically and with such clarity on paper. A teacher of Elizabeth Kubler-Ross beautifully stated "Should you shield the canyons from the windstorms, you would never see the beauty of their carvings" (16). By inquiring into the inner world of these children and helping them to put understanding and meaning into their plight, we are facilitating psychological movement, growth, and healing. Their works also become invaluable gifts to their parents. We thank all these children for allowing us to enter into their private thoughts, fears, and hopes. We thank them in their belief that they can touch your life as much as they have touched ours (16).

References

1. Lewis M, Lewis DO, Schonfeld DJ. Dying and death in childhood and adolescence. In: Lewis M, ed. Child and adolescent psychiatry. Baltimore: Williams & Wilkins, 1991:1051–1059.

2. Allen J. Inscapes of the child's world. Dallas: Spring Publications, 1988.

3. Coppolillo HP. Psychodynamic psychotherapy of children. Madison, CT: International Universities Press, 1987:9–10.

4. Allen J. Serial drawing: A therapeutic approach with young children. Can Counsellor 1978;12:223–228.

5. Bach SR. Spontaneous painting of severely ill patients: A contribution to psychosomatic medicine. Acta Paedopsychiatrica 1966;8:86–104.

6. Kiepenheuer K. Spontaneous drawings of a leukemic child: An aid for more comprehensive care of fatally ill children and their families. Psychosomatische Med 1980;9:21–32.

7. Furth GM. The use of drawings made at critical times in one's life. In: Kubler-Ross E, ed. Living with death and dying. New York: Macmillan, 1981:63–94.

8. Coppolillo HP. The use of play in psychodynamic psychotherapy. In: Lewis M, ed. Child and adolescent psychiatry. Baltimore: Williams & Wilkins, 1991:805–811.

9. Kramer E. Childhood and art therapy. Notes on theory and application. New York: Schodren Books, 1979.

10. Zambelli GC, DeRosa AP. Bereavement support groups for school-age children: Theory, intervention, and case examples. J Orthopsychiatry 1992; 62:484–493.

11. Heller D. The children's God. Chicago: University of Chicago Press, 1986.

12. Naumberg M. An introduction to art therapy. Studies of the "free" art expression of behavior problem children and adolescents as a means of diagnosis and therapy. New York: Columbia University Teachers College Press, 1973.

13. Alschuler RH, Hattwick LA. Significance of easel painting as compared to other media. In: Alschuler RH, Hattwick LW, eds. Painting and personality. Chicago: University of Chicago Press, 1969:119–143.

14. Linesch DG. Adolescent art therapy. New York: Brunner-Mazel, 1988.

15. Osterweis M, Solomon F, Green M. Bereavement: Reactions, consequences and care. Washington, DC: National Academy Press, 1984.

16. Kubler-Ross E. To live until we say good-bye. Englewood Cliffs, NJ: Prentice-Hall, 1978.

52
Health Care Perceptions and Needs of America's Poor

Reed Tuckson

As health professionals and American communities grapple with the specific challenges of preventing and managing human immunodeficiency virus (HIV) disease in our children, it is also important to consider the larger context from which this disease arises and which so often frustrates our best preventive and therapeutic efforts. The epidemiological descriptors of the etiology of AIDS in children clearly indicate that the most significant and intractable concerns are maternal intravenous drug abuse and ill-advised and/or inadequately protected sexual behavior by intravenous substance abusers and their associates. It is important to appreciate that these behaviors are the consequences of, and are contributors to, a larger mosaic of insults that produce and intensify a frightening experience with premature death, unnecessary illness, and preventable misery for millions of our children, their families, and their communities.

Mothers and children with HIV disease are most often African-American or Hispanic (1). They are very often poor and live in communities ravaged by poverty and the realities of race in American society. For them, the best advice of health educators has too often and for too long been overwhelmed by the daily struggle for survival. Medical care has too frequently been inaccessible.

Into this reality of unnecessary and inadequately addressed pain and suffering comes HIV disease with its additional and interconnected challenges for prevention and treatment. If HIV disease in children is to be successfully prevented and managed, health professionals must develop new insights, acquire additional skills, and form more effective partnerships with their colleagues and the communities from which their patients arise. Traditionally, narrow models of health promotion, disease prevention, and medical care are becoming increasingly unable to meet the complex demands presented by this disease.

PREEXISTING EPIDEMIOLOGICAL CHALLENGES

The health of poor Americans, and of Americans of color, is significantly worse than that of their countrymen and women. This is especially true for African-Americans. Throughout all age groups they experience more episodes of preventable illness, and they die prematurely (2–4). For example, in 1985, the Secretary's Task Force on Black and Minority Health estimated that 60,000 African-Americans died prematurely, in excess of what they would have, if their health status had been the same as that for white Americans. The ravages of cardiovascular disease and stroke, cancer, chemical dependency (as measured by deaths from cirrhosis), homicide and accidents, infant mortality, and diabetes accounted for 80% of these deaths (5). As a consequence of the emergence of HIV disease, and increases in the relative risk of death from illnesses associated with infancy,

963

homicide, accidents, heart disease, and diabetes, 75,000–80,000 excess premature deaths are now suffered each year by black Americans (2, 6).

These additional 20,000 excess deaths are a frightening and discouraging indicator of the further deterioration of many American communities and the health care systems that serve them. An important contextual perspective of the preexisting problems from which HIV disease has emerged is presented by 80,000 excess deaths.

Many of the details submerged in the excess mortality figures are particularly troubling. The health of black women has always been precarious and much worse than that of their white counterparts. They die younger and they suffer more. For example, their age-adjusted death rate for heart disease is much higher, as is that for stroke, which is double that of white women. Between 1980 and 1989, the age-adjusted death rate for breast cancer increased by 12% while remaining the same in white women. Breast cancer mortality was 14% higher in black women. Psychological distress has been self-reported in as many as 50% of black women aged 18–25 years. Violence, physical abuse, substance abuse, teenage pregnancy, and obesity are all issues that are disproportionately manifested in African-American women (3, 4).

For black males, life expectancy has declined steadily between 1984 and 1989 to a low of 64.8 years. This is almost 8 years lower than that for white males. Years of potential life lost, and the age-adjusted death rates from stroke and cancers of the lung and prostate, were all approximately twice as high for black males in 1989 compared with their white counterparts. Black males have higher rates of mental disorder than white males or black women (4).

Poor children of all races experience excess preventable death and disease. They die more often in infancy and suffer more often from fetal alcohol syndrome and the limiting effects of other drugs introduced during intrauterine development. Intentional and unintentional injury, asthma, abuse, immunizable preventable disease, and ear infections are just some of the threats that disproportionately afflict them (7). Perhaps no indicator better depicts the modern realities of health for America's poor and minorities than does violence. Violence has now come to be viewed as a public health problem as much as it is a criminal justice problem, in large measure because of the extraordinary toll that it takes on children and adolescents. It is now common in many communities to learn of children who have been killed by stray bullets passing through the windows or doors of their houses and apartments. Some children report that they prepare their homework in the family bathtub because that is their safest haven. Almost two million teenagers were victimized by violent crime in 1990 (8). Black adolescents are particularly at risk, with black males five to six times more likely, and black females two to three times more likely to become a homicide victim than their white counterparts (9).

The Hispanic community, perhaps to a much greater extent than the African-American community, is a complex and heterogeneous mixture of many different cultures, backgrounds, and socioeconomic experiences. It is difficult and unrealistic to summarize an "Hispanic" epidemiological profile. Also, far fewer data are available or collected for this population, particularly for poor Hispanic Americans who often must live "underground" because of their precarious legal status. However, in 1989, death rates for the Hispanic population aged 15–44 years were one-third greater than those for the white population (4). Homicide, suicide, accidents, and adverse effects account for much of this differential (4). The issues of poverty are significant obstacles for many Hispanic-Americans and their health status.

POVERTY AND HEALTH

A great deal more remains to be learned about the specific interrelationships between socioeconomic status and its attendants, race and ethnicity, and health. A persistent and pervasive link between socioeconomic status and disease exists. For a number of reasons, residents of poor communities are sicker than more affluent citizens. Their environment predisposes them to behaviors that are inconsistent with good health; it too often contains contaminants that are unhealthy; it exposes them to the adverse consequences of overcrowding and congestion; it overwhelms them with the debilitation that accompanies high levels of stress; and it does not contain the requisite health care and other resources necessary to prevent, cure, or manage disease adequately. Poor communities have high crime rates, pervasive violence, poor housing, inadequate transportation, less healthy food, and deficient schools (7, 10).

Perhaps the most important consequence of the combination of these factors for health in general, and pediatric AIDS in particular, is that poor communities are too often places without hope. An Arabian proverb says that "He who has health, has hope; and he who has hope, has everything." The Bible says that "where there is no hope, the people perish." Hopelessness ultimately destroys everything and health is one of the first things to go. Without hope, it is difficult to have health. Ultimately, the absence of the concept of a meaningful future for millions of our citizens prepares the soil for the seeds of substance abuse and risky sexual behaviors that become harvested as pediatric and maternal HIV disease.

Blacks and Latinos are overrepresented in the ranks of the poor and as residents of disadvantaged, disorganized communities. They are more frequently unemployed, incarcerated, institutionalized, victimized, uneducated, miseducated, disrespected, feared, and hated. They have a long history of being devalued and of having their illnesses labeled as, or dismissed as, deviance. They are frequently blamed for their own victimization by a frustrated and, too often, uncaring society. This produces further ostracization, marginalization, and exclusion that perpetuates the very conditions that entraps them (11). HIV disease has become only the most recent manifestation of this long present phenomenom.

Unfortunately, for millions of Americans, and especially for Americans of color and their children, this scenario is becoming even more bleak. In 1988, 13 million children lived with incomes below the federal poverty line, representing one-fifth of all children under age 18 years and two-fifths

of all poor people in the United States. They and their families then represented more than two-thirds of the poor (7). By 1990, with increases in out-of-wedlock births, teenage pregnancy, and family dissolution, there were 11 million female-headed households of which more than one-third were poor, and they accounted for half of all poor families (12). In fact, 55% of all black and Hispanic female-headed households with children younger than 18 years were poor. With median incomes of only $9000, compared with the American family median income of $30,000, these families comprise much of the poorest of the poor population (9). Being married did not necessarily immunize minority families from the realities of poverty. Almost 14% of black married couples and 20% of Hispanic married couples lived in poverty, compared with 8% of white families (9).

The tragic reality is that, based on 1991 data from the Children's Defense Fund,

> ... every sixth family with a child under 18 is poor. Every fifth child and every fourth preschooler is poor. Every third black and brown child is poor, and every second black preschooler is poor. Two out of every three preschoolers of any background are poor if they live in a female headed household (8).

These numbers do not capture the millions more who live in "near-poor" families who often have as much difficulty as those officially labeled as poor in purchasing food, obtaining shelter, and accessing basic medical care (13).

COMMUNITY AND FAMILY DISORGANIZATION

Complicating this growing trend of families and children living in poverty is the increased mobility and fragility of the contemporary family. Between 1985 and 1990, 40% of children aged 10–14 years moved to new homes. Almost half of them moved to new counties with the associated difficulties of adjusting to new people, different schools, and increasingly disorganized communities (9). This significantly compromises the work of health professionals and others who have come to appreciate the necessity of comprehensive and deeply rooted community supports in addressing the difficult challenges of health promotion, disease prevention, and illness management in fragile and multiply needy families.

As economic and other pressures increase on America's poor families, so also does homelessness. Families have become the fastest growing segment of the homeless population. An estimated 2.5 million children now live in domiciles other than homes. As many as 80% of homeless families are headed by a woman who is typically young, undereducated, and unemployed (5, 9). Almost 50% of them had their first child before age 20 years (5). Substance abuse with street drugs is common and is estimated to be between 13 and 52%. Many of these women struggle with mental health disorders and alcoholism as well. Issues of low self-esteem and extreme vulnerability are particularly prevalent in these women, especially for those who are also intravenous drug users (14).

Child abuse is yet another symptom, and consequence, of the intensification of forces on poor families. Nationwide, the number of children reported to be abused or neglected has tripled since 1980, increasing 40% between 1985 and 1991 (8). Data from the National Commission on Children show that, in 1991, 2.7 million children were reported to child protection agencies. Almost half of these cases were for neglect; 25% involved physical abuse; 15% alleged sexual abuse; and 6% cited emotional maltreatment. Tragically, almost 1400 children died from abuse or neglect in 1991, half of them 1 year old or younger (8). As states, counties, and cities experience escalations in serious human service demands, such as the abuse of children, their resources have either failed to grow proportionately or have been reduced. For a variety of reasons, not the least of which has been the financial impact of the flight of middle class citizens from urban communities to the suburbs, municipal tax bases have become inadequate to address these new demands. One state legislator testified to Congress in 1992 that only 39% of the children in confirmed cases of child abuse and neglect in his state received any services at all, and only half of reported cases were actually investigated (8). This is not atypical. Blaming victims, calculated indifference, and lack of confidence in the competencies of governments to solve complex problems further perpetuate the conditions of relative inaction on these and other related issues.

Unfortunately for those concerned with the prevention of HIV disease, given the cyclical nature, prevalence, and long-term psychological effects of abuse, failure to effectively prevent and manage it early results in very serious problems later. For example, data from the National Family Violence Survey suggest that between two and four million women are physically battered by their partners each year. Of the mothers of abused children, 45% are themselves battered women (3). Many of these women, as a result of their isolation, emotional pain, destroyed self-esteem, and other factors become predisposed to drug and alcohol abuse which often results in child abuse and vice versa. A cycle is created as the abused child becomes psychiatrically damaged, takes drugs to cope, and then abuses others as a result of the psychiatric and drug problems (15).

As with the abuse investigation system, there are distressingly few resources available to manage either the psychological disorders or the substance abuse problems of these women and children. Of equal importance is the even greater inability to address both diagnoses as the comorbidities that they, in reality, are. Too many women are unable to sleep at night because of the nightmares of the abuse they suffered as children and as adults. Too many of them become vulnerable to the tranquilization and escape provided by the ubiquitously present drugs. Too many of them have lost any sense of self or of esteem. As important as admonitions for personal responsibility are, "just say no" often becomes irrelevant in the context of such overwhelming pain.

In addition to the growing numbers of abused and homeless women and children are the increasing number of children who require foster care and other placements. In the early 1980s, approximately 270,000 children lived in foster family homes, group homes, or institutional settings (8). By 1988, that number had grown to an estimated 360,000, with 115,000 of them less than 6 years old (13). For 1991, the estimate is that 429,000 children resided in foster family homes, group homes, or institutional settings (8). How many of these children are from poor families is unknown, but in 1988, at least 123,000 of these children were removed from Aid to Families with Dependent Children (AFDC)-eligible families. A recent study of black children in foster care in five major cities found that AFDC was the primary source of income for 65% of the families before placement. Some 54% of the children were placed in foster care because of neglect and another 38% because of abuse (13). Parental substance abuse has been reported in 40–80% of cases. Traditionally, most placements for children occurred because of an unwillingness or inability of the mother to care for the child, rather than as a result of illness in the child (16). Like most other social service systems, the foster care system is straining to keep up with the demand. Obviously, as HIV disease incapacitates and kills more mothers, even more children will require foster placement. Many of them will require intense medical care for their HIV-related illnesses, and others will require extensive psychosocial support if they are to break the cycle of pain that reproduces the antecedents of infection.

HOPELESSNESS AND HIV PREVENTION

As increasing numbers of people confront ever more difficult circumstances without adequate support or resources, the ranks of those who have lost hope and trust in the future swells. If there is no concept of the possibility of a meaningful future, then many people will see little value in adopting those behaviors necessary to realize a healthy future. Many people will, and do, decide to live for the moment. Many others face such formidable daily challenges that there is no choice but to completely concern themselves with getting dinner on the table tonight and the kids off to school tomorrow. The health prevention agenda can seem somewhat distant in the context of bullets killing children while they play and sleep in their own homes. This is particularly true in disorganized communities where problems such as citizenship status, illiteracy, language barriers, undereducation, humiliating unemployment, excessive disease, and random violence can produce a fatalistic attitude of "if one thing doesn't get me, another will" (11).

Blacks and Latinos must also cope with the debilitating forces of racism and cultural insensitivities. Powerlessness and lowered self-esteem are particularly virulent forces; they produce behaviors that result in substance abuse and unhealthy sexual relationships, too often ending in HIV infection. This is particularly true for those whose low self-esteem, poverty, and limited options make them particularly vulnerable to unhealthy behavioral choices or economic exploitation by others (11). It is usual for male and female prostitutes to present these issues in the context of their HIV and/or drug therapy. It is also usual to hear a woman say, "I was desperate for love. I needed him. Yes, I've had negative things in my life, but I love him." Others express that, "Sometimes I had to do things just to put food on the table, just so my children wouldn't be naked ... I'm not proud of what I had to do. I just wanted to survive" (17). It is important to remind ourselves of the real life context of HIV disease if we are to preserve real lives.

For minority adolescents, and the health professionals and others who work with them, these issues are particularly challenging. If the leading cause of death for adolescents is homicide, and their most immediate concerns are with the walk to and from school because their neighborhoods have become what Marian Wright Edelman describes as "a no man's land peopled by armed gangs, drug dealers and nervous youthful gunslingers seeking to preempt death by first strike" (8), then admonitions about refraining from smoking cigarettes to prevent cancer or heart attacks at age 40 years can seem irrelevant. Combined with the limitations of impoverished and overwhelmed schools that often do not even offer the courses in higher math and science that are essential for the jobs of the deindustrialized future, it is not too surprising that each year 700,000 students drop out. In many urban communities, the dropout rates are as high as 50% (7).

Admonitions to avoid drugs and stay in school have difficulty penetrating the cacophony that accompanies the more than one in five 19- to 21-year-olds who do not have a high school diploma (18). Many of those who have managed a diploma can sense that it will not be enough to guarantee a secure future in the complex economy of the future.

Finally, many African-American and Latino adolescents receive precious little love or affection in their lives. The most common images of them in the society are with their hands tied behind their backs or their blood flowing red down the city streets on the evening news. Objects of fear and avoidance, they are rarely embraced, esteemed, or validated by the adults or the institutions of the larger society. As such, they increasingly turn to each other for the support that all humans, and especially children, require. They often organize themselves into "gangs" that serve the role traditionally provided by the extended family and that chart a pathway from childhood to adulthood. Convinced that their only method of controlling the world around them is through the two least common denominators of the human experience, violence and sex, they become increasingly violent and sexual. The boys and girls of their world are often all they have for the validation, nurturing, and ego development necessary for growth and development, no matter how superficial or undesirable. Messages to avoid sex until they are old enough to make mature and rational decisions, or to do so only in the context of a mutually monogamous relationship, often have little relevance for children who are in such need. As they often ask the health worker, "What do you have in trade?"

In many respects, the work of health professionals concerned with the prevention of disease and the promotion of health in poor and minority American communities is similar to sowing seeds in concrete. No wonder so little seems to grow. First, the soil needs to be tilled and then the seeds of health can be planted and nurtured. Health professionals are an important part, but only a part, of a comprehensive team of many other professionals—teachers, business persons, institutions, and community leaders—who require coordination around the survival needs of distressed communities and their citizens. To be successful, health professionals will require new skills, insights, sensitivities, and models in collaboration with their colleagues, patients, and communities.

ACCESS CHALLENGES IN MINORITY COMMUNITIES

As social and environmental conditions intensify behaviors that result in increased burdens of disease, the capacity of the traditional medical care system to diagnose, cure, and manage the health problems of traditionally underserved populations becomes further strained. Health professionals increasingly realize what the Ethical and Judicial Affairs Committee of the American Medical Association concluded in their statement, that "Blacks are more likely to require health care but are less likely to receive health care services" and that these disparities are "unjustifiable and must be eliminated" (17). Given the mixture and intensity of services required by women and children with HIV disease, many of whom already suffer from a variety of preexisting comorbidities, this goal will be difficult to achieve. In fact, the scenario that is too often played out within communities in need is for intense competition to occur between several priorities for the dwindling pool of resources. Unless rather profound changes are effected soon, the consequences will inevitably be similar to dropping an anvil called AIDS onto a system as fragile as wet tissue paper. Success in managing HIV disease could come at the expense of other underaddressed and equally serious health challenges.

As health care reform gains momentum in the national public policy debate, strategies for enhancing medical and health-related care for minority and poor Americans will, it is hoped, be much discussed. Unfortunately, even the most progressive reforms will take several years to make any substantial difference for many of our neediest communities. In the poorest areas, just getting a doctor may be all but impossible. Approximately 21 million Americans live in the 21 Health Professional Shortage Areas designated by the federal government. Combined with another estimated 16 million underserved Americans who do not live in officially designated shortage areas, at least 37 million people are considered medically underserved by the Department of Health and Human Services (19). Approximately 30–50% of these are children and women of childbearing age (3). Federal programs, especially the invaluable Community and Migrant Health Centers, whose patients are more than 60% minority and are overwhelmingly poor (19), address the primary care health needs of approximately 7.2 million of the underserved. Data are not yet available to determine how many of the almost 36 million underserved receive care in state and locally operated programs; however, 25 million people are conservatively estimated to be disenfranchised from a source of regular medical care (M. H. Gaston, personal communication, 1992). Given that the designation of an Health Professional Shortage Area is based upon the conservative ratio of one physician per 3000 patients, in contrast to the standard of one physician per 1500 patients used by many health maintenance organizations, there are considerably more than 37 million medically underserved Americans in need of urgent assistance.

For those with a regular source of care, much of that care occurs in institutional settings, such as hospital emergency rooms. Overall, 9.5 million children or 14.7% had no health insurance in 1991, and millions of others continue to be inadequately covered (20). The New York AIDS Advisory Commission estimates that 31% of poor adolescents and 35% of poor young adults have no insurance (21). Increasing numbers of poor children are now covered by Medicaid since the Omnibus Reconciliation Act of 1990 expanded eligibility requirements. While the percentage of poor children covered has improved from approximately 50% in 1988 to almost 66% for children in families with incomes below 100% of the poverty level in 1992, considerable numbers of children and women of childbearing age remain uncovered. For example, only 28.1% of children in families with incomes between 100 and 125% of poverty are currently covered by Medicaid.

Overall, only 40% of the poor received Medicaid coverage in 1992 (19, 23). Medicaid has been, and continues to be, a vital program for those who are enrolled. Unfortunately, for those concerned with comprehensive child health and with HIV disease in particular, it is inadequate to meet the enormous demands placed upon it. In 1990, two-thirds of the budget was spent on the purchase of health services for the care of institutionalized elderly, disabled, and mentally retarded patients. Only 18% of expenditures were for outpatient care, physician visits, and prescription drugs (23). The basic benefit packages are variable from state to state, and physicians in increasing numbers refuse to accept assignment altogether, or limit the number of patients that they do see (13), in part as a result of frustrations with reporting requirements, inadequate reimbursement rates, and liability concerns. Too often these patients receive their care in emergency rooms and public clinics where the continuity of care so necessary for people with complex comprehensive problems is difficult to achieve. Excessive waiting times for the relatively few providers and facilities that are available often result in delays in seeking or achieving care until disorders have become far advanced and difficult to overcome (7).

COMPREHENSIVE HEALTH CARE

As the political momentum builds for health reform, health advocates concerned with pediatric HIV disease must remain active in the debate for comprehensive, system-wide reforms. Insurance, as important as it is, will not be enough. Other barriers to care also exist and they include the following issues.

Service Capacity

There is an inadequate medical service capacity in many urban and rural communities that is manifested by an absolute and relative deficiency of physicians and other health professionals (19) and by insufficient availability of health care facilities. This condition has been worsened by the growing trend toward subspecialization by physicians, at the expense of primary care practice. Furthermore, the devastating assault over the past decade on the National Health Service Corps, which at its height provided 3000 scholarship-recipient physicians for poor communities, has had tragic consequences. In 1992, only 42 scholarship students were available for service (M. H. Gaston, personal communication, 1993). Thankfully, the program has been revived, but it will take years before the next generation of graduates will be available for service in the field.

As the medical and human service needs of poor and minority persons has increased, the capacity of many state and local jurisdictions to keep pace has actually decreased. In fact, many public health clinics and services either closed completely or severely curtailed their services. The tendency toward fragmentation of services that often accompanies categorical funding of programs has also posed difficult challenges in maximizing efficiency in the use of available resources.

Coordination of Services

Often the medical care and human services that are available are poorly coordinated, suffer from the absence of complimentary services, or are inaccessible to clients and patients. Transportation and child care services, which are often vital to successful health care delivery programs, are in short supply in many communities. Mental health and substance abuse therapy services, so vital to the prevention of HIV disease, are terribly inadequate to meet the demand. This is especially true for inpatient residential slots, which are so necessary for many women and their small children. It is rare for these programs to accept women, even rarer for them to accept poor women with Medicaid, and rarer still for them to accept women with children.

Drug and mental health treatment services are also often poorly coordinated with other primary care and maternity services. So too are nutrition counseling and supplemental food support programs, which, when available, are often off site or offered at limited hours. Well child care, child development, dental, vision, hearing, education,

and outreach workers are all in short supply and are often insufficiently coordinated.

Cultural Barriers

Cultural and language barriers between the patient and the providers of care often frustrate the provision of quality care. Quality is not only a function of the appropriate application of the medical science knowledge and the avoidance of inappropriate actions, but it also depends upon the ability of the practitioner and his or her patient to understand and communicate with each other. Often, poor and ethnically diverse patients become discouraged with the inability of their providers to understand the realities of their lives in the context of the prevention and management of disease. The increasing tendency for labeling, judging, and imposing the criminal justice system into the clinical arena, particularly in cases of maternal substance abuse, further complicates these issues.

HEALTH SYSTEM REFORM AND PEDIATRIC AIDS

Health care professionals and others who are seriously interested in the prevention and management of HIV disease in children must necessarily concern themselves with the broad etiologic and health care delivery system issues that have been presented in this chapter. The challenges of substance abuse prevention and achieving the requisite modifications in the sexual behaviors of poor and overwhelmed young adults require a connection of the traditional health care system to a much larger and more comprehensive set of resources. Similarly, the realization of the comprehensive medical and social supports necessary to adequately manage the full spectrum of HIV disease in children and families, who are not only ill with HIV virus but who are also ill in the context of a multiplicity of other health and social insults, requires the traditional health system and its providers to embrace new forms of practice. Providers need to develop new skills and become organized into more effective and coordinated multidisciplinary health teams (C. Callahan-Davis, personal communication, 1992).

In the last few years, a growing awareness of the need for both more primary care physicians and physicians who are better trained to cope with the rigorous demands of community-oriented primary care has developed. Movements such as the "Health of the Public" have spurred academic health sciences centers, with the support of major health foundations, to embrace new mission statements and new curricula designed to prepare the physician of the future more thoroughly to successfully address the complex health challenges presented by disadvantaged and ethnically diverse communities. Central to this effort has been the appreciation for the observation that the patient who presents for care does so as a member of a family that exists in the context of a community of people. The sociological, anthropological, and cultural characteristics of the patient's family and community have become increasingly important variables that the physician must learn to appreciate and to understand as he or she attempts to elicit the medical history and to communicate successfully and influence the therapeutic regimen.

Similarly, the skills of applied clinical epidemiology are becoming ever more vital to the intellectual work of making better informed diagnostic and therapeutic judgments. As more information is acquired about the population from which the individual patient arises, more precise disease probability determinations can be derived and more accurate therapeutic decisions can be achieved. Enhancements in the cost-effectiveness of medical practice are important byproducts and goals of this work.

Given the relative paucity of resources, and the magnitude of need in poor communities, medical decisions and practice must be much more informed so as to reach quality outcomes as efficiently as possible. As such, the disciplines of health services research and the evaluative sciences central to outcome and quality determinations assume a significant role in the training of health professionals. The urge to "do the right thing," combined with earnest effort on the front lines of health care, while commendable and unfortunately still rare, will not be enough to grapple successfully with the demands of pediatric HIV disease. Communities in need require professionals who are trained not only with commitment and compassion but who also have the skills to develop new knowledge in the context of more effective and efficient service. Their practices must be informed by new ideas and the efficient use of all available resources.

Physicians, nurses, a variety of allied health professionals, social workers, and community outreach workers will need to coordinate their work more completely among themselves and with their communities to deliver flexible and coherent care. Traditional medical care must increasingly be coordinated with outreach efforts such as telephone "hotlines" and mobile health van services; with case managers who concern themselves with the full array of supports necessary for many families to cope with the challenges of daily living; with early childhood assessment efforts and family psychological support systems that prepare the HIV-positive child and family to live with AIDS; and with the residential and foster care providers who will increasingly provide the housing for these mothers and their children. Fragmentation in successful programs has been overcome through staff versatility and by active collaboration across bureaucratic and professional boundaries. They take the time and have the training, skills, and desire to overcome communication barriers that often result from different terminology and educations. They support each other in building relationships of trust and respect with the children, families, and communities they serve (22).

Working successfully with communities requires skill, patience, and humility. Above all, it requires an appreciation of the reality that not all poor communities are alike, not all "Latino communities" are alike, nor are all "black communities" alike. Communities are often very different with varied social arrangements, traditions, histories, and learned behaviors (11). Their perspectives on and reactions to HIV disease in particular, and health problems in general, may be quite different. Successful community partnerships avoid the pitfalls of blaming the victim or of simplistic generalizing or labeling. Similarly, successful health workers interact with communities in such a manner that they assist the community without becoming indispensable or creating dependencies (11).

Much greater attention should be placed on the rebuilding of community infrastructures. Health professionals are encouraged to form innovative partnerships with the various agencies that provide services to children and families; the natural community support systems and information networks such as churches, barbershops, social clubs, restaurants, laundromats, youth centers, self-help groups, public housing developments, and supermarkets (11); and with the real community grassroots leadership. If the health care system is unsuccessful in developing these linkages, or is disinterested in trying because of a preoccupation with outdated concepts regarding the legitimate boundaries of "medical care," then it will be difficult to prevent or treat HIV disease successfully.

Communities will require resources and expertise as they are encouraged by health workers and others to accept their responsibilities for the promotion of health and the prevention of disease. Ultimately, successful AIDS prevention and the recruitment of the social supports necessary for the long-term management of women and children with AIDS requires community empowerment. The philosophy and technical elements of grantsmanship, in public and private programs, are important to this effort. It is very frustrating to observe the exploitation of small, poor, grassroots community organizations that are intimately in touch with the daily lives of disadvantaged people, by professional grant-writing middlemen who use them in the process of grantsmanship. Given the importance of developing a functional and intrinsic community-based competency, great care should be devoted to the direct nourishment of these often fragile organizations. As health care funding priorities change, comprehensive community-based programs should have a continuity of support as an important investment for the long-term struggle for health.

In the final analysis, the etiology of HIV disease in women and children of color is intimately and inextricably connected to the realities of the communities in which they live. So too are the forces that confound the early diagnosis and management

of HIV-related illness. Committed health professionals will increasingly be required to develop new competencies and relationships as they struggle with the comprehensive and complex issues presented by this virus. Be aware that communities of color are also busy with the process of organizing themselves to better address their responsibilities. How the health community behaves can either assist or impede these efforts that are so important to the survival of women and children of color. Ultimately, we are all in this together.

References

1. Centers for Disease Control. HIV/AIDS Surveillance. Atlanta: Department of Health and Human Services, 1991:9–14.
2. Braithwaite RL, Taylor SE. Health issues in the black community. San Francisco: Josse-Bass, 1992:6.
3. Office on Women's Health. Action plan for women's health. Washington, DC: Department of Health and Human Services, 1991:32, 33, 74–92.
4. Health United States 1991 and Prevention Profile. Hyattsville: Department of Health and Human Services, 1992:1–5, 121–302.
5. Anonymous. Report of the Secretary Task Force on Black and Minority Health, Executive Summary. Washington, DC: Department of Health and Human Services, 1985.
6. American's Health. Forgotten Americans (Special Report). New York: Pfizer, 1992:42.
7. Hamburg DA. Today's children creating a future for a generation in crisis. New York: Times Books, 1992:40, 43, 44, 46.
8. Anonymous. The state of America's children. Washington, DC: Children's Defense Fund, 1992: 9, 52, 62.
9. Hechinger F. Fateful choices: Healthy youth for the 21st century. New York: Hill and Wang, 1992:25, 29, 30.
10. Haan M, Kaplan GA, Camacho T. Poverty and health: Prospective evidence from the Alameda County Study. Am J Epidemiol 1987:997.
11. Cancela VDL. Minority AIDS prevention: Moving beyond cultural perspectives towards sociopolitical empowerment. New York: Guilford Press, 1989:144, 146.
12. Anonymous. Focus on children: The beat of the future. New York: Columbia Graduate School of Journalism, 1992:46.
13. National Center for Children in Poverty. Five million children: A statistical profile of our poorest young citizens. New York: Columbia University 1990:13,60, 61, 661.
14. Nyamathi A. Comparative study of factors relating to high risk level of black homeless women. J AIDS 1992:222.
15. Mirkatz IR, Thompson JE, et al. Perspective on prenatal care. New York: Elsevier, 1990:5306.

16. Anonymous. Report of the Surgeon General's Workshop on Children with HIV Infection and Their Families (AIDS). Rockville, MD: Department of Health and Human Services, 1987:41.

17. Grant Support Provided by Office of Minority Health, Department of Health and Human Services. Black women in crisis, mobilizing black women to prevent and reduce the spread of HIV disease. Washington, DC: Black Women's Agenda, 1991:18.

18. Gibbs JT. Black adolescents and youth: An endangered species. Am J Orthopsychiatr 1984:7.

19. Wiener JM, Engel J. Brookings dialogues on public policy. Improving access to health services for children and pregnant women. Washington, DC: The Brookings Institution, 1991:5, 40, 46.

20. Anonymous. Sources of health insurance and characteristics of the uninsured analysis of the Mar 1992 current population survey. (Special Report, SR-16) Washington, DC: Employee Benefit Research Institute, 1993:1, 61.

21. Dubler NN, Stern G. Illusions of immortality. The confrontation of adolescence and AIDS. New York: Ad Hoc Committee on Adolescents and HIV, a report to the New York State AIDS Advisory Council, 1991:20.

22. Meharry Medical College. Institute on Health Care for the Poor and Underserved. Health Care Poor and Underserved 1990;1:272.

23. Kent C. Medicaid: End it or mend it? Perspectives (a four page supplement to Medicine & Health Newsletter Dec 21, 1992). New York: Faulkner & Gray, 1992(suppl):20.

53

Expanding Access to Health Care for Infants, Children, and Adolescents

Paul H. Wise

The greater our clinical capability to modify the course of human immunodeficiency virus (HIV) infection, the greater is our collective burden to ensure access to it. This implies an essential interaction between the scope of clinical capacity and the requirements of clinical provision (1) and highlights the growing importance of access issues as the effectiveness of therapeutic approaches to pediatric HIV infection continues to expand.

Although access to health care remains a troubling issue for all segments of society, HIV infection in children casts a particularly harsh light on current delivery systems. The profound needs of these children coupled with the likelihood that they live in traditionally underserved communities has intensified the need for an expanded commitment to accessible service provision. This discussion is directed at how clinicians can confront this challenge in their own practices and work collaboratively with policymakers and community residents to ensure that children with HIV infection and their families have access to coordinated and comprehensive care.

DEFINING ACCESS

Access to care has been defined in various ways (2). However, for clinical purposes, access can be broadly outlined as the *provision of services based on need*. Although distinctions between availability, utilization, and access can, and have, been made, this discussion is based on the clinical reality that in any given case these distinctions may not be particularly relevant or even possible to discern. This is because many barriers to care may not be apparent to even the most astute clinicians. This can often lead clinicians to mistake a patient's lack of utilization as a lack of motivation. Hidden costs, dehumanizing prior contacts with the medical care system, cultural concerns, travel difficulties, multiple, uncoordinated service visits, lack of child care, and language barriers are just some of the powerful factors that can undermine the access claims of seemingly available clinical services. It is generally more useful to focus on the practical, operational character of service provision, on functional access, by struggling to ensure that the structure and content of clinical care responds seamlessly to the true dimensions of need.

FINANCING COORDINATED CARE

A central requirement of access is the assurance that appropriate care is not prohibited by inadequate financial resources (Table 53.1). In the United States, this financial requirement takes on special importance because of both the high cost of health care and the continued reliance on a highly fragmented system of private and public health insurance as the primary means of covering such costs. Together, these characteristics place a special burden on those who provide care for children with

975

Table 53.1.   Clinical Elements of Access to Care

Financial access
　Private health insurance
　Public health insurance
　Associated costs
Logistical access
　Transportation
　Safety of travel
　Child care
Cultural access
　Language
　Cultural understanding
　Community-based services
Intergrated access
　Program integration
　Case management
　Research and clinical care
　Special needs of adolescents
　Coordinated care for women

HIV to assess the adequacy of a family's capacity to cover the costs associated with optimal care.

Private Health Insurance

Children with HIV infection are less likely than other children to be covered by private insurers. However, because private insurance programs are so heterogeneous, it is important that one not assume that every patient covered by such programs will be protected from the financial implications of chronic illness. In general, the financial impact on families with private insurance will depend on five general issues: cost-sharing, cost cap, covered service, rating and availability, and associated costs.

Most private insurance plans will cover in-hospital costs. However, an increasing number of such plans may require substantial copayments by the child's family. Because hospital costs are so substantial, even relatively small copayment requirements, such as the traditional 20%, could ultimately result in large charges to the family. In addition, significant deductible payments may be required under some plans. Some private plans may offer coverage up to a designated cost or period of hospitalization. Once that cap has been reached, either an enhanced portion or even all of the subsequent costs are borne by the family.

The heterogeneity of private insurance plans becomes even more apparent when the range of covered services is examined. New procedures or therapeutic regimens may be considered "experimental" and, therefore, not accepted as covered services by many private insurers. Significantly, the designation of covered procedures and therapies may vary by insurer and can at times be based on rather arbitrary criteria. Outpatient services are commonly treated differently than inpatient care, often requiring larger copayments or full payment by patient families. This can have the effect of creating incentives for in-hospital care even if hospital discharge and ambulatory services are clinically more appropriate. Illness-related outpatient services, such as attendance at hospital-based subspecialty clinics, may have distinct coverage from well child or primary care. In general, primary care services are less likely to be covered fully than are specialized ambulatory or inpatient care. Certain medications and dental and optical care may not be covered even in programs with broad primary care coverage. In addition, social services, physical and occupational therapy, treatment for substance abuse, home visits, and mental health services often receive only limited coverage.

Perhaps the most catastrophic aspect of private insurance is the possibility that it can be terminated when patients and families need it most. Disturbingly, such occurrences have become more commonplace because of the growing practice of providing insurance on the basis of an individual's, rather than on a community's, risk for illness. Accordingly, it has become common for insurers to deny coverage to individuals for conditions that predated enrollment. This has created an environment in which parents of chronically ill children may find that they cannot change jobs for fear that the insurer at their new place of work will refuse coverage on the basis of their child's preexisting condition. The transition from foster care to adoption can involve difficult issues related to the transfer of health insurance. In some settings, particularly in small businesses, company premium costs may be increased in response to an employee's use of health care thereby creating incentives to limit employee benefits and even lay off employees deemed to be likely to require such services. The tragic implications of such practices have become the focus of considerable public concern and are being addressed under new proposals for health care reform.

The impact of a child's chronic illness on a family's daily life can generate several associated costs to families that can often be overlooked by health care providers. Even with adequate insurance coverage, time away from work may be both substantial and often unexpected; the lost pay and implications for advancement can alter the financial security of families for years to come. The cumulative effects of numerous small expenditures for transportation, household goods, or special foods can ultimately add to major expenses for the family.

The complexity of private health insurance plans coupled with the major costs associated with the care of children with HIV infection and their families require that care providers continue to assess the financial implications of their clinical decisions and develop a capacity to respond to identified areas of concern. Although the families of children covered by private insurance generally have greater financial resources than children covered by public programs, the financial impact of HIV infection in privately insured families can be substantial nevertheless and must, therefore, be addressed by any comprehensive clinical program.

Publicly Funded Health Insurance

The primary publicly funded health insurance program for children in the United States is Medicaid. Medicaid is an entitlement program, meaning that it is offered to all children who meet eligibility criteria and is jointly funded by federal and state governments. It is a financing program, not a health care delivery program, and relies upon local health care systems to provide services. Although the program's general structure is based on federal standards, considerable variation remains among the states regarding eligibility criteria and covered services. The most common mechanism by which children become eligible for Medicaid is as a dependent in a family receiving assistance through the Aid to Families with Dependent Children (AFDC) program, the primary welfare program in the United States.

Children with HIV infection may become eligible for Medicaid through the Supplemental Security Income program, which provides cash assistance to families with disabled children. Under some state provisions, Medicaid may be provided to children in foster care. Adolescents can be covered by Medicaid through these same mechanisms; however, in some states, income criteria for eligibility may be stricter for adolescents than for younger children. States may also provide Medicaid to adolescents age 21 years or younger who meet income criteria and live independently. Poor and near-poor pregnant women may be eligible for prenatal and delivery services under Medicaid. In addition, many states have initiated special presumptive eligibility programs in which the state assumes prenatal and delivery costs for uninsured pregnant women even if they are ultimately deemed ineligible for Medicaid.

Medicaid provides support for a core of essential services, including hospital care, ambulatory services, screening, and primary care. The foundation for the provision of preventive services under Medicaid is the Early and Periodic Screening, Diagnostic and Treatment (EPSDT) program. EPSDT provides funds for patient education, transportation, and basic health services including dental, hearing, and vision screening. In many states, however, the EPSDT program has had difficulty mounting effective outreach efforts and provider participation. In addition, the focus on basic services has meant that all too often EPSDT has not been effective in providing services to children with complex health and social needs. Some state Medicaid programs have attempted to extend basic Medicaid services through a range of expanded health and support services such as outreach programs, home-based services, and hospice care. Of special importance to providers concerned with pediatric HIV infection are the growing number of states that have implemented specific Medicaid programs to address the needs of persons infected with HIV. Enhanced case management efforts, psychosocial and other support services, extended coverage for HIV-infected children in foster care, and comprehensive home-based care have all been included in such state efforts.

Although Medicaid remains a critical resource for many families with HIV-infected children, it may neither fully facilitate access to requisite medical services nor protect such families from the major financial implications of a child with HIV infection. As for privately insured families, issues with cost caps, covered services, eligibility, and associated costs can create a debilitating financial burden even when Medicaid coverage is provided. Efforts to deal with inadequate funding for Medicaid have included caps on inpatient costs or lengths of stay. New procedures or therapies may not be covered by Medicaid even though they may have moved off experimental protocols. Some states have rather strict provisions regarding outpatient medications and support services, thereby making coordinated home-based care difficult. The rather tight linkage of Medicaid eligibility to income status can create major problems in maintaining the continuity of care when parents consider changes in their employment status or enhancing their earnings. In response to this concern, some states have adopted special federal provisions that continue a child's Medicaid coverage for a period despite a rise in family income above the Medicaid eligibility threshold.

Because some states have established eligibility criteria far below the official poverty line, many children in extreme need of publicly guaranteed health insurance have been excluded from the Medicaid program. Moreover, the many bureaucratic and logistical barriers to enrollment in Aid to Families with Dependent Children and Medicaid have left large portions of eligible children without program benefits. Recent federal and selected state initiatives have attempted to phase in extended income eligibility guidelines to encompass all poor and some near-poor children. However, large numbers of children, particularly older children and adolescents, remain without health insurance because of low family income. In addition, the dearth of health providers that accept Medicaid patients in many areas of the United States has meant that even when covered by Medicaid, many children lack functional access to health care. The associated costs of a child with HIV-related illness can also prove catastrophic for families with Medicaid coverage. Seemingly small items, such as bus fare to clinic visits or extra diapers for infants with diarrhea, can exhaust household funds and undermine a family's best efforts to meet basic needs. In such a setting of deprivation, financial access to care implies much more than health insurance; it requires a level of material well-being sufficient to ensure that the seeking of health care is not ultimately expressed as reduced food on the table.

In light of the complexity and considerable state-to-state variability of Medicaid eligibility criteria and covered services, it is essential that clinicians become familiar with the basic elements of the Medicaid program in their area. Medicaid is a dynamic program, continually being refashioned in response to changing funding levels and the evolving health needs of poor children and their families. Even providers who have considerable experience with local Medicaid provisions should specifically inquire about recent changes in coverage or special benefits for children with HIV infection.

Challenge and Opportunity of Managed Care

Both private and public insurance systems have increasingly implemented programs to control their beneficiaries' access to services through mandated approval and cost-sharing mechanisms. Generally referred to as "managed care," these efforts have had a significant impact on traditional patterns of clinical practice, particularly for patients with complex, chronic disorders. The necessity of multiple physician visits, specialty consultation, and frequent or prolonged hospitalizations may place major stresses on the functioning of managed care systems and can, therefore, place special requirements on those who must assure access to care for children with AIDS or HIV infection.

Cultural Understanding

Beyond language, clinicians must possess some basic understanding of the meaning of illness and traditions of healing in the communities they serve (4, 6). Given the strong link among health beliefs, health behaviors, and the use of health services, access to clinical services may often depend on how directly clinical programs relate to cultural perceptions of health and the utility of medical care. This can be particularly important in addressing AIDS, in light of the distinctions in how this illness is perceived by different ethnic and cultural groups. Athough cultural understanding helps determine access through the clinical sensitivity such insight generates, it also implies a level of practical competence in shaping clinical programs responsive to local perceptions and social institutions. This cultural competence not only ensures that recommended medical regimens will not be undermined by cultural influences but also that such clinical plans will take full advantage of the many great strengths that exist within culturally defined communities. Although such competence should be expected of all those providing care, clinical programs can benefit greatly from the purposeful inclusion of health workers and trained residents from the communities being served.

It is also critical for clinicians to recognize the power of social prejudice and racism to define access to care (7). Particularly when an illness is highly concentrated in minority populations, the potential for race and social position to determine a patient's experience with the health care system must be addressed. In addition, subtle institutional messages, such as dilapidated clinical settings for socially defined groups of patients can generate the kind of deep personal resentment that may ultimately affect clinical relationships. Strategies to confront these issues include the training and recruitment of minority health providers, ongoing training for all those interacting with patients and their families (including receptionists, security guards, billing personnel, as well as clinical providers), and active surveying of patients and family members regarding their experience at the clinical facility (7–9).

INTEGRATED ACCESS

True access for children and families with diverse clinical and social needs depends on the integration of services. A reliance on a multitude of isolated interventions will preclude comprehensive access even if each of these individual-programs is deemed available. The competing demands and disparate bureaucratic requirements of insular, categorical programs can all too often overwhelm even the most capable of families. Therefore, it is important that access be defined by the coordination of services as well as their singular provision.

Program Integration and Case Management

Coordinating services for children with HIV infection and AIDS can take the form of programmatic integration and clinical case management. Programmatic integration depends on the development of linkages between programs, particularly in unifying enrollment procedures, streamlining referral mechanisms, and coordinating service strategies (3). Clinical case management involves the use of program personnel to coordinate services for a panel of individual patients and their families. Together, programmatic integration and case management can greatly enhance both the utilization and effectiveness of diverse services.

A major challenge lies in financing integrative activities. The categorical nature of specialized health and social services for children in the United States has made integrative efforts both necessary and inadequately funded. However, recognition of the efficiency of coordinated services and the complex needs of persons with HIV infection and AIDS have generated several funding mechanisms for integrative services. The Ryan White Comprehensive AIDS Resources Emergency (CARE) Act of 1990 and the AIDS Pediatric Health Care Demonstration programs have provided some limited support for a range of integrative efforts in many communities affected by HIV infection and AIDS. In addition, Medicaid funding has been used to support case management and outreach services in some states (3).

Research and Clinical Care

The severe consequences of HIV infection coupled with the lack of a definitive cure have meant that the clinical care of children infected with HIV is intimately associated with investigative protocol. The convergence of this experimental requirement with the intense concentration of pediatric HIV infection in disadvantaged communities has created a disturbing reliance on research protocols for the delivery of high quality clinical services. Although troubling at many levels, this dependence on research programs for the delivery of clinical services places a special burden on the maintenance of access as children and infected family members move on and off of various investigative protocols. More fundamentally, the effort to provide care under current conditions should be coupled with a purposeful advocacy for programs and funding (including transportation, child care, respite, and hospice services) designed to more directly provide the necessary elements of high quality clincial care.

Special Needs of Adolescents

Although adolescents share with younger children many of the same basic requirements of functional access, they also raise a series of special concerns regarding their relationship with traditional mechanisms of health care delivery. Developmental struggles of adolescents are a central concern that may be expressed in various risk-taking and frankly self-destructive behaviors. Emphasis on the development of ongoing clinical relationships and integrated psychosocial support services may prove essential in this regard. When issues of adolescent sexuality emerge, programs may balk in providing access to clinically appropriate services. Complex legal issues may emerge regarding consent, confidentiality, and counseling because wide variation in relevant state statutes exists. In addition, the tragic likelihood that HIV-infected adolescents are living on the streets, in shelters, or in other nontraditional settings requires that access to care be redefined to address practical outreach and service delivery that such living environments entail.

Addressing Needs of Women

Of special concern is the need to coordinate services for children with those designed for infected women. Although issues regarding the care of both parents are always important in caring for children infected with HIV, there is a special requirement for the care of women. This stems from the tendency of pediatric programs to focus on maternal needs only to the extent that they affect the health of the newborn and child. This can be particularly problematic in settings where the interruption of vertical transmission in utero and in infancy is of central importance. Here, for example, efforts should be made to facilitate coordinated access to care when protocols that address vertical transmission exclude women postpartum, relying instead on quite separate programs for the care of non-pregnant women. It may also be useful to coordinate clinical programs through collaborative scheduling and integrated clinical services for women and their children. Without such purposeful attention, pediatric programs can serve to fragment the delivery of care to women with HIV infection, compounding their already difficult struggle for just treatment.

LEVELS OF CLINICIAN INVOLVEMENT

The complex needs of children with HIV infection present their clinical caretakers with an array of professional and personal challenges. First among these is the humane provision of direct clinical care. In this light, the commitment to ensure access to care to children with HIV infection should begin with a textured examination of the structure and content of one's current clinical practice. The needs of these children and their families, however, can never fully be met by clinical management alone. Indeed, for most experienced practitioners, the role of the clinician is defined by the dual appreciation of health care's utility and its inherent limitations. A clinician's effectiveness, therefore, may be enhanced by the purposeful coupling of direct clinical care with a broader commitment to service expansion and policy development.

Indeed, clinicians have been important in shaping a range of services and programs to meet local needs. Clinicians have served as local advocates, providing the technical expertise and professional legitimacy to help fashion effective community-based programs. Given the range of ambulatory and supportive care that children with HIV infection require, the innovative community-based programs should fill a critical void in the provision of needed services. Clinicians have also helped evaluate and disseminate these experiences so that this rich experience can be used and adapted in various community settings.

Clinicians have also been important in confronting the primary determinants of pediatric HIV infection and the scope of societal response through public advocacy and policy development. The continued public debate regarding health care reform in the United States could alter dramatically the nature and accessibility of health services to children infected with HIV. As this public deliberation moves forward, however, challenge will increasingly lie in ensuring that these emerging reforms draw on and ultimately reflect faithfully the caring intelligence and practical experience of all those who provide clinical care to children in need.

References

1. Wise PH, Lowe JA. Noise or fugue: Seeking the logic of child health indicators. Ment Retard 1992;30:323–329.
2. Dutton DB. Children's health care: The myth of equal access. The report of the select panel for the promotion of child health to the United States Congress and the Secretary of Health and Human Services. Better health for our children: A national strategy, Vol. IV, Washington, DC: Department of Health and Human Services, Publication 79-55071, 1981:357–440.
3. Surgeon General's report of panel on women, adolescents, and children with HIV infection and AIDS, A guide to family center comprehensive care for children with HIV, Aug, 1991.
4. Harwood A, Introduction. In: Harwood A, ed. Ethnicity and medical care. Cambridge, MA: Harvard University Press, 1981.
5. Putsch RW III, Cross-cultural communication. The special case of interpreters in health care. JAMA 1985;254:3344–3348.
6. Maduro R. Curanderismo and Latino views of disease and curing. West J Med 1983;139:868–874.
7. Council on Ethical and Judicial Affairs, Black-white disparities in health care. JAMA 1990;263:234.
8. Frank-Stromborg M. Changing demographics in the United States. Implications for health professionals. Cancer 1991;67:1772–1778.
9. Tatum BD. Talking about race, learning about racism: The application of racial identity development theory in the classroom. Harvard Educ Rev 1992:62:1–24.

Child Advocacy and Pediatric AIDS

Peggy Daly Pizzo

The purpose of this chapter is to inform the reader about 1) effective advocacy for children highly vulnerable to death or damage and 2) current developments in advocacy for children infected with human immunodeficiency virus (HIV). This chapter will define and discuss both legislative and administrative advocacy undertaken to help a class of United States citizens: children with HIV and their families. Legal advocacy for children with HIV, including test case litigation, is discussed elsewhere in this book (see Chapter 49).

The chapter will provide some background on the history and nature of child advocacy and the distinctions between professional child advocacy and parent advocacy for children. It will then discuss the central issues, agendas, goals and accomplishments of both professional child and parent legislative and administrative advocacy for children with HIV. It will explore a new model of parent advocacy that is being pioneered on behalf of children and families with HIV. The chapter will conclude with some reflections on implications for future combined advocacy efforts of both parents and professionals.

NATURE OF CHILD ADVOCACY

Child advocacy is the act of persuading individuals and institutions with decision making power over 1) legal protections, 2) financial and informational resources, and/or 3) services to assure that children in need receive these protections, resources, and services, consistent to the greatest extent possible with the rights of parents and the preservation of families. Child advocates work on behalf of children and families to prevent damage to children or to respond with help when children are being damaged. Child advocates try to promote the best possible response from powerful societal institutions when children experience the death of, serious disability of, or desertion by parents, the hardships of poverty, denial of justice, disease, injury, disability, abuse, or neglect.

For children living in families where a parent or parents are present and functional, child advocates do not (or should not) work in loco parentis, i.e., in the place of parents. For children living in families where there is no parent or the parent or parents are abusive or neglectful to the point that the child is endangered, child advocates do assume (typically with the consent of the courts) in loco parentis authority and responsibility for protection of the child. In such situations, child advocates will usually seek to have the children placed under the care and protection of individuals other than their parent(s).

There are two types of child advocacy: case advocacy and class advocacy. Case advocacy is protection and promotion of the rights and needs of an individual child (1). Class advocacy is protection and promotion of the rights and needs of children in general or of defined groups of children (1). This chapter focuses on class advocacy: advocacy for the class comprised of children with HIV and their family members.

Furthermore, there are several types of class advocacy: legislative advocacy (focusing on legislative branch enactment of laws and appropriations); administrative advocacy (focusing on executive branch regulatory and policy decisions, including the development of budget requests sent to the executive branch); and legal advocacy (focusing on judicial decisions, including those that set a precedent for future policy decisions in all three branches of government) (2).

PROFESSIONAL CHILD ADVOCACY

In professional child advocacy, individuals who typically have either training or experience in some aspect of services to children or families spend a substantial part of their time in child advocacy. This work might be paid or unpaid, but it is distinguished from part-time volunteer avocations in that the professional advocate expends a substantial amount of time at advocacy endeavors.

Professional child advocates involved in class advocacy typically organize their work around two goals: a different distribution of goods and services (e.g., an increase in or reallocation of funding amounts so that underserved populations receive needed services) or institutional reform (e.g., decrease in or elimination of discrimination against children on the basis of disability).

As a group, professional child advocates tend to emphasize egalitarianism and often eschew the classic characteristics of a profession. For example, entry into the activity of child advocacy is not limited only to individuals with certain formal credentials; child advocates do not have a formal creed of belief or practice "professed" by the members of the profession as a group, and there is no body of individuals either within or outside the profession set up to remove undesirable practitioners of child advocacy from practice. Formal training programs in child advocacy are extremely rare, and there is no degree considered to be a threshold qualifying degree for either legislative or administrative advocacy (as distinct from legal advocacy). Legal advocacy and test case litigation is usually undertaken only by child advocates trained as lawyers.

Individuals admitted to the bar are the best individuals to represent parents' and children's—or children's—interests in a court of law.

Although the work of child legislative and administrative advocacy does not require an entry degree, effectiveness at child advocacy requires the acquisition of a substantial degree of knowledge and skill. Acquisition of this knowledge and skill in turn requires considerable intelligence; sufficient literacy to be able to read and comprehend legislation, regulations, and policy documents; analytical and persuasive communication skills; and considerable expenditure of effort. But it does not require formal training in a college or university setting. One lesson that child advocates learned from early experiences with Head Start, for example, was that parents with little formal education could become effective advocates for children, if they could obtain the knowledge that they needed and increase their skills at advocacy through either parent to parent or professional to parent face-to-face mentoring, workshop, group meetings, and other mechanisms outside the formal education system (3–7).

Child advocates involved in class legislative or administrative advocacy are typically organized into or affiliated with two kinds of nonprofit groups: public interest policy and advocacy centers (e.g., the Childrens Defense Fund) or membership organizations whose members are usually either citizens deeply interested in childrens issues (e.g., the National Council of Jewish Women) or providers of a certain type of childrens service (e.g., the Child Welfare League).

The motivation for the kind of persistence needed for child advocacy is usually fueled by direct contact with children and families experiencing suffering. Consequently, among professionals, providers of direct care or services to children and families often have a strong motivation for persistent, long-term child advocacy. However, providers of care, particularly when they are paid for their services at levels that seem high to average citizens, are sometimes viewed with suspicion by policymakers when they engage in child advocacy. Some policymakers, for example, view provider advocacy for better financing of childrens services as a way to further the financial self-interest of the providers of these services, rather than the interests of children. Thus it becomes important in professional child advocacy to approach policymakers with all three types of organizations: the public interest policy and advocacy center, the citizen membership organizations, and the provider membership organizations.

PARENT ADVOCACY FOR CHILDREN AND FAMILIES

Parent advocacy for children is distinguished from professional child advocacy by two characteristics: 1) the fact of who practices this kind of advocacy and 2) its goals. Parent advocates engage in activities similar to (but not identical with) professional child advocates involved in legislative or administrative advocacy.

Like professional child advocates, parent advocates organize their activities around the goals of a different distribution of goods and services and institutional reform. But parent advocates seek reform of institutional practices that exclude or threaten harm to children *and* parents. The historical focus of child advocacy groups has been institutional reform that will benefit children. In recent decades, child advocates (e.g., those who promote increased funding for Head Start or similar early childhood programs) have consciously promoted services that respect and include parents in decision making about their children. However, with some notable exceptions, a strong emphasis on parents rights as well as childrens rights is still a more prominent characteristic of parent advocacy than it is of professional child advocacy. Parent advocates consciously organize their activities around the goal of greater support for parent participation in decision making about children within societal institutions of all types and at all levels of decision making. These include decisions about protections, resources, services, and training (8–10).

Furthermore, many parent advocacy organizations also organize their activities around the goal of providing mutual support to parents who are members of the group. All members of a parent advocacy group typically share a common experience with a certain medical or educational problem (e.g., childhood cancer or mental retardation in children), with a certain type of societal institution (e.g., hospitals, schools, or residential care institutions), or with a type of life event or life transition (e.g., adoption of a child or divorce of the parents). These shared experiences are often highly stressful ones in which parents confidence and sense of competence and self-worth has been impaired (8–10).

In addition, these shared experiences are often unusual or historically new experiences that are foreign to the life experiences of the parents own traditional support networks, e.g., extended family members, neighbors, work colleagues, or church groups. The mutual support activities of parent advocacy organizations include the development of new communities, some of them like "second families," in which parents exchange practical resources such as assistance with a dependent or information about the most effective sources of help. In these new communities, parents also repair damage to self-worth and help one another construct more positive images of themselves as individuals who are coping resourcefully with a stressful life experience (8–10).

In legislative and administrative advocacy, the effectiveness of parent advocates is enhanced by the often high regard in which they are held by policymakers. Parents concerned about the quality of schools or hospitals or community based health and social service agencies, for example, do not usually have to contend with policymaker suspicion of their motivations. Furthermore, parents bring an experientially based knowledge of public policies as they have been enacted in real life. Parent advocates know not just from individual but from shared experience which public policies have worked well for children and families and which have not. This actual direct experience with the effectiveness or ineffectiveness of public policy is respected by many policymakers. Concerned that public policy is too often constructed either from emotional arguments not well grounded in fact or from the findings of evaluations conducted by academics remote from the actual lives of children and families, many committed policymakers want to hear thoughtful appraisals of how well (or how poorly) policy has worked, directly from the people whom the policy was intended to benefit.

ACCOMPLISHMENTS OF PARENT AND PROFESSIONAL CHILD ADVOCACY

Over the last 25–30 years, professional child advocacy and parent advocacy have accomplished the enactment and preservation of many important services for children suffering from impoverishment, hunger, deprivation of health care, and unreported abuse and neglect. Among these accomplishments are authorization, funding, and expansion of food and nutrition programs; maternal and child health services; better laws requiring the reporting of child abuse and neglect; and improved access to educational opportunities within institutions that were once closed to children with special needs or low-income or minority children. Together, parent and professional child advocates have also obtained authorization of and expanded funding for Head Start; adoption assistance; health services and education for children with disabilities; early intervention services for children with developmental delay or likelihood of delay; and better laws emphasizing family preservation, wherever feasible, over hasty recourse to foster care placement.

CHILD ADVOCACY AND PEDIATRIC AIDS

The central challenges in child advocacy for children with pediatric AIDS are the identification of 1) the goals most essential to the well-being of children in general and in particular the child with HIV; 2) the primary obstacles to the realization of those goals; 3) the strategies most likely to be effective in overcoming those obstacles and achieving realization of those goals; and 4) actual outcomes from the implementation of public policy intended to further the well-being of children with HIV.

In this section, these issues will be explored within the context of each of three goals related to the well-being of the child with HIV. These are enhancement of participation in 1) treatment that leads toward a cure, 2) a family or family-like setting that

assures the daily care and protection of the child, and 3) the normal or nearly-normal experiences of childhood, whenever medically feasible. Within the context of these goals, the agendas, goals, and accomplishments of both professional child advocacy groups and parent advocates concerned about the child with HIV will be explored. A fourth goal, prevention of acquisition or further spread of HIV infection, will not be discussed here because of limitations of space.

GOAL I: PARTICIPATION IN TREATMENT THAT LEADS TOWARD A CURE
Background

Currently, children who have AIDS experience an inevitably fatal outcome. There is no cure at this time. Given the invariably fatal nature of pediatric AIDS, the goal of child advocates cannot be the simpler one of increasing access to existing effective treatment. Instead some child advocates are appropriately choosing to promote 1) biomedical research as a way to build a base of knowledge that will lead toward effective treatment, 2) increased access to research based treatment programs, and 3) increased access to therapeutic agents that may alleviate and eventually cure the disease.

Pediatric AIDS is characterized by neurodevelopmental degeneration caused by chronic encephalopathy (a degenerative disease of the brain). Children who have the disease regress motorically and mentally (see Chapter 23). Those who could walk before the disease takes hold may lose the ability to walk and then may lose the ability to crawl. Older children who could write or draw or trace figures may lose that ability and then may lose the ability to make any comprehensible marks with a writing or drawing instrument. Further, the disease is characterized in children by severe bacterial infections and lung disease that may require long periods of intensive medical care (see Chapters 13, 14, 16, 25). Some children experience gastrointestinal problems, including impairment of the ability to eat and severe discomfort (12). Death may be due to infections, progressive wasting or starvation, or organ damage.

Although there is no cure, there are treatment modalities that alleviate the symptoms. With sufficient research, further treatment approaches might be developed that will lead to long-term survival and eventual cure (see Chapter 35).

As of March 1993, 90% of the children acquire the disease from maternal transmission (11). The remaining children acquire the disease from infected blood transfusions, sexual abuse, drug abuse, or sexual intercourse. This has several implications for advocacy efforts to enhance participation in treatment. First, children with maternally transmitted HIV cannot always be expected to have biological parents who assure informed consent and other protections throughout their disease, even in situations where mothers are deeply attached to and involved with the care of their children. All children who acquired the disease from their mothers have biological mothers who currently face certain death from the same disease. Not every mother who is infected with HIV transmits the infection to her child; it appears that up to 75% of the children born to infected mothers may not be infected (see Chapter 10C). But currently every infected mother will die, and that death will gravely affect all surviving children, including those children with HIV who survive their parents. Additionally, an unknown number of children either have no father involved with their daily care or have a father who is himself infected with HIV and currently faces certain death. An unknown number of children have biological parents who are so dependent on drugs that they do not engage in the daily care and protection of their children.

Second, for the child with perinatally acquired HIV in particular, enhanced participation in treatment cannot always be achieved through clear diagnosis of the disease at a very early juncture after infection. New techniques make it possible to identify 30–50% of infected children at birth, but the remaining 50–70% of infected infants may not be identified until they are 3–6 months old, if they are reached by such diagnostic services (see also Chapters 10 and 11).

Infected mothers also make antibodies within their own bodies in response to the virus, and they transmit their antibodies through the placenta to the fetus in utero. These maternal antibodies remain in the child's blood for as long as 18 months after birth, even if the child does not have the disease. An estimated 25% of the babies will go on to have the disease, although this varies among institutions. The range of transmission rates is 10–40% (see Chapter 10C). Thus, in the early weeks after maternally transmitted HIV has been acquired, it is not always possible to distinguish between infected and noninfected children and to initiate treatment early.

Third, for many children and families, enhancing participation in treatment may not be possible without continuous, extensive, and competent emotional and financial support for the parents and other family members. For both the child with maternally acquired HIV infection and the child who acquired it through contact with infected blood or semen, the family stresses associated with the disease are perhaps the most severe currently faced in the treatment of seriously and/or chronically ill children. Families whose children acquired the disease from blood transfusions, for example, may have already struggled with years of life-threatening or serious illnesses such as cancer or hemophilia, with all the financial loss and emotional strain that those struggles entail. Families whose children have acquired the disease through maternal transmission may learn about both maternal and child infection (as well as possible paternal and sibling infection) simultaneously. In the wake of such catastrophic diagnoses, parents may have to make or remake wills that provide for the care of the child after the mothers (or the parents) death and undertake other tasks associated with planning for death.

Furthermore, many children and their families are members of low-income socioeconomic groups whose access to medical care and resources requiring financial well-being is fragile at best. Yet, for a chance at survival, the children must have access to medical care that is very expensive. The American Academy of Pediatrics estimates that treatment for a perinatally infected infant may cost, just in Medicaid funds, from $18,000 to $42,000 a year (13). Finally, many children and their families are members of ethnic and racial minority groups who have historically experienced rejection, exclusion, and discrimination by mainstream United States society. Both access to good medical care and levels of stress within a family are negatively affected by the continuing indifference or hostility of the white majority to people of color in the United States and to their condition.

In an unknown number of situations, these stresses are exacerbated by hostile rejection and even threats of physical harm from members of the affected families' previous support systems, who irrationally fear contagion from the affected family or view acquisition of the disease as a clear sign of wrongdoing on the part of the affected family. Neighborhoods, schools, child care programs, early intervention and special education centers, and even churches may attempt to bar both child and family from continued participation in their activities. These experiences of rejection are not universal nor do they occur across all support systems in a given community. However, the uncertainty about the extent and the depth of the rejection that must be anticipated by each family deepens family stress in the period after diagnosis when enhancement of participation in research based treatment depends on many difficult family decisions.

In sum, access to treatment that leads toward a cure depends on interconnecting factors. These include expansion of biomedical research in general related to pediatric AIDS; sufficient expansion of clinical trials so that adequate numbers of children can participate in treatment investigating possible cures; recruitment, training, and support of adequate biomedical research and clinical teams of scientists and professionals from various disciplines so that the research can actually be accomplished and sustained; expansion of health care financing so that children infected with HIV can receive good health care; the delivery and expansion of family centered, community based coordinated care so that child and family function can be well supported.

Issues

Advocates committed to enhancing participation of children with HIV in treatment that leads to a cure must deal with various issues that emerge in part from competing values and in part from still-scarce allocation of public resources for the financing of excellent research based treatment. These issues include the following:

- Advocacy support for a focused, unrelenting professional/parent spotlight on the need for pediatric HIV research so that children will not be voiceless in efforts to increase and allocate research funds vs. support for a comprehensive research agenda that speaks to adult and pediatric needs but may not effectively meet both needs well.
- Advocacy support for a coherent research agenda driven by a consensus around child and family needs vs. support for highly individualistic research agendas driven by the needs of persuasive researchers who may not possess a comprehensive overview of child and family needs.
- Advocacy support for increased and rapid access to therapeutic agents and treatment protocols still in investigational (experimental) stages vs. support for the protection of children from highly toxic experimental agents and treatment approaches whose benefits to the affected children are (or may seem) dubious or nonexistent.
- Advocacy support for highly sophisticated, centralized, and well controlled research based treatment, which will likely be best delivered in a tertiary care center remote from the child and family's community and other family members vs. support for the delivery of research based treatment in a highly dispersed community based manner, i.e., in medical centers located in the communities where the affected children actually live.
- Advocacy support for the conservation of limited fiscal and personnel resources principally for the achievement of rapid biomedical research breakthroughs achieved in settings that concentrate on the biological needs of the child vs. support for allocation of these limited resources to multidisciplinary comprehensive centers which provide or arrange for services that meet many psychosocial, educational, and other needs of the child.

• Advocacy support for family centered approaches to the treatment of pediatric AIDS vs. support for a child centered approach which realistically recognizes that an unknown number of the children will become bereft of families through parental disease, death, or, in a subset of the population, abandonment.

Advocacy Agenda, Goals, and Accomplishments

During the late 1980s, high-level policymakers within the Department of Health and Human Services identified critical policy issues and made some recommendations about the content, scope, and financing of research and care (14, 15). The treatment related recommendations reflected consensus within the agency on 1) the scope and content of a comprehensive research program, including clinical research, 2) enhanced access to investigational treatments consistent with ethical and legal standards for protection of the child and of the parent or custodial caretaker's right to informed consent, 3) the need for comprehensive, coordinated, culturally sensitive, community based, and family centered treatment programs, 4) outreach to at risk adolescents, 5) the recruitment of foster families, and 6) the financing of research and medical care (14, 15).

However, child and parent advocates remain concerned that, despite this consensus, child access to treatment leading toward a cure is still exceptionally limited. Thus, since the late 1980s, better access to researched based treatment has continued to be a high priority (although not an exclusive focus) for much child advocacy activity centered on pediatric AIDS. Activities have been undertaken by two sets of individuals in particular. One is the Pediatric AIDS Coalition, comprised of "thirty-eight national organizations advocating on behalf of children, adolescents, women and their families affected by HIV disease and AIDS" (16). Formed in 1987, the Coalition serves as the Pediatric Task Force for the National Organizations Responding to AIDS. The Pediatric AIDS Coalition is committed to ensuring that the unique needs of these populations are addressed in federal legislation and executive branch policy related to HIV/AIDS. In 1993, the Coalition called for Congressional action on 15 initiatives, many of which modified existing programs, to ensure that the special needs of HIV-infected women, children, and adolescents are met.

Child advocacy related particularly to the need for more research has been the principal focus of two individuals who are co-founders of the Pediatric AIDS Foundation but who do not represent the foundation when they engage in advocacy for increased research funding. These are Elizabeth Glaser and Susan De Laurentis. Ms. Glaser is infected with HIV. Having acquired the infection during a childbirth-related transfusion, she unknowingly transmitted it during breast feeding to the child born of that delivery (now deceased) and to a second child. Ms. De Laurentis, former businesswoman, mother of several children, and personal friend of the Glaser family, along with Susan Zeegen worked together with Ms. Glaser in founding the Pediatric AIDS Foundation. Both Ms. Glaser and Ms. De Laurentis are members of Hollywood's community of actors, actresses, and directors; both their spouses are prominent members of the film and television industry. Either singly or together, both women have sought and gained meetings with leadership in the federal government, including the President and many members of the House and Senate, to press the case for increased funds for research (E. Glaser, personal communication, 1990, 1993).

During 1988, child advocacy resulted in an increase in allocation of fiscal year 1989 funds for research. In 1989, these research related child advocacy efforts were further successful in achieving an allotment of an additional $10 million for biomedical research and an appropriation of $15 million for pediatric AIDS health care demonstration grants. Also in 1989, the drug, zidovudine was approved by the Food and Drug Administration under a treatment Investigational New Drug Application, making this therapeutic agent available to children with symptomatic infection. Since 1990, scientists across the country have been able to use the new pediatric AIDS research funds to initiate a broad range of both basic and clinical research studies.

Despite some impressive gains in understanding maternal and pediatric HIV therapeutic research, many basic biomedical research questions remain unanswered. For example, the epidemiology of HIV infection in pregnant women, infants, and children, the effectiveness of zidovudine in the treatment of infants and children, the degree of this drug's toxicity to the developing fetus, and the role of the placenta in viral transmission are among the areas where further study is needed. Additional diagnostic techniques for earlier detection of HIV in neonates, infants, and children is another area where further investigation is urgently needed (16).

For both 1992 and 1993, the Pediatric AIDS Coalition called on Congress to support increased funding for biomedical research and for pediatric AIDS clinical treatment trials sponsored by the National Institutes of Health. These trials constitute the principal opportunity for HIV-infected children, youth, and pregnant women in different parts of the country to access research based treatment (16).

The goal of facilitating child and family access to treatment that leads toward a cure, however, will be unattainable without increased financing of health care services for children infected with HIV. This implies health care reform and expansion of health care financing and coordinated, community based health services that combine health, developmental, and social services. Between 50 and 90% of the children with AIDS rely on Medicaid (17). During the late 1980s, child advocates persuaded Congress to mandate expansion of Medicaid coverage to all pregnant women, infants, and children younger than 6 with family incomes less than 133% of the federal poverty level, effective April 1, 1990 (17). In addition, Congress also phased in Medicaid coverage to children between the ages of 6 and 19, beginning with 6-year-olds in 1991 and expanding coverage each subsequent year to children in the next year of life, until all children between the ages of 6 and 19 are reached.

In 1990, Congress passed the Ryan White Comprehensive AIDS Resources Emergency Act, which provides health care and support services to individuals and families affected by HIV disease (18). Title II of this law provides grants to states. Not less than 15% of each state grant is reserved for infants, children, women, and families. However, a November 1991 survey of all lead state (and city) contacts showed that many states were not funding services for this population. Eleven states reported spending no funds on this population; 16 states could not give information regarding expenditures for this population (18). The Pediatric AIDS Coalition, which conducted this survey, recommends that the federal government evaluate and report on this set-aside for children and families, provide better technical assistance, and collect more in-depth data on the allocation of funds under this law. In 1993, the Pediatric AIDS Coalition called for appropriation of the full authorization ($875 million for the Ryan White CARE Act, including $20 million for Title IV) to increase participation in clinical trials by pregnant women, children, and adolescents and to ensure access to therapeutic drugs and services (16).

Finally, participation in research based treatment leading toward a cure should also be participation in *family centered* treatment. Children undergoing medical procedures and/or hospitalization should not be separated from their families, and a special effort should be made to help families strengthen their capacity to cope with this devastating disease. In 1988, Congress established a pediatric/family HIV health care demonstration grant program to promote collaborative, family centered prevention and treatment progress at the local level (19). In 1990, the National Pediatric HIV Resource Center was founded. Funded in part by the Maternal and Child Health Bureau of the Department of Health and Human Services, the Center promotes family centered care with consultation, technical assistance, and training for practitioners from the many different professional disciplines that work with HIV-infected children and their families (20).

Child advocacy efforts to obtain improved child and family access to treatment leading toward a cure have been among the most well organized. Although gains have been made, the need for further biomedical research breakthroughs and increased pediatric participation in research based treatment continues to be significant.

GOAL II: PARTICIPATION IN A FAMILY OR FAMILY-LIKE SETTING THAT ASSURES DAILY CARE AND PROTECTION OF THE CHILD

Background

Young children with HIV are fundamentally no different from all other children: they need to live within the context of a stable, reliable family deeply committed to assuring their care and protection. No other children in the United States, however, are more at risk of loss of permanent family than children whose mothers have HIV disease. Both infected and noninfected children of these mothers are at risk.

By the end of 1991, an estimated 18,500 children had been orphaned by the AIDS-related deaths of their mothers (the primary caretaker within HIV-affected families) (21). By the year 1995, the number of such orphans (comprising both infected and noninfected children born to HIV-infected mothers) is estimated to reach 45,700 (21). Further, an unknown additional number of children with HIV (or noninfected children whose mothers have HIV) are at risk of loss of a permanent family because either the disease or drug use causes parents to become severely dysfunctional. Thus, children may need child welfare services because they are infected or affected by this disease.

Even in a country with well developed child welfare policies and systems, pediatric AIDS poses challenges to assurance of the infected or affected child's continuous participation in a family or family-like setting. These problems include the following.

- The difficulties of sensitive and accurate assessment of the critical juncture when a child's biological family is not able to care for him or her, a problem exacerbated by cultural and class differences among many families exposed to HIV infection and the professionals called upon to make these difficult assessments (22–23).
- Culturally sensitive assessment of who the child's psychological family is. "Psychological family" means individuals who constitute the child's macrosystem of daily or very frequent face to face interactions, regardless of whether they are biologically related to the child (22–27).
- Responsible choice, when necessary, of the alternate care setting appropriate to this particular child and family from a range of program possibilities: foster family care, with specially trained foster parents; nontraditional foster family placements, such as with unmarried individuals; small community based congregate living facilities (28–30).

These assessments and choices are among the most difficult to make in societies with well developed, supportive child welfare systems. However, the child welfare system in the United States is not well developed. Consequently the obstacles to realizing the goal of assuring participation in a family or family-like setting are even more numerous and complicated.

Some of these obstacles have their policy origins in decisions made in the early 1980s. In the 1970s, many studies, commission reports, and scholarly analysis reaffirmed the importance of participation in a permanent, functional family to the well-being of children (31–33). This body of policy relevant literature was used by child advocates as a framework for the investigation of conditions in the lives of children without permanent loving families, primarily children whose parents were deceased, absent, or severely dysfunctional or who maltreated their offspring (34, 35).

The conditions documented were exceptionally adverse to child well-being. The federal government could not even give a reliable count of the number of children in foster care; it was estimated at 450,000. Children spent an average of 27 months in foster care, often in a series of one home after another, after removal from their biological families and before either reunification or placement with a permanent family. Foster care assistance payments through Title IV-E of the Social Security Act were paltry; and children who received Medicaid assistance while foster children were denied the same Medicaid coverage once they were adopted, even if they were adopted by their foster parents (36, 37).

The result of these investigations was a committed child advocacy effort to achieve reform of child welfare policies so that children could either be adopted by permanent families or reunited with their own biological families. In 1980, these child advocacy efforts culminated in passage of landmark legislation: the Adoption Assistance and Child Welfare Reform Act (PL 96-272). This law was designed to assure that children are not removed to foster care too hastily; that they are safeguarded while in foster care and either reunited with their biological families or placed with permanent families within a reasonable time; that adoption assistance payments be made available to families adopting children with special needs; and that Medicaid coverage would follow the child making the transition from federally funded foster care to adoption (36, 37).

Unfortunately, the severe retrenchment in social services and child welfare policies that characterized the Reagan administration meant that this landmark legislation was never much implemented (38–41).

During the 1980s, as the economy deteriorated and unemployment, homelessness, and substance abuse rose, reports of child abuse and neglect tripled (42). By 1991, 2.7 million cases of child abuse and neglect were reported (42). An estimated 429,000 children were in out of home care placements in 1991, an increase of 50% since 1986 (42) (Childrens Defense Fund, 1993). Thus, children with HIV became one of several child populations in deep need of family preservation and child welfare services. The pediatric AIDS crisis, however, has flared against a backdrop of failed child welfare reform policies and a skyrocketing need for improved child welfare services (38–43). Today the service system that these children and their families need teeters on fragile supports.

In 1992 Congress responded. The Child Welfare and Family Preservation Reforms were enacted, as part of the Urban Aid/Tax Bill, and subsequently vetoed by President Bush. In 1993, this bill was reintroduced by Senators Rockefeller and Bond as the Family Preservation and Child Protection Reform Act (S 596) (43). Family stability for children infected and affected by HIV is linked to the success of child welfare reform.

As in the research area, however, realization of the goal of enhanced participation in a family or family-like setting also depends on interlocking decisions: reform and expansion of improved child welfare and social services systems, adoption of policies that promote family support for children with HIV and their families in culturally sensitive, realistic ways, and recruitment, training, and retention of foster parents, child welfare workers, family support personnel, and social service professionals.

Issues: Child Advocacy

The issues surrounding realization of a family or family-like setting for every child with HIV include the following.

- Advocacy support for family preservation as the highest priority goal vs. support for the child's right to protection from likely or actual parental neglect caused by parental disease, disability, drug use, or death.
- Advocacy support for expansion and improvement of existing federal supports to child welfare services generally vs. support for the creation of new federal programs providing child welfare services specifically to children with HIV.
- Advocacy support for enhancement of child access to foster family care vs. support for enhancement of child access to family-like residential care settings.

Advocacy Agenda, Accomplishments, and Goals

During the late 1980s, child advocates focused on pediatric AIDS were less involved in advocating for child welfare policies that would assure children affected by HIV a permanent family than with the important advocacy agendas related to research and health care financing. Among the 32 recommendations of the Pediatric AIDS Coalition's 1990 legislative agenda, for example, there were no recommendations for improvements in the delivery of Title IV-E funds or expansion of and improvement in the delivery of general child welfare and social service funds.

In 1992 and 1993, however, the Pediatric AIDS Coalition called for passage of child welfare reform legislation and other measures that would provide more assurance of a permanent family to children whose lives have been affected by AIDS (16). In 1993, the Pediatric AIDS Coalition urged, for example, legislation that would "create a permanent entitlement for the financing of family preservation services intended to prevent unnecessary separation and facilitate family reunification" (16). In August 1993, Congress enacted such legislation. The Coalition also recommended the full authorization ($30 million) for the Abandoned Infants Assistance Act, "with special attention to the HIV-infected and substance-exposed populations" (16).

Advocates working to assure the HIV-infected (or affected) childs continuous participation in a family or family-like setting have struggled with many obstacles. Their efforts have been hampered by federal indifference to the mounting multiple crises within the child welfare system. To realize the goal of a family or a good family-like setting for every child with HIV, child advocacy within and outside of government should be expanded and intensified. Furthermore, both the executive and legislative branches of the federal government will need to make family preservation and permanent homes for children without families a high policy priority.

GOAL III: PARTICIPATION IN NORMAL OR NEARLY NORMAL EXPERIENCES OF CHILDHOOD WHENEVER MEDICALLY FEASIBLE

Background

In both public and private statements, parents of children with special needs emphasize that one of their most cherished goals for their children is participation in the mainstream of child, youth, and eventually adult life (42–45). For children, this means participation in neighborhood life, preschools and schools, child care programs, after school activities, churches and synagogues—all settings where other children play and learn.

One of the most significant obstacles to this kind of participation is discrimination against individuals with handicaps. This discrimination may be intentional or it may be institutional, i.e., discrimination resulting from the practices or policies of an institution that have the effect of discriminating even if this was not intended. Children who experience discrimination against the disabled are unfairly excluded from participation in the normal or nearly normal experiences of childhood. Thus children with special needs must bear the burden of their disease or handicap and the additional burden of exclusions, which assaults their emotional well-being.

Children with HIV are deeply vulnerable to discrimination. They have special health care needs, which frequently result in mental or motor disabilities. They are often members of racial or ethnic minorities who have historically been subjected to discrimination. They have a disease that is contagious (under certain conditions only) and fatal. There have been multiple and indeed even terrifying reprisals against children with HIV and their families, once the fact of their illness was known to neighbors or schoolmates. In short, protection of children with HIV and their families from unfair exclusion will depend on enforceable legal rights that ensure access on the part of children with HIV, their families, and their caretakers as well as safety on the part of nonaffected children, families and caretakers.

Issues: Child Advocacy

The issues surrounding civil rights protection of children with HIV include the following.

• Advocacy support for the rights of children with HIV, including children who do not have control over bodily secretions, to participate in schools, child care programs, recreational settings, and so forth vs. advocacy support for the rights of nonaffected children to be protected from transmission of this fatal disease.
• Advocacy that is focused on the rights of HIV-infected children vs. advocacy concerned with the civil rights of all individuals with disabilities, including HIV-infected children.

- Advocacy for rights of individuals with disabilities vs. advocacy for rights of citizens to be free from undue restriction on the exercise of their liberties or from undue burden to achieve the changes necessary to accommodate individuals with disabilities.

Advocacy Agenda, Accomplishments, and Goals

During the last decade, advocates have mobilized (or begun to mobilize) some new legal protections sufficient to allow disabled children and families to seek legal redress if discrimination is experienced. This has been done principally within the context of 1) a disabled child's right to education and 2) the civil rights of all individuals with disabilities generally. Although these advocacy accomplishments affect children with HIV, they were not motivated by nor designed around a specific concern for children with HIV. They respond to the needs of individuals with disabilities generally.

Parent and professional child advocates, for example, worked together to obtain enactment of a 1986 law that accorded disabled children older than 3 new legal protections vis a vis the United States public education system. Consequently, children older than 3 with HIV are protected under the Individuals with Disabilities Education Act (IDEA) from exclusion from public school education (46–48). In addition, in states that have participated in part H of IDEA for 4 or more years, children younger than 3 who are developmentally delayed or have a physical or mental condition likely to result in developmental delay are entitled to certain early intervention services. (At state option, children who are environmentally at risk are also entitled to these early intervention services, if the state has chosen to exercise this option.)

These protections have been buttressed, in the case of school age and nonneurologically handicapped children, by federal policy guidance from the Centers for Disease Control (CDC) (49). For preschool children and neurologically handicapped children, however, the statutory protections inherent in IDEA may have been weakened by the CDC guidelines (49).

IDEA assures children aged 3 and older of the right to participate in a free and appropriate public education in "the least restrictive setting". However, the CDC guidelines specifically call for a more restrictive environment for preschool and neurologically handicapped children with HIV. This could limit the rights of children aged 3 and older to the least restrictive environment. In addition, the CDC guidelines do not recommend reasonable ways to achieve a "more restrictive" environment, leaving the way open for unreasonable restrictions.

As described in Chapter 49, legal advocacy, together with parent advocacy, has resulted in judicial decisions that strengthen protections against unfair exclusion for all children with HIV (50). In addition, as described elsewhere in this text, the National Association of State Boards of Education has issued better guidelines for school and preschool participation by HIV-infected children, and the CDC has informally endorsed the Boards guidelines (see Chapters 48, 49). So too have the American Public Health Association and the American Academy of Pediatrics in their guidelines for child care (51). (The degree of actual risk of transmission in these populations and these settings is discussed in Chapter 48.)

Children younger than 3 years are not afforded the same type of protection in IDEA that children older than 3 have. Infants and toddlers are not afforded the right to a free appropriate public education. However, in states that have participated in IDEA for 4 years, this law does entitle infants and toddlers and their families to some benefits, including a comprehensive assessment, an Individualized Family Service Plan, and case management services. In states that are in this official fifth year of participation in IDEA, the law entitles infants and toddlers and their families to early intervention services that are named in the child's Individualized Family Service Plan. These protections will offer infants and toddlers with AIDS-related complex or AIDS enhanced opportunities to participate in some early intervention services. This in turn will help them better cope with their developmental disabilities; to play and learn; and thus to participate in the normal experiences of childhood (52, 53).

In addition, by clearing some obstacles to developmental and educational services, the new opportunities assured under IDEA for infants and toddlers as well as preschoolers have the potential of reducing some stress on families, thus contributing to a lessening of family breakup caused by severe strain. In turn, then, the goal of assuring participation in a family or family-like setting for the child with HIV may be better (if indirectly) realized with effective implementation of these new legislative protections against discrimination.

The legislative and administrative protections discussed above apply only to children and their rights to a free and appropriate public education. Two other statutes, Section 504 of the Rehabilitation Act of 1973 (as clarified in the Civil Rights Restoration Act of 1983) and the Americans with Disabilities Act, address the rights of persons with disabilities to protection from discrimination. These protections are well described elsewhere (see Chapter 49).

Like the goal of assuring participation in a family or family-like setting, the goal of assuring participation in the normal or nearly- normal experiences of childhood, wherever medically feasible, is an important area for child advocacy activities over the next few years. As implementation of IDEA and the Americans with Disabilities Act continues, administrative advocacy will be needed to ensure that children with HIV are well served by these statutes. In addition, better CDC guidelines are needed, particularly regarding the placement of preschool or neurologically handicapped children with HIV in care and education settings in "more restrictive environments" within those settings.

Child Advocacy and Pediatric AIDS: Implications for the Future

The suffering of children with HIV has attracted the attention of child advocates. HIV-specific legislative and administrative child advocacy has been principally undertaken by a coalition of national organizations concerned with children, youth, and families (the Pediatric AIDS Coalition) and by the personal work of a parent of a child with HIV, Elizabeth Glaser, and her colleagues,

Susan De Laurentis and Susan Zeegen. In addition, advocates for individuals with disabilities have successfully worked for passage of civil rights legislation that will protect rights of HIV-infected children as well.

In response, the federal government has authorized and appropriated some additional research funds and health care directed at prevention and treatment of HIV infection in children and their families. A major child welfare reform initiative has attracted some Congressional support. Children with HIV infection are better protected against discrimination. Yet still the children suffer and die. Still both infected and noninfected children witness the deaths of their mothers and other family members. And still children with HIV meet other children and adults who treat them with scorn and derision, or worse because they have a disease.

Certainly, much still needs to be done to fully realize the three goals of this chapter: enhanced participation in 1) treatment leading toward a cure, 2) a family or family-like setting deeply committed to daily care and protection of the child, and 3) the normal or nearly normal experiences of childhood, wherever medically feasible.

All professionals involved with the care and education of children with HIV and their families, and all parents of children with HIV, can contribute to the realization of these child advocacy goals. Active participation in child advocacy or disability rights organizations, in parent advocacy organizations concerned with children with special health care needs, or in coalitions can make a difference for HIV-infected children. Progress is possible. Committed and knowledgeable individuals can make that progress happen.

References

1. Westman J. Child advocacy: New professional roles for helping families. New York: Free Press, 1979.
2. Mnookin RH. In the interest of children: Advocacy law reform and public policy. New York: WH Freeman, 1985:38.
3. Greenberg P. The devil has slippery shoes: A biased biography of the child development group of Mississippi. Washington, DC: Youth Policy Institute, 1990.
4. Hubbell R, Aiken S, Jones G. A review of Head Start research since 1970. Washington, DC: Government Printing Office, 1984.

5. Robinson J, Choper W. Another perspective on program evaluation: The parents speak. In: Zigler E, Valentine J, eds. Project Head Start: A legacy of the war on poverty. New York: Free Press, 1979.

6. Schorr LB. Within our reach: Breaking the cycle of disadvantage. New York: Doubleday, 1988:179–200.

7. Valentine J, Stark E. The social context of parent involvement in Head Start. In: Zigler E, Valentine J, eds. Project Head Start: A legacy of the war on poverty. New York: Free Press, 1979.

8. Pizzo, P. Parent to parent: Working together for ourselves and our children. Boston: Beacon Press, 1983.

9. Pizzo, P. Parent to parent support groups: Advocates for social change. In: Kagan L, Powell D, Weissbourd B, Zigler E, eds. American family support programs. New Haven: Yale University Press, 1987:228–245.

10. Pizzo, P. Parent advocacy: A resource for early intervention. In: Meisels S, Shonkoff J, eds. Handbook of early childhood intervention. Cambridge: Cambridge University Press, 1990.

11. Centers for Disease Control and Prevention. HIV/AIDS Surveillance Rep Feb 1993.

12. Oleske J. Natural history of HIV infection II. Report of the Surgeon Generals workshop on children with HIV infection and their families. Washington, DC: Department of Health and Human Services, 1987.

13. American Academy of Pediatrics. Pediatric AIDS. In: Child health issues in the US Congress, 1990.

14. Department of Health and Human Services. Report of the Surgeon General's workshop on children with HIV infection and their families. Washington, DC: Department of Health and Human Services, 1987.

15. Novello A, Wise P, Willoughby A, Pizzo P. Final report of the United States Department of Health and Human Services secretary's work group on pediatric human immunodeficiency virus infection and disease: Content and implications. Pediatrics 1989;84:547–555.

16. Pediatric AIDS Coalition. 1993 legislative agenda. Washington, DC: 1993 (available from Pediatric AIDS Coalition, 1331 Pennsylvania Ave, NW, Suite 721 North, Washington, DC 20004).

17. Childrens Defense Fund. Memorandum to all interested persons from CDF Health Division re: news from Washington, DC, Jan 16, 1990 (available from Children's Defense Fund, 25 E St, NW, Washington, DC 20001).

18. Harvey D, Rathburn J, Leif E. Ryan White [AIDS] CARE act survey: Services funded for children and adolescents, 1991 (available from Pediatric AIDS Coalition, 1331 Pennsylvania Ave, NW, Suite 721 North, Washington, DC 20004).

19. National Pediatric HIV Resource Center. Pediatric/family health care demonstration grant program. Newark: National Pediatric HIV Resource Center, 1992.

20. National Pediatric HIV Resource Center. Summary of activities 1990–1991. Newark: National Pediatric HIV Resource Center, undated.

21. Michaels D, Levine C. Estimates of the number of motherless youth orphaned by AIDS in the United States. JAMA 1982;24:3456–3461.

22. Hearings before Select Committee on Children, Youth and Families, 100th Congress, 1st Session, 1987 (testimony of Manuel Laureano-Vega re: AIDS and young children in Florida).

23. Hearings before Select Committee on Children, Youth and Families, 100th Congress, 1st Session 1987 (testimony of Sylvia Villareal re: AIDS and young children: Emerging issues).

24. Bronfenbrenner U. Ecological systems theory. In: Vasta R, ed. Annals of child development. Greenwich, CT: Jai Press, 1989.

25. Hill R. The strengths of black families. New York: Emerson Hall, 1972.

26. McAdoo HP. Black families. Beverly Hills, CA: Sage Publications, 1981.

27. Stack C. All our kin: Strategies for survival in a black community. New York: Harper and Row, 1974.

28. Gitelson P, Emery LJ. Serving HIV-infected children, youth, and their families: A guide for residential group care providers. Washington, DC: Child Welfare League of America, 1989.

29. Granger M, Rosen S, Yokoyama J, Tasker M. Transitional group homes for children with HIV: Support for children, families and foster parents. Zero Three 1989;9:14–18.

30. Provence S. Infants in institutions revisited. Zero Three 1989;9:1–4.

31. Bane MJ. Here to stay: American families in the twentieth century. New York: Basic Books, 1976.

32. Keniston K. All our children: The American family under pressure. New York: Harcourt Brace Jovanovich, 1977.

33. National Research Council Advisory Committee on Child Development. Toward a national policy for children and families. Washington, DC: National Academy of Sciences, 1976.

34. Knitzer J, Allen M. Children without homes. Washington, DC: Childrens Defense Fund, 1978.

35. Steiner G. The futility of family policy. Washington, DC: Brookings Institution, 1981.

36. Title IV-E of Social Security Act, added by PL 96-272 (Adoption Assistance and Child Welfare Act of 1980) as amended 42 USC 670 et seq.

37. Joint hearing before Subcommittee on Children and Youth of Senate Labor and Public Welfare Committee and Subcommittee on Select Education of House Committee on Education and Labor, 94th Congress, 1st Session (Foster care: Problems and issues), 1976.

38. Hearings before Select Committee on Children, Youth and Families, 100th Congress, 1st Session, 1987 (testimony of George Miller re: continuing crisis in foster care: Issues and problems).

39. Hearings before Select Committee on Children, Youth and Families, 100th Congress, 1st Session, 1987 (testimony of Dodie Livingston re: continuing crisis in foster care).

40. Hearings before Select Committee on Children, Youth and Families, 100th Congress, 1st Session, 1987 (testimony of Linda Greenan re: continuing crisis in foster care: Issues and problems).

41. Miller G. Prepared statement in continuing crisis in foster care: Issues and problems. Hearing before Select Committee on Children, Youth, and Families, House of Representatives. Washington, DC: Government Printing Office, 1987:3–7.

42. Edge E, Pizzo P, eds. The four critical junctures: Support for parents of children with special needs. Washington, DC: National Center for Clinical Infant Programs, 1988.
43. National Center for Clinical Infant Programs. Equals in this partnership. Washington, DC: National Center for Clinical Infant Programs, 1985.
44. Turnbull AP, Turnbull HR, eds. Parents speak out: Growing with a handicapped child. Columbus: Merrill, 1988.
45. Turnbull AP, Turnbull HR, eds. Parents speak out: Then and now. Columbus: Merrill, 1985.
46. Part B of Education of the Handicapped ACT, added by PL 101-476 as amended (20 USC 1400-1485), 1990.
47. Part B of Education of Handicapped Act, added by PL 99-457 as amended (20 USC 1471 et seq), 1986.
48. Part B of Education of Handicapped Act, added by PL 94-142 as amended (20 USC 1411 et seq), 1975.
49. Education and foster care of children infected with human T-lymphotropic virus type III/lymphadenopathy-associated virus. Current Trends 1985;34:517–521.
50. Martinez v. School Board of Hillsborough County, Fla., 692 F Supp. 1293 (MD Fla 1988), vacated and remanded 861 F2d 1502 (11th Cir 1988); 711 F Supp. 1066 (MD Fla 1989).
51. Anonymous. Caring for our children. Washington, D.C.: American Public Health Association; Elk Grove Village, IL: American Academy of Pediatrics, 1989:231–236.
52. Meisels S, Shonkoff J. Handbook of early childhood intervention. New York: Cambridge University Press, 1990.
53. Woodruff G. The foundation for children with AIDS, 1990 (available from The Foundation for Children with AIDS, 77B Warren St., Brighton, MA 02135).

A Blueprint for Care, Treatment, and Prevention of HIV/AIDS in Children

Catherine M. Wilfert and Philip A. Pizzo

The preceding pages have documented the tragedy of human immunodeficiency virus (HIV) infection/AIDS in children and their families. They also describe the challenge of scientific inquiry and the excitement afforded by modern technologies that enable us to better answer questions posed by human diseases. We have conveyed the enormity of the problem of HIV infection, the expanding epidemiology, and the despair engendered by trying to contend with this ultimately fatal disease with a health care system that cannot meet the medical needs of our country.

We are watching this infection become increasingly acquired as a sexually transmitted disease in a heterosexual population. It has targeted our youth because the vast majority of infected persons are of reproductive age. Areas where the epidemic began continue to be overwhelmed by the tens of thousands of persons requiring care. Areas of the United States that were silent a few years ago now have been placed on the map of AIDS; e.g., the heterosexual spread of HIV infection is now occurring more rapidly in the southern United States than in any other part of our nation (1). Heterosexual transmission exacts an equal toll from men and women and creates an ever increasing proportion of infected children. Reported HIV infection in association with drug use by women constitutes a diminishing proportion of the total number of cases. It is not possible to define the majority of women at risk of acquiring HIV infection on the basis of self-described risk behaviors. This is because unprotected sexual intercourse is not a behavior perceived to place people at risk of acquiring HIV infection in the absence of promiscuity, multiple partners, bisexual activity, or drug use. Nevertheless, it is a fact that two-thirds of adolescent males and half of adolescent females initiate sexual intercourse by age 17 years. At least 25% of students report four or more sexual partners by the time they are in the twelfth grade. The average age of first sexual intercourse in the United States is 16 years (2). Young people view this behavior as normal, accepted by their peers, and deny that this constitutes a risk for acquisition of HIV infection and other sexually transmitted diseases. Clearly, we need national research on adolescent sexuality. Studies that were designed to define trends in adolescent sexuality were canceled by the federal government in 1992 because of opposition to explicit questions about sexual practices. We have not yet succeeded in altering the behavior of our youth, and without an appropriate information base, we cannot hope to be successful in this endeavor.

Infection with HIV continues its relentless worldwide progression. In the United States where priority has not been given to the health care or education of our children, HIV/AIDS has exposed our inadequacies. The United States and South Africa are alone among industrialized nations who fail to provide medical care and support services for all mothers either before or after delivery; 25% of pregnant women in the United States receive prenatal care either late in pregnancy or not at all. This deficiency in appropriate care increases by twofold the premature deliveries and complications of small for gestational age infants. The United States ranks 20th among all nations in infant mortality. Nine of every 1000 babies born will die before they reach their first birthday in the United States. All other industrialized nations have lower infant mortality rates than the United States. It is not surprising we cannot consistently recognize HIV infection in pregnant women. We must provide early access to prenatal care, include HIV counseling, and offer testing to all pregnant women to provide appropriate medical care to them, to their infants, and to their families. This has been done successfully in specific clinics and communities. For example, in seven counties in North Carolina counseling and testing offered uniformly to all pregnant women increased from <10% in each clinic to >80% for 7 months when a standardized unstigmatized approach to provide care was adopted. The American Academy of Pediatrics (3) and a consensus statement from the HIV resource center (4) have made this recommendation, and it must be implemented. "HIV counseling and HIV testing should be routinely offered by all health care providers to women of reproductive age. The offering of HIV antibody testing should be recommended as early as possible during the prenatal period. If women are not tested during pregnancy, counseling and testing should be offered during the postnatal period" (4).

All children in the U.S. should have access to health care. There are ~4.2 million births/year in the United States, and there are 65 million children younger than 18 years (5). Children comprise 26% of the United States population, but they comprise 40% of the poor in our nation. One in five of our children or 13 million are impoverished (6). Poor was defined in 1990 for a family of four as an income of <$13,359/year and for a single mother with one child as an income of <$9,000/year. Millions of impoverished United States citizens lack the resources to obtain medical care or even access to medical care. HIV infection disproportionately infects persons of lower socioeconomic status. The median family income of 350 children seen in a North Carolina population is $391.00/month. A lengthy and complex illness cannot be managed in the absence of resources. HIV/AIDS did not create the inequities, but it does highlight the deficiencies of our existing health care system.

Families with HIV/AIDS are in desperate need of health care. However, health insurance and care requires money. Thirty-two million people including 11 million women of reproductive age and 9 million children are without health insurance in the United States. Twenty-five million children are without insurance despite the fact that their parents are insured through their employers. Thus, in the United States, not only the children of the unemployed are uninsured, but it is quite likely that many children of parents who are themselves insured will not be covered by the parental insurance policy. Employees must be entitled to health care coverage for their dependent children themselves or spouses during pregnancy and after delivery. It is paradoxical that persons qualify for Medicaid assistance only if their income is below a state designated poverty level. If a family is employed at a job that makes their income exceed the minimum, or one which fails to provide insurance, they cannot qualify for Medicaid assistance unless they quit working. This does not encourage families to participate in their own support, and many financially disadvantaged persons cannot qualify for Medicaid. Medicaid has not solved the problem of appropriate access to medical care. We must also work to require that all health care providers honor the medical insurance for the poor to improve access to care.

Sadly, access to health care is unequal. Younger, lower income, uninsured, and nonwhite persons have diminished access to health care (7). They are more likely to utilize emergency rooms or community clinics to provide their care. Unfortunately, the Hispanic and African-American populations are two times less likely to have obtained needed medical care independent of income or insurance. Although optimal access to care may not exist for any population (including the elderly), insured, nonpoor working age adults have less access to medical care than do the elderly. A measure of inadequate access to health care by children is afforded by reviewing immunization rates. Half of all preschoolers are deficient in the requisite immunizations. Nonwhite children in the United States rank 70th in the world in immunizations received. This places them behind many developing nations.

The demographics of the epidemic tell us there now is a disproportionate representation of minority families who are infected with HIV. "The years of life lost per 100,000 population that were due to HIV was [sic] 177% higher for African-American males than white males and 796% higher for African-American females than white females" (13). These families lack health insurance and have more difficult access to health care, and this illness often involves more than one person in the family. This disease demands consistent, accessible support. These are the societal problems exposed by HIV infection of children and their families. The solution requires a nationwide universal health care system that places a priority on youth and does not penalize people of poor means but provides essential support services and medications.

The problems are further compounded by the fact that the three decades between 1960 and 1990 have seen a three-fold increase in married women who are working with children younger than 6 years (8). Additionally in 1990, over 74% of women whose youngest child was between 6 and 13 years were working (9). Simultaneously, there has been a doubling in divorced parents, and the number of children with only one parent has increased 2.5-fold. The number of babies born to single women has increased five-fold, and by 1988 more than 1 million infants were born out of wedlock (10, 12). Children living with single mothers are far more likely to be poor (11, 12). A significant number of HIV-infected women are single parents. The magnitude of the epidemic is demonstrated when it is realized that in the United States by 1995 12% of adolescents and 17% of children whose mothers die will have lost them to HIV/AIDS (13). By the end of 1995, 24,600 children and 21,000 adolescents will have been orphaned by HIV/AIDS, and the total number will reach 80,000 by the year 2,000

(13). These families must work but often cannot afford day care. HIV illness in the mother or child may remove all possibility of employment.

The litany of problems faced in the United States by our youth is impressive and demands correction. There are 22 homicides/100,000 of the population/year in the United States, placing us first in industrialized nations. This rate is four times that of Scotland, the country ranking second in homicides. Homicide is the number two cause of death in 15- to 24-year males in the United States and is the first cause of death of black males in this age group. It is not surprising that these risks of death are more immediate than acquisition of a disease, AIDS, that causes death years later. Hope for a better life including survival, quality education, and a chance to improve status must be provided if we are to alter drug use, decrease crime associated with acquisition of drugs, diminish dropping out of school, and improve acceptance of responsibility for sexual activity. These goals demand that the highest priority be given to the health and education of our children.

HIV infection/AIDS is a complex, ultimately fatal, communicable illness and can provide a paradigm for care in the 21st century. Available retroviral therapy prolongs life and improves the quality of life for children and adults. A child can reasonably expect to survive a median of 7–8 years with supportive care and antiretroviral therapy. We have every expectation that the duration of a life of quality will further increase. It is essential that care providers keep abreast of current recommendations for therapy of these children, and this involves collaboration with a tertiary medical center providing access to experimental therapies, sophisticated diagnostic methodology, and most importantly up to date information concerning state-of-the-art care. It is the responsibility of all medical care providers to willingly undertake the provision of care for these children and their families. It is unreasonable to expect that persons with HIV infection should travel long distances to obtain care for acute medical problems. Access to prompt and appropriate measures should be available with a consistent care provider who knows the family.

It is essential that we continue to advance our knowledge about treatment ultimately to encompass prevention of this infection. Carefully constructed randomized clinical trials form the backbone of the advancement of knowledge about treatment. Such studies must be efficiently designed to utilize the most modern methods, provide the current standard of care for study participants, and derive answers to the relevant questions utilizing the smallest possible number of infected persons. Children are an essential component of the clinical trials, and the pharmacology, safety, and tolerance of new agents must be as thoroughly tested in children as they are in adults. It is unacceptable to have a pediatric population with a fatal disease wait to benefit from successful therapies. These therapies must be developed in parallel with adult strategies, and this involves a collaboration between industry, the research establishment, and the regulatory agencies. There are no financial incentives for developing drugs for children. This must not deter drug development, and, if necessary, regulations should require or incentives be developed to ensure that promising therapies be appropriately investigated for all ages of persons sustaining the illness before approval is granted for use in adults.

The hope for the future is that transmission of this virus from women to their children and between sexual partners can be prevented. It is theoretically possible that specific antiviral agents could achieve prevention of infection in specific circumstances. Indeed, the investigation of interruption of transmission by administration of drug therapy is ongoing in maternal-infant trials. The goal of developing a vaccine that would successfully protect persons from acquiring disease caused by HIV upon exposure to this agent is laudable but years in the future. Vaccine trials must occur in the maternal-infant populations because this will provide the opportunity to demonstrate interruption of transmission. It is incumbent upon us to proceed expeditiously and not be stalled by perceived liability concerns or theoretical risks to mothers and their infants.

We are living with this epidemic of a communicable fatal illness at a time when our ability to solve scientific problems is greater than ever before. The crisis posed by our failures in health care delivery and education is formidable. We must continue to serve as child advocates and take on the added responsibility of providing a strong political voice to achieve these ends. The blueprint for the future places paramount importance on nurturing and promoting the health of our youth, which must include income security to families, quality education, and universal health care. Only then can we expect to successfully alter the spread of HIV, reach affected persons with therapy, and someday prevent this dreadful infection.

References

1. Centers for Disease Control Update. AIDS-United States, 1991. MMWR 1992;41:463–468.
2. Centers for Disease Control. Sexual behaviors among high school students. United States 1990. MMWR 1992;40:885–888.
3. Task Force on Pediatric AIDS. Perinatal HIV testing. Pediatrics 1992;89:791–793.
4. HIV Resource Center. Consensus statement. Pediatr Infect Dis J 1993;12:513–522.
5. Department of Commerce, Bureau of the Census, Current Population Reports, ser P-25, 1018. Projections of the population of the U.S. by age, sex and race: 1988–2080. Washington, DC: Government Printing Office, 1989:8.
6. Department of Commerce, Bureau of the Census, Current Population Reports, ser p-60, 168. Money, income and poverty status in U.S., 1989. Washington, DC: Government Printing Office, 1990:7,65.
7. Hayward RA, Shapiro MF, Freeman HI, Cooney CR. Inequities in health services among insured Americans. N Engl J Med 1988;318:1507–1512.
8. Bureau of Labor Statistics. March 1990 current population survey. Table 48. Washington, DC: Government Printing Office, 1990.
9. Bureau of Labor Statistics. March 1990 current population survey. Tables 14 and 15. Washington, DC: Government Printing Office, 1990.
10. Department Commerce, Bureau of the Census, Current Population Reports, ser P-20, 447. Household and family characteristics. Washington, DC: Government Printing Office, 1990:7.
11. Department Commerce, Bureau of the Census, Current Population Reports. ser P-60, 168. Money income, and poverty status in U.S., 1989. Washington, DC: Government Printing Office, 1990:61.
12. National Commission on Children. Beyond rhetoric. A new American agenda for children and families 1991. Washington, DC: Government Printing Office, 1991.
13. Michaels D, Levine C. Estimates of the number of motherless youth orphaned by AIDS in the United States. JAMA 1992;268:3456–3461.

Index

Page numbers in *italics* denote figures; those followed by "t" denote tables.